Instructional Course Lectures

Volume 44 1995

American Academy
of Orthopaedic Surgeons

Instructional Course Lectures

Volume 44 1995

Edited by
Douglas W. Jackson, MD
Medical Director
Southern California Center for Sports Medicine
Long Beach, California

With 442 illustrations

American Academy
of Orthopaedic Surgeons

American Academy of Orthopaedic Surgeons

Instructional Course Lectures
Volume 44

Director, Division of Education: Mark W. Wieting
Director, Department of Publications: Marilyn L. Fox, PhD
Senior Editor: Bruce Davis
Associate Senior Editors: Joan Abern, Jane Baque
Production Manager: Loraine Edwalds
Editorial Assistants: Sharon Duffy, Sophie Tosta, Sharon O'Brien
Publications Secretaries: Geraldine Dubberke, Em Lee Lambos

Design: James Buddenbaum Design, Wilmette, Illinois
Typesetting: Alexander Graphics, Indianapolis, Indiana
Printing and binding: Rand McNally, Taunton, Massachusetts
Stock: Influence Gloss

International Standard Book Number 0-89203-115-8
Library of Congress Catalog Card Number: 95-75249

Contributors

Paul Alan Anderson, MD, Clinical Associate Professor, Orthopaedic Surgery, University of Washington, Seattle, Washington

George Babikian, MD, Assistant Clinical Instructor, University of Vermont, Burlington, Vermont

James H. Beaty, MD, Associate Professor, University of Tennessee, Director of Orthopaedic Residency Program, Campbell Clinic, Memphis, Tennessee

Stephen K. Benirschke, MD, Associate Professor, Harborview Medical Center, University of Washington, Seattle, Washington

Mark Bernhardt, MD, Clinical Associate Professor, University of Missouri-Kansas City School of Medicine, St. Luke's Hospital, Kansas City, Missouri

Henry H. Bohlman, MD, Professor, Department of Orthopaedic Surgery, University Hospital, Case Western Reserve School of Medicine, Cleveland, Ohio

Lawrence B. Bone, MD, Director, Orthopaedic Trauma, Erie County Medical Center, Associate Professor, Orthopaedic Surgery, State University of New York, Buffalo, New York

Miguel E. Cabanela, MD, Professor of Orthopedics, Mayo Clinic, Rochester, Minnesota

S. Terry Canale, MD, Professor, University of Tennessee, Orthopaedic Department, Chief of Staff, Campbell Clinic, Memphis, Tennessee

James B. Carr, MD, Associate Professor of Orthopaedic Surgery, Medical College of Virginia Hospitals, Richmond, Virginia

Mark R. Colville, MD, Associate Professor, Division of Orthopaedics and Rehabilitation, Oregon Health Sciences University, Portland, Oregon

William P. Cooney III, MD, Professor of Orthopaedic Surgery, Mayo Medical School, Chair, Division of Hand Surgery, Department of Orthopaedics, Mayo Clinic, Rochester, Minnesota

Michael J. Coughlin, MD, Clinical Professor of Surgery, Division of Orthopaedics and Rehabilitation, Oregon Health Sciences University, Portland, Oregon

Alvin H. Crawford, MD, Professor of Pediatrics and Orthopaedic Surgery, Director of Pediatric Orthopaedic Surgery, Children's Hospital Medical Center, University of Cincinnati College of Medicine, Cincinnati, Ohio

Daniel Cummiskey, MD, Fort Wayne Orthopaedics, Fort Wayne, Indiana

Clive P. Duncan, MD, FRCSC Professor (PT) of Orthopaedics, Head, Division of Reconstructive Orthopaedics, Department of Orthopaedics, University of British Columbia, Vancouver, BC, Canada

Frank J. Eismont, MD, Professor & Vice Chairman, Department of Orthopaedics & Rehabilitation, Co-Director, Acute Spinal Cord Injury Unit, The University of Miami School of Medicine, Miami, Florida

Evan F. Ekman, MD, Department of Orthopaedic Surgery and Rehabilitation, The Bowman Gray School of Medicine, Wake Forest University, Winston-Salem, North Carolina

J. Whit Ewing, MD, Professor of Orthopaedics, Northeastern Ohio Universities College of Medicine, Akron, Ohio

Carol C. Frey, MD, Associate Clinical Professor of Orthopaedic Surgery, University of Southern California, Director, Orthopaedic Foot and Ankle Center, Los Angeles, California

Freddie H. Fu, MD, Executive Vice Chairman, Department of Orthopaedic Surgery, Professor of Orthopaedic Surgery, University of Pittsburgh, Pittsburgh, Pennsylvania

James R. Gage, MD, Medical Director, Gillette Children's Hospital, St. Paul, Minnesota

John Glaser, Vice President, Information Systems, Brigham and Women's Hospital, Boston, Massachusetts

Stuart A. Green, MD, Clinical Professor, Orthopaedic Surgery, University of California, Irvine, California

Lawrence P. Hanrahan, PhD, MS, Senior Epidemiologist, Wisconsin Division of Health, Bureau of Public Health, Madison, Wisconsin

Christopher D. Harner, MD, Associate Professor Orthopaedic Surgery, Chief, Division of Sports Medicine, Department of Orthopaedic Surgery, University of Pittsburgh School of Medicine, Pittsburgh, Pennsylvania

Robert N. Hensinger, MD, Professor of Surgery, Section of Orthopaedic Surgery, University of Michigan, Ann Arbor, Michigan

David S. Hungerford, MD, Professor of Orthopaedic Surgery, Johns Hopkins University School of Medicine, Baltimore, Maryland

Kirk S. Hutton, MD, Clinical Assistant Professor, University of Nebraska Medical Center, Staff Orthopaedic Surgeon, Sports Medicine Center, Omaha, Nebraska

Darren L. Johnson, MD, Assistant Professor of Orthopaedic Surgery, Section of Sports Medicine, Division of Orthopaedic Surgery, University of Kentucky, Lexington, Kentucky

Jesse B. Jupiter, MD, Director, Orthopaedic Trauma, Massachusetts General Hospital, Associate Professor, Orthopaedics, Harvard Medical School, Boston, Massachusetts

James R. Kasser, MD, Chief of Orthopaedics, Childrens Hospital, Harvard Medical School, Boston, Massachusetts

Mark Koris, MD, Clinical Instructor in Orthopaedic Surgery, Harvard Medical School, Boston, Massachusetts

Kenneth J. Koval, MD, Chief, Fracture Service, Hospital for Joint Diseases, New York, New York

Richard F. Kyle, MD, Chairman, Department of Orthopaedic Surgery, Hennepin County Medical Center, Associate Professor, University of Minnesota, Minneapolis, Minnesota

Melvin D. Law Jr, MD, Tennessee Spine Center, Nashville, Tennessee

Alan M. Levine, MD, Professor of Orthopaedic Surgery and Oncology, Consultant in Spinal Injury MIEMSS, University of Maryland, Baltimore, Maryland

David G. Lewallen, MD, Associate Professor, Mayo Graduate School of Medicine, Consultant, Orthopedic Surgery, Mayo Clinic/Mayo Foundation, Rochester, Minnesota

Henry J. Mankin, MD, Chief of the Orthopaedic Service, Massachusetts General Hospital, Edith M. Ashley Professor of Orthopaedics, Boston, Massachusetts

Richard A. Marder, MD, Associate Professor of Orthopaedic Surgery, University of California, Davis, School of Medicine, Sacramento, California

Bassam A. Masri, MD, Clinical Associate and Research Fellow, Division of Reconstructive Orthopaedics, University of British Columbia and Vancouver Hospital and Health Sciences Centre, Vancouver, BC, Canada

Paul C. McAfee, MD, Chief of Spinal Surgery, St. Joseph's Hospital, Baltimore, Maryland

Howard Mevis, Director, Electronic Media, American Academy of Orthopaedic Surgeons, Rosemont, Illinois

Mark D. Miller, MD, Associate Team Physician, Clinical Assistant Professor, Department of Orthopaedic Surgery, United States Air Force Academy, USAF Academy, Colorado

Bernard F. Morrey, MD, Professor and Chairman, Department of Orthopedics, Mayo Clinic, Rochester, Minnesota

Daniel J. Nagle, MD, Assistant Professor of Clinical Orthopaedic Surgery, Northwestern University Medical School, Chicago, Illinois

Tom F. Novacheck, MD, Director, Motion Analysis Laboratory, Gillette Children's Hospital, St. Paul, Minnesota

A. Lee Osterman, MD, Professor, Orthopaedic and Hand Surgery, Thomas Jefferson University, Philadelphia, Pennsylvania

David H. Palmer, MD, Clinical Assistant Professor, University of Minnesota, Department of Orthopaedic Surgery, Minneapolis, Minnesota

Gary G. Poehling, MD, Professor and Chairman, Department of Orthopaedic Surgery, Wake Forest University, Winston-Salem, North Carolina

Robert Poss, MD, Professor of Orthopaedic Surgery, Harvard Medical School, Brigham and Women's Hospital, Boston, Massachusetts

Thomas A. Russell, MD, Associate Professor of Orthopaedic Surgery, Department of Orthopaedic Surgery, University of Tennessee, Memphis, Tennessee

Marc R. Safran, MD, Fellow in Sports Medicine, Department of Orthopedics, University of Pittsburgh School of Medicine, Pittsburgh, Pennsylvania

Bruce J. Sangeorzan, MD, University of Washington, Harborview Medical Center, Seattle, Washington

Richard Santore, MD, Associate Professor of Orthopaedic Surgery, University of California, San Diego, School of Medicine, San Diego, California

Andrew H. Schmidt, MD, Attending Orthopaedic Surgeon, Hennepin County Medical Center, Minneapolis, Minnesota

Vladimir Schwartsman, MD, Associate Clinical Professor, Nevada School of Medicine, Las Vegas, Nevada

Karen S. Seale, MD, Assistant Clinical Professor, Department of Orthopaedic Surgery, University of Arkansas for Medical Sciences, Little Rock, Arkansas

Mitchell D. Seemann, MD, Orthopaedic Surgeon, Lakewood Orthopaedic Clinic, Lakewood, Colorado

Andrew Slucky, MD, Assistant Attending, Orthopaedic Surgery, The Hospital for Special Surgery, New York, New York

J. Richard Steadman, MD, Chairman, Medical Group US Ski Team, Orthopaedic Surgeon, Steadman Hawkins Clinic, Vail, Colorado

Philip Stegemann, MD, Clinical Assistant Professor, State University of New York, Buffalo, New York

Marc F. Swiontkowski, MD, Chief of Orthopaedics, Harborview Medical Center, Seattle, Washington

James Tasto, MD, Associate Clinical Professor, Orthopaedic Surgery, University of California, San Diego, California

Francesca M. Thompson, MD, Chief, Adult Orthopaedic Foot Clinic, St. Luke's-Roosevelt Hospital Center, New York, New York

Joe W. Tippett, MD, Southeast Orthopaedic Clinic, San Antonio, Texas

Vernon T. Tolo, MD, Head, Division of Orthopaedics, Childrens Hospital, Los Angeles, John C. Wilson, Jr, Professor of Orthopaedics, University of Southern California School of Medicine, Los Angeles, California

Major Daniel Veltri, MD, Chief of Orthopaedic Services, Luke Air Force Base, Litchfield Park, Arizona

Steven F. Viegas, MD, Professor and Chief, Division of Hand Surgery, Department of Orthopaedic Surgery and Rehabilitation, The University of Texas Medical Branch, Galveston, Texas

Mike Ward, Systems Designer, Information Systems, Brigham and Women's Hospital, Boston, Massachusetts

Russell F. Warren, MD, Hospital for Special Surgery, New York, New York

John H. Wedge, MD, FRCSC, Surgeon-in-Chief, The Hospital for Sick Children, University of Toronto, Toronto, Ontario, Canada

Terry L. Whipple, MD, Clinical Associate Professor, Orthopaedic Surgery, University of Virginia and Medical College of Virginia, Clinical Professor, Orthopaedic Surgery, The Bowman Gray School of Medicine, Richmond, Virginia

Augustus A. White, MD, Dr Med Sci, Professor of Orthopaedic Surgery, Beth Israel Hospital, Harvard Medical School, Boston, Massachusetts

Robert A. Winquist, MD, Clinical Professor of Orthopaedic Surgery, University of Washington, Seattle, Washington

Joseph D. Zuckerman, MD, Chairman, Department of Orthopaedic Surgery, Hospital for Joint Diseases, New York, New York

Preface

This 44th volume of the *Instructional Course Lectures* continues in the long tradition of bringing to its readership a current, up-to-date review of the topics orthopaedic surgeons deal with in treating their patients. These chapters, representing the work of 76 contributors, were chosen from the Instructional Course Lectures offered at the 61st Annual Meeting of the American Academy of Orthopaedic Surgeons, held in 1994 in New Orleans. These authors all met the deadlines necessary to allow this completed volume to be ready in time for the 1995 Annual Meeting. Besides the timely work and talent of the contributing authors, the resources of the Academy's Publications Department made the rapid turn-around required by this short-term deadline possible. Marilyn Fox, PhD, provided administrative support, Bruce Davis did excellent copy editing, follow-up and deadlines with authors were monitored by Sophie Tosta, and Loraine Edwalds headed up the production team. My personal secretary, Becky Yannatone, played a critical role in coordinating our office's efforts with those of the Academy.

Besides being representative of the 142 Instructional Course Lectures presented in 1994, the materials included in this volume are of the high quality that has distinguished the previous *Instructional Course Lectures* volumes and has contributed to our individual learning and educational experience. One way in which this volume demonstrates the continuing evolution of our post-graduate orthopaedic educational process is through the inclusion of our computer courses. In the years ahead, when orthopaedic surgeons look back at these chapters, they will wonder why such basic information about the application of computer technology was needed. The reason is simple. This volume serves the current continuing education of seasoned as well as young orthopaedic surgeons, and a number of our readers did not have the opportunity to use computers and experience hands-on interactive learning during their formal education.

As the Instructional Course Lectures have continued to expand to meet our educational needs, an additional manner of distributing a portion of this information has been implemented. Through a special agreement with *The Journal of Bone and Joint Surgery*, 15 of the 48 chapters in this volume have been published in that journal as Instructional Course Lectures. This cooperative arrangement has made it possible for us to reach a larger audience with selected current topics and has added additional review and editing to the material in this volume.

In spite of ongoing changes in the field of orthopaedics, the focus and charge of the Committee on Instructional Courses is to continue to bring you a wide range of cutting edge, practical, authoritative, multifaceted, timely topics. It is our hope that as you read these chapters you will expand your knowledge and find new challenges, both in your areas of particular interest and in the overall field of orthopaedics.

Douglas W. Jackson, MD
Long Beach, California
Chairman, Committee on Instructional Courses

W. Dilworth Cannon, MD
San Francisco, California

Richard H. Gelberman, MD
Saint Louis, Missouri

Douglas J. Pritchard, MD
Rochester, Minnesota

Michael Schafer, MD
Chicago, Illinois

Contents

SECTION V

SECTION VI

SECTION VII

Metabolic Bone Disease

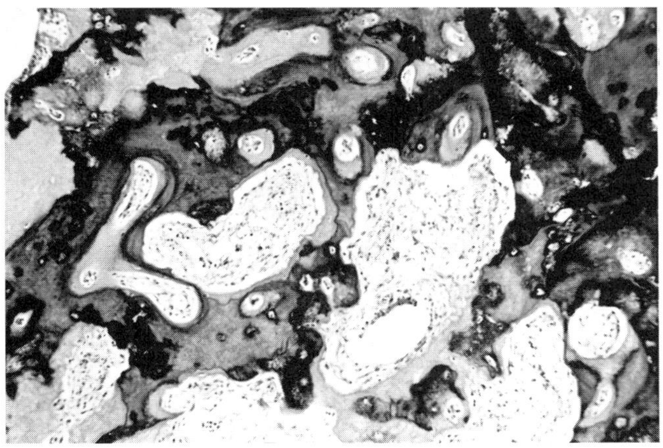

CHAPTER 1

Metabolic Bone Disease

Henry J. Mankin, MD

The purpose of this paper is to provide the orthopaedist, and especially the orthopaedic resident, with the basic information required to understand metabolic bone disease—those disorders of the skeleton associated with alterations in calcium and phosphorus homeostasis. Over the past few decades, great strides have been made in our knowledge of calcium and phosphorus metabolism and especially of the key elements and factors that control the homeostatic mechanisms. These important discoveries have led to a much clearer definition of metabolic bone disease and, more importantly, to new methods of treatment that are quite effective in some patients. These new findings and their value are the principal messages of this paper. Although orthopaedists do not ordinarily treat metabolic bone disease as such and, in fact, are not greatly intrigued by it, almost every time that they treat a patient with a distal radial or proximal femoral fracture they are entering the world of poor bone substance. If orthopaedists are to maintain their complete understanding (and control) of the normal and diseased skeletal system, they must be conversant with the basic knowledge of these disorders of bone metabolism.

In order to understand metabolic bone disease, we must first recognize that, in metabolic terms, bone is an illusion. Although it is concrete in substance (and hence has a finite and almost rigid structure that has a characteristic and specific shape), metabolically it is almost explosively active and serves as an extension and a reservoir for the extracellular space. The skeleton contains about one kilogram of calcium and a slightly lesser amount of phosphorus. It also contains a rather large amount of the body's pool of sodium and magnesium.[1] Because of the manner in which they are maintained in the tiny crystals of bone, these substances have a virtually free exchange with the same materials in the extracellular fluid space.[1,2]

Biomechanically, bone can be considered to be a two-phase composite. The organic phase consists of well-crosslinked, highly ordered, relatively insoluble type-I collagen fibers, which in large measure define the structure and shape of the bones.[2,3] Impregnated within those fibers at specific sites are tiny crystals of hydroxyapatite having the basic formula $Ca_{10}(PO_4)_6(OH)_2$.[2-4] The dimensions of the crystals are extraordinarily tiny—50 by 100 by 200 angstroms—which creates an enormous surface area.[2,4,5] If all of the calcium and phosphate of bone were combined into one crystal, the estimated surface area would be less than two square meters. In contrast, the crystalline polyhedral structure of the tiny segments of hydroxyapatite presents a reactive surface that, for a 60-kg person, is equivalent to the surface area of the lower half of Manhattan Island. If one also considers that the crystal has a hydration shell and unfilled surface spaces and is quite reactive,[3,5] it should be evident that these materials that are in direct contact with the extracellular space represent a highly reactive reservoir, both for deposition of excess minerals and for almost instantaneous recovery of minerals during periods of deficit.

In times of calcium deficit or need, the skeleton rapidly loses calcium salts to maintain the correct levels in the extracellular space. As such, it becomes a silent provider of these critical materials.[6] This is an effective means of solving even a severe deficiency until the structure of the bone becomes so weak that a pathological fracture develops. Before the fracture, it is unlikely that a patient, when asked the nature of his or her problem, will enunciate a chief complaint of "a declining concentration of calcium in the extracellular space." However, he or she certainly will notice a comminuted fracture of the weakened femur that occurred while stepping off of a curb.

Although the panoply of metabolic bone diseases must number in the hundreds, for the purpose of this paper, I will consider only four categories of causation of weakened bones: hyperparathyroidism, the rachitic syndromes (rickets, osteomalacia, and renal osteodystrophy), osteoporosis, and malignant diffuse skeletal disease (chiefly, multiple myeloma). The difficulty that a physician can have in distinguishing these diseases from each other on the basis of history, physical examination, and imaging is evident from the radiographs of the spine of four patients (Fig. 1), each with a different disease, who came to my office with the same complaint: the relatively recent onset of moderately severe pain in the back and no other symptoms. A simple system of further evaluation will be discussed later in this paper and the diagnoses will be provided.

Homeostatic Mechanisms for Calcium and Phosphorus

Before I discuss the causative mechanisms or define the resultant clinical syndromes included in this group of disorders, it is important to review briefly some of the principles of calcium and phosphorus homeostasis that are responsible for maintaining the necessarily narrow range of normal values for these substances. The rules that govern these homeostatic mechanisms are relatively simple and are based on three essential laws or, at least, truths: 1. The salt $CaHPO_4$ is not freely soluble in body fluids, and if the concentrations of Ca^{+2} or HPO_4^{-2} exceed the critical solubility product, ectopic calcification is likely to occur. Because all calcium salts are more soluble in an acid medium, a mild-to-moderate acidosis prevents precipitation of calcium, while an alkaline

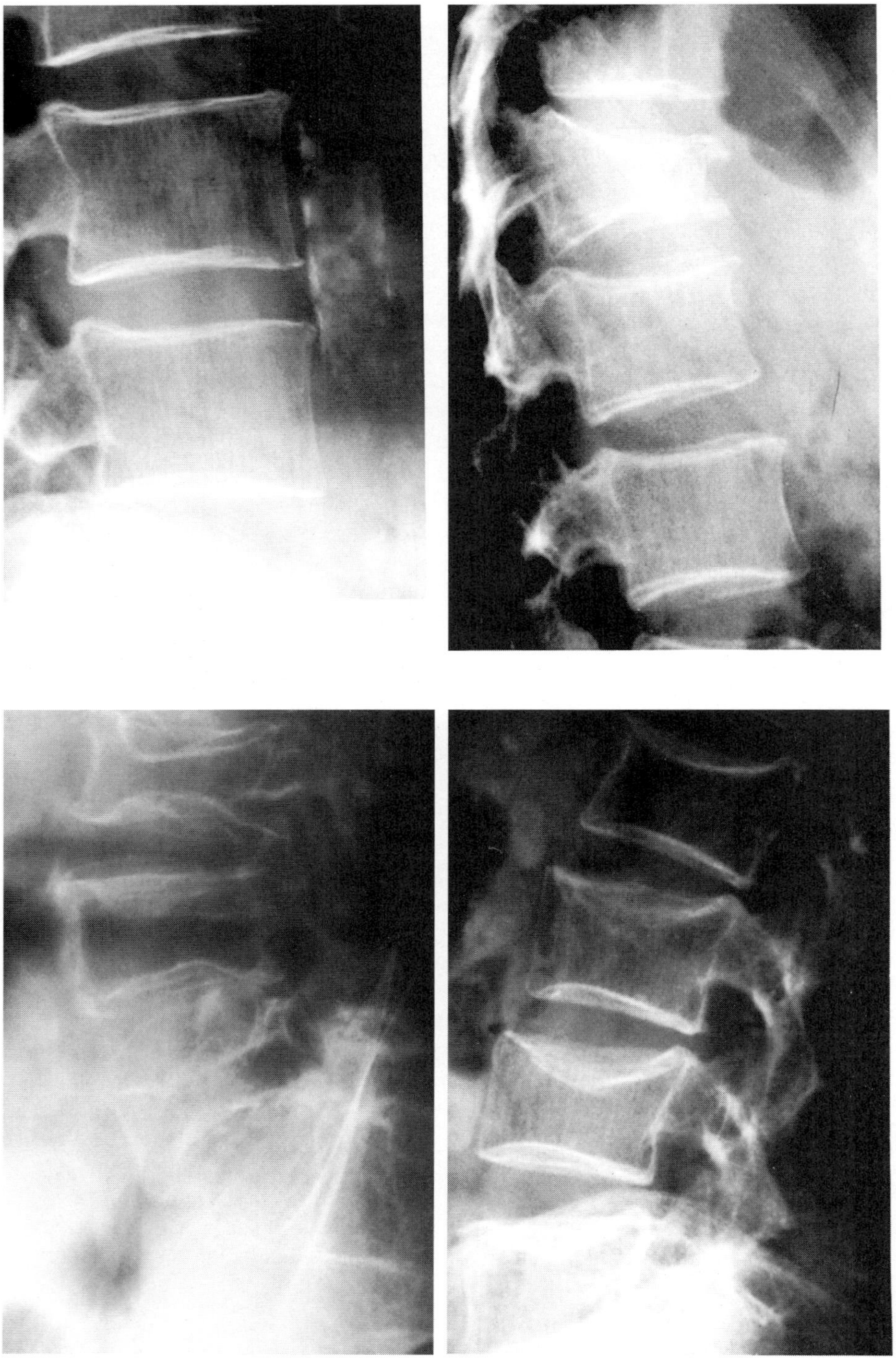

Fig. 1 Lateral radiographs of the lumbar spine of four patients who were seen in my office, over a period of several months, with moderately severe low-back pain without further localizing symptoms. Each of these patients had marked osteopenia, and all but one (top left) had compression fractures. Each patient had a different disorder.

substrate increases the likelihood of such an event. 2. The irritability and conductivity of nerve and the irritability and contractility of smooth and skeletal muscle are inversely proportional to the concentration of Ca^{+2}, whereas the irritability and contractility of cardiac muscle are directly proportional to the concentration of Ca^{+2}. All three of these relationships have a very narrow range of safety. Thus, when the serum calcium concentration is low, the patient becomes hypertonic and hyperreflexic, convulses, and dies in diastole. When the serum Ca^{+2} is elevated, the reverse is seen—that is, there is hypotonicity, hyporeflexia, obtundation, and coma, and death occurs in systole. 3. Calcium cannot cross a cell barrier without a transport system. The system, as defined, has two important components.[7-10] The first and principal of these components is 1,25-dihydroxyvitamin D, which acts to enhance the mRNA to increase synthesis of one or several calcium-binding proteins (calbindin or cholecalcin), which transport the calcium across the cell barrier to the extracellular space.[10-12] A second component is the cytosolic concentration of phosphate, which, if above a critical level, may "turn off" transport.[13-15] A third, less important, component is parathyroid hormone, which enhances the production of 1,25-dihydroxyvitamin D in the kidneys. The parathyroid hormone molecule binds to a receptor on the cell membrane and, through the action of adenyl cyclase and cyclic adenosine monophosphate, the hormone enhances the entry of calcium into the cell and may also activate the release of calcium by the mitochondria.[7,13,15]

The major material that controls the concentration of calcium and, to a lesser extent, phosphate is 1,25-$(OH)_2$-vitamin D. Phosphate exerts control only in the negative sense, in that turning off of calcium transport is protective against deposition of calcium salts (as defined in the first law). The role of parathyroid hormone is principally one of enhancement of the action of vitamin D.

Calcium absorption occurs at the level of the distal portion of the duodenum or the proximal portion of the jejunum and is dependent not only on the cellular mechanisms just described but also on the presentation of the calcium salt in an appropriate form.[14-18] If there are chelating agents, such as phytate or oxalate, in the gastrointestinal tract, or excessive concentrations of phosphate as a result of dietary intake or free fatty acids (such as occur in biliary disease or in some forms of chronic bowel disease), the calcium is either chelated or made less soluble and, thus, is rendered more difficult to absorb.[16-18] If these factors are not in excess, if dietary calcium intake is normal (approximately 1 g per day), and if sufficient concentrations of 1,25-dihydroxyvitamin D and parathyroid hormone are present, the calcium will be absorbed.[13,14,16] The ionic concentration of calcium in the serum is maintained by regulation of the renal glomerular filtration, by tubular reabsorption of calcium (also in large measure controlled by vitamin D and parathyroid hormone),[19-21] and by formation and resorption of bone (very much dependent on parathyroid hormone and, to a lesser extent, on vitamin D).[3,21,22]

If the ionic calcium concentrations in the serum and extracellular fluid are too low, the body's homeostatic mechanisms respond by increased synthesis and release of parathyroid hormone,[22,23] which increases the rate of production of 1,25-dihydroxyvitamin D.[23,24] Acting together, these two hormones increase absorption of calcium in the gut and increase tubular reabsorption of calcium in the kidneys, both of which processes increase the concentration of ionic calcium in the serum and extracellular fluid. Of equal importance, and critical to orthopaedic issues, is the fact that degradation of bone also is enhanced both by so-called crystallysis (release of mineral from the hydroxyapatite crystal) and by the much broader destruction of bone by osteoclasts.[25]

Of perhaps greater concern to the body, particularly in terms of such disorders as the hypercalcemia associated with various forms of malignancy, is the response (or lack of response) to an elevated calcium level in the serum and extracellular fluid. As noted in the second law described in this paper, the cardiac and neuromuscular sensitivity to hypercalcemia is exquisite and the margin of safety is narrow. In a chicken, the ultimobranchial body comes to the rescue with the elaboration of a material known as calcitonin,[26] which is believed to act by decreasing the absorption of calcium in the gastrointestinal tract, diminishing the tubular reabsorption of calcium, and immobilizing the osteoclast population of the bones. All of these processes lead to a decreased concentration of ionized calcium in the extracellular fluid.[26-29] Although the C cells of the human thyroid gland elaborate calcitonin, the autogenous output of calcitonin by human thyroid tissue appears to be insufficient to lower the serum calcium concentration markedly. However, when calcitonin is administered in greater than physiologic doses to patients with Paget disease or osteoporosis, the rate of bone-remodeling decreases markedly.[26]

The management of phosphate by the body is less complicated. Only ingestion of excessive calcium or aluminum (usually in the form of the hydroxide used as an antacid), or both, interfere with absorption.[16,30,31] Transport occurs more distally in the jejunum and is far less selective, with most of the ingested phosphate rapidly making its way into the extracellular space.[32] The relationship to the bone is an obligate one in that the breakdown or disorganization of the crystalline hydroxyapatite, $Ca_{10}(PO_4)_6(OH)_2$, requires an obligatory release of phosphate with either crystallysis or osteoclastic destruction. Conversely, synthesis of new crystals requires six phosphate ions for each ten calcium ions. The principal control mechanism for phosphate is renal, in that there is not only a tubular maximum (and hence a so-called spill) and tubular secretion but a very finely tuned tubular reabsorption mechanism for phosphate. This mechanism is affected by a number of factors but is principally under the control of parathyroid hormone.[33-35] Administration of parathyroid hormone causes a rapid decline in the percentage of tubular resorption of phosphate and a resultant phosphate diuresis.[22-35] Thus, conditions such as rickets, osteomalacia, or renal osteodystrophy, which cause an increase in parathyroid hormone release (principally in response to a lowered CA^{+2} concentration), cause a simultaneous decline in the percentage of tubular resorption of phosphate and a resultant hyperphosphaturia and hypophosphatemia.[22,36,37] Such a mechanism is clearly protective because, if both the ionic calcium and the phosphate concentrations rise, we are dangerously close to turning to stone!

The final element in this review of calcium and phosphorus homeostasis is the biology of vitamin D. Until 20 years ago, the most well-recognized of the D vitamins included provitamin D2 (ergosterol from certain plants and animal fat) and provitamin D3 (7-dehydrocholesterol synthesized in the liver and stored in the skin.[32,38-41] These and all of the vitamin-D metabolites are transported in the blood by a vitamin-D-binding protein, an alpha globulin synthesized in the liver.[38,39] With exposure to ultraviolet light at about 315 nm, these materials become active, converting the provitamins to vitamin D2 (calciferol) and vitamin D3 (cholecalciferol).[32,42] These vitamins are converted to 25-hydroxyvitamin D in the liver (under the direction of the enzyme vitamin D-25-hydrolase and Mg^{+2}) and are further converted in the proximal tubule of the kidney to several polar metabolites (1,25-dihydroxyvitamin D, 24,25-dihydroxyvitamin D, and 25,26-dihydroxyvitamin D), each through a specific enzyme system.[10,13,20,25,43,44] The most active of these metabolites is 1,25-dihydroxyvitamin D, which is as much as 12 times more active than the precursor 25-hydroxyvitamin D and seems to be one of the two major substances regulating calcium transport in the gut, the proximal renal tubule, and bone.[3,12,13,15,23,25,32] Receptor sites on these cells (and a number of other tissues) have been identified and purified,[9,45,46] and the gene error in several forms of rickets has been identified as occurring in the nuclear receptor for 1,25-dihydroxyvitamin D.[47,48] The actions of 1,25-dihydroxyvitamin D are somewhat broader than simply stimulation of calcium-binding proteins; they include activities that have an effect on osteocalcin production, osteoclastic resorption, monocytic maturation, myelocytic differentiation, skin growth, and insulin secretion.[9,25] In terms of mineral metabolism, however, the factors that favor the synthesis of 1,25-dihydroxyvitamin D rather than some of the other, less potent metabolites are an expression of biochemical need, signaled to the cells by reduced calcium-ion and phosphate concentrations and an increased serum parathyroid-hormone level.[32,44,49] In consideration of the entire picture, it is important also to consider the role of 24,25-dihydroxyvitamin D, which, although known to have some effect on calcium metabolism, is now thought to serve principally as an entry point to an alternative breakdown pathway for vitamin D.[25,32,50]

Primary Hyperparathyroidism

Having defined, at least in part, the homeostatic mechanisms, it is now possible to proceed to a discussion of each of the four disorders defined in the beginning of this paper. Primary hyperparathyroidism is a well-recognized entity that was, at least in part, identified more than a century ago by von Recklinghausen.[51] He and his coworkers are responsible for the descriptive term osteitis fibrosa cystica (generalisata).

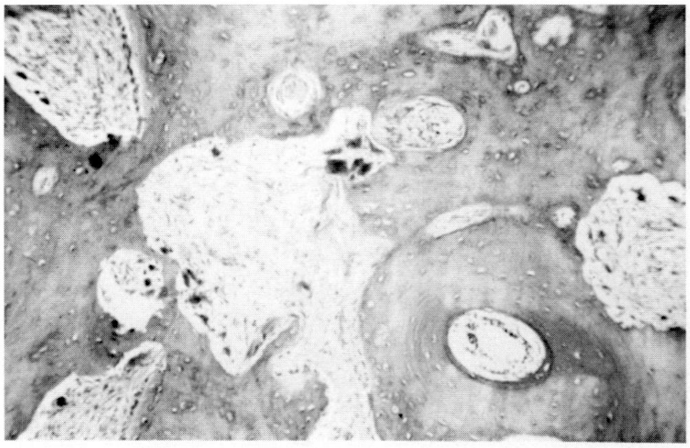

Fig. 2 Histologic findings in a patient who had primary hyperparathyroidism. Note especially the fibrous replacement of the marrow (osteitis fibrosa) and the osteoclastic resorption of the osseous trabeculae along with simultaneous osteoblastic rimming and new-bone formation (hematoxylin and eosin, × 100).

The histologic changes are quite distinctive and, in florid disease, consist of fibrous replacement of the marrow, osteoclastic resorption of the bone, osteoblastic rimming on new and often incompletely mineralized lamellar bone trabeculae, and so-called brown tumors—areas of granulation tissue, inflammatory cells, and giant cells with virtually no bone at all (Fig. 2).[52] The disease results from an excessive secretion of parathyroid hormone that occurs in response to an adenoma; hyperplasia; or, in rare cases, a carcinoma of a single parathyroid gland.[53-56] Because the parathyroid gland output of parathyroid hormone is believed to be almost entirely dependent on the serum and extracellular fluid values of calcium, the implication is that the diseased gland fails to recognize the signal and does not turn off in response to the high levels of Ca^{+2} and hence becomes a "runaway train," pouring out the parathyroid hormone and not obeying or even recognizing the critical message sent by the excessive calcium levels.[57,58]

The effect of primary hyperparathyroidism on the serum values for calcium as well as on the skeleton is consistently predictable (Fig. 3). The increased concentration of parathyroid hormone acts to enhance the synthesis of 1,25-dihydroxyvitamin D, and together the two substances work at the level of the intestinal cell to increase gastrointestinal absorption of calcium and at the level of the glomerulus to increase tubular reabsorption of calcium,[22,23,53,54] rendering the patient intermittently hypercalcemic.[57,58] Bone breakdown occurs partly as a result of destruction of hydroxyapatite crystals but more importantly as a result of osteoclastic resorption, which produces holes in the bone.[27,59-61] These holes fill in with fibrous tissue (hence the name osteitis fibrosa) and, at times, become confluent, to produce a large defect known as a brown tumor.[52,54,59,60] Because there

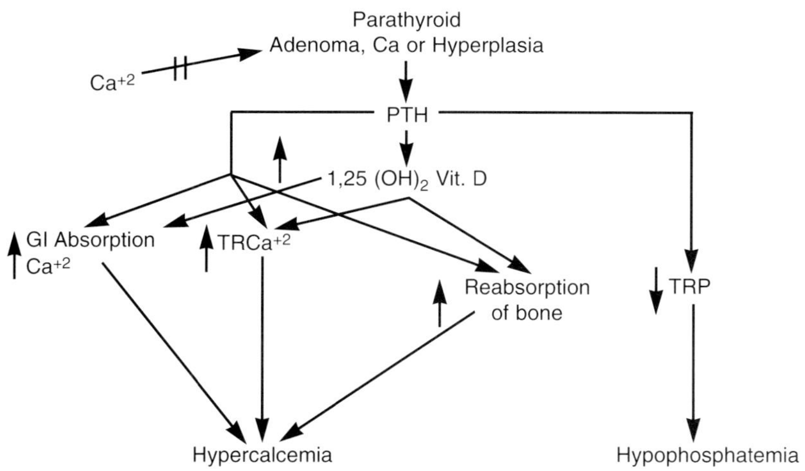

Fig. 3 Diagram showing the mechanism of the development of the biochemical and osseous findings of primary hyperparathyroidism. PTH = parathyroid hormone, GI = gastrointestinal, and TR = tubular resorption.

is also a simultaneous decrease in the percentage of tubular resorption of phosphate, a phosphate diabetes ensues and the patient becomes hyperphosphaturic.[53,54] The chemical findings, then, are an elevated level of serum calcium, a lowered level of serum phosphate, an elevated level of serum alkaline phosphatase (because bone formation occurs in response to the destruction), and an elevated level of serum urate (reflecting tissue breakdown.[62] Patchy increased activity on a bone scan, combined with elevated serum uric acid, a diminished percentage of tubular resorption of phosphate, and an increased level of urinary calcium all point to the presumptive diagnosis. However, to be certain, particularly in the face of the many other causes of hypercalcemia,[53,63] an analysis of the concentration of parathyroid hormone is required. It has been proposed that the principal test at present is immunoassay for parathyroid hormone 1-84, the greatest value of which is its ability to distinguish the hypercalcemia of malignancy from that of hyperparathyroidism.[53,54,63,64]

Early in the course of the disease, pathologic examination of bone specimens is likely to show small islands of fibrous tissue replacing the normal marrow and evidence of increased osteoclastic resorption coupled with an increase in bone formation.[52,54,60] The latter finding is characterized by new trabeculae that may not be completely mineralized (narrow osteoid seams) with osteoblastic rimming (Fig. 2). With advancing disease or in sites of more severe involvement, the osteoclastic resorption may become so overwhelming that no bone at all is seen. Instead, there is a granulation tissue with fibroblasts, giant cells, inflammatory cells, and macrophages, containing hemosiderin in many cases. This finding is characteristic of a brown tumor of hyperparathyroidism.

When imaging studies are performed on patients who have primary hyperparathyroidism, they show osteopenia of the skeletal structures that is asymmetrical and that seems to affect one or several sites more than it does others. Some of the remarkable radiographic features of this disorder are so-called salt-and-pepper skull (Fig. 4), loss of the lamina dura, erosion of the outer centimeter of the clavicle (Fig. 5), marked osteopenia of the medial aspect of the tibia, and subperiosteal resorption of the digital tufts and phalanges (which, for some unknown reason, is usually more marked on the radial than on the ulnar side of the hand) (Fig. 6). These changes are usually associated with a diffuse osteopenia and sometimes with compression fractures, particularly in the vertebrae. Occasionally, in severe or neglected cases, brown tumors and pathological fractures occur. Because the level of serum calcium is high, a temporary rise in the level of serum phosphorus may cause calcification to occur in the soft tissues—as described in the first law presented earlier in this paper.[65,66] Renal calculi are the rule,[53,67] but, in addition, calcifications in the connective tissues are not uncommon.[53,65,66] Special sites of affinity for calcification include the triangular ligament in the distal radioulnar articulation, the menisci, and the articular cartilages.

Decades ago, these florid and easily noticeable changes on the imaging studies were the usual presentation of primary hyperparathyroidism. The picture was defined by the term "stones, bones, and groans."[53,61,68] The term bones referred to the osseous changes just described, but it was also an indication of the fact that, in those days, most patients were seen with diffuse bone pain and sometimes tenderness. The term stones describes the common occurrence of renal calculi. Indeed, in untreated cases, the calculi sometimes caused renal failure.[53,54,61,67,68] The term groans was in part related to the second law enunciated earlier in this paper. Individuals with a serum calcium level of greater

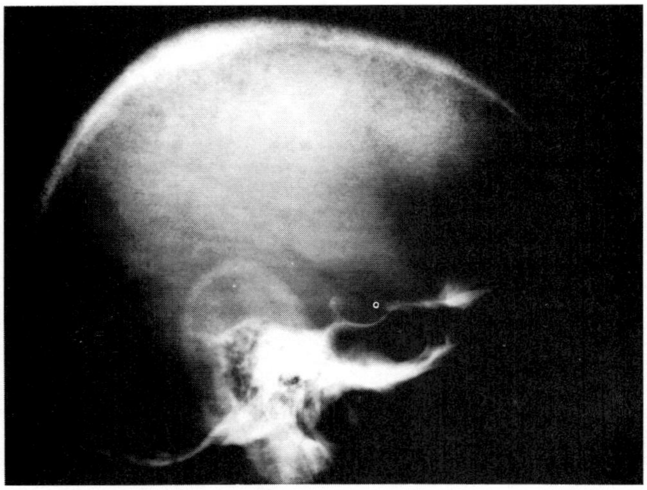

Fig. 4 The so-called salt-and-pepper appearance of the skull in a patient with florid osteitis fibrosa cystica from primary hyperparathyroidism.

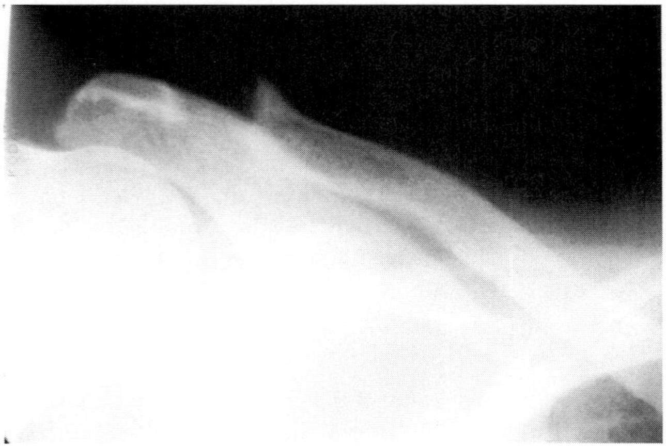

Fig. 5 Erosion of the lateral aspect of the clavicle, a classic finding in patients with hyperparathyroidism.

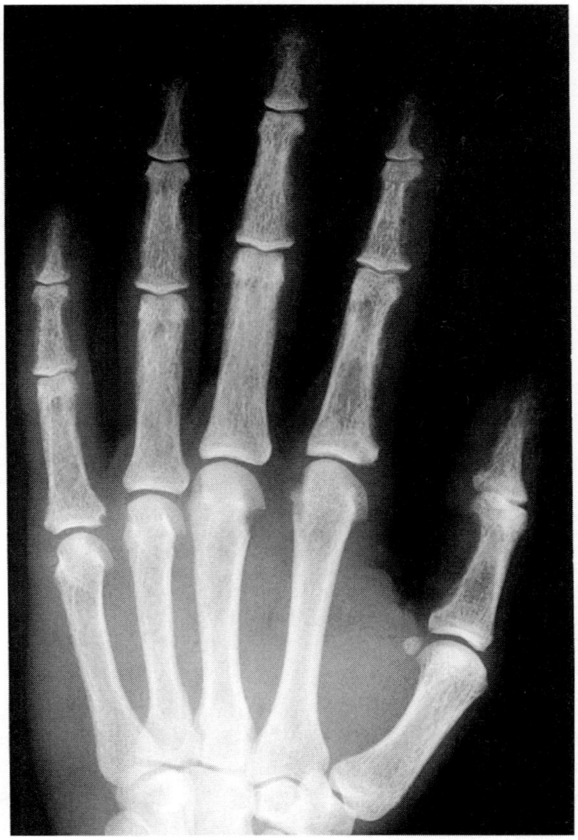

Fig. 6 Typical radiographic changes in the hand of a patient with severe primary hyperparathyroidism. Note the erosion of the tufts, the diffuse osteopenia, and the distinctive subperiosteal resorption of the phalanges, which is more marked on the radial side.

than 12 mg/dl (2.99 mM/l) have mental aberrations and sometimes fairly evident confusion and dementia.[53,54,69,70] Gastric ulcers and pancreatitis rounded out the full-blown clinical picture.[71,72] Without a competent assay for parathyroid hormone or effective methods of imaging of the glands, the diagnosis of primary hyperparathyroidism was a difficult challenge to the practitioner in those days.[53,54,59,64,65,68]

Today—for reasons probably related to the widespread use of rapid, automated laboratory screening systems—the presentation of the disorder has changed to a much blander and often much more subtle picture.[73-77] One rarely encounters the full-blown clinical syndrome and, most often, the patient either is asymptomatic or has, at worst, low-back pain, a mild increase in thirst and urination, and perhaps evidence of osteopenia on radiographs. The occurrence of renal calculi, formerly said to affect more than 50% of patients, has now been reduced to less than 10%,[76] and florid bone lesions (especially brown tumors) are rarely if ever seen.[59,73,75,76] Because the disorder is considerably more frequent in women and because the prevalence increases with advanced age, the potential for confusion with osteoporosis is great. Because localization of the diseased gland or glands is now much easier with the use of modern imaging technology[78] and surgical treatment has now progressed to the point at which eradication of the lesion is a reasonable certainty,[73,75] most patients can be treated before orthopaedic problems develop. Today, more and more of the management is medical, and considerable experience has been gained with the use of such agents as phosphate, bisphosphonates, and estrogen, making surgery unnecessary in many asymptomatic patients.[63,73]

The principal role of the orthopaedist in the management of patients with hyperparathyroidism is that of a case-finder. A high index of suspicion in the management of patients with bone pain coupled with a compression fracture or even just radiographic evidence of osteopenia should stimulate the physician to obtain serum chemistry studies (determinations of the levels of calcium, phosphorus, blood urea nitrogen, and alkaline phosphatase). The diagnosis is easily confirmed by appropriate immunoassays for parathyroid hormone.[64,73] Once the diagnosis has been made, the patient should be managed by physicians who are skilled in the treatment of metabolic bone disease and by surgeons with experience in the removal of adenomatous parathyroid glands.

Rickets, Osteomalacia, and Renal Osteodystrophy

In 1974, I wrote a two-part review article on rickets, osteomalacia, and renal osteodystrophy that summarized the knowledge to that time and cited the then-current literature.[36,37] A more recent update was added in 1990.[79] It is not the purpose of the present paper to repeat either of those works, although they are liberally quoted in the text. An attempt will be made to provide a brief summary of the subject with special emphasis on the differential diagnosis of the osteopenic bone conditions in adults. Several sources[9,16,36,37,79-83] can provide more in-depth information on specific areas within the field, and I especially recommend one that offers a review of the subject in the form of the extraordinary artwork of the late Frank H. Netter.[84]

Although the history of rickets, osteomalacia, and renal osteodystrophy is almost as long as that of any other disorder (having been recognized since the middle of the 17th century) and, in many ways, is remarkable for scientific progress during virtually every generation, far more progress has been made in our understanding and management of these disorders in the past 30 years than in the previous 300 years. The earliest recognized forms of the disease—vitamin D-deficient osteomalacia and rickets[36,37,81]—are now far less commonly encountered in the United States, principally because of the recognition of the importance of dietary calcium and vitamin D and the improved general nutrition of the well population. Now, the previously less common and even rare forms are more prevalent. These include the vitamin D-resistant and vitamin D-dependent disorders as well as renal osteodystrophy.[80,82,83]

In previous years, little effective treatment was available to patients with the resistant, dependent, or renal osteodystrophic forms, and little could be done to ameliorate the process or even to diminish its osseous ravages. Most of our efforts were directed at recognition of the disease, provision of inadequate treatment (mostly huge doses of vitamin D), and performance of surgery that often proved less than satisfactory. The extraordinary scientific discoveries of the previous 20 years have not only materially increased our knowledge of the pathogenesis of these disorders but have provided potent agents for treatment. These discoveries include the remarkable definition of the biochemistry of calcium transport by selected cells[9-12] and the outstanding scientific exploration of the nature and role of the polar metabolites of vitamin D, not only in transport but in other body systems as well.[9,13,20,25] These scientific efforts have not only increased our understanding of the cause and mechanism by which these diseases develop but have also greatly improved the capacity of clinicians to diagnose and to treat the various clinical syndromes.[25]

There are many different causes of the rachitic and osteomalacic syndromes, but all have a central theme: the lack of available calcium or phosphorus (or both) for mineralization of newly formed osteoid. Because the disorders have a final common pathway (defects in the mineralization of the bones), children with rickets and adults with osteomalacia present with sometimes strikingly similar findings. This stereotypic presentation is such a remarkable feature that the clinician is sometimes hard-pressed to distinguish one type from another on the basis of physical examination or imaging studies alone and must sometimes resort to a highly sophisticated laboratory analysis, some components of which were not available until quite recently.[64,85-87]

The Causes of Rickets and Osteomalacia

Although there are many causes for the rachitic and osteomalacic syndromes, they fall principally into five major categories: deficiency states, gastrointestinal causes, renal tubular causes, unusual causes, and renal osteodystrophy (Table 1).

Deficiency States

The mechanism of vitamin D-deficient rickets or osteomalacia (Fig. 7) is as follows. Reduced vitamin-D intake causes a diminution in the absorption of calcium from the gastrointestinal tract. Insufficient absorption leads to a lowering of the serum calcium level, which in turn causes a secondary hyperparathyroidism and a resultant increase of the serum Ca^{+2} concentration to low normal and a phosphate diuresis.[16,36,37,81] The chemical changes in the blood and urine that reflect this finding are almost invariably a lowering of the levels of serum calcium, serum phosphate, and urinary calcium; a reduced percentage of tubular resorption of phosphate; and an increased level of serum alkaline phosphatase. The concentrations of both 25-hydroxyvitamin D and 1,25-dihydroxyvitamin D are reduced and the level of parathyroid hormone is modestly elevated (Table 1). The combination of a reduced amount of mineral (both ionized calcium and phosphate) and secondary hyperparathyroidism is presumed to be the principal factor responsible for the pathological changes in the epiphyseal plates (in rickets) and bones and the resultant alterations in radiographic images.

Table 1
Biochemical Findings in the Rachitic and Osteomalacic Syndromes

Category	Serum Calcium	Serum Phosphate	Serum Alkaline Phosphatase	Parathyroid Hormone	25-Hydroxyvitamin D	1,25-Dihydroxyvitamin D	Tubular Resorption of Phosphate (%)	Urinary Calcium	Miscellaneous Findings
Deficiency states									
Vitamin-D deficiency	Low to normal	Low	High	High	Low	Low	Low	Low	
Phosphate deficiency	Normal	Low	High	Normal	Normal	Normal	High	Normal	
Gastrointestinal	Low	Low	High	High	Low to normal	Low to normal	Low	Low	
Vitamin-D resistant									
Phosphaturic	Normal	Low	High	Normal	Normal	Normal	Low	Normal	Glycosuria, aminoaciduria, etc. (Fanconi-I syndrome)
Type-I dependent	Low	Low	High	High	Normal	Low	Low	Low	
Type-II dependent	Low	Low	High	High	Normal to high	Normal to high	Low	Low	
Renal tubular acidosis	Low	Low	High	High	Normal to high	Normal to high	Low	High	Low levels of sodium and potassium; high levels of chloride acidosis and alkaline urine
Renal osteodystrophy	Low	High	High	High	Low	Low	?	Low	High levels of blood urea nitrogen and creatinine

(Adapted with permission from Mankin H J: Rickets, osteomalacia, and renal osteodystrophy: An update. *Orthop Clin North Am* 1990;21:81-96.)

Vitamin-D Deficiency This is the classic form of the disease (Fig. 7). It usually results from a deficiency in dietary intake of vitamin D, often coupled with inadequate exposure to sunlight. Children with this disorder usually show the abnormality by the age of 1 year or, in florid cases, even earlier. They may display severe weakness, the inability to walk, and remarkable deformities of the skeleton.[36,37,88-90] Adults, in contrast, have few localizing symptoms or findings. They may complain of malaise, easy fatigability, bone pain and tenderness, weakness, or a combination of these symptoms. Physical findings in the adult are sparse but may include a Trendelenburg gait and tenderness over osseous prominences. The great concern, particularly in dealing with an elderly patient, is that the osteopenia or fracture may be attributed to osteoporosis when, in fact, it represents a nutritional osteomalacia.[1,81,91-94,150]

Chelators in the Diet These are rarely a cause of the rachitic syndromes and are seen as a problem only in individuals who have a very unusual or bizarre diet. The major dietary inclusions that can bind calcium and render it unabsorbable in the ionized state are phytate (from some coarse cereals), oxalate (present principally in spinach), and an excess of phosphate.[7,13,16,17,81]

Phosphorus Deficiency This is very unusual in any but the most extraordinary of diets but can occur with the introduction into the diet of beryllium (as an industrial toxic material) or, much more commonly, aluminum, which is present as $Al(OH)_3$ in many antacid preparations. Both of these materials cause precipitation of the insoluble beryllium or aluminum phosphates[16,31-33,81]

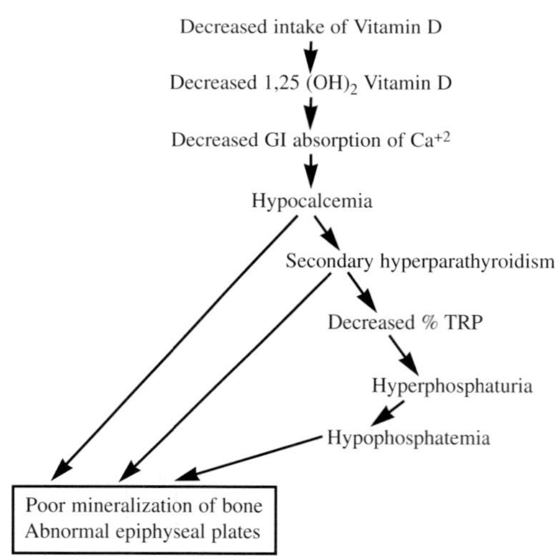

Fig. 7 Diagram depicting the mechanism of the development of the biochemical and osseous changes in patients with vitamin D-deficient rickets and osteomalacia. GI = gastrointestinal and TRP = tubular resorption of phosphate. (Reproduced with permission from Zaleske DJ, Doppelt SH, Mankin HJ: Metabolic and endocrine abnormalities of the immature skeleton, in Lovell WW, Winter RB (eds): *Pediatric Orthopaedics*, ed 2. Philadelphia, PA, JB Lippincott, 1986, vol 1, pp 81-145.)

and render the ingested phosphate non-absorbable. Ingested aluminum itself may cause an osteomalacic-like state by interfering with bone formation at the mineralization front.[17,24,79,95]

Gastrointestinal Causes

Gastric Rickets or Osteomalacia An unusual entity, this disorder has rarely been seen since the decline in frequency of gastric operations for duodenal ulcers. In years past, following a Polya or Billroth II gastrectomy, an osteomalacia developed that was quite subtle and only revealed itself by increasing muscle weakness or a pathological fracture.[79,96,97] The cause of this syndrome is not well understood, but it is believed to result from a diminished acid content in the stomach (all calcium salts are more soluble in an acid medium) and an excessively rapid transit of the gastrointestinal contents through the duodenum and the proximal part of the jejunum (the so-called dumping syndrome).[18,36,37]

Biliary Rickets or Osteomalacia The cause of this disorder is abnormal fat metabolism, usually associated with failure of the emulsifying action of bile salts or the presence of free fat in the intestinal tract. Vitamin D is a fat-soluble vitamin,[20,98,99] and absorption is reduced in the presence of excessive fat in the bowel contents.[9,81] In addition, a recent study has demonstrated a reduced concentration of vitamin D in the serum of obese individuals.[38,100] Ionized calcium may serve as the counter-ion for free fatty acids and thus produce a so-called calcium soap, a material that is grossly insoluble in the body fluids. Classic vitamin-D-deficiency disease has been described in patients with biliary cirrhosis and in alcoholics,[101-104] further confirming the importance of an intact hepatic mechanism in the handling of vitamin D and calcium in the gastrointestinal tract.

Enteric Rickets or Osteomalacia This is usually associated with some diffuse injury to the wall of the small bowel, as occurs with inflammatory processes such as celiac disease, Crohn disease, or disorders associated with a short loop (shunts or fistulae) or rapid transit (gluten-sensitive enteropathy and other sprue-like syndromes).[7,98,105-109] In recent years, total parenteral nutrition has been associated with an osteomalacic syndrome that can be quite severe in patients on prolonged therapy.[110,111]

Renal Tubular Causes of Rachitic Syndromes

In the more than 50 years since the first recognition of rickets resistant to normal doses of vitamin D by Albright and associates,[112] a large group of acquired or genetic renal tubular reabsorptive defects has been described, all of which result in rickets or osteomalacia. The syndromes are not only dissimilar in terms of the extent of the defect in the proximal or distal tubular reabsorptive system but are sometimes confusing as a result of the relatively frequent application of eponyms, often based on a rather colorful history of discovery, each with their own various manifestations and distinguishing diagnostic studies.[36,37,79] However, current thinking suggests that all of the syndromes can be included in four separate and generally quite disparate categories.

Hypophosphatemic Rickets or Osteomalacia (Albright Syndrome, Phosphate Diabetes, and Classic Vitamin-D-Deficient Rickets) This most frequently encountered form of the disease consists of a genetic or acquired fault in the handling of phosphate in the proximal tubule.[113-117] A detailed family history aids in the diagnosis. The signs and symptoms of rickets rarely are manifest before the age of 3 years. The most prevalent form, first described by Albright and associates[112] in 1937, is transmitted as an X-linked dominant condition and is confined to a diminished tubular reabsorption of phosphate. In other cases, the proximal tubular defect may be more extensive and may result not only in hyperphosphaturia and a diminished percentage of tubular resorption of phosphate but in glycosuria and aminoaciduria as well.[36,37,79,80] If defects in the absorption of all three substances (phosphate, glucose, and amino acids) are present, the syndrome is known as Fanconi proximal tubular vitamin-D-deficient rickets, or Fanconi-I syndrome. (It should be noted that a broader defect—also involving the distal tubule and a failure to reabsorb water, fixed base, and hydrogen—is present in Fanconi-II [Debré-de Toni-Fanconi] syndrome,[36,37,118] and the latter state combined with deposition of cystine crystals in various organs is known as Lignac-Fanconi syndrome, or systemic cystinosis.[36,37,119] Administration of vitamin D even in toxic doses (as was done in the past) has little beneficial effect on these lesions. Instead, it is more appropriate to manage these patients with neutral phosphate orally[120,121] and 1,25-dihydroxyvitamin D. If patients are given oral phosphate supplements alone, secondary hyperparathyroidism may result. Recently, some additional forms of the primary hypophosphatemic entity have been described. These include hypophosphatemic osteomalacia in adults (often acquired)[80,122] and a rare genetic entity in which the hypophosphatemia is associated with hypercalcuria.[123,124] A major breakthrough in the definition of the cause of hypophosphatemic osteomalacia occurred when the gene locus was discovered for a rare X-linked syndrome associated with alopecia. This disorder is believed to result from a gene-directed alteration in the vitamin-D receptor site.[47,48,95,125-127]

Type-I Vitamin-D-Dependent Rickets or Osteomalacia A failure of conversion of 25-hydroxyvitamin D to 1,25-dihydroxyvitamin D is the cause of this disorder. The defect is not clearly understood but may be a deficiency or an abnormality of the renal 1-hydroxyvitamin D-25-hydrolase, believed necessary for the conversion of 1-hydroxyvitamin D to 1,25-dihydroxyvitamin D.[80,120,128,129] The disorder is considered to be a pseudodeficiency state in which the patient does not respond to even large doses of orally administered vitamin D, despite a rise in the amount of 25-hydroxyvitamin D generated by the liver (Fig. 7). In some cases the defect can be overcome with large doses of vitamin D, but more importantly it can be completely eliminated by physiologic doses of 1,25-dihydroxyvitamin D.[80,120,129]

Type-II Vitamin-D-Dependent Rickets or Osteomalacia This is believed to represent an end-organ insensitivity to autogenous 1,25-dihydroxyvitamin D. The pathogenesis is obscure but the cause appears to be a genetic error that results in the failure of the gut (and other) cells to recognize autogenous 1,25-dihydroxyvitamin D. The patients become rachitic despite normal or high serum concentrations of 25-hydroxyvitamin D and 1,25-dihydroxyvitamin D and remain rachitic despite high doses of vitamin D or calcitriol in the diet.[128-130] Some part of this syndrome may be analogous to the previously described sex-linked hypophosphatemic rickets with alopecia in which the nuclear receptor for 1,25-dihydroxyvitamin D in the gut cell is genetically altered.[48,125-127] Patients with type-II vitamin-D-dependent osteomalacia sometimes respond to exogenously administered synthetic 1,25-dihydroxyvitamin D but may need additional calcium administered orally or by infusion for the control of symptoms.[121,128-132]

Renal Tubular Acidosis This may occur as a primary genetic or acquired syndrome or as a component of some other disorder.[36,37] It may also be a component of another renal tubular syndrome, such as the Debré-de Toni-Fanconi syndrome (which includes not only renal tubular acidosis but also phosphate-wasting, glycosuria, aminoaciduria, and loss of fixed base), Lignac-Fanconi syndrome (similar to Fanconi-II syndrome but with the addition of cystine crystals in a variety of organs), Lowe syndrome (some of the just described characteristics as well as neurologic findings, glaucoma, and mental retardation), or superglycine syndrome (some of the just described findings as well as muscle weakness and extraordinary glycinuria).[36,37,80,119,133-136] The syndrome of renal tubular acidosis, regardless of etiology, is thought to be caused by a failure to substitute hydrogen ion for fixed base or bicarbonate wastage and results in a hyperchloremic, hyponatremic, hypokalemic acidosis with an alkaline urine and a notable loss of fixed base including calcium ion. This results in rachitic or osteomalacic findings and sometimes renal calculi.[137] The rachitic part of the syndrome is sometimes overshadowed by the other manifestations of the disease (especially the Fanconi-II group). The renal tubular acidosis in the various syndromes cannot be treated effectively with vitamin D, calcitriol, or phosphate, alone or in combination, but requires alkalinization of the extracellular fluid with the use of sodium bicarbonate or other alkaline solutions.[133,138]

Unusual Causes of Rickets and Osteomalacia

Fibrous Dysplasia or Neurofibromatosis Osteomalacia and rickets are rare osteoendocrine or neuroendocrine manifestations of florid fibrous dysplastic or neurofibromatous disease. Although the two primary disorders appear to be unrelated, they share some features (café-au-lait spots, osseous deformities, and pseudarthroses), but the form of vitamin D-deficient rickets is similar; it is often very severe and resistant to therapy.[36,37,79]

Bone and Soft-Tissue Tumors Very rarely, severe and intractable vitamin-D-deficient rickets develops in patients with certain benign, usually fibrous, connective-tissue tumors.[139-142] It is thought that the cause is the synthesis of a rachitogenic factor or an antagonist to vitamin D.[139,143] Several attempts to identify the material have suggested that it may not be identical for all lesions. Resection of the primary osseous or soft-tissue tumor results in the disappearance of the clinical and laboratory manifestations of the vitamin D-deficient rickets, while recurrence of the tumor promptly results in the reappearance of the often very resistant rachitic syndrome.

Chronic Use of Anticonvulsant Medication Rickets or osteomalacia may occur with use of almost all of the drugs currently prescribed for the control of seizures.[144-148] The cause, although disputed, is believed to be an alteration in the microsomal P450 enzymes in the liver, which changes the mechanism of conversion of vitamin D to its more active 25-hydroxy polar metabolite. The rachitic disease may be mild, and there may be only minor manifestations. The syndrome is dangerous because of the increased sensitivity of the central nervous system that occurs with lowering of the serum Ca^{+2} concentration. The disorder is believed to be very common and may be present in some degree in as many as 15% of patients being managed with chronic anticonvulsant drug maintenance. The disorder can be corrected by administration of either vitamin D in excess or physiologic doses of 1,25-dihydroxyvitamin D.[145,148]

Anatomic and Radiographic Changes in Rickets and Osteomalacia

The anatomic and pathologic changes that occur with rickets or osteomalacia differ principally according to the age of the patient and the severity of the disorder. Rickets is a disease of the growing skeleton and thus affects the epiphyseal plates as well as the bones of children. By definition, osteomalacia occurs only in adults and thus has no effect on the growth cartilage. The osseous changes in osteomalacia are similar to those in children but are much less evident because the adult skeleton is metabolically less active. The osseous changes in both adults and children reflect the fact that either ionized calcium or phosphate, or both, is insufficient in concentration to mineralize the skeleton fully. There is less mineralized bone per unit volume of bone. Some or all of the trabeculae and, indeed, the cortex not only have less bone, but what bone there is, is surrounded by a layer of unmineralized bone, known as an osteoid seam (Fig. 8).[36,37,80,83] Although osteoid seams are not pathognomonic of rickets or osteomalacia (they may also be seen in hyperparathyroidism, fibrous dysplasia, and bone-forming tumors), they are highly suggestive of osteomalacia, and osteomalacia can be associated with seams of a width that are unlikely to occur in any other disorder (Fig. 8).[79] When the pathogenesis of the disease is being considered, it is important to understand that almost all patients with rickets or osteomalacia, regardless of the cause, have similar histologic features of bone; thus, the diagnosis of the correct syndrome cannot be made on the basis of a biopsy or of histomorphometry.

Osseous changes in the rapidly growing skeleton of a young child with florid rickets were formerly thought to cause such severe softening of the bones as to result in bowing deformities.[36,37] It is more likely, however, that the rachitic skeleton is less resistant to bending or shearing moments than is the normal skeleton. As a consequence, stress fractures with resultant deformities occur more readily. Regardless of cause, however, the end result is bones that are defective in strength and have characteristic deformities.[36,37,83,90] Radiographs of the bones (Fig. 9) show thin cortices and indistinct, fuzzy trabeculae that assume an almost ground-glass appearance as a result of the prevalence of the widened osteoid seams.[36,37,83] Focal collections of osteoid may produce ribbon-like transverse zones of incomplete radiolucency, particularly notable on the concave side of the long bones, the medial side of the femoral neck, the ischial and pubic rami, the ribs, the clavicles, and the axillary border of the scapulae (Fig. 10). These Milkman pseudofractures or Looser lines usually show increased activity on bone scans and may, under stress, propagate to become true fractures.[80,81,82,84,90] In adults with osteomalacia, the osteopenic bone changes may dominate the picture; osteomalacic alterations may be very subtle and, unless a Looser line is present, the picture can be mistaken easily for osteoporosis.

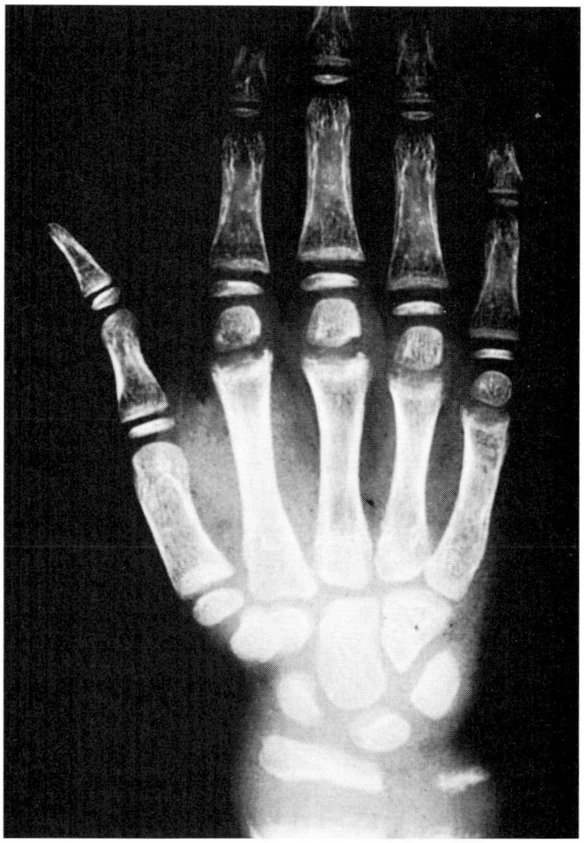

Fig. 9 Radiograph of a hand of a child with florid rickets. Note the increase in the axial height, the cupping and flaring of the distal radial epiphysis, the fuzzy and indistinct trabeculae, and the cortical thinning. (Reproduced with permission from Mankin HJ: Rickets, osteomalacia, and renal osteodystrophy: Part I. *J Bone Joint Surg* 1974;56A:101-128.)

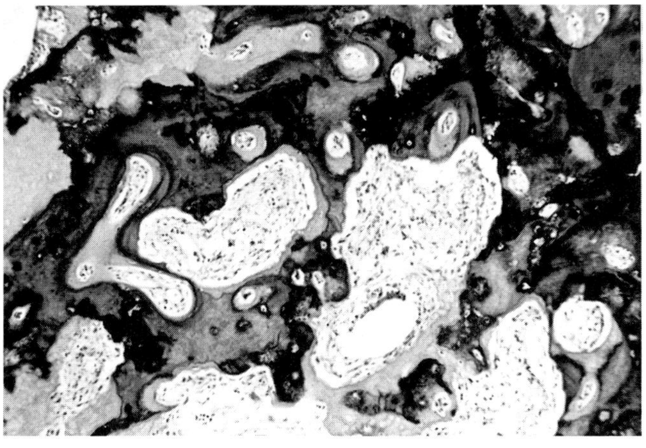

Fig. 8 Histologic section showing the osteoid seams of osteomalacic trabecular bone. The mineralized portion is deeply stained, centrally located, and surrounded by a considerably less well-stained wide zone of osteoid. This finding, although not pathognomonic, is highly characteristic of rickets and osteomalacia (hematoxylin and eosin, × 100).

Clinical Manifestations of Rickets and Osteomalacia

Most children who have florid rickets, regardless of etiology, have some stunting of growth, and the height sometimes falls far below the normal range.[36,37,80,83,88,90] Children with extensive disease are apathetic and irritable and often are hypokinetic, preferring to sit rather than to stand or to walk. Because of this apathy and an enlarged abdomen (the rachitic potbelly), they are

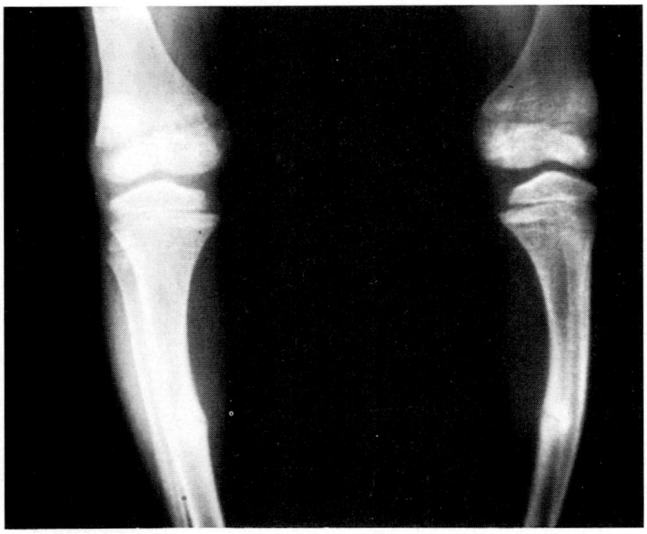

Fig. 10 Looser lines (pseudofractures) symmetrically located on the concave side of the middle of the tibiae. These occur in about 20% of patients with florid rickets or osteomalacia and are considered to be very characteristic of the disease.

spoken of as assuming a Buddha-like appearance. Examination of the skull in very young children may show softening (craniotabes) and prominence of the suture lines (hot-cross-bun skull) and the frontal bones (frontal bossing). Defects of the dental enamel and extensive caries are common. Examination of the thorax may show prominence of the costochondral junctions (rachitic rosary) and, not uncommonly, pectus carinatum. Indentation of the lower part of the rib cage, at the insertion of the diaphragm, is referred to as Harrison groove. Examination of the spine frequently shows a thoracic kyphosis (the rachitic cat-back).[36,37,80,83,88,90] Examination of the extremities is likely to show rather marked enlargement of the wrists, ankles, knees, and elbows and bowing deformity of the long bones, especially of the lower limbs.[36,37] Fractures are common in children with rickets and in those with renal osteodystrophy. Slipped capital femoral epiphysis is sometimes a serious problem.[36,37,90,149]

Of greater importance to the theme of this paper are the findings of adult osteomalacia, which are often much more subtle. Historical data and physical findings in patients with adult osteomalacia are much more difficult to elicit.[83,88,150] These patients generally complain of easy fatigability, malaise, and bone pain. The pain is diffuse and poorly localized and is accompanied by a general tenderness of the bones,[88] such that pressing on a femur, a tibia, a humerus, or a forearm bone elicits an "ouch" and a grimace of pain from the patient. The complaints and rather bizarre findings of bone tenderness may give the examiner the impression that the patient has a mental aberration. In patients with extensive disease, proximal muscle weakness is evident and often is reflected in a bilateral Trendelenburg gait. A fracture in an elderly individual that is thought to be the result of osteoporosis may be the first sign of osteomalacia, and these patients must be evaluated carefully. Several investigators have noted that an unusually high percentage of the elderly population in urban communities have some degree of osteomalacia.[92,93,150] All symptomatic elderly patients should be screened for occult disease.[151,152]

Renal Osteodystrophy

The syndrome of renal osteodystrophy is much less common today than it was in previous years, partly because of the improved management of patients with chronic renal disease.[153,154] The remarkable advancement in the biochemical management of patients with end-stage renal disease, dialysis systems, and the increased success of renal transplantation have led to a decline in the frequency and severity of the osseous changes that were among the most serious consequences of renal failure.[155]

It is understandable that metabolic bone disease results from damage to the kidneys. The kidney plays a pivotal role in the homeostatic mechanisms for calcium, phosphorus, and magnesium.[33,34,82] The kidney is the site of synthesis of 1,25-dihydroxyvitamin D,[9,25] is a target organ for the action and degradation of parathyroid hormone,[24] and also provides the normal mechanism for ridding the system of aluminum.[95]

The mechanism by which renal osteodystrophy occurs in patients with glomerular failure (Fig. 11) begins with the failure of filtration that occurs with damage to the glomerular apparatus, which results in phosphate retention. Hyperphosphatemia[56,82,153,156,157] plays a key role in the development of the syndrome of renal osteodystrophy as well as in that of ectopic calcification. The combination of a reduced tubular mass and an increased serum phosphate concentration causes a reduction in the synthesis of 1,25-dihydroxyvitamin D. Those changes and the increase in phosphate in the cytosol of the gastrointestinal cell cause a marked reduction in calcium absorption. Despite adequate oral intake of calcium and vitamin D, virtually no calcium is absorbed. The profound reduction in serum Ca^{+2} promotes a marked secondary hyperparathyroidism, usually a clear-cell hyperplasia affecting all four glands (one, several, or all of which, on occasion, become autonomous).[36,37,82,130] As a result, the serum Ca^{+2} rises partially to nearer-normal values, obviously at the expense of the bones. The rise in ionic calcium places the patient at risk for ectopic calcification and, less often, for ossification by exceeding the critical solubility product for $CaHPO_4$, even in the face of acidosis.[36,37,82,158] Such ectopic calcification principally occurs in the conjunctivae (the red eyes of renal failure), the blood vessels (medial and muscularis deposits), the skin (an occasional cause of intractable itching), and the peri-

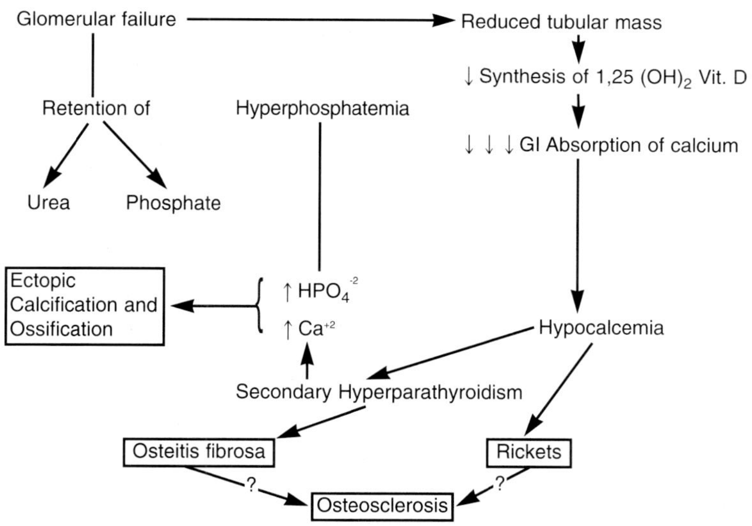

Fig. 11 Diagram depicting the mechanism that leads to the biochemical and osseous alterations in renal osteodystrophy. GI = gastrointestinal. (Reproduced with permission from Zaleske DJ, Doppelt SH, Mankin HJ: Metabolic and endocrine abnormalities of the immature skeleton, in Lovell WW, Winter RB (eds): *Pediatric Orthopaedics*, ed 2. Philadelphia, PA, JB Lippincott, 1986, vol 1, pp 81-145.)

articular tissues (leading to so-called frozen joints).[36,37,82,159]

Three other syndromes may affect patients with chronic renal disease. Some of these patients are quite ill and undernourished, and severe nutritional osteoporosis may develop.[159] Aluminum toxicity may develop in some others. Aluminum hydroxide gels are taken orally by these patients to diminish the concentration of phosphate in the blood. The aluminum is normally excreted by the kidneys but, in patients with renal failure, it is retained and deposited in the brain and the bones. Aluminum alone can produce a neurodepressant or an osteomalacic-like syndrome, or both, and each is refractory to treatment and may require the use of chelating agents such as desferrioxamine to diminish the body's concentration of the metal.[95,160-163] The third possible complicating metabolic bone disorder is seen when hyperplastic parathyroid glands continue to produce and secrete parathyroid hormone beyond the level needed to maintain a normal serum calcium concentration (tertiary hyperparathyroidism). Such individuals, in whom the serum calcium concentration exceeds 12 mg/dl (2.99 mM/l), are at risk for the development of progressive extraskeletal calcification or even calciphylaxis (ischemic lesions of the soft tissues due to small-vessel calcification) and may require partial parathyroidectomy for control.[164,165]

It is now possible to define the clinical syndrome of renal osteodystrophy as a combination of rickets (Fig. 12) and osteomalacia, sometimes with slipped capital femoral epiphysis, often with severe secondary hyperparathyroidism (Fig. 13), and occasionally with bizarre ectopic calcification and ossification (Fig. 14). One other feature, which is present in about 20% of patients, is a patchy osseous sclerosis of unknown cause that can at times be quite dramatic and in fact is misleading on skeletal radiographic imaging (Fig. 15).[36,37,82,159]

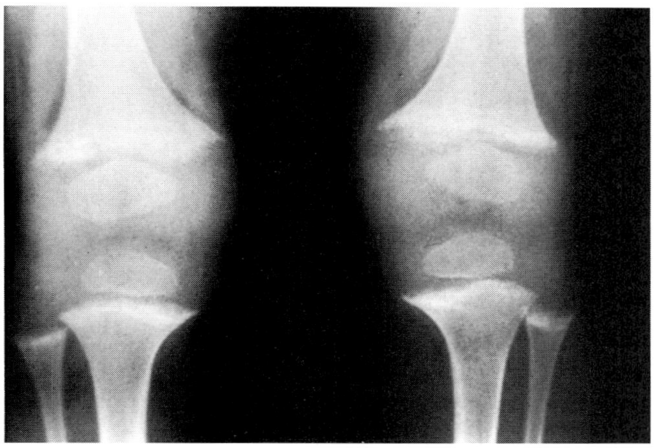

Fig. 12 Classic rickets of the distal aspects of the femora and the proximal aspects of the tibiae in a 7-year-old patient with chronic renal osteodystrophic disease. Note the thin cortices, the increase in the axial height of the physes, and the moderate cupping and flaring. (Reproduced with permission from Mankin HJ: Rickets, osteomalacia, and renal osteodystrophy: Part I. *J Bone Joint Surg* 1974;56A:101-128.)

Management of Patients with Rickets, Osteomalacia, and Renal Osteodystrophy

The role of the orthopaedist in the care of patients with rickets, osteomalacia, and renal osteodystrophy has changed considerably over the years. In the past, the orthopaedist was the diagnostician and caretaker, particularly in children's hospitals throughout the country.[36,37,115] Braces were prescribed for bowed extremities and multiple osteotomies were performed to treat

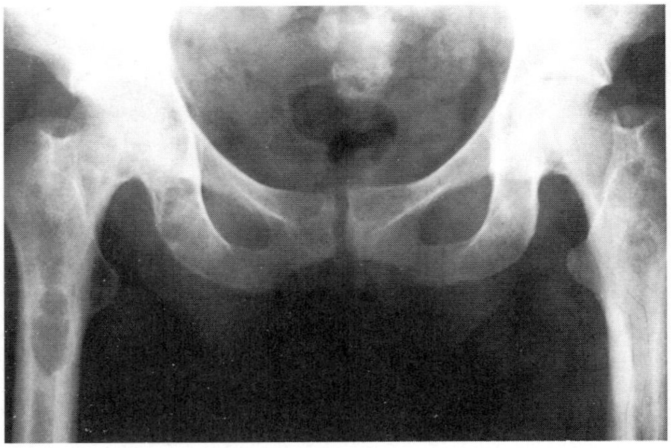

Fig. 13 Secondary hyperparathyroidism in an adult with chronic renal disease. Note the presence of several so-called brown tumors, particularly in the femoral shaft, and the poor definition of the cortices and medullary bone. (Reproduced with permission from Mankin HJ: Rickets, osteomalacia, and renal osteodystrophy: Part I. *J Bone Joint Surg* 1974;56A:101-128.)

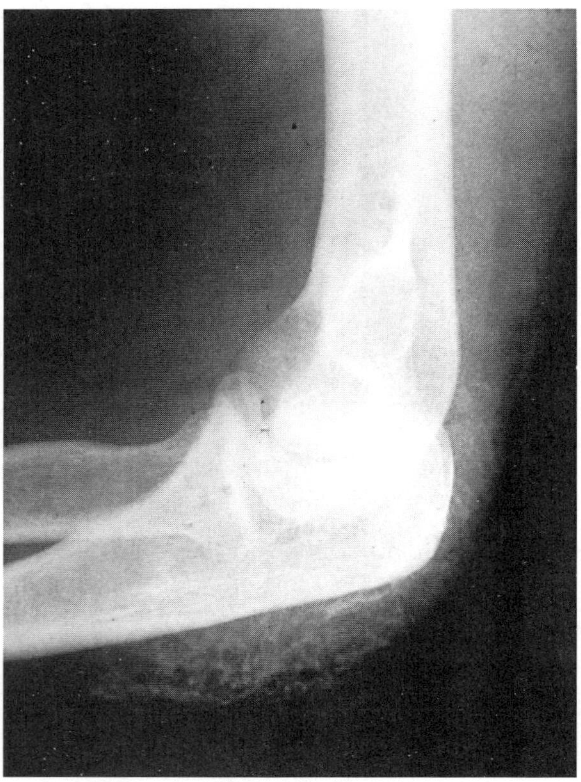

Fig. 14 Ectopic calcification or, less likely, ossification about the elbow in a 35-year-old patient with chronic renal disease. The critical solubility product of $CaHPO_4$ was exceeded at some point during the treatment.

the principal skeletal manifestations of the disorders.[36,37,115] Children with vitamin D-deficient rickets were often overdosed with vitamin D and calcium (and

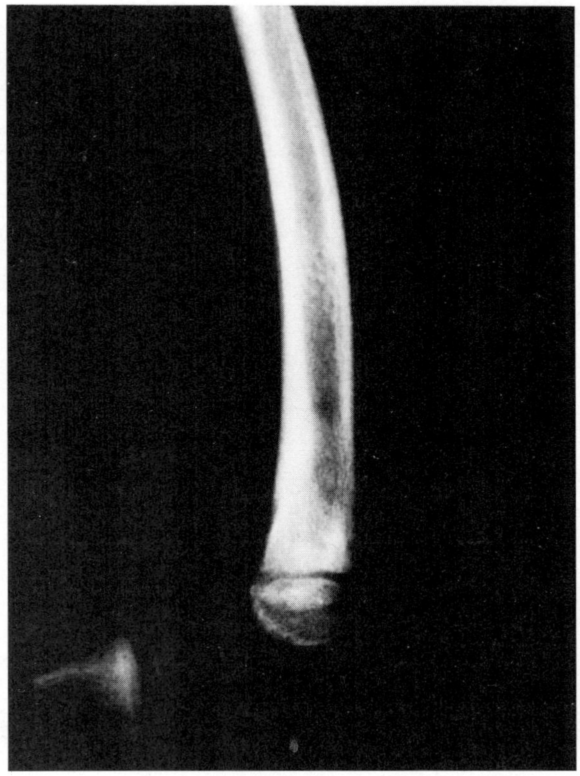

Fig. 15 Approximately 20% of patients with renal osteodystrophy show an increase in bone density that is patchy and irregular in outline. This change is seen in the posterior aspect of the femur in an immature patient with chronic renal disease. (Reproduced with permission from Mankin HJ: Rickets, osteomalacia, and renal osteodystrophy: Part II. *J Bone Joint Surg* 1974;56A:368.)

occasionally renal calculi or chronic renal failure developed as a result), because the underlying metabolic disorder of renal phosphate wasting had not yet been discovered and therefore was not being treated.

Children were maintained in spica casts for years, and the overall management did not prevent dwarfing or deformity. Patients with renal osteodystrophy were considered to have such a poor prognosis for life that only limited attempts were made to control the disorder. As a result, extensive musculoskeletal disability often rendered the children or adults chair-ridden or bedridden.

The picture has changed remarkably. In terms of prophylaxis, all physicians, regardless of medical specialty, should strongly support the development of programs that are designed to prevent diseases that result from deficiency states. Avoidance of food fads, adoption of appropriate diets (particularly by the elderly, pregnant and lactating women, and chronically ill individuals), addition of prophylactic calciferol to the diet, and recommendations regarding exposure to sunlight can often prevent mineral and vitamin D-deficient states and their consequences.[81,83,92,93,150]

On the other hand, the management of patients with established rickets, osteomalacia, or renal osteodystrophy has become much more complex than in the past and has become the responsibility of the endocrinologist or nephrologist. The treatment armamentarium is much broader than in former years and contains such agents and techniques as vitamin D, an array of calcium supplements, 1,25-dihydroxyvitamin D, 1 alpha-hydroxyvitamin D, calcium infusions, neutral phosphate, $Al(OH)_3$, calcitonin, and, when indicated, dialysis, renal transplantation, and subtotal parathyroidectomy. Early diagnosis and aggressive medical treatment can prevent or slow the progression of many of the late musculoskeletal manifestations of these disorders. For this group of patients, the orthopaedist's principal roles are those of suspecting and establishing the diagnosis and of serving as the treating physician for the osseous and soft-tissue complications. Fractures must be treated effectively; slipped capital femoral epiphyses must be fixed; bowing deformities must be treated with braces or corrected by osteotomy; and joints that are damaged late in the course of the disease must be realigned or replaced. In dealing with these complications in patients with rickets, osteomalacia, or renal osteodystrophy, the orthopaedist must maintain an awareness of the patient's underlying disease and be concerned about the effect of the orthopaedic treatment on the impaired calcium homeostatic mechanisms.

Osteoporosis

Osteoporosis is a disease of uncertain etiology that has been assigned a number of putative causes. The disease was recognized by Hippocrates in his writings. Cooper,[166] in 1824, described the disorder by stating that "the regular decay of nature which is called old age is attended by changes. . . . One of the principal of these is found in the bones for they become thin in their shell and spongy in their texture." There are many causes of osteoporosis,[167] but in most patients, it is primary or idiopathic, and clearly osteoporosis is a major health hazard in the elderly population.[168-170]

In terms of definition, I prefer the venerable but very descriptive one first enunciated by Albright and Reifenstein[171] in 1948. They defined osteoporosis as the condition of having too little bone, but what bone there is, is normal. As an example, a biopsy specimen from the proximal end of the femur of a 65-year-old woman with severe idiopathic osteoporosis (Fig. 16) reveals normal fat in the marrow spaces. The bone that is present is lamellar in character and without osteoid seams, resorption cavities, or osteoblastic or osteoclastic activity. Again, the bone is normal, but there is too little of it.

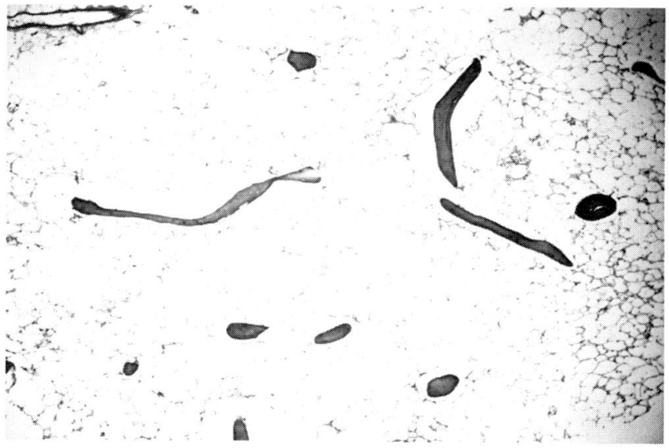

Fig. 16 Histologic section of a biopsy specimen from the proximal end of the femur in a 65-year-old woman with severe osteoporosis. Note the normal fatty marrow, the sparse trabeculae that are normal in texture and appearance with no evidence of osteoclastic resorption, the increased synthesis, and the osteoid seams (hematoxylin and eosin, × 100).

Elaboration of the causes of osteoporosis can provide a very long list of entities that range from genetic disturbances such as osteogenesis imperfecta, Ehlers-Danlos disease, or Turner syndrome;[172-174] to inflammatory states such as rheumatoid arthritis or systemic mastocytosis;[175-179] to endocrine disorders such as hyperthyroidism or adrenal disorders;[180-184] to the use (or abuse) of such drugs as heparin,[185,186] alcohol, vitamin A,[187,188] or corticosteroids;[189-194] to such mechanically directed disorders as disuse or the weightlessness of space travel.[167,195-197] Although many of these conditions are fascinating in their genesis and display special and sometimes very unusual mechanisms, altogether they account for less than 5% of the osteoporotic syndromes seen in common practice and, for the most part, are viewed as entities to be ruled out in what can be an impressive (and costly) differential diagnosis.[167] The syndrome that is seen in the elderly population with far greater regularity and that commands the bulk of our medical resources is the idiopathic form. This form is divided into two basic types: type I, which affects postmenopausal women, is believed to be associated with a greater decline in the medullary bone and better preservation of the cortex, and type II, which affects a more elderly group of both men and women, is associated with equal depletion of the cortex and the medulla.[168,169,198]

Idiopathic osteoporosis is a common condition. It is by far the most prevalent of the metabolic bone diseases.[170,198] Most elderly women and many older men have the disorder, and it has been postulated that one of three women older than 60 will have a vertebral fracture and one of three women and one of six men older than 70 will have a proximal femoral fracture because of osteoporosis.[199,200] Although there has been considerable study and research during the last 100 years, the mechanism and cause of osteoporosis remain speculative. Perhaps the most attractive theory is related to the concept that bone formation and destruction are closely coupled in a healthy person.[201-204] Hence, if either the production or the destruction of bone is increased, a compensatory increase is noted in the opposite function to offset the change, while a decline in either function results in a similar decline in the opposite process. This mechanism is believed to be highly conserved in nature and, presumably, serves to maintain the status of bone mass, which by and large is the protective system for the higher-order animal structure, either in terms of a shield for vital organs or as a mechanism of ambulation or prehension to avert danger.

What appears to be a characteristic of osteoporosis is an uncoupling of the osteoblastic and osteoclastic processes; presumably, this is at least in part a result of aging, but many other factors must play a role.[170,202-204] There is ample evidence to support the concept that bone formation is diminished in postmenopausal women and elderly men and, similarly, osteoclastic resorption appears to be modestly increased. Over many years (or sometimes a shorter period), these aberrations take their toll on the skeleton, silently but substantially decreasing the bone mass until fractures occur.[131,132,166,198] Fracture more frequently occurs in the vertebrae, the distal aspect of the radius, and the intertrochanteric region of the femur in type-I osteoporosis and in the vertebrae and the femoral neck in type-II osteoporosis.[198,199]

Perhaps the most extraordinary aspect of the syndrome is its relationship to menopause.[205-206] It has been postulated, on the basis of considerable study, that the skeleton continues to accrete bone until the age of 30 but that after the age of 40, both men and women begin to lose bone at a rate of about 0.3% per year.[170,199] For men, this steady state is maintained so that it can be estimated that, at the age of 60, the skeleton has undergone a 10% reduction in mass or more. For women, the pattern is identical until menopause, at which time the rate of skeletal loss increases by a factor of ten, to about 3% per year.[152,207-214] Heaney and associates[168,169] demonstrated a decline in calcium absorption in the gut and an increase in calcium excretion in the urine of menopausal woman. In addition, estrogen is thought to stimulate the production of transforming growth-factor beta, insulin-like growth-factor 1, and insulin-like growth-factor 2, all of which are known to increase the synthesis of bone,[215,216] while loss of estrogen stimulates the production of interleukin-1 and interleukin-6, which may increase bone resorption.[217,218] Over the first 8 to 10 years after menopause, all of these factors can cause a woman to lose as much as 30% of the skeletal mass and become severely osteoporotic. At the magical time of 8 to 10 years after menopause, the loss once again reverts to the lower rate, and then elderly men and women are equal in their 0.3% annual decline in bone mass. There is little doubt that this accelerated decrease is related to estrogen concentrations and that it can, at least to some degree, be diminished by administration of that hormone,[219-221] but not without a substantially increased risk of the development of certain neoplasms.[222-225]

An attractive alternative theory is the possible sex-hormone-related or, in men, age-related decline in 1-alpha-hydrolase activity in the kidneys. Such a decline would decrease the amount of 1,25-dihydroxyvitamin D that is synthesized.[226] This theory is supported by the finding of a reduction in 1,25-dihydroxyvitamin-D concentrations both with increasing age and with menopause.[227,228] As a result, with the advent of menopause or increased age, the gut is not as efficient in responding to a low calcium intake. The role of calcium intake has not been fully clarified, but carefully recorded dietary histories of osteoporotic patients strongly support the concept of a chronic calcium deficit, particularly in elderly women.[168,169,229,230]

Diagnosis

The diagnosis of osteoporosis is not difficult. White women of English, Scandinavian, or northern European origin have the highest prevalences.[167,170,200,224] The disease is considerably less frequent in black, Hispanic, and Oriental individuals. The typical patient is slender, physically inactive, and a cigarette smoker and will often describe either nulliparity or an early menopause. Patients with widespread osteoarthrotic disease, particularly of the spine and hips, usually have little if any osteoporosis.[231,232] Typically, the major clinical symptom that the patient describes is a progressive decline in height (in association with the development of a so-called dowager's hump in the upper thoracic spine). Spinal compression fractures are insidious and are indicated only by modest back pain early in the course of the disease. Hip fractures are the principal problem, however, and once these occur function is severely compromised, not only because of the disability of that injury but also because of the attendant disuse osteopenia that results from immobilization, bed rest, or just limitation of active exercise.[170,179,210,232]

Radiographic imaging most often helps to confirm the diagnosis, but it cannot be depended on to provide any degree of quantitation[233] or sense of certainty as to the cause of the osteoporosis. (The diagnosis of osteoporosis is generally made by exclusion of other possible causes.) Radiographs of the spine show loss of the horizontal trabeculae and thinning of the cortices of the vertebral end-plates, which are finely delineated in contrast with the typically fuzzy and indistinct markings associated with osteomalacia or hyperparathyroidism (Fig. 17).[233,234] Radiographs of the hip may show prominence of the trabeculae that constitute the Ward triangle (Fig. 18).[235] Radiographic studies of other parts show a similar pattern of fine cortical and cancellous markings with a decrease in the numbers of

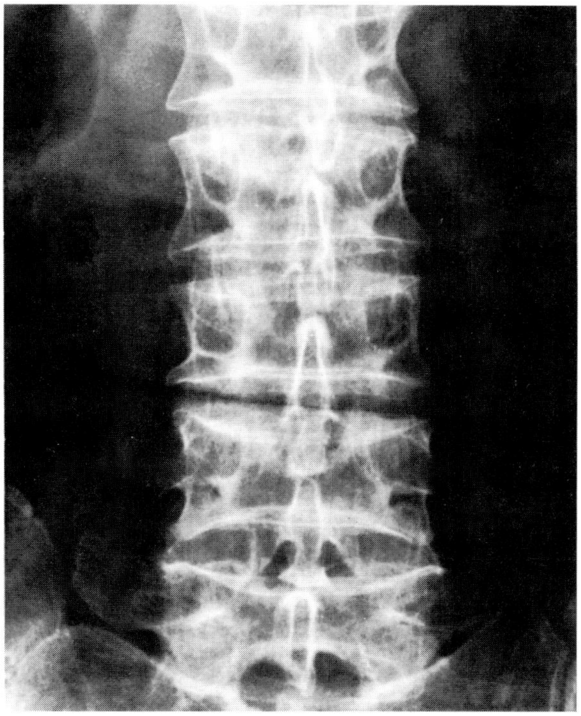

Fig. 17 Radiograph of the spine of a 46-year-old woman with severe osteoporosis. Note the medullary bone loss with preservation of the vertical trabeculae and the sharp and distinct osseous end-plates in the unfractured segments.

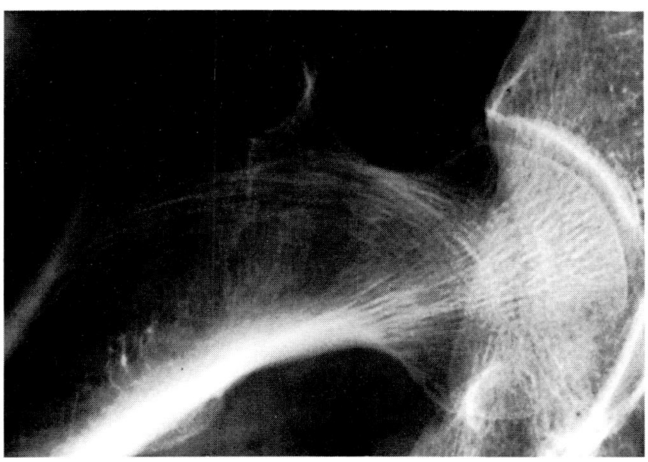

Fig. 18 Radiograph of the proximal end of the femur in a 78-year-old man, showing severe changes of osteoporosis. The trabeculae are present and, in some respects, accentuated by the relative loss of the bone between them.

trabeculae, particularly the horizontal ones. Bone scans usually show no increase in radionuclide uptake unless a fracture has occurred.

Quantitation of bone mineral density provides the ability to study patients serially, to determine the extent of bone loss, and to monitor the efficacy of prevention and treatment modalities. The earliest methodology used to define the extent of the disease quantitatively was based on a comparison of bone density on radiographs against an aluminum wedge that had been added to standardize the system.[236] Soon thereafter, special studies of cortical thickness on radiographs (usually of the hand) followed and, later, single-photon absorptiometry of the wrist or elbow was used.[236,237] These techniques were somewhat cumbersome and difficult to apply, but they were considered to be reasonably accurate. Over the past 15 years, newer procedures have replaced them, including dual-energy x-ray absorptiometry, which can be performed at more central sites such as the hip or spine; quantitative digital radiography; and quantitative computed tomography.[213,236-238] All of these modalities have the advantages of accuracy and reproducibility and therefore can not only define the disease state with a 3% to 5% accuracy but can also be used to assess changes in bone density over time. One of the more provocative uses of these newer systems is the prediction of fracture risk. These predictions are based on tabular data and clearly do not take into account the patient's medical history, level of vigor, balance, or lifestyle.[170] They may cause consternation on the part of both the patient with osteoporosis and the physician, particularly in view of the fact that no really safe and effective therapy has as yet been developed.

Until recently, laboratory studies for patients with idiopathic osteoporosis have been thought to be of little value.[170,198] The levels of serum calcium, phosphorus, alkaline phosphatase, urinary calcium, parathyroid hormone, and 25-hydroxyvitamin D and 1,25-dihydroxyvitamin D, as well as the percentage tubular resorption for phosphate, have all been, for the most part, normal in these patients. Recently, biologic markers have been introduced that, although as yet not fully tested, may provide some definition of the extent of disease but, more importantly, create an opportunity to assess the effect of treatment. Biologic markers of bone formation include levels of bone-specific alkaline phosphatase, serum osteocalcin, and serum type-I collagen extension peptides.[86,239,240] Bone destruction can now be assessed crudely by measurements of levels of urinary hydroxyproline and somewhat more accurately by study of urinary pyridinoline cross-links of type-I collagen and plasma tartrate-resistant acid phosphatase.[170,239,240] Studies are currently in progress in a number of centers to validate these markers, to use them to identify populations at risk for fracture, and to follow the course of patients who are being treated with various agents.

Treatment

The treatment of osteoporosis is complex in some patients, and, for severely affected patients or for those in whom there is some concern about the diagnosis, it should be reserved for the endocrinologist. The orthopaedist's role is one of diagnosing the problem, referring the patient to the appropriate physician or clinic, and managing fractures if they occur. Regrettably, sufficient numbers of interested endocrinologists are not always available to treat the vast numbers of patients who are seen with back pain or with a wrist or hip fracture, and the orthopaedic surgeon, sometimes somewhat reluctantly, becomes the primary physician. It is therefore critical that he or she be at least conversant with the major approaches to treatment.

The first important task is to rule out hyperthyroidism because it represents the only truly reversible form of the disease.[181-184] The other methods of treatment include exercise, which has been shown to increase skeletal mass (or at least to slow the decline). This can and should be prescribed by the orthopaedist and should, in general, be for toning rather than specific.[170,224,241] Patients should avoid swimming (during which they are weightless) and concentrate on gravitational programs such as walking, hiking, or stair-climbing.[195,196] Vitamin-D and calcium supplements have been shown to be effective in the prevention of some degree of loss of the skeleton and to decrease the likelihood of fracture.[224,242-245] These supplements can easily be added to the patient's normal diet, providing there is no evidence of renal failure. The orthopaedist may wish to treat all severely osteoporotic patients with calcium and vitamin-D supplementation because, even in the presence of established osteoporosis, they are effective in the prevention of hip fractures in elderly women.

Administration of estrogen or estrogen and progestin is logical treatment for patients with postmenopausal osteoporosis, and these substances have many advocates.[219,221,224,243] Orthopaedists are unlikely to prescribe these drugs, because they have little knowledge of their side effects, nor should they take the responsibility for monitoring patients for the development of tumors and other serious side effects. Calcitonin has recently been shown to be an effective agent in the management of patients with osteoporosis, although the drug is expensive and difficult to administer.[224,244,246-248] The use of the drug in an inhalant form may make it a more feasible option.[249] Such newer agents as low-dose parathyroid hormone,[224] growth hormone,[250] calcitriol,[251] modified androgens,[170] and electromagnetic fields[252] remain experimental.

Cyclic etidronate appears to be an effective drug if given appropriately, but it may lose some of its effectiveness after several years of treatment.[170,253-256] Fluoride, formerly advocated as a treatment agent, has been withdrawn pending additional studies on its efficacy and safety.[257,258] It is highly likely that new methods of treatment involving bone growth factors or mediators will be introduced in the not-too-distant future, and the orthopaedist should at least attempt to assess the logic behind their use.[257,259,260]

There is little doubt that the numbers of patients with osteoporosis will grow as the longevity of the population increases and that the orthopaedic manifestations of this disorder will be seen even more frequently than they are today. We as orthopaedic surgeons must be prepared to offer these patients a careful diagnostic review of their problem and, when needed, to help with their pain and the treatment of their injuries. We should also be able to provide simple treatment in the form of exercise programs and supplementation with vitamin D and calcium when appropriate.

Multiple Myeloma and Other Diffuse Malignancies

It is not the purpose of this review to provide an exhaustive description of all of the malignant processes that affect bone or even to discuss in detail multiple myeloma, the one tumor that occasionally presents with diffuse osteopenia and thus masquerades as a metabolic bone disease. In any discussion of diffuse bone loss, however, one must include myeloma and the other monoclonal gammopathies as possible causes.

Monoclonal gammopathies include multiple disorders of varying severity, including malignancy. All are associated with abnormalities of the plasma cell. Under the stimulus of some other condition such as Gaucher disease or lupoid hepatitis or de novo, a clonal abnormality develops, with the slow production of abnormal cells that produce a monoclonal immunoglobulin product that can be detected on serum protein or immunoelectrophoretic studies.[261-263] In addition to the monoclonal gammopathies associated with specific disorders, Waldenström macroglobulinemia may have osteopenia as a feature.[261] However, of all of these gammopathies, the most frequently encountered and the most pernicious is multiple myeloma, which is believed by many to be a primary malignancy of bone and far exceeds in frequency of occurrence all other primary bone tumors, including osteosarcoma.[262,263]

Myeloma is a malignant disorder in which a single clone of plasma cells undergoes neoplastic conversion to so-called myeloma cells. From a primary single site (or even perhaps from multiple separate sites), the myeloma spreads to involve virtually the entire bone marrow, producing a specific symptom complex and almost always leading to the death of the patient.[262,264] Myeloma is considered to be a small round-cell tumor, and hence it may be localized to one area and may present as a fairly discrete permeative lesion. It may also be generalized throughout the bone marrow and, on imaging, its features may resemble those of the osteopenic states already described. Thus, it is included in this paper on metabolic bone disease.

Clinically, patients with generalized multiple myeloma are in their middle 50s or older and generally complain of fatigue, malaise, and feeling ill. They may be intermittently febrile and describe night sweats. They may complain of weight loss and poor appetite and often have poorly localized bone pain in the back, shoulders, or lower extremities.[262,265] A pathological fracture of the spine or the femur may be the heralding event. On physical examination, the patients appear pale and chronically ill, and many complain of diffuse bone tenderness, particularly over the sternum and pelvis. Standard radiographs may show a diffuse osteopenia with one fracture or more in the spine (Fig. 19).[265] Bone-scanning, although likely to show increased activity at the site of a fracture, shows no increase even at the site of a discrete lesion in 25% of patients. For this reason, most orthopaedic oncologists and experienced radiologists advocate a radiographic skeletal survey to search for foci of myeloma.[262,266] Special imaging studies may disclose more extensive disease than can be appreciated on plain radiographs. A magnetic resonance image of the spine is especially useful, because it is likely to show evidence of patchy areas, consistent with marrow element disease.

As the radiographic lesions of myeloma progress with time, they change from a diffuse osteopenia to a more permeative pattern to a so-called moth-eaten destruction to complete dissolution of the bone, often with considerable cortical expansion (Fig. 20). Only rarely is a soft-tissue mass discernible on imaging studies of these advanced lesions.

The laboratory findings in patients with myeloma can be extraordinary and may be very useful in the diagnosis. Most patients with diffuse disease and associated osteopenia have a fairly profound normocytic, normochromic anemia, often with a hematocrit of less than 30%. The sedimentation rate is usually more than 100 mm/hr. These two tests are often very helpful as a screen for the disease. There may be many other laboratory abnormalities. Platelet deficiency, a high level of uric acid (secondary gout), abnormal renal function, an increased level of hydroxyproline peptides in the urine, and an abnormal result of serum protein electrophoresis or, more appropriately, serum immunoelectrophoresis provide almost certain evidence of the disease.[267-269] The finding of an abnormal protein peak migrating with the IgA or IgG fraction is virtually diagnostic of myeloma. If the bone marrow shows greater than 20% plasma cells (as much as 8% is normal and between 10% and 20% is a presumptive diagnosis), there is no need to biopsy the bone lesion or lesions for a diagnosis (Fig. 21).[262,263,266] Bence Jones proteinuria, once a valuable diagnostic test, has been recognized as occurring in less than 50% of patients. A urinary immunoelectrophoresis may have a substantially higher yield for IgG light chains excreted in the urine.[151]

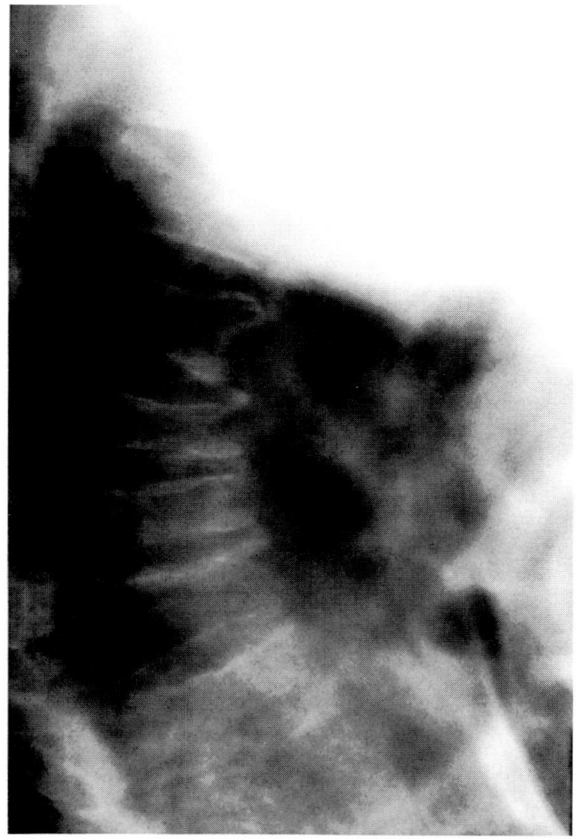

Fig. 19 Severe diffuse osteopenia and multiple compression fractures of the spine in a patient with multiple myeloma.

Screening for Metabolic Bone Disease

Many patients who are initially seen with non-specific symptoms of low-back pain and who have diffuse osteopenia with or without a compression fracture on standard radiographs represent a puzzle to the orthopaedic surgeon to whom they turn for help (Fig. 1). The problem that faces clinicians is how one screens for the presence or absence of hyperparathyroidism, osteomalacia, osteoporosis, or myeloma. Some imaging studies are useful but are relatively nonspecific. Laboratory studies are of greater help, but it should be understood that the current ease with which one can obtain an entire battery of laboratory screening tests does not free the clinician from the need to seek the tests that specifically relate to the diagnosis of the entities that I have described. The differentiation is sometimes subtle and difficult but, with the help of the studies that will be described, the diagnosis can often be not only suspected but also confirmed.

The metabolic (and neoplastic) screening studies include: a history and physical examination, radiographs of the spine and pelvis (and of the hands and the lateral aspect of the skull if indicated), posteroanterior and right lateral radiographs of the chest, bone

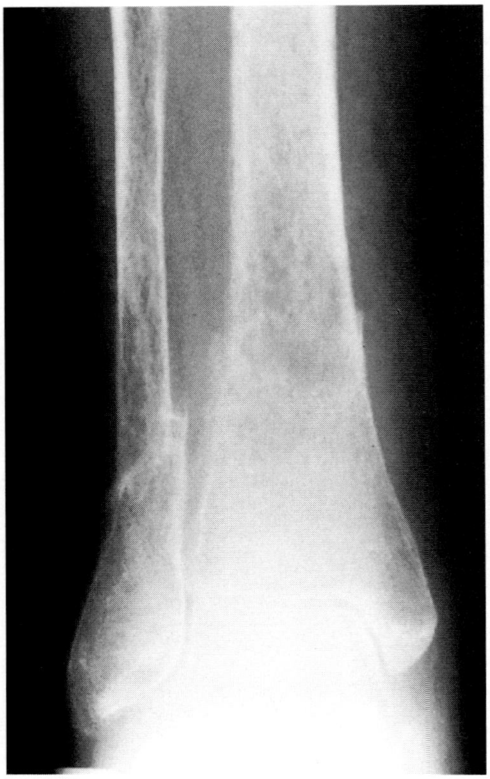

Fig. 20 Although the lesions of myeloma, particularly in the spine, may suggest osteoporosis, there may be in the same patient discrete lesions that, in turn, may result in pathological fractures. Note the lesions in both the tibia and the fibula.

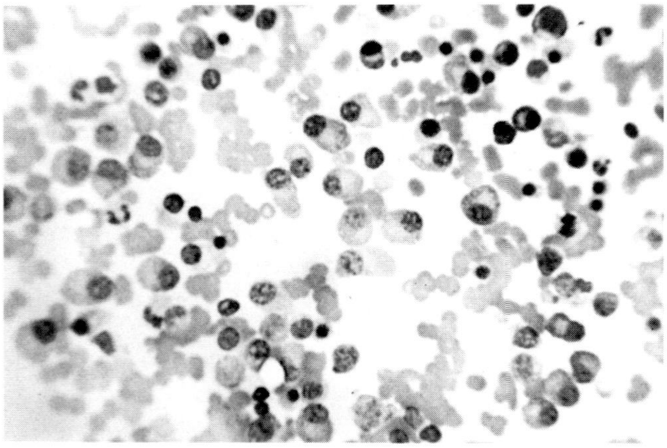

Fig. 21 Diffuse myelomatosis of the bone marrow with few normal cells. Most of the cells are myeloma cells (plasma cells) (Wright stain, × 300).

scans, and laboratory screens. The so-called big-10 laboratory tests (in fact, a total of 13 tests) are: complete blood-cell count; erythrocyte sedimentation rate; levels of blood urea nitrogen and creatinine, sugar, calcium, phosphorus, alkaline phosphatase, serum glutamic oxaloacetic transaminase, and thyroxin (T3 and T4); serum immunoelectrophoresis; and urinalysis. If a patient with metabolic bone disease has enough osteopenia for it to be visible on routine radiographs of the spine (with or without compression fractures) or the pelvis, the tests may be used to distinguish the various disorders.

Hyperparathyroidism

The calcium level is elevated, the phosphorus level is diminished, the alkaline phosphatase level is elevated, and the bone scan and radiographs of the hands and skull may show specific types of lesions. Second-order tests for this group of patients should include determinations of the levels of calcium in 24-hour collection of urine, parathyroid hormone, uric acid, pyridinoline cross-links of type-I collagen, and plasma tartrate-resistant acid phosphatase (the last two tests are designed to assess the rate of bone destruction). In addition, it is not unreasonable to invite radiologic consultation to help one to decide how best to demonstrate an enlarged parathyroid gland by magnetic resonance imaging.

Osteomalacia (All Types)

The calcium level is likely to be low or low-normal and, except in renal osteodystrophy, the phosphorus level is low or very low depending on the type of osteomalacia. In renal osteodystrophy, the blood urea nitrogen and creatinine levels should reveal the nature of the process, but the phosphorus level is almost invariably high and the calcium level is quite low. The alkaline phosphatase level is usually elevated in all forms of osteomalacia (except hypophosphatasia) and is occasionally elevated in chronic renal disease. Second-order screens for this group of disorders include determinations of the levels of electrolytes, parathyroid hormone, 25-hydroxyvitamin D and 1,25-dihydroxyvitamin D, serum osteocalcin, and urinary pyridinoline cross-links. A determination of the level of calcium in a 24-hour collection of urine is very helpful, as is urinalysis for the level of sugar, amino acids, and fixed base and determination of the percentage tubular reabsorption for phosphate. A bone biopsy is often confirmatory, particularly for the presence of wide osteoid seams.

Myeloma

A complete blood-cell count almost always shows a normocytic, normochromic anemia, and the erythrocyte sedimentation rate is likely to be more than 100 mm/hr. Serum immunoelectrophoresis displays an abnormal protein migrating with the IgG or IgA bond in about 90% of patients. The level of serum calcium may be elevated. Second-order confirmatory studies include urinary immunoelectrophoresis, a skeletal survey, and a bone-marrow biopsy to search for a high concentration of plasma cells (greater than 20%).

Osteoporosis

This disorder is the most difficult of all to diagnose because the results of all of the tests generally are normal. The exceptions are the thyroid function tests (for the only so-called curable form of osteoporosis) and determination of the blood sugar level (some patients with diabetes have serious osteoporosis). Bone scans almost never show increased activity except in the presence of a fracture. Secondary screens for osteoporosis include determinations of the levels of bone-specific alkaline phosphatase, serum osteocalcin, and serum type-I collagen extension peptides, all of which measure synthesis, and determinations of the levels of urinary pyridinoline cross-links and tartrate-resistant acid phosphatase, which measure bone destruction. To map and trace the degree of the disease, various forms of non-invasive bone densitometry may be used. A transiliac bone biopsy is often helpful in assessing the extent of skeletal remodeling.

Illustrative Case Reports

Case 1 A 58-year-old woman (Fig. 1, *top left*) was initially seen because of increasing low-back pain of several months' duration. Additional historical data and physical findings did not help in the determination of which metabolic bone disorder she had. However, the laboratory studies demonstrated a calcium level of 12.5 mg/dl (3.12 mM/l), a phosphorus level of 1.5 mg/dl (0.48 mM/l), and an alkaline phosphatase level that was twice normal. Additional imaging studies supported the diagnosis of hyperparathyroidism, and several weeks later an adenocarcinoma of one of the parathyroid glands was discovered.

Case 2 A 59-year-old man (Fig. 1, *top right*) lifted a garage door and felt sudden pain in the back. He had no abnormal neurologic findings but radiographs showed marked osteopenia and compression fractures. When questioned further about his symptoms, he admitted to easy fatigability and weight loss. On physical examination, he appeared chronically ill and the conjunctivae appeared moderately pallid. Bone-scanning showed increased activity not only at the fracture site but also in multiple locations, and a skeletal survey showed permeative lesions in multiple sites. The hematocrit was only 0.32, the sedimentation rate was 125 mm/hr, and the level of calcium was slightly elevated. The results of immunoelectrophoresis were classic for a myeloma, with a large spike migrating with the IG band. The patient was treated for the myeloma, but he died within a year and a half after the diagnosis.

Case 3 A 64-year-old woman (Fig. 1, *bottom left*) had had surgical treatment for Crohn disease years before being seen in my office. The bowel had become asymptomatic, but she had had increasingly severe back pain over the previous 3 years and had also noted bone tenderness. The results of the physical examination were normal, with the exception of a slight Trendelenburg gait. Bone-scanning showed modestly increased activity over multiple sites, and the serum calcium level was 8.1 mg/dl (2.02 mM/l), the phosphorus level was 2.3 mg/dl (0.74 mM/l), and the alkaline phosphatase level was about one and a half times normal. Additional studies, including a bone biopsy, confirmed that she had osteomalacia, presumably on the basis of an absorptive defect. She was treated effectively with vitamin D and calcium and became asymptomatic.

Case 4 A 55-year-old woman (Fig. 1, *bottom right*) had had back pain of long duration. The history revealed no relevant findings except for an early, surgically induced menopause; a 40-year history of smoking; and excessive alcohol intake at one point in her life. Bone-scanning showed increased activity at several sites of fracture, and all screening laboratory tests revealed normal findings. She was seen before the introduction of the newer tests for bone formation and destruction in osteoporosis. She was treated with an exercise program, told to stop smoking (which she did not do), and given vitamin D (50,000 units per week) and calcium carbonate (1.5-1.8 g per day). She remained moderately symptomatic but had had no new fractures at the most recent (12-year) examination.

Concluding Comments

For reasons that are not entirely clear, metabolic bone disease as an academic interest appears only occasionally in the research and teaching agendas of the orthopaedic units of universities and resident-training programs. The subject tissue, bone, is clearly germane to what orthopaedists do. Indeed, the end-result of a failure of calcium and phosphorus homeostatic mechanisms is quite frequently an orthopaedic disaster that requires all of an orthopaedist's ingenuity and talent to repair. Yet, orthopaedists as a group (at least among the current generation), have, with rare exception, abrogated their interest in metabolic bone disease to pediatric and adult endocrinologists and sometimes to rheumatologists, all of whom see patients with these problems far less commonly than do orthopaedists. The reason for this relative lack of enthusiasm probably, at least currently, lies principally in orthopaedists' limited knowledge of, and interest in, such subjects as cellular transport mechanisms, parathyroid function, polar metabolites of vitamin D, and bone synthesis and degradative activities and their controlling mediators.

I have presented a limited summary of the current knowledge of metabolic bone disease. It is hoped that orthopaedic scientists and students will be encouraged not only to read some of the key references but will also become interested in, and perhaps fascinated by, this important field. There are many questions still unanswered and many that have not been asked. Bone is the birthright of the orthopaedist, and he or she should know as much about it as possible. I think that it is essential that orthopaedists as a group continue to have an active interest in the subject of metabolic bone disease. They must not only follow closely the discoveries and treatment protocols advanced by endocrinologists, but they must produce more experts and investigators who can not only understand the disorders and their genesis but also have the distinct advantage of being very familiar with the tissue, the patients' needs, and the treatment of the consequences of the diseases.

References

1. Broadus AE: Physiologic functions of calcium, magnesium, and phosphorus, in Favus MJ (ed): *Primer on the Metabolic Bone Diseases and Disorders of Mineral Metabolism.* Kelseyville, CA, American Society for Bone and Mineral Research, 1990, pp 29-30.
2. Glimcher MJ: The nature of the mineral component of bone and the mechanism of calcification, in Coe FL, Favus MJ (eds): *Disorders of Bone and Mineral Metabolism.* New York, NY, Raven Press, 1992, pp 265-286.
3. Rodan GA: Introduction to bone biology. *Bone* 1992;13 (suppl1):S3-6.
4. Landis WJ, Glimcher MJ: Electron diffraction and electron probe microanalysis of the mineral phase of bone tissue prepared by anhydrous techniques. *J Ultrastruct Res* 1978;63:188-223.
5. Boskey AL: Mineral-matrix interactions in bone and cartilage. *Clin Orthop* 1992;281:244-274.
6. Silverberg SJ: The distribution and balance of calcium, magnesium and phosphorus, in Favus MJ (ed): *Primer on the Metabolic Bone Diseases and Disorders of Mineral Metabolism.* Kelseyville, CA, American Society for Bone and Mineral Research, 1990, pp 30-32.
7. Karbach U: Mechanism of intestinal calcium transport and clinical aspects of disturbed calcium absorption. *Dig Dis* 1989;7:1-18.
8. Brautbar N, Levine BS, Walling MW, et al: Intestinal absorption of calcium: Role of dietary phosphate and vitamin D. *Am J Physiol* 1981;241:G49-G53.
9. Reichel H, Koeffler HP, Norman AW: The role of the vitamin D endocrine system in health and disease. *N Engl J Med* 1989;320:980-991.
10. Wasserman RH, Brindak ME, Buddle MM, et al: Recent studies on the biological actions of vitamin D on intestinal transport and the electrophysiology of peripheral nerve and cardiac muscle. *Prog Clin Biol Res* 1990;332:99-126.
11. Wasserman RH, Chandler JS, Meyer SA, et al: Intestinal calcium transport and calcium extrusion processes at the basolateral membrane. *J Nutr* 1992;122(Suppl 3):662-671.
12. Gross M, Kumar R: Physiology and biochemistry of vitamin D-dependent calcium binding proteins. *Am J Physiol* 1990; 259:F195-F209.
13. Bronner F: Current concepts of calcium absorption: An overview. *J Nutr* 1992;122(Suppl 3):641-643.
14. Charles P: Calcium absorption and calcium bioavailability. *J Intern Med* 1992;231:161-168.
15. Bronner F: Intestinal calcium transport: The cellular pathway. *Miner Electrolyte Metab* 1990;16:94-100.
16. Birge SJ, Avioli LV: Pathophysiology of calcium and phosphate absorptive disorders, in Avioli LV, Krane SM (eds): *Metabolic Bone Disease and Clinically Related Disorders.* Philadelphia, PA, WB Saunders, 1990, pp 196-221.
17. Heaney RP, Weaver CM: Oxalate: Effect on calcium absorbability. *Am J Clin Nutr* 1989;50:830-832.
18. Recker RR: Calcium absorption and achlorhydria. *N Engl J Med* 1985;313:70-73.
19. Wright FS, Bomsztyk K: Calcium transport by the proximal tubule. *Adv Exper Med Biol* 1986;208:165-170.
20. Kumar R: Vitamin D metabolism and mechanisms of calcium transport. *J Am Soc Nephrol* 1990;1:30-42.
21. Friedman PA, Gesek FA: Calcium transport in renal epithelial cells. *Am J Physiol* 1993;264:181-198.
22. Rizzoli R, Ferrari SL, Pizurki L, et al: Actions of parathyroid hormone and parathyroid hormone-related protein. *J Endocrinol Invest* 1992;15(Suppl 6):51-56.
23. Boden SD, Kaplan FS: Calcium homeostasis. *Orthop Clin North Am* 1990;21:31-42.
24. Segre GV: Secretion, metabolism and circulating heterogeneity of parathyroid hormone, in Favus MJ (ed): *Primer on the Metabolic Bone Diseases and Disorders of Mineral Metabolism.* Kelseyville, CA, American Society for Bone and Mineral Research, 1990, pp 43-44.
25. DeLuca HF: New concepts of vitamin D functions. *Ann NY Acad Sci* 1992;669:59-69.
26. Martin TJ, Moseley JM: Calcitonin, in Avioli LV, Krane SM (eds): *Metabolic Bone Disease and Clinically Related Disorders,* ed 2. Philadelphia, PA, WB Saunders, 1990, pp 131-154.
27. Raisz LG: Mechanisms and regulation of bone resorption by osteoclastic cells, in Coe FL, Favus MJ (eds): *Disorders of Bone and Mineral Metabolism.* New York, NY, Raven Press, 1992, pp 287-311.
28. Care AD: The regulation of the secretion of calcitonin. *Bone Miner* 1992;16:182-185.
29. Matthews JL: Effect of calcitonin on bone cell ultrastructure. *Bone Miner* 1992;16:178-181.
30. Lemann J Jr: Intestinal absorption of calcium, magnesium and phosphorus, in Favus MJ (ed): *Primer on the Metabolic Bone Diseases and Disorders of Mineral Metabolism.* Kelseyville, CA, American Society for Bone and Mineral Research, 1990, pp 32-35.
31. Cross HS, Debiec H, Peterlik M: Mechanism and regulation of intestinal phosphate absorption. *Miner Electrolyte Metab* 1990; 16:115-124.
32. Henry HL, Norman AW: Metabolism of vitamin D, in Coe FL, Favus MJ (eds): *Disorders of Bone and Mineral Metabolism.* New York, NY, Raven Press, 1992, pp 149-162.
33. Jacobson H, Knochel JP: Renal handling of phosphate in health and disease, in Brenner BM, Rector FC Jr (eds): *The Kidney,* ed 3. Philadelphia, PA, WB Saunders, 1986, pp 619-662.
34. Lemann J Jr: The urinary excretion of calcium, magnesium and phosphorus, in Favus MJ (ed): *Primer on the Metabolic Bone Diseases and Disorders of Mineral Metabolism.* Kelseyville, CA, American Society for Bone and Mineral Research, 1990, pp. 36-42.
35. Yanagawa N, Lee DBN: Renal handling of calcium and phosphorus, in Coe FL, Favus MJ (eds): *Disorders of Bone and Mineral Metabolism.* New York, NY, Raven Press, 1992, pp 3-40.
36. Mankin HJ: Rickets, osteomalacia, and renal osteodystrophy: Part I. *J Bone Joint Surg* 1974;56A:101-128.
37. Mankin HJ: Rickets, osteomalacia, and renal osteodystrophy: Part II. *J Bone Joint Surg* 1974;56A:352-386.
38. Cooke NE, Haddad JG: Vitamin D binding protein (Gc globulin). *Endocrine Rev* 1989;10:294-307.
39. Haddad, JG Jr: Clinical aspects of measurements of plasma vitamin D sterols and the vitamin D binding protein, in Coe FL, Favus MJ (eds): *Disorders of Bone and Mineral Metabolism.* New York, NY, Raven Press, 1992, pp 195-216.
40. Holick MF: Skin: Site of the synthesis of vitamin D and a target tissue for the active form, 1,25-dihydroxyvitamin D3. *Ann NY Acad Sci* 1988;548:14-26.

41. Mawer EB, Backhouse J, Holman CA, et al: The distribution and storage of vitamin D and its metabolites in human tissues. *Clin Sci* 1972;43:413-431.
42. Webb AR, Holick MF: The role of sunlight in the cutaneous production of vitamin D3. *Ann Rev Nutr* 1988;8:375-399.
43. Henry HL: Vitamin D hydroxylases. *J Cell Biochem* 1992;49:4-9.
44. Fraser DR: Regulation of the metabolism of vitamin D. *Physiol Rev* 1980;60:551-613.
45. Pike JW: Molecular mechanisms of cellular response to the vitamin D3 hormone, in Coe FL, Favus MJ (eds): *Disorders of Bone and Mineral Metabolism.* New York, NY, Raven Press, 1992, pp 163-193.
46. Baker AR, McDonnell DP, Hughes M, et al: Cloning and expression of full-length cDNA encoding human vitamin D receptor. *Proc Nat Acad Sci USA* 1988;85:3294-3298.
47. Hochberg Z, Benderli A, Levy J, et al: 1,25-Dihydroxyvitamin D resistance, rickets, and alopecia. *Am J Med* 1984;77:805-811.
48. Malloy PJ, Hochberg Z, Tiosano D, et al: The molecular basis of hereditary 1,25-dihydroxyvitamin D3 resistant rickets in seven related families. *J Clin Invest* 1990;86:2071-2079.
49. Garabedian M, Holick MF, DeLuca HF, et al: Control of 25-hydroxycholecalciferol metabolism by parathyroid glands. *Proc Nat Acad Sci USA* 1972;69:1673-1676.
50. Kappelle JW, Raymakers JA, Bosch R, et al: No short-term effects of 24,25-dihydroxycholecalciferol in healthy subjects. *Bone* 1989;10:397-399.
51. von Recklinghausen FD: Die fibrose oder deformierende Ostitis, die Osteomalazie und die Osteoplastische Carcinose in ihren gegenseitigen Beziehungen. *Fortschr. Virchow* 1891;1-45.
52. Jaffe HL (ed): *Metabolic, Degenerative, and Inflammatory Diseases of Bones and Joints.* Philadelphia, PA, Lea & Febiger, 1972, pp 301-331.
53. Bilezikian JP: Hypercalcemic states: Their differential diagnosis and acute management, in Coe FL, Favus MJ (eds): *Disorders of Bone and Mineral Metabolism.* New York, NY, Raven Press, 1992, pp 493-521.
54. Habener JF, Potts JT Jr: Primary hyperparathyroidism, in Avioli LV, Krane SM (eds): *Metabolic Bone Disease and Clinically Related Disorders,* ed 2. Philadelphia, PA, WB Saunders, 1990, pp. 475-545.
55. Wynne AG, van Heerden J, Carney JA, et al: Parathyroid carcinoma: Clinical and pathologic features in 43 patients. *Medicine (Baltimore)* 1992;71:197-205.
56. Obara, T, Fujimoto Y: Diagnosis and treatment of patients with parathyroid carcinoma: An update and review. *World J Surg* 1991;15:738-744.
57. Ladenson JH: Calcium determination in primary hyperparathyroidism. *J Bone Miner Res* 1991;6(Suppl 2):S33-S41.
58. Spiegel AM: Pathophysiology of primary hyperparathyroidism. *J Bone Miner Res* 1991;6(Suppl 2):S15-S17.
59. Hayes CW, Conway WF: Hyperparathyroidism. *Radiol Clin North Am* 1991;29:85-96.
60. Parisien M, Silverberg SJ, Shane E, et al: Bone disease in primary hyperparathyroidism. *Endocrinol Metab Clin North Am* 1990;19:19-34.
61. Heath DA: Primary hyperparathyroidism: Clinical presentation and factors influencing clinical management. *Endocrinol Metab Clin North Am* 1989;18:631-646.
62. Scott JT, Dixon AS, Bywaters EG: Association of hyperuricaemia and gout with hyperparathyroidism. *Br Med J* 1964;1:1070-1073.
63. Lafferty FW: Differential diagnosis of hypercalcemia. *J Bone Miner Res* 1991;6(Suppl 2):S51-S59.
64. Nussbaum SR, Potts JT Jr: Immunoassays for parathyroid hormone 1-84 in the diagnosis of hyperparathyroidism. *J Bone Miner Res* 1991;6(Suppl 2):S43-S50.
65. Grahame R, Sutor, DJ, Mitchener MB: Crystal deposition in hyperparathyroidism. *Ann Rheum Dis* 1971;30:597-604.
66. Dodds WJ, Steinbach HL: Primary hyperparathyroidism and articular cartilage calcification. *Am J Roentgenol* 1968;104:884-892.
67. George JM, Rabson AS, Ketcham A, et al: Calcareous renal disease and hyperparathyroidism. *Q J Med* 1965;34:291-301.
68. Cope O: The study of hyperparathyroidism at the Massachusetts General Hospital. *N Engl J Med* 1966;274:1174-1182.
69. Numann PJ, Torppa AJ, Blumetti AE: Neuropsychologic deficits associated with primary hyperparathyroidism. *Surgery* 1984;96:1119-1123.
70. Patten BM, Bilezikian JP, Mallette LE, et al: Neuromuscular disease in primary hyperparathyroidism. *Ann Intern Med* 1974;80:182-193.
71. Ostrow JD, Blanshard G, Gray SJ: Peptic ulcer in primary hyperparathyroidism. *Am J Med* 1960;29:769-779.
72. Kelly TR: Relationship of hyperparathyroidism to pancreatitis. *Arch Surg* 1968;97:267-274.
73. Breslau NA, Pak CYC: Asymptomatic primary hyperparathyroidism, in Coe FL, Favus MJ (eds); *Disorders of Bone and Mineral Metabolism.* New York, NY, Raven Press, 1992, pp 523-538.
74. Heath H III, Hodgson SF, Kennedy MA: Primary hyperparathyroidism: Incidence, morbidity, and potential economic impact in a community. *N Engl J Med* 1980;302:189-193.
75. Harrison BJ, Wheeler MH: Asymptomatic primary hyperparathyroidism. *World J Surg* 1991;15:724-729.
76. Heath H III: Clinical spectrum of primary hyperparathyroidism: Evolution with changes in medical practice and technology. *J Bone Miner Res* 1991;6(Suppl 2):S63-S70.
77. Mundy GR, Cove DH, Fisken R: Primary hyperparathyroidism: Changes in the pattern of clinical presentation. *Lancet* 1980;1:1317-1320.
78. Doppman JL, Miller DL: Localization of parathyroid tumors in patients with asymptomatic hyperparathyroidism and no previous surgery. *J Bone Miner Res* 1991;6(Suppl 2):S153-S158.
79. Mankin HJ: Rickets, osteomalacia, and renal osteodystrophy: An update. *Orthop Clin North Am* 1990;21:81-96.
80. Econs MJ, Drezner MK: Bone disease resulting from inherited disorders of renal tubule transport and vitamin D metabolism, in Coe FL, Favus MJ (eds): *Disorders of Bone and Mineral Metabolism.* New York, NY, Raven Press, 1992, pp 935-950.
81. Bikle DD: Bone disease due to nutritional, gastrointestinal, and hepatic disorders, in Coe FL, Favus MJ (eds): *Disorders of Bone and Mineral Metabolism.* New York, NY, Raven Press, 1992, pp 951-976.
82. Slatopolsky E, Delmez J.: Bone disease in chronic renal failure and after renal transplantation, in Coe FL, Favus MJ (eds): *Disorders of Bone and Mineral Metabolism.* New York, NY, Raven Press, 1992, pp 905-934.
83. Parfitt AM: Osteomalacia and related disorders, in Avioli LV, Krane SM (eds): *Metabolic Bone Disease and Clinically Related Disorders,* ed 2. Philadelphia, PA, WB Saunders, 1990, pp 329-396.
84. Netter FH, Mankin HJ: Rickets, osteomalacia, and renal osteodystrophy, in Netter FJ (ed): *The Ciba Collection of Medical Illustrations.* Summit, NJ, Ciba Geigy Corporation, 1987, vol 8, pp 205-215.
85. Clemens TL; Adams JS, Nolan JM, et al: Measurement of circulating vitamin D in man. *Clin Chim Acta* 1982;121:301-308.
86. Tohme JF, Seibel MJ, Silverberg SJ, et al: Biochemical markers of bone metabolism. *Z Rheumatol* 1991;50:133-141.
87. Holick MF: The use and interpretation of assays for vitamin D and its metabolites. *J Nutr* 1990;120(Suppl 11):1464-1469.
88. Doppelt SH: Vitamin D, rickets, and osteomalacia. *Orthop Clin North Am* 1984;15:671-686.
89. Garabedian M, Vainsel M, Mallet E, et al: Circulating vitamin D metabolite concentrations in children with nutritional rickets. *J Pediatr* 1983;103:381-386.
90. Zaleske DJ, Doppelt SH, Mankin HJ: Metabolic and endocrine abnormalities of the immature skeleton, in Lovell WW, Winter RB (eds): *Pediatric Orthopaedics,* ed 2. Philadelphia, PA, JB Lippincott, 1986 vol 1, pp 81-145.
91. Tucker GS, Middha VP, Sural A, et al: Incidence of osteomalacia in fractures of the proximal end of femur. *Injury* 1988;19:89-92.

92. Hordon LD, Peacock M: Vitamin D metabolism in women with femoral neck fracture. *Bone Miner* 1987;2:413-426.
93. Parfitt AM, Gallagher JC, Heaney RP, et al: Vitamin D and bone health in the elderly. *Am J Clin Nutr* 1982;36(Suppl 5):1014-1031.
94. Slovik DM, Adams JS, Neer RM, et al: Deficient production of 1,25-dihydroxyvitamin D in elderly osteoporotic patients. *N Engl J Med* 1981;305:372-374.
95. Gokal R: Renal osteodystrophy and aluminum bone disease in CAPD patients. *Clin Nephrol* 1988;30(Suppl 1):S64-S67.
96. Tovey FI, Karamanolis DG, Godfrey J, et al: Screening for early post-gastrectomy osteomalacia. *Practitioner* 1987;231:817,822.
97. Klein KB, Orwoll ES, Lieberman DA, et al: Metabolic bone disease in asymptomatic men after partial gastrectomy with Billroth II anastomosis. *Gastroenterology* 1987;92:608-616.
98. Favus MJ: Factors that influence absorption and secretion of calcium in the small intestine and colon. *Am J Physiol* 1985;248:G147-G157.
99. Felsenfeld A, Llach F: Vitamin D and metabolic bone disease: A clinicopathologic overview. *Pathol Annu* 1982;17:383-410.
100. Liel Y, Ulmer E, Shary J, et al: Low circulating vitamin D in obesity. *Calcif Tissue Int* 1988;43:199-201.
101. Bengoa JM, Sitrin MD, Meredith S, et al: Intestinal calcium absorption and vitamin D status in chronic cholestatic liver disease. *Hepatology* 1984;4:261-265.
102. Lalor BC, France MW, Powell D, et al: Bone and mineral metabolism and chronic alcohol abuse. *Q J Med* 1986;59:497-511.
103. Herlong HF, Recker RR, Maddrey WC: Bone disease in primary biliary cirrhosis: Histologic features and response to 25-hydroxyvitamin D. *Gastroenterology* 1982;83:103-108.
104. Schnitzler CM, Solomon L: Bone changes after alcohol abuse. *S Afr Med J* 1984;66:730-734.
105. Hey H, Stokholm KH, Lund B, et al: Vitamin D deficiency in obese patients and changes in circulating vitamin D metabolites following jejunoileal bypass. *Int J Obes* 1982;6:473-479.
106. Franck WA, Hoffman, GS, Davis JS, et al: Osteomalacia and weakness complicating jejunoileal bypass. *J Rheumatol* 1979;6:51-56.
107. Driscoll RH Jr, Meredith SC, Sitrin M, et al: Vitamin D deficiency and bone disease in patients with Crohn's disease. *Gastroenterology* 1982;83:1252-1258.
108. Haddad JG: Inherited and acquired disorders of vitamin D metabolism. *Adv Exp Med Biol* 1982;151:341-354.
109. Hessov I, Mosekilde L, Melsen F, et al: Osteopenia with normal vitamin D metabolites after small-bowel resection for Crohn's disease. *Scand J Gastroenterol* 1984;19:691-696.
110. Shike M, Harrison JE, Sturtridge WC, et al: Metabolic bone disease in patients receiving long-term total parenteral nutrition. *Ann Intern Med* 1980;92:343-350.
111. Klein GL, Coburn JW: Metabolic bone disease associated with total parenteral nutrition. *Adv Nutr Res* 1984;6:67-92.
112. Albright F, Butler AM, Bloomberg E: Rickets resistant to vitamin D therapy. *Am J Dis Child* 1937;54:529-547.
113. Balsan S, Tieder M: Linear growth in patients with hypophosphatemic vitamin D-resistant rickets: Influence of treatment regimen and parental height. *J Pediatr* 1990;116:365-371.
114. Brunette MG: The X-linked hypophosphatemic vitamin D resistant rickets: Old and new concepts. *Int J Pediatr Nephrol* 1985;6:55-62.
115. Evans GA, Arulanantham K, Gage JR: Primary hypophosphatemic rickets: Effect of oral phosphate and vitamin D on growth and surgical treatment. *J Bone Joint Surg* 1980;62A:1130-1138.
116. Frymoyer JW, Hodgkin W: Adult-onset vitamin D-resistant hypophosphatemic osteomalacia: A possible variant of vitamin D-resistant rickets. *J Bone Joint Surg* 1977;59A:101-106.
117. Hardy DC, Murphy WA, Siegel BA, et al: X-linked hypophosphatemia in adults: Prevalence of skeletal radiographic and scintigraphic features. *Radiology* 1989;171:403-414.
118. Baran DT, Marcy TW: Evidence for a defect in vitamin D metabolism in a patient with incomplete Fanconi syndrome. *J Clin Endocrinol Metab* 1984;59:998-1001.
119. Schulman JD: Cystinosis. *Prog Clin Biol Res* 1989;305:137-144.
120. Chan JC: Renal hypophosphatemic rickets: A review. *Int J Pediatr Nephrol* 1982;3:305-310.
121. Glorieux FH, Marie PJ, Pettifor JM, et al: Bone response to phosphate salts, ergocalciferol, and calcitriol in hypophosphatemic vitamin D-resistant rickets. *N Engl J Med* 1980;303:1023-1031.
122. Dent CE, Stamp TC: Hypophosphataemic osteomalacia presenting in adults. *Q J Med* 1971;40:303-329.
123. Tieder M, Modai D, Samuel R, et al: Hereditary hypophosphatemic rickets with hypercalciuria. *N Engl J Med* 1985;312:611-617.
124. Tieder M, Modai D, Shaked U, et al: "Idiopathic" hypercalciuria and hereditary hypophosphatemic rickets: Two phenotypical expressions of a common genetic defect. *N Engl J Med* 1987;316:125-129.
125. Balsan S, Garabedian M, Liberman UA, et al: Rickets and alopecia with resistance to 1,25-dihydroxyvitamin D: Two different clinical courses with two different cellular defects. *J Clin Endocrinol Metal* 1983;57:803-811.
126. Takeda E, Kuroda Y, Saijo T, et al: 1 alpha-hydroxyvitamin D3 treatment of three patients with 1,25-dihydroxyvitamin D-receptor-defect rickets and alopecia. *Pediatrics* 1987;80:97-101.
127. Scriver CR, Tenenhouse HS: X-linked hypophosphataemia: a homologous phenotype in humans and mice with unusual organ-specific gene dosage. *J Inherit Metab Dis* 1992;15:610-624.
128. Brooks MH, Bell NH, Love L, et al: Vitamin-D-dependent rickets type II: Resistance of target organs to 1,25-dihydroxyvitamin D. *N Engl J Med* 1978;298:996-999.
129. Silver J, Landau H, Bab I, et al: Vitamin D-dependent rickets types I and II: Diagnosis and response to therapy. *Isr J Med Sci* 1985;21:53-56.
130. Reade TM, Scriver CR, Glorieux FH, et al: Response to crystalline 1alpha-hydroxyvitamin D3 in vitamin D dependency. *Pediatr Res* 1975;9:593-599.
131. Weisman Y, Bab I, Gazit D, et al: Long-term intracaval calcium infusion therapy in end-organ resistance to 1,25-dihydroxyvitamin D. *Am J Med* 1987;83:984-990.
132. Sakati N, Woodhouse NJ, Niles N, et al: Hereditary resistance to 1,25-dihydroxyvitamin D: Clinical and radiological improvement during high-dose oral calcium therapy. *Horm Res* 1986; 24:280-287.
133. Cunningham J, Fraher LJ, Clemens TL, et al: Chronic acidosis with metabolic bone disease. Effect of alkali on bone morphology and vitamin D metabolism. *Am J Med* 1982;73:199-204.
134. Chan JC, Alon U: Tubular disorders of acid-base and phosphate metabolism. *Nephron* 1985;40:257-279.
135. Schoen EJ, Young G: "Lowe's syndrome": Abnormalities in renal tubular function in combination with other congenital defects. *Am J Med* 1959;27:781-792.
136. Kallmeyer J, Dunea G, Schwartz FD: Hypophosphatemic osteomalacia with hyperglycinuria. *Ann Intern Med* 1967;66:136-141.
137. Brenner RJ, Spring DB, Sebastian A, et al: Incidence of radiographically evident bone disease, nephrocalcinosis, and nephrolithiasis in various types of renal tubular acidosis. *N Engl J Med* 1982;307:217-221.
138. Kraut JA, Gordon EM, Ransom JC, et al: Effect of chronic metabolic acidosis on vitamin D metabolism in humans. *Kidney Int* 1983;24:644-648.
139. McClure J, Smith PS: Oncogenic osteomalacia. *J Clin Pathol* 1987;40:446-453.

140. Ryan EA, Reiss E: Oncogenous osteomalacia: Review of the world literature of 42 cases and report of two new cases. *Am J Med* 1984;77:501-512.
141. Weidner N, Santa-Cruz D: Phosphaturic mesenchymal tumors: A polymorphous group causing osteomalacia or rickets. *Cancer* 1987;59:1442-1454.
142. Siris ES, Clemens TL, Dempster DW, et al: Tumor-induced osteomalacia: Kinetics of calcium, phosphorus, and vitamin D metabolism and characteristics of bone histomorphometry. *Am J Med* 1987;82:307-312.
143. Drezner MK, Feinglos MN: Osteomalacia due to 1alpha, 25-dihydroxycholecalciferol deficiency: Association with a giant cell tumor of bone. *J Clin Invest* 1977;60:1046-1053.
144. Richens A, Rowe DJ: Disturbance of calcium metabolism by anticonvulsant drugs. *Br Med J* 1970;4:73-76.
145. Hunt PA, Wu-Chen ML, Handal NJ, et al: Bone disease induced by anticonvulsant therapy and treatment with calcitriol (1,25-dihydroxyvitamin D3). *Am J Dis Child* 1986;140:715-718.
146. Barden HS, Mazess RB, Chesney RW, et al: Bone status of children receiving anticonvulsant therapy. *Metab Bone Dis* 1982;4:43-47.
147. Weinstein RS, Bryce GF, Sappington LJ, et al: Decreased serum ionized calcium and normal vitamin D metabolite levels with anticonvulsant drug treatment. *J Clin Endocrinol Metab* 1984;58:1003-1009.
148. Davie MW, Emberson CE, Lawson DE, et al: Low plasma 25-hydroxyvitamin D and serum calcium levels in institutionalized epileptic subjects: Associated risk factors, consequences and response to treatment with vitamin D. *Q J Med* 1983;52:79-91.
149. Goldman AB, Lane JM, Salvati E: Slipped capital femoral epiphyses complicating renal osteodystrophy: A report of three cases. *Radiology* 1978;126:333-339.
150. Hoikka V, Alhava EM, Savolainen K, et al: Osteomalacia in fractures of the proximal femur. *Acta Orthop Scand* 1982;53:255-260.
151. Ganeval D, Lacour B, Chopin N, et al: Proteinuria in multiple myeloma and related diseases. *Am J Nephrol* 1990;10(Suppl 1):58-62.
152. Genant HK, Block JE, Steiger P, et al: Appropriate use of bone densitometry. *Radiology* 1989;170:817-822.
153. Cushner HM, Adams ND: Review: Renal osteodystrophy—pathogenesis and treatment. *Am J Med Sci* 1986;291:264-275.
154. Sutton RA, Cameron EC: Renal osteodystrophy: Pathophysiology. *Semin Nephrol* 1992;12:91-100.
155. Lee DB, Goodman WG, Coburn JW: Renal osteodystrophy: Some new questions on an old disorder. *Am J Kidney Dis* 1988;11:365-376.
156. Baker LR: Prevention of renal osteodystrophy. *Miner Electrolyte Metab* 1991;17:240-249.
157. Coburn JW, Henry DA: Renal osteodystrophy. *Adv Intern Med* 1984;30:387-424.
158. Cohen-Solal M, Sebert JL: Renal osteodystrophy and hypercalcemia. *Curr Opin Rheumatol* 1993;5:357-362.
159. Teitelbaum SL: Renal osteodystrophy. *Hum Pathol* 1984;15:306-323.
160. Ackrill P, Day JP, Garstang FM, et al: Treatment of fracturing renal osteodystrophy by desferrioxamine. *Proc Eur Dial Transplant Assoc* 1983;19:203-207.
161. Alfrey AC, LeGendre GR, Kaehny WD: The dialysis encephalopathy syndrome: Possible aluminum intoxication. *N Engl J Med* 1976;294:184-188.
162. Malluche HH, Smith AJ, Abreo K, et al: The use of deferoxamine in the management of aluminum accumulation in bone in patients with renal failure. *N Engl J Med* 1984;311:140-144.
163. Ward MK, Feest TG, Ellis HA, et al: Osteomalacic dialysis osteodystrophy: Evidence for a water-borne aetiological agent, probably aluminium. *Lancet* 1978;1:841-845.
164. Wilson RE, Hampers CL, Bernstein DS, et al: Subtotal parathyroidectomy in chronic renal failure: A seven-year experience in a dialysis and transplant program. *Ann Surg* 1971;174:640-654.
165. Katz AD, Kaplan L: Parathyroidectomy for hyperplasia in renal disease. *Arch Surg* 1973;107:51-55.
166. Cooper AP (ed): *A Treatise on Dislocations and on Fractures of the Joints*, ed 4. London, Longman, Hurst, Rees, Orme, Brown and Green, 1824.
167. Marcus R: Secondary forms of osteoporosis, in Coe FL, Favus MJ (eds): *Disorders of Bone and Mineral Metabolism.* New York, NY, Raven Press, 1992, pp 889-904.
168. Heaney RP, Recker RR, Saville PD: Calcium balance and calcium requirements in middle-aged women. *Am J Clin Nutr* 1977;30: 1603-1611.
169. Heaney RP, Recker RR, Saville PD: Menopausal changes in calcium balance performance. *J Lab Clin Med* 1978;92:953-963.
170. Lindsay R, Cosman F: Primary osteoporosis, in Coe FL, Favus MJ (eds): *Disorders of Bone and Mineral Metabolism.* New York, NY, Raven Press, 1992, pp 831-888.
171. Albright F, Reifenstein, EC Jr (eds): Metabolic bone disease: Osteoporosis, in *The Parathyroid Glands and Metabolic Bone Disease.* Baltimore, MD, Williams & Wilkins, 1948, pp 145-204.
172. Barr DG: Proceedings: Bone deficiency in Turner's syndrome measured by metacarpal dimensions. *Arch Dis Child* 1974;49:821-822.
173. Herman TE, McAlister WH: Inherited diseases of bone density in children. *Radiol Clin North Am* 1991;29:149-164.
174. Kivirikko KI: Collagens and their abnormalities in a wide spectrum of diseases. *Ann Med* 1993;25:113-126.
175. Bardin T, Lequesne M: The osteoporosis of heparinotherapy and systemic mastocytosis. *Clin Rheumatol* 1989;8(Suppl 2):119-123.
176. Chines A, Pacifici R, Avioli LA, et al: Systemic mastocytosis and osteoporosis. *Osteoporos Int* 1993;3(Suppl 1):147-149.
177. Kennedy AC, Smith DA, Buchanan WW, et al: Bone loss in patients with rheumatoid arthritis. *Scand J Rheumatol* 1975;4:73-79.
178. Reid DM, Kennedy NS, Smith MA, et al: Total body calcium in rheumatoid arthritis: Effects of disease activity and corticosteroid treatment. *Br Med J* 1982;285:330-332.
179. Saville PD, Kharmosh O: Osteoporosis of rheumatoid arthritis: Influence of age, sex and corticosteroids. *Arthritis Rheum* 1967;10:423-430.
180. Aloia JF, Roginsky M, Ellis K, et al: Skeletal metabolism and body composition in Cushing's syndrome. *J Clin Endocrinol Metab* 1974;39:981-985.
181. Bayley TA, Harrison JE, McNeill KG, et al: Effect of thyrotoxicosis and its treatment on bone mineral and muscle mass. *J Clin Endocrinol Metab* 1980;50: 916-922.
182. Eriksen EF, Mosekilde L, Melsen F: Trabecular bone remodeling and bone balance in hyperthyroidism. *Bone* 1985;6:421-428.
183. Fraser SA, Anderson JB, Smith DA, et al: Osteoporosis and fractures following thyrotoxicosis. *Lancet* 1971;1:981-983.
184. Smith DA, Fraser SA, Wilson GM: Hyperthyroidism and calcium metabolism. *Clin Endocrinol Metab* 1973;2:333-354.
185. Aarskog D, Aksnes L, Markestad T, et al: Heparin-induced inhibition of 1,25-dihydroxyvitamin D formation. *Am J Obstet Gynecol* 1984;148:1141-1142.
186. Frame B, Nixon RK: Bone-marrow mast cells in osteoporosis of aging. *N Engl J Med* 1968;279:626-630.
187. Frame B, Jackson CE, Reynolds WA, et al: Hypercalcemia and skeletal effects in chronic hypervitaminosis A. *Ann Intern Med* 1974;80:44-48.
188. Hough S, Avioli LV, Muir H, et al: Effects of hypervitaminosis A on the bone and mineral metabolism of the rat. *Endocrinology* 1988;122:2933-2939.
189. Adachi JD, Bensen WG, Hodsman AB: Corticosteroid-induced osteoporosis. *Semin Arthritis Rheum* 1993;22:375-384.

190. Als OS, Gotfredsen A, Christiansen C: The effect of glucocorticoids on bone mass in rheumatoid arthritis patients: Influence of menopausal state. *Arthritis Rheum* 1985;28:369-375.
191. Crilly RG, Marshall DH, Nordin BE: Metabolic effects of corticosteroid therapy in post-menopausal women. *J Steroid Biochem* 1979;11:429-433.
192. Jowsey J, Riggs BL: Bone formation in hypercortisonism. *Acta Endocrinol* 1970;63:21-28.
193. Rickers H, Deding A, Christiansen C, et al: Corticosteroid-induced osteopenia and vitamin D metabolism: Effect of vitamin D2, calcium phosphate and sodium fluoride administration. *Clin Endocrinol* 1982;16:409-415.
194. Seeman E, Kumar R, Hunder GG, et al: Production, degradation, and circulating levels of 1,25-dihydroxyvitamin D in health and in chronic glucocorticoid excess. *J Clin Invest* 1980;66:664-669.
195. Anderson SA, Cohn SH: Bone demineralization during space flight. *Physiologist* 1985;28:212-217.
196. Carter DR: Mechanical loading history and skeletal biology. J Biomech 1987;20:1095-1109.
197. Krolner B, Toft B: Vertebral bone loss: An unheeded side effect of therapeutic bed rest. *Clin Sci* 1983;64:537-540.
198. Riggs BL, Melton LJ III: Involutional osteoporosis. *N Engl J Med* 1986;314:1676-1686.
199. Christiansen C: Prevention and treatment of osteoporosis with hormone replacement therapy. *Int J Fertil Menopausal Stud* 1993; 38(Suppl1):45-54.
200. Melton LJ III, Sampson JM, Morrey BF, et al: Epidemiologic features of pelvic fractures. *Clin Orthop* 1981;155:43-47.
201. Eriksen EF, Melsen F, Mosekilde L: Reconstruction of the resorptive site in iliac trabecular bone: A kinetic model for bone resorption in 20 normal individuals. *Metab Bone Dis* 1984;5:235-242.
202. Parfitt AM: Age-related structural changes in trabecular and cortical bone: Cellular mechanisms and biomechanical consequences. *Calcif Tissue Int* 1984;36(Suppl1):S123-S128.
203. Recker RR, Kimmel DB, Parfitt AM, et al: Static and tetracycline-based bone histomorphometric data from 34 normal postmenopausal females. *J Bone Miner Res* 1988;3:133-144.
204. Steiniche T, Hasling C, Charles P, et al: A randomized study on the effects of estrogen/gestagen or high dose oral calcium on trabecular bone remodeling in postmenopausal osteoporosis. *Bone* 1989;10:313-320.
205. Aitken JM, Hart DM, Anderson JB, et al: Osteoporosis after oophorectomy for non-malignant disease in premenopausal women. *Br Med J* 1973;2:325-328.
206. Richelson LS, Wahner HW, Melton LJ III, et al: Relative contributions of aging and estrogen deficiency to postmenopausal bone loss. *N Engl J Med* 1984;311:1273-1275.
207. Ettinger B, Genant HK, Cann C: Menopausal bone loss can be prevented by low dose estrogen with calcium supplements. *J Comput Assist Tomog* 1985;9:633-634.
208. Genant HK, Cann CE, Ettinger B, et al: Quantitative computed tomography of vertebral spongiosa: A sensitive method for detecting early bone loss after oophorectomy. *Ann Intern Med* 1982;97:699-705.
209. Geusens P, Dequeker J, Verstraeten A, et al: Age-, sex-, and menopause-related changes of vertebral and peripheral bone: Population study using dual and single photon absorptiometry and radiogrammetry. *J Nucl Med* 1986;27:1540-1549.
210. Meema HE, Meema S: Postmenopausal osteoporosis: Simple screening method for diagnosis before structural failure. *Radiology* 1987;164:405-410.
211. Melton LJ III, Chrischilles EA, Cooper C, et al: Perspective: How many women have osteoporosis? *J Bone Miner Res* 1992;7:1005-1010.
212. Nilas L, Christiansen C: Bone mass and its relationship to age and the menopause. *J Clin Endocrinol Metab* 1987;65:697-702.
213. Riis BJ, Christiansen C: Measurement of spinal or peripheral bone mass to estimate early postmenopausal bone loss? *Am J Med* 1988;84:646-653.
214. Riis B, Thomsen K, Christiansen C: Does calcium supplementation prevent postmenopausal bone loss? A double-blind, controlled clinical study. *N Engl J Med* 1987;316:173-177.
215. Ernst M, Heath JK, Rodan GA: Estradiol effects on proliferation, messenger ribonucleic acid for collagen and insulin-like growth factor-I, and parathyroid hormone-stimulated adenylate cyclase activity in osteoblastic cells from calvariae and long bones. *Endocrinology* 1989;125:825-833.
216. Gray TK, Mohan S, Linkhart TA, et al: Estradiol stimulates in vitro the secretion of insulin-like growth factors by the clonal osteoblastic cell line, UMR106. *Biochem Biophys Res Commun* 1989;158:407-412.
217. Pacifici R, Rifas L, Teitelbaum S, et al: Spontaneous release of interleukin 1 from human blood monocytes reflects bone formation in idiopathic osteoporosis. *Proc Nat Acad Sci USA* 1987;84:4616-4620.
218. Stock JL, Coderre JA, McDonald B, et al: Effects of estrogen in vivo and in vitro on spontaneous interleukin-1 release by monocytes from postmenopausal women. *J Clin Endocrinol Metab* 1989;68:364-368.
219. Ettinger B, Genant HK, Cann CE: Long-term estrogen replacement therapy prevents bone loss and fractures. *Ann Intern Med* 1985;102:319-324.
220. Gallagher JC, Riggs BL, DeLuca HF: Effect of estrogen on calcium absorption and serum vitamin D metabolites in postmenopausal osteoporosis. *J Clin Endocrinol Metab* 1980;51:1359-1364.
221. Quigley ME, Martin PL, Burnier AM, et al: Estrogen therapy arrests bone loss in elderly women. *Am J Obstet Gynecol* 1987;156:1516-1523.
222. Brinton LA, Hoover R, Fraumeni JF Jr: Menopausal oestrogens and breast cancer risk: An expanded case-control study. *Br J Cancer* 1986;54:825-832.
223. Hulka BS, Fowler WC Jr, Kaufman DG, et al: Estrogen and endometrial cancer: Cases and two control groups from North Carolina. *Am J Obstet Gynecol* 1980;137:92-101.
224. Mitlak BH, Nussbaum SR: Diagnosis and treatment of osteoporosis. *Annu Rev Med* 1993;44:265-277.
225. Nomura AM, Kolonel LN, Hirohata T, et al: The association of replacement estrogens with breast cancer. *Int J Cancer* 1986;37:49-53.
226. Riggs BL, Melton LJ III, Wahner HW: Heterogeneity of involutional osteoporosis: Evidence for two distinct osteoporosis syndromes, in Frame B, Potts JT Jr (eds): *Clinical Disorders of Bone and Mineral Metabolism*. Amsterdam, Excerpta Medica, 1983, pp 337-342.
227. Gallagher JC, Riggs BL, Eisman J, et al: Intestinal calcium absorption and serum vitamin D metabolites in normal subjects and osteoporotic patients: Effect of age and dietary calcium. *J Clin Invest* 1979;64:729-736.
228. Tsai KS, Heath H III, Kumar R, et al: Impaired vitamin D metabolism with aging in women: Possible role in pathogenesis of senile osteoporosis. *J Clin Invest* 1984;73:1668-1672.
229. Alevizaki CC, Ikkos DG, Singhelakis P: Progressive decrease of true intestinal calcium absorption with age in normal man. *J Nucl Med* 1973;14:760-762.
230. Heaney RP, Gallagher JC, Johnston CC, et al: Calcium nutrition and bone health in the elderly. *Am J Clin Nutr* 1982;36(Suppl 5):986-1013.
231. Dequeker J, Goris P, Uytterhoeven R: Osteoporosis and osteoarthritis (osteoarthrosis): Anthropometric distinctions. *JAMA* 1983;249:1448-1451.

232. Cummings SR, Kelsey JL, Nevitt MC, et al: Epidemiology of osteoporosis and osteoporotic fractures. *Epidemiol Rev* 1985;7:178-208.
233. Siegelman SS: The radiology of osteoporosis, in Barzel US (ed): *Osteoporosis.* New York, NY, Grune & Stratton, 1970, pp 68-79.
234. Genant HK, Vogler JB, Block JE: Radiology of osteoporosis, in Riggs BL, Melton LJ III (eds): *Osteoporosis: Etiology, Diagnosis and Management.* New York, NY, Raven Press, 1988, pp 181-220.
235. Singh M, Nagrath AR, Maini PS: Changes in trabecular pattern of the upper end of the femur as an index of osteoporosis. *J Bone Joint Surg* 1970;52A:457-467.
236. Barnett E, Nordin BEC: The radiological diagnosis of osteoporosis: A new approach. *Clin Radiol* 1960;11:166-174.
237. Ostlere SJ, Gold RH: Osteoporosis and bone density measurement methods. *Clin Orthop* 1991;271:149-163.
238. Grampp S, Jergas M, Gluer CC, et al: Radiologic diagnosis of osteoporosis: Current methods and perspectives. *Radiol Clin North Am* 1993;31:1133-1145.
239. Delmas PD: Biochemical markers of bone turnover for the clinical investigation of osteoporosis. *Osteoporos Int* 1993;3(Suppl 1):81-86.
240. McGowan JA: Osteoporosis: Assessment of bone loss and remodeling. *Aging* 1993;5:81-93.
241. Snow-Harter C, Marcus R: Exercise, bone mineral density, and osteoporosis. *Exerc Sport Sci Rev* 1991;19:351-388.
242. Heaney RP: Lifelong calcium intake and prevention of bone fragility in the aged. *Calcif Tissue Int* 1991;49(Suppl):S42-S45.
243. Lobo RA: The role of progestins in hormone replacement therapy. *Am J Obstet Gynecol* 1992;166:1997-2004.
244. Wallach S: The role of calcitonin treatment in postmenopausal osteoporosis. *Orthop Rev* 1992;21:1034-1042;1130-1131.
245. Wardlaw GM: Putting osteoporosis in perspective. *J Am Diet Assoc* 1993;93:1000-1006.
246. Avioli LV: Calcitonin therapy in osteoporotic syndromes. *South Med J* 1992;85:2S17-2S21.
247. Nordin BE, Morris HA: Osteoporosis and vitamin D. *J Cell Biochem* 1992;49:19-25.
248. Reginster JY: Effect of calcitonin on bone mass and fracture rates. *Am J Med* 1991;91(Suppl 5B):19S-22S.
249. Reginster JY: Calcitonins: Newer routes of delivery. *Osteoporos Int* 1993;3(Suppl 2):S3-S7.
250. Brixen K, Kassem M, Eriksen EF, et al: Growth hormone (GH) and adult bone remodeling: The potential use of GH in treatment of osteoporosis. *J Pediatr Endocrinol* 1993;6:65-71.
251. DeLuca HF: Osteoporosis and the metabolites of vitamin D. *Metabolism* 1990;39(Suppl 1):3-9.
252. Aaron RK, Ciombor DM: Therapeutic effects of electromagnetic fields in the stimulation of connective tissue repair. *J Cell Biochem* 1993;52:42-46.
253. Kanis JA, McCloskey EV, Sirtori P, et al: Rationale for the use of clodronate in osteoporosis. *Osteoporos Int* 1993;3(Suppl 2):S23-S28.
254. Kleerekoper M, Balena R: Fluorides and osteoporosis. *South Med J* 1992;85:2S34-2S42.
255. Lombardi A, Santora AC: Clinical trials with bisphosphonates. *Ann Ital Med Int* 1992;7(Suppl 3):158S-165S.
256. Papapoulos SE, Landman JO, Bijvoet OL, et al: The use of bisphosphonates in the treatment of osteoporosis. *Bone* 1992;13(Suppl 1):S41-S49.
257. de-Vernejoul MC, Cohen-Solal M, Orcel P: Bone cytokines. *Curr Opin Rheumatol* 1993;5:332-338.
258. Licata AA: Therapies for symptomatic primary osteoporosis. *Geriatrics* 1991;46:62-63;66-67.
259. Bab IA, Einhorn TA: Regulatory role of osteogenic growth polypeptides in bone formation and hemopoiesis. *Crit Rev Eukaryot Gene Expr* 1993;3:31-46.
260. Mundy GR: Visions for the future in osteoporosis research. *Osteoporos Int* 1993;3(Suppl 2):S29-S34.
261. Waldenström JG: Benign monoclonal gammapathy. *Acta Med Scand* 1984;216:435-447.
262. Campanacci M (ed): Plasmacytoma, in *Bone and Soft Tissue Tumors.* Wien, Springer-Verlag, 1990, pp 559-574.
263. Goodman MA: Plasma cell tumors. *Clin Orthop* 1986;204:86-92.
264. Kyle RA: Monoclonal gammopathy and multiple myeloma in the elderly. *Baillieres Clin Haematol* 1987;1:533-557.
265. Jackson A, Scarffe JH: Prognostic significance of osteopenia and immunoparesis at presentation in patients with solitary myeloma of bone. *Eur J Cancer* 1990;26:363-371.
266. Kyle RA: Diagnostic criteria of multiple myeloma. *Hematol Oncol Clin North Am* 1992;6:347-358.
267. Dimopoulos MA, Moulopoulos A, Delasalle K, et al: Solitary plasmacytoma of bone and asymptomatic multiple myeloma. *Hematol Oncol Clin North Am* 1992;6:359-369.
268. Kyle RA, Garton JP: Laboratory monitoring of myeloma proteins. *Semin Oncol* 1986;13:310-317.
269. Vaickus L, Ball ED, Foon KA: Immune markers in hematologic malignancies. *Crit Rev Oncol Hematol* 1991;11:267-297.

Spine

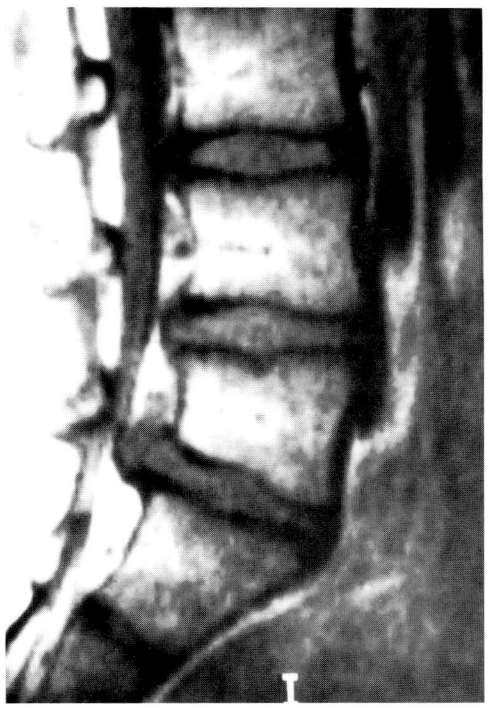

CHAPTER 2

Evaluation and Emergent Treatment of Patients with Thoracolumbar Trauma

Alan M. Levine, MD
Paul C. McAfee, MD
Paul A. Anderson, MD

Trauma to the spine and to the spinal cord is a devastating injury that can have debilitating long-term effects. The ultimate function of patients with these injuries is dependent on the ability to reconstruct the spine as well as on residual neurologic function. Thoracolumbar spinal cord injuries range from high thoracic injuries (which are quite similar in the degree of devastation and disability to those in the low cervical spine) to those at the thoracolumbar junction (which, although they still keep the patient wheelchair-bound, allow more truncal balance and ability to function). Interestingly, there are not great differences in the degree of disability between complete neurologic injuries at the thoracolumbar junction and the low lumbar spine until the top of the sacrum is reached. Wheelchair dependence can be the sequela of injury at almost any level in the thoracolumbar junction or the lumbar spine. Those patients with absence of bowel, bladder, and sexual function but the ability to walk clearly experience a psychologically devastating injury. There are approximately 10,000 survivors of new spinal cord injuries every year. An additional undetermined number die of spinal cord injuries (predominantly in the high cervical spine).[1-3] The number of patients with thoracolumbar injuries who have neurologic deficit is approximately 15% to 20%. This is considerably less than that seen in the cervical spine injuries (40%).[4]

Most patients with spinal cord injuries are male, and their mean age is in the middle 20s. The most common causes of these injuries are motor vehicle accidents (approximately 45%), falls (20%), sports injuries (15%), acts of violence (15%), and other causes (5%).[3-5] The survival rate of patients with spinal cord injuries decreases dramatically after age 50.[6] For many patients, the associated injuries that accompany the spinal cord injury, such as severe chest trauma (especially in high thoracic paraplegics), may be life threatening. Many long-term problems of the musculoskeletal, genitourinary, and nervous systems develop after the initial treatment.[7-11] In addition, the psychological problems associated with spinal cord injury and its rehabilitation are well documented.[12] More than 50% of all spinal cord injuries occur in patients who are under the influence of alcohol or drugs at the time of the incident, meaning that many of these patients are dysfunctional prior to their injury. This is aggravated by their subsequent feelings of inadequacy, loss of self-esteem and body image, and inability to care for themselves.

Recently, advances have been made in the care of patients with spinal cord injuries in the following areas: initial evaluation, resuscitation, imaging, treatment, and management of complications. The concept of spinal cord injury centers was developed by Sir Ludwig Guttman during World War II at Stoke Mandeville Hospital, subsequently in Toronto, Canada, and later in the United States at Rancho Los Amigos Hospital and the Veterans Administration. In the 1970s and 1980s, regional spinal cord injury centers were developed, both to care for patients and to educate health professionals and the public about ways to help improve care and prevent spinal cord injury. The major benefits these centers provide to patients are (1) improved neurologic function, (2) reduced secondary complications, and (3) extended life expectancy.

However, in a multicenter study, Marshall and associates[13] documented that, in spite of spinal cord injury centers, approximately 6% of all patients with spinal cord injuries had some deterioration of function during the course of their treatment. At the same time, due to advances in transport and early care, the percentage of patients whose spinal cord injuries are partial, rather than complete, has increased steadily over the last 20 years. The rate of neurologic deterioration is probably more significant for those patients treated in institutions unaccustomed to dealing with a spinal cord injury patient, although the documentation is not complete. In addition, in centers currently established to care for spinal injury, physical therapy, self catheterization of the bladder, and other adjunctive modalities begin immediately, thus saving overall rehabilitation time, shortening hospitalization, and decreasing complications.[14]

The advent of newer treatment modalities has shortened hospital time and lowered costs. In the 1950s and into the 1960s, nonsurgical treatment of spinal cord injuries was the norm, requiring prolonged periods of hospitalization and bed rest with attendant complications. Today, adequate stabilization can be achieved for even the most unstable injuries, thus placing the spinal cord in the optimal situation for recovery and allowing rapid mobilization of the patient. Early mobilization can be critical for polytrauma spine patients, in whom recumbency is associated with increased morbidity and mortality. Several studies have documented that patients with spinal cord injuries stabilized within 48 hours have a significantly shorter hospital stay and less morbidity than patients whose treatment is delayed.[15-17]

Transport and Immobilization

Accident victims with suspected injury to the spine, significant contusions over the spine, or transient neurologic symptoms are placed immediately on a backboard by paramedics and are transported to the evaluation center on the backboard. It is then the responsibility of the treating center to determine the type of immobilization during the evaluation. Although there are several types of backboards, the one-piece rigid wooden backboard is the one most commonly used. The scoop backboard is more effective and makes it easier to transport patients from place to place. Backboards constructed of plastics allow satisfactory images in plain radiography, computed tomography (CT), and magnetic resonance imaging (MRI). Patients with thoracolumbar trauma, especially those with neurologic deficit, are at risk for decubitus ulceration unless the patient's position is changed every 2 hours. However, log rolling is associated with significant fracture site motion.[18,19] Therefore, we recommend rapid patient evaluation and early definitive treatment.

Initial Assessment

As in all polytrauma patients, the standard primary considerations of (1) airway, (2) breathing, and (3) circulation are paramount.[20] At presentation, thoracolumbar spine trauma patients may be hemodynamically unstable as a result of associated chest, abdominal, or pelvic injuries. Specific systemic injuries are commonly associated with certain patterns of spinal fractures. Patients with T2-T10 thoracic spine fractures resulting in paraplegia have a high association of severe chest injuries. Because of the biomechanical effects of the rib cage, large forces are required to cause significant thoracic spine trauma. These forces frequently result in multiple rib fractures, costovertebral dissociations, and injury to the lung parenchyma. In addition, patients with displaced translational shear injuries at these levels may have partial aortic disruptions. Any widening of the mediastinum must be carefully investigated with aortography. Sixty percent of the patients with flexion-distraction injuries caused by seatbelts have intra-abdominal trauma, usually to the bowel.[21-23] In those patients with lower lumbar fractures, there is an associated incidence of pelvic injury, as well as lower extremity injury.

Secondary Assessment

Once the patient is stabilized, a secondary evaluation of the patient is necessary. This evaluation includes a history of the injury, a general medical history, a physical examination encompassing the spine, and the appropriate radiographic examination. For those patients who are awake, information about the mechanism of injury will frequently aid in their evaluation. It is critical to know how patients were injured, that is, whether as a belted passenger or by being ejected from the car, and if they remember anything about the way that they struck the pavement once ejected. Clearly those patients being ejected and landing on their chest will be more likely to have thoracic injuries, whereas belted passengers will more frequently have thoracolumbar junction injuries. Patients falling or jumping from a height frequently have lower extremity and low lumbar or sacral fractures. Patients with hyperextension injuries, such as lumberjack injuries, will have characteristic fracture patterns associated with the mechanism. The patients' subjective feelings at the time of injury should be noted. Although they may be neurologically intact, if they had either paresthesias or momentary paralysis from which they recovered slowly over several minutes, the severity of the injury may be more significant.

To perform a physical examination of the spine, the patient should be rolled carefully into a semi-lateral position. The spine is palpated to determine areas of tenderness, and to identify areas of skin abrasion. Finally, evident gaps in the interspinous ligament between the spinous processes or, in patients with bilateral facet dislocations, step-offs or sharp areas of kyphosis allow the immediate localization of the injury site. It is important to evaluate the entire spine because multiple spinal injuries occur in 10% to 15% of cases.[24]

The neurologic examination of patients with thoracolumbar trauma should begin cranially with the trapezius and deltoid and progress distally to the hand intrinsics, because these patients may have associated cervical spine fractures and/or brachial plexus injuries.[25] The chest and abdomen are checked for sharp/dull discrimination to pin prick to determine any sensory level. Levels of normal sensation, transitional sensation, and absence of sensation should be noted as should any difference between the right and left sides. Sensation around the rectum must be tested as this may be the only residual of sparing in conus injuries.[26] A digital rectal exam should be performed to determine tone, ability to voluntarily contract the anal sphincter and pelvic floor, and to check the bulbocavernosus reflex. Finally, the lower extremity motor function should be carefully assessed beginning at the hip flexors and again working distally.

Prompt recording of the examination in the medical record is critical to the patient's care and for future analysis of the data on spinal injury. Spinal injury assessment instruments have been published to attempt to better quantify degrees of injury and allow serial comparisons. Sensations to pain (pin prick) and light touch are scored (0 = absent; 1 = impaired; 2 = intact) and recorded for each dermatome. A motor score ranging from 0 to 100 is determined by summating standard manual muscle grades (range 0 to 5) of the following ten muscle groups: elbow flexors, wrist extensors, elbow extensors, finger flexors, finger intrinsics,

Table 1
American Spinal Injury Association (ASIA) Impairment Scale

A Complete	No preservation of motor or sensory function below level of neurologic injury
B Incomplete	Sensory but no motor function is preserved below level of neurologic injury
C Incomplete	Sensory and motor function are preserved below level of neurologic injury. The majority of key muscle groups have less than grade 3 strength.
D Incomplete	Sensory and motor function are preserved below level of neurologic injury. The majority of key muscle groups have greater than grade 3 strength.
E Normal	Sensory and motor function are normal.

(Adapted with permission from the American Spinal Injury Association: *Standards for Neurological and Functional Classification of Spinal Cord Injury,* revised. Chicago, IL, American Spinal Injury Association, 1992.)

hip flexors, knee extensors, ankle dorsiflexors, long toe extensors, and ankle plantiflexors.[27] Voluntary anal contraction is also recorded. The form recommended by the American Spinal Injury Association (ASIA) is given in Figure 1. ASIA defines the level of neurologic injury as the most caudal level with at least grade 3 motor function. The modified Frankel impairment scale evaluates the integrity of the cross-sectional components of the spinal cord.[25,28] Frankel A refers to complete absence of distal motor/sensory function. Frankel B has some sensation but no distal motor function. Frankel C has distal sensation and some (functionless) motor function. Frankel D has distal sensation and useful motor function. Frankel E is neurologically intact but patients may have spasticity (Table 1).

Radiographic Assessment

The patient with an injured spine or any patient with major deceleration injuries should have lateral cervical spine, anteroposterior chest, and pelvic radiographs. These radiographs should be complemented by plain

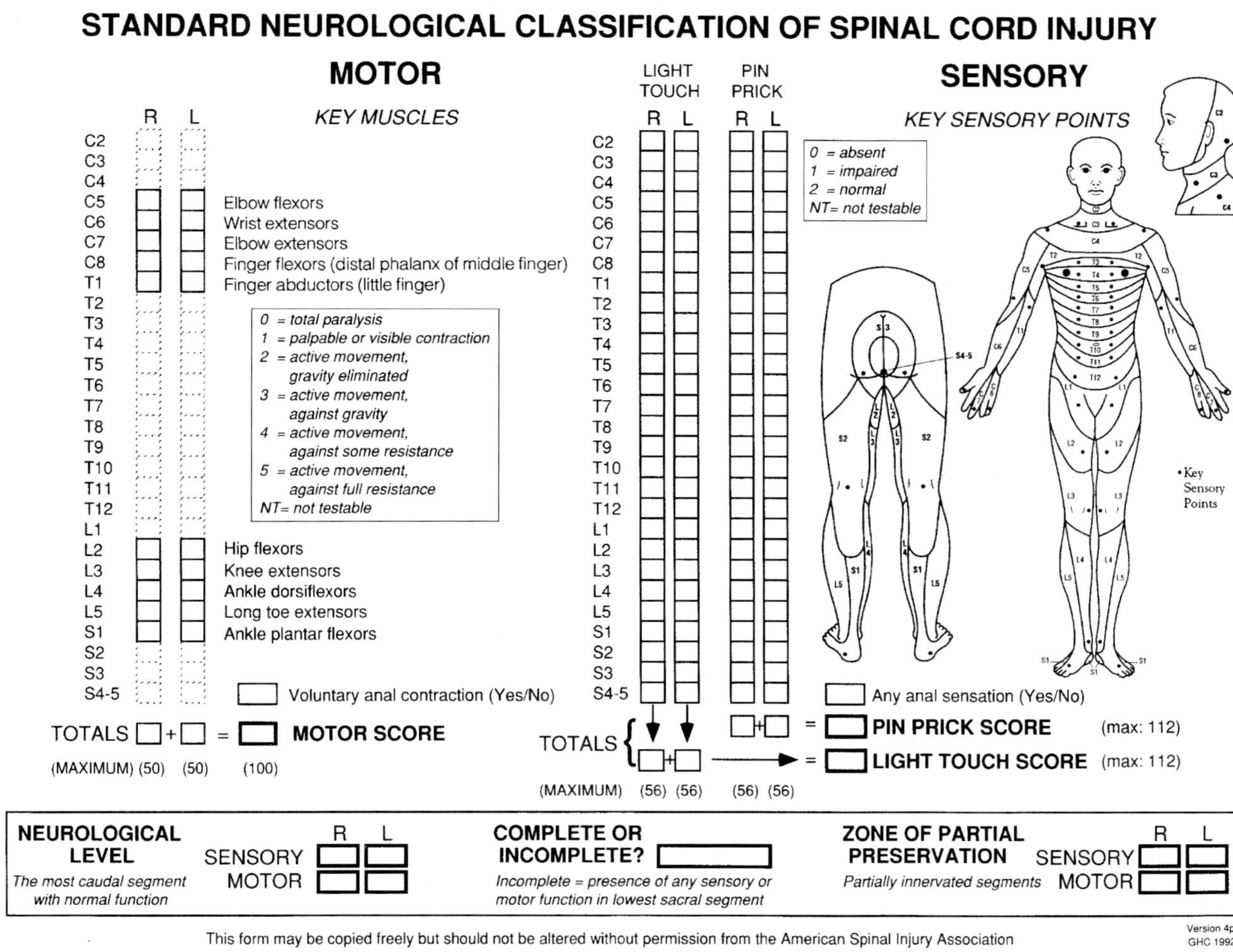
STANDARD NEUROLOGICAL CLASSIFICATION OF SPINAL CORD INJURY

MOTOR

KEY MUSCLES

	R	L	
C2			
C3			
C4			
C5			Elbow flexors
C6			Wrist extensors
C7			Elbow extensors
C8			Finger flexors (distal phalanx of middle finger)
T1			Finger abductors (little finger)
T2			
T3			
T4			
T5			
T6			
T7			
T8			
T9			
T10			
T11			
T12			
L1			
L2			Hip flexors
L3			Knee extensors
L4			Ankle dorsiflexors
L5			Long toe extensors
S1			Ankle plantar flexors
S2			
S3			
S4-5			Voluntary anal contraction (Yes/No)

0 = total paralysis
1 = palpable or visible contraction
2 = active movement, gravity eliminated
3 = active movement, against gravity
4 = active movement, against some resistance
5 = active movement, against full resistance
NT= not testable

TOTALS ☐+☐ = ☐ MOTOR SCORE
(MAXIMUM) (50) (50) (100)

SENSORY

LIGHT TOUCH R L — PIN PRICK R L

KEY SENSORY POINTS

C2, C3, C4, C5, C6, C7, C8, T1, T2, T3, T4, T5, T6, T7, T8, T9, T10, T11, T12, L1, L2, L3, L4, L5, S1, S2, S3, S4-5

0 = absent
1 = impaired
2 = normal
NT= not testable

☐ Any anal sensation (Yes/No)

TOTALS ☐+☐ = ☐ PIN PRICK SCORE (max: 112)
☐+☐ = ☐ LIGHT TOUCH SCORE (max: 112)
(MAXIMUM) (56) (56) (56) (56)

• Key Sensory Points

NEUROLOGICAL LEVEL — The most caudal segment with normal function — SENSORY R L, MOTOR R L

COMPLETE OR INCOMPLETE? — Incomplete = presence of any sensory or motor function in lowest sacral segment

ZONE OF PARTIAL PRESERVATION — Partially innervated segments — SENSORY R L, MOTOR R L

This form may be copied freely but should not be altered without permission from the American Spinal Injury Association

Version 4p
GHC 1992

Fig. 1 American Spinal Injury Association (ASIA) Spinal Cord Injury Assessment Form. (Reproduced with permission from the American Spinal Injury Association: *Standards for Neurological and Functional Classification of Spinal Cord Injury,* revised. Chicago, IL, American Spinal Injury Association, 1992.)

roentgenograms of the suspected area, as determined from the patient's physical and neurologic examination. Once the level of injury is established, centered cone-down biplane views should be obtained. These are most commonly taken in the supine position, with the patient still immobilized on the spine board. If a spinal injury is identified, complete spine radiographs of the cervical, thoracic, and lumbar spine should be obtained.

A CT scan is indicated in the majority of patients with plain radiologic evidence of injury. In a blinded study, orthopaedic surgeons and radiologists were only 50% accurate in distinguishing burst from compression fractures.[29] CT slice thicknesses at 3 mm intervals provide high sensitivity and allow quality sagittal reconstructions. Axial sections allow visualization of the percent of canal compromise, the degree of comminution of the vertebral body, and posterior element involvement. For certain fractures, such as low lumbar burst fractures, midsagittal splits of the spinous processes accompanied by high-grade neurologic deficit, and high-grade canal compromise indirectly suggest the presence of a dural tear.

MRIs are rarely required for the management of thoracolumbar injury. Their most common application is for the patient in whom a fracture is not visualized but who has neurologic deficit (especially a child) or the patient who has a fracture in which the level of bony injury does not correlate with the level of the neurologic injury. MRI can be used to evaluate the posterior ligamentous complex. Increased signal intensity on fat-suppressed images in these soft tissues indicates ligamentous disruption.[30]

Classification of Thoracolumbar Fractures

The classification of thoracolumbar injuries is used to decide (1) which injuries are stable, (2) which injuries benefit from spinal cord decompression, and (3) which injuries require surgical stabilization. The type of spinal stabilization should directly correlate with the mechanism of injury. Different classification systems have been developed based on the concept of stability, morphologic features, and fracture mechanisms. Nicoll[31] first described stable versus unstable fractures. He defined stable fractures as those that did not progress and allowed patients to return to work. A currently accepted definition of spinal instability is that the unstable spine has the potential for neurologic injury, increasing spinal deformity, and long-term pain and disability when the spinal column is subjected to physiologic loads. It is often difficult to assess the severity of injury at the time of injury and, unfortunately, sometimes instability is discovered only by following the patient over time.

Holdsworth[32] and Whitesides and Shah[33] popularized the idea that the spine acts as two columns. The anterior vertebral bodies and disks resist compressive loads, and the posterior osseoligamentous structures resist tensile load. Instability exists when both columns are injured. A significant advance in patient management and determination of spinal stability of traumatic fractures was the development of the "three column theory" of Denis.[34] The anterior column comprised three structures—the anterior longitudinal ligament, the anterior portion of the vertebral body, and the anterior portion of the annulus fibrosis (Fig. 2). The middle osteoligamentous column comprises the posterior longitudinal ligament, the posterior aspect of the vertebral body, and the posterior aspect of the annulus fibrosis. The third longitudinal column of spinal stability comprises the posterior elements such as the posterior facet joints and facet joint capsules, the ligamentum flavum, the interspinous ligaments, and the posterior aspect of the neural arch. McAfee and associates[35] described six main categories of injury based on the mechanism of injury of the middle osteoligamentous column (Table 2).

Types of Injury

Wedge Compression Fracture The wedge compression fracture is caused by hyperflexion or compressive failure of the anterior column (Fig. 3). There is no posterior ligamentous injury and no failure of the middle osteoligamentous column. The wedge compression fracture is therefore a stable injury and rarely requires internal fixation except when the degree of compression exceeds 50%.

Table 2
McAfee classification of thoracolumbar fractures

1 Wedge compression fracture	Compression failure of only the anterior column.
2 Stable burst fracture	Compression failure of the anterior and middle columns. The posterior column is intact.
3 Unstable burst fracture	Compression failure of the anterior and middle columns. The posterior column is disrupted in either compression or distraction.
4 Flexion-distraction injury	The anterior column fails in compression and the posterior column in distraction. Frequently the fulcrum is at the middle column.
5 Chance-type fracture	Tension failure of all three columns. The injury may occur through bone, ligaments or combinations.
6 Translational shear injury	The alignment of the neural canal is disrupted. At the affected level one part of the spinal canal is displaced in the transverse plane. All three columns are injured usually from shear, hyperflexion or rotational forces.

(Reproduced with permission from McAfee PC, Yuan HA, Fredrickson BE, et al: The value of computed tomography in thoracolumbar fracture: An analysis of one-hundred consecutive cases and a new classification. *J Bone Joint Surg* 1983;65A:461-473.)

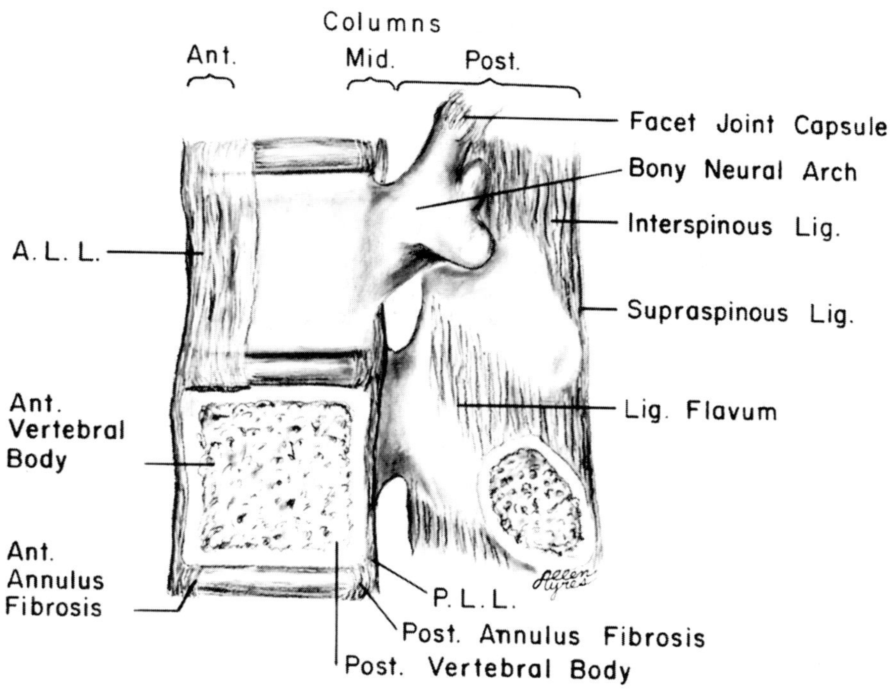

Fig. 2 The Denis three-column spine. The anterior column is composed of the anterior two-thirds of the vertebral body, disk and annulus, and anterior longitudinal ligament. (A.L.L. = anterior longitudinal ligament). The middle column consists of the posterior third of the vertebral body, disk and annulus, and posterior longitudinal ligament (P.L.L. = posterior longitudinal ligament). The posterior column includes all posterior osseous and ligamentous structures including the pedicles.

Stable Burst Fracture A stable burst fracture is defined as failure of the anterior and middle longitudinal columns, secondary to an axial load (Fig. 4). Because by definition there is no disruption of the posterior elements, these injuries are stable and do not normally require interior fixation. CT will demonstrate intact facet articulations. Bony retropulsion is usually less than 50% and kyphosis less than 15°. These fractures can usually be managed successfully nonoperatively.

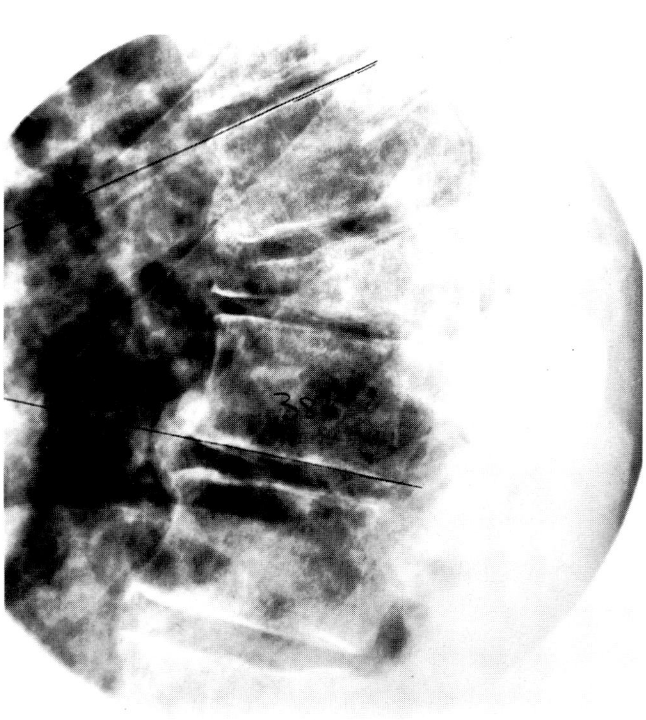

Fig. 3 Wedge compression fracture. Failure of only the anterior column secondary to hyperflexion or axial loading. The middle and posterior columns are intact.

Unstable Burst Fracture The unstable burst fracture is an injury from compressive axial failure of the anterior and middle columns which also involves complete disruption of the posterior column (Fig. 5). The posterior column can fail either under distraction or compression. These injuries are extremely unstable and are best managed with internal fixation to prevent further compression of the spine. As the vertebral bodies compress, owing to axial load, the bone fragments from the vertebral bodies are retropulsed against the neural structures. The posterior structures are damaged by rupturing of the interspinous ligaments, fracturing of pedicles at their bases, disruption of the facet joints, or displacement of laminar fractures.

Denis[34] described five subtypes of unstable burst fractures: (A) Predominant superior and inferior endplate fracture; (B) Superior endplate fracture and retropulsion of the posterosuperior aspect of the vertebral body into the spinal canal (most common subtype); (C) Lower endplate comminution and retropulsion; (D) Lateral collapse; and (E) Rotation.

Gaines and associates[36] developed a quantitative method based on a point system to predict the degree

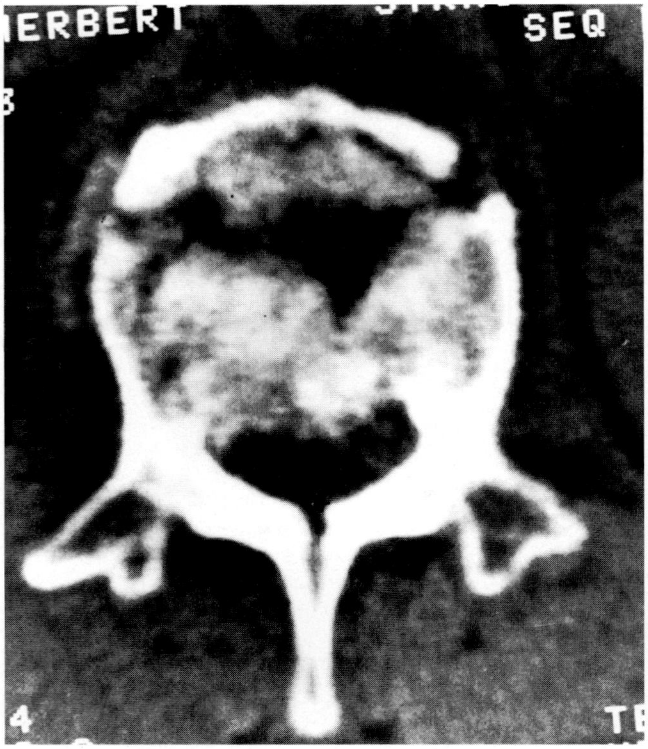

Fig. 4 Stable burst fracture. Compression failure of the anterior and middle columns secondary to hyperflexion or axial loading. The posterior column is intact. Patients are neurologically intact and generally have less than 50% canal compromise, no greater than 15° of kyphosis and no greater than 40% vertebral body wedging.

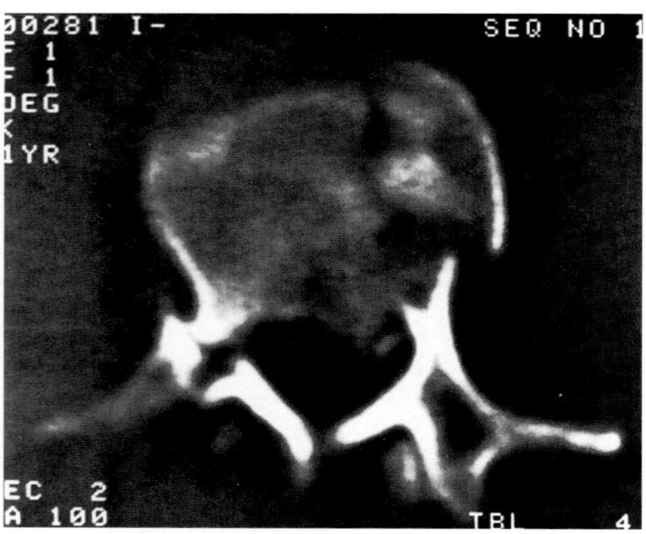

Fig. 5 Unstable burst fracture. Compression failure of the anterior and middle columns secondary to hyperflexion or axial loading. Additionally, the posterior column is disrupted in either compression or distraction.

of subsequent vertebral body collapse. This approach to classifying burst fractures was intended to determine

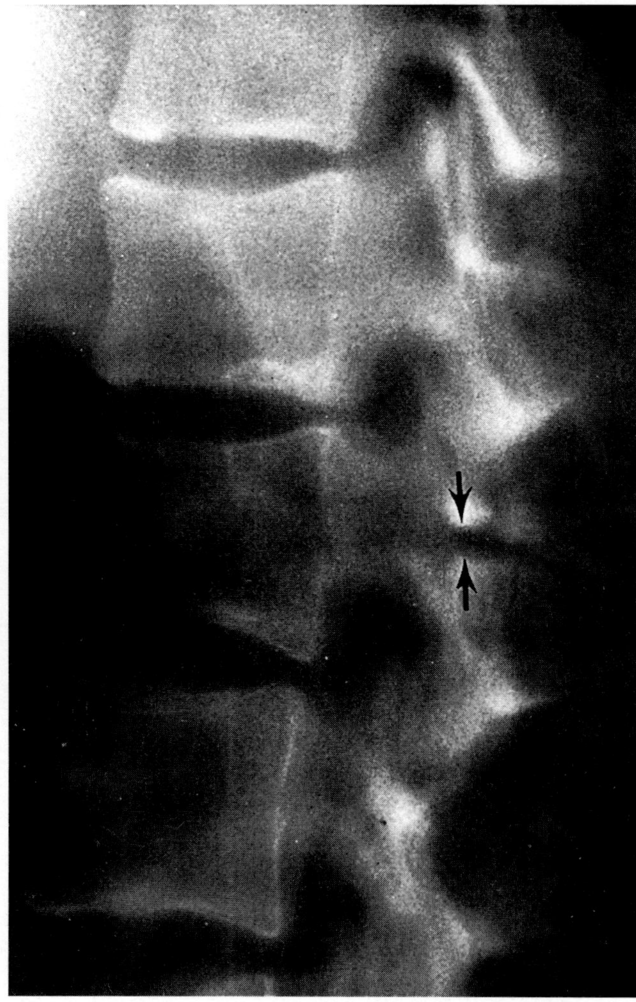

Fig. 6 Chance-type fracture. Transverse avulsion injury through all three columns secondary to hyperflexion with the center of rotation anterior to the anterior longitudinal ligament. All three columns are distracted. The injury may be bony, ligamentous, or a combination.

which cases require posterior instrumentation alone versus anterior load-sharing using anterior corpectomy strut grafts.

Chance-Type Fracture A Chance fracture occurs due to distraction forces of the posterior and middle columns (Fig. 6). This is a characteristic injury in the lumbar and the lower thoracic areas, usually secondary to a seatbelt injury. Rapid deceleration over a seatbelt in a motor vehicle crash causes a distraction force to be transmitted to the posterior aspect of the thoracic spinal column. Initially the posterior structures fail in tension, followed by progressive failure of the middle and anterior columns. In the classic Chance fracture a transverse bony avulsion fracture is present through all three columns. Other patterns include pure diskoligamentous injuries and combinations of bone and ligament injuries.

Flexion-Distraction Injury A flexion-distraction injury is unstable, involving ligamentous disruption of the posterior elements and compression failure of the anterior column (Fig. 7). A flexion-distraction injury is created during hyperflexion when the posterior elements fail under tension and the anterior column under compression. Frequently, the fulcrum is at the middle column. Clinically, patients with flexion-distraction injuries have dorsal swelling and tenderness and a palpable gap between spinous processes. Lateral radiographs may only demonstrate an innocent compression fracture. The anteroposterior views will have a wide separation between spinous process indicative of the flexion-distraction of Chance-type fractures.

Translation Injury A translation injury is defined as any injury of the thoracolumbar spine that results from a shearing failure of the middle osteoligamentous column (Fig. 8). Holdsworth,[32] who originally described this injury, termed it a "slice" fracture. This is the most unstable of all spinal injuries, and it is associated with the highest incidence of paraplegia and complete neurologic deficit. There is often a complete loss of continuity of the patient's spinal canal, and ligamentous discontinuity from one vertebral level to the next.

Gertzbein[37] has modified the AO/ASIF system of classification (Table 3). Magerl and associates[38] originally described a mechanistic classification system including over 20 subtypes of fractures. This made the classification very good for descriptive terms, but it provided more subtypes than there were alternatives for treatment. Gertzbein's modified classification is being tested in large multicenter studies sponsored by the Scoliosis Research Society, the International Society for Study of the Lumbar Spine, the Cervical Spine Research Society, the North American Spine Society, and the Orthopaedic Trauma Association. The modified classification has three main categories: Type A, compression injuries involving the vertebral body primarily; Type B, distraction injuries affecting both the

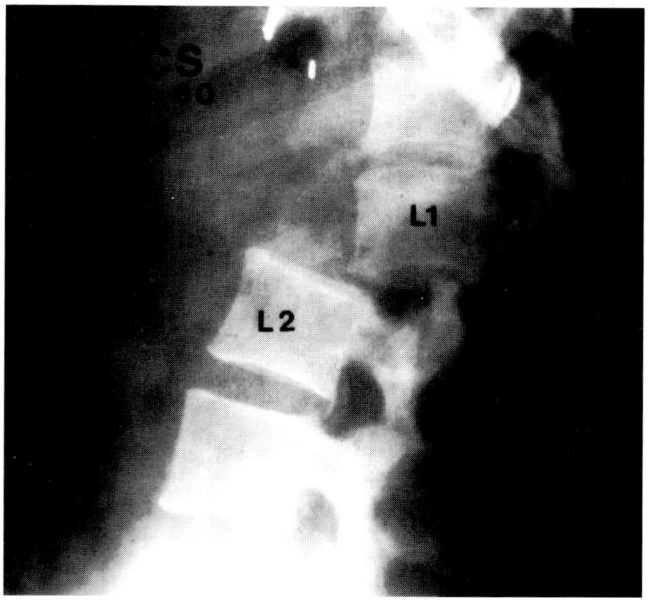

Fig. 8 Translational shear injury. Loss of continuity between two adjacent vertebral levels. Usually secondary to facet fracture dislocations as a result of hyperflexion, shear, or rotational forces.

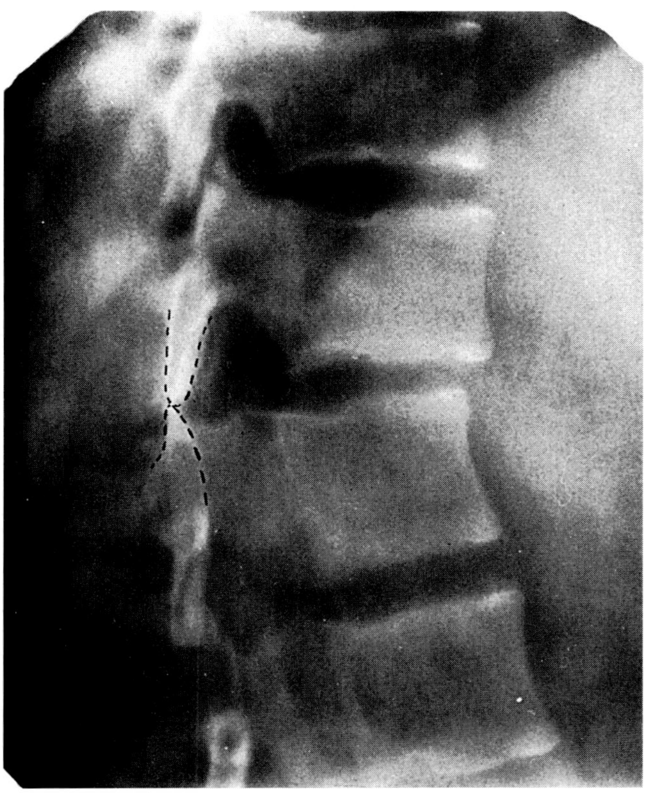

Fig. 7 Flexion-distraction injury. Similar mechanism to the Chance-type fracture. In this injury the anterior column is compressed and the middle and posterior columns are distracted. Radiographically, an innocent anterior compression fracture is seen. Dorsally, a separation of the posterior column is present.

Table 3
Comprehensive classification of thoracic and lumbar fractures

Type	Group
A Compression	1 Impaction (wedge)
	2 Split (coronal)
	3 Burst (complete burst)
B Distraction	1 Through the soft tissues posteriorly (subluxation)
	2 Through the arch posteriorly (Chance fracture)
	3 Through the disk anteriorly (extension spondylosis)
C Multidirectional with translation	1 Anteroposterior (dislocation)
	2 Lateral (lateral shear)
	3 Rotational (rotational burst)

(Reproduced with permission from Gertzbein SD (ed): Classification of thoracic and lumbar fractures, in *Fractures of the Thoracic and Lumbar Spine*. Baltimore, MD, Williams & Wilkins, 1992, pp 25-57.)

anterior and posterior elements; and Type C, multidirectional injuries with translation also affecting the anterior and posterior elements of the spinal column (Fig. 9). The classification is arranged by increasing severity of bony and soft-tissue disruption. It includes an increased association of comminution and displacement as well as an increasing number of planes of deforming forces. The fractures are more unstable as one progresses through the classification and the neurologic deficit also increases as one progresses from Type A to Type C.

Because of progressive instability, the further down it is in the classification, the more likely a fracture is to be treated surgically. The principles of management of the fractures can be established by understanding the forces that caused the injury and the planes of disruption. For example, in Type A injuries caused by axial load with compression, reversal of the forces (distraction) will lead to restoration of alignment. In Type B injuries, where distraction is the primary mechanism, corrective forces of compression will be required. And finally, for Type C injuries with multiplanar instability, the most unstable category, additional stabilizing techniques will be necessary, such as fixation of the vertebrae two or more levels above and below the injury (instead of only at one level above and below), or a combined approach of anterior and posterior stabilization may be warranted.

The merits of this newer classification are that it arranges spinal injuries into an order of progressive severity consistent with instability and neurologic injury. It determines planes of disruption and mechanisms of injury, which in turn can be used as a guideline for management.

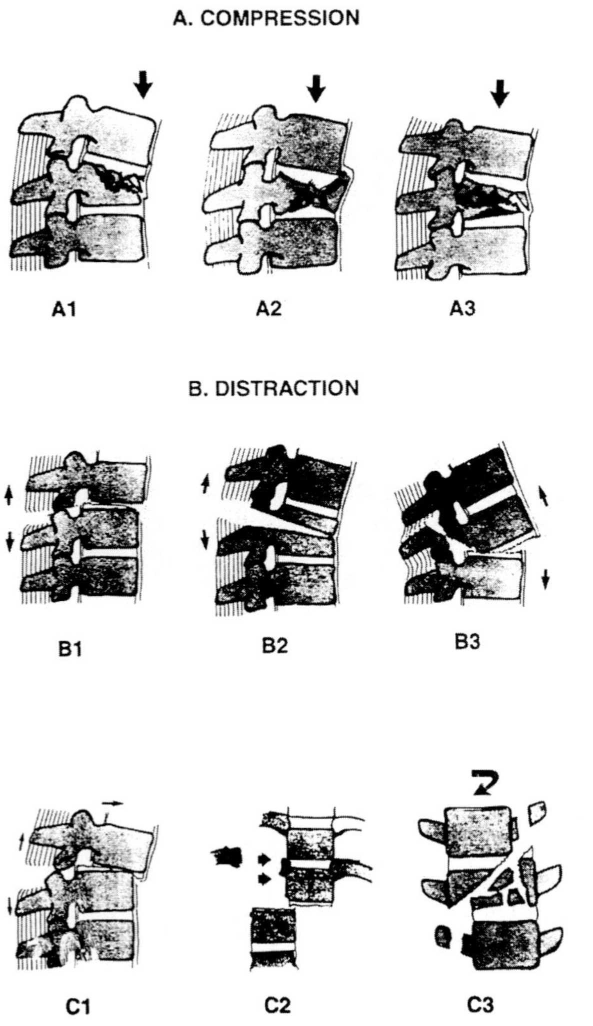

Fig. 9 AO classification of thoracolumbar injuries. (Reproduced with permission from Gertzbein SD (ed): Classification of thoracic and lumbar fractures, in *Fractures of the Thoracic and Lumbar Spine.* Baltimore, MD, Williams & Wilkins, 1992, pp 25-57.)

Acute Management of Patients with Spinal Cord Injuries

In patients with neurologic injuries, specific treatments within the first few hours of injury may result in significant recovery and enhancement of long-term function. It is, therefore, important that prompt evaluation and radiologic studies be performed to allow early treatment. An understanding of the pathophysiology of spinal cord injuries is required so that the treating physician can address the abnormal processes that occur following injury and can create an environment for maximal neurologic recovery.

Pathophysiology of Spinal Cord Injury

Spinal cord trauma can be categorized into primary and secondary injuries. The primary injury is the initial trauma, which is usually applied to the ventral aspect of the cord secondary to compressive and distractive forces. In animal investigation, the clinical and histologic effect of spinal cord injury is directly related to the energy absorbed at the time of injury.[39,40] Assenmacher and Ducker[39] created reversible injuries in Rhesus monkeys with a 300 gm/cm force. Animals subjected to a 500 gm/cm force sustained irreversible neurologic deficits. In humans, we are unable to determine the magnitude of forces causing a spinal cord injury, although radiographs may imply force direction and quantity. However, in in vitro experiments, Chang and associates[41] demonstrated that residual radiographic findings did not correlate with the canal compromise or vertebral deformation that occurred at the time of injury.

In spinal cord trauma, the spinal cord is rarely severed. Instead, a gradual, progressive process of neuronal necrosis and axonal separation occurs over the first few days following injury.[40,42-45] Immediately, there is a disruption of information transmitted through the axons. This disruption may be caused by an immediate depolarization of axonal membranes secondary to failure of repolarization as a result of potassium leakage.[46] Also, decreased spinal cord blood flow may create ischemic conditions resulting in impaired conduction.[47-49]

Immediate pathologic examination following trauma reveals greater injury in the gray matter than the white myelinated tissue.[40] Within 3 to 5 minutes, petechial hemorrhages are present in the gray matter. By 30 minutes, neural hemorrhages are seen centrally, and glial and neuronal necrosis is present. At this time, the nerve fibers are swollen, but structurally intact axons are noted in the white matter. By 4 hours, marked gray matter necrosis is present. In the white matter, increases in necrotic oligodendroglia are noted, but the main histologic feature is axonal swelling.[42] By 8 hours, maximal axonal swelling is present and axonal necrosis has begun. Ultrastructurally, vesicular degeneration of myelin is noted.[42] These findings correlate with the known differences between gray and white matter blood flow that occur following trauma.

Experimental evidence that the spinal cord undergoes progressive changes following injury and that the changes are less in myelinated axonal tracts than in gray matter has important therapeutic considerations. These progressive changes have been termed the secondary injury.[44,45] At one time, the secondary injury was thought to have been caused by ischemia, but other biochemical events have since been implicated.

Following injury, adenosine triphosphate (ATP) storages are depleted, causing failure of calcium-dependent enzymes and membrane transport systems.[44,45,50,51] Under these conditions, uncontrolled intracellular influx of calcium is observed. The mitochondrial calcium pump is overloaded, which uncouples oxidative phosphorylization and further decreases production of ATP. Calcium-dependent phospholipase A2 is activated, which breaks down membranes and releases arachidonic acid. Arachidonic acid is metabolized into a variety of substances, which can decrease local spinal cord blood flow, cause release of lysosomal enzymes, mediate platelet aggregation, and generate peroxide free radicals. The peroxide free radicals are released into the cytosol where they can break down cellular membranes, creating more free radicals. Disruption of cellular membranes by peroxidation and hydrolytic enzymes is thought to be an important component of the secondary injury following spinal cord trauma. Recently, researchers have focused on pharmacologic techniques to limit lipid peroxidation, thereby decreasing the secondary injury.[52-55]

Experimental Treatment of Spinal Cord Injuries

Methylprednisolone succinate is a corticosteroid that has a significantly greater effect than dexamethasone on decreasing lipid peroxidation.[53-55] Animal studies confirm that methylprednisolone given in high doses decreases lipid peroxidations, preserves the integrity of neuronal structures, and improves outcome following experimental spinal cord injuries. Large doses (30 mg/kg) of the drug are required and must be administered within 8 hours of injury. The efficacy of methylprednisolone in humans has been confirmed by the National Spinal Cord Injury Study 2 (NSCIS 2).[54] This double-blind, randomized study of 476 patients compared placebo, naloxone, and methylprednisolone in patients with spinal cord injuries.

Statistically significant improvement of motor and sensory scores occurred in the groups given methylprednisolone compared to placebo and naloxone. However, the degree of overall motor improvement was small. Actual functional recovery was not measured in this study. Patients with incomplete as well as complete cord injuries benefited if the drug was given within 8 hours of injury. Complications such as wound infection and gastrointestinal bleeding were greater in the methylprednisolone group, but not to a statistically significant level. Lesions of the conus medullaris and cauda equina were not evaluated.

Triliazoid is an aminosteroid that does not have glucocorticoid activity but is a potent inhibitor of lipid peroxidation.[52] This drug has been demonstrated to promote functional recovery in experimental spinal cord injury models.[52] It is currently being investigated in the NSCIS 3.

Gangliosides are large glycolipid molecules that are found on the outer surface of most cell membranes.[56] They are thought to be involved in immunologic processes and other cellular membrane properties such as binding and transport. Gangliosides are highly concentrated in neural tissues. In cell culture, they induce nerve cytogenesis and have a trophic effect on nerve cells. In experimental traumatic brain injuries, they have been shown to reduce cerebral edema and speed recovery. Geisler and associates[57] reported a statistically significant increase in functional recovery in patients with spinal cord injuries who were given GM-1 ganglioside compared to placebo. Unlike methylprednisolone, this drug can be administered effectively up to 3 days following injury. Although encouraging, gangliosides are considered experimental and are currently undergoing a multicenter investigation.

Mechanical Factors in Spinal Cord Injuries

Residual mechanical factors may play a role in the pathogenesis of spinal cord injury. Following trauma, spinal instability may lead to recurrent injury, exacerbating the neural damage. Ducker and associates,[58] who evaluated the therapeutic effect of a variety of pharmacologic agents, found that immobilization of the injured primate had the greatest effect on neurologic recovery. Prevention of fracture-site motion in humans with unstable thoracolumbar injuries is difficult except by surgical means. Nursing techniques such as log rolling or turning on the roto-rest bed have been shown to cause significant fracture-site motion.[18]

Breig[59] studied the anatomic effect of residual kyphotic deformity and spinal cord compression. He found that abnormal tension of axonal tracts was created and that these tensile forces were eliminated by anatomic positioning. In kyphotic states, the intramedullary blood vessels were narrowed and displaced outward. Spinal cord compression displaced anterior tracts laterally and posteriorly, creating increased tension. He recommended immediate anatomic reduction to minimize these adverse tensile forces.

Böhler[60] hypothesized that many patients with spinal cord injuries have extrinsic cord compression that prevents return of neural function. He correctly noted that fracture reduction rather than laminectomy would relieve this compression. Numerous other attempts have been made to understand the significance of residual neural compression.[61-63] Rivlin and Tator[64] compressed the spinal cords of rats from 0 to 5 minutes and demonstrated a linear correlation between the log of compression time and the animal's clinical outcome. Bohlman and associates[65] developed a chronic anterior compression dog model. They found that functional recovery occurred after anterior decompression performed as late as 2 months after injury. Numerous clinical studies document the efficacy of anterior decompression in spinal cord injured patients.[66]

Surgical Treatment of Spinal Cord Injuries

The goals of treatment are to reduce fractures, stabilize the spinal column, and decompress the neural element. Unlike the cervical spine, where these goals can be accomplished by traction, reduction of thoracolumbar injuries usually requires surgical intervention. The efficacy of surgical management of thoracolumbar spinal cord injuries has remained elusive. The majority of investigations that have compared surgical and nonsurgical treatment have failed to demonstrate any impact on neurologic recovery that resulted from surgery. The results of these studies are difficult to interpret because they lack patient randomization, use outmoded surgical techniques, and do not achieve full decompression or stabilization of the spine.

However, recent studies by Edwards and Levine,[67] Krengel and associates,[68] and Kaneda and associates[69] indicate that complete spinal canal decompression and stabilization may lead to better neurologic recovery than nonsurgical treatment. The major adverse effect of surgical treatment is the potential for neurologic deterioration. This has rarely been reported in series of patients with thoracolumbar fractures treated surgically. However, McAfee and Bohlman[70] document five patients whose condition deteriorated following Harrington rod instrumentation. This deterioration resulted from overdistraction or from displacement of posterior elements into the spinal canal.

Marshall and associates[13] prospectively studied 283 patients with acute spinal cord injuries, 14 of whom deteriorated neurologically following hospital admission. Five of the 129 patients with thoracolumbar fractures deteriorated. One patient worsened while immobilized on a regular hospital bed, one while prone on a Stryker bed, one during roto-bed rotation, and one, who already had neurologic deterioration, following laminectomy. No patients had neurologic complications related to spinal instrumentation of thoracolumbar fractures, whereas four patients deteriorated following cervical surgery. Because the four patients had surgery before 5 days following injury, these researchers recommended a 4- to 5-day delay before surgical treatment. However, analysis of these results clearly demonstrated that deterioration during nonsurgical treatment occurred more frequently than that related to surgery, especially in patients with thoracolumbar injuries. These findings confirm the investigation of Ducker and associates,[58] who found that immobilization was essential for optimal neurologic recovery.

The timing of surgical intervention remains controversial. Animal studies by Rivlin and Tator,[64] Bohlman and associates,[65] and Delamarter and associates[61] confirm that neurologic recovery is inversely related to time from injury to decompression. Delamarter and associates[61,62] recently studied the effect of time of "decompression" in canine spinal cords on neurologic outcome. Constricting bands were placed around the spinal cord and were then removed either immediately, at 1 hour, at 6 hours, or at 24 hours. Six weeks later the animals "decompressed" at time zero and at one hour were clinically normal, whereas animals decompressed at 6 or 24 hours remained completely paraplegic. This study identified a specific time period during which spinal cord injuries are reversible, and it correlates with histopathologic studies that show minimal changes in cord axonal structure during the first few hours following spinal cord injuries. We and others hypothesize that treatment to protect neuronal structures, improve the microcirculation, and relieve adverse mechanical factors can significantly diminish irreversible neuronal tissue loss.

Krengel and associates[68] studied the efficacy of early treatment within 24 hours of injury on neurologic recovery in 13 patients with incomplete thoracic (T3-11) spinal cord injuries. Initially all patients were Frankel B or C paraplegics. At follow-up, 11 of 13 were Frankel D or E and had become ambulatory. The average improvement in Frankel grade was 2.2 per patient. These results compared favorably to an average improvement of 0.9 Frankel grades per patient when treated by postural reduction.[28] Also, this rate of recovery was greater than that reported for delayed posterior instrumentation or anterior decompression. Kahmann and associates[71] reported the results of acute anterior decompression in 35 patients with incomplete spinal cord injury from burst fractures. The average time from injury to surgery was 12.3 days. All patients improved at least one Frankel grade and 41% improved two Frankel grades. Edwards and Levine[67] assessed neurologic recovery in patients treated by the rod-sleeve method. They found that patients surgically treated within 9 hours of injury had 72% improvement of their initial deficit, compared to 57% if surgery was performed after 10 to 21 hours. These results correlated with an increased ability to achieve indirect spinal canal decompression if the patients were operated on in the first 2 days following injury. Although these reports suggest that improved neurologic outcome can be achieved by early surgery, no well-controlled human study is available to answer this question of timing.

Current Recommendations for Thoracolumbar Spinal Cord Injuries

Patients with thoracolumbar spinal cord injuries are initially immobilized on backboards to stabilize the fracture and to facilitate transport to and within the hospital. Once the initial diagnostic studies and resuscitation have been completed, the patient should be placed in a supine position on a firm mattress and log rolled every 2 hours. Decubitus ulceration can occur within 2 hours, especially in patients with insensate skin who are left on backboards for prolonged periods of time. Supplemental oxygen should be administered at 4 l/minute, unless contraindicated.

Injured spinal cords lose their ability to autoregulate and maintain spinal cord blood flow despite changes in systemic blood pressure. Therefore, the systolic blood pressure should be maintained to at least 90 mm Hg. Neurogenic shock following spinal cord injury is associated with low blood pressure and bradycardia. Treatment of hypotension due to spinal shock consists of vasopressors, atropine and, on rare occasions, the use of a pacemaker.

Methylprednisolone is administered as a 30 mg/kg loading and 5.4 mg/kg/hr maintenance dose for 23 hours to patients with spinal cord injuries who are seen within 8 hours of injury. No scientific data is available on the use of methylprednisolone in patients with conus medullaris or cauda equina injuries or in spinal cord injuries associated with penetrating trauma. We currently favor the use of methylprednisolone for these injuries. Patients with incomplete neural deficits and neural compression, translation, or kyphotic deformity should have emergent surgical treatment. Those patients with progressive neurologic deterioration are also candidates for emergent surgery following appropriate diagnostic testing. The aims of surgery are to reduce the fracture, stabilize the spine, and decompress the spinal canal either indirectly or directly. The approach and techniques are based on fracture pattern, injury level, age of patient, and associated injuries. Patients with complete thoracic cord injuries do not appear to benefit neurologically from immediate surgery and, therefore, stabilization can be delayed for 1 to 2 days, if warranted.

References

1. Ergas Z: Spinal cord injury in the United States: A statistical update. *Cent Nerv Sys Trauma* 1985;2:19-32.
2. Fine PR, Kuhlemeier KV, DeVivo MJ, et al: Spinal cord injury: An epidemiologic perspective. *Paraplegia* 1979;17:237-250.
3. Stover SL, Fine PR (eds): *Spinal Cord Injury: The Facts and Figures.* Birmingham, AL, University of Alabama at Birmingham, 1986, pp 13-29.
4. Riggins RS, Kraus JF: The risk of neurologic damage with fractures of the vertebrae. *J Trauma* 1977;17:126-133.
5. Bosch A, Stauffer ES, Nichel VL: Incomplete traumatic quadriplegia: A ten-year review. *JAMA* 1971;216:473-478.
6. Geisler WO, Jousse AT, Wynne-Jones M, et al: Survival in traumatic spinal cord injury. *Paraplegia* 1983;21:364-373.
7. Freehafer AA, Hazel CM, Becker CL: Lower extremity fractures in patients with spinal cord injury. *Paraplegia* 1981;19:367-372.
8. Igram RR, Suman RK, Freeman A: Lower limb fractures in the chronic spinal cord injured patient. *Paraplegia* 1989;27:133-139.
9. Katz RT: Management of spasticity. *Am J Phys Med Rehab* 1988; 67:108-116.
10. Sobel JW, Bohlman HH, Freehafer AA: Charcot's arthropathy of the spine following spinal cord injury: A report of five cases. *J Bone Joint Surg* 1985;67A:771-776.
11. Williams B: Post-traumatic syringomyelia: An update. *Paraplegia* 1990;28:296-313.
12. Kettl P: Prevalence of suicidal ideation after spinal cord injury. *J Am Para Soc* 1991;14:62.
13. Marshall LF, Knowlton S, Garfin SR, et al: Deterioration following spinal cord injury: A multicenter study. *J Neurosurg* 1987;66:400-404.
14. Apple DF: Regional spinal cord injury centers, in Hochschuler SH, Cotler HB, Guyer RD (eds): *Rehabilitation of the Spine: Science and Practice.* St. Louis, MO, CV Mosby, 1993, pp 294-299.
15. Lewis B, Alpert B, Tucker W, et al: Early versus delayed fixation of thoracolumbar spine in polytrauma patients. Proceedings of the Orthopaedic Trauma Association 6th Annual Meeting, Toronto, Canada, 1990, p 39.
16. Schlegel J, Yuan H, Frederickson B, et al: Timing of operative intervention in the management of acute spinal injuries. Proceedings of the Orthopaedic Trauma Association 6th Annual Meeting, Toronto, Canada, 1990, p 38.
17. Wilberger JE: Diagnosis and management of spinal cord trauma. *J Neurotrauma* 1991;8(suppl 1):S21-S30.
18. McGuire RA, Neville S, Green BA, et al: Spinal instability and the log-rolling maneuver. *J Trauma* 1987;27:525-531.
19. Slabaugh PB, Nickel VL: Complications with use of the Stryker frame. *J Bone Joint Surg* 1978;60A:1111-1112.
20. American College of Surgeons: *Advanced Trauma Life Support Manual.* Chicago, IL, American College of Surgeons, 1992.
21. Dehner JR: Seatbelt injuries of the spine and abdomen. *Am J Roentgenol Rad Therapy Nucl Med* 1971;111:833-843.
22. Garrett JW, Braunstein PW: The seat belt syndrome. *J Trauma* 1962;2:220-238.
23. Haddad GH, Zickel RE: Intestinal perforation and fracture of lumbar vertebra caused by lap-type seat belt. *NY J Med* 1967; 67:930-932.
24. Keenen TL, Antony J, Benson DR: Non-contiguous spinal fractures. *J Trauma* 1990;30:489-491.

25. American Spinal Injury Association (ed): *Standards for Neurological and Functional Classification of Spinal Cord Injury*, revised. Chicago, IL, American Spinal Injury Association, 1992.
26. Schrader SC, Sloan TB, Toleikis JR: Detection of sacral sparing in acute spinal cord injury. *Spine* 1987;12:533-535.
27. Lucas JT, Ducker TB: Motor classification of spinal cord injuries with mobility, morbidity and recovery indices. *Am Surg* 1989;45: 151-158.
28. Frankel HL, Hancock DO, Hyslop G, et al: The value of postural reduction in the initial management of closed injuries of the spine with paraplegia and tetraplegia. *Paraplegia* 1969;7:179-192.
29. Ballock RT, Mackersie R, Abitbol JJ, et al: Can burst fractures be predicted from plain radiographs? *J Bone Joint Surg* 1992;74B:147-150.
30. Brightman RP, Miller CA, Rea GL, et al: Magnetic resonance imaging of the trauma to the thoracic and lumbar spine: The importance of the posterior longitudinal ligament. *Spine* 1992; 17:541-550.
31. Nicoll EA: Fractures of the dorso-lumbar spine. *J Bone Joint Surg* 1949;31B:376-394.
32. Holdsworth F: Fractures, dislocations, and fracture-dislocations of the spine. *J Bone Joint Surg* 1970;52A:1534-1551.
33. Whitesides TE Jr, Shah SGA: On the management of unstable fractures of the thoracolumbar spine: Rationale for use of anterior decompression and fusion and posterior stabilization. *Spine* 1976;1:99-107.
34. Denis F: Spinal instability as defined by the three-column spine concept in acute spinal trauma. *Clin Orthop* 1984;189:65-76.
35. McAfee PC, Yuan HA, Fredrickson BE, et al: The value of computed tomography in thoracolumbar fracture: An analysis of one-hundred consecutive cases and a new classification. *J Bone Joint Surg* 1983;65A:461-473.
36. Gaines RW Jr, McCormack T, Maurizi M: A classification to predict screw breakage when using short segment instrumentation with pedicle screws: The load-sharing classification of spinal fractures. *Orthop Trans* 1993;17:131.
37. Gertzbein SD (ed): Classification of thoracic and lumbar fractures, in *Fractures of the Thoracic and Lumbar Spine*. Baltimore, MD, Williams & Wilkins, 1992, pp 25-57.
38. Magerl F, Harms J, Gertzbein SD, et al: A new classification of spinal fractures. Presented at the Societe Internationale Orthipedie et Traumatologie Meeting, Montreal, Canada, September 9, 1990.
39. Assenmacher DR, Ducker TB: Experimental traumatic paraplegia: The vascular and pathological changes seen in reversible and irreversible spinal-cord lesions. *J Bone Joint Surg* 1971;53A:671-680.
40. Ducker TB, Kindt GW, Kempf LG: Pathological findings in acute experimental spinal cord trauma. *J Neurosurg* 1971;35:700-708.
41. Chang DG, Tencer AF, Ching RP, et al: Geometric changes in the cervical spinal canal during impact. *Spine* 1994;19:973-980.
42. Balentine JD: Pathology of experimental cord trauma: II. Ultrastructure of axons and myelin. *Lab Invest* 1978;39;254-266.
43. Dohrmann GJ, Wagner FC Jr, Bucy PC: Transitory traumatic paraplegia: Electron microscopy of early alterations in myelinated nerve fibers. *J Neurosurg* 1972;36:407-415.
44. Yashon D: Pathogenesis of spinal cord injury. *Orthop Clin North Am* 1978;9:247-261.
45. Young W: Secondary injury mechanisms in acute spinal cord injury. *J Emerg Med* 1993;11(suppl 1):13-22.
46. Anderson TE: Spinal cord contusion injury: Experimental dissociation of hemorrhagic necrosis and subacute loss of axonal conduction. *J Neurosurg* 1985;62:115-119.
47. Balentine JD: Pathology of experimental spinal cord trauma: I. The necrotic lesion as a function of vascular injury. *Lab Invest* 1978;39:236-253.
48. Fried LC, Goodkin R: Microangiographic observations of the experimentally traumatized spinal cord. *J Neurosurg* 1971;35:709-714.
49. Sandler AN, Tator CH: Review of the effect of spinal cord trauma on the vessels and blood flow in the spinal cord. *J Neurosurg* 1976;45:638-646.
50. Ikata T, Iwasa K, Morimoto K, et al: Clinical considerations and biochemical basis of prognosis of cervical spinal cord injury. *Spine* 1989;14:1096-1101.
51. Jansen L, Hansebout RR: Pathogenesis of spinal cord injury and newer treatments: A review. *Spine* 1989;14:23-32.
52. Anderson DK, Braughler JM, Hall ED, et al: Effects of treatment with U-74006F on neurological outcome following experimental spinal cord injury. *J Neurosurg* 1988;69:562-567.
53. Bracken MB, Collins WF, Freeman DF, et al: Efficacy of methylprednisolone in acute spinal cord injury. *JAMA* 1984;251:45-52.
54. Bracken MB, Shepard MJ, Collins WF, et al: A randomized, controlled trial of methylprednisolone or naloxone in the treatment of acute spinal-cord injury: Results of the Second National Acute Spinal Cord Injury Study. *N Engl J Med* 1990;322:1405-1411.
55. Hall ED: Effects of the 21-aminosteroid U74006F on posttraumatic spinal cord ischemia in cats. *J Neurosurg* 1988;68:462-465.
56. Rodden FA, Wiegandt H, Bauer BL: Gangliosides: The relevance of current research to neurosurgery. *J Neurosurg* 1991;74:606-619.
57. Geisler FH, Dorsey FC, Coleman WP: Recovery of motor function after spinal-cord injury: A randomized, placebo-controlled trial with GM-1 ganglioside. *N Engl J Med* 1991;324:1829-1838.
58. Ducker TB, Salcman M, Daniell HB: Experimental spinal cord trauma: III. Therapeutic effect of immobilization and pharmacologic agents. *Surg Neurol* 1978;10:71-76.
59. Breig A: The therapeutic possibilities of surgical bio-engineering in incomplete spinal cord lesions. *Paraplegia* 1972;9:173-182.
60. Böhler L (ed): *The Treatment of Fractures*, ed 4. Baltimore, MD, W. Wood & Co, 1935.
61. Delamarter RB, Sherman J, Carr JB: Spinal cord injury: The pathophysiology of spinal cord damage and subsequent recovery following immediate or delayed decompression. Proceedings of the 21st Annual Meeting of the Cervical Spine Research Society, New York, NY, Dec 1-4, 1993, pp 32-33.
62. Delamarter RB, Sherman JE, Carr JB: 1991 Volvo Award in experimental studies: Cauda equina syndrome: Neurologic recovery following immediate, early, or late decompression. *Spine* 1991;16:1022-1029.
63. Dolan EJ, Tator CH, Endrenyi L: The value of decompression for acute experimental spinal cord compression injury. *J Neurosurg* 1980;53:749-755.
64. Rivlin AS, Tator CH: Effect of duration of acute spinal cord compression in a new acute cord injury model in the rat. *Surg Neurol* 1978;10:38-43.
65. Bohlman HH, Bahniuk E, Raskulinecz G, et al: Mechanical factors affecting recovery from incomplete cervical spinal cord injury: A preliminary report. *Johns Hopkins J* 1979;145:115-125.
66. McAfee PC, Bohlman HH, Yuan HA: Anterior decompression of traumatic thoracolumbar fractures with incomplete neurological deficit using a retroperitoneal approach. *J Bone Joint Surg* 1985; 67A:89-104.
67. Edwards CC, Levine AM: Early rod-sleeve stabilization of the injured thoracic and lumbar spine. *Orthop Clin North Am* 1986; 17:121-145.
68. Krengel WF III, Anderson PA, Henley MB: Early stabilization and decompression for incomplete paraplegia due to a thoracic-level spinal cord injury. *Spine* 1993;18:2080-2087.
69. Kaneda K, Abumi K, Fujiya M: Burst fractures with neurologic deficits of the thoracolumbar-lumbar spine: Results of anterior decompression and stabilization with anterior instrumentation. *Spine* 1984;9:788-795.

70. McAfee PC, Bohlman HH: Complications following Harrington instrumentation for fractures of the thoracolumbar spine. *J Bone Joint Surg* 1985;67A:672- 686.
71. Kahmann RD, Bradford DS, Ogilvie JW, et al: Acute anterior decompression of thoracic and lumbar spine fractures with neurologic involvement. Presented at the 57th Annual Meeting of the American Academy of Orthopaedic Surgeons, New Orleans, LA, February 1990.

CHAPTER 3

Surgical Management of Thoracolumbar Fractures

Paul C. McAfee, MD
Alan M. Levine, MD
Paul A. Anderson, MD

The goals of surgical treatment for thoracolumbar injury are anatomic reduction of the fracture, rigid fixation, neural decompression when necessary, and, long-term, a functional painless spinal column. For each patient, the goals must be clearly defined and appropriate treatment methods employed. Thus, the trauma patient who has a marked sagittal or coronal deformity of the spine (traumatic kyphosis, axial compression, and/or translation) but no neurologic deficit requires only correction of alignment and rigid fixation, with no need for canal decompression. However, the patient who has kyphosis and displacement of bone fragments into the neural tissues and an incomplete neurologic deficit requires spinal realignment, canal decompression, and stabilization.

The most important biomechanical consideration for the use of implants in spinal trauma is that the strengths of the system must be matched to the instabilities of the injury.[1,2] Thus, for any injury with axial compression, the implant must be able to apply axial distraction to correct the deformity, to maintain alignment, and to resist axial compression in the erect position. Similarly, for the flexion component of an injury there must be a component of the instrumentation that can apply extension centered at the level of injury, and it must be able to resist subsequent loss of reduction in flexion. For injuries caused by axial distraction, the implant must be able to apply axial compressive forces and resist further axial distraction. In some cases, the applied construct may not be able to counteract a deforming force directly, but, if the force is part of a coupled motion, the correctly applied hardware may be able to resist a coupled motion by resisting the force partner. Finally, for injuries that have a significant shear injury and have bi-directional instability, the hardware system must be able to reduce the deformity progressively and then lock in the corrected position, resisting displacement in all three planes of motion.

Controversies persist regarding the indications for the anterior approach versus the posterior approach for management of thoracolumbar injuries. This controversy has centered on the ability to achieve neural decompression and limit the length of fixation.

Posterior Instrumentation

Indications

The indications for the posterior approach may be divided into absolute indications, relative indications, and contraindications. An absolute indication is for the patient with a complete neurologic deficit and an upper thoracic injury. These patients need rapid stabilization that will allow them to be mobilized and diminish the risk of pulmonary complications. In a patient with a complete neurologic deficit, posterior instrumentation is the most reasonable approach, because it can achieve axial realignment and rigid stabilization, and it allows rapid patient mobilization. In the multiply injured patient with chest trauma, the goals of the surgery are to stabilize and realign the spine but not necessarily to decompress the neural tissues. A second indication for posterior instrumentation is for a patient with a low lumbar burst fracture and dural lacerations. The traumatic dural lacerations are posterior, and they frequently have extravasation of the roots into the laminar fracture. An anterior approach would not allow repair nor is fixation to the fifth lumbar vertebra or sacrum ideal through an anterior approach.[3,4] The third group of patients who should have a posterior reduction and stabilization are those who have segment deformity without neural deficit at the thoracolumbar junction (either early or late). Correction of this deformity is more easily accomplished and maintained by the posterior approach.

The relative indications for posterior instrumentation are broad and include treatment of neurologically intact patients who have unstable fractures. If the surgical goal is the reduction of the deformity and rigid stabilization, it is best accomplished by posterior surgery and instrumentation, carried out within 4 to 6 weeks following the initial injury. Other patients with relative indications for posterior instrumentation are patients with neural deficit and canal compromise who were injured less than 48 hours earlier. Indirect decompression by ligamentotaxis and reduction of deformity is most effective in that time frame.[5-9] In these patients, the goal of the surgery is realignment, rigid fixation to protect the cord, and indirect neural decompression.

In approximately 85% of patients, posterior stabilization and reduction is sufficient to give adequate canal decompression in the neurologically compromised patient. If satisfactory decompression is not attained, a second-stage anterior decompression is indicated. Patients with low lumbar fractures are also more easily decompressed and stabilized from a posterior approach. Patients with unstable flexion distraction injuries and Chance-type fractures who have significant ligamentous injuries are best treated surgically with posterior instrumentation. Finally, patients with shear injuries require segmental posterior instrumentation.

Contraindications to posterior instrumentation are patients who were injured more than 10 days earlier and who have an incomplete neurologic deficit and canal compromise. These patients are best treated by direct canal decompression using an anterior approach.[8] Also, indirect decompression is not as satisfactory for patients in whom computed tomography (CT) demonstrates minimal axial compression or sagittal plane deformity but significant canal retropulsion, or in whom the posterior fragment of the wall is turned around so that the cancellous portion is facing posteriorly into the canal, which indicates that the posterior longitudinal ligament is disrupted. In such cases, anterior decompression can yield a better result than posterior instrumentation. In patients with retropulsion localized to one side, posterior decompression through a transpedicular route can be effective, but indirect decompression is generally not effective.[10,11]

Posterior Instrumentation Systems

Harrington rod instrumentation was the first effective system for treatment of thoracolumbar fractures.[9,12-16] The rods apply a progressive reduction force in a single plane, either axial distraction or axial compression. With additional distraction increased kyphosis is produced due to lengthening of the posterior column. Harrington rods provide no rotational correction nor are they able to correct or stabilize the flexion component of the deformity. To be effective, Harrington rods require intact longitudinal ligaments and instrumentation of two to three levels above and below the injury. In shear injuries these ligaments have usually failed and, in such cases, distraction instrumentation may result in iatrogenic overlengthening of the spinal column.[17]

Contouring of square-ended Harrington rods allows application of both a distraction force and extension moment to correct the traumatic kyphosis. The amount of lordosis in the rod is difficult to control and maintain. Also, the rods provide little or no rotational stability. The relatively loose fit between the proximal hook and the rod tends to create kyphosis at the upper end of the construct. Segmental fixation with sublaminar wires applied to Luque rods or Harrington instrumentation poorly controls axial height and, therefore, has little role in the management of spinal fractures.

The rod-sleeve method, based on either Harrington distraction rods or Universal rods, allows the application of a distractive force by the rod and a lordotic force by sleeves placed at the appropriate level.[8,18-20] Lordosing forces are applied directly to the pedicles at the apex of the kyphosis in compression and burst-type fractures when the pedicles and posterior elements are intact. The sleeves can be placed in a bridging fashion at the pedicle above and below the injury to create a three-point fixation for patients who require a laminectomy, who have comminution of the posterior elements, or who have fracturing of the pedicles (Denis Type A fractures).

The rod-sleeve method also allows application of the lordotic force without compromising the proximal hook site. If the angle of the lamina is such that application of a straight rod will create excessive kyphosis at the proximal segment, slight contouring can be achieved at that level without sacrificing the overall lordotic force applied by the rod. In addition, because the sleeves wedge between the facets and spinous processes, they impart a degree of rotational stability. Thus, they are used in compression fractures and burst-type fractures to provide axial distraction and lordosis. For bilateral facet dislocations, a special application of the construct is required. Once the facets have been reduced, an interspinous wire is placed across the facet dislocation as a tension band posteriorly to hold reduction. A lordotic force is imparted at the apex, and distraction is used to restore the disk height with the rod sleeve. In bony flexion-distraction injuries, a compression construct can be used with the same system, again using sleeves to impart lordosis. This rod-sleeve technique as a pure hook-rod-sleeve system does not provide adequate stabilization for shear injuries.

Segmental hook-rod methods, including Cotrel-Dubousset (CD), Texas Scottish Rite Hospital (TSRH), and ISOLA, are useful in many spinal injury patterns.[21] After all of the hooks have been seated, distraction forces can be applied to the rods to relieve axial compression. The rods can be prebent or bent in situ to reduce kyphosis. The rotational stability of segmental-hook rod methods is excellent, especially with the use of crosslocking devices. These devices are useful in patients with high thoracic injuries in whom segmental fixation avoids the use of external immobilization. For increased correction of kyphotic deformities, stiffer rods, which will better resist the flexion forces, are available in most systems. The disadvantage of segmental fixation is the increased length of instrumentation. Attempts to shorten the instrumentation by applying two hooks at the same lamina (either proximally or distally) have resulted in a higher failure rate.

The use of pedicle screw constructs remains controversial. Accurate placement of pedicle screws becomes increasingly difficult above L-1.[22,23] In younger individuals, the pedicles at T10, T11, T12, and L1 are elliptical,

Table 1
Correction of kyphosis

Author (Year)	Surgical Technique	Mean follow-up (in months)	Number of Patients	Mean kyphosis in degrees		
				Preop	Postop	Follow-up
Convery (1978)[35]	Harrington Rods	16	24	17	5	15
McEvoy (1985)[37]	Harrington Rods	12	53	16		16
Edwards (1986)[8]	Rod-sleeve	12	135	14	0	0.5
Floman (1986)[36]	Harrington Rod	36	36	28	10	14
Kinnard (1986)[48]	Plates	24	21	loss of correction greater than 10° in 5 patients		
Aebi (1987)[40]	Fixateur	12	30	15.8	3.5	7.1
Karlström (1990)[47]	Olerud	24	37	11.0	-2.0	7.0
Crutcher (1991)[6]	Jacobs		44	13.3	-1.0	?
Daniaux (1991)[44]	VSP plate	38	172		mean loss of correction of 9.3°	
Ebelke (1991)[45]	VSP plate	17	21	12.7	0.0	7.4
Esses (1991)[28]	Fixateur	17	89	18.8	2.7	?
Lindsey (1991)[29]	Fixateur	35	80	17	6.0	14.5
Sasso (1991)[52]	Plates	20	23	10.8	6.2	13.0
Chang (1992)[43]	RF System	24	33	21	0.0	0.0
Hardaker (1992)[10]	Harrington	43	58	15	5	8
Sim (1992)[22]	Fixateur	25	27	8.6	-2.7	6.4
Willen (1992)[54]	Harrington	12	26	18	7	?
McLain (1993)[25]	CD screws	15	19		mean loss of correction of 7.4°	

with a width too narrow to accommodate pedicle screws.[24] Smaller screws are not strong enough to withstand the loads and are subject to fatigue failure. Short segment pedicle screw constructs a single level above and below the fracture at the thoracolumbar junction may be inadequate to correct and withstand the applied forces.[25] Some systems have a coupled mechanism that requires both axial distraction and lordosis to be secured at the same time, which will lead to incomplete reductions. In addition, because the normal alignment at the thoracolumbar junction is slight kyphosis (0° to 5°), the weightbearing axis lies anterior to the linkage of the device. The excessive bending forces applied to the screws have resulted in frequent screw fracture, bending, and device loosening.[25,26] Anterior fracture comminution increases bending and is more likely to result in failure of the plate/screw system. Cantilever (fixation) systems similarly have a high rate of loss of fixation and screw failure when applied at the thoracolumbar junction.[25,27-29] Because of the higher complication rate and the difficulty of inserting large enough screws within the pedicles at the thoracolumbar junction, the use of screws at that level is less advantageous and carries a higher risk than the use of a rod sleeve or a segmental rod-hook system. In the lower lumbar spine, the importance of saving levels and preserving open motion segments is critical. Also, distal hook fixation is tenuous, and, therefore, pedicle screw systems are more advantageous. Here larger screws can be inserted into the pedicles, and the weightbearing axis falls posterior to the vertebral body. Depending on the screw-rod linkage, pedicle screws can be used for the distal end of constructs, with hooks used at the proximal end. Multiple pedicle screws may also be used to reduce and stabilize shear injuries.

Length of Arthrodesis

The optimal length of fixation and number of fused segments remains controversial. Two predominant theories are "rod long, fuse short" and arthrodesing over the entire length of instrumentation, while attempting to minimize the number of levels instrumented, especially in the lumbar spine.[30,31] Disadvantages of the rod long, fuse short technique are: (1) requirement for two surgical procedures; (2) insufficient data determining the optimal time for removal of the hardware (long enough for the fusion mass to mature and short enough to avoid damaging the joints that have been immobilized); (3) difficulty with hook placement without disruption of facet capsules and the ligamentous structures at adjacent levels; (4) temporary immobilization of facet joints, which can lead to degenerative changes.[32] Although recent studies show adequate functional outcome,[33,34] this technique must be distinguished from reduction of the fracture without arthrodesis. This technique is often associated with collapse of the injury segment following hardware removal. The more common approach is to limit the number of levels of posterior stabilization and arthrodesis of the entire length of fixation. The number of segments instrumented is determined by the lever arms necessary to reduce the fracture. With straight Harrington rods, because the forces were poorly concentrated and could not be applied specifically to the injured areas of the spine, two to three levels of instrumentation above and two levels below the fracture were necessary. Improved instrumentation systems, such as pedicle screw systems and the rod-sleeve system, allow specific forces to be applied in concentrated areas, which means that a shorter construct can be used. With the rod-sleeve system, the construct can be shortened to one level below and one to two interspaces above the injury. The segmental hook-rod systems generally instrument two normal levels above and below the fractured level. In the thoracic spine, this may be an appropriate exchange for the increased rigidity.

Outcomes of Posterior Instrumentation

Comparison of the results of Harrington instrumentation,[6,7,10,15,16,35-37] rod sleeves,[8,18-20,38,39] and pedicle screw systems[5,23,25,28,29,40-54] is given in Table 1. The factors compared include the preoperative angular deformity and translation, the adequacy of correction, the maintenance of correction, and the rate of fusion. At long-term follow-up, Harrington rod and Luque rod systems were seen to have lost the correction achieved intraoperatively. This problem occurred less frequently with rod sleeves and segmental hook-rod systems. The pedicle screw systems similarly also showed a high rate of early failure when used at the thoracolumbar junction. In the lower lumbar spine, the degree of correction and fusion as well as maintenance of correction was satisfactory.[55]

Adjunctive Decompression

Decompression of the spinal canal is an important goal in the surgical treatment of thoracolumbar fractures. Previously, it was recommended that patients who were neurologically intact with 30% canal compromise should have anterior decompression to prevent symptoms related to spinal stenosis. However, there have been no reported cases of spinal stenosis in patients who had reduction and stabilization of fractures. In most cases in which late secondary decompressions were performed, patients had residual kyphosis deformities at the time of initial reduction. Long-term follow-up studies in patients treated both surgically and nonsurgically demonstrate that significant remodeling of the residual bone occurs.[20,56]

Adjunctive posterior decompression at the time of initial surgery is occasionally recommended. Indirect canal decompression is less effective in patients with low lumbar burst fractures. Because restoration of lordosis decreases the tension in the posterior longitudinal ligament, there is a decreased effect of ligamentotaxis.[57] In addition, the larger spinal canals in the low lumbar spine afford easier access to the retropulsed fragments from the posterior approach. Therefore, in patients with a specific root deficit and a large retropulsed fragment on preoperative CT scan, a posterior decompression is easily accomplished. At the thoracolumbar junction, a transpedicular posterolateral decompression is an accepted technique if there is significant deformity and a unilateral retropulsion of either a free fragment or of a large contained fragment.[10,38,58] The use of intraoperative ultrasound has been effective in gauging the adequacy of reduction. Alternatively, a postoperative CT scan is obtained to determine if neural compression is present. If the patient does not show adequate recovery, a second-stage anterior decompression is indicated.

Patients with bilateral facet dislocations as a result of flexion-distraction injury may have associated intravertebral disk disruption.[59] If compression forces are applied, extravasation of the disk material into the spinal cord may occur with resultant neurologic injury.[39] Several treatment strategies are possible to avoid this complication. First, the fracture can be stabilized by a neutralization construct (after reduction) to prevent further axial compression of the disk space. Second, placement of a rod sleeve system converts the deformity into a coupled force.[39] Once the facet dislocation is reduced, an intraspinous wire is placed and a rod sleeve system is located directly over the dislocated facets creating local lordosis. The rods can then be used to apply distraction and restore the height of the disk. Further dislocation is prevented, because both the wire and the rod sleeve prevent flexion. Finally, prophylactic diskectomy can be performed and a compression construct applied. In the low lumbar spine, in order to preserve levels, a pedicle screw construct is recommended.

Postoperative Orthosis

Postoperatively, the majority of patients should use a brace. The type of brace depends on fracture pattern, level, and instrumentation system. The use of either a total contact orthosis (TCO) for fractures between T6 and L4 or the use of a TCO with a leg extension for those with fixation extending to the sacrum is recommended. Patients are rapidly mobilized out of bed but are maintained in braces for 4 to 6 months. The use of orthoses results in lower rates of instrumentation failure, pseudarthrosis, and loss of correction. In segmental hook-rod systems, especially in the upper thoracic fractures, an orthosis is not required. The use of TCO, even in patients with paraplegia, is well tolerated with few complications. Patients are able to learn transfers, self-catheterization, and, eventually, driving. Floor-to-chair transfers and several other limited activities are completed when the TCO is removed.

Anterior Decompression and Arthrodesis

Rationale for Anterior Decompression

The goal of anterior spinal decompression is to provide an optimal environment for recovery from incomplete neural deficits by achieving reduction and complete decompression of the spinal canal.[58,60,61] In 90% of unstable burst fractures, the offending agent is the posterior superior corner of the comminuted vertebral body. Posterior instrumentation attempts "ligamentotaxis" or indirect closed reduction of the spinal canal by distracting the posterior longitudinal ligament or the disk annulus. Often, if the surgery is performed more than 48 hours after injury, posterior distraction rods do not alleviate continued compression from displaced fragments of bone or disk within the spinal canal.[6,8,9] The rationale for anterior surgery is to perform an "open reduction of the spinal canal" under direct vision either through a retroperitoneal (L1 to L4) anterior approach or a thoracotomy (T2 to T12).

Surgical Technique

The retroperitoneal approach through the periosteal envelope of the 12th rib can be used for exposure from the 11th thoracic to the 4th lumbar vertebrae without entering the pleural cavity.[58,62] Access can also be provided through the periosteal envelope of the 11th rib, but there is a greater chance of inadvertently violating the parietal pleura. The description of the decompression of a burst fracture of the first lumbar vertebrae follows.

The patient is placed in the lateral decubitus position, left side up. The 12th rib is centered over the hinged portion of the operating table to provide maximum working space between the thorax and the left iliac crest when the table is flexed. The skin incision is made along the left 12th rib, which is then dissected subperiosteally, with care taken not to violate the parietal pleura or diaphragm. The rib is disarticulated from its costotransverse attachment with a Cobb periosteal elevator. As the transversalis fascia is bluntly dissected from the left psoas muscle, the posterior renal fascia, perinephric fat, left kidney, and peritoneal contents are safely retracted anteriorly with a large abdominal pad. This maneuver exposes the left crus of the diaphragm and the origin of the left psoas muscle, and facilitates ligation of the segmental vertebral vessels. A Finochietto rib-retractor is placed between the 11th rib and the iliac crest. The aorta can be mobilized anteriorly and protected throughout the procedure with a malleable retractor. After subperiosteal dissection of the crus of the diaphragm superiorly and the psoas muscle inferiorly, the comminuted fragments of the first lumbar vertebra are visualized. Visualization of the thecal sac is accomplished by following the left 12th intercostal nerve toward the neural foramen of the 12th thoracic-1st lumbar area. The left 1st lumbar transverse process can be palpated and removed with a rongeur. The upper and lower margins of the left 1st lumbar pedicle are then clearly delineated with a small elevator. The pedicle is removed in its entirety using a 45°-angle Kerrison rongeur while protecting the first lumbar nerve root. Once the pedicle has been removed, the first lumbar nerve can be traced to the thecal sac and the bone fragments of the 1st lumbar vertebrae are visualized. For experienced spinal surgeons, and provided the surgeon is well-oriented, the step of removal of the ipsilateral pedicle can be skipped. There are abundant epidural venous anastomoses around the neuroforamen so this step can cause moderate hemorrhaging. An alternative method of becoming oriented to the direction and depth of the compromised spinal canal is to perform a complete excision of the T12-L1 and L1-L2 intervertebral disks. These are avascular structures and they must be meticulously excised in their entirety to achieve a solid fusion in any case. The bulk of the vertebral body is removed with a high speed burr and osteotomes. A diamond burr and long curettes are used to remove the displaced posterior part of the vertebral body from the anterior aspect of the thecal sac. The posterior longitudinal ligament is often found to be disrupted or attenuated as a result of the original injury. The decompression is not complete until the base of the opposite pedicle of L1 is visualized and the dural tube is expanded anteriorly.

Seating holes for an iliac-strut graft are made in the inferior end-plate and body of the 12th thoracic vertebra and in the superior end-plate and body of the 2nd lumbar vertebra. This can usually be accomplished with a medium-sized curette, but if the end-plates are sclerotic, particularly during a late decompression, a high-speed burr can be used. The seating holes should be large enough to allow insertion of the surgeon's fingertip approximately half the length of the distal phalanx. A malleable probe is required to determine the precise height of the iliac graft. An oscillating saw is used to obtain the iliac-crest graft, and the graft is fashioned into a T shape similar to that described for use in the cervical spine. The tricortical iliac graft is locked into place, with the rounded cortical edge of the iliac crest directed toward the patient's right side, oriented in the coronal plane. Additional portions of cancellous graft are placed anteriorly and a gelatin sponge is placed over the dura to provide hemostasis. The transversalis fascia, underlying peritoneum, and parietal pleura are examined for tears. The wound is closed over a suction drain.

Beginning on the 4th postoperative day, the patient is permitted to sit or stand while wearing a thoracolumbosacral orthosis. The orthosis is removed for bathing only, during which time the patient must be log-rolled and kept recumbent. The orthosis is used until fusion is confirmed radiographically, usually after 3 months. At this time, if doubt arises concerning the adequacy of fusion, lateral flexion-extension tomograms are made. Depending on the radiographic appearance, use of the orthosis may be required for as long as 6 months.

Anterior Instrumentation

It is beyond the scope of this text to describe in great detail the technique of anterior instrumentation. Currently marketed devices include the Kaneda device, Z-plate, CASP plate, and Thoracolumbar Locking Plate.[60,61] Several principles are common to these devices so they will be emphasized. First and foremost, anterior instrumentation is a much more exacting procedure than posterior spinal instrumentation. All metal should be kept away from the great vessels to avoid vascular erosion by leaving a screw in juxtaposition to the iliac vein, aorta, or vena cava. Anterior instrumentation devices are load-sharing implants. Meticulous detail is required in sizing and shaping a tricortical iliac strut graft so that its parallel surfaces are press-fit against the adjacent vertebral bodies.[63] In the transverse plane, the vertebral screws need to be directed in a triangular configuration to provide maximum resistance to pull-out. Finally, when the Kaneda paravertebral rods or other devices are attached to the vertebral screws, they need to apply a compressive force across the long axis of the iliac strut graft. Once both rods or plates are inserted properly, the graft is compressed. The importance of this maneuver cannot be overemphasized. Anterior instrumentation devices rely directly on load transmission through a healthy strong tricortical graft for secure fixation and for long-term healing. If firm compression of the graft is not provided during instrumentation, the construct will fail.

Outcome of Anterior Decompression and Arthrodesis

McAfee, Bohlman, and Yuan[58] reported the neurologic recovery of 70 patients who had undergone anterior decompression for thoracolumbar fractures. At a minimum follow-up of 2 years, no patient lost further cord or cauda equina function. Of 42 patients who had a motor deficit, 37 improved by at least one class (Eismont grading system) in motor strength. Fourteen of the 30 patients whose quadriceps and hamstrings were too weak to permit walking regained full independent walking ability. Twelve of the 32 patients who had a conus medullaris injury demonstrated recovery from neurogenic bowel and bladder incontinence.

Kaneda[60] documented the most comprehensive outcome study evaluating thoracolumbar spinal injuries treated by anterior decompression. One hundred ten consecutive patients (average age 43.5 years, range 14 to 79 years) were followed for a minimum of 4 years postoperatively. Because the Kaneda procedures were performed at Hokkaido University, an island, and the stability of the island's population, 100% follow-up of the patients was achieved. The recovery of motor function was: 11 patients improved two or more Frankel levels; 46 patients improved one Frankel level; 17 patients were unchanged. Using the McBride modified evaluation, 12 patients in this group improved from D1 to D2 or from D2 to D3.[21] Thirty-six patients who were intact remained normal at follow-up.

Using the Motor Index Scale (maximum total 50 points) the average preoperative score was 26.[64] After the anterior decompression and Kaneda instrumentation, the motor index was 49.4. Of 42 patients in the Japanese series who had neurogenic bladder injury (lesion of the conus medullaris), 28 demonstrated recovery of bladder function. The restoration of anterior spinal stability was also achieved at a high rate. In 106 of 110 procedures (96.4%), a stable fusion was achieved by the primary procedure. Four failures of anterior instrumentation occurred and will be discussed in the complication section.

Currently we believe anterior decompression and fusion can be performed as a primary procedure for patients with neurologic defects and burst-type fractures from T11-L4. In acute cases anterior instrumentation can be added except for fractures at L4 or L5. Alternatively, anterior decompression and fusion can follow a posterior instrumentation when there is residual cord or root compression and persistent neurologic deficits.

Complications of Instrumentation

Complications of treatment of patients with thoracolumbar trauma have been reported frequently. Many are due to lack of understanding of the patients' altered spinal mechanics; others are due to poor technique or choice of instrumentation. In this section complications of instrumentation will be discussed.

McAfee and Bohlman[17] reviewed 40 patients with failure of Harrington instrumentation for fractures of the thoracolumbar spine. This series currently includes 120 cases of failure of posterior instrumentation in trauma patients. Forty-two patients had dislodgement or disengagement of the instrumentation with loss of fixation. Harrington distraction instrumentation requires intact ligaments for stability, and overdistraction is a complication more likely in translational injuries. The use of a claw-type configuration of pointing hooks placed in a segmental fashion towards each other decreases the incidence of loss of fixation. Twenty patients were referred with iatrogenic neurologic deficits. Nine patients had inadequate reduction of translational injuries. Twenty patients had persistent unrecognized neurologic compression. If primary posterior "indirect" reduction techniques are attempted for incomplete neurologic deficits, it is mandatory to perform a CT-myelogram postoperatively to determine if a second-stage anterior corpectomy is indicated.

At the time of this writing, all pedicle instrumentation procedures are considered investigational by the FDA. However, 95% of the membership in the North American Spine Society have answered a survey saying "pedicle instrumentation is the state-of-the-art in the treatment of some patients in my clinical practice." Steffee and Brantigan performed a prospective multicentered study of 250 patients done under an FDA-approved protocol.[65] Overall fusion success was achieved in 186 of 200 (93%) with no statistical difference when comparing the numbers of levels fused. There were 21 device-related complications (8.4%). These included ten wound infections; three hematomas; three patients who developed leg pain or weakness; three patients who lost bowel or bladder control; and one patient who had a spinal cord infarction. The spinal cord infarction occurred in an 85-year-old patient who remained paraplegic postoperatively. Non-device related complications were reported on 16 occasions for 15 patients (6.4%). These included ileus (6); atelectasis (3); chronic obstructive pulmonary disease (1); myocardial infarction (1); deep venous thrombosis (2); urinary tract infection (1); and idiopathic neuritis (1). Screw breakage occurred in 33 screws of 1,314 screws implanted in 31 patients.

West reported 124 consecutive cases of Vertebral Spinal Plating (VSP) instrumentation and described complications in 33 patients (27%).[66] Unfortunately, this study (and others on pedicle instrumentation) combined the medical postoperative complications with the complications specific to the pedicle screw. Neurologic deficit developed in 7 patients (6%). In five of them, the deficit was due to manipulation and reduction of the neural elements.

McAfee and associates[67] reported a survivorship analysis of pedicle instrumentation in 120 consecutive pedicle instrumentation cases (78 VSP procedures and 42 procedures that used Cotrel-Dubousset instrumentation). Survivorship analysis was used to calculate a predicted cumulative rate of success for this series of patients over 10 years postoperative follow-up. Out of 526 pedicle screws, there were 22 problem screws (22/526 = 4.18%). In most patients, the hardware failure was an incidental radiographic finding. Only five patients had screw breakage associated with a pseudoarthrosis. Actuarial analysis predicted the survivorship of solid posterolateral fusion at 90% after 10 years. This survivorship rate is similar to those predicted at 10 years for other more widely used orthopaedic surgical implants, such as total hip arthroplasty components.[68] To reduce the incidence of complications in this series, the technique of "probing" rather than "drilling" the pedicle was used.

Pedicle screws are the instrumentation of choice in the posterior stabilization of lower lumbar (L4 or L5) unstable burst fractures. If pedicle instrumentation is applied in fractures across the thoracolumbar junction, it is important to supplement the pedicle screws with anterior structural bone grafting—placed via either an anterior or a posterolateral approach. Akbarnia and associates[69] reported a multi-center study of over 100 VSP used in thoracolumbar fractures. Anterior load-sharing was necessary with pedicle instrumentation to prevent an unacceptably high rate of screw breakage and failure.

McAfee[70] studied the incidence of complications from 1984 to 1990 in 185 anterior thoracolumbar procedures (thoracotomies, transthoracic-retroperitoneal, and retroperitoneal approaches). A complete listing of the complications encountered is shown in Table 2. There were no cases of iatrogenic neurologic deficit. There were also no deep wound infections. One patient died 1 week postoperatively due to disseminated intravascular coagulopathy. None of the five patients with pseudoarthrosis of the anterior corpectomy graft required repeat anterior

Table 2
Complications of anterior thoracolumbar decompression, instrumentation and fusion[70]

	Total Procedures 185
Iatrogenic spinal neurologic deficits	0
Lumbar plexus neuropraxia	3
Retraction of psoas muscle against transverse processes of L4 and L5	
Deep wound infections	0
Meningitis resolved with 6 weeks antibiotics	1
Pseudarthrosis	5
Graft displacement requiring additional posterior surgery	1
Pulmonary complications	
Postoperative pneumothorax	2
Pneumonia	2
Tension hemopneumothorax	1
Pleural effusion requiring thoracentesis	1
Inadvertent detachment of the diaphragm off of chest wall requiring intraoperative repair	1
Instrumentation Failures	
Dwyer-Hall rod bending (275 lb patient) 10 days postoperatively	1
Axial slipping of Dwyer-Hall rod requiring posterior CD instrumentation	1
Dwyer-Hall rod breaking requiring revision of anterior stabilization using Kaneda system	1
Breakage of Kaneda screws requiring posterior CD instrumentation	2
L2 vertebral body screw in spinal canal neurologically intact	1
Death	
41 units post-op blood loss following L3 corpectomy for *Mycobacterium tuberculosis* and *Escherichia coli* infection secondary to abdominal gunshot wound and pancreatitis—patient developed disseminated intravascular coagulopathy	1
Total complications	24
Incidence of complications: 24 of 185 (12.9%)	

surgery. All five cases were successfully revised with posterior Cotrel-Dubousset instrumentation and posterior spinal fusion.

In a similar finding, Kaneda[60] did not have to remove any of the 110 anterior instrumentation devices. The four cases with anterior pseudoarthrosis or anterior implant failures were successfully stabilized by posterior spinal fusion and instrumentation (Kaneda paravertebral rod breakage—1 patient, Kaneda vertebral screw breakage—1 patient). In one patient, the inferior vena cava ruptured during exposure of an untreated burst fracture with severe kyphosis. One postoperative death occurred at 2 weeks from pneumonia in a patient with diabetes, two patients had superficial wound infections, and five patients had postoperative atelectasis. In our experience, there have been more postoperative pulmonary problems with the contralateral lung than with the lung on the side of the anterior approach, probably because of dependency during surgery.

Conclusion

The goals of surgical treatment are to protect the neural structures from further injury, reduce fractures and dislocations, stabilize the spine and, long term, have a stable painless spine. The surgeon must accurately identify the fracture pattern and plan a technique that best reverses the abnormal biomechanics. The specific procedure should reduce the malalignment in all three planes and provide sufficient stability to allow fracture and bone graft healing without redisplacement. This goal should be accomplished with a minimal number of levels fused. Postoperative braces are used in most cases, although patients are rapidly mobilized. Second-stage decompressive or stabilization procedures are indicated to maximize neurologic recovery or maintain alignment. Complications are avoided by meticulous technique, selection of appropriate procedures, and careful postoperative care.

References

1. Gurwitz GS, Dawson JM, McNamara MJ, et al: Biomechanical analysis of three surgical approaches for lumbar burst fractures using short-segment instrumentation. *Spine* 1993;18:977-982.
2. Krag MH: Biomechanics of thoracolumbar spinal fixation: A review. *Spine* 1991;16(suppl 3):S84-S99.
3. Cammisa FP Jr, Eismont FJ, Green BA: Dural laceration occurring with burst fractures and associated laminar fractures. *J Bone Joint Surg* 1989;71A:1044-1052.
4. Levine AM: Dural lacerations associated with low lumbar burst fractures. *Orthop Trans* 1992.
5. Cigliano A, de Falco R, Scarano E, et al: A new instrumentation system for the reduction and posterior stabilization of unstable thoracolumbar fractures. *Neurosurgery* 1992;30:208-217.
6. Crutcher JP Jr, Anderson PA, King HA, et al: Indirect spinal canal decompression in patients with thoracolumbar burst fractures treated by posterior distraction rods. *J Spinal Disord* 1991;4:39-48.
7. Doerr TE, Montesano PX, Burkus JK, et al: Spinal canal decompression in traumatic thoracolumbar burst fractures: Posterior distraction rods versus transpedicular screw fixation. *J Orthop Trauma* 1991;5:403-411.
8. Edwards CC, Levine AM: Early rod-sleeve stabilization of the injured thoracic and lumbar spine. *Orthop Clin North Am* 1986; 17:121-145.
9. Willén J, Lindahl S, Irstam L, et al: Unstable thoracolumbar fractures: A study by CT and conventional roentgenology of the reduction effect of Harrington instrumentation. *Spine* 1984;9:214-219.
10. Hardaker WT Jr, Cook WA Jr, Friedman AH, et al: Bilateral transpedicular decompression and Harrington rod stabilization in the management of severe thoracolumbar burst fractures. *Spine* 1992;17:162-171.
11. Viale GL, Silvestro C, Francaviglia N, et al: Transpedicular decompression and stabilization of burst fractures of the lumbar spine. *Surg Neurol* 1993;40:104-111.
12. Dickson JH, Harrington PR, Erwin WD: Results of reduction and stabilization of the severely fractured thoracic and lumbar spine. *J Bone Joint Surg* 1978;60A:799-805.
13. Harrington PR: Surgical instrumentation for management of scoliosis. *J Bone Joint Surg* 1960;42A:1448.
14. Karjalainen M, Aho AJ, Katevuo K: Operative treatment of unstable thoracolumbar fractures by the posterior approach with the use of Williams plates or Harrington rods. *Int Orthop* 1992; 16:219-222.
15. Riebel GD, Yoo JU, Fredrickson BE, et al: Review of Harrington rod treatment of spinal trauma. *Spine* 1993;18:479-491.
16. Rosenthal RE, Lowery ER: Unstable fracture-dislocations of the thoracolumbar spine: Results of surgical treatment. *J Trauma* 1980;20:485-490.
17. McAfee PC, Bohlman HH: Complications following Harrington instrumentation for fractures of the thoracolumbar spine. *J Bone Joint Surg* 1985;67A:672-686.
18. Edwards CC: Thoracolumbar trauma: Posterior reduction and fixation with a modular spinal system. *Semin Spine Surgery* 1990;2:8-18.
19. Eismont FJ, Garfin SR, Abitbol JJ: Thoracic and upper lumbar spine injuries, in Browner BD, Jupiter JB, Levine AM, et al (eds): *Skeletal Trauma: Fractures, Dislocations, Ligamentous Injuries.* Philadelphia, PA, WB Saunders, 1992, vol 1, chap 29, pp 729-803.
20. Levine AM: Lumbar and sacral spine trauma, in Browner BD, Jupiter JB, Levine AM, et al (eds): *Skeletal Trauma: Fractures, Dislocations, Ligamentous Injuries.* Philadelphia, PA, WB Saunders, 1992, vol 1, chap 30, pp 805-848.
21. McBride GG: Cotrel-Dubousset rods in surgical stabilization of spinal fractures. *Spine* 1993;18:466-473.
22. Sim E: Location of transpedicular screws for fixation of lower thoracic and lumbar spine: Computed tomography of 45 fracture cases. *Acta Orthop Scand* 1993;64:28-32.
23. Simpson JM, Ebraheim NA, Jackson WT, et al: Internal fixation of the thoracic and lumbar spine using Roy-Camille plates. *Orthopedics* 1993;16:663-672.
24. Sjostrom L, Jacobsson O, Karlstrom G, et al: CT analysis of pedicles and screw tracts after implant removal in thoracolumbar fractures. *J Spinal Disord* 1993;6:225-231.
25. McLain RF, Sparling E, Benson DR: Early failure of short-segment pedicle instrumentation for thoracolumbar fractures: A preliminary report. *J Bone Joint Surg* 1993;75A:162-167.
26. Benson DR, Burkus JK, Montesano PX, et al: Unstable thoracolumbar and lumbar burst fractures treated with the AO fixateur interne. *J Spinal Disord* 1992;5:335-343.
27. Carl AL, Tromanhauser SG, Roger DJ: Pedicle screw instrumentation for thoracolumbar burst fractures and fracture-dislocations. *Spine* 1992;17(suppl 8):S317-S324.

28. Esses SI, Botsford DJ, Wright T, et al: Operative treatment of spinal fractures with the AO internal fixator. *Spine* 1991;16(suppl 3):S146-S150.
29. Lindsey RW, Dick W: The fixateur interne in the reduction and stabilization of thoracolumbar spine fractures in patients with neurologic deficit. *Spine* 1991;16(suppl 3):S140-S145.
30. Broom MJ, Jacobs RR: Update 1988: Current status of internal fixation of thoracolumbar fractures. *J Orthop Trauma* 1989;3:148-155.
31. Jacobs RR, Casey MP: Surgical management of thoracolumbar spinal injuries: General principles and controversial considerations. *Clin Orthop* 1984;189:22-35.
32. Kahanovitz N, Bullough P, Jacobs RR: The effect of internal fixation without arthrodesis on human facet joint cartilage. *Clin Orthop* 1984;189:204-208.
33. Dekutoski MB, Conlan ES, Salcicioli GG: Spinal mobility and deformity after Harrington rod stabilization and limited arthrodesis of thoracolumbar fractures. *J Bone Joint Surg* 1993;75A:168-176.
34. Jacobs RR, Montesano PX: Development of the locking hook spinal rod system. *Orthopedics* 1988;11:1415-1421.
35. Convery FR, Minteer MA, Smith RW, et al: Fracture-dislocation of the dorsal-lumbar spine: Acute operative stabilization by Harrington instrumentation. *Spine* 1978;3:160-166.
36. Floman Y, Fast A, Pollack D, et al: The simultaneous application of an interspinous compressive wire and Harrington distraction rods in the treatment of fracture-dislocation of the thoracic and lumbar spine. *Clin Orthop* 1986;205:207-215.
37. McEvoy RD, Bradford DS: The management of burst fractures of the thoracic and lumbar spine: Experience in 53 patients. *Spine* 1985;10:631-637.
38. Garfin SR, Mowery CA, Guerra J Jr, et al: Confirmation of the posterolateral technique to decompress and fuse thoracolumbar spine burst fractures. *Spine* 1985;10:218-223.
39. Levine AM, Bosse M, Edwards CC: Bilateral facet dislocations in the thoracolumbar spine. *Spine* 1988;13:630-640.
40. Aebi M, Etter C, Kehl T, et al: Stabilization of the lower thoracic and lumbar spine with the internal spinal skeletal fixation system: Indications, techniques, and first results of treatment. *Spine* 1987;12:544-551.
41. Berlanda P, Bassi G: Surgical treatment of traumatic spinal injuries with cord damage: Clinical review of 12 years of experience with the Roy-Camille technique. *Ital J Orthop Traumatol* 1991;17:491-498.
42. Blumenthal S, Gill K: Complications of the Wiltse Pedicle Screw Fixation System. *Spine* 1993;18:1867-1871.
43. Chang KW: A reduction-fixation system for unstable thoracolumbar burst fractures. *Spine* 1992;17:879-886.
44. Daniaux H, Seykora P, Genelin A, et al: Application of posterior plating and modifications in thoracolumbar spine injuries: Indication, techniques, and results. *Spine* 1991;16(suppl 3):S125-S133.
45. Ebelke DK, Asher MA, Neff JR, et al: Survivorship analysis of VSP spine instrumentation in the treatment of thoracolumbar and lumbar burst fractures. *Spine* 1991;16(suppl 8):S428-S432.
46. Greenfield RT III, Grant RE, Bryant D: Pedicle screw fixation in the management of unstable thoracolumbar spine injuries. *Orthop Rev* 1992;21:701-706.
47. Karlström G, Olerud S, Sjöstrom L: Transpedicular fixation of thoracolumbar fractures. *Contemp Orthop* 1990;20:285-300.
48. Kinnard P, Ghibely A, Gordon D, et al: Roy-Camille plates in unstable spinal conditions: A preliminary report. *Spine* 1986; 11:131-135.
49. Lemons VR, Wagner FC Jr, Montesano PX: Management of thoracolumbar fractures with accompanying neurological injury. *Neurosurgery* 1992;30:667-671.
50. Roy-Camille RL: Posterior screw plate fixation in thoracolumbar injuries, in Eilert RE (ed): *Instructional Course Lectures 41*. Park Ridge, IL, American Academy of Orthopaedic Surgeons, 1992, pp 157-163.
51. Roy-Camille R, Saillant G, Mazel C: Plating of thoracic, thoracolumbar, and lumbar injuries with pedicle screw plates. *Orthop Clin North Am* 1986;17:147-159.
52. Sasso RC, Cotler HB, Reuben JD: Posterior fixation of thoracic and lumbar spine fractures using DC plates and pedicle screws. *Spine* 1991;16(suppl 3):134-139.
53. Sim E, Stergar PM: The fixateur interne for stabilising fractures of the thoracolumbar and lumbar spine. *Int Orthop* 1992;16:322-329.
54. Willen J: Unstable thoracolumbar injuries. *Orthopedics* 1992; 15:329-335.
55. An HS, Simpson JM, Ebraheim NA, et al: Low lumbar burst fractures: Comparison between conservative and surgical treatments. *Orthopedics* 1992;15:367-373.
56. Mumford J, Weinstein JN, Spratt KF, et al: Thoracolumbar burst fractures: The clinical efficacy and outcome of nonopoerative management. *Spine* 1993;18:955-970.
57. Harrington RM, Budorick T, Hoyt J, et al: Biomechanics of indirect reduction of bone retropulsed into the spinal canal in vertebral fracture. *Spine* 1993;18:692-699.
58. McAfee PC, Bohlman HH, Yuan HA: Anterior decompression of traumatic thoracolumbar fractures with incomplete neurological deficit using a retroperitoneal approach. *J Bone Joint Surg* 1985;67A:89-104.
59. Gellad FE, Levine AM, Joslyn JN, et al: Pure thoracolumbar facet dislocation: Clinical features and CT appearance. *Radiology* 1986;161:505-508.
60. Kaneda K: Anterior approach and Kaneda instrumentation for lesions of the thoracic and lumbar spine in Bridwell KH, DeWald RL, Lubicky JP, et al (eds): *The Textbook of Spinal Surgery*. Philadelphia, PA, JB Lippincott, 1991, vol 2, chap 38, pp 959-990.
61. Kaneda K, Abumi K, Fujiya M: Burst fractures with neurologic deficits of the thoracolumbar-lumbar spine: Results of anterior decompression and stabilization with anterior instrumentation. *Spine* 1984;9:788-795.
62. Bohlman HH, Eismont FJ: Surgical techniques of anterior decompression and fusion for spinal cord injuries. *Clin Orthop* 1981;154:57-67.
63. Gurr KR, McAfee PC, Shih CM: Biomechanical analysis of anterior and posterior instrumentation systems after corpectomy: A calf-spine model. *J Bone Joint Surg* 1988;70A:1182-1191.
64. Lucas JT, Ducker TB: Motor classification of spinal cord injuries with mobility, morbidity and recovery indices. *Am Surg* 1979;45:151-158.
65. Steffee AD, Brantigan JW: The VSP spinal fixation system: Report of a prospective study of 250 patients enrolled in FDA clinical trials. *Orthop Trans* 1994;18:250.
66. West JL III, Ogilvie JW, Bradford DS: Complications of the variable screw plate pedicle screw fixation. *Spine* 1991;16:576-579.
67. McAfee PC, Weiland DJ, Carlow JJ: Survivorship analysis of pedicle spinal instrumentation. *Spine* 1991;16(suppl 8):S422-S427.
68. Jinnah RH, Amstutz HC, Tooke SM, et al: The UCLA Charnley experience: A long-term follow-up using survival analysis. *Clin Orthop* 1986;211:164-172.
69. Akbarnia BA, Mardjetko SM, Kostial PN: Results of anterior spinal fusion and Kaneda instrumentation using tricorticate iliac allograft, a two-year follow-up. *Orthop Trans* 1993;17:123.
70. McAfee PC: Complications of anterior approaches to the thoracolumbar spine: Emphasis on Kaneda instrumentation. *Clin Orthop* 1994;306:110-119.

Nonsurgical Treatment of Patients with Thoracolumbar Fractures

Paul A. Anderson, MD

Introduction

The goals of treatment for patients with spinal fractures are to protect the neural tissues, to create an environment for maximal neurologic recovery, and to provide a stable, painless spine. Early mobilization of patients is important to minimize costs of treatment and allow early return to function. Nonsurgical treatment can be successful in the majority of patients but often requires extended periods of recumbency or prolonged external immobilization. Today, patients and physicians have many alternative treatment options. The choice of treatment is fundamentally based on fracture type and neurologic state. Other important considerations are level of injury; patient's age, occupation, and body habits; and physician's skill.

Historically, controversies regarding indications and techniques of closed management of thoracolumbar fractures are well documented. Hippocrates rebuked charlatans who created a spectacle by strapping the upper torso of an injured patient to a ladder and then raising the ladder to allow gravity to reduce the fracture.[1] He advocated prone positioning and longitudinal traction applied in opposite directions to the legs and upper arms by turnbuckles. Once spinal length was restored, the physician reduced the gibbous deformity by pushing downward with his bare foot. Alternatively, the physician could sit on the patient's back or apply downward pressure with a lever. Ambroïse Paré advocated fracture reduction and developed the use of vertical suspension.[2] Wagner and Staples applied downward hand pressure on the prone patient who was suspended.[2] At the same time, traction was applied by assistants pulling on the arms and legs. Following reduction, the patients were maintained in traction by a head halter and adhesive straps applied to the legs for 4 to 6 weeks.

Conflicting views arose regarding the necessity for reduction in patients who were neurologically intact. Magnes[3] recommended functional treatment without reduction. He felt prolonged extension and immobilization would allow stiffening of the joints and weakening of the spinal muscles. Böhler[2] emphasized the need for fracture reduction and maintenance during healing. He felt reduction of the angular deformity was essential to produce a normal gait pattern without hyperextension of the hips or hyperlordosis of adjacent areas of the spinal column. In the United States, Davis[4] was the first to document successful radiographic outcome of a closed reduction. Reduction was obtained by hyperextension and was maintained by nursing the patient in extension in plaster shells. Disadvantages of fracture reduction, as pointed out by Nicoll,[5] include risk of paralysis, stiffness secondary to immobilization of damaged soft tissues in a shortened position, and increased likelihood of nonunion due to the disimpaction of vertebral body bone fragments that occurs with hyperextension. In an excellent functional outcome study of 132 injured miners, he was unable to demonstrate any correlation between long-term result and the degree of spinal deformity.

Nonsurgical treatment is indicated in the majority of patients with thoracolumbar spine fractures, because it limits the number of permanently fused motion segments, avoids complications related to surgery (such as infection, anesthetic risk, hardware failure, pseudoarthrosis), and may be less costly. However, the risk of neurologic deterioration is not limited to patients treated surgically. Marshall and associates[6] documented five cases of neurologic deterioration in 129 patients with spinal cord injury of the thoracolumbar spine. Four patients deteriorated prior to surgical treatment, and one patient had a preoperative progressive neurologic deficit that became complete after laminectomy. No patient worsened following posterior instrumentation. In contradistinction, the advantages of surgical treatment include early mobilization of the patient, elimination of fracture disease (atrophy and osteoporosis), decreased hospitalization time and cost, improved spinal alignment, and reduction of complications related to recumbency, such as pneumonia, deep venous thrombosis, and decubitus ulceration.[7-9] In the multiply injured patient, early surgical treatment appears to decrease morbidity and the mortality associated with trauma.[10]

Spinal Cord Injuries

Prior to the institution of comprehensive rehabilitation in the 1940s, the prognosis for patients with spinal cord injury was poor. Surgical treatment, ie, laminectomy, did not remedy the situation and often hastened the demise of the patient. Magnes[3] felt that the paralysis was caused by hematomyelia or cord transection and, therefore, laminectomy was unnecessary. Böhler[2] described an alternative mechanism of spinal cord injury that could be reversible. He felt that it might be pressure from displaced bone fragments, not cord crushing, that was preventing recovery. He correctly hypothesized that fracture reduction would "reestablish lumina of the neural canal and then paralysis would recede if the spinal cord was not crushed but merely subjected to pressure from the bone fragments." He recommended that the reduction should proceed quickly in contradistinction to the treatment for the chronic kyphotic conditions such as tuberculosis. Davis[4] reported cases of neurologic recovery following closed reduction using traction, hyperextension, and immobilization on plaster shells. He also concluded that recovery resulted from decompression through reduction of the bony deformity and removal of pressure on the spinal cord.

Postural reduction for patients with spinal cord injury was developed by Sir Ludwig Guttman at Stoke Mandeville Hospital.[11-13] This method involves prolonged recumbency on rotating beds. By careful placement of pillows, fracture reduction is achieved in the supine, prone, or lateral positions. Patients are maintained recumbent for an average of 10 to 13 weeks. Frankel and associates[12] retrospectively reported the long-term outcome of 394 patients with thoracolumbar fractures and neurologic injury treated by this technique. Although the anatomic radiographic results were not reported, only two patients developed late instability that required surgery. Ten percent of complete paraplegic patients made significant motor recovery. Of patients with incomplete injuries (Frankel grades B and C), 68% made recovery of at least one Frankel grade. Overall, improvement of an average of 0.9 Frankel grades per patient was observed. No significant correlation between fracture reduction and neurologic recovery was present. Limitations of this study include a failure to document the incidence of complications and the length of hospitalization. Also, 70 patients were excluded from analysis because they had died within 3 months of injury, perhaps as a result of the prolonged recumbent treatment.

Jacobs and associates[9] compared the neurologic recovery of 55 patients treated using Harrington rods with the recovery of 32 patients who were treated nonsurgically. Neurologic recovery was measured as the percent possible recovery based on Frankel score. The average neurologic improvement was 53% in the Harrington rod group compared to 44% in the conservatively treated group. The anatomic results were better, time of rehabilitation was shortened, and overall complication rate was lower in the surgically treated patients. However, Burke and Murray[14] found no difference in neurologic recovery between groups of surgically and nonsurgically treated patients who had incomplete neurologic deficits. Radiographic outcome was not reviewed, although three of 89 patients in the conservatively treated group later developed instability. Chronic pain was more prevalent in the surgically treated group, although this pain may have been related to the inadequate fixation of Meurig William's plates. Willén and associates[15] compared 24 patients treated conservatively and 26 patients treated with Harrington rods. No difference in neurologic recovery was noted between the groups. Radiographic parameters, time of mobilization, and length of hospitalization were decreased in the surgically treated group. By 3 months, the rehabilitation index (level of independence) was equal between the two groups. Soreff and associates[16] similarly compared surgically and nonsurgically treated groups. There was no difference in neurologic outcome, but they did demonstrate a reduction in hospitalization time, a lower incidence of complications, and improved anatomic results in the surgically managed patients.

More recent studies demonstrate greater neurologic recovery in incomplete paraplegic patients treated with early stabilization and decompression compared to the historic control groups. Krengel and associates[17] reviewed 14 patients with Frankel B or C paraplegia treated with early decompression and stabilization. Eleven of 13 survivors improved to at least Frankel D. There was an overall neurologic improvement of 2.2 Frankel grades, which exceeded the 0.9 documented by Frankel. Edwards and associates[18] evaluated 38 patients with partial deficits who were treated by the rod-sleeve method. Neurologic improvement occurred in 88% of patients and averaged an increase of 1.25 Frankel grades. Surprisingly, ten of 41 patients with complete motor sensory paraplegia on admission made functional recovery. Kahmann and associates[19] documented improvement in 96% of 35 patients treated by acute anterior decompression. Although these more recent investigations did not have control groups, they all document a higher degree of neurologic recovery compared to nonsurgically treated groups reported previously. In the current United States health care system, it is considered impractical to hospitalize neurologically impaired patients for the period of time required to allow sufficient healing. A major aim of treatment should be rapid mobilization, so that neurologically impaired individuals can successfully participate in rehabilitation.

The most efficacious means to achieve maximum neurologic recovery in spinal cord patients is fracture reduction. Unlike those of the cervical spine, closed reduction of thoracolumbar fractures is difficult and is rarely performed today on patients with neurologic deficits. The surgical goals in these patients are to restore alignment, stabilize the spinal column, and decompress the neural elements. Unfortunately, patients with complete paraplegia from T2 to T11 did not appear to benefit neurologically from surgical treatment.[7-9,20] In this patient population, surgery is reserved for those with unstable fractures which are likely to cause increased deformity.

Nonsurgical Treatment Options

Patients with fractures of the thoracolumbar spine can be treated nonsurgically by a variety of methods. The choice of treatment depends on the fracture type

Outline 1
Methods for nonsurgical treatment of patients with thoracolumbar fractures

1. Prolonged recumbency
2. Ambulation with serial observation without orthosis
3. Minimal orthoses, eg lumbosacral corset
4. Orthotic immobilization: Controlling motion in a single plane, eg Jewett brace
5. Orthotic immobilization: Controlling motion in multiple planes, eg total contact custom molded orthoses
6. Hyperextension reduction and casting

and stability, level of injury, associated injuries, body habitus, and age of patient.[21] Treatment options are presented in Outline 1.

Orthotic Biomechanics

The goals of brace treatment are to limit overall trunk motion; decrease muscular activity; increase intra-abdominal pressure, thereby stabilizing the spine; decrease the loads in the spinal column; and limit intersegmental motion. Lantz and Schultz[22] evaluated the lumbosacral corset, chair-back brace, and custom-molded orthosis and found that all braces limited overall trunk rotation, with the custom-molded orthosis having the greatest effect. These braces had an unpredictable effect on muscular activity. Fidler and Plasmans[23] studied the effects of bracing on intersegmental motion. Braces were most effective at their center with increased intersegmental motion seen in areas adjacent to the ends of the brace. Lumbosacral corsets, the Rainey flexion jacket, and the Baycast jacket limited intersegmental motion to 50% to 60% of normal. A Baycast jacket with leg spica reduced L4-5 and L5-S1 motion to 12% and 8% of normal, respectively.

Norton and Brown[24] found that longer braces, while achieving excellent fixation on the thorax, would increase lumbosacral motion, especially if the brace was not well fixed to the pelvis. Similarly, short braces with good pelvic fixation were associated with increased motion in the upper lumbar spine. Nachemson and associates[25] evaluated the effect of bracing on intradiskal and intra-abdominal pressures.[22] Lumbar spine compression was found to decrease by 33% during flexion when the patient was wearing a brace. No significant effect of intra-abdominal pressure was observed. Nagel and associates[26] evaluated the effectiveness of the Taylor-Knight brace, Jewett hyperextension brace, and body cast in immobilizing an L1-2 ligamentous injury. The Taylor-Knight brace was effective in reducing flexion and lateral bending but had little effect on axial rotation. The Jewett brace reduced flexion by 40% but had little effect on lateral bending or rotation. The body cast was effective in reducing intersegmental motion in all planes and was more effective than Harrington rods.

Treatment by Prolonged Recumbency

Treatment of patients with thoracolumbar fractures by strict bed rest has been practiced throughout recorded history as discussed above. Outcome studies document that the majority of patients without neurologic deficit heal their injuries and return to work.[2,5,27] Factors associated with treatment failure are severe comminution of the vertebral body, diskoligamentous injuries, fracture dislocations, and patients treated with laminectomy. Böhler,[2] as early as 1935, recognized the increased frequency of poor outcome in compensation cases.

Currently, prolonged hospitalization for recumbent treatment is usually not cost effective. However, some patients may be managed by early hospital discharge and home bed rest, using home health care services. This is appropriate for children and young adult patients with low lumbar fractures in whom surgical alternatives would result in multiple segment fusion of the lumbar spine. Complications related to bed rest, such as thromboembolic disease and skin breakdown, should be prevented during any recumbent treatment.

Treatment by Serial Observation

Patients with stable injuries, such as thoracic compression fractures, do not require any specific form of immobilization and may be treated by early ambulation. Weitzman[28] reviewed 107 patients with stable thoracolumbar fractures treated by ambulation and exercise without immobilization. The average follow-up was 3.6 years. Only 10% of the patients developed increased deformity, and none required further treatment. Young[29] reviewed 116 patients with stable fractures who were claimants of the Workers' Compensation Board of Ontario. Persistent symptoms occurred in 72% of patients and incapacitating symptoms in 21%. He found a strong correlation of residual symptoms in patients who were treated with "active rehabilitation." Of patients treated without rehabilitation, 90% had returned to former work compared to only 47% treated with some form of rehabilitation. No correlation of outcome to fracture severity, degenerative changes, level of injury, or age of patient was present.

Concerns of treatment by serial observation include risks of progressive deformity and development of chronic pain. Medical and legal issues may arise in a patient who develops a poor outcome after treatment without an orthosis. Also, some physicians and patients feel that treatment is required for any fracture and, therefore, use an orthosis in order to do something. When nonsurgical treatment has been recommended, the physician must recognize that the initial assessment of fracture stability may have been inaccurate and, therefore, the fracture may have developed progressive deformity. White and Panjabi[30] have recommended that routine, follow-up physical examinations and radiographic studies be performed at 3 weeks, 6 weeks, 3 months, 6 months, and 1 year to allow early detection of late instability.

Treatment by Minimal Bracing

Lumbosacral corsets and elastic bands are frequently prescribed to diminish pain and decrease mobility of the lumbar spine.[31] These braces decrease overall upper trunk motion, but have little effect on intersegmental motion or spinal loads.[22] Corsets have been shown to decrease low back pain, primarily because they act as a reminder to patients to avoid excessive forward or lateral bending.[31] Increased motion at L5-S1 can occur as a result of these braces. Corset use should be restricted to patients with stable fracture patterns or to elderly patients with osteoporosis. The potential adverse effects of corsets are disuse muscle atrophy, increased osteoporosis, psychological dependency, and concentration of forces at the lumbosacral junction. When prescribing corsets, it is useful to encourage an active exercise program, including paraspinal and abdominal strengthening and cardiovascular fitness training.

Treatment by Orthoses that Control Motion in a Single Plane

The Jewett hyperextension brace immobilizes the spine by providing three-point fixation—anteriorly at the sternum and pubis, and posteriorly at the thoracolumbar junction. Nagel and associates[26] demonstrated that the Jewett brace reduced intersegmental motion and flexion at the thoracolumbar junction. Because this brace has no pelvic support, lateral and axial rotation were not affected. Outcome studies of patients treated by Jewett braces are not available.

I recommend the Jewett brace when treating patients who have injuries between T6 and L3 that are unstable only in flexion. Patwardhan[32] evaluated the Jewett hyperextension brace using a finite element analysis that simulated three severities of thoracolumbar injury. He found that the Jewett brace restored stiffness to normal values in injuries simulating one- and two-column fractures. For three-column injuries, which had greater than 85% loss of normal stiffness, the Jewett brace was ineffective.

Treatment by Orthoses that Control Motion in Multiple Planes

The advantages of custom-molded total contact orthoses are: distribution of forces over a large surface area; improved fixation of the pelvis and thorax, thereby controlling lateral bending and axial rotation; better patient and nursing acceptance; and ability to obtain unobscured radiographs.[33] Also, theoretically, deformities can be corrected by patient positioning during the molding process. In insensate patients, a total contact orthosis offers a substantial advantage because of the ability to monitor the skin and readily adjust areas of excessive pressure.

Reid and associates[34] reported 21 patients with thoracolumbar burst fractures treated by early ambulation in a custom-molded orthosis. No complication occurred as a result of the brace and none of the patients required surgery for brace failure or development of a neurologic deficit. Cantor and associates[35] and Mumford and associates[36] report similar good and excellent results with no complications for patients with thoracolumbar burst fractures treated with custom orthoses.

The total contact orthosis is the most effective orthosis for immobilization of patients with a thoracolumbar fracture.[32] This brace is indicated for patients who have instabilities in more than a single plane, in patients with impaired skin sensation, or in patients with multiple osteoporotic compression fractures. A total contact orthosis is not indicated for the very obese patient or patients who are likely to be noncompliant. The brace must be fabricated by a skilled orthotist. After fitting, the skin should be checked for excessive pressure and, if present, the brace should be modified. Molding for the orthosis should be delayed if patients have abdominal distension or excessive weight gain from fluid retention. Patients with spinal cord injuries or multiple injuries may have significant weight change and may require reassessment of the fit of the total contact orthosis. Occasionally, patients with significant weight change may require fabrication of a second brace.

Protocols for brace use vary. I recommend that patients wear braces full time, including at night. Patients may shower and swim in the orthosis, but they must then lie flat in bed until the orthosis dries and can be reapplied. Standard total contact orthoses or other braces do not immobilize below L4 or above T5-6 and may increase loads and range of motion at these levels. To immobilize L4 and below, a rigid thigh extension in 15° to 30° of hip flexion is required. Injuries above T5-6 are immobilized by adding chin and occipital pads to the custom-molded orthosis.

Treatment by Hyperextension Reduction and Casting

Closed reduction and hyperextension casting affords the ability to achieve and maintain fracture reduction until consolidation. Biomechanically, the cast is more effective than any orthosis.[24,26] Nagel and associates[26] found that the body cast was more effective at limiting L2-3 motion than were Harrington rods. Additionally, because casting is enforced, it is not as dependent on patient cooperation. Disadvantages of casting include cast weight, pressure sores, inability to monitor skin, neurapraxia of the lateral femoral percutaneous nerve, deep venous thrombosis secondary to groin pressure, and poor patient acceptance. Cast syndromes in trauma patients are rare.

Closed reduction is performed on a fracture table using Goldwaithe Irons or on a Risser table. The patient lies supine on the fracture table and reduction is performed by bringing the table sections together, which increases the bending in the Goldwaithe Irons and creates hyperextension of the spine. When using the Risser table, a vertically oriented localizing strap can be used to lift the spine upward, thus reducing the fracture. Following reduction, an underarm body cast is applied. Cast trimming ensures an adequate abdominal fenestration, full shoulder range of motion, and 90° of hip flexion. The cast should be trimmed posteriorly to allow the patient to sit. Three-point molding on the sternum, over the pubis, and posteriorly at the fracture site is essential. Additionally, molding over the iliac crest prevents pistoning of the cast during ambulation. Böhler and Watson-Jones methods of reduction may be used but are less controlled.[2,37] The cast is worn for 3 to 5 months.

Recent reports regarding the efficacy of cast treatment are not available. However, Cantor and associates,[35] Reid and associates,[34] and Mumford and associates[36] reported excellent outcomes of patients with stable burst fractures treated by total contact orthoses, indicating that fracture reduction in these patients may not be that essential. Radiographically, the majority of patients ended with residual deformities similar to those seen on initial radiographs.

Closed reduction casting is indicated in younger patients with two- and three-column injuries who have significant deformity, in patients who are likely to be noncompliant, and when reduction is required, such as in patients with Chance type fractures.

Indication for Nonsurgical Treatment

The choice of treatment for patients with thoracolumbar fractures is based on fracture stability as determined by fracture type. Nonsurgical treatment is recommended for most patients who are neurologically intact and have stable fracture patterns. Patients with neurologic injury and unstable fractures should be treated surgically. However, some patients with complete thoracic paraplegia can be managed with a total contact orthosis after a short period of bed rest.[38] Nonsurgical treatment is indicated for compression fractures, stable burst fractures, and some seatbelt-related injuries. Patients with significant anterior column injury and posterior osteoligamentous disruption are not candidates for nonsurgical treatment.

Patient Assessment

Patient assessment is described above. In evaluating patients for nonsurgical treatment, careful attention should be directed to the examination of the spine. Patients with obvious gibbous deformities may not be candidates for surgical treatment. A large dorsal hematoma may indicate the presence of significant posterior ligamentous injury. Uncontrolled pain in patients who are turned supine and lateral may indicate pending neurologic deficit or the presence of an unstable fracture. The presence of a dermatologic condition or associated injuries may preclude nonsurgical treatment.

Rehabilitation

Böhler[2] described a detailed calisthenics program that patients perform during cast treatment. He felt that the rehabilitation process should begin immediately, and his goal was to have patients in better physical condition than prior to injury. Nicoll[5] recommended functional treatment for stable fractures by early ambulation and exercise. Weitzman[28] noted poorer results in patients with stable fractures who were immobilized by cast or braces than in those prescribed early ambulation and extension exercises. By necessity, patients treated by Guttmann's postural treatment performed an extensive exercise program that involved all the extremities as well as the axial musculature.[12,13] Young,[29] however, compared the outcomes of patients treated with and without formal rehabilitation. Those who received more treatment had greater disability and longer time to return to work.

Surprisingly, the long-term effects of spinal bracing have not been investigated to my knowledge. Contraction of soft tissue, muscle atrophy, decreased joint range of motion, decreased bone mass, increased fatigability of posture muscles, and diminished cardiovascular endurance are potential consequences. Trunk strengthening and cardiovascular exercise have been shown to be of benefit in patients with other low back conditions.

We recommend that patients treated nonsurgically be instructed in fundamental body biomechanics (back school), perform isometric trunk-strengthening exercises, and be aerobically trained to achieve a pulse rate of 130/min sustained for 30 minutes. The exercise programs should begin once pain from the injury is resolved. Patients treated surgically also benefit from this rehabilitation program. Once healing has commenced, a stretching program is instituted to restore spinal motion.

Nonsurgical Management of Specific Fracture Types

Compression Fractures

Compression or wedge compression fractures are thought to be stable injuries resulting from hyperflexion forces. The injury is localized to the anterior vertebral body only. The posterior osseoligamentous complex is intact. Compression injuries in the thoracic spine may have increased stability due to the biomechanical effects of the rib cage. Fractures of the thoracolumbar junction or lumbar spine are subjected to greater bending loads and are more likely to develop increased kyphosis.

Hazel and associates[39] reviewed the long-term outcome of 25 patients with compression fractures. Treatment methods were poorly defined but included a cast or brace in some patients. Eight patients had no pain, 11 patients had occasional back pain without restriction of activity, five patients required modifications of activity, and one patient was disabled secondary to pain. No correlation was found between severity of initial injury and development of degenerative changes on radiographic examination. Three patients were found to have previously undetected fractures and seven patients had a wedging increase of greater than 10%. Young[29] reviewed 116 patients with stable fractures, of whom 75% had continuing symptoms. The presence of symptoms did not correlate to the fracture severity, fracture deformity, or other radiographic features.

The treatment of compression fractures is dictated by the level involved. Patients are initially treated with bed rest for 2 to 3 days until pain and/or ileus are resolved. Injuries of the upper thoracic spine (T2 to T10) are generally more stable and can be treated by serial observation. Fractures at the thoracolumbar junction and lumbar spine are treated with a Jewett brace or total contact orthosis. I do not recommend thigh extension for compression fractures at L4 or below. Multiple contiguous levels of compression fractures are often present, especially in the thoracic spine. These injuries may require more rigid forms of immobilization, such as a cast or total contact orthosis. Surgery is indicated when overall kyphosis is greater than 60° or in patients who develop progressive deformities.

Stable Burst Fractures

Stable burst fractures are characterized by compression failure of the anterior and middle column with retropulsion of the vertebral body into the spinal canal. The posterior column is intact, although a nondisplaced vertical laminar or spinous fracture may be present.[40] Biomechanically, further axial shortening does not occur during treatment because of the intact posterior column. Proper orthotic management or extension casting using three-point fixation can prevent progressive kyphosis. An unstable burst fracture with an associated posterior column injury does not have sufficient residual stiffness to withstand weight-bearing loads without deformation.[32] These fractures may also be unstable in rotation or lateral bending.

Radiographic criteria of stable burst fractures have been arbitrarily defined. Fredrickson and associates[41] felt that stable fractures occurred in patients who were intact and had less than 25° kyphosis and less than 50% stenosis. Reid and associates[34] classified stable burst fractures as those who had less than 35° kyphosis, less than 60% vertebral crush, and injuries primarily of the anterior and middle column. Cantor's criteria were neurologically intact patients with less than 30° kyphosis and less than 50% anterior vertebral height loss.[35]

Denis and associates[42] retrospectively compared 13 patients with burst fractures treated surgically to 39 patients treated nonsurgically. Pain, work status, and deformity were significantly worse in the nonsurgically treated group. Six of the 39 patients treated nonsurgically developed neurologic deficits. They concluded that prophylactic stabilization of burst fractures in neurologically intact patients was a viable alternative. Recent investigations by Reid and associates,[34] Cantor and associates,[35] and Mumford and associates[36] contradict these results. Mumford and associates[36] reviewed 41 patients with burst fractures who were treated nonsurgically by bed rest for an average of 30 days and were then mobilized into a total contact orthosis. At minimum 2 year follow-up, 66% of patients had good or excellent results, and 90% had returned to work. Radiographically, bony deformity progressed marginally. Based on serial computed tomographic (CT) examination, a mean 22% canal remodeling occurred. No correlation of outcome and preoperative severity of injury or residual deformity was present. Cantor and associates[35] reviewed 18 patients with stable thoracolumbar junction burst fractures treated by custom molded orthoses and early ambulation. Fifteen of 18 had little or no pain and returned to prior activities. An average increase of only 1° of deformity and no greater than 5% wedging was observed. A minimum of 50% canal remodeling occurred in the eight patients who had follow-up CT. Reid and associates[34] reported identical clinical and radiographic results.

Thus, stable burst fractures can be successfully treated nonsurgically in the majority of cases. Candidates for this treatment are those who are neurologically intact, have less than 25° of kyphosis, less than 40% to 50% vertebral height loss, less than 50% canal stenosis, and intact posterior elements. The patient should not be severely obese, have skin conditions precluding bracing, or have an associated injury that would interfere with brace management. Additionally, the patient should be expected to be compliant. Both hyperextension casting and total contact orthoses appear to give excellent results in patients with stable burst fractures. Patients with more significant deformities or who are noncompliant may benefit from hyperextension reduction and casting. The choice between total contact orthosis and hyperextension casting is based on physician preference and the patient's wishes and degree of injury.

Low lumbar burst fractures present a different treatment challenge. Fracture patterns are significantly different than at the thoracolumbar junction and often are not associated with an apparent kyphotic deformity.[43] High-grade spinal stenosis may be present and often is associated with displaced laminar fractures, which can be entrapping the dura and caudal equina.[44] An and associates[45] compared outcomes of patients with low lumbar burst fractures (L3-L5) treated by body cast immobilization, Harrington rods, Luque rods, and vertebral spinal plates. Poor results correlated with loss of lumbar lordosis and long instrumented fusions. Good results were seen in patients treated nonsurgically who had minimal height loss or angulation and who were initially neurologically intact. Finn and Stauffer[46] reported seven cases of L5 burst fractures treated with body cast including a leg spica. Patients were neurologically intact except for two who had grade 3-4 strength of lower extremity muscles at the time of injury. Canal compromise ranged from 0 to greater than 90%. Further collapse or neurologic deficit did not occur. Clinical results were good, although all patients complained of occasional back pain. Mick and associates[47] reviewed 11 patients with L5 burst fractures who were treated successfully nonsurgically, although radiculopathies did not resolve in two of the patients.[40] They concluded that nonsurgical treatment was successful in neurologically intact patients, but surgical decompression stabilization was appropriate for those with neurologic deficits.

I concur with these findings and recommend nonsurgical treatment for patients with low lumbar burst fractures and stable pattern. If significant displacement or comminution of the posterior elements is present, the patient should be treated either with prolonged bed rest or surgically with laminectomy and pedicle screw instrumentation. I have observed neurologic deterioration following extension casting of a patient with an L3 burst fracture due to laceration of the roots trapped in the lamina fracture. Orthotic treatment of patients with a lower lumbar burst fracture should include immobilization of at least one hip.

Flexion Distraction and Chance Type Fractures

Flexion distraction and Chance type fractures usually result from hyperflexion of the torso over a lap belt, which acts as a fulcrum.[48] These injuries are occurring with increased frequency due to the higher percentage of restrained passengers in automobile crashes.[49] The pediatric population has been reported to be at increased risk.[49]

In flexion distraction injuries, the center of rotation is within the vertebral body so that the anterior column fails in compression and the posterior and middle columns fail in distraction. In the Chance type fracture, all three columns fail in tension or distraction.[48] Both of these injuries may have bony injury, ligamentous injury, or a combination thereof. However, at surgery, even in injuries that radiographically appear to be exclusively a bony injury, significant soft-tissue injury is present, including rupture of the thoracodorsal fascia, avulsion of the ligamentum flavum, torn paraspinal musculature and stripping of facet joint capsules.[48] The extensive soft-tissue injury may account for the frequent failures of nonsurgical management in these patients.

Anderson and associates[49] reviewed 20 patients with seatbelt injuries. Seven patients with less severe injuries were treated by extension casting or bracing. Thirteen patients with ligamentous injuries or associated multiple trauma were managed with posterior instrumentation. Four of seven conservatively managed patients had poor outcomes, compared to only one of 13 treated surgically. The average kyphosis increased from 10° to 16° in patients treated without surgery, while kyphosis decreased from 16° to 4° in the surgical group. Glassman and associates[50] evaluated 12 pediatric patients with seatbelt-related injuries. Seven patients with ligamentous injuries had nonsurgical treatment. Four of these patients had greater than 20° of kyphosis and all failed brace management. LeGay and associates[51] similarly found that patients treated nonsurgically had poor outcome if there was facet involvement or greater than 17° of initial kyphotic angulation. Biomechanically, these injuries involve all three columns and have loss of the posterior tension band and, therefore, are at risk for progressive deformity. If the injury primarily involves the bony structure and can be held in a reduced position, then a satisfactory outcome by nonsurgical means can be expected.[50,51]

Indications for nonsurgical treatment of flexion distraction and Chance fractures are in bony injuries with less than 10° to 15° of kyphosis. I recommend hyperextension in a custom molded orthosis or body cast. Patients with fractures at L4 and below require the addition of a hip spica. In patients with associated abdominal injury, I recommend surgical rather than closed treatment because of the difficulty of maintaining a brace or cast in these multiply injured patients.

Translational Injuries

Translational injuries result from severe hyperflexion, rotation, or shear forces. The injuries result in extensive ligamentous disruption of all three spinal columns.[42] Translation is usually anterior with facet fracture and/or dislocations. These injuries are highly unstable and, therefore, should rarely be treated nonsurgically. Patients who are neurologically intact are at high risk for deterioration and, therefore, should be treated with open reduction and stabilization. Translation injuries in the lumbar spine are associated with significant deformities that can affect sitting balance. However, thoracic fracture dislocations may not have kyphotic deformity and are generally more stable. Bohlman and associates[38] found that paraplegic patients became "stable" after 4 to 6 weeks of bed rest and could then be mobilized. Thus, for patients with translation injuries, nonsurgical treatment is not indicated except in patients with upper thoracic injuries whose associated injuries preclude surgical stabilization.

Conclusion

Nonsurgical treatment is appropriate for the majority of patients with thoracolumbar injuries. This treatment is indicated for patients with stable fracture patterns and absence of neurologic injuries. An important goal in today's cost conscious health care system is early mobilization and hospital discharge. Orthoses decrease intersegmental range of motion and overall trunk motion but do not decrease axial loads across the intervertebral disks. To have maximum effect, the central point of the orthoses must be centered at the injury site. After placement of the orthoses, serial upright radiographs are assessed for fracture alignment. During healing, isometric trunk-strengthening exercises and aerobic training are performed so that the patient may have an early return to motion.

References

1. Adams F (ed): *The Genuine Works of Hippocrates.* Baltimore, MD, Williams & Wilkins, 1939, pp 231-243.
2. Böhler L (ed): *The Treatment of Fractures,* 4th ed (English), Groves EWH (translator). Baltimore MD, W Wood & Co, 1935.
3. Magnes G: Die Behandlung and Begutachtung von Wirbelbruchen. Munchener Medizinische Wochenschrift Jahrgang 76, Marz 1929.
4. Davis AG: Fractures of the spine. *J Bone Joint Surg* 1929;11:133-156.
5. Nicoll EA: Fractures of the dorso-lumbar spine. *J Bone Joint Surg* 1949;31B:376-394.
6. Marshall LF, Knowlton S, Garfin SR, et al: Deterioration following spinal cord injury: A multicenter study. *J Neurosurg* 1987;66:400-404.
7. Dickson JH, Harrington PR, Erwin WD: Results of reduction and stabilization of the severely fractured thoracic and lumbar spine. *J Bone Joint Surg* 1978;60A:799-805.
8. Flesch JR, Leider LL, Erickson DL, et al: Harrington instrumentation and spine fusion for unstable fractures and fracture-dislocations of the thoracic and lumbar spine. *J Bone Joint Surg* 1977;59A:143-153.
9. Jacobs RR, Asher MA, Snider RK: Thoracolumbar spinal injuries: A comparative study of recumbent and operative treatment in 100 patients. *Spine* 1980;5:463-477.
10. Schlegel J, Yuan H, Fredrickson B, et al: Timing of surgical decompression and fixation of acute spinal fractures. *Orthop Trans* 1992;16:688.
11. Bedbrook GM: Spinal injuries with teraplegia and paraplegia. *J Bone Joint Surg* 1979;61B:267-284.
12. Frankel HL, Hancock DO, Hyslop G, et al: The value of postural reduction in the initial management of closed injuries of the spine with paraplegia and tetraplegia: Part 1. *Paraplegia* 1969; 7:179-192.
13. Guttmann L: I. Organization of spinal units: History of the National Spinal Injuries Centre, Stoke Mandeville Hospital, Aylesbury. *Paraplegia* 1967;5:115-126.
14. Burke DC, Murray DD: The management of thoracic and thoracolumbar injuries of the spine with neurological involvement. *J Bone Joint Surg* 1976;58B:72-78.
15. Willén J, Lindahl S, Nordwall A: Unstable thoracolumbar fractures: A comparative clinical study of conservative treatment and Harrington instrumentation. *Spine* 1985;10:111-122.
16. Soreff J, Axdorph G, Bylond P, et al: Treatment of patients with unstable fractures of the thoracic and lumbar spine: A follow-up study of surgical and conservative treatment. *Acta Orthop Scand* 1982;53:369-381.
17. Krengel WF III, Anderson PA, Henley MB: Early stabilization and decompression for incomplete paraplegia due to a thoracic-level spinal cord injury. *Spine* 1993;18:2080-2087.
18. Edwards CC, Levine AM: Early rod-sleeve stabilization of the injured thoracic and lumbar spine. *Orthop Clin North Am* 1986; 17:121-145.
19. Kahmann RD, Bradford DS, Ogilvie JW, et al: Acute anterior decompression of thoracic and lumbar spine fractures with neurologic involvement. Presented at the 57th Annual Meeting of the American Academy of Orthopaedic Surgeons, New Orleans, LA, 1990, Paper No. 331, p 188.
20. Waters RL, Yakura JS, Adkins RH, et al: Recovery following complete paraplegia. *Arch Phys Med Rehabil* 1992;73:784-789.
21. Stauffer ES (ed): *Thoracolumbar Spine Fractures Without Neurologic Deficit.* Rosemont, IL, American Academy of Orthopaedic Surgeons, 1993.
22. Lantz SA, Schultz AB: Lumbar spine orthosis wearing. *Spine* 1986; 11:834-842.
23. Fidler MW, Plasmans CMT: The effect of four types of support on the segmental mobility of the lumbosacral spine. *J Bone Joint Surg* 1983;65A:943-947.
24. Norton PL, Brown T: The immobilizing efficiency of back braces: Their effect on the posture and motion of the lumbosacral spine. *J Bone Joint Surg* 1957;39A:111-139.
25. Nachemson A, Schultz AB, Andersson GBJ: Mechanical effectiveness of lumbar spine orthoses. *Scand J Rehab Med* 1983;(Suppl 9):139-149.
26. Nagel DA, Koogle TA, Piziali RL, et al: Stability of the upper lumbar spine following progressive disruptions and the application of individual internal and external fixation devices. *J Bone Joint Surg* 1981;63A:62-70.
27. Holdsworth F: Fractures, dislocations, and fracture-dislocations of the spine. *J Bone Joint Surg* 1970;52A:1534-1551.
28. Weitzman G: Treatment of stable thoracolumbar spine compression fractures by early ambulation. *Clin Orthop* 1971;76:116-122.
29. Young MH: Long-term consequences of stable fractures of the thoracic and lumbar vertebral bodies. *J Bone Joint Surg* 1973; 55B:295-300.
30. White AA III, Panjabi MM: The problem of clinical instability in the human spine: A systematic approach, in White AA III, Panjabi MM (eds): *Clinical Biomechanics of the Spine,* ed 2. Philadelphia, PA, JB Lippincott, 1990, pp 277-378.
31. Ahlgren SA, Hansen T: The use of lumbosacral corsets prescribed for low back pain. *Prosthet Orthot Int* 1978;2:101-104.
32. Patwardhan AG, Li SP, Gavin T, et al: Orthotic stabilization of thoracolumbar injuries: A biomechanical analysis of the Jewett hyperextension orthosis. *Spine* 1990;15:654-661.
33. Van Hanswyk EP, Yuan HA, Eckhardt WA: Orthotic management of thoraco-lumbar spine fractures with a "total-contact" TLSO. *Orthotics and Prosthetics* 1979;33:10-19.
34. Reid DC, Hu R, Davis LA, et al: The nonsurgical treatment of burst fractures of the thoracolumbar junction. *J Trauma* 1988; 28:1188-1194.
35. Cantor JB, Lebwohl NH, Garvey T, et al: Nonsurgical management of stable thoracolumbar burst fractures with early ambulation and bracing. *Spine* 1993;18:971-976.
36. Mumford J, Weinstein JN, Spratt KF, et al: Thoracolumbar burst fractures: The clinical efficacy and outcome of nonsurgical management. *Spine* 1993;18:955-970.
37. Watson-Jones R (ed): *Fractures and Joint Injuries,* ed 4. Baltimore, MD, Williams & Wilkins, 1955, vol 2.
38. Bohlman HH, Freehafer A, Dejak J: The results of treatment of acute injuries of the upper thoracic spine with paralysis. *J Bone Joint Surg* 1985;67A:360-369.

39. Hazel WA Jr, Jones RA, Morrey BF, et al: Vertebral fractures without neurological deficit: A long-term follow-up study. *J Bone Joint Surg* 1988;70A:1319-1321.
40. McAfee PC, Yuan HA, Fredrickson BE, et al: The value of computed tomography in thoracolumbar fractures: An analysis of one hundred consecutive cases and a new classification. *J Bone Joint Surg* 1983;65A:461-473.
41. Fredrickson BE, Yuan HA, Bayley JC: The nonsurgical treatment of thoracolumbar injuries. *Semin Spine Surg* 1990;2:70-78.
42. Denis F, Armstrong GWD, Searls K, et al: Acute thoracolumbar burst fractures in the absence of neurologic deficit: A comparison between operative and nonsurgical treatment. *Clin Orthop* 1984; 189:142-149.
43. Levine AM: The surgical treatment of low lumbar fractures. *Semin Spine Surg* 1990;2:41-53.
44. Cammisa FP Jr, Eismont FJ, Green BA: Dural laceration occurring with burst fractures and associated laminar fractures. *J Bone Joint Surg* 1989;71A:1044-1952.
45. An HS, Vaccaro A, Cotler JM, et al: Low lumbar burst fractures: Comparison among body cast, Harrington rod, Luque rod, and Steffee plate. *Spine* 1991;16(suppl 8):S440-S444.
46. Finn CA, Stauffer ES: Burst fracture of the fifth lumbar vertebra. *J Bone Joint Surg* 1992;74A:398-403.
47. Mick CA, Carl A, Sachs B, et al: Burst fractures of the fifth lumbar vertebra. *Spine* 1993;18:1878-1884.
48. Anderson PA, Henley MB, Rivara FP, et al: Flexion distraction and Chance injuries to the thoracolumbar spine. *J Orthop Trauma* 1991;5:153-160.
49. Anderson PA, Rivara FP, Maier RV, et al: The epidemiology of seatbelt-associated injuries. *J Trauma* 1991;31:60-67.
50. Glassman SD, Johnson JR, Holt RT: Seatbelt injuries in children. *J Trauma* 1992;33:882-886.
51. LeGay DA, Petrie DP, Alexander DI: Flexion-distraction injuries of the lumbar spine and associated abdominal trauma. *J Trauma* 1990;30:436-444.

CHAPTER 5

Treatment of Acute Injury of the Cervical Spine

Andrew V. Slucky, MD
Frank J. Eismont, MD

Acute injury of the cervical spine presents the treating physician with numerous diagnostic and management issues. Successful long-term treatment is contingent on early recognition of the injury, prompt resuscitation of the patient, stabilization of the injury, prevention of additional neurologic injury, and avoidance of complications.

The improvement of emergency medical procedures, including the education of pre-hospital personnel with an emphasis on the recognition and stabilization of spinal injury at the trauma scene, combined with the development of centers for the treatment of acute spinal-cord injuries, has proved to be of benefit in the management of patients who have such an injury.[1-5] Tator and associates[5,6] compared a regional group of 351 patients managed before and 201 patients managed after the establishment of a unit for the treatment of acute spinal-cord injuries. After the establishment of the unit, the proportion of complete spinal-cord injuries decreased from 65% to 46%, and overall mortality decreased from 20% to 9%. Similar results were reported by Meyer and Carle,[3] with the proportion of neurologically complete injuries decreasing from 50% to 39% after the development of the Midwest Regional Spinal Cord Injury Care System.[3,7]

The expense to society of spinal-cord injuries is overwhelming, with average hospitalization costs, in 1987 dollars, of $50,000 to $90,000 for patients who had low-level paraplegia and $170,000 to $250,000 for those who had high-level quadriplegia and were respirator-dependent.[1,8] The individual tragedy and the cost of lost productivity are immeasurable and underline the need for a systematic approach to the treatment of acute injuries of the cervical spine.

Epidemiology

The National Head and Spinal Cord Injury Statistical Center estimated that 14,000 spinal-cord injuries occur each year, with 10,000 individuals surviving the initial accident.[9-11] The reported annual incidence has varied, with most studies demonstrating a rate of 3.2 to 5.3 new spinal-cord injuries per 100,000 persons at risk in the United States.[11,12] The peak months of occurrence of the injury are the late spring and summer months.[13,14]

The injury has a bimodal distribution in terms of the age of occurrence, with the highest prevalence in people who are between 15 and 24 years of age and a second, smaller peak in people who are older than 55.[14] Spinal-cord injury is more frequent in boys and men than in girls and women, with several studies demonstrating variable male-to-female ratios ranging from 0.8:1 to 3.5:1, and there is a slightly higher prevalence in black people than in white people, a finding that is consistent with the higher accidental death rate observed among black people.[12,14]

The causes of spinal-cord injury vary regionally; however, with few exceptions, most spinal-cord injuries result from motor-vehicle accidents (42% to 56%), falls from a height (19% to 30%), gunshots (12% to 21%), and sports-related activities (6% to 7%) (primarily diving) (Table 1).[11,13,15] The mechanism of injury varies with age; motor-vehicle and water sports-related accidents account for most of the injuries in individuals who are younger than 30, while falls and gunshots are more common causes in individuals who are older than 35.[9] In recent years, gunshot wounds have accounted for an increasing number of spinal-cord injuries in younger patients.[16]

Table I
Causes of Spinal Cord Injury in Other Studies*

Cause of Injury	Kraus et al[11] (1975)	Fine et al[13] (1979)	Fife and Kraus[15]† (1986)	Total
Motor-vehicle accident	338 (56)	152 (42)	259 (47) [169]	749 (50)
Fall	116 (19)	106 (30)	120 (22) [64]	342 (23)
Gunshot wound	74 (12)	76 (21)	73 (13) [27]	223 (15)
Recreational accident	43 (7)	25 (7)	33 (6) [32]	101 (7)
Other	33 (5)	—	65 (12) [39]	98 (6)
Total	604 (100)	359 (100)	550 (100) [331]	1513 (100)

*The numbers in each column indicate the number of injuries in each study, with the percentage given in parentheses.
†The numbers in brackets indicate the number of patients who had an injury of the cervical spine.

The anatomic location of the spinal-cord injury bears a distinct relationship to the cause and mechanism of the injury. Fife and Kraus[15] reviewed the cause and anatomic location of 550 fatal and non-fatal spinal-cord injuries; 331 (60%) of these injuries involved the cervical spine (Table 1). Of 259 injuries sustained in a motor-vehicle accident, 169 (65%) involved the cervical spine; of 120 injuries sustained in a fall from a height, 64 (53%) were cervical injuries; and of 73 gunshot wounds, only 27 (37%) were cervical injuries. Although diving accidents accounted for less than 10% of the spinal-cord injuries, those injuries had the highest rate of involvement of the cervical spine (32 [97%] of 33 injuries). Within the cervical region, the greatest frequency of injury is at the level of the first cervical vertebra, followed by the fifth, sixth, and seventh cervical vertebrae.[15] Injuries from a motor-vehicle accident are most frequent at the levels of the first, fifth, sixth, and seventh cervical vertebrae, while injuries resulting from a fall or a diving accident predominantly involve the caudad cervical regions (the fifth, sixth, and seventh cervical vertebrae). Gunshot injuries have a random distribution. Given these findings, the mechanism of injury and the age of the patient should alert the physician to the probable level of the injury.

Pathophysiology

Injury Mechanism

The spinal cord is particularly prone to injury in the cervical region because of the coupling of a large mass, the head, to a lever arm of great flexibility, the cervical spine. The spinal cord is injured when the ligaments, muscles, and osseous structures between the skin and the spinal cord fail to dissipate the energy of impact.[17,18] The spinal cord can be injured directly, by means of excessive flexion, extension, rotation, or axial loading, or indirectly, by the impact of a displaced disk or bone fragments, or both. Fracture-dislocation is the most common cause of cervical spinal-cord injury;[19] however, the spinal cord also can be injured without radiographic evidence of injury to the vertebral column. This latter condition is called spinal-cord injury without radiographic abnormality, and it typically occurs in very young patients or in older individuals who have cervical spondylosis.[4]

The biomechanics of injury of the cervical spine have been studied extensively. Allen and associates[20] classified closed, indirect fracture-dislocations of the cervical spine into six groups that were based on the mechanism of injury: compressive flexion, distractive flexion, vertical compression, compressive extension, distractive extension, and lateral flexion. Each of these groups then was subdivided according to the severity of the injury on the basis of radiographic findings. White and associates[21] further defined cervical instability on the basis of disrupted anatomy, radiographic signs of malalignment (sagittal-plane translation, rotation, or distraction), clinical signs (spinal-cord or nerve-root damage), or the anticipation of dangerous loading after the injury (for example, in an interior lineman on a professional football team). Typically, unstable fracture patterns include bilateral facet dislocations, fracture-dislocations, or cervical vertebral fractures with more than 11.5° of angular rotation compared with adjacent levels, or 3.5 mm of sagittal translation, and clinical signs of injury of the medulla or of at least one nerve root.

The risk of spinal-cord injury with damage to cervical vertebrae is greater in individuals who have narrow spinal-canal diameters.[22,23] Patients who have a narrow midsagittal spinal-canal diameter have an increased chance of sustaining a severe neurologic injury in association with a given spinal fracture or dislocation, or both, compared with patients who have a larger midsagittal canal diameter.[22] Patients at risk include those who have cervical stenosis radiographically and who had an episode of neurapraxia in association with an event of axial compression of the cervical spine (for example, during a competitive dive from a 10-m height).[23] According to Torg and associates,[23] a patient has cervical stenosis when the ratio of the diameter of the cervical canal to the width of the cervical body is less than 0.8 as seen on the lateral radiograph.

Spinal-Cord Injury

Transmission of the energy of impact to the cervical spinal cord results in microhemorrhage in the central gray matter and loss of neuroconduction in the adjacent white matter. Following this primary injury event, there is a deleterious secondary-injury pattern that is characterized by a biochemical cascade that destabilizes the neurologic membrane of the axon, with a resultant progressive and heretofore irreversible pattern of spinal-cord cystic degeneration and neurolysis.[18,24-26]

There are two theories on how this spinal-cord lesion progresses. A *vascular theory* suggests that reduced or interrupted blood flow secondary to microvascular endothelial damage and thrombus formation results in ischemia in the central gray matter. The ischemia in the gray matter and an associated loss of vascular autoregulation contribute to ischemic changes in the adjacent white matter.[25,27-30] A *neuronal theory* postulates a traumatic distortion of the neurologic membrane of the axon at the instant of injury, with resultant paraplegia and the initiation of a secondary injury cascade.[31] This theory is supported by studies of focal blood flow in experimental animals that had functional paraplegia, which have shown increased post-injury blood flow to the lateral axon tracts of the white matter.[31,32]

Despite the uncertainty regarding the exact etiology, it is clear that the primary injury produces a complex cascade of metabolic abnormalities, which results in secondary injury to the neurologic tissues within minutes to hours after the initial insult (Fig. 1).[18,24-26] Within an ischemic environment, adenosine triphosphate stores are depleted, leading to an inactivation of calcium-dependent adenosine triphosphatase. This factor, as well as the fact that the neuronal membrane is depolarized by potassium and sodium fluxes following similar inactivation of the membrane-bound sodium and potassium adenosine triphosphatase pump, leads to an uncontrolled influx of calcium ions, with resultant uncoupling of mitochondrial oxidative phosphorylation, further loss of adenosine triphosphate production, and exacerbation of ischemia caused by local vasospasm.[18,26,33]

In addition, the uncontrolled influx of calcium ions promotes the activation of calcium-dependent phospholipase A_2, with resultant liberation of membrane phospholipid arachidonic acid, generation of free radicals, and peroxidation of membrane lipids, leading to membrane degradation.[26] Additional generation of free radicals occurs from hemorrhagic products, which release ferrous ions and hemoproteins into the cellular environment.

The primary cord injury leads to altered autonomic tone, loss of autoregulation, depressed cardiovascular function, and hypotension, thus promoting ischemia in the area of the injury.[18,26,30] Additionally, the inflammatory response to the injury, modulated by the migration of polymorphonuclear leukocytes and coupled with the generation of free radicals, contributes to further neuronal necrosis and edema.[25,34] After a spinal-cord injury has occurred, the current pharmacologic treatment is concerned with minimizing the deleterious effects of this secondary injury biochemical cascade.

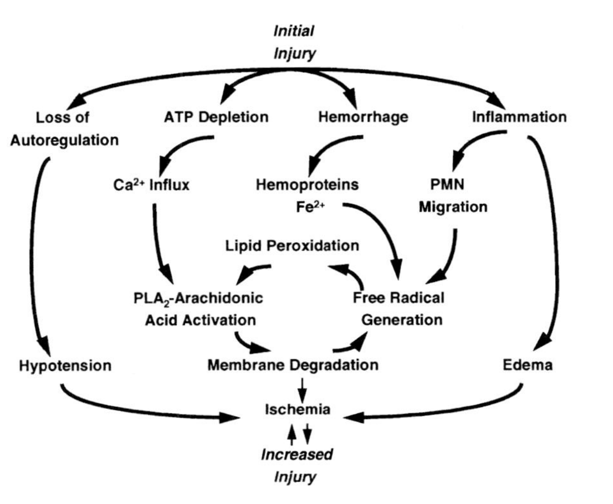

Fig. 1 Biochemical cascade effect following primary spinal-cord injury. ATP = adenosine triphosphate, PMN = polymorphonuclear leukocytes, and PLA_2 = phospholipase A_2.

Neurologic Classification

Spinal cord lesions are classified as complete or incomplete. A patient who has a complete cord injury has no sensory or motor function caudad to the level of the injury. If the lesion is complete and remains so for 48 hours, no return of sensation or motor function will occur.[35] In a review of the cases of 359 patients who had been managed consecutively at an acute spinal-cord-injury unit, Fine and associates[13] reported a neurologically complete lesion in 77 (46%) of 169 patients who had a cervical injury.

Anterior Cord Syndrome This is the loss of neurologic function in the anterior two-thirds of the spinal cord. Affected regions include the spinothalamic (pain and temperature) and corticospinal (motor function) tracts. Patients have complete loss of sharp pain and temperature sensation and of motor function, but they retain proprioception and the ability to sense vibration and deep pressure.[35,36] This syndrome usually is associated with a flexion injury, a fracture-dislocation, or a burst fracture. The prognosis is poor, with a chance of recovery of one nerve-root level of motor function and a minimum chance of a return of functional walking.[35,37,38] Preservation of the spinothalamic tract (retained pinprick sensation) conveys a better prognosis.[39]

Central Cord Syndrome This syndrome typically results from a hyperextension injury with pinching of the spinal cord between the ligamentum flavum and the intervertebral disk and posterior vertebral body bone spurs. Central cord injury and hemorrhage occur with compression of adjacent white-matter tracts. The syndrome is characterized by a mixed upper and lower-motor-neuron lesion, with flaccid paralysis of the upper extremities (indicative of involvement of the lower motor neurons) and spastic paralysis of the lower extremities (indicative of involvement of the upper motor neurons).[39] The more peripheral positioning of the lower extremity axons within the spinal cord tracts accounts for the injury pattern. The prognosis for recovery is fair; in one series, 23 (59%) of 39 patients achieved functional walking.[35]

Brown-Séquard Syndrome This syndrome results from hemitransection of the spinal cord with unilateral damage to the spinothalamic and corticospinal tracts and resultant loss of ipsilateral motor and dorsal column function and of contralateral pain and temperature sensation. Common injury mechanisms include penetrating trauma or unilateral facet fracture or dislocation. Little and Halar,[40] in a review of the literature, noted a substantial recovery of voluntary strength of the lower extremities and functional walking in 55 (93%) of 59 patients within a period of 6 months after the injury.

Posterior Cord Syndrome This rare syndrome is characterized by the loss of dorsal column function (deep pressure and proprioception). The prognosis is good, as motor function is preserved; however, walking is extremely difficult or impossible because of persistent impairment of proprioception.[35,39]

Cervical Root Syndrome This is an isolated deficit in a specific nerve root. It commonly is associated with acute disk protrusion or facet dislocation, often with associated vertebral-body rotation.[39]

The extent of a spinal-cord injury is classified according to functional criteria. The level of the injury is defined as the most caudad nerve root that innervates muscles that demonstrate at least antigravity strength, provided that the next cephalad level is normal. The classification system of Frankel and associates[41] subdivides injuries according to sensory loss and the amount of preserved motor function. The American Spinal Injury Association Motor Scale is based on a numeric strength score for specific bilateral motor groups of both the upper and the lower extremities and is the classification system most often recommended for current studies (Fig. 2).[42]

Immediate Patient Care

Accident Scene Management

The first step in the management of a patient who has an injury of the cervical spine is the recognition or suspicion of cervical injury. In a review of the cases of 300 patients who had been hospitalized because of an injury of the cervical spine, Bohlman[43] reported a delayed or missed diagnosis in 100 patients (33%). In another multiregional study, 33% of 371 patients who had an injury of the cervical spine were transferred from the field to the hospital with only a soft collar or no cervical immobilization.[44] Factors leading to delayed diagnosis have included concurrent head injury, an altered state of consciousness, and poor radiographic

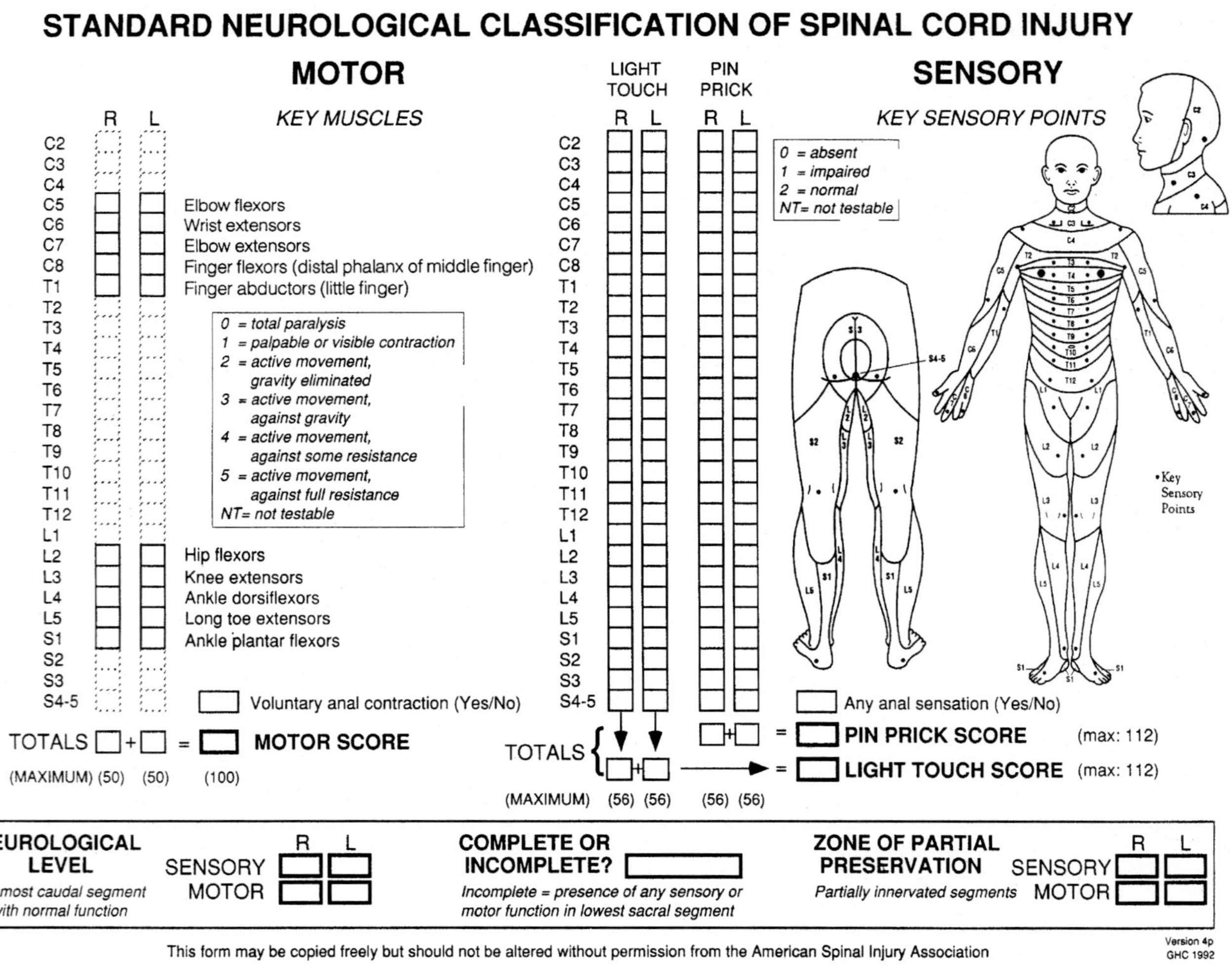

Fig. 2 Scoring diagram of the American Spinal Injury Association Motor Scale[42] for spinal-cord injury.

visualization in the hospital setting.[45] In many patients, multiple injuries may mask the spinal-cord injury; conversely, spinal-cord injury can mask other injuries, such as visceral rupture or long-bone fracture.[2,46]

Evaluation of the patient begins with general observation. Abrasions, lacerations, or deformities of the upper part of the thorax, neck, or head suggest that substantial force vectors were applied to the cervical region. Pain or tenderness should be evaluated only by palpation—not by movement—of the neck or spine.[2] An abbreviated neurologic examination should be specific for motor signs (weakness or paralysis of the extremities or trunk muscles), sensory signs (absence or alteration of sensation of the trunk or extremities), and incontinence (loss of control of the bladder or bowel, or both).[2] Patients who are unconscious or inebriated should be considered to have a spinal cord or spinal column injury until it has been proved otherwise.[2,45] Bohlman[43] noted that 14 of 100 patients who had a misdiagnosed cervical injury had been intoxicated due to alcohol or drugs. Other investigators have noted similar alcohol or drug involvement.[6,44,47]

With recognition of the potential for an injury of the cervical spine, primary treatment should then focus on the ABC's of resuscitation: airway, breathing, and circulation.

Airway and Breathing

An unobstructed airway is necessary in all patients. Aspiration of gastric contents and shock are the two most common causes of prehospital death in patients who have a spinal-cord injury.[48] In a patient who is awake, a standard cut-off oral airway or tongue-blade wrapped in tape will suffice. In a patient who is unconscious, a full standard oral airway or esophageal obturator should be inserted. In the event of emesis in the acute setting, the oral cavity should be suctioned until clear. The neck should never be moved out of position in order to establish an airway in any patient suspected of having a spinal injury.

If insertion of a device into the airway does not improve ventilation as determined by lung auscultation, the patient should be intubated. Use of an esophageal obturator (that is, pharyngeal intubation) or blind nasotracheal intubation is preferable at the accident scene because of the comparative ease of placement without the need to hyperextend the head or neck.[2,9] In the event of insufficient ventilation or respiratory excursion, artificial assistance should be initiated immediately. Paralysis of intercostal muscles or diaphragm muscles, or both; atelectasis; aspiration; and chest trauma all act to compromise ventilation.

Patients who have a spinal-cord injury should receive supplemental oxygen at all times during the acute-care and transportation sequence. The physiologic effects of cervical spinal-cord injury, including the loss of sympathetic tone, bradycardia, hypotension, and decreased respiratory excursion, all act to compromise oxygenation despite the appearance of adequate breathing. Uncorrected hypoxia further compounds the localized ischemia at the level of the cord injury.[49,50] In the acutely injured patient, the goal should be to maintain a minimum PaO_2 of at least 100 torr (13.3 kPa) and a $PaCO_2$ of less than 45 torr (6.0 kPa).[2,51]

Circulation and Shock

Active bleeding should be controlled with direct pressure. Objects that have penetrated the head or neck should not be removed until the patient is in a more controlled, hospital setting. If necessary, a penetrating object may be shortened at the point of entry, with great care taken not to manipulate the object or the head or neck.

The maintenance of adequate circulation and cardiac function is essential and minimizes secondary spinal-cord injury.[49,50,52] In specific instances of asystole or arrhythmia, manual cardiopulmonary resuscitation and defibrillation is necessary to maintain adequate cardiac and neurologic perfusion.[2] Care must be taken to avoid manipulation of the neck during ventilation attempts.[53]

Depending on the associated injuries, patients who have a spinal-cord injury may be in neurogenic shock or hemorrhagic shock, or both. Both types of shock are characterized by hypotension and decreased body temperature. The keys to differentiation of the two types are the rate and character of the pulse. Bradycardia (a pulse of less than 60 beats per minute) and a regular pulse are characteristic of neurogenic shock, while tachycardia (a pulse of more than 100 beats per minute) and an irregular pulse are indicative of hemorrhagic shock.[2]

Neurogenic shock associated with a cervical spinal-cord injury is due to the loss of peripheral sympathetic vascular tone, with resultant pooling of blood in the extremities and inadequate central venous return. Bradycardia results from a loss of sympathetic stimulation, which allows the parasympathetic effects of the vagus nerve to predominate. Patients in neurogenic shock typically have a systolic blood pressure of 70 mm Hg (9.3 kPa) or less and a pulse of less than 60 beats per minute.

Resuscitation from neurogenic shock begins with the placement of the patient in the Trendelenburg position, which immediately reduces pooling of peripheral blood and increases central venous return. Such positioning also reduces the chance of aspiration of gastric contents with emesis. A pneumatic counterpressure suit also can be used to complement central venous return, provided that the application of the suit does not compromise the positioning of the spine.[51,54] Intravenous administration of atropine (0.4 mg) helps to block the dominant vagal effects causing the bradycardia. The overriding consideration must be to maintain perfusion to the vital organs, including the spinal cord, during the early minutes or hours after the injury.[2] Fluid resuscitation must proceed with caution, because blood volume is sufficient in patients in neurogenic shock, which is instead a problem with blood distribution. The administration of a large volume of intravenous fluid in an attempt to increase central venous return may cause congestive heart failure.

Immobilization and Extrication

After medical stabilization, acute-care efforts should be directed toward immobilization of the injured spine, preferably before the removal of the patient from the injury scene (for example, from the water after a diving injury). Regardless of the posture in which the patient was found after the accident, the patient should be placed in a neutral supine position and a splint should be applied from the top of the head to the bottom of the buttocks.[2] When the patient is being moved, the head must be held in neutral position with respect to the long axis of the body, and great care must be taken to avoid flexion, extension, or rotation of the neck. Very gentle traction can be applied, with the hands of the rescue worker locked under the jaw and neck of the patient to help move the head into the neutral body plane. Once the neck is in neutral position, a cervical collar can be placed for additional support. Recently developed two-piece cervical collars allow placement without undue motion of the neck. Traction with weights should not be used in the field because of the risk of overdistraction of certain cervical injuries. Once in neutral position, the patient is ready for transfer to a rigid splint (backboard). Previously advocated transfer maneuvers, including the log-roll or four-man lift, are discouraged. Recent cadaveric and human studies have demonstrated that such transfers do not offer any marked degree of stability.[55] Currently, it is recommended that a scoop-style stretcher be used to lift and transfer the patient to a backboard, with both elements then being secured for complete support. The head and neck then are stabilized with sandbags. The thorax and extremities are secured with straps, with care being taken not to compromise respiratory excursion. When a patient who has an injury of the spinal cord is to be moved, the most important factors are the evaluation at the accident scene and the development of an organized extrication plan.[2]

Transportation

As with all critical-care transport, emphasis should be placed on life support and on the stability of the patient as opposed to unwarranted rapid transport. Patients should be transported in the Trendelenburg position to maximize cardiovascular function and to avoid aspiration of gastric contents with emesis.[48] In the ambulance, the patient should be positioned with the feet facing forward so as to avoid inadvertent cervical injury from the forward momentum of a sudden stop.

Selection of the transport vehicle depends on a combination of factors: patient stability, equipment availability, and the logistics of time, distance, weather, and local conditions. Recommended guidelines are as follows: use of an ambulance for distances of less than 50 miles (81 km), although a helicopter may be used at peak traffic periods or when associated injuries require more rapid transport; use of a helicopter for distances of between 50 and 150 miles (81 and 242 km); and use of a fixed-wing aircraft for distances of more than 150 miles (242 km).[39] Before prolonged transport, the placement of intravenous lines, a nasogastric tube, and a Foley catheter is recommended.[2,39]

The selection of hospital destination is contingent on patient stability. For patients who have concurrent destabilizing injuries, transport to the nearest emergency facility is necessary for resuscitation, stabilization, and immobilization. Secondary transport to an appropriate facility then should be initiated as soon as possible. It is recommended that patients in whom the spinal-cord injury is physiologically stable be transferred directly to a level-I trauma center or a similar tertiary-care facility within a reasonable transport distance (that is, one that is less than 1 hour away).[7,18]

Hospital Management

Resuscitation

On arrival at the appropriate emergency facility, the respiratory and circulatory status of the patient must be reevaluated. For patients who have concurrent injuries of the cervical spine and spinal cord, peripheral or central venous access should be obtained. The levels of blood gases and electrolytes and the hematocrit should be evaluated and corrected as necessary. A nasogastric tube and a Foley catheter should be inserted. Appropriate respiratory and cardiovascular support should be initiated to maintain adequate systemic and spinal-cord perfusion.

Assessment and Physical Examination

After resuscitation and stabilization, a thorough assessment and complete physical examination of the patient should be carried out. Particular attention should be directed toward the accident history, the mechanism of injury, and any change in the condition of the patient during transport. The detailed neurologic examination must include an assessment of cranial nerve function, sensory and motor function, and rectal tone, as well as testing of reflexes, including the bulbocavernosus reflex.

Spinal shock represents a condition of altered spinal-cord conduction with transient loss of all motor, sensory, and reflex function caudad to the level of the injury; it can persist for 48 hours and occasionally longer. The definitive neurologic status cannot be assessed until the cessation of spinal shock. The return of a bulbocavernosus or anal wink reflex signals the end of spinal shock and allows an accurate classification of the neurologic injury.

An accurate physical examination cannot be performed for an unconscious patient. In this situation, suspicion of an injury of the cervical spine must be confirmed by radiographic evaluation.

Radiographic Examination

The evaluation of a patient who has had cervical trauma should follow an orderly progression of diagnostic steps (Fig. 3). Radiographic examination of the cervical spine is indicated for all alert, sober patients who have neck pain or tenderness; for patients who have a neurologic deficit, polytrauma, or craniofacial injuries; and for all inebriated or unconscious patients who have sustained trauma.[56-58] The standard radiographic study is the five-view series, in which lateral, anteroposterior, odontoid, and right and left oblique radiographs are made. The lateral radiograph should be made first, as an initial assessment. A standard target-to-film distance of 72 inches (183 cm) eliminates magnification distortion. Every attempt must be made to visualize the entire lateral part of the cervical spine to the cervicothoracic junction. A substantial number of patients who have an injury of the cervical spine demonstrate additional fractures at other levels of the cervical spine.[59] When the cervicothoracic junction cannot be seen on the routine lateral radiograph, a so-called swimmer's (Twinning) radiograph will allow evaluation of the cervicothoracic junction.[60] Additional radiographs of the thoracic spine, the lumbar spine, and extremities in which an injury is suspected should be made for all patients who have multiple injuries, who are unconscious, or who have neurologic compromise. In one review, 39 (10%) of 372 consecutive patients had noncontiguous vertebral injuries, typically at the cervicothoracic or thoracolumbar juncture.[61] Patients who have a spinal-cord injury often have concurrent osseous injury.[9,51,62] Soderstrom and Brumback[51] reported the additional diagnosis of a thoracic, pelvic, or long-bone fracture in 87 (21%) of 408 patients who had cervical spine trauma.

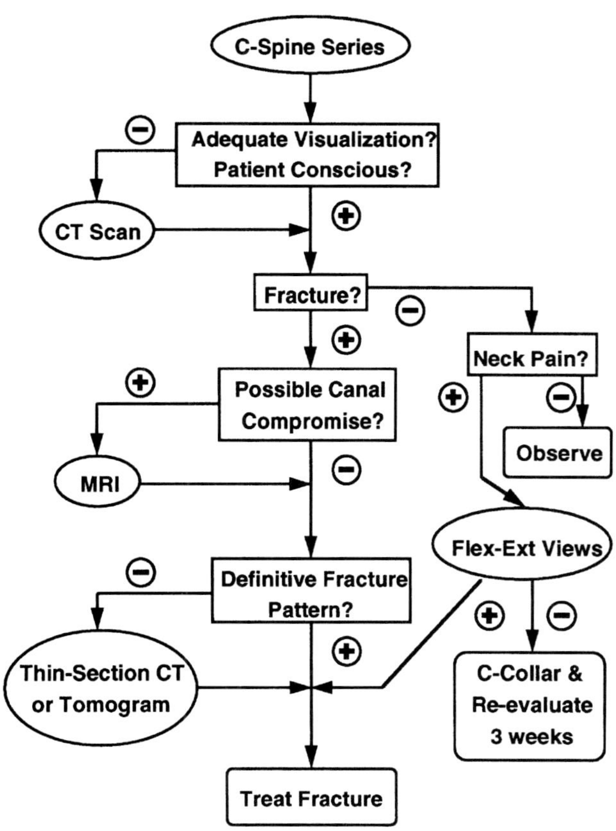

Fig. 3 Diagram of diagnostic steps to be taken in the evaluation of cervical trauma. C = cervical, CT = computed tomography, and MRI = magnetic resonance imaging.

Computed Tomography

If available, a computed tomographic scan is warranted for an unconscious patient and for a patient who has suspicious or inadequate cervical radiographic findings. The standard tomographic evaluation includes 5-mm sections in a spiral format. Suspect areas on standard radiographs should be evaluated with a high-resolution, thin-section (2 to 3-mm), nonspiral format to minimize the image-averaging artefact. Thin-section acquisition also allows for sagittal reconstruction in select patients.[18,58]

Magnetic Resonance Imaging

In recent years, because of improved technique and availability, magnetic resonance imaging (MRI) has played an expanding role in the assessment of acute injuries of the cervical spine. The advantages of MRI include excellent visualization of spinal soft-tissue structures and clear definition of canal compromise, when it exists, as well as demonstration of areas of hemorrhage and extraspinal soft-tissue edema.[58,63,64] In addition, studies have shown a direct relationship of the pathological characteristics of spinal-cord injury with image changes seen on MRI.[64,65]

The disadvantages of MRI include its limited availability, high expense, poor resolution due to motion of the patient (typically due to coughing by a patient who has respiratory compromise), and the requirement of compatible (nonferrous) equipment (such as graphite Gardner-Wells tongs) and shielded cardiac-monitoring devices.

MRI is indicated for patients who have a complete or incomplete neurologic deficit, for assessment of the degree of spinal-cord compression; for patients whose neurologic status has deteriorated; and for patients in whom there is a suspicion of disk retropulsion with canal compromise or possible posterior ligamentous injury (Fig. 4).[66] Several studies have demonstrated the

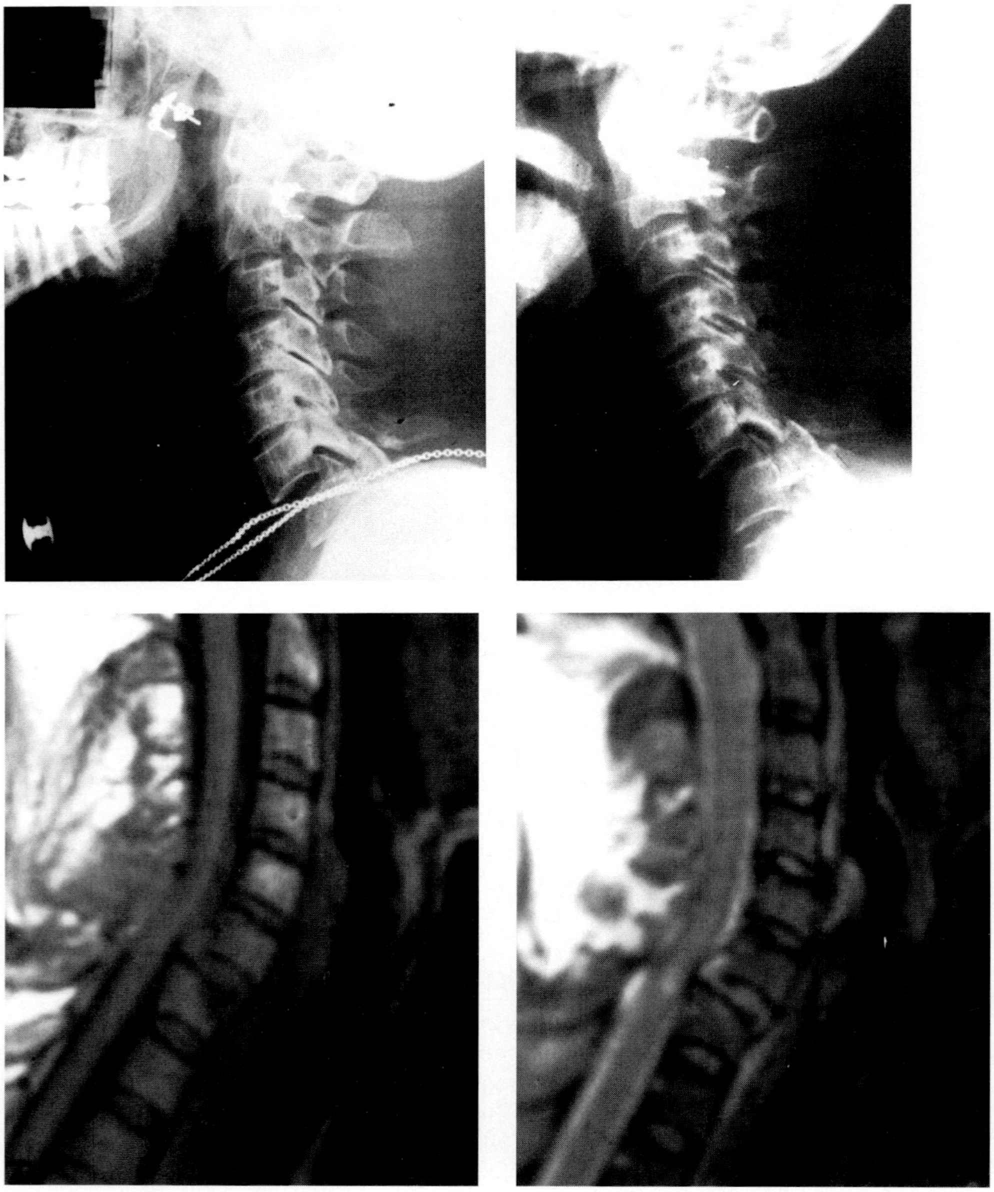

Fig. 4 A 65-year-old woman fell and struck her head after a syncopal episode. The patient was seen in the emergency room because of bilateral weakness and paresthesias of the upper extremity. Physical examination showed weakness (grade 3 of 5) of the triceps, wrist flexors, finger extensors and flexors, and intrinsic muscles of both hands. The strength of the other muscles in the arms and lower extremities was normal. The lower extremities were hyperreflexic. **Top left,** Lateral cervical radiograph demonstrating a unilateral dislocation of the sixth and seventh facets. **Top right,** Lateral radiograph made with the patient in traction. T1-weighted (**bottom left**) and T2-weighted (**bottom right**) mid-sagittal MRI demonstrating herniated disk material behind the body of the sixth cervical vertebra.

herniation of intervertebral disks in association with fracture or dislocation, or both, and subsequent catastrophic compression of the spinal cord during reduction and realignment.[67,68] This problem is associated with such injuries as facet dislocations (unilateral or bilateral) and flexion-compression patterns. MRI is contraindicated for patients who have a pacemaker, aneurysm clips, metallic fragments in the eye or spinal cord, or severe claustrophobia.[66]

Tomograms

Tomograms can be used to evaluate patients who have a slightly displaced horizontal fracture of the odontoid process, to assess the extent of a facet or a lateral mass injury, or as a complement to thin-section computed tomographic sagittal reconstructions.

Flexion-Extension Radiographs

Flexion-extension radiographs are useful in the evaluation of patients who have neck pain despite normal neurologic and plain radiographic findings. Flexion-extension radiographs for these patients should be made under the supervision of a physician, with the patient moving the head and neck through a pain-free range of motion. No attempt at forced motion should be made. If these radiographs are normal, it is recommended that the patient be managed with a cervical collar and reevaluated with flexion-extension radiographs after three weeks; Herkowitz and Rothman[69] reported on several patients who had a late onset of cervical instability despite initially normal radiographic findings.

Immobilization and Realignment

In patients who have instability of the cervical spine, initial immobilization is achieved with skeletal traction. Gardner-Wells tongs that are compatible with MRI are applied 1 cm above the tips of the ears and in line with the external auditory meatus. Shaving of the skin is not necessary. After placement of the tongs, the patient is transferred to a rotating bed (Rotorest; Kinetic Concepts, San Antonio, Texas) by means of the transport backboard. Ten pounds (4.5 kg) of weight then is gently applied to the tongs, with close attention being paid to the maintenance of neutral alignment of the head and neck. The patient must be monitored closely for any change in neurologic condition. Post-traction alignment must be confirmed immediately by a lateral radiograph. Overdistraction should be avoided.

Closed reduction should be attempted for all patients who have an injury of the cervical spine associated with malalignment.[41,66] Before reduction, the injury mechanism must be assessed. Certain injury patterns, particularly facet dislocations, frequently are accompanied by marked disk herniation into the anterior part of the spinal canal. In patients who have such an injury, catastrophic compression of the spinal cord can result from an uncontrolled facet reduction. Eismont and associates[67] reported intervertebral disk herniation with marked protrusion of disk material into the spinal canal in six (9%) of 68 patients who had subluxation or dislocation of a cervical facet. MRI is recommended for such patients before reduction or surgical intervention is attempted.

Reduction must be done under the supervision of a physician, with close monitoring of the neurologic and radiographic status of the patient, preferably when the patient is awake and alert. Skeletal traction, patient positioning, and postural bumps assist in reduction. Traction weight is added incrementally, with radiographs being made after each addition. As a general rule, 10 lb (4.5 kg) is added for the occiput, and an additional 5 lb (2.3 kg) for each vertebra to the level of the injury (for example, a fracture at the level of the fifth cervical vertebra would require 35 lb [15.8 kg] of traction). The maximum amount of traction weight that can be applied safely is unknown.[66] Generally, as much as 20 lb (9.1 kg) can be applied in the upper cervical region (first and second cervical vertebrae) and as much as 50 lb (22.5 kg) can be applied in the lower cervical region (third through seventh cervical vertebrae) with close supervision;[70] however, some authors have recommended that a much greater force be used.[71] Attempts at closed reduction should be discontinued when reduction is achieved, when more than 1 cm of distraction occurs at the site of the injury or at any other level, when the neurologic status of the patient deteriorates, or when it is evident that reduction cannot be achieved safely with this method.[66] Once reduction has been achieved, the traction weight can be reduced to 20 lb (9.1 kg) or less to maintain alignment.[66]

Pharmacologic Treatment

Recently, clinical studies have demonstrated the potential benefits of pharmacologic treatment as an adjunct to the principles of stabilization and reduction of a spinal injury. The treatment is directed toward interruption of the pathway of the secondary injury mechanism associated with spinal-cord damage.

Methylprednisolone

Numerous animal studies and a multicenter clinical trial of 487 patients have demonstrated the benefit of high-dose methylprednisolone in the treatment of acute spinal-cord injury.[72-75] Its mechanisms of action are believed to be the reduction of edema, an anti-inflammatory effect, and the protection of neuronal membranes by the scavenging of oxygen free radicals.[76] Bracken and associates,[74] in the multicenter National Acute Spinal Cord Injury Study (Phase 2), at the time of follow-up 6 months after the treatment, reported improvement in the motor scores of 47 patients who had an incomplete motor lesion and who had been managed within 8 hours after the injury with high-dose methylprednisolone compared with those of similar patients who had been managed with naloxone (37 patients) or a placebo (46 patients). No significant difference was noted between treatment groups, consisting of 337 patients, managed 8 hours after the injury. Complications after treatment with steroids included an increased, although not significantly so, prevalence of wound infection (8%, 3%, and 4% for patients given methylprednisolone, naloxone, and placebo, respectively [$p = 0.21$]) and gastrointestinal hemorrhage (5%, 2%, and 3% for patients given methylprednisolone, naloxone, and placebo, respectively [$p = 0.44$]). Criticisms of the study have included the lack of control for subsequent surgical intervention in the long-term follow-up period, stratification of the patient population, use of summed motor scores, and absence of functional assessment with respect to improvement in motor scores.[77] In a subsequent review of the data after a 1-year follow-up interval, Young and Bracken[78] addressed several of the shortcomings of the design. At 1 year, the number of surgical approaches and overall patient mortality did not significantly differ among the three treatment groups. At 6 weeks after the injury, the odds ratio for patients who had been managed with methylprednisolone to improve from one motor category to a better one was 2.04 (95% confidence interval, 0.81 to 5.21).[74] At 1 year after the injury, the probability of improved motor function was greater in patients who had been managed with methylprednisolone (odds ratio, 1.29; 95% confidence interval, 0.64 to 3.03) than in patients who had received a placebo.[78] Separate analysis of the lumbosacral segments revealed significantly improved motor scores (11.8%; 95% confidence interval, 2.9% to 25.5%) for the patients who had received methylprednisolone within 8 hours compared with those of the patients who had received a placebo. These results suggest that the beneficial effects of methylprednisolone were not limited to segments close to the site of the injury.

Despite uncertainty regarding the ultimate role of high-dose methylprednisolone in the treatment of cervical spine injuries, the current recommendation is intravenous administration of a bolus of 30 mg/kg of body weight over 15 minutes, followed by an infusion of 5.4 mg/kg of body weight per hour for 23 hours for all patients who are managed within 8 hours after blunt trauma involving the spinal cord.

GM-1 Ganglioside

Gangliosides are complex acidic glycolipids that are present in high concentration in the cells of the central nervous system; they form a major component of the cell membrane, predominantly in the outer leaflet of the lipid bilayer of the membrane.[79,80] In a small prospective, randomized, placebo-controlled clinical trial, the administration of GM-1 ganglioside was shown to markedly enhance neurologic motor function at a 1-year follow-up.[79] Thirty-four patients were given either 100 mg of GM-1 ganglioside or a placebo intravenously each day for 18 to 32 days, with the first dose being taken within 72 hours after the injury. All patients also received a bolus of 250 mg of methylprednisolone followed by intravenous administration of 125 mg of methylprednisolone every 6 hours for 72 hours. The improvement was attributed to the return of useful motor strength to initially paralyzed muscles rather than to the strengthening of paretic muscles. This finding was derived from studies of experimental injuries in which an increase in axonal survival, from less than 3% to more than 6%, at the site of the injury allowed neurologic function to return caudad to the site of the injury (that is, paralyzed muscles regained normal movement).[81] It has been postulated that the mechanism of GM-1 ganglioside is the facilitation of neurite growth, the attenuation of retrograde neurologic degeneration, the modulation of glutamate-mediated endotoxicity and protein-kinase activity, or a combination of these actions.[79,80,82] Studies of larger patient populations are planned.[79]

A controversial issue is the concurrent use of GM-1 ganglioside and high-dose methylprednisolone in the acute setting. Recent studies have demonstrated that GM-1 ganglioside induces a blockade of the lipocortin-mediated anti-inflammatory effects of high-dose methylprednisolone.[82] Additional investigations, of the use of interval dosing to maximize the acute injury protective effects of high-dose methylprednisolone and the potential neuronal recovery effects of GM-1 ganglioside, are warranted.

21-Aminosteroids (Tirilizad Mesylate-U74006F)

Clinical trials of 21-aminosteroid compounds are currently in progress. This is a group of methylprednisolone analogs without the 11-beta-hydroxyl function that is known to be essential for glucocorticoid-receptor binding.[83] The presumed mechanism of action is through an anti-oxidant protective effect. These drugs lack the drawbacks of the glucocorticoid-modulated systemic effects.[84] Many studies of animals that had an acute spinal-cord injury have shown a substantial neuroprotective effect, with a greater anti-oxidant efficacy than is achieved with high-dose methylprednisolone.[83,85-87]

Naloxone and Thyrotropin-Releasing Hormone

Both naloxone and thyrotropin-releasing hormone are opiate-receptor antagonists. The theoretic benefit of the compounds is the blockade of the release of endogenous spinal-cord opioids with a reversal of injury-induced systemic hypotension and its coupled decrease in spinal-cord blood flow. Despite controversial success in animal studies, the inclusion of naloxone in the National Acute Spinal Cord Injury Study (Phase 2), demonstrated no apparent clinical benefit.[72-74,78] Recent work with other opiate receptors has suggested that kappa receptor-mediated mechanisms may be protective of spinal cord blood flow after an acute spinal-cord injury.[88,89]

Thyrotropin-releasing hormone is a pituitary tripeptide that has many physiologic effects, including the ability to act in vivo as a partial physiologic opiate antagonist. Thyrotropin-releasing hormone differs pharmacologically from naloxone in that it does not act as an opiate receptor and it reverses opioid autonomic and behavioral effects while maintaining opioid analgesic effects.[90] In several animal models, thyrotropin-releasing hormone and associated analogs have been shown to improve neurologic recovery from experimental spinal-cord injury, suggesting that it has therapeutic clinical potential.[91,92]

Other Pharmacologic Agents

Vitamin E Preinjury treatment with vitamin E (alpha tocopherol) has been shown to reduce morbidity after a spinal-cord injury in experimental models.[93] The presumed mechanism of action is through an anti-oxidation effect and phospholipid membrane stabilization. Clinical shortcomings include the need for preinjury treatment, thus limiting the benefit in the treatment of acute injuries.

Calcium-Channel Blockers The benefit of calcium- channel agents with regard to posttraumatic spinal-cord ischemia is controversial. The presumed mechanism of action is through stabilization of postinjury calcium influx, minimizing the deleterious calcium-modulated elements of the secondary injury cascade. Numerous calcium-channel blockers (nifedipine, nimodopine, and flunarizine) have decreased posttraumatic spinal-cord ischemia in some models[94,95] and not in others.[96,97]

Osmotic Diuretics Despite experimental success with these edema-reducing agents, including mannitol, glycerol, and low-molecular- weight dextran, there has been no compelling evidence of clinical effectiveness with regard to posttraumatic spinal-cord ischemia.[25,26]

Physical Approaches

Hypothermia

Cooling of traumatized spinal-cord segments has been shown to be of some benefit.[26,98,99] A combined review of 11 clinical trials demonstrated that 28 (45%) of 62 patients who had an injury of the spinal cord with no motor or sensory sparing had neurologic improvement and ten (16%) regained the ability to walk.[98] These results can be compared with the historically poor results of conventional treatment, in which only 2% to 10% of patients who had a complete injury on presentation exhibited substantial distal motor function after the period of spinal shock.[35,37,100] However, the clinical results of cord-cooling have been clouded by the concurrent use of steroids in many of the studies. The theoretic mechanism of action of cord-cooling is a local decrease of spinal cord metabolism and oxygen consumption, with a resultant reduction of edema and the blockade of the secondary injury biochemical cascade. Mathematic modeling studies have suggested that additional benefit is derived from cerebrospinal fluid convection within injured spinal levels.[101]

Controversy exists with regard to the degree and duration of cooling that is required for benefit. Recent experimental studies have demonstrated moderate temperature decreases of 1° to 3° C to be of value.[99]

Cooling has serious disadvantages: the need for acute surgical intervention in a traumatized patient, the need for a wide multilevel laminectomy and prolonged surgical exposure, and the technical difficulties inherent in the currently available cooling devices.[25,98,99] At this time, the clinical role of cord-cooling is experimental.

Indications for Acute Surgical Treatment

The value of late surgical decompression of cervical spine nerves has been well documented in the literature.[70,102] The role of acute surgical decompression (within 48 hours after the injury) is more controversial and less clear. The theoretic benefits include removal of mechanical compression, correction of malalignment, and improved neurologic circulation. Opponents think that the maximum damage to the cervical spinal cord occurs at the time of the injury and with the secondary injury biochemical cascade, and that no substantial benefit can be achieved by acute surgical intervention.[103,104]

In a recent multicenter study, neurologic deterioration was noted in four of 26 patients who had had surgery within 5 days after a spinal-cord injury, but in none of the 108 patients who had had an operation after the fifth day.[105] In 44 patients who had been managed consecutively because of a cervical injury, Wagner and Chehrazi[106] noted no difference in long-term neurologic recovery whether decompression had been early (within 8 hours after the injury) or late (9 to 48 hours after the injury).

Current recommendations for the treatment of acute injuries of the cervical spinal cord stress patient resuscitation, immobilization, and skeletal traction for fracture reduction and alignment. In our experience, approximately 40% of these injuries have been most appropriately treated nonsurgically. Surgical treatment plays a role in decompression and stabilization in the elective setting, after patient stabilization. Most surgeons would agree that an absolute indication for emergent surgical intervention is progressive neurologic deterioration in the presence of irreducible canal compromise.[107] Other relative indications for an operation include a stable neurologic deficit with irreducible canal compromise, an incomplete lesion with initial improvement and a subsequent early plateau, and grossly unstable osseous or ligamentous injury patterns. A contraindication to surgical treatment is deteriorating neurologic status without evidence of canal compromise; this condition suggests irreversible ascending necrosis of the cord.[43]

Future Directions

Future research trends in the treatment of spinal-cord injury include efforts at blocking the secondary injury biochemical cascade, direct manipulation of central nervous-system regeneration and plasticity, and enhancement of neuronal function after the injury. Numerous efforts are underway with regard to axonal regeneration[61,108] and neurologic tissue transplantation.[108-112] For example, the ability of 4-aminopyridine to enhance conduction in demyelinated nerve fibers in patients who have chronic spinal-cord injury recently has been documented.[113-115]

Despite encouraging research and improvements in treatment, successful treatment of cervical spinal-cord injuries rests with prevention. Public awareness campaigns, injury-prevention programs, promotion of automotive safety devices, and civil legislation with regard to seat-belt laws, alcohol abuse, and gun-control enforcement are the most effective ways to reduce the costs, to the individual and society, of this devasting injury.

References

1. De Vivo MJ, Kartus PL, Stover SL, et al: Benefits of early admission to an organised spinal cord injury care system. *Paraplegia* 1990;28:545-555.
2. Green BA, Eismont FJ, O'Heir JT: Pre-hospital management of spinal cord injuries. *Paraplegia* 1987;25:229-238.
3. Meyer PR, Carle TV: Midwestern Regional Spinal Cord Injury Care System. Northwestern University and Rehabilitation Institute of Chicago Progress Report No. 9. Chicago, Northwestern University, 1980.
4. Tator CH: Spine-spinal cord relationships in spinal cord trauma. *Clin Neurosurg* 1983;30:479-494.
5. Tator CH, Duncan EG, Edmonds VE, et al: Abstract: Demographic analysis of 552 patients with acute spinal cord injury in Ontario, Canada, from 1948 to 1981. *Paraplegia* 1988;26:112-113.
6. Tator CH, Duncan EG, Edmonds VE, et al: Changes in epidemiology of acute spinal cord injury from 1947 to 1981. *Surg Neurol* 1993;40:207-215.
7. Gunby I: New focus on spinal cord injury. *JAMA* 1981;245:1201-1206.
8. Whiteneck GG, Menter RR, Charlifue SW, et al: Abstract: Initial and long-term costs of spinal cord injury. *Paraplegia* 1988;26:135.
9. Garfin SR, Shackford SR, Marshall LF, et al: Care of the multiply injured patient with cervical spine injury. *Clin Orthop* 1989;239:19-29.
10. Kalsbeek WD, McLaurin RL, Harris BS III, et al: The national head and spinal cord injury survey: Major findings. *J Neurosurg* 1980;53(suppl):S19-S31.
11. Kraus JF, Franti CE, Riggins RS, et al: Incidence of traumatic spinal cord lesions. *J Chronic Dis* 1975;28:471-492.
12. Stover SL, Fine PR: The epidemiology and economics of spinal cord injury. *Paraplegia* 1987;25:225-228.
13. Fine PR, Kuhlemeier KV, DeVivo MJ, et al: Spinal cord injury: An epidemiologic perspective. *Paraplegia* 1979;17:237-250.
14. Kraus JF: A comparison of recent studies on the extent of the head and spinal cord injury problem in the United States. *J Neurosurg* 1980;53(suppl):S35-S43.
15. Fife D, Kraus J: Anatomic location of spinal cord injury: Relationship to the cause of injury. *Spine* 1986;11:2-5.
16. Capen DA, Nelson RW, Nagelberg S, et al: Etiology of spinal cord injuries: Significant changes over ten years. *Orthop Trans* 1994;17:1035.
17. Bunegin L, Hung TK, Chang GL: Biomechanics of spinal cord injury. *Crit Care Clin* 1987;3:453-470.
18. Sonntag VK, Douglas RA: Management of cervical spinal cord trauma. *J Neurotrauma* 1992;9(suppl 1):S385-S396.
19. Riggins RS, Kraus JF: The risk of neurologic damage with fractures of the vertebrae. *J Trauma* 1977;17:126-133.
20. Allen BL Jr, Ferguson RL, Lehmann TR, et al: A mechanistic classification of closed, indirect fractures and dislocations of the lower cervical spine. *Spine* 1982;7:1-27.
21. White AA, Southwick WO, Panjabi MM: Clinical instability in the lower cervical spine: A review of past and current concepts. *Spine* 1976;1:15-27.
22. Eismont FJ, Clifford S, Goldberg M, et al: Cervical sagittal spinal canal size in spine injury. *Spine* 1984;9:663-666.
23. Torg JS, Pavlov H, Genuario SE, et al: Neurapraxia of the cervical spinal cord with transient quadriplegia. *J Bone Joint Surg* 1986; 68A:1354-1370.
24. Bauer RD, Errico TJ, Waugh TR, et al: Evaluation and diagnosis of cervical spine injuries: A review of the literature. *Cent Nerv Sys Trauma* 1987;4:71-93.
25. de la Torre JC: Spinal cord injury: Review of basic and applied research. *Spine* 1981;6:315-335.
26. Janssen L, Hansebout RR: Pathogenesis of spinal cord injury and newer treatments: A review. *Spine* 1989;14:23-32.
27. Collins WF, Piepmeier J, Ogle E: The spinal cord injury problem: A review. *Cent Nerv Syst Trauma* 1986;3:317-331.
28. Nelson E, Gertz SD, Rennels ML, et al: Spinal cord injury: The role of vascular damage in the pathogenesis of central hemorrhagic necrosis. *Arch Neurol* 1977;34:332-333.
29. Senter HJ, Venes JL: Loss of autoregulation and posttraumatic ischemia following experimental spinal cord trauma. *J Neurosurg* 1979;50:198-206.
30. Tator CH: Hemodynamic issues and vascular factors in acute experimental spinal cord injury. *J Neurotrauma* 1992;9:139-141.
31. Kobrine AI, Doyle TF, Martins AN: Local spinal cord blood flow in experimental traumatic myelopathy. *J Neurosurg* 1975;42:144-149.
32. Locke GE, Yashon D, Feldman RA, et al: Ischemia in primate spinal cord injury. *J Neurosurg* 1971;34:614-617.
33. Clendenon NR, Allen N, Gordon WA, et al: Inhibition of Na+-K+-activated ATPase activity following experimental spinal cord trauma. *J Neurosurg* 1978;49:563-568.
34. Anderson DK: Chemical and cellular mediators in spinal cord injury. *J Neurotrauma* 1992;9:143-146.
35. Bosch A, Stauffer ES, Nickel VL: Incomplete traumatic quadriplegia: A ten-year review. *JAMA* 1971;216:473-478.
36. Anderson PA: Spinal cord injuries, in Hansen ST Jr, Swiontkowski MF (eds): *Orthopaedic Trauma Protocols.* New York, NY, Raven Press, 1993, pp 193-198.
37. Ducker TB, Russo GL, Bellegarrique R, et al: Complete sensorimotor paralysis after cord injury: Mortality, recovery, and therapeutic implications. *J Trauma* 1979;19:837-840.
38. Stauffer ES: Neurologic recovery following injuries to the cervical spinal cord and nerve roots. *Spine* 1984;9:532-534.
39. Meyer PR Jr, Rosen JS, Hamilton BB, et al: Fracture-dislocation of the cervical spine: Transportation, assessment, and immediate management, in Evans EB (ed): *American Academy of Orthopaedic Surgeons Instructional Course Lectures XXV.* St. Louis, MO, CV Mosby, 1976, pp 171-183.
40. Little JW, Halar E: Temporal course of motor recovery after Brown-Séquard spinal cord injuries. *Paraplegia* 1985;23:39-46.
41. Frankel HL, Hancock DO, Hyslop G, et al: The value of postural reduction in the initial management of closed injuries of the spine with paraplegia and tetraplegia: Part I. *Paraplegia* 1969; 7:179-192.
42. Lucas JT, Ducker TB: Motor classification of spinal cord injuries with mobility, morbidity, and recovery indices. *Am Surg* 1979; 45:151-158.
43. Bohlman HH: Acute fractures and dislocations of the cervical spine: An analysis of three hundred hospitalized patients and a review of the literature. *J Bone Joint Surg* 1979;61A:1119-1142.
44. Garfin SR, Marshall LF, Eisenberg HM, et al: Abstract: Spinal cord injury in three regions in the United States. *Paraplegia* 1988;26:113.
45. Bohlman HH: The neck, in D'Ambrosia RD (ed): *Musculoskeletal Disorders, Regional Examination and Differential Diagnosis,* ed 2. Philadelphia, PA, JB Lippincott, 1986, pp 219-286.
46. Soderstrom CA, McArdle DQ, Ducker TB, et al: The diagnosis of intra-abdominal injury in patients with cervical cord trauma. *J Trauma* 1983;23:1061-1065.
47. Ersmark H, Dalen N, Kalen R: Cervical spine injuries: A follow-up of 332 patients. *Paraplegia* 1990;28:25-40.
48. Green BA, Callahan RA, Klose KJ, et al: Acute spinal cord injury: Current concepts. *Clin Orthop* 1981;154:125-135.
49. Ducker TB, Salcman M, Perot PL Jr, et al: Experimental spinal cord trauma: I. Correlations of blood flow, tissue oxygen and neurologic status in the dog. *Surg Neurol* 1978;10:60-63.

50. Ducker TB, Salcman M, Lucas JT, et al: Experimental spinal cord trauma: II. Blood flow, tissue oxygen, evoked potentials in both paretic and plegic monkeys. *Surg Neurol* 1978;10:64-70.
51. Soderstrom CA, Brumback RJ: Early care of the patient with cervical spine injury. *Orthop Clin North Am* 1986;17:3-13.
52. Rawe SE, Lee WA, Perot PL Jr: The histopathology of experimental spinal cord trauma: The effect of systemic blood pressure. *J Neurosurg* 1978;48:1002-1007.
53. Mesard L, Carmody A, Mannarino E, et al: Survival after spinal cord trauma: A life table analysis. *Arch Neurol* 1978;35:78-83.
54. Rockwell DD, Butler AB, Keats TE, et al: An improved design of the pneumatic counter-pressure trousers. *Am J Surg* 1982;143:377-379.
55. McGuire RA, Neville S, Green BA, et al: Spinal instability and the log-rolling maneuver. *J Trauma* 1987;27:525-531.
56. Clark CR, Igram CM, el-Khoury GY, et al: Radiographic evaluation of cervical spine injuries. *Spine* 1988;13:742-747.
57. Harris JH Jr: Radiographic evaluation of spinal trauma. *Orthop Clin North Am* 1986;17:75-86.
58. Kaye JJ, Nance EP Jr: Cervical spine trauma. *Orthop Clin North Am* 1990;21:449-462.
59. Vaccaro AR, An HS, Lin SS , et al: Non-contiguous injuries of the spine. *J Spinal Disord* 1992;5:320-329.
60. Ballinger PW (ed): *Merrill's Atlas of Radiographic Positions and Radiologic Procedures*, ed 7. St. Louis, MO, Mosby-Year Book, 1991, vol 1, pp 318-319.
61. Schwab ME: Regeneration of lesioned CNS axons by neutralization of neurite growth inhibitors: A short review. *J Neurotrauma* 1992;9(suppl 1):S219-S221.
62. Meinecke FW: Frequency and distribution of associated injuries in traumatic paraplegia and tetraplegia. *Paraplegia* 1968;5:196-209.
63. Beers GJ, Raque GH, Wagner GG, et al: MR imaging in acute cervical spine trauma. *J Comput Assist Tomog* 1988;12:755-761.
64. Goldberg AL, Rothfus WE, Deeb ZL, et al: The impact of magnetic resonance on the diagnostic evaluation of acute cervicothoracic spinal trauma. *Skeletal Radiol* 1988;17:89-95.
65. Weirich SD, Cotler HB, Narayana PA, et al: Histopathologic correlation of magnetic resonance imaging signal patterns in a spinal cord injury model. *Spine* 19990;15:630-638.
66. Rizzolo SJ, Cotler JM: Unstable cervical spine injuries: Specific treatment approaches. *J Am Acad Orthop Surg* 1993;1:57-66.
67. Eismont FJ, Arena MJ, Green BA: Extrusion of an intervertebral disc associated with traumatic subluxation or dislocation of cervical facets: Case report. *J Bone Joint Surg* 1991;73A:1555-1560.
68. Pratt ES, Green DA, Spengler DM: Herniated intervertebral discs associated with unstable spinal injuries. 1990;15:662-666.
69. Herkowitz HN, Rothman RH: Subacute instability of the cervical spine. *Spine* 1984;9:348-357.
70. Bohlman HH, Anderson PA: Anterior decompression and arthrodesis of the cervical spine: Long-term motor improvement: Part I. Improvement in incomplete traumatic quadriparesis. *J Bone Joint Surg* 1992;74A:671-682.
71. Colter JM, Herbison GJ, Nasuti JF, et al: Closed reduction of traumatic cervical spine dislocation using traction weights up to 140 pounds. *Spine* 1993;18:386-390.
72. Bracken MB, Holford TR: Effects of timing of methylprednisolone or naloxone administration on recovery of segmental and long-tract neurological function in NASCIS 2. *J Neurosurg* 1993;79:500-507.
73. Bracken MB, Shepard MJ, Collins WF, et al: Methylprednisolone or naloxone treatment after acute spinal cord injury: 1-year follow-up data. Results of the Second National Acute Spinal Cord Injury Study. *J Neurosurg* 1992;76:23-31.
74. Bracken MB, Shepard MJ, Collins WF Jr, et al: A randomized, controlled trial of methylprednisolone or naloxone in the treatment of acute spinal-cord injury: Results of the Second National Acute Spinal Cord Injury Study. *N Engl J Med* 1990;322:1405-1411.
75. Xu J, Qu ZX, Hogan EL, et al: Protective effect of methylprednisolone on vascular injury in rat spinal cord injury. *J Neurotrauma* 1992;9:245-253.
76. Hall ED, Braughler JM, McCall JM: Antioxidant effects in brain and spinal cord injury. *J Neurotrauma* 1992;9(suppl 1):S165-S172.
77. Bohlman HH, Ducker TB: Spine and spinal cord injuries, in Rothman RH, Simeone FA (eds): *The Spine*, ed 3. Philadelphia, PA, WB Saunders, 1992, pp 973-1103.
78. Young W, Bracken MB: The Second National Acute Spinal Cord Injury Study. *J Neurotrauma* 1992;9(suppl 1):S397-S405.
79. Geisler FH, Dorsey FC, Coleman WP: Recovery of motor function after spinal-cord injury: A randomized, placebo-controlled trial with GM-1 ganglioside. *N Engl J Med* 1991;324:1829-1838.
80. Geisler FH, Dorsey FC, Coleman WP: GM-1 ganglioside in human spinal cord injury. *J Neurotrauma* 1992;9(suppl 1):S407-S416.
81. Young W: Recovery mechanisms in spinal cord injury: Implications for regenerative therapy, in Seil FJ (ed): *Neural Regeneration and Transplantation, Frontiers of Clinical Neurosciences*. New York, NY, Alan R. Liss, 1989, vol 6, pp 157-169.
82. Constantini S, Young W: The effects of methylprednisolone and the ganglioside GM1 on acute spinal cord injury in rats. *J Neurosurg* 1994;80:97-111.
83. Hall ED, Yonkers PA, Andrus PK, et al: Biochemistry and pharmacology of lipid antioxidants in acute brain and spinal cord injury. *J Neurotrauma* 1992;9(suppl 2):S425-S442.
84. Hall ED: Effects of the 21-aminosteroid U74006F on posttraumatic spinal cord ischemia in cats. *J Neurosurg* 1988;68:462-465.
85. Anderson DK, Hall ED, Braughler JM, et al: Effect of delayed administration of U74006F (tirilazad mesylate) on recovery of locomotor function after experimental spinal cord injury. *J Neurosurga* 1991;8:187-192, 1991.
86. Francel PC, Long BA, Malik M, et al: Limiting ischemic spinal cord injury using a free radical scavenger 21-aminosteroid and/or cerebrospinal fluid drainage. *J Neurosurg* 1993;79:742-751.
87. Hall ED, Braughler JM, McCall JM: New pharmacological treatment of acute spinal cord trauma. *J Neurotrauma* 1988;5:81-89.
88. Faden AI: Opioid and nonopioid mechanisms may contribute to dynorphin's pathophysiological actions in spinal cord injury. *Ann Neurol* 1990;27:67-74.
89. Hall ED, Wolf DL, Althaus JS, et al: Beneficial effects of the kappa opioid receptor agonist U-50488H in experimental acute brain and spinal cord injury. *Brain Res* 1987;435:174-180.
90. Faden AI, Jacobs TP, Holaday JW: Thyrotropin-releasing hormone improves neurologic recovery after spinal trauma in cats. *N Engl J Med* 1981;305:1063-1067.
91. Faden AI: TRH analog YM-14673 improves outcome following traumatic brain and spinal cord injury in rats: Dose-response studies. *Brain Res* 1989;486:228-235.
92. Faden AI, Jacobs TP, Smith MT: Thyrotropin-releasing hormone in experimental spinal injury: Dose response and late treatment. *Neurology* 1984;34:1280-1284.
93. Anderson DK, Waters TR, Means ED: Pretreatment with alpha tocopherol enhances neurologic recovery after experimental spinal cord compression injury. *J Neurotrauma* 1988;5:61-67.
94. De Ley G, Leybaert L: Effect of flunarizine and methylprednisolone on functional recovery after experimental spinal injury. *J Neurotrauma* 1993;10:25-35.
95. Pointillart V, Gense D, Gross C, et al: Effects of nimodipine on posttraumatic spinal cord ischemia in baboons. *J Neurotrauma* 1993;10:201-213.
96. Faden AI, Jacobs TP, Smith MT: Evaluation of the calcium channel antagonist nimodipine in experimental spinal cord ischemia. *J Neurosurg* 1984;60:796-799.
97. Shi RY, Lucas JH, Wolf A, et al: Calcium antagonists fail to protect mammalian spinal neurons after physical injury. *J Neurotrauma* 1989;6:261-278.
98. Hansebout RR, Tanner JA, Romero-Sierra C: Current status of spinal cord cooling in the treatment of acute spinal cord injury. *Spine* 1984;9:508-511.

99. Martinez-Arizala A, Green BA: Hypothermia in spinal cord injury. *J Neurotrauma* 1992;9(suppl 2):S497-S505.
100. Hansebout RR: A comprehensive review of methods of improving cord recovery after acute spinal cord injury, in Tator CH (ed): *Seminars in Neurological Surgery: Early Management of Acute Spinal Cord Injury.* New York, NY, Raven Press, 1982, pp 181-196.
101. Goetz T, Romero-Sierra C, Ethier R, et al: Modeling of therapeutic dialysis of cerebrospinal fluid by epidural cooling in spinal cord injuries. *J Neurotrauma* 1988;5:139-150.
102. Anderson PA, Bohlman HH: Anterior decompression and arthrodesis of the cervical spine: Long-term motor improvement: Part II. Improvement in complete traumatic quadriplegia. *J Bone Joint Surg* 1992;74A:683-692.
103. Guttmann L (ed): *Spinal Cord Injuries: Comprehensive Management and Research.* Oxford, Blackwell Scientific, 1973, pp 122-157.
104. Ikata T, Iwasa K, Morimoto K, et al: Clinical considerations and biochemical basis of prognosis of cervical spinal cord injury. *Spine* 1989;14:1096-1101.
105. Marshall LF, Knowlton S, Garfin SR, et al: Deterioration following spinal cord injury: A multicenter study. *J Neurosurg* 1987;66:400-404.
106. Wagner FC Jr, Chehrazi B: Early decompression and neurological outcome in acute cervical spinal cord injuries. *J Neurosurg* 1982;56:699-705.
107. Ducker TB, Bellegarrigue R, Salcman M, et al: Timing of operative care in cervical spinal cord injury. *Spine* 1984;9:525-531.
108. Bunge RP, Bunge MB: Prospects for treatment of chronic human neural injury. *J Neurotrauma* 1993;10(suppl):S123.
109. Anderson DK, Reier PJ: Transplantation and spinal cord repair in higher vertebrates. *J Neurotrauma* 1993;10(suppl):S117.
110. Kuhlengel KR, Bunge MB, Bunge RP: Implantation of cultured sensory neurons and Schwann cells into lesioned neonatal rat spinal cord: I. Methods for preparing implants from dissociated cells. *J Compar Neurol* 1990;293:63-73.
111. Kuhlengel KR, Bunge MB, Bunge RP, et al: Implantation of cultured sensory neurons and Schwann cells into lesioned neonatal rat spinal cord: II. Implant characteristics and examination of corticospinal tract growth. *J Compar Neurol* 1990;293:74-91.
112. Reier PJ, Anderson DK, Thompson FJ, et al: Neural tissue transplantation and CNS trauma: Anatomical and functional repair of the injured spinal cord. *J Neurotrauma* 1992;9(suppl 1):S223-S248.
113. Blight AR, Toombs JP, Bauer MS, et al: The effects of 4-aminopyridine on neurological deficits in chronic cases of traumatic spinal cord injury in dogs: A phase I clinical trial. *J Neurotrauma* 1991;8:103-119.
114. Hansebout RR, Blight AR, Fawcett S, et al: 4-aminopyridine in chronic spinal cord injury: A controlled, double-blind, crossover study in eight patients. *J Neurotrauma* 1993;10:1-18.
115. Waxman SG: Aminopyridines and the treatment of spinal cord injury. *J Neurotrauma* 1993;10:19-24.

CHAPTER 6

Cervical Spondylosis and Myelopathy

Henry H. Bohlman, MD

Introduction

The clinical entity of cervical spondylotic myelopathy (CSM) became well recognized in the 1950s through the work of Brain and associates,[1-3] as well as that of Clarke and Robinson,[4] who specifically identified CSM as arising from the spondylotic process rather than from just an acute herniated disk. As early as 1928, Stookey[5] described a syndrome of bilateral and ventral cord compression resulting in the Brown-Séquard syndrome. Brain and associates[3] further discussed the importance of impaired blood supply of the spinal cord in chronic cervical spondylosis producing myelopathy and the ultimate clinical and neurologic manifestations of cervical spondylosis, including radicular as well as myelopathic signs. In 1956, Clarke and Robinson[4] published a review of 120 patients with CSM in which they noted that spontaneous regression was clinically observed in two. However, 75% of this group of patients had recurring episodes, and new symptoms of myelopathy and neurologic deterioration occurred in approximately 66%. In 5% of the 120 patients, there was rapid onset of symptoms followed by a long period of neurologic plateau. These authors also described the clinical onset of cervical myelopathy as being manifested by leg spasticity and weakness, which most often was gradual and occurred at around 50 years of age. The disease was more common in men, especially those exposed to occupational trauma, and the progression, which was often slow, included neurologic signs of both cervical cord and root impairment. They additionally pointed out that nonsurgical treatment, including immobilization and bed rest, could significantly improve the myelopathy.

In 1967, Brain and Wilkinson[1] published a monograph on cervical spondylosis. They defined it as progressive degeneration of the cervical disks and all of the surrounding structures, including the zygoepiphyseal joints and the joints of Luschka, as well as the formation of chondro-osseous spurs and thickening with infolding of the ligamentum flavum.

In 1977, Robinson and associates[6] published an article on the etiology and treatment concepts of CSM, in which they pointed out that the basic pathology of spondylosis was the production of chondro-osseous spurs. These spurs remain and grow as long as the degenerative disk material remains in the disk space, even with reduced motion. Secondly, neck motion was also a factor in the activation of symptoms and signs of CSM, not only in the long-term spur formation but also in the presence of disk degeneration. They noted that when cervical spondylosis reduced the already narrow sagittal diameter of the spinal canal and the foramen, the myelopathy progressed. After reviewing the literature, Robinson and associates[6] outlined a combination of pathologic factors that included the initial size of the cervical spinal canal, progression of the spondylosis with spur formation, interruption of the intrinsic arterial supply of the spinal cord, and motion, which in conjunction with the spurs produced irritation and compression of the spinal cord.

Breig[7] published a monograph describing the biomechanics of the cervical spinal cord and their relationship to the cervical spinal canal. He noted that, in flexion, mechanical flattening of the spinal cord occurred, with narrowing of the lumina of the anterior sulcal and transverse arteries. Other authors have noted that compression of the spinal cord in the anteroposterior direction caused stretching of the transverse vessels and of the terminations of the anterior spinal artery, thereby producing ischemia of the anterior two-thirds of the gray matter.

Pathophysiology

The pathophysiology of cervical myelopathy is probably multifactorial, in that it is related to an initial congenital cervical spinal stenosis, progressive cervical spondylosis, and direct spinal cord compression, as well as impairment of the blood supply to the spinal cord. In addition, mechanical factors play a significant role.[8] Since the 1950s and 1960s many authors have written about the sagittal diameter of the spinal canal, the subarachnoid space, the diameter of the spinal cord, and the significance of these in association with CSM.[9,10] Most authors agree that the common diameter of the spinal canal is approximately 17 to 18 mm between C3 and C7, with slight variation between sexes. In 1955, Arnold[10] pointed out, in a pathologic study, that there was a high correlation between the sagittal diameter of the spinal canal, cervical spondylosis, and the production of myelopathy. He found that a sagittal diameter of 12 mm or less was critical in the production of myelopathy. In 1971, Adams and Logue[11] identified three groups of spondylosis patients, and in the myelopathy group the sagittal diameter was 11.8 mm with a range of 9 to 15 mm. In order to accurately measure the sagittal diameter of the cervical spinal canal on normal radiographs, the tube-to-film distance had to be the standard 6 feet. The mean sagittal diameter from C3 to T1 will be 17 mm plus or minus 5 mm. If the diameter of the spinal canal is less than 13 mm, the canal is stenotic by definition.

The sagittal diameter of the cervical spinal cord from C1 to C7 has been documented by a number of authors with very little variation. The average diameter is 10 mm and the range is from 8.5 to 11.5 mm.[12-17] In my opinion, almost all patients who present with CSM have congenital cervical stenosis with superimposed spondylosis or other pathologic problems.[18-28]

Mechanical factors play a major role in the production of cervical myelopathy.[29-33] A number of authors have pointed out that when the cervical spinal canal diameter has reduced the amount of room available for the spinal cord, the functional diameter may be reduced to a critical level, or even narrower, with hyperextension as well as flexion of the cervical spine. Hyperextension causes the ligamentum flavum to buckle posteriorly, whether or not disk protrusion anterior to the cervical spinal cord further compromises the canal.[34] In 1972, Nurick,[35,36] who measured plain radiographs and myelograms to study CSM, pointed out that the minimum sagittal diameter for the spinal cord was 11.3 mm in men and 9.9 mm in women. Bohlman,[37] in 1977, pointed out the dynamic problem of pathologic compensatory subluxation of the upper cervical spine above stiff spondylotic segments that produces cord compression and myelopathy. Of the 17 patients so reported with severe myelopathy (Nurick's grades 3 to 5), 12 had degenerative subluxation of the cervical spine with instability, and, in addition, all of the patients had a stenotic spinal canal. It was pointed out that anterior cervical fusion[37] as an internal stabilizer, as well as external support by a rigid orthosis, improved neurologic recovery and protected the spinal cord.[38]

Other mechanical factors may play a role in the production of cervical myelopathy. Kyphotic deformities cause the cervical spinal cord to be drawn into a flexion mode, which produces direct neural compression and flattening of the spinal cord.[39]

There is significant evidence in the literature to indicate that impairment of the blood supply to the spinal cord plays a major role in CSM.[40-44] Interruption of the vascular supply can occur in a variety of ways. First, a large chondro-osseous spur or mass, in conjunction with a congenitally narrow canal, may produce direct neural compression and deformity of the spinal cord with flattening in the anteroposterior direction. With direct spinal cord compression, the sulcal and terminal vessels of the anterior spinal artery become interrupted and, therefore, the anterior two thirds of the spinal cord become ischemic.[45,46] If impairment of the blood supply becomes chronic, the ischemia ultimately produces demyelinization and nerve cell damage as well as loss of axoplasmic flow. Although no author has conclusively demonstrated pathologically that there is a thrombosis of the anterior spinal artery, there is a large volume of evidence experimentally and pathologically to indicate that it is the sulcal and terminal vessels of the anterior spinal artery that become impaired with compression.

The second mechanism of vascular ischemia to the spinal cord is a result of tethering and compression of the foraminal or radicular feeder arteries to the cord, which may occur by encroachment into the foramen by osteophytes and by thickening of the ligamentum flavum. In 1964, Taylor[47] compared these pathologic features with other obstructive vascular lesions of the spinal cord that produce spinal cord anoxia through occlusion of extrinsic vessels. The clinical signs were comparable with those associated with myelopathy and cervical spondylosis. He describes the motor elements of the spinal cord as being the most seriously affected. In 1952, Allen[48] noted that the cervical cord in a patient with a spondylitic cervical spine blanched when it was flexed during a laminectomy. Other authors, including Holt and Yates,[49] noted a correlation between perineural fibrosis of the nerve roots with demyelination and cystic changes of the spinal ganglia in the intervertebral foramen. In 1953, Mair and Druckman[33] described pathologic findings in the spinal cord situated in the area of the distribution of the anterior spinal artery—that is, the anterior two thirds of the cord. Gooding and associates,[41] in 1975, and also Hukuda and associates[50] and Hoff and associates[42] published experimental studies of anterior cord compression in conjunction with ligation of feeder arteries. In these studies, there was an additive effect of ischemia on spinal cord compression with increasing neurologic deficit. Pathologic analysis of the spinal cords of dogs demonstrated extensive demyelination involving the white matter, with the cortical spinal tract being the area most severely injured. However, there was no gliosis or infarction of the gray matter and no clotting of the intermedullary vessels. The authors, therefore, believe that these neurologic lesions may be recoverable. In 1973, Gledhill and associates[51] reported on the correlation between the degree of demyelinization following spinal cord compression and the actual clinical neurologic deficit. They and Gooding and associates[41] concluded that demyelinization was a major pathologic finding but that neurologic recovery could occur. These studies indicated that the Schwann type cells that produce the myelin sheath for the axon of the neuronal cell are very sensitive to either pressure or vascular impairment and that the neuronal cells themselves could remain viable. In 1975, Doppman[40] studied compression of the spinal cord using a Fogerty balloon catheter to compress the anterior, posterior, and lateral cord. Anterior compression affected the sulcal arteries and, therefore, the transverse arterioles in the compressed spinal cord, but when compression occurred posteriorly, there was no perfusion of the intramedullary branches of the central gray matter. He noted also that anteroposterior compression of the cord produced flattening and widening, which stretched the intrinsic transverse vessels or terminal branches of the anterior spinal artery.

In 1977, Hoff and associates[42] studied microangiographic data from an animal model in which ischemia produced cervical myelopathy and concluded that both compression and ischemia of the cord were causes of myelopathy in man. Earlier, Shimomura and associates[44] published an experimental study of ischemic damage in conjunction with compression of the cervical cord in dogs. They found that blood flow through the vertebral and radicular arteries at their origin had little relationship to cervical ischemic myelopathy and, furthermore, that occlusion of the anterior spinal artery alone produces pathologic change only in the ventral one third of the spinal cord and not in the lateral pyramidal tract. They concluded that obstruction of the arteries on the surface of the spinal cord as well as of the intermedullary arteries produces the pathologic process. Hukuda and Wilson,[43] in 1972, published further on the effects on the canine cervical cord of combined anterior cord compression and ischemia indicating that both of these etiologies were additive in production of clinical CSM in patients.

There have been a number of pathologic studies of animals as well as humans, which demonstrated the findings in CSM.[52-57] My coworkers and I[52] studied a canine model of graded chronic anterior cervical cord compression with and without long-term decompression. Spinal cord monitoring with cortical evoked potentials demonstrated a decreased amplitude and increased latency in the chronically compressed cord. The alteration in evoked potentials correlated with the degree of paralysis during compression as well as after decompression and with resultant recovery of neurologic function. Pathologic analysis of the spinal cord revealed a variety of alterations, including central cyst formation in the gray matter, demyelinization of the lateral columns, and ascending necrosis of the posterior columns, which indicate degeneration of the ascending sensory tracks. Some of the animals that developed quadriparesis following anterior cord compression demonstrated normal spinal cords at autopsy, which indicated a significant ischemic factor. Most of these animals recovered neurologically from their chronic compressive lesion if anterior decompression was carried out. This study appeared to indicate etiologically both an ischemic event and neurapraxia of the spinal cord with chronic compression, which was reversible.

There have been few pathologic studies of CSM in humans until recent years. In 1967, Jellinger[58] published a series of 1,037 necropsies in which the spinal cord was analyzed for arteriosclerotic change and vascular fibrosis. He found arteriosclerotic changes in major spinal arteries in 12.7% of the total group, in 22.2% of those patients over 41 years, and in 21.7% of those over 61 years of age. Approximately 10.5% showed intimal fibrosis and hypertrophy of the internal elastic lamina without a great deal of narrowing of the lumen. In addition, 2.2% of the entire series revealed severe spinal cord atheromatosis without a correlation of sclerotic changes in the rest of the body. Changes in the small intermedullary vessels of the cord were much more frequent than changes in the major spinal arteries. In 1977, Ono and associates[55] described the pathology of five patients whose cervical myelopathy and neurologic deficits had been documented before death, and whose spinal cords were recovered at autopsy. Compression of the spinal cord was associated with extensive destruction of both gray and white matter and ascending and descending demyelinization. They described a ratio of the anteroposterior diameter to the lateral diameter of the spinal canal, which was called the anteroposterior compression ratio and which was measured on each cross-sectional image of the spinal cord and spine to evaluate the degree of anterior compression. There was a good correlation between the measured anteroposterior compression ratios and the areas of most severe infarction of the spinal cord. Spastic paralysis was predominant in the lower extremities, and profound sensory loss in the upper and lower extremities was believed to be secondary to descending pyramidal tract lesions and ascending posterior funicular lesions, respectively. Ono and associates[55] also noted sparing of the anterior white column from infarction as a common pathologic feature.

In 1983, Ogino and associates[54] published a description of nine patients, which included data from premorbid neurologic examinations and pathologic studies at the time of death. They found that the degree of cord destruction correlated with the anteroposterior compression ratio. The posterolateral white columns (lateral corticospinal tracts) suffered first from minor compression, and anterior horn cell loss and localized infarction of the gray matter were associated more with severe cord compression and an anteroposterior canal ratio below 20%. An infarction eventually extended to the entire gray matter, then the entire lateral white columns were destroyed but the anterior white columns remained preserved. Four patients with mild to moderate cord compression exhibited mainly lower extremity long tract signs, whereas four patients with severe cord compression demonstrated a more classic spastic quadriparesis, which included marked disability of the hands and fingers accompanied by intrinsic hand wasting with evidence of upper as well as lower motion neuron signs.

It is apparent from both clinical experience and experimental studies that multiple factors are involved in the pathophysiology and pathogenesis of CSM.[59] In my experience, most patients with this disease present with a variation of the anterior cord syndrome without loss of the posterior column modalities of position and vibration sense. These symptoms indicate that early in the disease process the major pathologic problems are anterior cord compression and ischemia in conjunction with congenital cervical stenosis.[60,61] There is little doubt that electrophysiologic changes occur and alteration of evoked potentials increases as the disease becomes moderately severe.[62-66] Most likely, therefore, a number of other intrinsic changes occur within the spinal cord; these include blockage of axoplasmic flow, distortion of the cord tissue, stretching of the intrinsic transverse terminations of the anterior spinal artery, and, in more severe advanced cases, tissue destruction with demyelinization of the white matter in both the ascending and descending tracks. In more severe cases, there is gliosis and scarring as well as ultimate neuronal cell loss as an end stage. Finally, cystic degeneration and total destruction of the spinal cord may occur. The pathologic findings appear to be correlated with the clinical severity of the disease.

Etiology

As previously mentioned, I have found that almost all of the patients who present with CSM have congenital cervical stenosis. From there, it is a progression of myelopathy secondary to other influencing factors. In its simplest form, CSM may be produced by a herniated nucleus pulposus in a narrow spinal canal with severe cord compression (Figs. 1 and 2). The myelopathy may be insidious or acute with precipitous ataxia. Most commonly, a spondylotic bar has formed over a period of years and may involve more than one cervical level. This is usually a combination of hard disk protrusion and posterior osteophyte formation anterior to the spinal cord in conjunction with thickening and infolding of the ligamentum flavum, posteriorly. If the chondro-osseous spur or mass becomes large enough and the spinal cord compression severe enough, then myelopathy ensues and in most instances is progressive (Fig. 3).

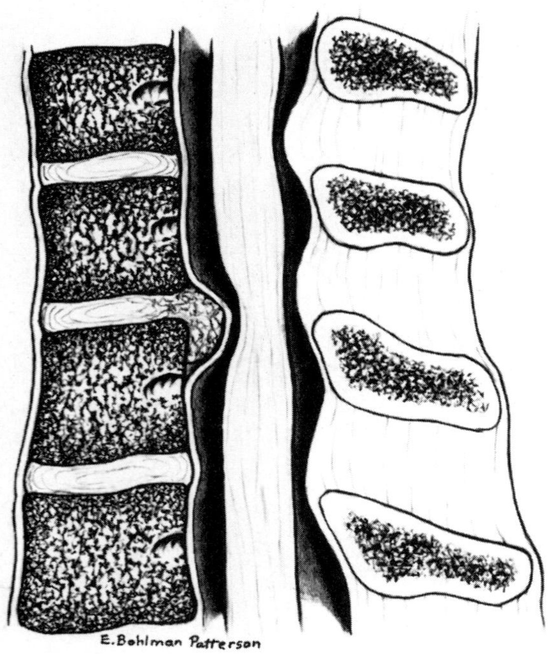

Fig. 1 Illustration demonstrating association of soft disc protrusion as spondylosis with a narrow spinal canal. The cervical disk is usually anterior to the posterior longitudinal ligament, but some disk material may protrude posterior to the vertebral body. (Reproduced with permission from Bohlman HH: Cervical spondylosis with moderate to severe myelopathy. *Spine* 1977;2:151-162.)

Degenerative osteoarthritic anterior subluxation with or without disk protrusion may produce CSM. It ordinarily begins with neck pain, which is then followed by nerve root signs and, ultimately, if the subluxation compromises the spinal canal by 13 mm or greater, myelopathy may ensue.[67] This frequently is above preexisting spondylotic levels that have fused spontaneously or become immobile (Figs. 4 and 5). The osteoarthritic process destroys the facet joints above and causes their incompetency and, hence, the forward luxation. In rare circumstances, degenerative arthrosis may produce a retrolisthesis (Fig. 6) by narrowing of the disk space and settling of the vertebrae, with osteophytes compressing the spinal cord in conjunction with inbuckling of the ligamentum flavum. This is not infrequently seen with hyperextension injuries secondary to minor or major trauma in which there is disruption of the anterior and posterior longitudinal ligaments as well as the degenerative disk (Figs. 7 and 8).

Kyphotic deformity of approximately 40° or greater can be associated with and productive of cervical myelopathy in conjunction with spondylosis. Kyphosis may be produced secondary to severe degenerative arthrosis in which the facets and posterior ligament structures become incompetent in association with degenerative disk disease anteriorly and wedging of the vertebral bodies (Figs. 9 and 10). Iatrogenic kyphosis is caused by cervical laminectomy, with or without facetectomy, in which the ligament structures have been removed and the capsules of the facet joints have been violated.[68,69]

Another less common cause of CSM in this country, although it is very frequent in Japan, is ossification of the posterior longitudinal ligament (OPLL). Isolated or segmental OPLL may produce radiculopathy or myelopathy;[70] although, as many Japanese authors have pointed out, OPLL may form a solid mass over the entire cervical spine producing severe anterior spinal cord compression.[71-73]

History, Physical Examination, and Neurologic Examination

Patients with cervical spondylosis and myelopathy usually present complaining mainly that they are having difficulty with walking and balance, with or without weakness. They often have trouble grasping objects

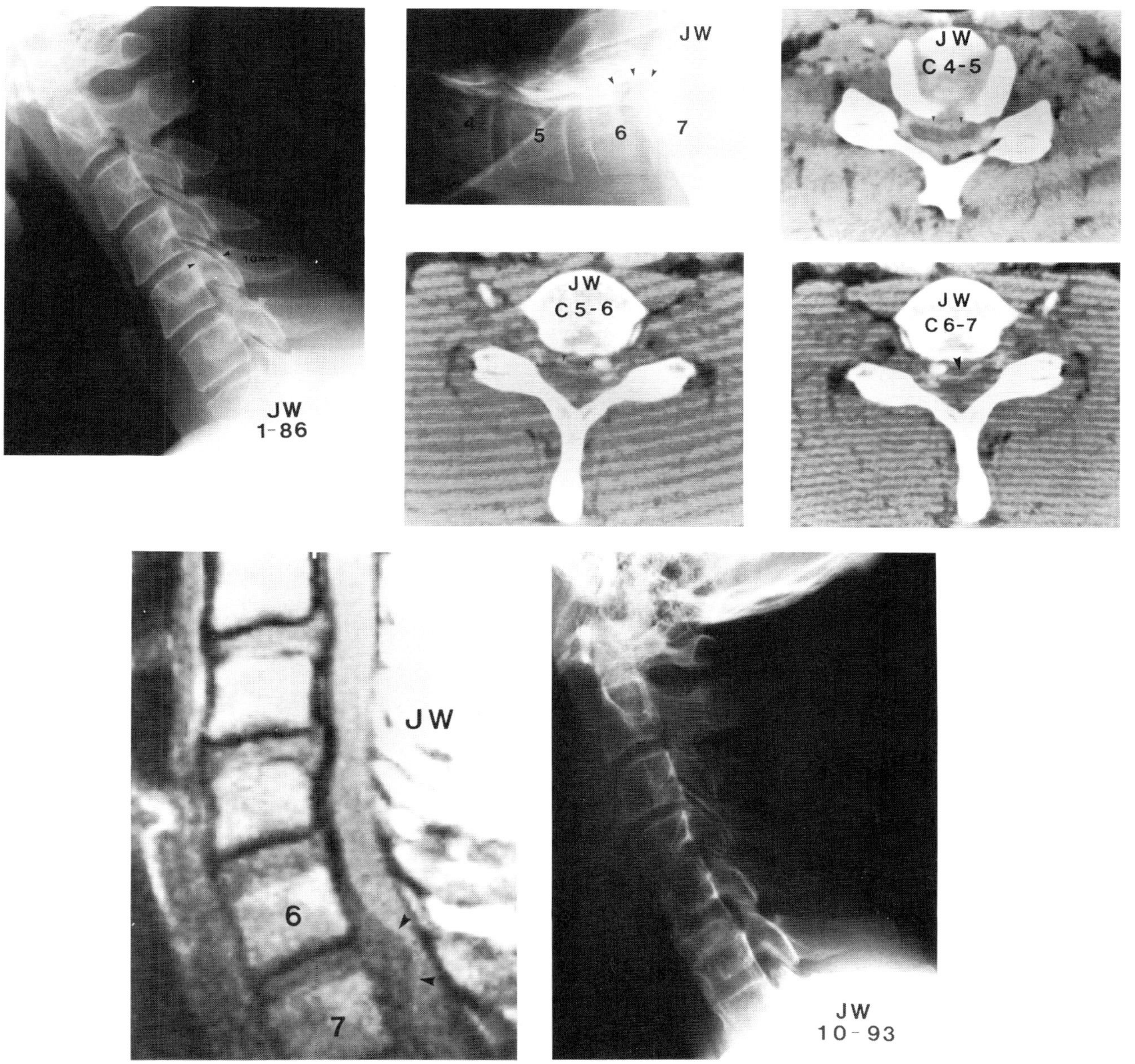

Fig. 2 **Top left,** Lateral radiograph demonstrating congenital cervical spinal stenosis in a 34-year-old man who presented with cervical radiculopathy and myelopathy. Note that the inner laminar cortex is adjacent to the facet cortex indicating very little anteroposterior diameter of the spinal canal. There is very little evidence of cervical spondylosis with the exception of slight narrowing of the disk space at C4-5. **Top center,** Lateral view of the cervical myelogram demonstrating disk protrusions at three levels C4-5, C5-6, and the largest at C6-7. **Top right,** Enhanced computed tomographic (CT) scan demonstrating marked compression of the spinal cord by soft disk protrusion at C4-5. **Center left,** Enhanced CT scan demonstrating severe spinal cord compression by calcified soft disk protrusion. Note very little dye surrounding the spinal cord at C5-6. **Center right,** Enhanced CT scan demonstrating calcified soft disk protrusion severely compressing the spinal cord at the C6-7 level. **Bottom left,** Lateral magnetic resonance imaging (MRI) scan demonstrating marked spinal cord compression at three levels, most severely at the C6-7 level secondary to herniated disks. **Bottom right,** Lateral radiograph of the patient 7 years after surgery demonstrating complete incorporation of the bone graft. The patient was asymptomatic with neurologic recovery.

with their hands; they specifically have difficulty with small objects, such as buttons on their clothing, because of impaired sensation and dexterity. Loss of motion of the cervical spine is very common, and the patient may have noted this before examination. Other complaints include paresthesias of the upper as well as lower extremities, and patients with severe cord compression may have a Lhermitte's sign, in which flexion or extension of the neck produces arm, leg, and body paresthesias. All of these signs and symptoms may occur without any neck or arm pain. Of interest is that almost all patients with cervical CSM have a combination of upper as well as lower motor neuron signs; that is, they will present with atrophy and fasciculations of the

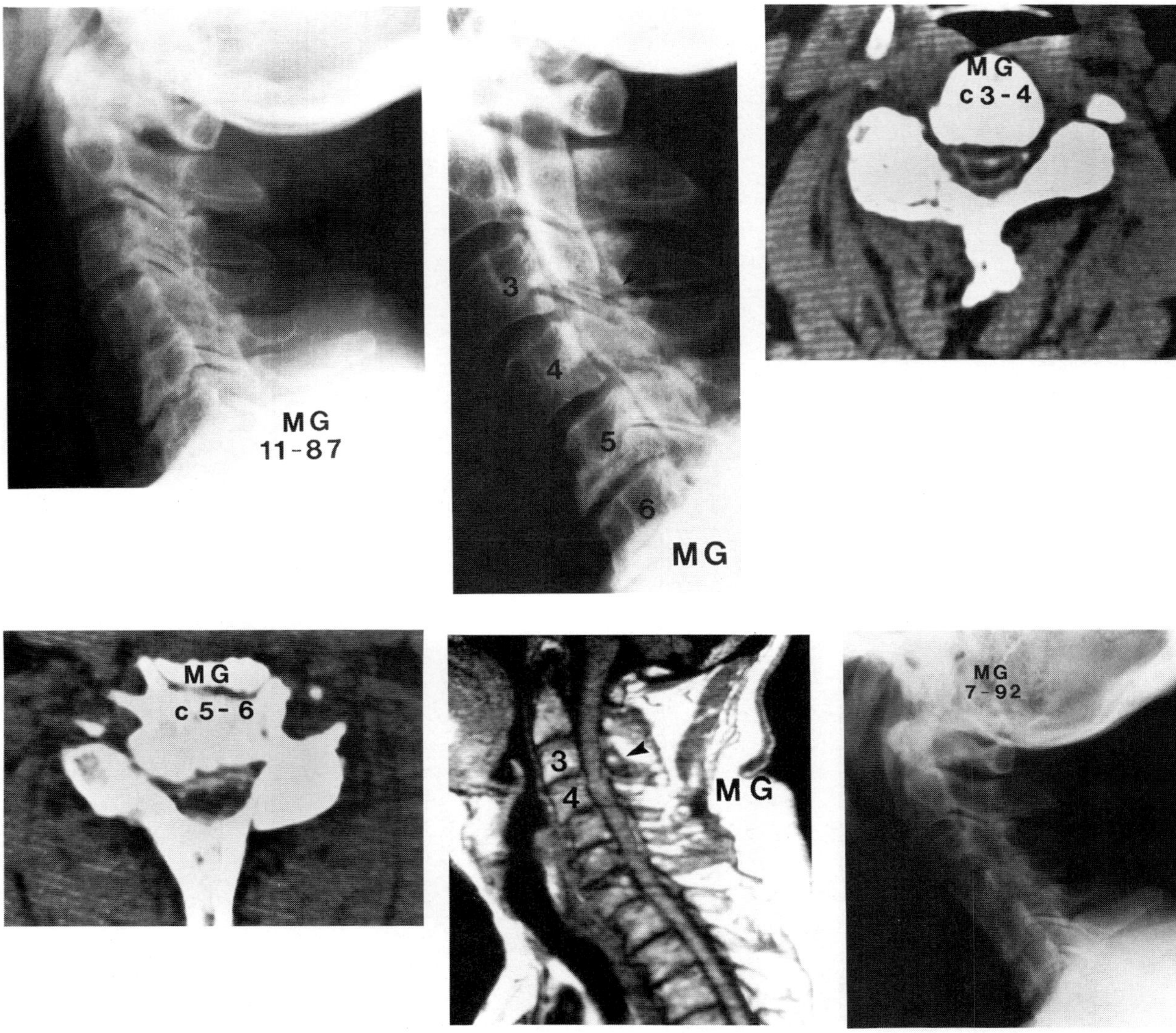

Fig. 3 **Top left,** Lateral roentgenogram of a very active 81-year-old man with multiple levels of cervical spondylosis and severe Nurick Grade IV myelopathy. He had no intrinsic function of his hands and was barely able to walk with a walker. **Top center,** Lateral view of the cervical myelogram demonstrating severe spinal cord compression with flattening at the C3-4 level. **Top right**, Enhanced computed tomography (CT) scan of C5-6 level revealing cord compression. **Bottom left,** Enhanced CT scan demonstrating marked spinal cord compression by an osteophyte at the C3-4 level. Note the very small amount of dye surrounding the spinal cord. **Bottom center,** Lateral view of the cervical magnetic resonance imaging (MRI) scan demonstrating multiple levels of spinal cord compression and absence of a thecal space surrounding the spinal cord from C3 to C7. **Bottom right,** Lateral radiograph 4 years and 7 months following an anterior cervical corpectomy of C4,5, and 6 to decompress the spinal cord, followed by a fibular strut fusion from C3 to C7. Note the complete incorporation of the fibular graft. The patient had completely recovered his neurologic function to Nurick Grade I, including recovery of intrinsic hand function.

shoulder girdle and upper extremity or hands in conjunction with hyperreflexia and other signs of upper motor neuron impairment.[74-79] In my experience, loss of bladder and bowel control as well as loss of position and vibration sense occurs late in the disease and usually indicates severe myelopathy and a poor prognosis for recovery of function. Sensory loss is usually radicular in pattern but may extend over the shoulder girdle and arms involving multiple root levels in conjunction with upper extremity weakness. One spinal cord syndrome that occurs with CSM is the central cord lesion, in which the patients have upper extremity paralysis, which is greater than that of the lower legs, and varying degrees of sensory loss with sparing of posterior column sensations. In milder forms of CSM, patients present with an anterior cord syndrome; that is, hyperreflexia and spasticity with gait impairment and less motor deficit. However, when motor deficit occurs, the pattern is one of lower extremity paralysis greater than that of the upper extremities, with preservation of posterior column functions.[74] Less commonly, patients may have a Brown-Séquard syndrome with

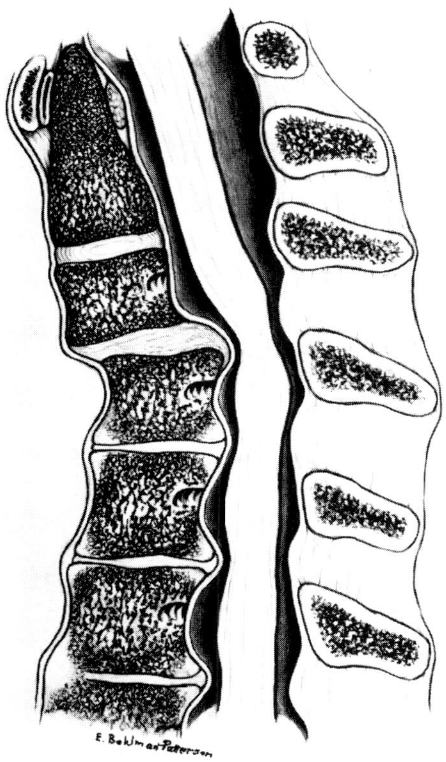

Fig. 4 Diagrammatic illustration of compensatory anterior subluxation of the third on fourth cervical vertebrae secondary to degenerative osteoarthritis and above the stiff spondylitic segments. (Reproduced with permission from Bohlman HH: Cervical spondylosis with moderate to severe myelopathy. *Spine* 1977;2:151-162.)

motor impairment on one side and a dissociated sensory loss of pain and temperature on the contralateral side. This syndrome occurs only with a unilateral spinal cord compression. Reflexes are universally hyperactive unless a patient has a superimposed lower motor neuron disease, such as severe lumbar spinal stenosis or peripheral neuropathy, in which case the hyperreflexia is lost or does not occur in the lower extremities.[77] Brain and Wilkinson[1] have described an inverted radial reflex in which the brachioradialis reflex produces an involuntary grasp of the fingers, which is supposed to indicate C6 level spinal cord disease.

It is critically important to document an exact neurologic examination in the office as well as during hospitalization and at follow-up in order to determine progression of the disease as well as recovery after surgical intervention. My coworkers and I use the standard motor grading system, with grades 0 to 5 of all muscle groups, as well as a body sensory diagram and specific documentation of position and vibratory sense. Reflexes are graded from 0 to 4, with specific identification of all pathologic reflexes. It is important to document the jaw jerk and its grade because if the latter is hyperreflexic, this indicates a lesion above the level of the pons rather than in the cervical spinal cord.

Table 1
Nurick's classification of disability in spondylotic myelopathy

Grade	Description*
Grade I	Signs of cord involvement, normal gait
Grade II	Mild gait impairment, ADL normal, able to be employed
Grade III	Gait abnormality that prevents employment and normal ADL
Grade IV	Able to ambulate only with assistance
Grade V	Chairbound or bedridden

* ADL = activities of daily living

There are a number of neurologic grading systems that can be incorporated to document functional ability of both the upper and lower extremities. The Nurick grading system is basically one of demonstrating myelopathy with the ability to walk and function in activities of daily living (ADL)[35,36] (Table 1). It is not specific as far as arm and hand function are concerned. Nurick grade I indicates hyperreflexia and no impairment of ADL or walking. Grade II indicates hyperreflexia, no impairment of ADL, and slight impairment in gait. Nurick grade III indicates impairment in both ADL and gait; whereas, grade IV indicates impairment of ADL and inability to walk without aid. Finally, Nurick grade V indicates the patient is unable to walk and is chairbound or bedridden. The Japanese grading system (Table 2)[71] is much more specific with regard to hand and arm function as well as gait function, and my coworkers and I have incorporated it partially in our current grading system.

Diagnostic Studies

When a patient with suspected CSM is seen in the office, anteroposterior, lateral, flexion, and extension lateral as well as oblique radiographs of the cervical spine are obtained. In this way, it is possible to identify immediately many pathologic processes, such as degenerative subluxation, congenital stenosis, spondylotic stenosis, and rigid spine segments, as well as intraforaminal narrowing. If signs of cervical myelopathy are present on neurologic examination, the next step is a cervical magnetic resonance imaging (MRI) scan as a screening study to determine the severity of spinal cord compression and canal compromise.[80] The patient with identifiable CSM should be placed in a soft collar initially, with the narrow portion anteriorly to prevent hyperextension. My coworkers and I occasionally use somatosensory evoked potential and cortical evoked potential monitoring if we believe the patient is becoming more severely impaired, and the myelopathy is progressive. Electromyographic studies are useful in differentiating peripheral nerve compression in the upper extremities, which may be producing atrophy and weakness, as well as neuropathies that may be present in conjunction with CSM. If it appears as though the patient has progressed enough in the

Table 2
The assessment scale proposed by the Japanese Orthopaedic Association

Dysfunction	Score*
Motor dysfunction of the upper extremity	0 = Unable to feed oneself
	1 = Unable to handle chopsticks, able to eat with spoon
	2 = Handle chopsticks with much difficulty
	3 = Handle chopsticks with slight difficulty
	4 = None
Motor dysfunction of the lower extremity	0 = Unable to walk
	1 = Walk on flat floor with walking aid
	2 = Up and/or down stairs with handrail
	3 = Lack of stability and smooth reciprocation
	4 = None
Sensory deficit	
Upper extremity	0 = Severe sensory loss of pain
	1 = Mild sensory loss
	2 = None
Lower extremity	0 = Severe sensory loss of pain
	1 = Mild sensory loss
	2 = None
Trunk	0 = Severe sensory loss of pain
	1 = Mild sensory loss
	2 = None
Sphincter dysfunction	0 = Unable to void
	1 = Marked difficulty in micturition (retention strangury)
	2 = Difficulty in micturition (pollakiuria, hesitation)
	3 = None

* Maximum points = 17

disease and is impaired, and if surgical intervention is contemplated, then we proceed with a cervical myelogram and enhanced computed tomography (CT) scan.[81] Although the MRI can reveal spinal cord compression and intrinsic spinal cord signal change, we believe that the myelogram is very useful in determining the degree of nerve root compression and bony architecture in relationship to the spinal cord compression. Occasionally, tomography is useful in determining the bony architecture, especially in patients with ossification of the posterior longitudinal ligament or large chondro-osseous spurs. In addition, dynamic views of the cervical spine are important in determining whether a lordotic or kyphotic deformity is fixed or flexible.[82]

Treatment Methods

Nonsurgical Treatment

As mentioned above, immobilization of the neck with an orthosis and intermittent bed rest can offer some relief for myelopathic symptoms and signs. Immobilization diminishes the neural irritation and compression, and isometric exercises can be used in conjunction with the cervical immobilization.[83] If patients have cervical and radicular pain, immobilization can provide relief. However, if patients are having difficulty walking and their MRIs and other radiographs indicate severe spinal cord compression,[84] then I believe a more aggressive approach should be carried out; that is, surgical decompression and stabilization. I do not believe that epidural steroids have proven to be beneficial in this disease. In addition, I do not recommend the use of cervical traction, because it could create further hyperextension and additional spinal cord compression.

Surgical Treatment

Historically, the most common surgical treatment of CSM was by laminectomy at one or more levels.[85-87] It has been well documented that there may be significant immediate or delayed impairment of neural function following this procedure.[88,89] Brain and associates[3] found impairment of neural function in 19% of patients who had been treated with laminectomy. Crandall and Gregorius,[88] after long-term follow-up, reported that nine of 15 patients treated by laminectomy were worse postoperatively. The causes of loss of neural function with cervical laminectomy probably are related to intraoperative manipulation of the spinal cord, failure to treat the causes of anterior compression, and loss of stability of the spine. The long-term results of laminectomy alone are believed to be very poor, and this procedure should not be performed in most situations. Japanese surgeons and others in this country have treated cervical myelopathy with laminoplasty, which does not manipulate the spinal cord and increases the size of the spinal canal from a posterior approach.[89-91] Laminoplasty is contraindicated in patients with kyphosis or loss of normal lordosis and in patients with large anterior chondro-osseous masses, which produce anterior spinal cord compression.[92] The major indication for laminoplasty appears to be in the rare patient with a solid, long OPLL that spans multiple levels. The other more common indication would be in a patient with multiple levels of mild cervical spondylosis in conjunction with severe cervical stenosis, in which case the end results appear to be quite good as far as neurologic recovery is concerned.

In most situations, anterior decompression and fusion at one or more levels appears to be an extraordinarily safe and reliable procedure that has stood the test of time.[93-101] The technique and type of anterior decompression used depend on the etiology, the degree of spinal cord compression, the number of levels involved, and the spinal deformity. Other factors, such as a previous laminectomy or osteoporosis in an elderly person, may determine the type of operation.

Most patients present with ataxia, hyperreflexia, and varying degrees of weakness, with either an anterior or central cord type syndrome.[102] In addition, it is extraordinarily rare to have loss of posterior column function. Because preoperative studies, including myelography and CT as well as MRI, ordinarily show the major spinal cord and nerve root compression to be from the anterior direction, anterior decompression and autogenous fusion are believed to be the surgical procedure of choice in the majority of patients with cervical myelopathy.[103] If, indeed, the pathology is a single or

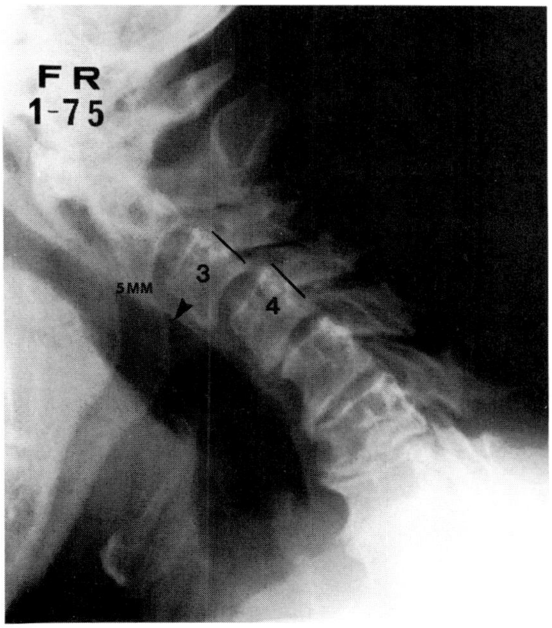

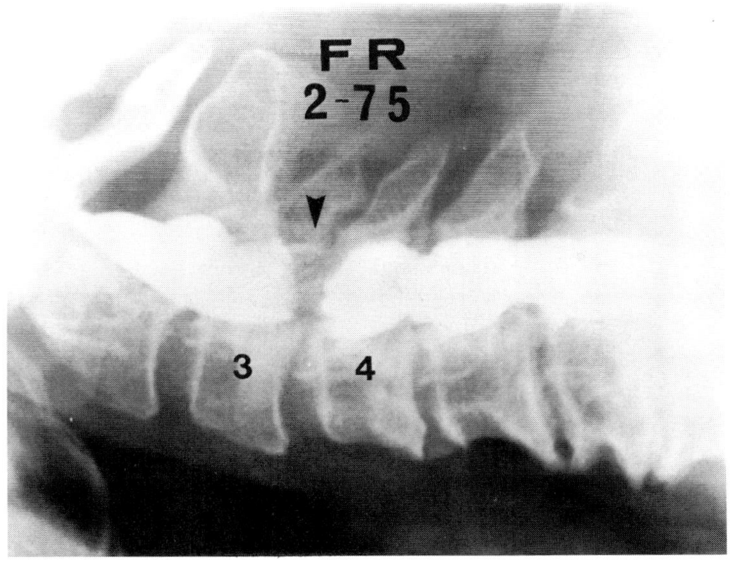

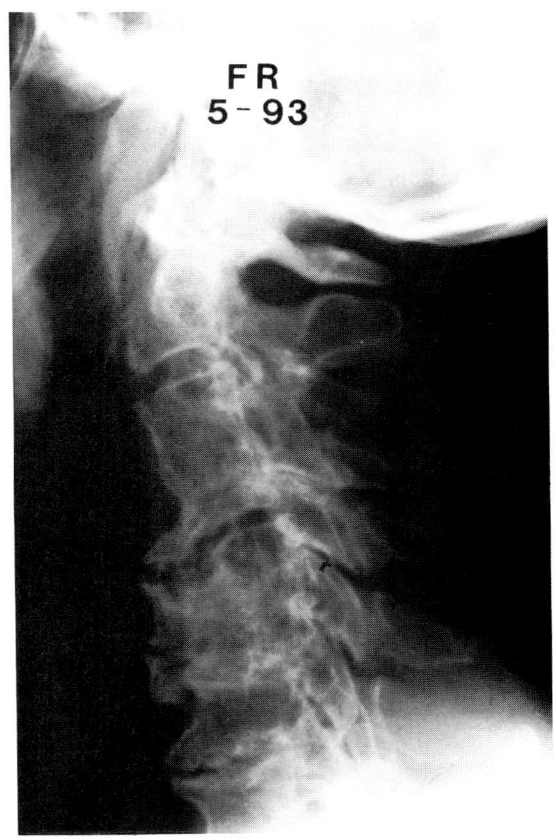

Fig. 5 **Top left,** Lateral radiograph of a 59-year-old male who presented with severe cervical myelopathy after being admitted for a total hip replacement. He was unable to walk without a walker and had a spastic quadriparesis with central cord syndrome. Note the anterior subluxation of C3 on 4 above the stiff spondylitic levels. **Top right,** Lateral view of the cervical myelogram demonstrating severe spinal cord compression at the C3-4 level. Note the relatively good filling of the dye column at the lower cervical spine where spontaneous fusion had occurred. (Reproduced with permission from Bohlman HH: Cervical spondylosis with moderate to severe myelopathy. *Spine* 1977;2:151-162.) **Bottom,** Lateral radiograph 18 years postoperatively demonstrating complete incorporation of the graft at C3-4 and some progression of the cervical spondylosis below. However, the patient was completely asymptomatic and was functioning normally with the lack of osteophyte formation at the solidly fused level.

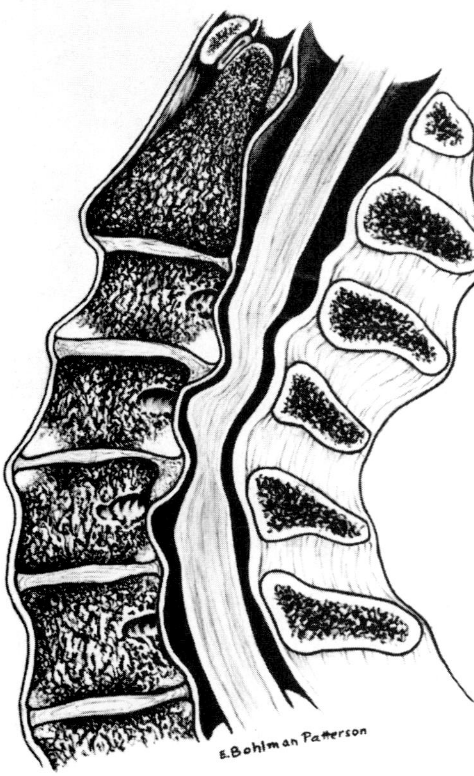

Fig. 6 Diagrammatic illustration of retrolisthesis or posterior subluxation which causes anterior spinal cord compression. Although there may be buckling of the ligamentum flavum posteriorly, these patients usually present with anterior cord compression syndromes without loss of posterior column function. (Reproduced with permission from Bohlman HH: Cervical spondylosis with moderate to severe myelopathy. *Spine* 1977;2:151-162.)

multiple level with a transverse bar or a soft disk herniation, then an anterior diskectomy and decompression with fusion should be carried out. The long-term neurologic results have been reported to be quite good with the standard Smith-Robinson decompression and fusion (Fig. 2).[37,104] If, however, a patient has a very large chondro-osseous mass compressing the spinal cord, then a wider decompression should be performed; that is, resection of a third of the vertebral body above and below followed by arthrodesis with iliac crest graft. In some more severely myelopathic patients, there will be multiple levels of spinal cord compression demonstrated on the preoperative studies. In that situation, anterior cervical corpectomies may be carried out, with resection of osteophytes from one to five levels. The extent of decompression is based on the preoperative neurologic examination as well as the cervical myelogram and CT scan. All pathologic levels that have demonstrated cord compression and deformity are resected. Technically speaking, if a two-level corpectomy is performed, then an iliac bone graft can be used. However, when the length of decompression is greater, my coworkers and I use autogenous fibular grafts.

A more complex situation arises when a patient presents with severe cervical myelopathy and cervical kyphosis after having had a previous laminectomy at multiple levels. In this situation, the kyphotic deformity frequently is rigid and it is necessary not only to do anterior decompression at appropriate levels but also to correct the kyphotic deformity[68] (Fig. 9). In addition, these patients may require posterior stabilization and arthrodesis, which can be carried out on the same day, using either a facet fusion or facet plates posteriorly with fusion. All patients treated by anterior corpectomy and fusion have intraoperative spinal cord monitoring and are treated with intraoperative skeletal traction, either by halo ring or Gardner-Wells tongs.

Presurgical Care

As mentioned, all patients have a cervical myelography and enhanced CT scan before surgery to define completely the various levels and extent of pathology and neural compression. Presurgically, cortical evoked potentials are carried out as a baseline against potentials determined intraoperatively, especially on all corpectomies, and then postoperatively before discharge and at long-term follow-up. Although not mandatory, spinal cord monitoring is believed to be useful in identifying various factors that may affect spinal cord function intraoperatively. Such factors include various anesthetic agents and manipulation of the spinal cord by skeletal traction with extension, and they provide neurologic evidence of recovery of function. It is important during surgery to maintain blood pressure and, therefore, spinal cord blood flow, because a severely compromised spinal cord, which is atrophic, can be damaged by ischemia if spinal cord perfusion is not maintained. Once the procedure is completed, the patients are placed in a rigid two-poster orthosis unless they have had a previous laminectomy or are osteoporotic or in some way deemed to be unstable, in which case they are placed in a halo vest. The orthosis or halo is worn for 6 weeks, at which time the devices are removed and the patient is placed in a soft collar for 2 more weeks. If a high-level corpectomy is performed or multiple-level corpectomies are necessary, the patient is placed routinely in the surgical intensive care unit and kept intubated until the anesthesiologist deems the soft-tissue swelling is sufficiently reduced and that the airway is sufficient. The anesthesiologist periodically examines the oral pharynx and the external neck and also deflates the endotracheal cuff to see if air is blowing by the tube.[105] My coworkers and I have begun recently to use steroids during surgery as well as 24

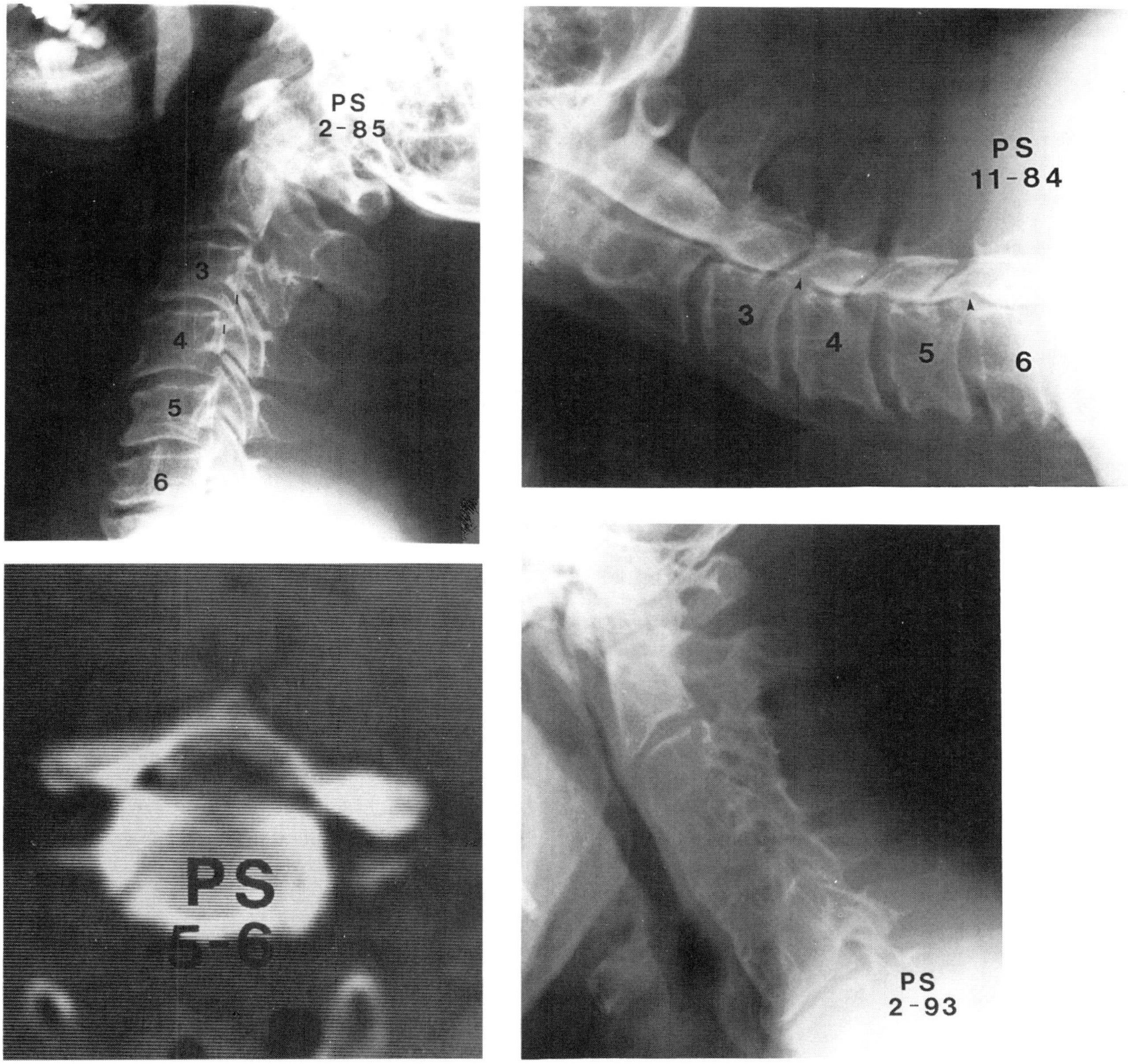

Fig. 7 **Top left,** Lateral radiograph of the cervical spine in a 48-year-old orthopaedic surgeon who fell forward off of his bicycle in November 1983, sustaining a hyperextension injury and central cord quadriparesis. Initially he was Nurick Grade V and was unable to walk. Note the congenital cervical stenosis at all levels and the retrolisthesis of C3 on C4. **Top right,** Lateral view of the cervical myelogram demonstrating multiple levels of cervical stenosis with disk protrusions at C3-4, C4-5, and C5-6. At this point, 1 year after injury, the patient had regained ambulatory status but had residual arm and hand weakness as well as some 4/5 grade leg weakness. He was unable to practice. **Bottom left,** Enhanced computed tomography (CT) scan of the patient at the C5-6 level demonstrating severe spinal cord compression. **Bottom right,** Lateral radiograph of the patient 8 years following anterior diskectomies and fusions at C3-4, C4-5, and C5-6. The patient recovered complete neurologic function and was able to practice nonoperative orthopaedics and play the piano.

hours postsurgically to decrease soft-tissue swelling. Although there is no absolute evidence in the literature that this is truly effective, it is widely used by head and neck surgeons at the hospitals in which I perform surgery, and these surgeons believe it to be quite helpful.

Complications

Complications may be related to the bone graft, soft-tissue structures of the neck, and the neurologic system. Pseudoarthroses have occurred rarely when iliac grafts were used for cervical corpectomies, but a

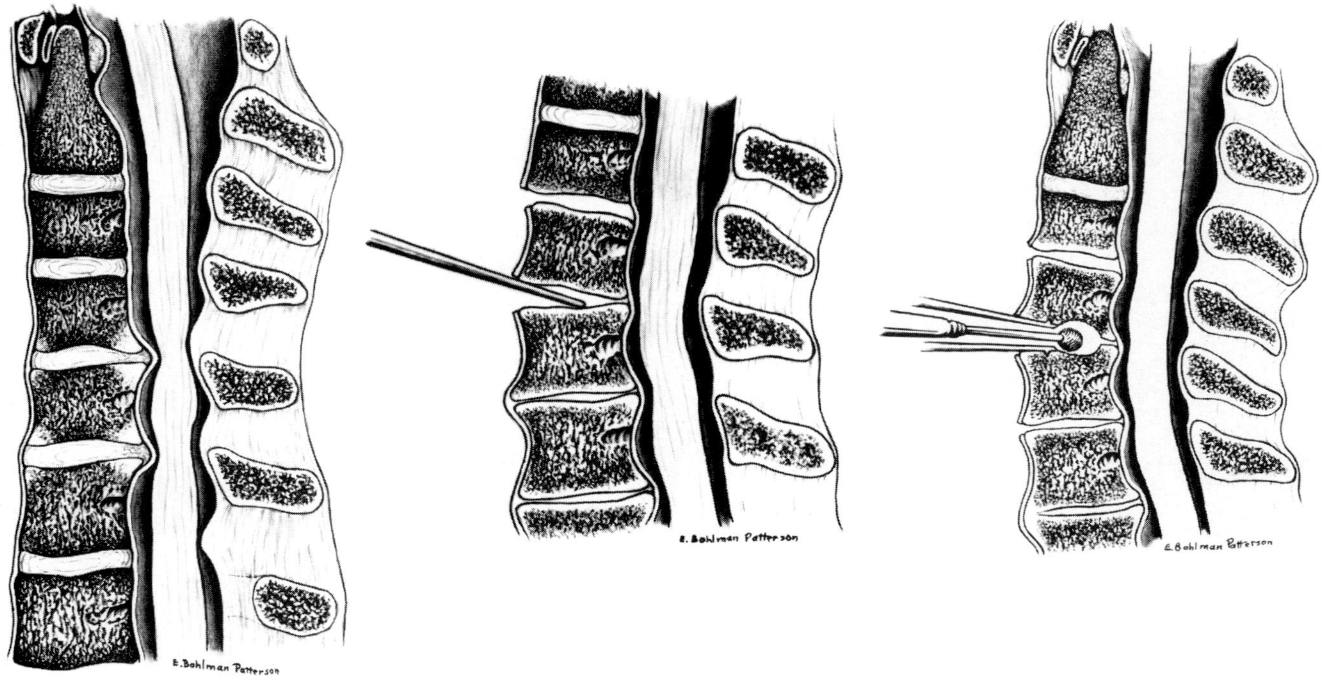

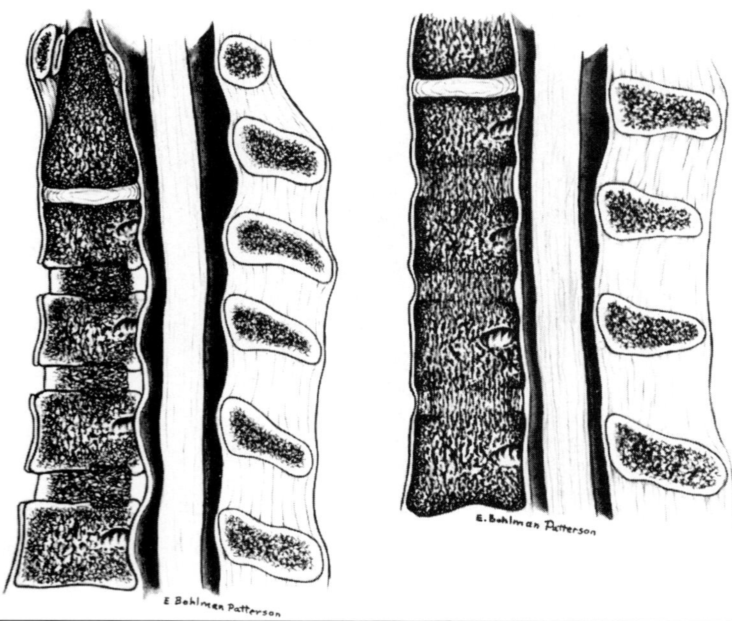

Fig. 8 **Top left,** Cervical spondylitic spine demonstrating a narrow canal, decreased height of the disk space, posterior osteophytes, and disk protrusions with buckled posterior longitudinal ligaments and ligamentum flavum. **Top center,** Technique used to pry apart the narrow disk space and allow acceptance of a graft 5 mm or greater in height. Smaller grafts may collapse and absorb. **Top right,** Technique of removing the sclerotic bony endplates with a power burr in order to have a more vascular bed to accept the bone graft and to seat the graft more accurately. This technique has also enhanced the fusion rate. **Bottom left,** Bone blocks in place and properly countersunk. The entire disk has been removed at each level without violating the posterior longitudinal ligament. Distraction straightens the redundant posterior longitudinal ligament and ligamentum flavum and immediate decompression and stability are achieved. **Bottom right,** Incorporation of the bone grafts, loss of osteophytes by normal bone remodeling, and no further redundancy of the ligamentous structures. The pathologic segments have been stabilized. (Reproduced with permission from Bohlman HH: Cervical spondylosis with moderate to severe myelopathy. *Spine* 1977;2:151-162.)

current review of patients did not reveal a pseudarthrosis when a fibular graft was used. Grafts may extrude if they are not seated properly or, in the case of fibular grafts, they may fracture through the anterior vertebral body and extrude, usually distally.[68] This problem is more common in elderly osteoporotic patients, but it can occur in younger individuals. One patient extruded an iliac graft, which perforated the esophagus and produced an abscess that had to be drained with replacement of the graft and esophageal repair. Recurrent laryngeal nerve palsy is reported as a complication with anterior cervical fusions; however, in my patients, this has not occurred as a permanent problem in 20 years.[104] The majority of my procedures are carried out from the left side purposely to avoid the aberrant course of the nerve on the right side. Vertebral artery injuries have been reported, and I have seen one occurrence of this. Ordinarily, clipping or ligation of the artery is necessary if it is lacerated. This complication will have no effect on brain function unless there is an aplastic artery on the opposite side.

The patients who are at higher risk for neurologic injury are those who have a preexisting atrophic spinal cord with long-standing spinal cord compression. My

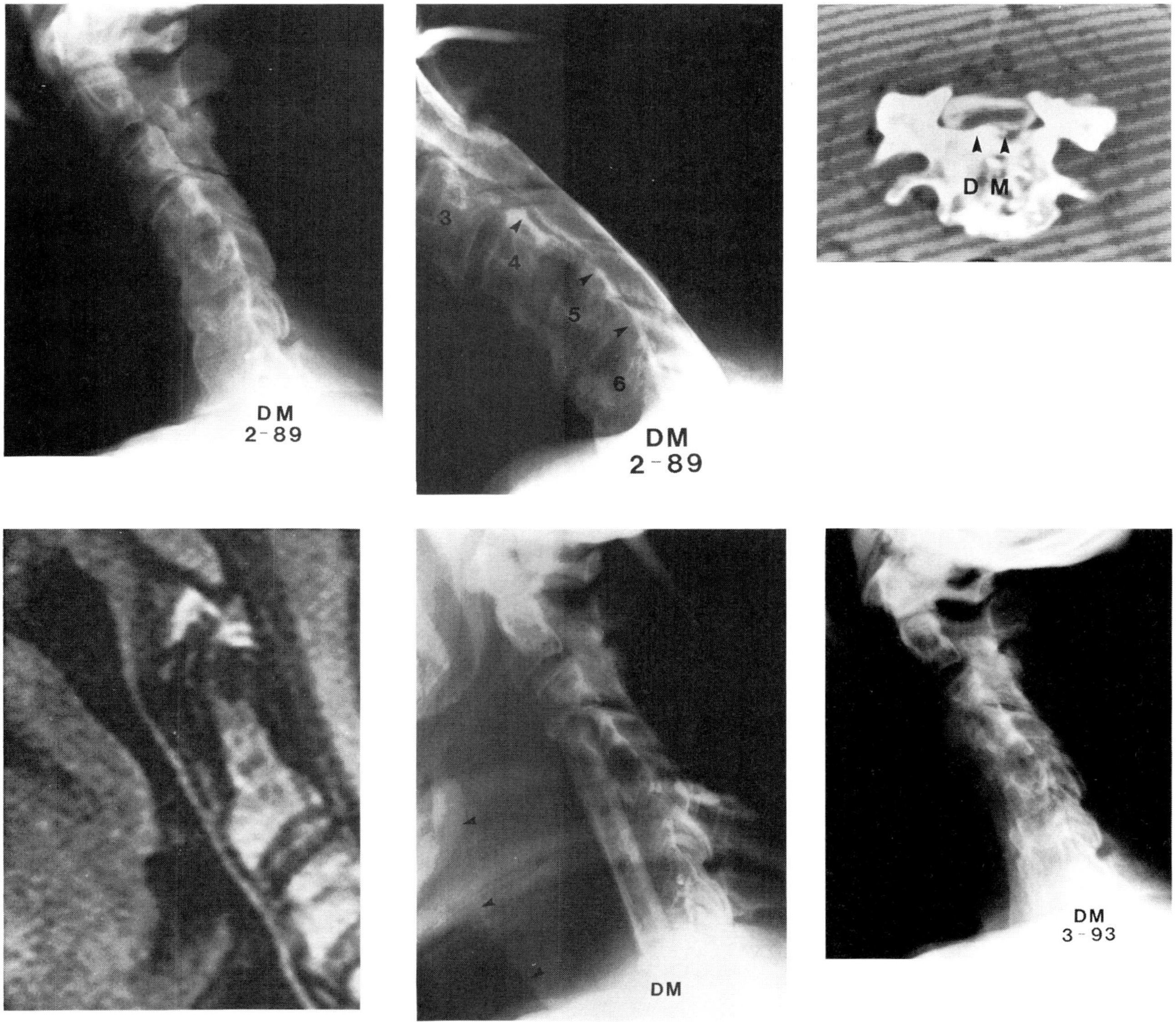

Fig. 9 **Top left,** Lateral cervical radiograph of a 56-year-old man who presented with Nurick Grade IV cervical myelopathy. He had a history of a remote laminectomy from C3 through C6, followed by individual anterior cervical fusions with progressive kyphotic deformity and myelopathy. He was unable to walk without aid. **Top center,** Lateral myelogram demonstrating marked anterior cord compression over multiple levels because of the kyphotic deformity and residual spondylosis. **Top right,** Enhanced computed tomography (CT) scan demonstrating marked flattening and anterior compression of the spinal cord by osteophytes at the kyphotic deformity. Note that the previous laminectomy has done nothing to correct the anterior cord compression. **Bottom left,** Sagittal view of the cervical magnetic resonance imaging scan demonstrating marked anterior cord compression at the kyphotic deformity. Note the atrophy and signal change of the spinal cord in the mid-cervical level. **Bottom center,** The patient underwent an anterior cervical corpectomy of C3,4,5, and 6, decompressing the spinal cord followed by insertion of a fibular strut graft from C3-C7. Note the immediate postoperative radiograph demonstrating a large hematoma formation, which can cause respiratory obstruction. To avoid this, the endotracheal tube is retained for the first few days following surgery. This patient spontaneously drained his hematoma without respiratory distress, but he did have dysphasia. **Bottom right,** Lateral radiograph of the cervical spine 4 years following surgery. Note the totally incorporated fibular graft. The patient recovered neurologic function to a Nurick Grade I and was fully ambulatory without aid.

coworkers and I have had two patients in 20 years who had C5 root palsy. The patient who had this problem immediately following the procedure recovered; and the one in whom it occurred late, 5 weeks following an extensive anterior multiple-level corpectomy and corrections of kyphosis, recovered incompletely following posterior foraminotomy. In addition, one patient with preoperative severe myelopathy developed hypotension during the surgical procedure; this resulted in a complete quadriplegia, which was permanent. This patient had a very atrophic and severely compressed spinal cord. Intraoperative spinal cord monitoring docu-

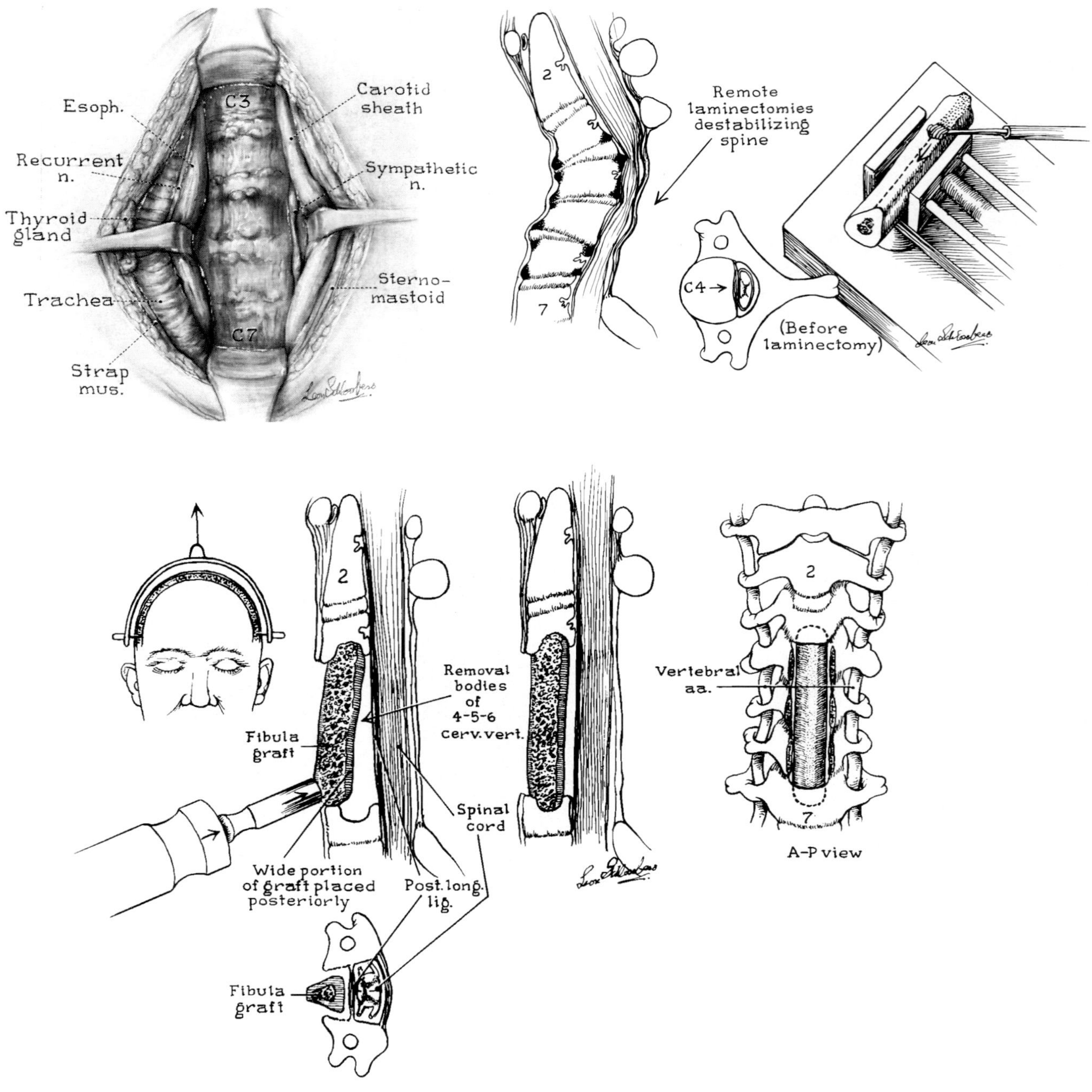

Fig. 10 **Top left,** The surgical approach, including anterior transverse incision and dissection between the carotid sheath and the trachea and esophagus to expose the anterior aspect of the spine. **Top right,** Marked compression of the spinal cord from posterior osteophytes despite a laminectomy. After the fibular strut is harvested it is shaped by using a burr. A small vise facilitates preparation of the bone graft. **Bottom,** The steps of the procedure performed following anterior corpectomy and decompression. Skeletal traction is increased to reduce the kyphosis. Extension of the neck may also be needed. Seating holes are made in the endplates of the superior and inferior intact vertebral bodies with a burr. The ends of the graft are then rounded, and the graft is impacted into place. When the traction is released, the graft is locked into place. (Reproduced with permission from Zdeblick TA, Bohlman HH: Cervical kyphosis and myelopathy: Treatment by anterior corpectomy and strut grafting. *J Bone Joint Surg* 1989;71A:170-182.)

mented loss of spinal cord function during the procedure, which was a two-level corpectomy and iliac fusion.[106]

Spinal fluid fistula may occur secondary to absence of the dura, especially in cases of ossification of the posterior longitudinal ligament.[107-110] We attempt to

Table 3
Neurologic recovery of motor function—111 patients

	Number of patients	
Nurick Grade	Presurgical	Postsurgical
I	13	86
II	31	15
III	27	4
IV	25	5
V	15	1
Total patients	111	111

repair the defect during surgery when the dura is absent because of long-standing compression. If absence of the dura is suspected presurgically, it is recommended that a lumbar spinal fluid drain be placed so that this drain can be used during surgery when the dural defect is encountered. At that time, the spinal fluid drainage is begun and my coworkers and I attempt to patch the defect by sewing a piece of muscle fascia with a stint to cover the defect. We then use fibrin glue to seal off the repair before placement of the bone graft. If the dural defect cannot be repaired with a suture and patch, we then place an onlay muscle fascial graft over the defect, seal it with fibrin glue, and place gelatin sponge on top of that repair. Following these procedures, the lumbar spinal fluid drain is kept activated for approximately 3 days. The patient is kept sedated, recumbent, on antibiotics and, once the drain is removed, the patient is then ambulated.

The only postoperative wound infection that we have had in patients with cervical myelopathy was in the one individual mentioned above whose esophagus was perforated. Although we do not use intraoperative antibiotics in less extensive decompressions, with multiple-level corpectomies it is our policy to use a broad-spectrum antibiotic for 3 days.

Results of Treatment

By and large, the long-term results of treatment of cervical myelopathy with anterior decompression and fusion have been excellent. I have carried out this procedure on more than 120 patients in 20 years to treat varying degrees of pathology causing cervical myelopathy. Of the 111 patients analyzed to date, motor function recovery has been superb even for those with severe Nurick grades of paralysis (Table 3).

References

1. Brain L, Wilkinson M (eds): *Cervical Spondylosis and Other Disorders of the Cervical Spine*, ed 1. Philadelphia, PA, WB Saunders, 1967.
2. Brain WR: Discussion on rupture of the intervertebral disc in the cervical region. *Proc R Soc Med* 1948;41:509-516.
3. Brain WR, Northfield D, Wilkinson M: The neurological manifestations of cervical spondylosis. *Brain* 1952;75:187-225.
4. Clarke E, Robinson PK: Cervical myelopathy: A complication of cervical spondylosis. *Brain* 1956;79:483-510.
5. Stookey B: Compression of the spinal cord due to ventral extradural cervical chondromas: Diagnosis and surgical treatment. *Arch Neurol Psychiat* 1928;20:275-291.
6. Robinson RA, Afeiche N, Dunn EJ, et al: Cervical spondylotic myelopathy: Etiology and treatment concepts. *Spine* 1977;2:89-99.
7. Breig A (ed): *Adverse Mechanical Tension in the Central Nervous System; An Analysis of Cause and Effect: Relief by Functional Neurosurgery*, ed 2. New York, NY, Wiley & Sons, 1978.
8. Breig A, Turnbull I, Hassler O: Effects of mechanical stresses on the spinal cord in cervical spondylosis. *Brain* 1952;75:187-225.
9. Alker G: Neuroradiology of cervical spondylotic myelopathy. *Spine* 1988;13:850- 853.
10. Arnold JG Jr: The clinical manifestations of spondylochondrosis (spondylosis) of the cervical spine. *Ann Surg* 1955;141:872-889.
11. Adams CB, Logue V: Studies in cervical spondylotic myelopathy: II. The movement and contour of the spine in relation to the neural complications of cervical spondylosis. *Brain* 1971;94:568-586.
12. Burrows EH: The sagittal diameter of the spinal canal in cervical spondylosis. *Clin Radiol* 1963;14:77-86.
13. Edwards WC, LaRocca H: The developmental segmental sagittal diameter of the cervical spinal canal in patients with cervical spondylosis. *Spine* 1983;8:20-27.
14. Epstein BS, Epstein JA, Jones MD: Cervical spinal stenosis. *Radiol Clin North Am* 1977;15:215-226.
15. Epstein JA, Carras R, Hyman RA, et al: Cervical myelopathy caused by developmental stenosis of the spinal canal. *J Neurosurg* 1979;51:362-367.
16. Hayashi H, Okada K, Hamada M, et al: Etiologic factors of myelopathy: A radiographic evaluation of the aging changes in the cervical spine. *Clin Orthop* 1987;214:200-209.
17. Hinck VC, Hopkins CE, Savara BS: Sagittal diameter of the cervical spinal canal in children. *Radiology* 1962;79:97-108.
18. LaRocca H: Cervical spondylotic myelopathy: Natural history. *Spine* 1988;13:854-855.
19. Lees F, Turner JWA: Natural history and prognosis of cervical spondylosis. *Br Med J* 1963;2:1607-1610.
20. Moiel RH, Raso E, Waltz TA: Central cord syndrome resulting from congenital narrowness of the cervical spinal canal. *J Trauma* 1970;10:502-510.
21. Murone I: The importance of the sagittal diameters of the cervical spinal canal in relation to spondylosis and myelopathy. *J Bone Joint Surg* 1974;56B:30-36.
22. Nordqvist L: The sagittal diameter of the spinal cord and subarachnoid space in different age groups: A roentgenographic post-mortem study. *Acta Radiol (Suppl)* 1964;227:1-96.
23. Parke WW: Correlative anatomy of cervical spondylotic myelopathy. *Spine* 1988;13:831-837.
24. Pavlov H, Torg JS, Robie B, et al: Cervical spinal stenosis: Determination with vertebral body ratio method. *Radiology* 1987;164:771-775.
25. Payne EE, Spillane JD: The cervical spine: An anatomico-pathological study of 70 specimens (using a special technique) with particular reference to the problem of cervical spondylosis. *Brain* 1957;80:571-596.
26. Torg JS: Pavlov's ratio: Determining cervical spinal stenosis on routine lateral roentgenograms. *Contemp Orthop* 1989;18:153-160.
27. Wilkinson M: The morbid anatomy of cervical spondylosis and myelopathy. *Brain* 1960;83:589-617.
28. Wolf BS, Khilnani M, Malis L: The sagittal diameter of the bony cervical spinal canal and its significance in cervical spondylosis. *J Mt Sinai Hosp* 1956;23:283-292.

29. Penning L, Zwaag P van der: Biomechanical aspects of spondylotic myelopathy. *Acta Radiol* 1966;5:1090-1103.
30. Bailey P, Casamajor L: Osteo-arthritis of the spine as a cause of compression of the spinal cord and its roots, with reports of five cases. *J Nerv Ment Dis* 1911;38:588-609.
31. Bedford PD, Bosanquet FD, Russell WR: Degeneration of the spinal cord associated with cervical spondylosis. *Lancet* 1952;2:55-59.
32. Fujiwara K, Yonenobu K, Hiroshima K, et al: Morphometry of the cervical spinal cord and its relation to pathology in cases with compression myelopathy. *Spine* 1988;13:1212-1216.
33. Mair WGP, Druckman R: The pathology of spinal cord lesions and their relation to the clinical features in protrusion of cervical intervertebral discs: A report of four cases. *Brain* 1953;76:70-91.
34. Kang JD, Figgie M, Bohlman HH: Sagittal measurements of the cervical spine in subaxial fractures and dislocations: An analysis of 288 patients with and without neurologic deficits. *J Bone Joint Surg* 1994;76A:1617-1628.
35. Nurick S: The natural history and the results of surgical treatment of the spinal cord disorder associated with cervical spondylosis. *Brain* 1972;95:101-108.
36. Nurick S: The pathogenesis of the spinal cord disorder associated with cervical spondylosis. *Brain* 1972;95:87-100.
37. Bohlman HH: Cervical spondylosis with moderate to severe myelopathy: A report of seventeen cases treated by Robinson anterior cervical discectomy and fusion. *Spine* 1977;2:151-162.
38. Johnson RM, Hart DL, Simmons EF, et al: Cervical orthoses: A study comparing their effectiveness in restricting cervical motion in normal subjects. *J Bone Joint Surg* 1977;59A:332-339.
39. Bailey RW, Badgley CE: Stabilization of the cervical spine by anterior fusion. *J Bone Joint Surg* 1960;42A:565-594.
40. Doppman JL: The mechanism of ischemia in anteroposterior compression of the spinal cord. *Invest Radiol* 1975;10:543-551.
41. Gooding MR, Wilson CB, Hoff JT: Experimental cervical myelopathy: Effects of ischemia and compression of the canine cervical spinal cord. *J Neurosurg* 1975;43:9-17.
42. Hoff J, Nishimura M, Pitts L, et al: The role of ischemia in the pathogenesis of cervical spondylotic myelopathy: A review and new microangiographic evidence. *Spine* 1977;2:100-108.
43. Hukuda S, Wilson CB: Experimental cervical myelopathy: Effects of compression and ischemia on the canine cervical cord. *J Neurosurg* 1972;37:631-652.
44. Shimomura Y, Hukuda S, Mizuno S: Experimental study of ischemic damage to the cervical spinal cord. *J Neurosurg* 1968; 28:565-581.
45. Suh TH, Alexander L: Vascular system of the human spinal cord. *Arch Neurol Psychiatry* 1939;41:659-677.
46. Turnbull IM: Microvasculature of the human spinal cord. *J Neurosurg* 1971;35:141-147.
47. Taylor AR: Vascular factors in the myelopathy associated with cervical spondylosis. *Neurology* 1964;14:62-68.
48. Allen KL: Neuropathies caused by bony spurs in the cervical spine with special reference to surgical treatment. *J Neurol Neurosurg Psychiatry* 1952;15:20-36.
49. Holt S, Yates PO: Cervical spondylosis and nerve root lesions: Incidence at routine necropsy. *J Bone Joint Surg* 1966;48B:407-423.
50. Hukuda S, Mochizuki T, Ogata M, et al: Operations for cervical spondylotic myelopathy: A comparison of the results of anterior and posterior procedures. *J Bone Joint Surg* 1985;67B:609-615.
51. Gledhill RF, Harrison BM, McDonald WI: Demyelination and remyelination after acute spinal cord compression. *Exp Neurol* 1973;38:472-487.
52. Bohlman HH, Bahniuk E, Raskulinecz G, et al: Mechanical factors affecting recovery from incomplete cervical spinal cord injury: A preliminary report. *Johns Hopkins Med J* 1979;145:115-125.
53. Nugent GR: Clinicopathologic correlations in cervical spondylosis. *Neurology* 1959;9:273-281.
54. Ogino H, Tada K, Okada K, et al: Canal diameter, anteroposterior compression ratio, and spondylotic myelopathy of the cervical spine. *Spine* 1983;8:1-15.
55. Ono K, Ota H, Tada K, et al: Cervical myelopathy secondary to multiple spondylotic protrusions: A clinicopathologic study. *Spine* 1977;2:109-125.
56. Panjabi M, White A III: Biomechanics of nonacute cervical spinal cord trauma. *Spine* 1988;13:838-842.
57. Peet MM, Echols DH: Herniation of the nucleus pulposus: A cause of compression of the spinal cord. *Arch Neurol Psychiatry* 1934;32:924-932.
58. Jellinger K: Spinal cord arteriosclerosis and progressive vascular myelopathy. *J Neurol Neurosurg Psychiatry* 1967;30:195-206.
59. Bohlman HH, Emery SE: The pathophysiology of cervical spondylosis and myelopathy. *Spine* 1988;13:843-846.
60. Bernhardt M, Hynes RA, Blume HW, et al: Cervical spondylotic myelopathy. *J Bone Joint Surg* 1993;75A:119-128.
61. Schneider RC: The syndrome of acute anterior spinal cord injury. *J Neurosurg* 1955;12:95-122.
62. Cusick JF: Monitoring of cervical spondylotic myelopathy. *Spine* 1988;13:877-880.
63. Leblhuber F, Reisecker F, Boehm-Jurkovic H, et al: Diagnostic value of different electrophysiologic tests in cervical disk prolapse. *Neurology* 1988;38:1879-1881.
64. Shinomiya K, Komori H, Matsuoka T, et al: Neuroradiologic and electrophysiologic assessment of cervical spondylotic amyotrophy. *Spine* 1994;19:21-25.
65. Yiannikas C, Shahani BT, Young RR: Short-latency somatosensory-evoked potentials from radial, median, ulnar, and peroneal nerve stimulation in the assessment of cervical spondylosis: Comparison with conventional electromyography. *Arch Neurol* 1986; 43:1264-1271.
66. Yu YL, Jones SJ: Somatosensory evoked potentials in cervical spondylosis: Correlation of median, ulnar and posterior tibial nerve responses with clinical and radiological findings. *Brain* 1985;108(Pt 2):273-300.
67. Boden SD, Dodge LD, Bohlman HH, et al: Rheumatoid arthritis of the cervical spine: A long-term analysis with predictors of paralysis and recovery. *J Bone Joint Surg* 1993;75A:1282-1297.
68. Zdeblick TA, Bohlman HH: Cervical kyphosis and myelopathy: Treatment by anterior corpectomy and strut-grafting. *J Bone Joint Surg* 1989;71A:170-182.
69. Raynor RB, Pugh J, Shapiro I: Cervical facetectomy and its effect on spine strength. *J Neurosurg* 1985;63:278-282.
70. McAfee PC, Regan JJ, Bohlman HH: Cervical cord compression from ossification of the posterior longitudinal ligament in non-orientals. *J Bone Joint Surg* 1987;69B:569-575.
71. Hirabayashi K, Miyakawa J, Satomi K, et al: Operative results and postoperative progression of ossification among patients with ossification of cervical posterior longitudinal ligament. *Spine* 1981;6:354-364.
72. Hirabayashi K, Satomi K, Sasaki T: Ossification of the posterior longitudinal ligament in the cervical spine, in The Cervical Spine Research Society Editorial Committee (eds): *The Cervical Spine,* ed 2. Philadelphia, PA, JB Lippincott, 1989, pp 678-692.
73. Yonenobu K, Fuji T, Ono K, et al: Choice of surgical treatment for multisegmental cervical spondylotic myelopathy. *Spine* 1985; 10:710-716.
74. Bohlman HH: The neck, in D'Ambrosia RD (ed): *Musculoskeletal Disorders: Regional Examination and Differential Diagnosis,* ed 2. Philadelphia, PA, JB Lippincott, 1986, pp 219-286.
75. Brown BM, Schwartz RH, Frank E, et al: Preoperative evaluation of cervical radiculopathy and myelopathy by surface-coil MR imaging. *AJR Am J Roentgenol* 1988;151:1205-1212.

76. Clark CR: Cervical spondylotic myelopathy: History and physical findings. *Spine* 1988;13:847-849.
77. Epstein NE, Epstein JA, Carras R, et al: Coexisting cervical and lumbar spinal stenosis: Diagnosis and management. *Neurosurg* 1984;15:489-496.
78. Keegan JJ: The cause of dissociated motor loss in the upper extremity with cervical spondylosis: A case report. *J Neurosurg* 1965;23:528-536.
79. Matsunaga S, Sakou T, Imamura T, et al: Dissociated motor loss in the upper extremities: Clinical features and pathophysiology. *Spine* 1993;18:1964-1967.
80. Modic MT, Ross JS, Masaryk TJ: Imaging of degenerative disease of the cervical spine. *Clin Orthop* 1989;239:109-120.
81. Penning L, Wilmink JT, van Woerden HH, et al: CT myelographic findings in degenerative disorders of the cervical spine: Clinical significance. *AJR Am J Roentgenol* 1986;146:793-801.
82. Epstein JA, Carras R, Epstein BS, et al: Myelopathy in cervical spondylosis with vertebral subluxation and hyperlordosis. *J Neurosurg* 1970;32:421-426.
83. Murphy MJ, Lieponis JV: Nonoperative treatment of cervical spine pain, in Cervical Spine Research Society Editorial Committee (ed): *The Cervical Spine*, ed 2. Philadelphia, PA, JB Lippincott, 1989, pp 670-677.
84. Epstein NE, Hyman RA, Epstein JA, et al: Dynamic MRI scanning of the cervical spine. *Spine* 1988;13:937-938.
85. Epstein JA, Epstein NE: The surgical management of cervical spinal stenosis, spondylosis, and myeloradiculopathy by means of the posterior approach, in The Cervical Spine Research Society Editorial Committee (ed): *The Cervical Spine*, ed 2. Philadelphia, PA, JB Lippincott, 1989, pp 625-643.
86. Epstein JA, Janin Y, Carras R, et al: A comparative study of the treatment of cervical spondylotic myeloradiculopathy: Experience with 50 cases treated by means of extensive laminectomy, foraminotomy, and excision of osteophytes during the past 10 years. *Acta Neurochir* 1982;61:89-104.
87. Ishida Y, Suzuki K, Ohmori K, et al: Critical analysis of extensive cervical laminectomy. *Neurosurg* 1989;24:215-222.
88. Crandall PH, Gregorius FK: Long-term follow-up of surgical treatment of cervical spondylotic myelopathy. *Spine* 1977;2:139-146.
89. Gregorius FK, Estrin T, Crandall PH: Cervical spondylotic radiculopathy and myelopathy: A long-term follow-up study. *Arch Neurol* 1976;33:618-625.
90. Herkowitz HN: A comparison of anterior cervical fusion, cervical laminectomy, and cervical laminoplasty for the surgical management of multiple level spondylotic radiculopathy. *Spine* 1988; 13:774-780.
91. Herkowitz HN: The surgical management of cervical spondylotic radiculopathy and myelopathy. *Clin Orthop* 1989;239:94-108.
92. Hirabayashi K, Satomi K: Operative procedure and results of expansive open-door laminoplasty. *Spine* 1988;13:870-876.
93. White AA III, Panjabi MM: Biomechanical considerations in the surgical management of cervical spondylotic myelopathy. *Spine* 1988;13:856-860.
94. Boni M, Cherubino P, Denaro V, et al: Multiple subtotal somatectomy: Technique and evaluation of a series of 39 cases. *Spine* 1984;9:358-362.
95. Connolly ES, Seymour RJ, Adams JE: Clinical evaluation of anterior cervical fusion for degenerative cervical disc disease. *J Neurosurg* 1965;23:431-437.
96. Emery SE, Bolesta MJ, Banks MA, et al: Robinson anterior cervical fusion: Comparison of the standard and modified techniques. *Spine* 1994;19:660-663.
97. Hanai K, Fujiyoshi F, Kamei K: Subtotal vertebrectomy and spinal fusion for cervical spondylotic myelopathy. *Spine* 1986;11:310-315.
98. Simmons EH, Bhalla SK: Anterior cervical discectomy and fusion: A clinical and biomechanical study with eight-year follow-up. *J Bone Joint Surg* 1969;51B:225-237.
99. Smith GW, Robinson RA: The treatment of certain cervical-spine disorders by anterior removal of the intervertebral disc and interbody fusion. *J Bone Joint Surg* 1958;40A:607-624.
100. White AA III, Southwick WO, Deponte RJ, et al: Relief of pain by anterior cervical-spine fusion for spondylosis: A report of sixty-five patients. *J Bone Joint Surg* 1973;55A:525-534.
101. Bernard TN Jr, Whitecloud TS III: Cervical spondylotic myelopathy and myeloradiculopathy: Anterior decompression and stabilization with autogenous fibula strut graft. *Clin Orthop* 1987;221:149-160.
102. Whitecloud TS III: Anterior surgery for cervical spondylotic myelopathy: Smith-Robinson, Cloward, and vertebrectomy. *Spine* 1988;13:861-863.
103. Ferguson RJ, Caplan LR: Cervical spondylitic myelopathy. *Neurol Clin* 1985;3:373-382.
104. Zdeblick TA, Ducker TB: The use of freeze-dried allograft bone for anterior cervical fusions. *Spine* 1991;16:726-729.
105. Bohlman HH, Emery SE, Goodfellow DB, et al: Robinson anterior cervical discectomy and arthrodesis for cervical radiculopathy: Long term follow-up of one hundred and twenty-two patients. *J Bone Joint Surg* 1993;75A:1298-1307.
106. Emery SE, Smith MD, Bohlman HH: Upper-airway obstruction after multilevel cervical corpectomy for myelopathy. *J Bone Joint Surg* 1991;73A:544-551.
107. Flynn TB: Neurologic complications of anterior cervical interbody fusion. *Spine* 1982;7:536-539.
108. Smith MD, Bolesta MJ, Leventhal M, et al: Postoperative cerebrospinal-fluid fistula associated with erosion of the dura: Findings after anterior resection of ossification of the posterior longitudinal ligament in the cervical spine. *J Bone Joint Surg* 1992;74A:270-277.
109. Emery SE, Bolesta MJ, Bohlman HH: Anterior decompression and fusion for cervical spondylotic myelopathy: 2-17 year follow-up. Presented at the 61st Annual Meeting of the American Academy of Orthopaedic Surgeons, New Orleans, LA, 1994.
110. Saunders RL, Bernini PM, Shirreffs TG Jr, et al: Central corpectomy for cervical spondylotic myelopathy: A consecutive series with long-term follow-up evaluation. *J Neurosurg* 1991; 74:163-170.

CHAPTER 7

Evaluation and Management of Cervical Spondylotic Myelopathy

Melvin D. Law Jr, MD
Mark Bernhardt, MD
Augustus A. White III, MD, Dr Med Sci

Cervical spondylotic myelopathy (CSM) is defined as spinal cord dysfunction secondary to extrinsic compression of the cord or its vascular supply, or both,[1] that is caused by degenerative disease of the cervical spine. It is the most common type of spinal cord dysfunction in patients who are older than 55 years of age.[2,3] Cervical spondylotic myelopathy frequently is underdiagnosed and undertreated, often leading to increased disability. The key to the initial diagnosis is a careful neurologic examination. The physical findings may be subtle; thus, a high index of suspicion is important.

Pathophysiology

CSM may be associated with congenital or developmental stenosis of the cervical canal. The problem begins with degenerative changes in the disk,[1] which produce secondary changes in the adjacent osseous and soft-tissue structures. Encroachment on the available space in the spinal canal results from osteophytic spurring of the facet and uncovertebral joints (Fig. 1). Soft-tissue compression of the spinal cord results from intervertebral disk herniation and invagination of the ligamentum flavum into the canal. This invagination is thought to result from a decrease in disk height and a loss of elasticity of the ligamentum flavum.[4] Thickening of the ligamentum flavum also may occur.[4-6] Ligamentous laxity resulting from degenerative changes, inflammatory disease, or trauma may allow anterior or posterior subluxation of the cervical vertebrae and pinching of the cord between the vertebral bodies.[2,6,7] Even without subluxation, normal motion of the neck can produce a pincer mechanism when there are morphologic changes of the posterior aspect of the vertebral body (spurring) and protrusion of the anterior aspect of the lamina or ligamentum flavum into the canal.[5,8-14]

Clinical Evaluation

The clinical evaluation includes a history, a physical examination, and a radiographic examination. Magnetic resonance imaging (MRI) or myelography (or both) followed by computed tomographic (CT) scanning is most useful for surgical planning.[2,15] Electrophysiologic studies usually are not necessary for the diagnosis, but they may be useful for following the patient's progress.[16] A careful and complete evaluation is necessary in order to make the diagnosis and to rule out other causes of spinal cord dysfunction, such as cerebrovascular disease, arteriovenous malformation, demyelinating disease, syringomyelia, intracranial tumor, hydrocephalus, tabes dorsalis, myopathy, peripheral neuropathy, and metabolic or alcoholic encephalopathy.[2]

History

Characteristically, patients who have CSM have neck pain, difficulty walking, and unsteadiness on the feet. Pain, numbness, paresthesias, weakness, and loss of dexterity of the upper extremities are common findings. Frequently, there is coexisting compression of cervical nerve roots, which causes radicular symptoms as well. Bladder dysfunction may occur, but it is not common. Coexisting lumbar spinal stenosis is common;[17] there-

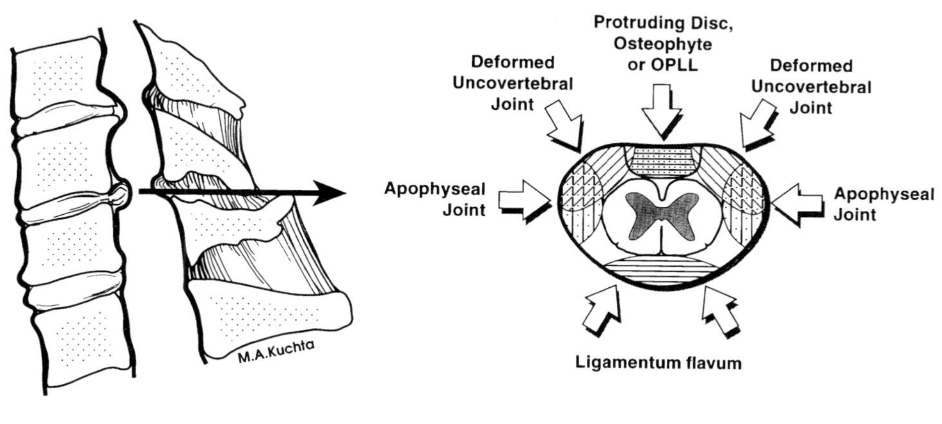

Fig. 1 Schematic drawings showing various structures that can contribute to the pathological anatomy of cervical spondylotic myelopathy. (OPLL = ossification of the posterior longitudinal ligament)

fore, patients who have severe lumbar stenosis should have a careful evaluation in order to rule out CSM.

Physical Examination

Upper motor neuron findings occur in the lower extremities and lower motor neuron findings occur in the upper extremities at the level of the compressive lesion. This combination can be remembered by the phrase "uppers in the lowers and lowers in the uppers." Upper motor neuron findings also may occur in the upper extremities caudad to the level of the lesion; thus, deep tendon reflexes may be hyperactive in both the upper and the lower limbs. The Hoffmann reflex, the inverted radial reflex,[18] the Lhermitte sign, and clonus are indicative of myelopathy. The Hoffmann reflex or sign is present when the ipsilateral interphalangeal joints of the thumb and index finger flex when the volar surface of the terminal phalanx of the long finger is flicked. Extension of the neck by the patient or the examiner during testing increases the sensitivity of the Hoffmann sign.[19]

The inverted radial reflex is spontaneous flexion of the digits when the examiner attempts to elicit the brachioradialis reflex. When present, this sign is virtually pathognomonic of CSM because it indicates spondylotic compression of the cord at the fifth and sixth cervical level, which is where CSM most commonly occurs. A large spur or disk interferes with the reflex arc (brachioradialis) at the sixth cervical level and compresses the cord, causing an upper motor neuron lesion with spontaneous (spastic) contraction of the finger flexors, which are innervated caudad to the sixth cervical level.

Flexion or extension of the neck may produce the Lhermitte sign (paresthesias or electric shock-like sensations, usually occurring in the legs). This sign is seen more often with the neck in flexion. Abnormal plantar responses (the Babinski sign) usually do not occur until myelopathy becomes severe.[18] Sensory examination may reveal changes in the reaction to pain, temperature, and light touch, but the more specific findings are changes in position and vibratory sensation. The earliest findings are disdiadochokinesia (slow or uncoordinated rapid alternating movements), difficulty with tandem gait, and subtle deficits in fine motor function. The Hoffmann and Lhermitte signs may be seen both early and late (Table 1).

Table 1
Physical findings associated with cervical spondylotic myelopathy

Early Findings	Late Findings
Disdiadochokinesia	Spasticity
Difficulty with tandem gait	Difficulty with routine gait
Fine motor deficits	Gross motor deficits
Mildly increased reflexes	Markedly increased reflexes
Clonus (mild and unsustained)	Clonus (sustained)
Decreased proprioception	Gross difficulty with balancing

Diagnostic Studies

Plain anteroposterior, oblique, and lateral radiographs often show narrowing of the disk space. Posterior, foraminal, and uncovertebral osteophytes also may be seen. The lateral radiograph may show spondylolisthesis, lordosis, or kyphosis.

Lateral radiographs made with the spine in flexion and extension are a useful test for instability.[4] On the lateral radiograph, the presence of developmental stenosis can be identified by measurement of the Pavlov ratio (the anteroposterior diameter of the spinal canal divided by the anteroposterior diameter of the vertebral body at the same level) (Fig. 2).[20,21] This ratio is not affected by variations in radiographic magnification; therefore, it is a better guide than direct measurement of the size of the canal on a radiograph. A ratio of 1.0 is normal and a ratio of less than 0.8 indicates a developmentally narrow canal.

MRI should be used to evaluate the soft-tissue structures and the spinal cord.[22] The T2-weighted gradient-echo image may show increased signal intensity, indicating injury to the spinal cord. So-called dynamic MRI scans (scans obtained with the neck in flexion and in extension) can document dynamic cord compression,[5] which may occur even though osseous instability is not demonstrated on flexion and extension radiographs. These magnetic resonance images may show compression of the cord by a hypotonic ligamentum flavum or by dynamic annular bulging.[11,13,14] Myelography followed by CT scanning can be an adjunct to MRI, and it helps to distinguish disk material from osteophytes.[22] The myelogram is superior for determination of compression of the spinal cord by the vertebral body when

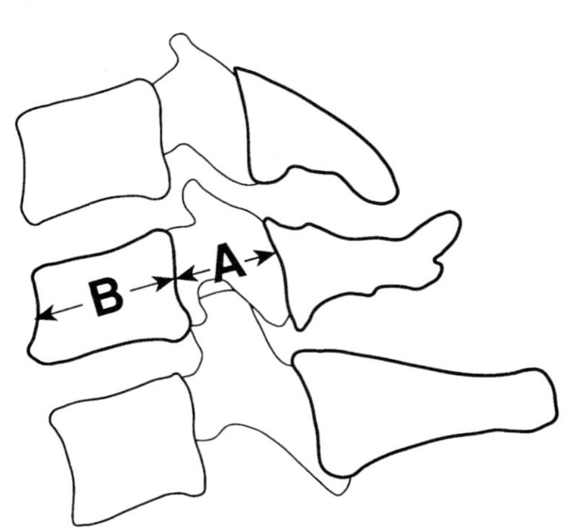

Fig. 2 The Pavlov ratio, which is the anteroposterior diameter of the spinal canal (A) divided by the anteroposterior diameter of the vertebral body at the same level (B), as measured on a lateral radiograph. It is normally about 1.0; a ratio of less than 0.8 indicates a developmentally narrow cervical canal.

subluxation is present, and post-myelographic CT is superior for evaluation of ossification of the posterior longitudinal ligament.[23,24]

A useful measurement that can be made on the axial MRI or the post-myelographic CT scan is the compression ratio (Fig. 3).[6,25] The compression ratio is measured by dividing the smallest anteroposterior dimension of the spinal cord (the sagittal diameter) by the broadest transverse diameter at the same level. A compression ratio of less than 0.4 after decompression, especially when myelopathy has been present for more than 6 months, portends a guarded prognosis for recovery.[25] Conversely, an increase in the compression ratio to 0.4 or more postoperatively or an increase in the transverse area of the spinal cord to more than 40 mm^2 correlates with clinical recovery.[25,26] The measurement of the transverse area of the spinal cord at the affected level on the post-myelographic axial CT has been shown to be the most accurate predictor of neurologic recovery from CSM and ossification of the posterior longitudinal ligament.

Treatment

The natural history of CSM has not been thoroughly defined and documented. Almost all patients worsen clinically if left untreated, and most studies have demonstrated a high proportion (more than 50%) of patients who have progressed to severe disability.[27-34] Catastrophic neurologic deterioration has developed rapidly in some patients, but there is no known method of identifying these patients beforehand.[30] Although the prognosis for the recovery of spinal cord function postoperatively is variable, the best results have been obtained for those who were managed with decompression within 6 months to 1 year after the onset of symptoms; those who had early, mild myelopathic findings;[26,35] and those in whom the transverse area of the spinal cord was greater than 40 mm^2 postoperatively.[25,26]

Nonsurgical Treatment

The nonsurgical treatment of CSM consists of cervical immobilization in a firm orthosis, the use of anti-inflammatory medications, physical therapy emphasizing isometric muscle strengthening, and other symptom-relieving measures such as the application of heat or ice and massage. Patients who are managed nonsurgically should be monitored closely and taught to look for the progression of weakness, spasticity, imbalance, or a combination of these symptoms. We suggest that patients have follow-up examinations every 6 to 12 weeks initially, and then every 6 months if the neurologic deficit has not progressed. We advise against the use of traction because it can make the condition worse.[36] Manipulation is contraindicated because extension of the neck causes narrowing of the spinal canal[8-11,13,14] and the foramina.[37] Manipulation can also irritate the facet joints, causing further swelling of the soft tissues with encroachment on the spinal cord. For patients who have a high surgical risk or serious comorbid factors, as do many elderly patients, cervical epidural steroid injections may help to control symptoms.[38]

Surgical Indications

Because the natural history of CSM is not well understood, there is debate over the indications for surgical treatment. Absolute indications for surgery are the progression of a neurologic deficit or the failure of neurologic findings to improve with nonsurgical treatment, especially if CSM has been present for 6 months or longer. Because of the less favorable prognosis for recovery for patients who have a compression ratio of less than 0.4, a transverse spinal cord area of 40 mm^2 or less, or increased signal intensity of the spinal cord on the T2-weighted MRI, we recommend that surgical treatment be undertaken before this degree of spinal cord compromise occurs.

Patients who are older than 70 years of age and who have neurologic deficits and serious medical problems should be considered individually for surgical management. The risk of an operation should be weighed against the neurologic findings and the potential for disability resulting from progression of the myelopathy.[39,40]

For patients who have coexisting CSM and lumbar stenosis, it usually is preferable to decompress the

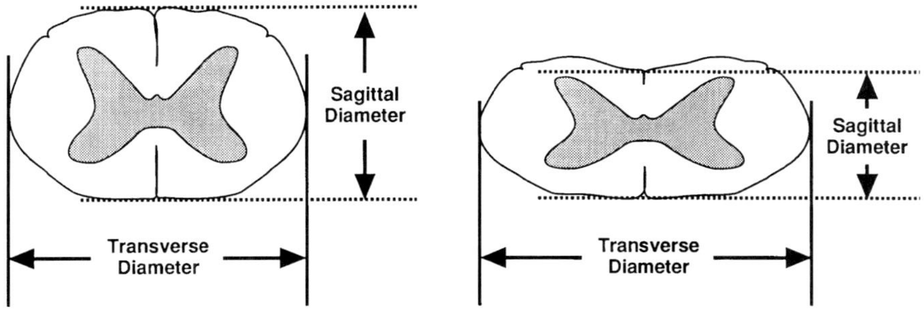

Fig. 3 The compression ratio, which is the smallest anteroposterior diameter (sagittal diameter) of the spinal cord divided by the broadest transverse diameter at the same level, is a good indicator of pathological changes of the spinal cord. This ratio can be measured on axial MRIs or on post-myelographic CT images.

cervical spine first in order to decrease the risk of intubation during the lumbar procedure. In addition, lower-extremity pain and spasticity of myelopathic origin may improve after cervical decompression; however, the neurogenic claudication caused by cauda equina compression will not be affected and may even worsen.[17]

Decompression may be achieved using an anterior, a posterior, or a combined approach. Each patient has unique clinical conditions that require individualized treatment. An algorithm, based on our clinical experience, the previously stated goals, and the current literature, can serve as a guideline for surgical decision-making (Fig. 4). The specific steps of this algorithm are described in subsequent sections of this lecture.

Presurgical Considerations

All nonsteroidal anti-inflammatory medication should be discontinued 1 to 2 weeks before the operation. The patient should be prepared for the performance of a fiberoptic intubation while he or she is awake. The positioning of the patient on the operating table should avoid hyperextension of the cervical spine. If the patient also has symptoms of lumbar stenosis, lumbar extension should be avoided as well.

For the anterior approach, we prefer for the patient to be in the supine position; an interscapular and low posterior neck roll is used to support the lower cervical spine in a neutral position. The head is secured with a head halter with 3 to 5 lb (1.4 to 2.3 kg) of cervical traction, and it is turned slightly to the right to facilitate a left-sided approach. We prefer the left-sided approach because it minimizes the potential for injury to the recurrent laryngeal nerve.[41] For the posterior approach, the patient is placed in the prone position, with the head secured by a Mayfield three-pin head holder and with the neck positioned in neutral.

Pneumatic compression stockings and a urinary catheter should be used. Intravenous administration of methylprednisolone (125 mg) should be considered presurgically and again 4 to 6 hours after the first dose; theoretically, this lessens the chance of intrinsic and extrinsic cord swelling. Antacids and H-2 receptor blockers should be given when corticosteroids are used. In order to minimize bleeding when a patient is managed with the posterior approach, as much as 250 ml of 1:500,000 epinephrine solution should be used to infiltrate the skin, subcutaneous tissues, and muscles before the skin is incised. It is important that the needle be directed 45° caudad, in order to avoid its entering the spinal canal.

Bone Graft Technique

A controversial point is the type of graft (allograft or autograft) to be used for anterior interbody arthrodesis. Although there is morbidity at the donor site, we prefer iliac-crest autograft to allograft. Several studies have documented substantially higher rates of nonunion and collapse and slower rates of fusion when allograft was used.[42,43] When the arthrodesis has included more than one spinal motion segment, the rate of nonunion has been reported to be as high as 63% when allograft was used compared with 17% when autograft was used.[44]

The Smith-Robinson interbody graft should be thick enough to provide at least 2 mm more distraction compared with the baseline disk height and even more distraction when the baseline disk height is less than 3.5 mm.[45] The graft should be tricortical and harvested with an oscillating saw instead of an osteotome, because saw-harvested grafts have substantially greater strength.[46]

Lesions Involving One or Two Intervertebral Disk Levels

Soft-Disk Herniation

Soft-disk herniations usually occur in younger patients. Osteophytic spurring contributes little if any to this disorder.[47] Because the spinal cord compression is caused by the soft disk and an adequate reserve space remains in the spinal canal, the rate of recovery after decompression is more rapid than that after decompression for CSM or ossification of the posterior longitudinal ligament, irrespective of the transverse area of the spinal cord, the compression ratio, or the duration of symptoms.[26] Nonsurgical treatment often is effective for the treatment of soft-disk herniations, and absolute surgical indications should be limited to the failure of nonsurgical therapy with continued neurologic findings for 6 months or the presence of progressive myelopathy with correlative diagnostic studies demonstrating the herniated disk.

When surgical treatment is indicated, the MRI should be reviewed carefully in order to identify a free fragment of disk material lying behind the posterior longitudinal ligament (PLL). The disk should be resected back until the vertical fibers of the PLL are seen. Then, the PLL should be inspected carefully for a defect, and any disk material that may have herniated through the defect should be removed. Routine removal of the PLL and inspection of the space behind it is not recommended if the MRI does not reveal a free fragment and careful intrasurgical inspection of the PLL does not show a defect.

Satisfactory short-term results have been obtained with the use of simple decompression without arthrodesis for the treatment of a soft-disk herniation involving one level.[47,48] These studies had limited clinical follow-up and only small numbers of patients who had myelopathy. The long-term likelihood of kyphotic collapse or spondylosis developing at the level of the diskectomy is not known; therefore, we do not recommend this procedure when myelopathy is present. We suggest the use of the arthrodesis technique described by Smith and Robinson[49] because it provides the most stable con-

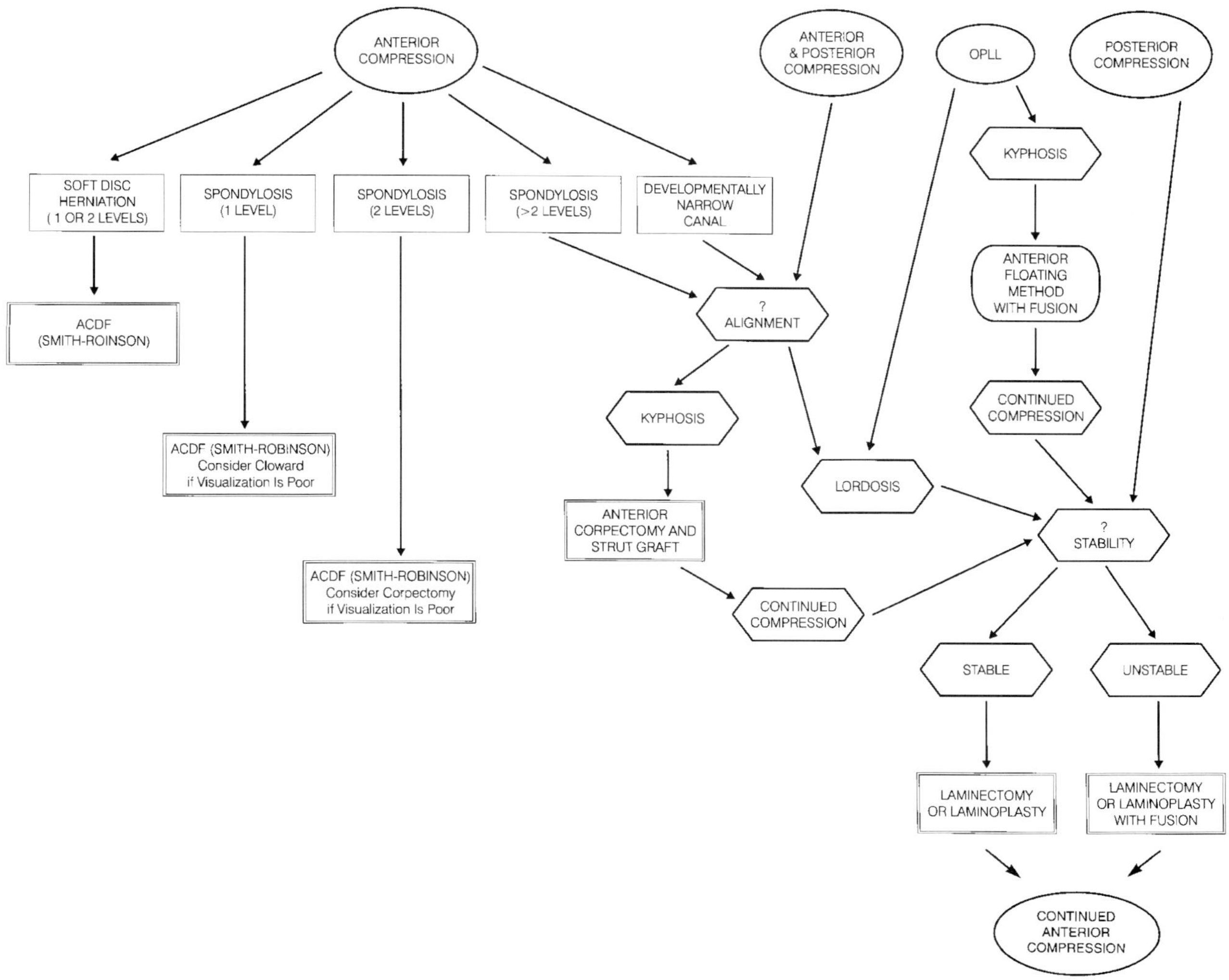

Fig. 4 Algorithm for the surgical treatment of CSM. (ACDF = anterior cervical diskectomy and fusion; OPLL = ossification of the posterior longitudinal ligament)

struct, it is the least likely to collapse, and it allows for distraction if disk-space narrowing has occurred.

Degenerative Disk Disease (Spondylosis)

Cervical spondylosis, with its associated disk-space narrowing, disk herniation, and osteophyte formation, is the most common cause of CSM (Fig. 5). Although osteophytes resorb in most patients after a solid fusion is achieved,[7] they can impede recovery or even cause late deterioration of results.[50] For these reasons, prominent osteophytes or those associated with a developmentally narrow canal should be removed in order to ensure that adequate space is available for the spinal cord. After the disk has been removed back to the PLL, the osteophyte on the posterior part of the body should be ground down to a thin cortical shell and left attached to the PLL. The cortical shell then can be cracked off and removed with a microcuret or a small Kerrison rongeur.

We recommend the Smith-Robinson technique for anterior interbody arthrodesis (Fig. 5), because it provides distraction of the collapsed disk, thereby opening the foramina and decompressing the nerve roots, and because it provides the most stable construct. Another benefit of distraction is that tension is placed on the ligamentum flavum, thereby reducing invagination of this structure into the canal. Excessive distraction should not be attempted because it can result in harmful tension on the spinal cord.[4,51]

The Smith-Robinson technique has some limitations. It is difficult to decompress the nerve root directly in the foramen through the anterior approach. A second disadvantage is the limited visibility posteriorly for osteophyte removal. An operating microscope may be helpful in this situation. The Cloward procedure[52] also may provide improved visualization; when this procedure is used, however, the fusion is less stable,[53] there is

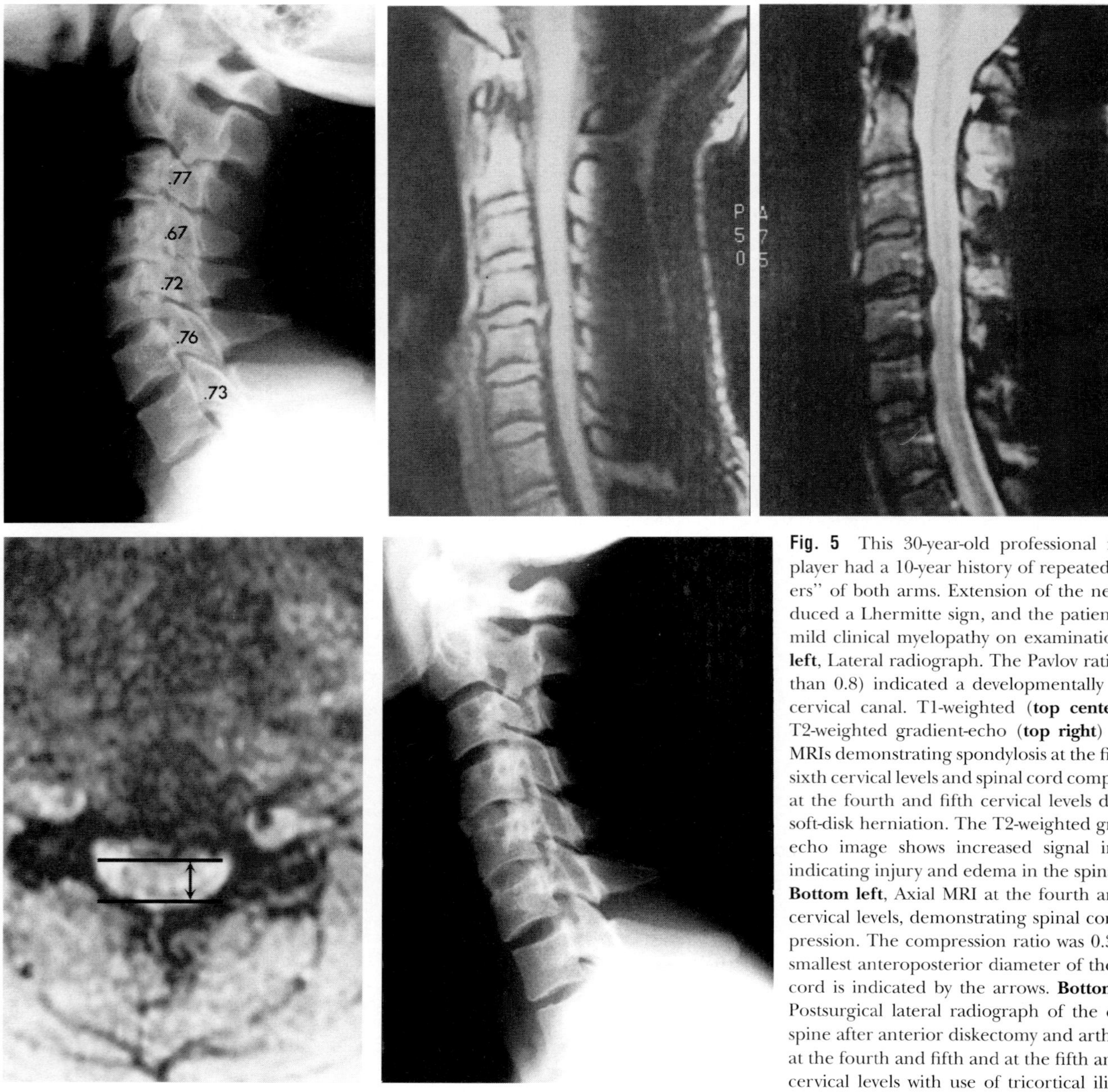

Fig. 5 This 30-year-old professional football player had a 10-year history of repeated "stingers" of both arms. Extension of the neck produced a Lhermitte sign, and the patient had a mild clinical myelopathy on examination. **Top left**, Lateral radiograph. The Pavlov ratios (less than 0.8) indicated a developmentally narrow cervical canal. T1-weighted (**top center**) and T2-weighted gradient-echo (**top right**) sagittal MRIs demonstrating spondylosis at the fifth and sixth cervical levels and spinal cord compression at the fourth and fifth cervical levels due to a soft-disk herniation. The T2-weighted gradient-echo image shows increased signal intensity indicating injury and edema in the spinal cord. **Bottom left**, Axial MRI at the fourth and fifth cervical levels, demonstrating spinal cord compression. The compression ratio was 0.33. The smallest anteroposterior diameter of the spinal cord is indicated by the arrows. **Bottom right,** Postsurgical lateral radiograph of the cervical spine after anterior diskectomy and arthrodesis at the fourth and fifth and at the fifth and sixth cervical levels with use of tricortical iliac-crest autologous graft.

no distraction, and there is a greater potential for postsurgical collapse because the vertebral end plates are removed. (In the Cloward procedure, a large drill is directed through the disk, which is removed along with a semicircle of bone from the vertebrae cephalad and caudad to the disk. A dowel-shaped graft then is inserted into the space in order to achieve an interbody fusion.) For two-level involvement, vertebral corpectomy provides the best visualization, but this is a very destabilizing procedure and it has a higher rate of complications than do other techniques.[54]

One or Two-Level Spondylosis with Mild Developmental Narrowing of the Canal

We define mild developmental narrowing of the canal as a Pavlov ratio of between 0.8 and 1.0. If the compression is purely anterior in the stenotic canal and the adjacent levels are without spondylosis, a successful result can be expected from anterior decompression and arthrodesis. If the adjacent levels have degenerative changes, the patient is at risk for the development of stenosis adjacent to the level of the anterior arthrodesis,[50] and consideration should be given to posterior decompression and arthrodesis. We prefer the anterior approach, especially for younger patients, when it is apparent that enough space will be available for the cord after decompression (that is, when there is an absence of facet joint or ligamentum flavum hypertrophy in the developmentally narrow canal). This approach is recommended because it limits the operation to the involved levels and addresses the lesion directly. If there is no progressive improvement of the myelopathy within 3 to 6 months after the anterior decompression and arthrodesis, and postsurgical imaging studies show continued compression of the spinal cord without a substantial increase in the transverse area of the cord, we recommend posterior decompression. This approach is controversial, because the prognosis and the time for recovery after the operation are variable and have not been well defined.

One or Two-Level Spondylosis with Developmental Narrowing of the Canal or Posterior or Combined Anterior and Posterior Compression

When there is posterior compression, combined anterior and posterior compression, or a developmentally narrow canal (a Pavlov ratio of less than 0.8), a posterior approach usually is preferable.[55,56] The anterior approach in this situation may increase the risk of injury to the spinal cord because the dura and spinal cord are pressed against the PLL in the stenotic canal. The posterior decompression should extend one or two levels cephalad and one or two levels caudad to the level of the anterior pathological changes in order to allow the dura and cord to migrate dorsally.[55] The decision to decompress one level or two levels is based on the amounts of stenosis and anterior compression; the more severe the lesion, the greater the amount of decompression needed. We suggest that any level should be decompressed if the compression ratio at the adjacent level is 0.5 or less. Assessment of the adequacy of decompression can be difficult intrasurgically. Intrathecal instillation of water-soluble contrast medium may help the surgeon to identify an inadequate decompression intrasurgically.[57] When the adequacy is in doubt, it is preferable to err on the side of more levels of decompression.

Involvement of More than Two Intervertebral Disk Levels

When disks at more than two levels are compressing the cord, we recommend a posterior approach (Figs. 6 and 7). This recommendation is somewhat controversial, because successful results have been obtained with use of the anterior approach.[23,54,58] The disadvantages of the anterior approach in this situation are destabilization of the spine, the difficulty involved in the achievement of a fusion of multiple levels, and the risk of strut graft dislodgment.[24,59] There is also a higher rate of late CSM at adjacent segments when more than two levels are fused (Fig. 6).[60] The advantages of the posterior approach are that it provides direct visualization of the nerve roots[61] and it allows avoidance of multiple levels of fusion.

Another controversy involves the selection of a laminaplasty or a laminectomy for the posterior decompression.[55,62-67] Laminectomy has the potential disadvantage of destabilizing the spine and allowing kyphosis to occur, but post-laminectomy kyphosis is uncommon except in the skeletally immature cervical spine.[55,66-69] A well-designed, controlled, prospective study with a 5-year follow-up revealed no difference between the results of laminectomy and those of laminaplasty,[66] as did another study.[69] Several laminaplasty techniques have been described,[62,64-66,67,69] but their relative advantages have not yet been determined.

The facet joints are very important for spinal stability. Resection of as little as 25% of a facet can result in cervical instability. If a destabilizing facet resection is needed in order to decompress the cord, a posterior arthrodesis should be done. Laminaplasty results in less damage to the facet joints and thus preserves more stability.[70] When the lesion of the facet joints has caused instability at some of the levels, laminaplasty at the stable levels combined with arthrodesis at the unstable level or levels may be considered.

Laminaplasty results in a loss of cervical motion, especially in extension; however, this limitation may help to prevent the progression of spondylosis and the development of deformity. Another potential disadvantage of laminaplasty is that recurrent stenosis can be caused by excessive bone formation at the laminaplasty site.

Cervical lordosis must be present for a successful posterior decompression. After decompression, a bowstring effect occurs as the spinal cord migrates dorsally away from the anterior structures, thereby providing decompression.[55] This migration also decreases the axial tension on the cord and improves the perfusion of the cord.[55] Kyphotic deformity of the cervical spine is a contraindication to posterior decompression, because the spinal cord cannot be expected to migrate away from the anterior compressing structures in the kyphotic position.[55,71]

For laminectomy, we suggest a technique similar to the open-door laminaplasty technique.[64] A high-speed burr and a small Kerrison rongeur are used to thin out and cut the lateral aspect of the lamina. Instead of hinging open the opposite side, as one would do in a classic laminaplasty, the same technique of cutting the lamina is used on both sides. The lamina then can be lifted free from the underlying dura and excised. This technique avoids having to place instruments beneath the lamina into the canal.

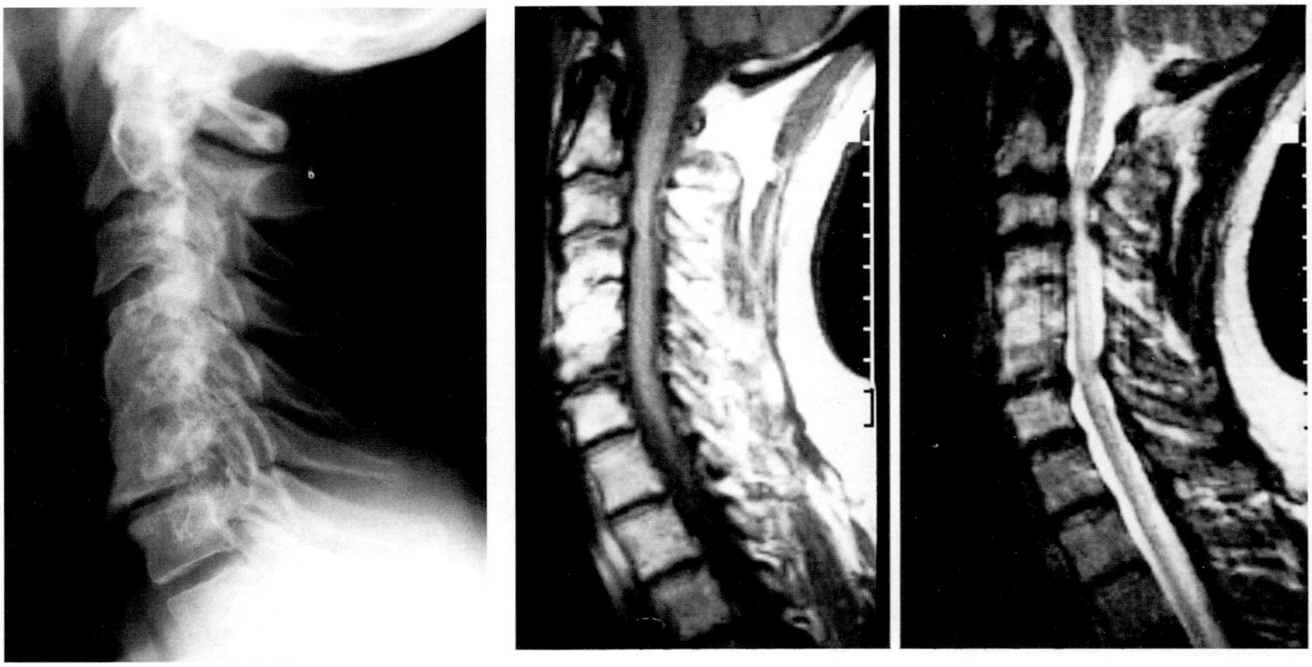

Fig. 6 Imaging studies of the cervical spine of a 43-year-old diabetic man who had a three-month history of severe, left-sided pain in the neck, shoulder, and arm and who had been unable to walk for three weeks. Eight years earlier, he had been managed successfully, for radiculopathy, with anterior diskectomy and arthrodesis at the fourth and fifth and at the fifth and sixth cervical levels. Examination revealed a left nerve root deficit at the seventh cervical level and severe clinical myelopathy. **Left**, Lateral radiograph. T1-weighted (**center**) and T2-weighted gradient-echo (**right**) sagittal MRIs showing spinal cord compression at the second and third cervical levels, severe compression at the third and fourth cervical levels, and spondylosis at the sixth and seventh cervical levels.

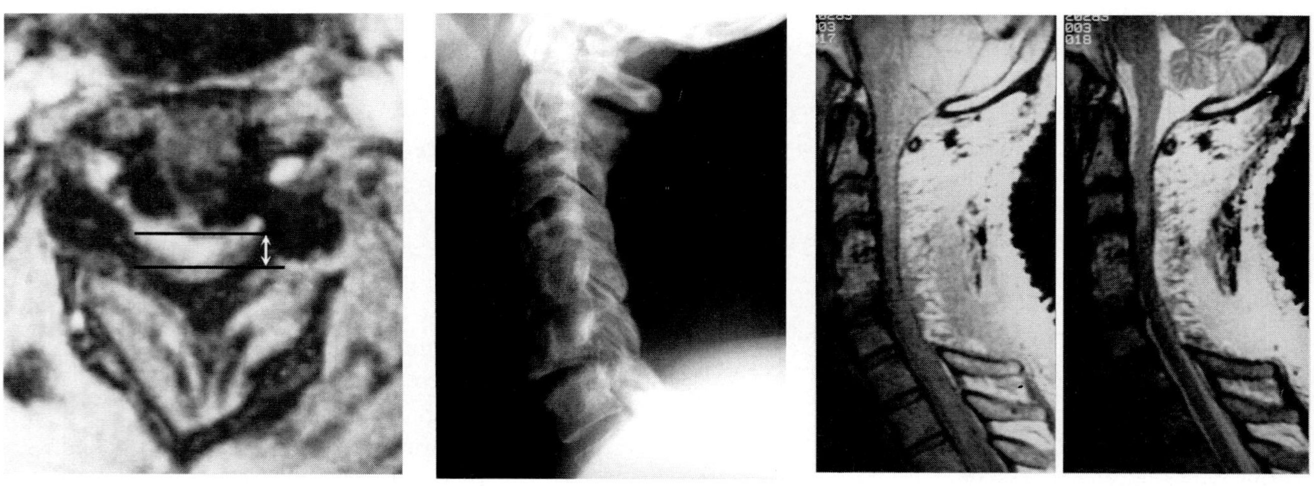

Fig. 7 Same patient as Fig. 6. **Left,** Axial magnetic resonance image at the third and fourth cervical levels, revealing severe compression of the spinal cord. The compression ratio was 0.25. The smallest anteroposterior diameter of the spinal cord is indicated by the arrows. **Left center,** Postsurgical lateral radiograph of the cervical spine after an en bloc laminectomy at the second through the seventh cervical levels and a left foraminotomy at the seventh cervical level. Postsurgical T1-weighted (**right center**) and T2-weighted gradient-echo (**right**) sagittal MRIs after laminectomy at the second through the seventh cervical levels, showing resolution of the spinal cord compression. The patient had prompt relief of the radicular pain in the left arm and regained the ability to walk independently over a 3-week period postsurgically.

It is useful to point out that, during the surgical procedure, the erector spinae muscles should not be dissected laterally beyond the facets. This is recommended to avoid denervation of the posterior cervical muscles, a condition that may cause postsurgical kyphosis.[55] Finally, a 5-mm-thick free fat graft should be placed over the exposed dura in order to minimize adhesions or the formation of a postlaminectomy membrane, a condition that may cause postsurgical neurologic deterioration.[72]

Kyphosis and CSM

The preferred approach when a kyphotic deformity is present is anterior corpectomy and strut-grafting (Fig. 8).[59,62] The lateral borders of the vertebral body should be preserved. For two disk levels, an iliac-crest strut graft is adequate; for more than two levels, a fibular strut graft is superior.[58,59] For defects longer than 7 cm, a vascularized fibular strut graft may be advantageous.[50] Postsurgical use of halo immobilization minimizes the probability of graft dislodgment, spinal malalignment, and pseudarthrosis. In the unusual situation of spondylosis with kyphosis and posterior compression, a combined anterior and posterior decompression should be considered.

When there is kyphosis and CSM associated with developmental narrowing of the canal, an anterior corpectomy with fibular strut-grafting is recommended. To decompress the cord adequately, the trough should be at least 16 mm wide.[50] The adequacy of the decompression can be assessed with intrasurgical ultrasound.

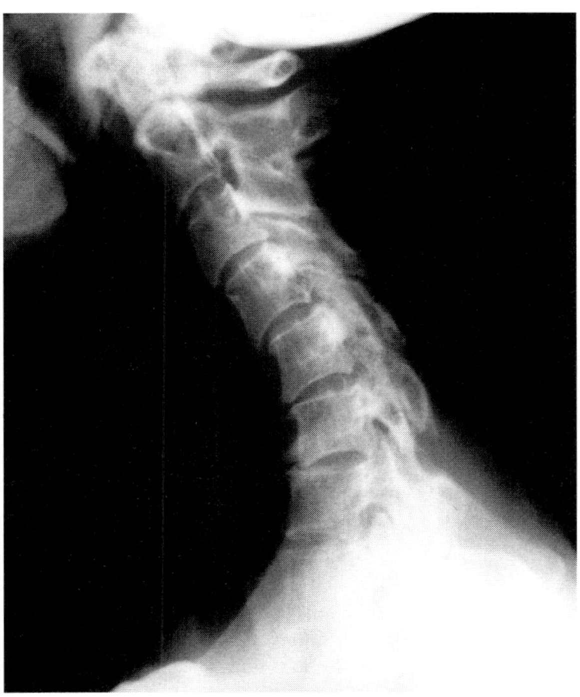

Fig. 8 Lateral radiograph of the cervical spine of a 58-year-old woman, showing a postsurgical kyphotic deformity 18 months after a laminectomy was performed at the third through the sixth cervical levels because of CSM. She had severe, constant neck pain and paresthesias. The patient was managed with anterior release and arthrodesis with a fibular strut graft followed by posterior arthrodesis. The neck pain and paresthesias resolved postsurgically.

Instability and CSM

When cervical instability is present, an arthrodesis is indicated. Treatment should be individualized on the basis of the levels affected and the degree of instability. For patients who have severe instability or instability with kyphosis, combined anterior and posterior approaches for decompression, arthrodesis, and stabilization should be considered.[36]

Anterior Decompression and Arthrodesis

Bone grafts should be sized appropriately and fashioned to create the most stable construct.[58,73,74] Attention to sagittal alignment is important. Care should be taken to maintain physiologic lordosis at the segment or segments involved in the arthrodesis, both during surgery and during the postsurgical course until a solid fusion is obtained.[60] A long-standing localized angular kyphosis resulting from inadequate bone-grafting or graft subsidence may lead to recurrence of myelopathy from stenosis at adjacent levels.[60]

After corpectomy, halo immobilization can be used to maintain the proper position. Catastrophic neurologic injury can result from strut graft dislodgment;[59,74,75] unfortunately, graft displacement has been reported even with use of the halo.[74]

The theoretical advantages of internal fixation are that it maintains spinal alignment, improves the stability of the graft construct, and possibly eliminates the need for a halo in selected patients.[76,77] The anterior plate fixation system developed by Morscher and associates[78] is particularly appealing because the screws do not need to penetrate to the posterior cortex in order to provide secure fixation. Furthermore, the screws are locked into the plate, minimizing the risk of the screw loosening, backing out, and causing esophageal erosion or other complications. Although internal fixation may help to maintain alignment in multiple-level arthrodeses, one animal study has suggested that the rate of fusion is not substantially higher when anterior instrumentation is used,[79] and further study is necessary before recommendations can be made regarding its routine use.

Posterior Decompression and Arthrodesis

If the facets are intact and will hold wire fixation after posterior decompression, the posterior cervical wiring technique described by Robinson and Southwick[80] is a useful procedure that adds little to the surgical risk. When the facets are deformed by the disease or have been removed during the decompression, the use of posterior cervical plates or rods with screws that provide fixation to the lateral masses is a reasonable option that is being employed more frequently for posterior cervical arthrodeses.[76,81] This technique carries the risk of injury to nerve roots or the vertebral artery;[76] therefore, a thorough knowledge of the anatomy and a careful, precise application of well-practiced technique is required to avoid these complications. Cancellous bone graft from the posterior aspect of the iliac crest should be applied to the decorticated posterior elements in order to obtain a solid fusion.

Ossification of the PLL

Ossification of the PLL previously was thought to occur only in Asian patients;[24,65] however, it has been reported with increasing frequency and identical clinical, radiographic, and histologic features in non-Asian patients.[24] About one-half of the patients who have had ossification of the PLL have had diffuse idiopathic skeletal hyperostosis (Forestier disease), which is seen readily on plain radiographs.[24,82] Enhanced axial CT scanning is the best method to confirm the diagnosis of ossification of the PLL.[24] The PLL ossifies and thickens, causing anterior compression of the spinal cord. At the time of presentation, there may be few levels of involvement; however, the disease may progress to involve the PLL at multiple levels.[23,83]

The recommended surgical procedure for treatment of this condition is a posterior decompression. Stability actually may be quite good, because the ossified PLL may enhance stability, allowing a more extensive decompression.[6] With anterior decompression, a serious and potentially fatal complication can occur.[6,24,75] Because the dura may be absent[75] or the ossified PLL may be adherent to the dura, attempts to remove the ligament can result in major dural injuries that are often difficult or impossible to repair.[24] Many complications were reported in a series of 22 patients who underwent anterior decompression. Three of the patients had serious postoperative neurologic deficits that were thought to be directly related to the manipulation of the ossified PLL during surgical decompression.[24] Anterior decompression is indicated when ossification of the PLL is associated with kyphosis. The anterior floating method, in which the disk and a portion of the vertebral body are removed in order to allow the ossified PLL to be pulled forward gently without actually being removed,[84,85] has had an acceptable rate of success, but the rate of complications has been higher than that associated with posterior decompression.[84] A recent study of the anterior floating method, using 18- to 20-mm-wide diskectomy or corpectomy troughs, an operating microscope, and evoked-potential monitoring, demonstrated a lower rate of complications and a higher rate of neurologic recovery compared with those obtained with use of laminectomy for the treatment of ossification of the PLL.[86] Awareness that ossification of the PLL occurs in non-Asian patients and careful presurgical evaluation of all patients who have CSM can help to avoid catastrophic surgical complications.[6,24,75]

Conclusion

When CSM is mild, nonprogressive, and of relatively short duration, the appropriate method of treatment is controversial. More prospective, controlled studies are needed in order to provide the information that is required to make definitive decisions about which patients should have surgery and which procedure should be done.[87,88] Severe, progressive myelopathy should be treated with surgical decompression and stabilization. Decompression of the spinal cord should be accomplished with the least possible surgical risk and the least possible disruption of the structural integrity of the spinal column.

Acknowledgments

The authors thank the Daniel E. Hogan Spine Fellowship, Beth Israel Hospital, Boston, Massachusetts, for financial support of the preparation of this manuscript and the fellowship training of the two junior authors, Mark Bernhardt and Melvin D. Law, Jr. They also thank the Division of Research Support, St. Luke's Hospital of Kansas City, Kansas City, Missouri, for financial support and photographic services.

References

1. Parke WW: Correlative anatomy of cervical spondylotic myelopathy. *Spine* 1988;13: 831-837.
2. Bernhardt M, Hynes RA, Blume HW, et al: Current concepts review: Cervical spondylotic myelopathy. *J Bone Joint Surg* 1993;75A:119-128.
3. Whitecloud TS III: Anterior surgery for cervical spondylotic myelopathy: Smith-Robinson, Cloward, and vertebrectomy. *Spine* 1988;13:861-863.
4. White AA III, Panjabi MM (eds): *Clinical Biomechanics of the Spine*, ed 2. Philadelphia, PA, JB Lippincott, 1990, pp 314, 511-528.
5. Epstein NE, Hyman RA, Epstein JA, et al: "Dynamic" MRI scanning of the cervical spine. *Spine* 1988;13:937-938.
6. White AA III, Panjabi MM: Biomechanical considerations in the surgical management of cervical spondylotic myelopathy. *Spine* 1988;13:856-860.
7. White AA III, Southwick WO, DePonte RJ, et al: Relief of pain by anterior cervical-spine fusion for spondylosis. A report of sixty-five patients. *J Bone Joint Surg* 1973;55A:525-534.
8. Adams CB, Logue V: Studies in cervical spondylotic myelopathy: I. Movement of the cervical roots, dura and cord, and their relation to the course of the extrathecal roots. *Brain* 1971;94:557-568.
9. Adams CB, Logue V: Studies in cervical spondylotic myelopathy: II. The movement and contour of the spine in relation to the neural complications of cervical spondylosis. *Brain* 1971;94:568-586.
10. Adams CB, Logue V: Studies in cervical spondylotic myelopathy: III. Some functional effects of operations for cervical spondylotic myelopathy. *Brain* 1971;94:587-594.

11. Gruninger W, Gruss P: Stenosis and movement of the cervical spine in cervical myelopathy. *Paraplegia* 1982;20:121-130.
12. Panjabi M, White A III: Biomechanics of nonacute cervical spinal cord trauma. *Spine* 1988;13: 838-842.
13. Penning L: Some aspects of plain radiography of the cervical spine in chronic myelopathy. *Neurology* 1962;12: 513-519.
14. Reid JD: Effects of flexion-extension movements of the head and spine upon the spinal cord and nerve roots. *J Neurol Neurosurg Psychiatry* 1960;23:214-221.
15. Alker G: Neuroradiology of cervical spondylotic myelopathy. *Spine* 1988;13:850-853.
16. Cusick JF: Monitoring of cervical spondylotic myelopathy. *Spine* 1988;13:877-880.
17. Epstein NE, Epstein JA, Carras R, et al: Coexisting cervical and lumbar spinal stenosis: Diagnosis and management. *Neurosurgery* 1984;15:489-496.
18. Simeone FA, Rothman RH: Cervical disc disease, in Rothman RH, Simeone FA (eds): *The Spine*, ed 2. Philadelphia, PA, WB Saunders, 1982, pp 440-499.
19. Denno JJ, Meadows GR: Early diagnosis of cervical spondylotic myelopathy: A useful clinical sign. *Spine* 1991;16:1353-1355.
20. Pavlov H, Torg JS, Robie B, et al: Cervical spinal stenosis: Determination with vertebral body ratio method. *Radiology* 1987;164: 771-775.
21. Torg JS: Pavlov's ratio: Determining cervical spinal stenosis on routine lateral roentgenograms. *Contemp Orthop* 1989;18:153-160.
22. Brown BM, Schwartz RH, Frank E, et al: Presurgical evaluation of cervical radiculopathy and myelopathy by surface-coil MR imaging. *AJR* 1988;151:1205-1212.
23. Jamjoom A, Williams C, Cummins B: The treatment of spondylotic cervical myelopathy by multiple subtotal vertebrectomy and fusion. *Br J Neurosurg* 1991;5:249-255.
24. McAfee PC, Regan JJ, Bohlman HH: Cervical cord compression from ossification of the posterior longitudinal ligament in non-Orientals. *J Bone Joint Surg* 1987;69B:569-575.
25. Fujiwara K, Yonenobu K, Ebara S, et al: The prognosis of surgery for cervical compression myelopathy: An analysis of the factors involved. *J Bone Joint Surg* 1989;71B:393-398.
26. Koyanagi T, Hirabayashi K, Satomi K, et al: Predictability of surgical results of cervical compression myelopathy based on presurgical computed tomographic myelography. *Spine* 1993;18:1958-1963.
27. Clarke E, Robinson PK: Cervical myelopathy: a complication of cervical spondylosis. *Brain* 1956;79:483-505.
28. Epstein JA, Janin Y, Carras R, et al: A comparative study of the treatment of cervical spondylotic myeloradiculopathy: Experience with 50 cases treated by means of extensive laminectomy, foraminotomy, and excision of osteophytes during the past 10 years. *Acta Neurochir* 1982;61:89-104.
29. Gregorius FK, Estrin T, Crandall PH: Cervical spondylotic radiculopathy and myelopathy: A long-term follow-up study. *Arch Neurol* 1976;33:618-625.
30. LaRocca H: Cervical spondylotic myelopathy: Natural history. *Spine* 1988;13:854-855.
31. Lees F, Aldren-Turner JW: Natural history and prognosis of cervical spondylosis. *Br Med J* 1963;92:1607-1610.
32. Montgomery D M, Brower RS: Cervical spondylotic myelopathy: Clinical syndrome and natural history. *Orthop Clin North Am* 1992;23:487-493.
33. Nurick S: The natural history and the results of surgical treatment of the spinal cord disorder associated with cervical spondylosis. *Brain* 1972;95: 101-108.
34. Symon L, Lavender P: The surgical treatment of cervical spondylotic myelopathy. *Neurology* 1967;17:117-127.
35. Lesoin F, Bouasakao N, Clarisse J, et al: Results of surgical treatment of radiculomyelopathy caused by cervical arthrosis based on 1000 operations. *Surg Neurol* 1985;23:350-355.
36. Cusick JF: Pathophysiology and treatment of cervical spondylotic myelopathy. *Clin Neurosurg* 1991;37:661-681.
37. Yoo JU, Zou D, Edwards WT, et al: Effect of cervical spine motion on the neuroforaminal dimensions of human cervical spine. *Spine* 1992;17:1131-1136.
38. Murphy MJ, Lieponis JV: Nonsurgical treatment of cervical spine pain, in The Cervical Spine Research Society Editorial Committee (ed): *The Cervical Spine*, ed 2. Philadelphia, PA, JB Lippincott, 1989, pp 670-677.
39. Ono K, Ota H, Tada K, et al: Cervical myelopathy secondary to multiple spondylotic protrusions: A clinicopathologic study. *Spine* 1977;2:109-125.
40. Taylor J, Johnston RA, Caird FI: Surgical treatment of cervical spondylotic myelopathy in elderly patients. *Age Ageing* 1991; 20:407-412.
41. Hoppenfeld S, DeBoer P (eds): *Surgical Exposures in Orthopaedic Surgery: The Anatomic Approach*. Philadelphia, PA, JB Lippincott, 1984, pp 258-269.
42. Brown MD, Malinin TI, Davis PB: A roentgenographic evaluation of frozen allografts versus autografts in anterior cervical spine fusions. *Clin Orthop* 1976;119:231-236.
43. Fernyhough JC, White JI, LaRocca H: Fusion rates in multilevel cervical spondylosis comparing allograft fibula with autograft fibula in 126 patients. *Spine* 1991;16(suppl 10):S561-S564.
44. Zdeblick TA, Ducker TB: The use of freeze-dried allograft bone for anterior cervical fusions. *Spine* 1991;16:726-729.
45. An HS, Evanich CJ, Nowicki BH, et al: Ideal thickness of Smith-Robinson graft for anterior cervical fusion: A cadaveric study with computed tomographic correlation. *Spine* 1993;18:2043-2047.
46. Jones AA, Dougherty PJ, Sharkey NA, et al: Iliac crest bone graft: Osteotome versus saw. *Spine* 1993;18:2048-2052.
47. Selladurai BM: Cervical myelopathy due to nuclear herniations in young adults: Clinical and radiological profile, results of microdiscectomy without interbody fusion. *J Neurol Neurosurg Psychiatry* 1992;55:604-608.
48. Rosenorn J, Hansen EB, Rosenorn MA: Anterior cervical discectomy with and without fusion: A prospective study. *J Neurosurg* 1983;59:252-255.
49. Smith GW, Robinson RA: The treatment of certain cervical-spine disorders by anterior removal of the intervertebral disk and interbody fusion. *J Bone Joint Surg* 1958;40A:607-624.
50. Goto S, Mochizuki M, Kita T, et al: Anterior surgery in four consecutive technical phases for cervical spondylotic myelopathy. *Spine* 1993;18:1968-1973.
51. Breig A, el-Nadi AF: Biomechanics of the cervical spinal cord: Relief of contact pressure on and overstretching of the spinal cord. *Acta Radiol* 1966;4:602-624.
52. Cloward RB: The anterior approach for removal of ruptured cervical disks. *J Neurosurg* 1958;15: 602-617.
53. White AA III, Jupiter J, Southwick WO, et al: An experimental study of the immediate load bearing capacity of three surgical constructions for anterior spine fusions. *Clin Orthop* 1973;91:21-28.
54. Saunders RL, Bernini PM, Shirreffs TG Jr, et al: Central corpectomy for cervical spondylotic myelopathy: A consecutive series with long-term follow-up evaluation. *J Neurosurg* 1991;74:163-170.
55. Epstein JA: The surgical management of cervical spinal stenosis, spondylosis, and myeloradiculopathy by means of the posterior approach. *Spine* 1988;13:864-869.
56. Epstein JA, Epstein BS, Lavine LS: Cervical spondylotic myelopathy: The syndrome of the narrow canal treated by laminectomy, foraminotomy, and the removal of osteophytes. *Arch Neurol* 1963;8:307-317.
57. Walker J, Gillespie R, Davis J, et al: Water-soluble contrast medium for intrasurgical evaluation of anterior cervical discectomy: Technical note. *J Neurosurg* 1988;68:491-492.
58. Bernard TN Jr, Whitecloud TS III: Cervical spondylotic myelopathy and myeloradiculopathy: Anterior decompression and stabilization with autogenous fibula strut graft. *Clin Orthop* 1987;221:149-160.

59. Zdeblick TA., Bohlman HH: Cervical kyphosis and myelopathy. Treatment by anterior corpectomy and strut-grafting. *J Bone Joint Surg* 1989;71A:170-182.
60. Baba H, Furusawa N, Imura S, et al: Late radiographic findings after anterior cervical fusion for spondylotic myeloradiculopathy. *Spine* 1993;18:2167-2173.
61. Raynor RB: Anterior or posterior approach to the cervical spine: An anatomical and radiographic evaluation and comparison. *Neurosurgery* 1983;12: 7-13.
62. Herkowitz HN: A comparison of anterior cervical fusion, cervical laminectomy, and cervical laminoplasty for the surgical management of multiple level spondylotic radiculopathy. *Spine* 1988;13:774-780.
63. Herkowitz HN: The surgical management of cervical spondylotic radiculopathy and myelopathy. *Clin Orthop* 1989;239:94-108.
64. Hirabayashi K, Satomi K: Operative procedure and results of expansive open-door laminoplasty. *Spine* 1988;13:870-876.
65. Hirabayashi K, Miyakawa J, Satomi K, et al: Operative results and postsurgical progression of ossification among patients with ossification of cervical posterior longitudinal ligament. *Spine* 1981;6:354-364.
66. Hukuda S, Ogata M, Mochizuki T, et al: Laminectomy versus laminoplasty for cervical myelopathy: Brief report. *J Bone Joint Surg* 1988;70B:325-326.
67. Yoshida M, Otani K, Shibasaki K, et al: Expansive laminoplasty with reattachment of spinous process and extensor musculature for cervical myelopathy. *Spine* 1992;17:491-497.
68. Jenkins DH: Extensive cervical laminectomy: Long-term results. *Br J Surg* 1973;60:852-854.
69. Nakano N, Nakano T, Nakano K: Comparison of the results of laminectomy and open-door laminoplasty for cervical spondylotic myeloradiculopathy and ossification of the posterior longitudinal ligament. *Spine* 1988;13:792-794.
70. Nowinski GP, Visarius H, Nolte LP, et al: A biomechanical comparison of cervical laminaplasty and cervical laminectomy with progressive facetectomy. *Spine* 1993;18:1995-2004.
71. Tencer A, Allen BL Jr, Ferguson RL: A biomechanical study of thoracolumbar spinal fractures with bone in the canal: Part I. The effect of laminectomy. *Spine* 1985;10:580-585.
72. Oiwa T, Hirabayashi K, Uzawa M, et al: Experimental study on postlaminectomy deterioration of cervical spondylotic myelopathy: Influences of intradural surgery and persistent spinal block. *Spine* 1985;10: 717-721.
73. Ripa DR, Kowall MG,Meyer PR Jr, et al: Series of ninety-two traumatic cervical spine injuries stabilized with anterior ASIF plate fusion technique. *Spine* 1991;16:S46-S55.
74. Stauffer ES, Kelley EG: Fracture-dislocations of the cervical spine: Instability and recurrent deformity following treatment by anterior interbody fusion. *J Bone Joint Surg* 1977;59A:45-48.
75. Smith MD, Bolesta MJ, Leventhal M, et al: Postsurgical cerebrospinal-fluid fistula associated with erosion of the dura: Findings after anterior resection of ossification of the posterior longitudinal ligament in the cervical spine. *J Bone Joint Surg* 1992;74A: 270-277.
76. Montesano PX, Juach EC, Anderson PA, et al: Biomechanics of cervical spine internal fixation. *Spine* 1991;16(suppl 3):S10-S16.
77. Ulrich C, Woersdoerfer O, Kalff R, et al: Biomechanics of fixation systems to the cervical spine. *Spine* 1991;16:S4-S9.
78. Morscher E, Sutter F, Jenny H, et al: Anterior plating of the cervical spine with the hollow screw-plate system of titanium. *Chirurg* 1986;57:702-707.
79. Zdeblick TA, Cooke ME, Wilson D, et al: Anterior cervical discectomy, fusion, and plating: A comparative animal study. *Spine* 1993;18:1974-1983.
80. Robinson RA, Southwick WO: Surgical approaches to the cervical spine, in Reynolds FC (ed): *American Academy of Orthopaedic Surgeons Instructional Course Lectures Volume XVII.* St. Louis, MO, CV Mosby, 1960, pp 299-330.
81. Anderson PA, Henley MB, Grady MS, et al: Posterior cervical arthrodesis with AO reconstruction plates and bone graft. *Spine* 1991;16:S72-S79.
82. Pouchot J, Watts CS, Esdaile JM, et al: Sudden quadriplegia complicating ossification of the posterior longitudinal ligament and diffuse idiopathic skeletal hyperostosis. *Arthritis Rheum* 1987;30:1069-1072.
83. Epstein NE: Ossification of the posterior longitudinal ligament in evolution in 12 patients. *Spine* 1994;19:673-681.
84. Kamikozuru M: Significance of the anterior floating method for cervical myelopathy due to the ossification of the posterior longitudinal ligament. *Nippon Seikeigeka Gakkai Zasshi* 1991;65:431-440.
85. Tsuyama N: Ossification of the posterior longitudinal ligament of the spine. *Clin Orthop* 1984;184:71-84.
86. Epstein NE: The surgical management of ossification of the posterior longitudinal ligament in 43 North Americans. *Spine* 1994;19: 664-672.
87. Rowland LP: Surgical treatment of cervical spondylotic myelopathy: Time for a controlled trial. *Neurology* 1992;42:5-13.
88. White AA III: Introduction: Symposium on cervical spondylotic myelopathy. *Spine* 1988;13:829-830.

Acute Back Pain in Children

Robert N. Hensinger, MD

It is uncommon for a child to complain of pain in the back. Unlike the adult population, in whom back pain seems to be part of everyday life, relatively few children have symptoms serious enough to warrant a visit to a physician. For most of those who do seek care, the problems respond to simple measures. Several years ago, we reviewed 100 children who were presented to the pediatric orthopaedic clinic with the complaint of back pain.[1] The children's problems were divided into three categories: (1) developmental (35%), predominantly caused by kyphosis or, to a lesser extent, scoliosis; (2) traumatic (35%), the majority of which were spondylolysis of L5-S1; and (3) spontaneous onset (15%), usually caused by tumor or infection. The remaining 15% were originally undetermined, but the etiology for several of these was determined later. Thus, nearly 90% had objective problems, and, importantly, the vast majority of these problems could be successfully diagnosed and managed with a very satisfactory outcome.

Clinical Findings

The fact that children are not very specific in their complaints can be disconcerting to the examining physician. Children are poor at localizing pain and tend to be more global in their description. They usually complain of pain in the entire back rather than a more discreet complaint limited to the lumbosacral or dorsal lumbar junction. The complaint of leg pain may represent simple hamstring tightness and night cramps, or it may be the radicular pain of a herniated disk. These are very typical complaints of children which in an adult might suggest a strong emotional overlay.

Because children are less familiar with the glossary of terms associated with illness, such as numbness, tingling, and weakness, they find it difficult to express these complaints. Similarly, the fact that children have difficulty remembering and describing the specifics of their activity or injury mechanisms can be frustrating and confusing to the examiner.

The mechanism or circumstance of injury is often an important clue to the diagnosis. A spondylolysis should be suspected if the onset of the pain is during athletics such as diving, during a back walkover in gymnastics, or while performing a racing turn or the butterfly stroke in swimming.[2,3] Similarly, increasing pain with repetition may indicate the onset of a stress reaction in the pars interarticularis.[3,4] The high rate of occurrence of spondylolysis among family members and certain ethnic groups is often an important clue to the correct diagnosis.[5] Night pain and the relief of symptoms with aspirin (or Naprosyn) should lead one to suspect an osteoid osteoma or osteoblastoma (Fig. 1).[6-8] Morning stiffness may represent the beginning of juvenile ankylosing spondylitis.

The dangerous signs of childhood back pain are persistent pain unrelieved by rest or immobilization, increasing pain, unexplained fever, and symptoms of systemic illness, weight loss, general malaise or simply "not feeling well" (Fig. 2). Neurologic signs, complaints of nerve root irritation, radicular pain, numbness, and tingling are uncommon accompaniments to childhood back pain and, when found, suggest that a serious problem is in progress, which demands immediate evaluation. Similarly, bladder and bowel dysfunction or perineal hypoesthesia would justify extensive investigation.

An intraspinal tumor must be considered in young children (commonly, those younger than 4 years of age) who complain of recurrent back pain. The differential is extensive, including a malignant astrocytoma, benign tumors such as dermoid cysts, lipomas, intramedullary cysts, diastematomyelia and syringomelia.[9-11] Cutaneous abnormalities, such as a hairy patch, nevi, or dermal sinus, suggest the presence of an intraspinal anomaly. The examiner should search carefully for a subtle gait

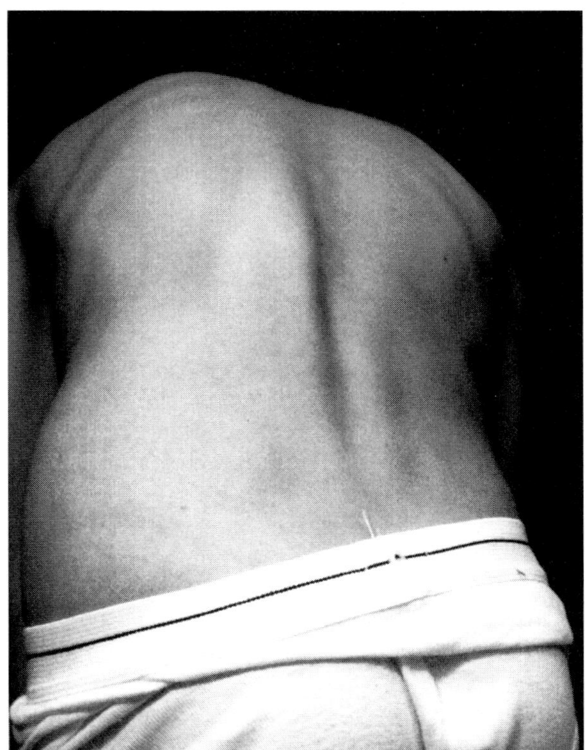

Fig. 1 An 11-year-old male with extreme back pain and guarding caused by an osteoid osteoma of L4. Forward bending demonstrates a curvature of the spine, which resolved with removal of the tumor.

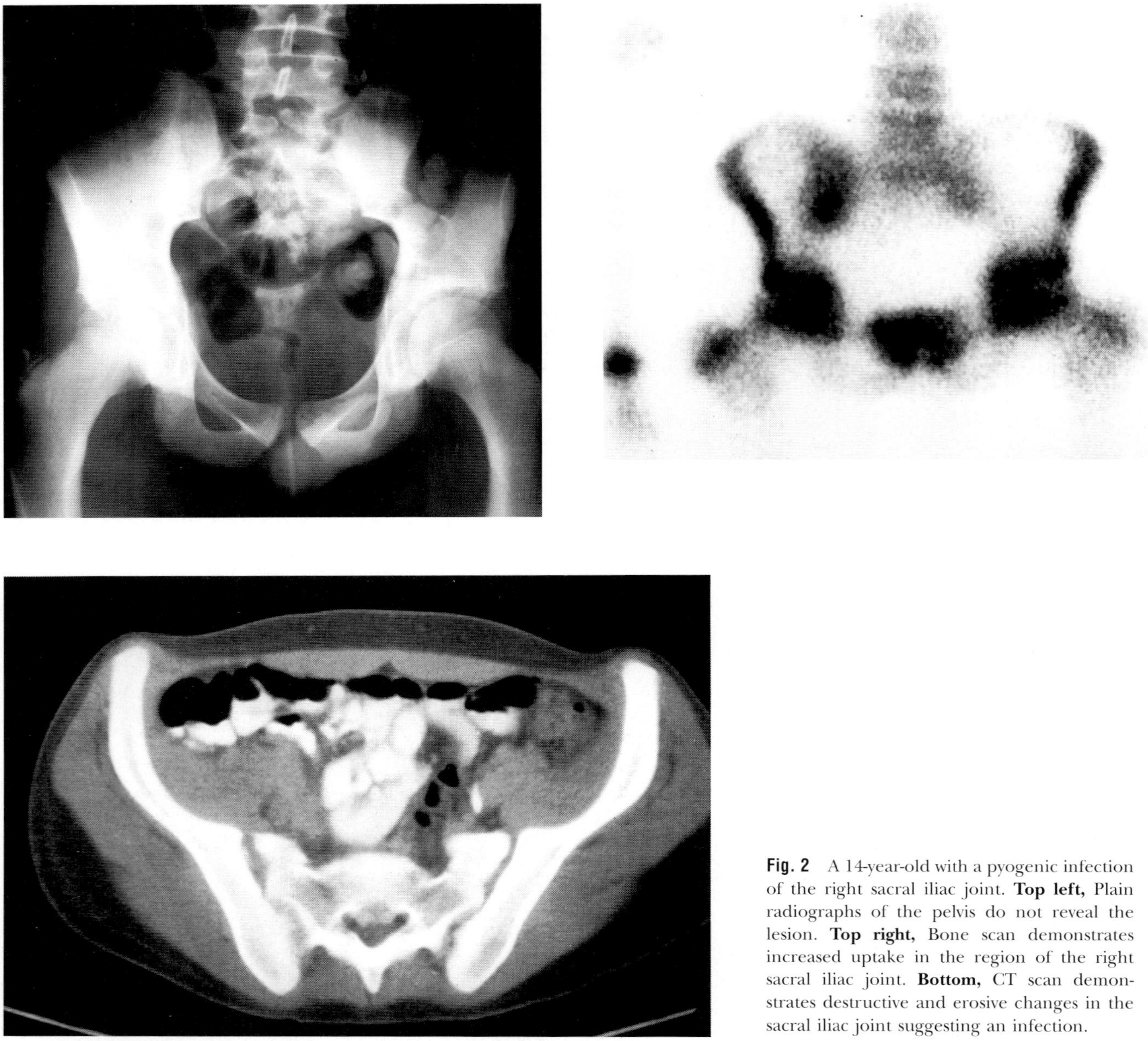

Fig. 2 A 14-year-old with a pyogenic infection of the right sacral iliac joint. **Top left,** Plain radiographs of the pelvis do not reveal the lesion. **Top right,** Bone scan demonstrates increased uptake in the region of the right sacral iliac joint. **Bottom,** CT scan demonstrates destructive and erosive changes in the sacral iliac joint suggesting an infection.

alteration, limp, leg or arm weakness, and such neurologic findings as hyperreflexia or a positive Babinski.[12] These findings usually precede the onset of back pain. Bowel and bladder dysfunction are frequent, but these can be difficult to evaluate in a young child who has only been recently trained in toileting.

It is uncommon for a child with idiopathic scoliosis to complain of back pain. If the pain is persistent, one should exclude other causes, such as tumor, infection, or spondylolysis.[8] Spondylolysis occurs with the same frequency (5%) in children with idiopathic scoliosis as in the general population. Conversely, a spondylolisthesis may be the cause of a lumbar scoliosis. One should be particularly sensitive to a spine curvature that does not follow the typical right thoracic left lumbar pattern of idiopathic scoliosis (Fig. 3). If the family history is negative or the curvature progresses rapidly (particularly in the male), a careful search for another etiology should be conducted.[13]

Physical examination should include routine inspection of the spine with forward bending to examine for scoliosis. Stiffness and guarding can be extreme and forward bending at the hips may be severely limited by hamstring tightness. Because the child's spine is much more flexible than an adult's, severe posturing and spine curvature is a common finding (Fig. 1).[8,14] Movements of the spine such as hyperextension or side-to-side bending may point to the etiology of the

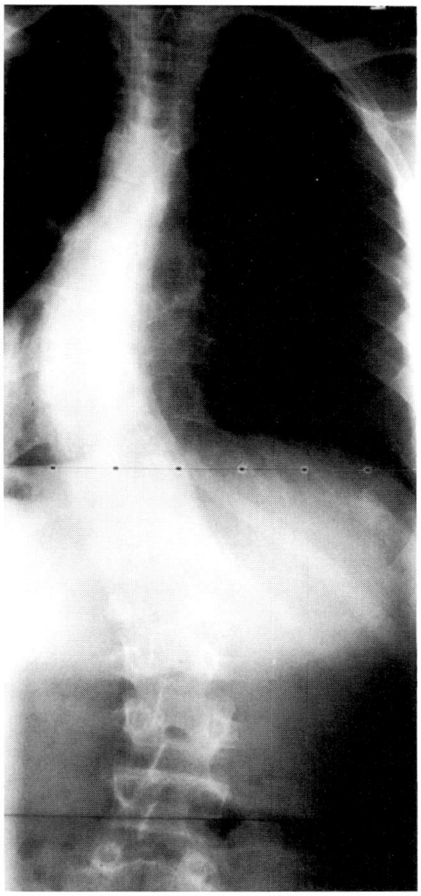

Fig. 3 A 12-year-old with a left thoracic right lumbar curvature caused by a spinal cord tumor. This pattern is the reverse of that associated with typical idiopathic scoliosis. In addition, the patient had a negative family history for scoliosis and the curvature had progressed rapidly, which would support another etiology.

problem. Spondylolysis can be particularly uncomfortable with backward extension. Children with Scheuermann's dorsal lumbar kyphosis find forward bending accentuates the problem. The neurologic examination should include a careful search for muscle weakness and nerve root impingement. Limitation of straight leg raising is very common in children with low back complaints, particularly spondylolysis and spondylolisthesis.[15]

Radiologic Investigation

The most important radiographs are a standing anteroposterior (AP) and a lateral of the entire spine. As children are not precise in localizing the area of discomfort, the long (36-in) films used for scoliosis and kyphosis are very helpful. The study should show the spine well above and below the area of the suspected problem. The standing film often accentuates scoliosis, lordosis, or spondylolysis.[16] If the history or physical exam suggests a spondylolysis, oblique films should be obtained, because 20% of the defects will be missed if only AP and lateral films are used.[17] The flexion-extension views, particularly of the lumbosacral and dorsolumbar junctions, can be helpful in the young child to demonstrate instability or highlight a small defect in the pars interarticularis or to document the restricted motion and stiffness caused by an inflammatory lesion. The vertebral canal should be examined for widening of the interpedicular distance, which suggests an intraspinal mass or the bone spike of a diastematomyelia.

When plain films do not provide the information needed for diagnosis, bone scans are recommended as a second level of testing.[3,18,19] The bone scan is not recommended as a routine study unless the problem has been persistent or the child exhibits findings suggesting a tumor or infection (Fig. 2). A bone scan is excellent for detecting the reactive process associated with recent trauma, repetitive stress, tumor, and inflammatory conditions that involve the spine and/or pelvis. Single photon emission computed tomography (SPECT) is a more sensitive imaging technique when a stress reaction of bone is suspected.[20]

Newer imaging techniques such as computed tomography (CT) can be helpful once the anatomic location of the problem has been identified. Magnetic resonance imaging (MRI) is an important aid in evaluating disk problems, lesions contained within the spinal canal, and the relationship between the neural structures and bony vertebral elements.

Spondylolysis/Spondylolisthesis

Spondylolysis is a common cause of acute back pain in children,[1] particularly those involved in sports, such as gymnastics, weight-lifting, and tennis, that emphasize hyperextension of the spine.[21] Spondylolysis is found after walking age but rarely before the age of 5. It gradually increases to age 20, when it reaches the adult incidence of 5%.[22,23] Because there is a genetic predisposition, many children will have a positive family history.[5]

The origin of spondylolysis as a stress or fatigue fracture of the pars interarticularis has been substantially documented.[4,23,24] It has been postulated that lumbar lordosis is accentuated by the normal flexion contractures of the hip in childhood, and that this posture focuses the force of weightbearing on the pars interarticularis.[4,23] Anatomic studies have suggested that shear stresses on the pars interarticularis are greater when the lumbar spine is extended.[4] In young people, the pars interarticularis is thin, the neural arch has not reached its maximum strength, and the intervertebral disk is less resistant to shear.[25] A fatigue fracture of the pars interarticularis can occur at physiologic loads during cyclic flexion-extension motion of the lumbar spine.[4] These stresses may be further accentuated by lateral flexion movements on the extended spine, as can occur during a back walk-over in gymnastics, when the weight of the lower limb causes extreme hyperextension of the lumbar spine.[2,26,27] Jackson and associates[2] noted that the incidence of spondylolysis was 11% (4 times higher than normal) in female gymnasts. An increased incidence of acute spondylolysis has also been noted in young people such as weightlifters and football linemen who engage in strenuous physical activity.[21]

An increased incidence (from 32% to 50%) has been noted in adolescents who have thoracolumbar Scheuermann's disease.[28,29] In this condition, which is now believed to be caused by excessive and repetitive mechanical loading on the immature spine, thoracolumbar kyphosis is often associated with a compensatory increase in lumbar lordosis.[28,29]

Clinical Findings

Most children first develop symptoms during the adolescent growth spurt, at approximately 11 to 14 years of age. The pain, which is very characteristic, is usually in the low back and radiates to the posterior thighs. Pain is seldom noted below the knees or in the foot.[30] Symptoms are usually initiated or aggravated by strenuous activity, particularly repetitive flexion-extension of the spine. Symptoms are decreased by rest or limitation of activity.[3,4] Unlike adults, children seldom have objective signs of nerve root compression, such as motor weakness, decrease reflexes, or a sensory deficit.[30] Physical examination, however, should include a careful search for sacral anesthesia and dysfunction of the bladder, which suggests a cauda equina syndrome.

The results of physical examination may be normal in a child who has spondylolysis or mild (Grade I or II) spondylolisthesis. If the posture or gait is abnormal, restricted flexion of the hips, caused by tight hamstrings, may be the only finding.[31] Eighty percent of symptomatic patients have tight hamstrings; some have considered this to be a sign of nerve root irritation, but there is no objective evidence to support that opinion.[21] Tightness of the hamstrings, which may be found in patients who have spondylolysis or any grade of spondylolisthesis, is seldom accompanied by neurologic signs.[21,30] The tightness may be so extreme that the child cannot bend forward at the hips or that, during the straight leg-raising test, the examiner is unable to lift the foot more than a few centimeters from the examining table.

Radiologic Findings

The term spondylolysis refers to a radiolucent defect of the pars interarticularis. If the defect is large, it can be seen on nearly all views of the lumbar spine (Fig. 4). However, if it is unilateral, as it is in 20% to 25% of patients, or if it is not accompanied by spondylolisthesis, it can be a very subtle finding.[17] Oblique radiographs of the lumbar spine are often necessary to view this area in relief, apart from the overlying osseous elements (Fig. 5). It has been found that the diagnosis

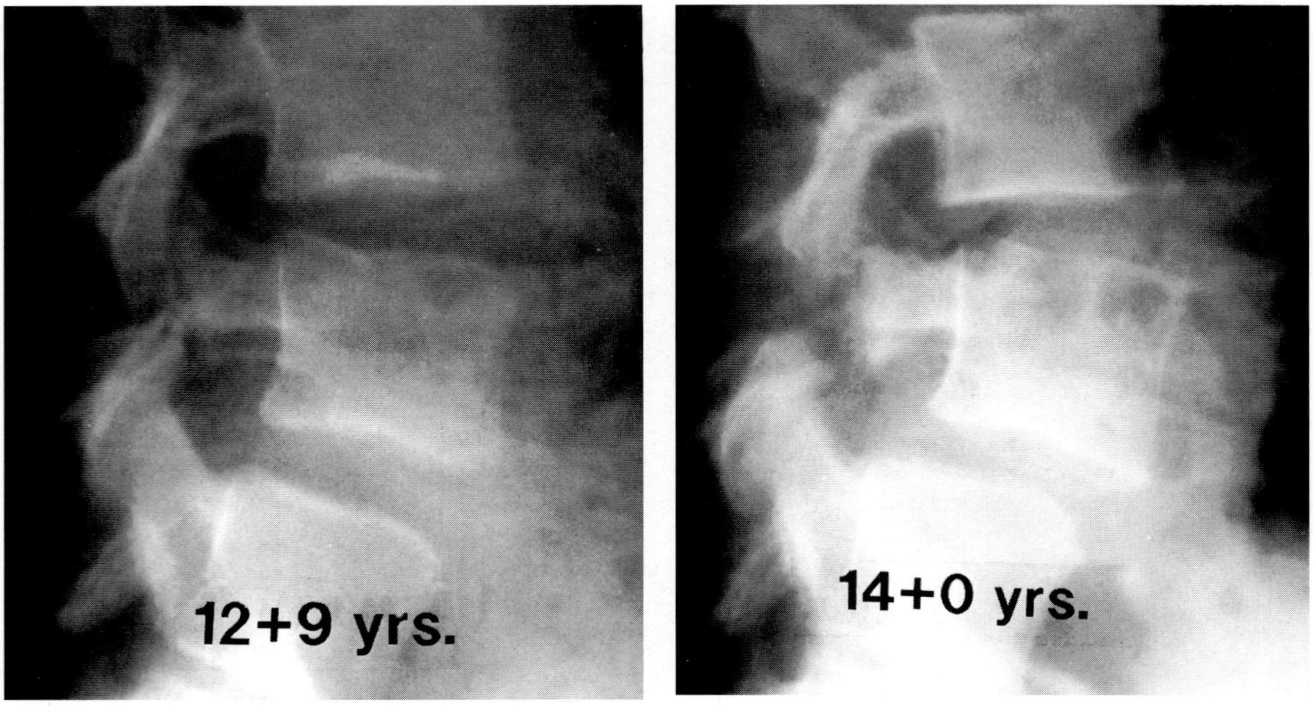

Fig. 4 Spondylolysis. **Left,** At 12 years, 9 months, a small break is seen in the pars interarticularis. **Right,** At age 14, radiographs of the same patient now demonstrate a widening of the defect in the pars interarticularis and Grade I spondylolisthesis. The patient is asymptomatic.

will be missed in 20% of young symptomatic patients if oblique radiographs are not made.[17] The so-called Scotty-dog sign of Lachapele, with the defect appearing as a collar around the dog's neck, is a helpful visual aid for those who are inexperienced in interpreting oblique radiographs. In a patient who has an acute injury, the gap is narrow and has irregular edges, whereas in a patient who has a long-standing lesion, the edges are smooth and rounded, suggesting a pseudarthrosis. The width of the gap depends on the amount of resorption of bone after the fracture and on the degree of spondylolisthesis. Confusion can occur when spondylolisthesis develops without spondylolysis, as dysplastic (Type I) spondylolisthesis does.[21] About a third of symptomatic patients have spondylolisthesis without spondylolysis.[30] In this condition, in which there is no gap or defect in the pars interarticularis, the fifth lumbar facets appear to subluxate ventrally on the sacral facets. If the slip continues, the pars interarticularis may become attenuated, like pulled taffy (the so-called greyhound sign of Hensinger).[30]

Sherman and associates[32] described the unusual occurrence of reactive sclerosis and hypertrophy of one pedicle and lamina as well as contralateral spondylolysis in the same vertebral segment (Fig. 6). They suggested that this finding is a physiologic response to the stress of repeated trauma in the presence of an unstable neural arch and that the problem will respond satisfactorily to symptomatic treatment.[4,32] Radiographically, the appearance may be confused with the reactive sclerosis that is associated with osteoid osteoma. This becomes an important concern, because excision of the sclerotic pars interarticularis and/or pedicle associated with a contralateral spondylolysis may increase the instability of L5/S1. The presence of a nidus on CT should confirm the diagnosis of an osteoid osteoma. A bone scan may not be helpful in differentiating between the two lesions, because in both increased bone activity causes uptake of the isotope.

Bone Scans

Spondylolysis that is suspected clinically but cannot be confirmed radiographically, or that is seen early in the stress-reaction stage before fracture (pre-spondylolytic), may be detected by radioactive bone-scanning (Fig. 7).[3,18] Single photon emission computed tomography (SPECT) is a very sensitive method of confirming the diagnosis when a stress reaction is suspected.[20] Bone scans can demonstrate increased uptake in patients who have had symptoms for only 5 to 7 days.[3,20] Small or partial fractures may be overlooked on radiographs, but scintigrams can demonstrate the areas of increased bone turnover at the site of healing fractures.[3] Later, bone scans are helpful in distinguishing between patients who have an established nonunion and those in whom healing is still progressing and who thus may benefit from immobilization.[17,19] Bone scans are not recommended for patients who have had symptoms for more than a year or for those who are asymptomatic.[19]

Bone scans are particularly helpful in the treatment of young athletes whose activities, such as gymnastics, are known to be associated with spondylolysis.[16] Early detection of the stress reaction can lead to appropriate

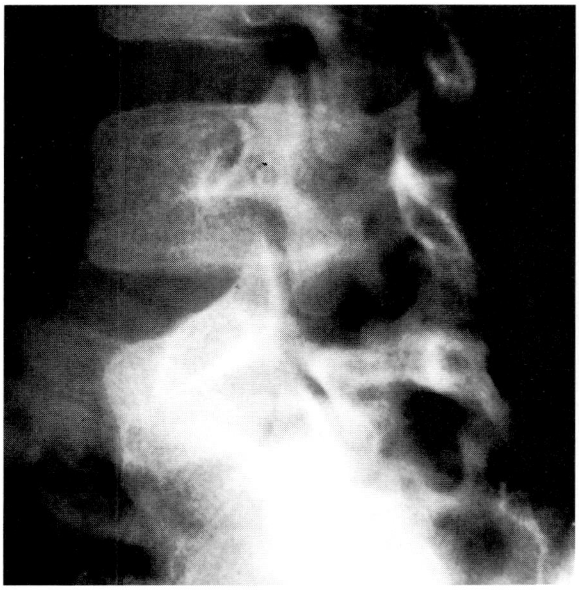

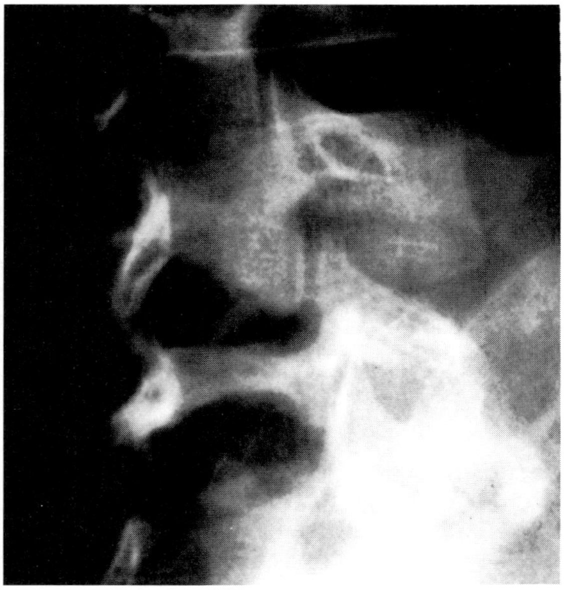

Fig. 5 **Left,** A 9-year old male with low back pain demonstrates a unilateral spondylolysis. Oblique views demonstrate spondylolysis in the left pars interarticularis. If obliques are not obtained, the lesion could be missed in 20%. The narrow, irregular appearance suggests a recent injury. **Right,** This patient can expect with time that the opposite pars interarticularis will fracture.

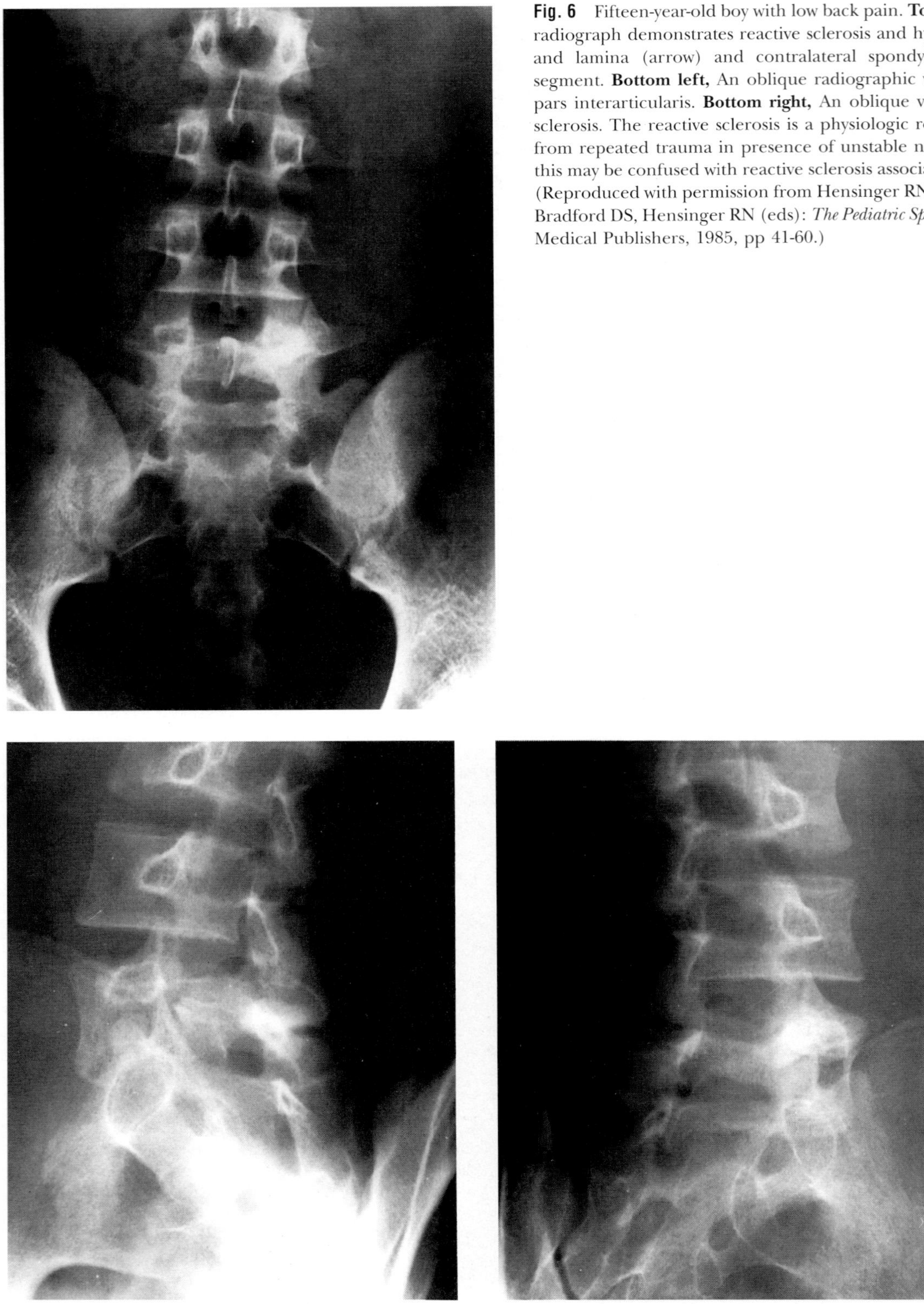

Fig. 6 Fifteen-year-old boy with low back pain. **Top left,** An anteroposterior radiograph demonstrates reactive sclerosis and hypertrophy of one pedicle and lamina (arrow) and contralateral spondylolysis of same vertebral segment. **Bottom left,** An oblique radiographic view shows a break in the pars interarticularis. **Bottom right,** An oblique view demonstrates reactive sclerosis. The reactive sclerosis is a physiologic response to stress resulting from repeated trauma in presence of unstable neural arch. Radiologically, this may be confused with reactive sclerosis associated with osteoid osteoma. (Reproduced with permission from Hensinger RN: Back pain in children, in Bradford DS, Hensinger RN (eds): *The Pediatric Spine.* New York, NY, Thieme Medical Publishers, 1985, pp 41-60.)

treatment and, as a consequence, may shorten the recovery period. Similarly, bone scans can be used to assess recovery and to determine when an athlete can return to competition.[26]

Treatment of Spondylolysis

Several authors have reported healing of a spondylolytic defect in children and young adults after treat-

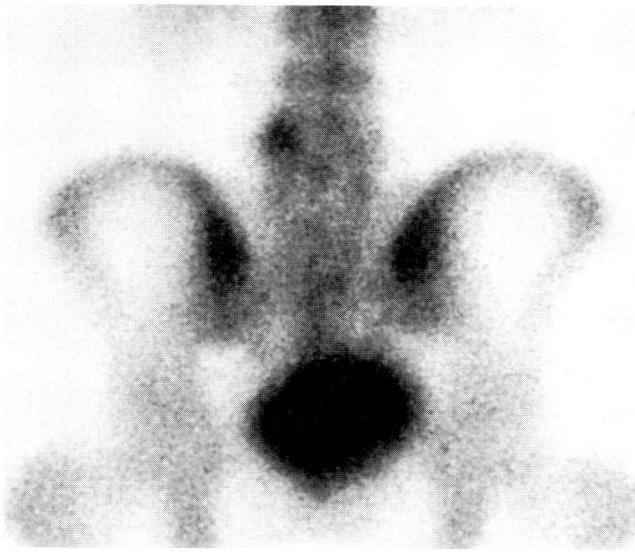

Fig. 7 A positive bone scan from a 16-year-old male with a unilateral spondylolysis. Such scans are positive by approximately 1 week after fracture and continue so for 1 year.

ment with a cast or a thoracolumbosacral orthosis (TLSO).[3,4,23,33] Typically, the children in these studies had had an acute onset of symptoms and the episode of injury was clearly documented.[17,33] Unilateral defects are more likely to heal than are bilateral ones.[17] Unfortunately, not all defects heal after treatment with immobilization, but such treatment should be considered if the injury can be proved to have been recent.[23] A bone scan may be helpful to determine whether osseous repair is continuing and is likely to result in healing, or if pseudarthrosis has been established.[4]

Although, in children and teen-agers, spondylolysis of long duration is not likely to heal, a clinical response to simple nonsurgical measures can be expected.[21,30] Restriction of vigorous activities and strengthening exercises for the muscles of the back and abdomen are usually successful in controlling symptoms in patients who have mild backache and tight hamstrings.[26] Tightness of the hamstrings is an excellent clinical guide to the success or failure of treatment. Patients who have more severe or persistent complaints may need bed rest, immobilization in a cast or throacolumbosacral orthosis, and nonnarcotic analgesics.[33] Most children will have excellent relief of symptoms, and can expect to return to unrestricted activities.[26] A small percentage of young people who have spondylolysis do not respond to nonsurgical measures or are unwilling to curtail their activities, and they may require surgical stabilization.[34]

Children who, in addition, have spondylolisthesis grade I or II usually will respond to symptomatic treatment but will need continued follow-up during the growth years to observe for progression.[35,36] This is especially true for children who are younger than 10 years of age. I do not advise children or adolescents who have asymptomatic spondylolysis or minimal symptoms to restrict their activities. As 5% of the adult population reportedly have a defect of the pars interarticularis, and relatively few of them have persistent symptoms, it does not seem justified to limit the activity of an asymptomatic child or adolescent.[21,35,37]

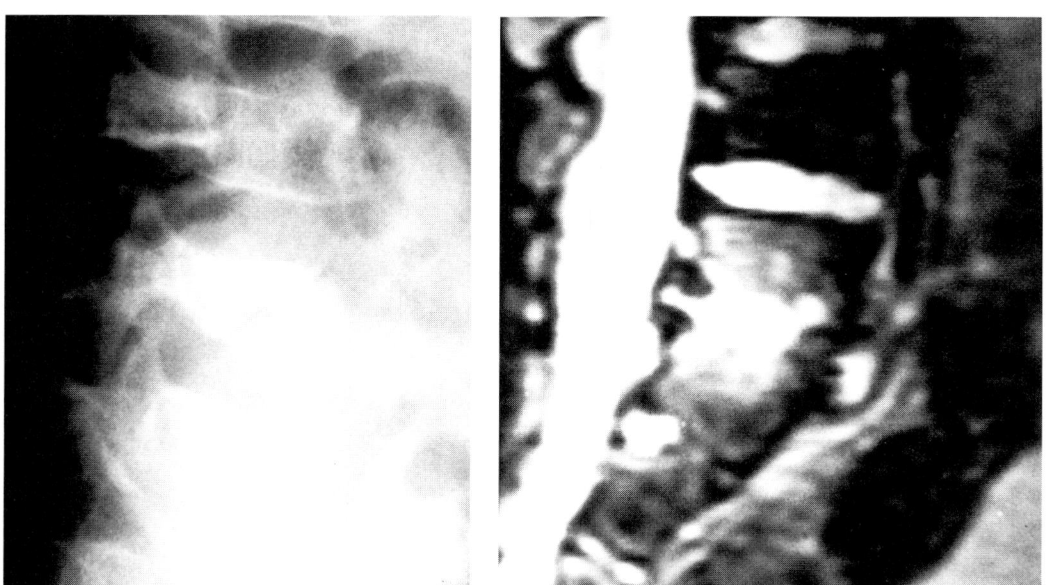

Fig. 8 A 5-year-old with severe low back pain. **Left,** Radiograph of the lumbosacral junction demonstrates mild erosive changes of L5. **Right,** MRI demonstrates extensive involvement of the disk space and edema in the vertebral bodies. This inflammatory process is suggestive of diskitis of childhood.

Disk Problems

Diskitis of Childhood

Of the causes of acute back pain in children, perhaps the most unsettling is that of the vertebral diskitis. This is usually of sudden onset, often accompanied by systemic signs of sepsis, fever, and elevated sedimentation rate. Many of these patients will have a history of a recent febrile illness such as a sore throat or earache.[13,38-40] Usually any motion of the spine is extremely painful and weightbearing, including sitting, may be uncomfortable. The young child (younger than 3 years of age) will refuse to walk or stand.[40] The lumbar spine is usually involved and paravertebral muscle spasm and limited back motion are characteristic. This condition is believed to be caused by a bacterial infection, with the inflammatory response starting at the vertebral endplate and spreading to the disk space.

Plain radiographs of the spine early in the course of the disease are typically not diagnostic (Fig. 8). If the problem is long-standing (2 to 4 weeks), the radiographs will demonstrate disk space narrowing and irregularity of the vertebral endplates. The bone scan is very helpful and usually demonstrates increased uptake early in the course of the illness.[40] Szalay and associates[41] reported that magnetic resonance imaging studies were more sensitive than bone scans in demonstrating early development of the process (Fig. 8).

In the young child, aspiration of the disk space and needle biopsy of the vertebrae, blood cultures, and other measures to document a bacterial infection are usually unsuccessful.[38,39,42,43] However, aspiration or biopsy is indicated for children who fail to respond to nonsurgical management and for the older child and adolescent in whom organisms are more typically identified (Fig. 9).[44]

Most children respond to bed rest and antibiotics. Immobilization in a cast or orthosis can be very helpful in controlling back pain. Crawford and associates[45] recommended that antibiotics be used only after failure of symptomatic treatment, such as immobilization. Interestingly, the authors found that in 36 consecutive children with diskitis the infection healed satisfactorily regardless of treatment.[45]

Disk Herniation

Although it is not as common as in the adult, disk herniation can occur in children as young as 12 years of age, with similar signs and symptoms.[46-51] The onset of symptoms is usually less dramatic in children, and not as frequently associated with trauma (36%).[47] DeOrio[48]

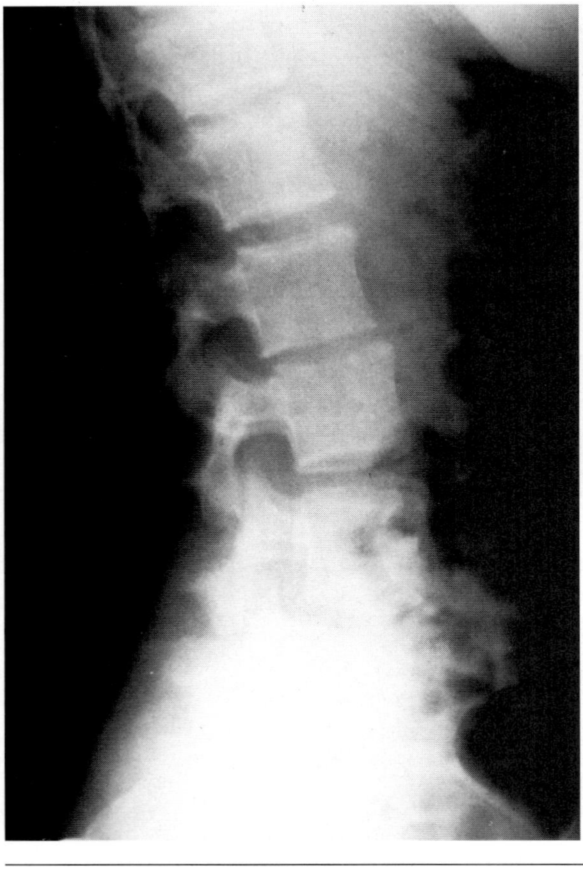

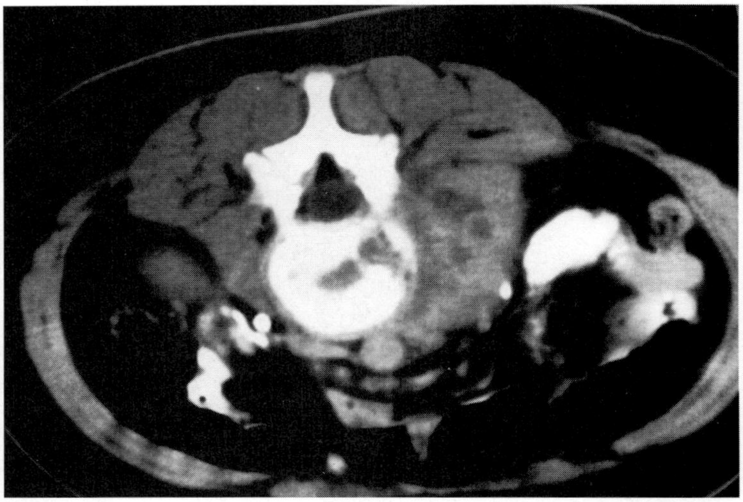

Fig. 9 A 13-year-old female with a 2-month history of back pain following a urinary tract infection. **Left,** A plain lateral radiograph of the lumbar spine shows some decrease in the disk height of L3 and L4. **Right,** A CT reveals a marked erosive change in vertebral body and disk space, suggesting a pyogenic vertebral osteomyelitis.

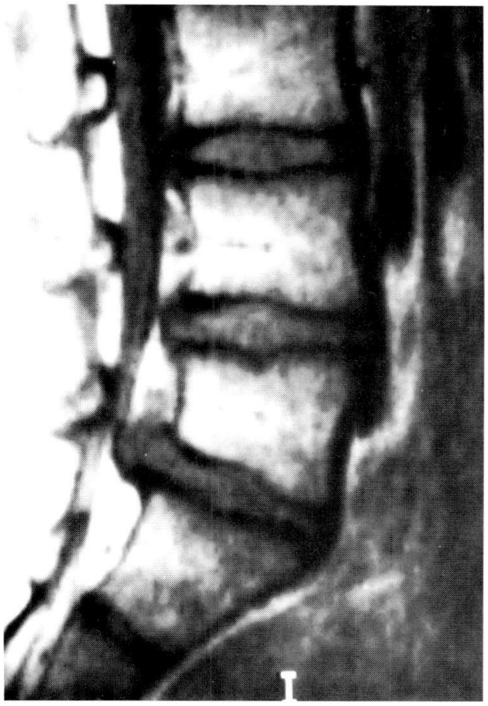

Fig. 10 This MRI of a 12-year-old female with back pain demonstrates a herniated disk at L5-S1, with almost complete extrusion of the disk.

suggests that disk herniation in children is more likely to be related to cumulative trauma than to a single event. In the adolescent, back pain is a predominant finding, and symptoms are typically increased with activity and relieved by recumbency.[48,49,52] Coughing and sneezing may increase the pain, and local tenderness is inconsistent. A high percentage (85%) have positive straight leg raising, and 85% to 90% have sciatica.[47,51] The incidence of decreased deep tendon reflexes (22%) and decrease in sensation (21%) and muscle weakness (40%) is less than what would be expected in a similar adult population.[53]

The muscle spasm commonly causes splinting, scoliosis, and gait disturbances.[47,49,51,53] As in the adult, herniation at the L4-5 and L5-S1 levels is by far the most common.[49,51] Disk space narrowing is uncommon and plain films are typically normal in appearance, thus, diagnosis will frequently require confirmation by CT or MRI (Fig. 10).[52,53] Children with documented disk herniation usually require surgical removal.[53] Those who underwent surgical excision had a 91% good to excellent result. The nonsurgical group had 25% good to excellent and 75% poor results.[53]

Slipped Vertebral Apophysis

Slipped vertebral apophysis was previously believed to be uncommon, but, with new imaging techniques,

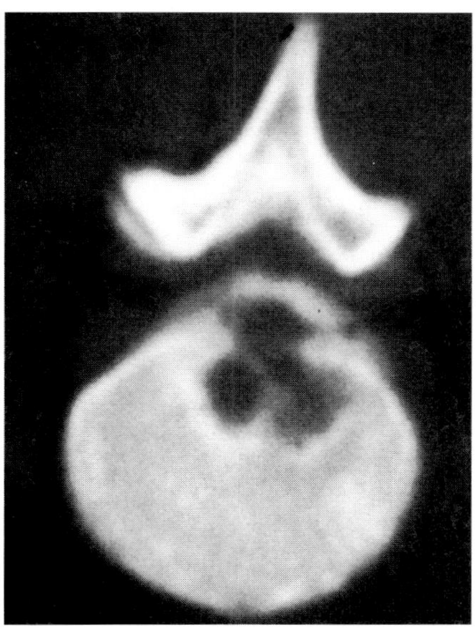

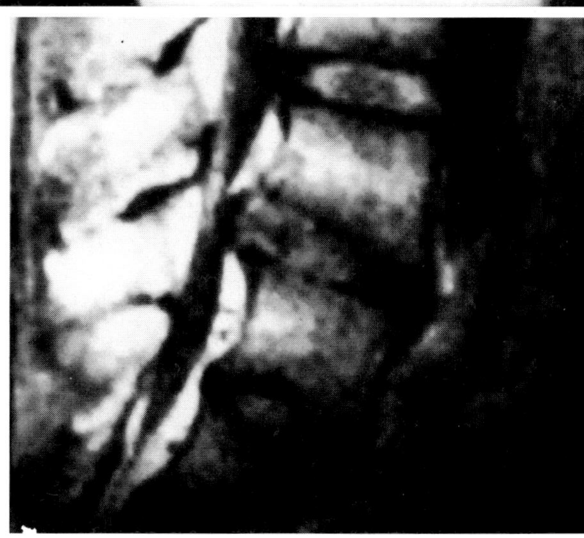

Fig. 11 A 15-year-old male with a slipped vertebral apophysis had a 1-year history of back pain, radiating into the lower extremities. **Top left,** This CT demonstrates a posterior defect of the vertebral body at the point of a Schmorl's node. **Top right,** A CT reconstruction again demonstrates the Schmorl's node and the bony projection into the spinal canal. **Bottom right,** MRI demonstrates extrusion of disk and bone into the canal.

the problem has been more frequently recognized.[54-58] The growth plate of the vertebral body, apophysis, is similar to the epiphysis in the long bone. Just as one can displace the proximal femoral epiphysis, the same problem can occur with the apophysis of the vertebral body. This typically involves the inferior rim of L4, but it can occur at any location. Clinically, the signs and symptoms are similar to those of a herniated disk. However, with this injury, both the bony rim and disk project into and narrow the spinal canal and lead to symptoms of spinal stenosis. On plain films this injury is seen as a very small fleck of calcification adjacent to the disk, but CT and MRI can successfully delineate its extent (Fig. 11).

Disk Space Calcification

This rare clinical syndrome of uncertain etiology usually involves the cervical spine, but it can also occur in the thoracic and lumbar region.[59-61] Boys are affected twice as often as girls, commonly around 7 years of age. The child presents with pain, stiffness, and local tenderness. There may be signs of inflammation, with an elevated temperature, increased sedimentation rate, and leukocytosis. The condition is self-limited and usually responds quickly to symptomatic treatment. Occasionally, the involved disk is weakened by the process and can herniate into the spinal canal, in which case plain radiographs will usually reveal a hazy calcification of the disk.[62,63]

Kyphosis

A frequent cause of back complaints in children is Scheuermann's dorsal lumbar kyphosis.[64] Scheuermann, in his original article, described two forms of kyphosis. The first of these, kyphosis involving a long segment of the thoracic spine, is usually painless in onset. Scheuermann's description was further refined by Sorenson, who noted a familial tendency and described the classic radiographic findings of three consecutive vertebrae wedged 5° or greater.[65] Endplate irregularity, Schmorl's node formation, and narrowing of the disk space were common accompaniments but were not in themselves diagnostic.[65,66] The second type of kyphosis described by Scheuermann is localized to the dorsal lumbar junction and involves fewer vertebrae and more acute angulation. This kyphosis is always associated with vertebral wedging, endplate irregularity, and Schmorl's node formation. This condition is painful and is commonly found in children who perform heavy physical activity, such as shoveling clay or lifting weights (Fig. 12).[3,67,68]

There is strong clinical and experimental evidence to suggest a traumatic origin of Scheurmann's dorsal lumbar kyphosis.[3,69,70] The apophyseal ring is thinner in its center than at the periphery and increased pressure may force the intervertebral disk through the endplate and into cancellous bone, with narrowing of the disk space.[70] Endplate rupture, which has been reproduced in the laboratory by increasing the force on the spine, is believed to be analogous to the mechanism that leads to Schmorl's nodes.[69] Heavy lifting, especially when seated or bending forward, can double interdiskal pressure.[69] Micheli[3] noted that the force of flexion-extension seen with rowers, weightlifters, and gymnasts approaches the lower end of the range demonstrated experimentally to induce vertebral endplate fractures in normal vertebral specimens.[69]

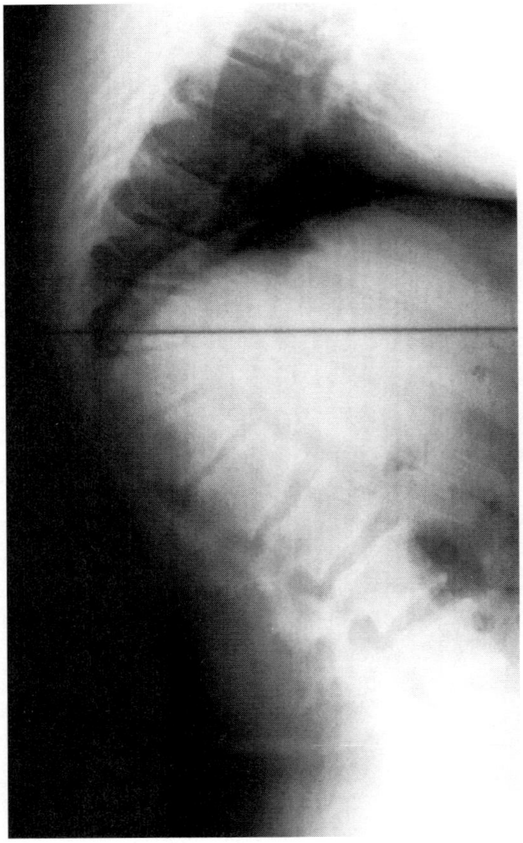

Fig. 12 This radiograph of a 14-year-old demonstrates severe kyphosis centered at the dorsolumbar junction secondary to lumbar Scheuermann's disease. Note the endplate changes, wedging, and narrowing of the disk spaces. Schmorl's node formation can be seen as well in adjacent lumbar vertebrae.

In some children, the disk material passes peripherally (usually anterior), submarginally beneath the apophyseal ring (Fig. 13).[28] Radiologically there will be separation of a triangular, smooth bone fragment from the vertebral body, which represents the ring apophysis.[28] The vertebral changes progress slowly toward healing during the time of remaining growth. However, the Schmorl's node formation and disk space narrowing generally persist and the fragment of the ring apophysis typically remains separate from the vertebral body.[71]

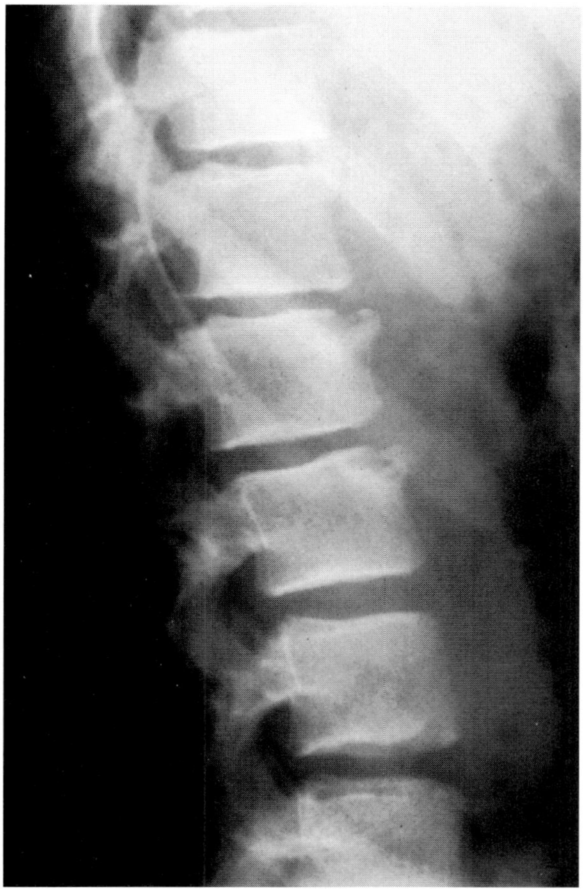

Fig. 13 This 15-year-old recreational weight lifter had persistent back pain at the dorsolumbar junction. The routine lateral film demonstrates anterior Schmorl's node formation and disk space narrowing at T11-12 and T12 - L1.

Symptoms may be of sudden onset, associated with a specific activity. They gradually become more persistent over time and are accentuated with forward bending. The acute phase involves sudden herniation of the disk into the vertebral body, or there can be gradual repetitive injury to the spine with a refractive process leading to the disk expulsion. This kyphosis is often accompanied by spondylolysis. The close association of the two conditions suggests that hyperlordosis, compensating for the kyphosis, increases the likelihood of stress on the pars interarticularis and that the two conditions may be related to the repetitive nature of particular sports.[28]

This condition can be managed quite successfully by simple symptomatic treatment, including immobilization and rest, which allows the vertebrae to heal. When the child is comfortable, gradual resumption of activities is permitted along with physical therapy to strengthen the back musculature. Until rehabilitation is completed, the patient must learn to avoid the specific activities that initiated the problem (Fig. 14).[28,71] Typically, these activities involve repetitive forceful flexion of the dorsal lumbar spine, such as occur during weight lifting, rowing, and gymnastics.

Benign Neoplasm

Osteoid osteoma and osteoblastoma are the most common benign tumors of the spine. Children with these tumors usually present with back pain and scoliosis. The osteoid osteoma usually involves the pedicles and posterior elements. Typically, there is a large sclerotic bone response to a small nidus, best seen on the CT scan (Fig. 15).[7,72] Osteoblastomas usually cause

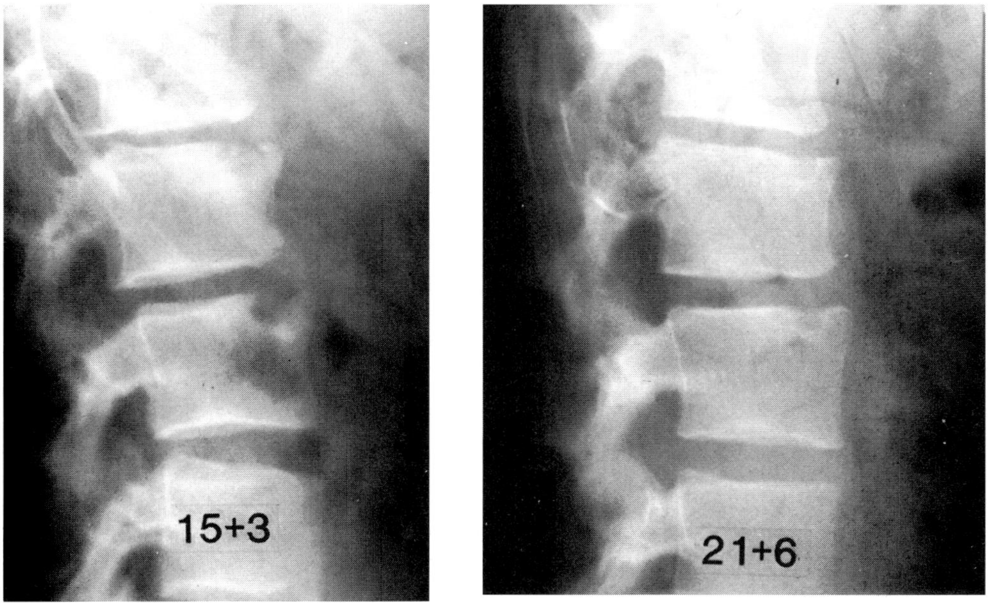

Fig. 14 **Left,** At 15 years and 3 months, back pain due to kyphosis was treated symptomatically. **Right,** Note healing changes in vertebrae at age 21. (Reproduced with permission from Green TL, Hensinger RN, Hunter LY: Back pain and vertebral changes simulating Scheuermann's disease. *J Pediatr Orthop* 1985;5:1-7.)

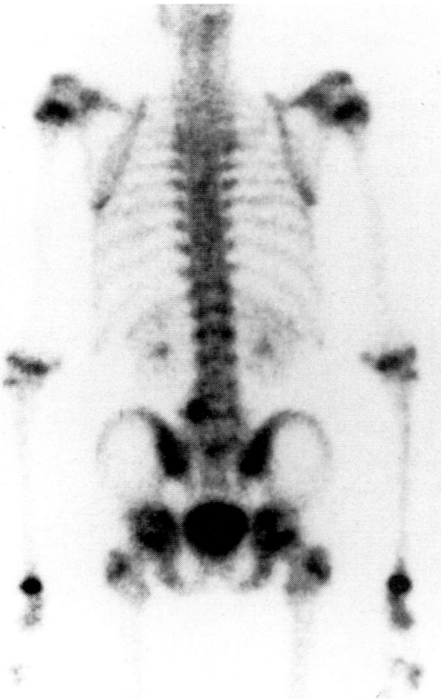

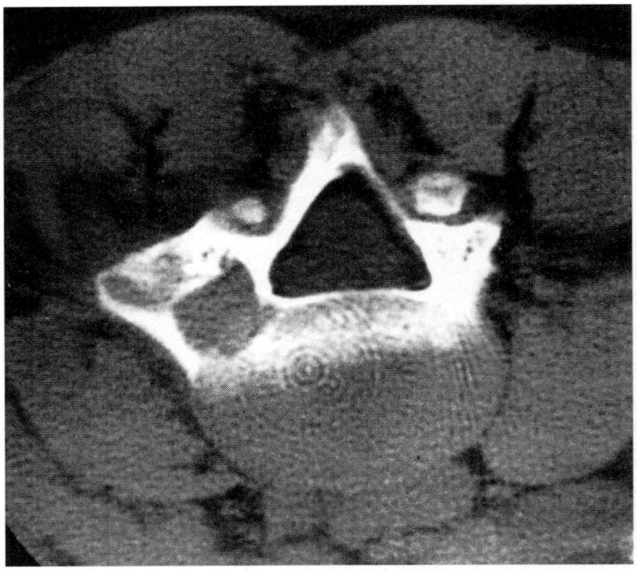

Fig. 15 A 13-year-old male with back pain. **Left,** Bone scan reveals an increased uptake in the region of L4. **Right,** CT demonstrates an osteoid osteoma in the pedicle of L4. (Reproduced with permission from Hensinger RN: Back pain in children, in Andersson GBJ, McNeill TW (eds): *Lumbar Spine Syndromes: Evaluation and Treatment.* Berlin, Springer-Verlag, 1989, pp 126-152.)

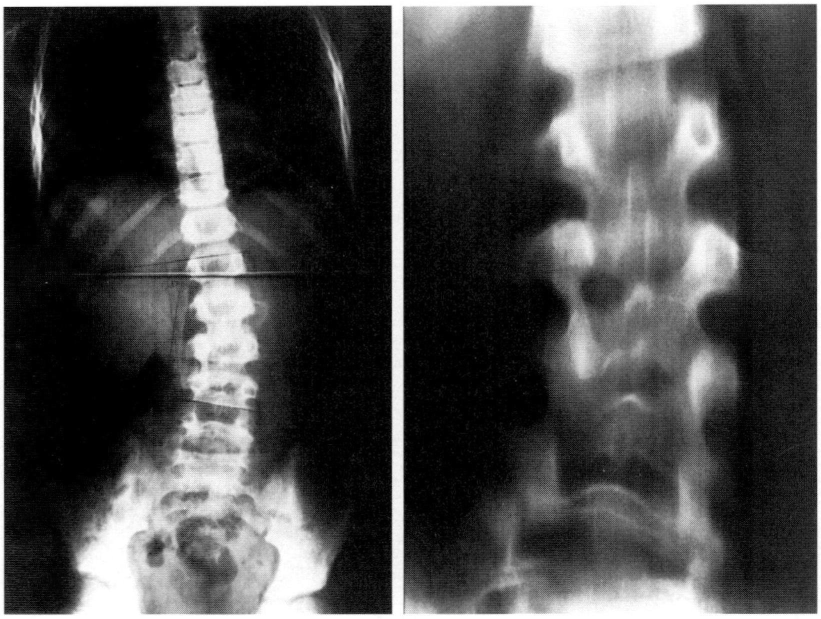

Fig. 16 A 7-year-old with an osteoblastoma. **Left,** Routine radiographs demonstrate a significant lumbar scoliosis, but the lesion could not be identified on this view. **Right,** A laminagram demonstrates erosion of the lamina of L3. (Reproduced with permission from Hensinger RN: Back pain in children, in Bradford DS, Hensinger RN: *The Pediatric Spine.* New York, NY, Thieme Medical Publishers, 1985, pp 41-60.)

the same clinical findings, but they are typically larger and more destructive (Fig. 16). Osteoblastomas can compress the spinal cord, particularly in the cervical and thoracic spine. The tumors are usually symptomatic and the pain is quite characteristic; it is often nocturnal and is relieved by aspirin or naprosyn. The tumors are best localized with the bone scan, followed by definitive identification of the nidus with CT (Figs. 15 and 16).

Eosinophilic granuloma leads to a gradual replacement of the vertebral body and gradual weakening. A trivial injury can precipitate a sudden collapse and bleeding initiating the onset of pain (Fig. 17).[73] Plain films usually reveal the classic radiographic findings of vertebral plana. MRI can confirm the diagnosis. However, in some patients, the radiographic appearance may be confused with Ewing's sarcoma. In such cases, definitive diagnosis requires biopsy. Occasionally, the tumor herniates posteriorly into the spinal canal, causing spinal cord compression, but paraplegia is a rare complication.

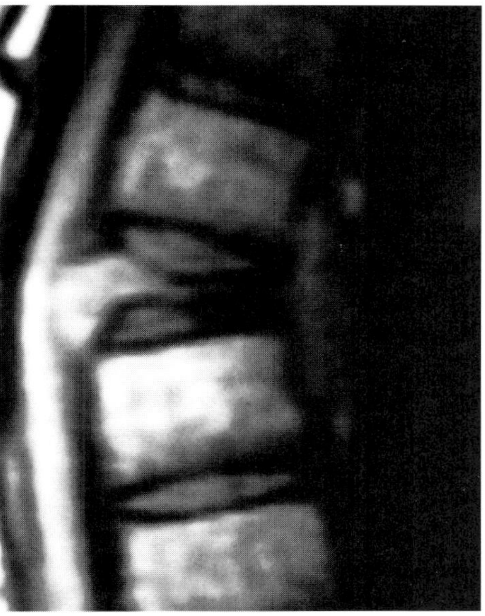

Fig. 17 A 14-year-old male with an eosinophilic granuloma. MRI demonstrates protrusion into the canal posteriorly. The patient was hyperreflexic and the lesion was removed and bone grafted.

The aneurysmal bone cyst may be present for a long period without causing symptoms. The onset of symptoms and discovery is triggered by a fracture through the weakened bone, collapse, and spontaneous hemorrhage. These cysts generally occur in the thoracic or lumbar vertebral body and sacrum but are occasionally found in posterior structures (Fig. 18). Exploration and bone grafting usually resolves the problem.

Malignant Neoplasms

Primary malignant tumors are rare in the spine, the most common being Ewing's sarcoma, leukemia, and lymphoma.[74] More commonly, such lesions are metastatic and represent spread from a distant primary site, usually from bone or bone marrow. In children, the most common skeletal metastases to the spine are neuroblastomas and rhabdomyosarcomas. Less common are teratoma, teratocarcinoma, Wilm's tumor, and osteogenic sarcoma.[74-76] Depending on the series reported, up to 70% of patients with neuroblastoma will have metastatic skeletal disease at the time of their initial diagnosis or during the course of their treatment.[75,77] The spine is typically involved. The diffuse permeative destruction of bone resembles the changes seen in the metaphyseal areas of long bones, with cortical destruction and variable amounts of periosteal reaction.[77] Rhabdomyosarcoma is the most common soft-tissue malignancy in children, and spine metastases occur in 30% to 50% of patients.[78] The abnormal cells displace the normal bone-forming elements, and the vertebra becomes structurally weak and collapses with

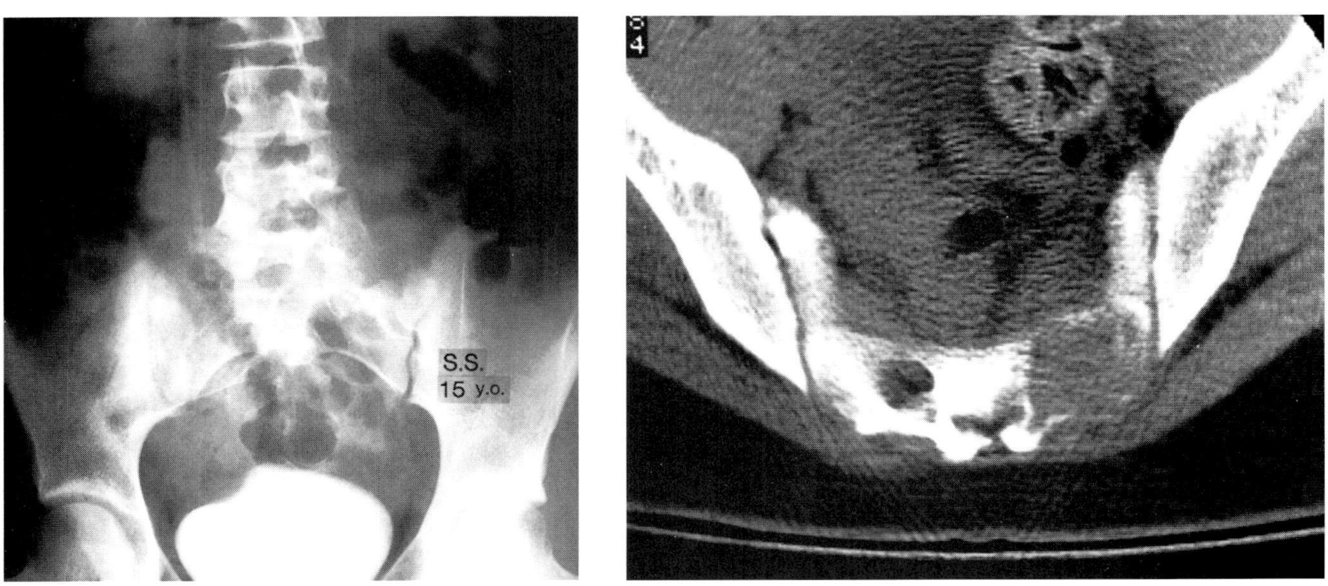

Fig. 18 Aneurysmal bone cyst in the sacrum of a 15-year-old girl. **Left**, An anteroposterior radiograph of the pelvis. Overlying gas shadows and material in the bowel prevent complete examination of the sacrum. **Right,** CT reveals a large aneurysmal bone cyst in the sacrum. (Reproduced with permission from Hensinger RN: Back pain in children, in Bradford DS, Hensinger RN (eds): *The Pediatric Spine*. New York, NY, Thieme Medical Publishers, 1985, pp 41-60.)

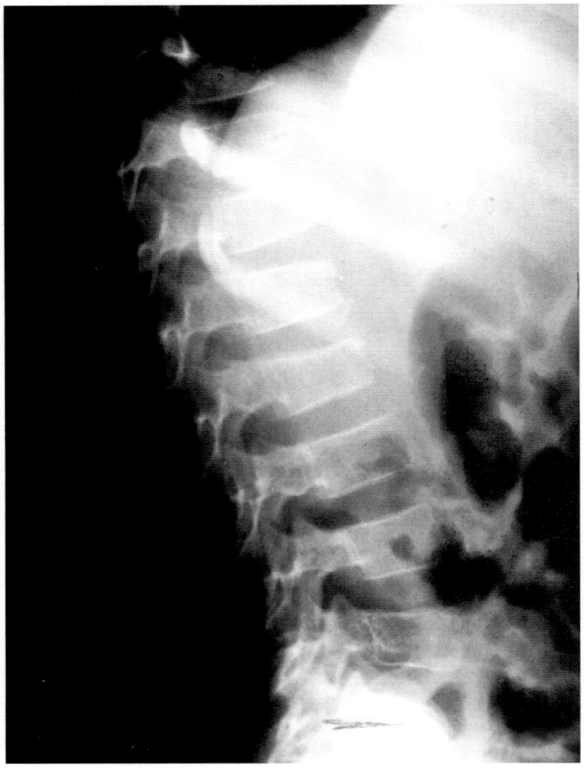

Fig. 19 Radiograph of a 4-year-old with acute lymphatic leukemia and no history of injury demonstrates multiple compression fractures of the lumbar spine. The presenting symptom was back pain. (Reproduced with permission from Hensinger RN: Back pain in children, in Bradford DS, Hensinger RN (eds): *The Pediatric Spine.* New York, NY, Thieme Medical Publishers, 1985, pp 41-60.)

minor trauma.[76,79] Back pain is a common initial complaint, usually in the region of the collapse, and neurologic complications can occur.[9,75] The bone scan is the most sensitive method for diagnosis of a metastasis or primary bone tumor, and in children is more sensitive than skeletal surveys.[75,80] Many children with a leukemia or lymphoma will have involvement of the viscera, as well as the skeleton at other sites in addition to the spine (Fig. 19).

Conclusion

Back pain in children is serious. It is uncommon, and children who have this complaint should be evaluated promptly. Most conditions can be diagnosed with simple measures, such as routine radiographs and bone scan. A few may require more extensive measures, such as CT and MRI. A vast majority will be found to have an objective disease that can be managed quite successfully.

Physicians evaluating acute back pain in children should be particularly alert for those who have persistent pain. Most problems during childhood are relieved with rest and decrease in activity. If there is persistent pain and/or increasing pain, fever, or such neurologic signs as bladder incontinence or nerve root compression, the evaluation should be swift and persistent until the etiology has been determined.

References

1. Hensinger RN: Back pain in children, in Bradford DS, Hensinger RN (eds): *The Pediatric Spine.* New York, NY, Thieme, 1985, pp 41-60.
2. Jackson DW, Wiltse LL, Cirincione RJ: Spondylolysis in the female gymnast. *Clin Orthop* 1976;117:68-73.
3. Micheli LJ: Low back pain in the adolescent: Differential diagnosis. *Am J Sports Med* 1979;7:362-364.
4. Letts M, Smallman T, Afanasiev R, et al: Fracture of the pars interarticularis in adolescent athletes: A clinical-biomechanical analysis. *J Pediat Orthop* 1986;6:40-46.
5. Wynne-Davies R, Scott JHS: Inheritance and spondylolisthesis: A radiographic family survey. *J Bone Joint Surg* 1979;61B:301-305.
6. Keim HA, Reina EG: Osteoid-osteoma as a cause of scoliosis. *J Bone Joint Surg* 1975;57A:159-163.
7. Kirwan EO, Hutton PAN, Pozo JL, et al: Osteoid osteoma and benign osteoblastoma of the spine: Clinical presentation and treatment. *J Bone Joint Surg* 1984;66B:21-26.
8. Mehta MH, Murray RO: Scoliosis provoked by painful vertebral lesions. *Skeletal Radiology* 1977;1:223-230.
9. Conrad EU III, Olszewski AD, Berger M, et al: Pediatric spine tumors with spinal cord compromise. *J Pediatr Orthop* 1992;12:454-460.
10. Hood RW, Riseborough EJ, Nehme AM, et al: Diastematomyelia and structural spinal deformities. *J Bone Joint Surg* 1980;62A:520-528.
11. McMaster MJ: Occult intraspinal anomalies and congenital scoliosis. *J Bone Joint Surg* 1984;66A:588-601.
12. Rasool MN, Govender S, Naidoo KS, et al: Foot deformities and occult spinal abnormalities in children: A review of 16 cases. *J Pediatr Orthop* 1992;12:94-99.
13. Coonrad RW, Richardson WJ, Oakes WJ: Left thoracic curves can be different. *Orthop Trans* 1985;9:126-127.
14. Winter RB, Lipscomb PR Jr.: Back pain in children. *Minnesota Med* 1978;61:141-147.
15. Turner PG, Green JH, Galasko CSB: Back pain in childhood. *Spine* 1989;14:812-814.
16. Lowe RW, Hayes TD, Kaye J, et al: Standing roentgenograms in spondylolisthesis. *Clin Orthop* 1976;117:80-84.
17. Libson E, Bloom RA, Dinari G: Symptomatic and asymptomatic spondylolysis and spondylolisthesis in young adults. *Internat Orthop* 1982;6:259-261.
18. Papanicolaou N, Wilkinson RH, Emans JB, et al: Bone scintigraphy and radiography in young athletes with low back pain. *Am J Roentgenol* 1985;145:1039-1044.
19. van den Oever M, Merrick MV, Scott JHS: Bone scintigraphy in symptomatic spondylolysis. *J Bone Joint Surg* 1987;69B:453-456.
20. Bodner RJ, Heyman S, Drummond DS, et al: The use of single photon emission computed tomography (SPECT) in the diagnosis of low-back pain in young patients. *Spine* 1988;13:1155-1160.
21. Hensinger RN: Spondylolysis and spondylolisthesis in children and adolescents. *J Bone Joint Surg* 1989;71A:1098-1107.
22. Baker DR, McHollick W: Spondyloschisis and spondylolisthesis in children. *J Bone Joint Surg* 1956;38A:933-934.
23. Wiltse LL, Widell EH Jr, Jackson DW: Fatigue fracture: The basic lesion in isthmic spondylolisthesis. *J Bone Joint Surg* 57A:17-22, 1975.
24. Krenz J, Troup JD: The structure of the pars interarticularis of the lower lumbar vertebrae and its relation to the etiology of

spondylolysis, with a report of a healing fracture in the neural arch of a fourth lumbar vertebra. *J Bone Joint Surg* 1973;55B:735-741.

25. Cyron BM, Hutton WC: Variations in the amount and distribution of cortical bone across the partes interarticulares of L5: A predisposing factor in spondylolysis? *Spine* 1979;4:163-167.
26. Jackson DW: Low back pain in young athletes: Evaluation of stress reaction and discogenic problems. *Am J Sports Med* 1979;7:364-366.
27. Micheli LJ: Back injuries in dancers. *Clin Sports Med* 1983;2:473-484.
28. Greene TL, Hensinger RN, Hunter LY: Back pain and vertebral changes simulating Scheuermann's disease. *J Pediat Orthop* 1985;5:1-7.
29. Ogilvie JW, Sherman J: Spondylolysis in Scheuermann's disease. *Spine* 1987;12:251-253.
30. Hensinger RN, Lang JR, MacEwen GD: Surgical management of spondylolisthesis in children and adolescents. *Spine* 1976;1:207-216.
31. Phalen GS, Dickson JA: Spondylolisthesis and tight hamstrings. *J Bone Joint Surg* 1961;43A:505-512.
32. Sherman FC, Wilkinson RH, Hall JE: Reactive sclerosis of a pedicle and spondylolysis in the lumbar spine. *J Bone Joint Surg* 1977;59A:49-54.
33. Steiner ME, Micheli LJ: Treatment of symptomatic spondylolysis and spondylolisthesis with the modified Boston brace. *Spine* 1985;10:937-943.
34. Seitsalo S, Österman K, Poussa M, et al: Spondylolisthesis in children under 12 years of age: Long-term results of 56 patients treated conservatively or operatively. *J Pediart Orthop* 1988;8:516-521.
35. Pizzutillo PD, Hummer CD III.: Nonoperative treatment for painful adolescent spondylolysis or spondylolisthesis. *J Pediatr Orthop* 1989;9:538-540.
36. Seitsalo S, Osterman K, Hyvarinen H, et al: Progression of spondylolisthesis in children and adolescents: A long-term follow-up of 272 patients. *Spine* 1991;16:417-421.
37. Frennered AK, Danielson BI, Nachemson AL: Natural history of symptomatic isthmic low-grade spondylolisthesis in children and adolescents: A seven-year follow-up study. *J Pediatr Orthop* 1991;11:209-213.
38. Menelaus MB: Discitis: An inflammation affecting the intervertebral discs in children. *J Bone Joint Surg* 1964;46B:16-23.
39. Spiegel PG, Kengla KW, Isaacson AS, et al: Intervertebral disc-space inflammation in children. *J Bone Joint Surg* 1972;54A:284-296.
40. Wenger DR, Bobechko WP, Gilday DL: The spectrum of intervertebral disc-space infection in children. *J Bone Joint Surg* 1978;60A:100-108.
41. Szalay EA, Green NE, Heller RM, et al: Magnetic resonance imaging in the diagnosis of childhood discitis. *J Pediatr Orthop* 1987;7:164-167.
42. Boston HC Jr, Bianco AJ Jr, Rhodes KH: Disk space infections in children. *Orthop Clin North Am* 1975;6:953-964.
43. Smith RF, Taylor TKF: Inflammatory lesions of intervertebral discs in children. *J Bone Joint Surg* 1967;49A:1508-1520.
44. McNeill TW: Spinal infections, in Greene, WB (ed): *Instructional Course Lectures, Volume XXXIX.* Park Ridge, Illinois, The American Academy of Orthopaedic Surgeons, 1990, pp 515-524.
45. Crawford AH, Kucharzyk DW, Ruda R, et al: Diskitis in children. *Clin Orthop* 1991;266:70-79.
46. Borgesen SE, Vang PS: Herniation of the lumbar intervertebral disk in children and adolescents. *Acta Orthop Scand* 1974;45:540-549.
47. Bradford DS, Garcia A: Herniations of the lumbar intervertebral disk in children and adolescents: A review of 30 surgically treated cases. *JAMA* 1969;210:2045-2051.
48. DeOrio JK, Bianco AJ Jr: Lumbar disc excision in children and adolescents. *J Bone Joint Surg* 1982;64A:991-996.
49. Epstein JA, Epstein NE, Marc J, et al: Lumbar intervertebral disk herniation in teenage children: Recognition and management of associated anomalies. *Spine* 1984;9:427-432.
50. Garrido E, Humphreys RP, Hendrick EB, et al: Lumbar disc disease in children. *Neurosurgery* 1978;2:22-26.
51. Kurihara A, Kataoka O: Lumbar disc herniation in children and adolescents: A review of 70 operated cases and their minimum 5-year follow-up studies. *Spine* 1980;5:443-451.
52. Takata K, Takahashi K: Hamstring tightness and sciatica in young patients with disc herniation. *J Bone Joint Surg* 1994;76B:220-224.
53. DeLuca PF, Mason DE, Weiand R, et al: Excision of herniated nucleus pulposus in children and adolescents. *J Pediatr Orthop* 1994;14:318-322.
54. Handel SF, Twiford TW Jr, Reigel DH, et al: Posterior lumbar apophyseal fractures. *Radiology* 1979;130:629-633.
55. Keller RH: Traumatic displacement of the cartilagenous vertebral rim: A sign of intervertebral disc prolapse. *Radiology* 1974;110:21-24.
56. Lippitt AB: Fracture of a vertebral body end plate and disk protrusion causing subarachnoid block in an adolescent. *Clin Orthop* 1976;116:112-115.
57. Lowrey JJ: Dislocated lumbar vertebral epiphysis in adolescent children: Report of three cases. *J Neurosurg* 1973;38:232-234.
58. Techakapuch S.: Rupture of the lumbar cartilage plate into the spinal canal in an adolescent: A case report. *J Bone Joint Surg* 1981;63A:481-482.
59. Melnick JC, Silverman FN: Intervertebral disk calcification in childhood. *Radiology* 1963;80:399-408.
60. Schechter LS, Smith A, Pearl M: Intervertebral disk calcification in childhood. *Am J Dis Child* 1972;123:608-611.
61. Sonnabend DH, Taylor TKF, Chapman GK: Intervertebral disc calcification syndromes in children. *J Bone Joint Surg* 1982;64B:25-31.
62. McCartee CC Jr, Griffin PP, Byrd EB: Ruptured calcified thoracic disc in a child: Report of a case. *J Bone Joint Surg* 1972;54A:1272-1274.
63. Peck FC Jr: A calcified thoracic intervertebral disk with herniation and spinal cord compression in a child: Case report. *J Neurosurgery* 1957;14:105-109.
64. Scheuermann H: Kyphosis dorsalis juvenilis. *Ztschr Orthop Chir* 1921;41:305-317.
65. Sörenson KH: Scheuermann's juvenile kyphosis: Clinical appearances, radiography, aetiology and prognosis. Copenhagen, Munksgaard, 1964.
66. Bradford DS, Moe JH, Montalvo FJ, et al: Scheuermann's kyphosis and roundback deformity: Results of Milwaukee brace treatment. *J Bone Joint Surg* 1974;56A:740-758.
67. Edgren W, Vainio S: Osteochondrosis juvenilis lumbalis. *Acta Chir Scand* 1957;227(suppl):1-47.
68. Wassmann K: Kyphosis juvenilis Scheuermann: An occupational disorder. *Acta Orthop Scand* 1951;21:65-74.
69. Jayson MIV, Herbert CM, Barks JS: Intervertebral discs: Nuclear morphology and bursting pressures. *Ann Rheum Dis* 1973;32:308-315.
70. Resnick D, Niwayama G: Intravertebral disk herniations: Cartilaginous (Schmorl's) nodes. *Radiology* 1978;126:57-65.
71. Lowe TG: Scheuermann's disease. *J Bone Joint Surg* 1990;72A:940-945.
72. Gitelis S, Schajowicz F: Osteoid osteoma and osteoblastoma. *Orthop Clin North Am* 1989;20:313-325.
73. Nesbit ME, Kieffer S, D'Angio GJ: Reconstitution of vertebral height in histiocytosis X: A long-term follow-up. *J Bone Joint Surg* 1969;51A:1360-1368.
74. Young JL Jr, Miller RW: Incidence of malignant tumors in U.S. children. *J Pediatr* 1975;86:254-258.
75. Leeson MC, Makley JT, Carter JR: Metastatic skeletal disease in the pediatric population. *J Pediatr Orthop* 1985;5:261-267.
76. Ogden JA, Ogden DA: Skeletal metastasis: The effect on the immature skeleton. *Skeletal Radiology* 1982;9:73-82.

77. Fernbach DJ, Williams TE, Donaldson MH: Neuroblastoma, in Sutow WW, Vietti TJ, Fernbach DJ (eds): *Clinical Pediatric Oncology*, ed 2. St Louis, MO, CV Mosby, 1977, pp 506-537.
78. Maroteaux P: Malignant tumors, in Maroteaux P (ed): *Bone Diseases of Children*. Philadelphia, PA, JB Lippincott, 1979, pp 397-420.
79. Rogalsky RJ, Black GB, Reed MH: Orthopaedic manifestations of leukemia in children. *J Bone Joint Surg* 1986;68A:494-501.
80. Gilday DL, Ash JM, Reilly BJ: Radionuclide skeletal survey for pediatric neoplasms. *Radiology* 1977;123:399-406.

Wrist

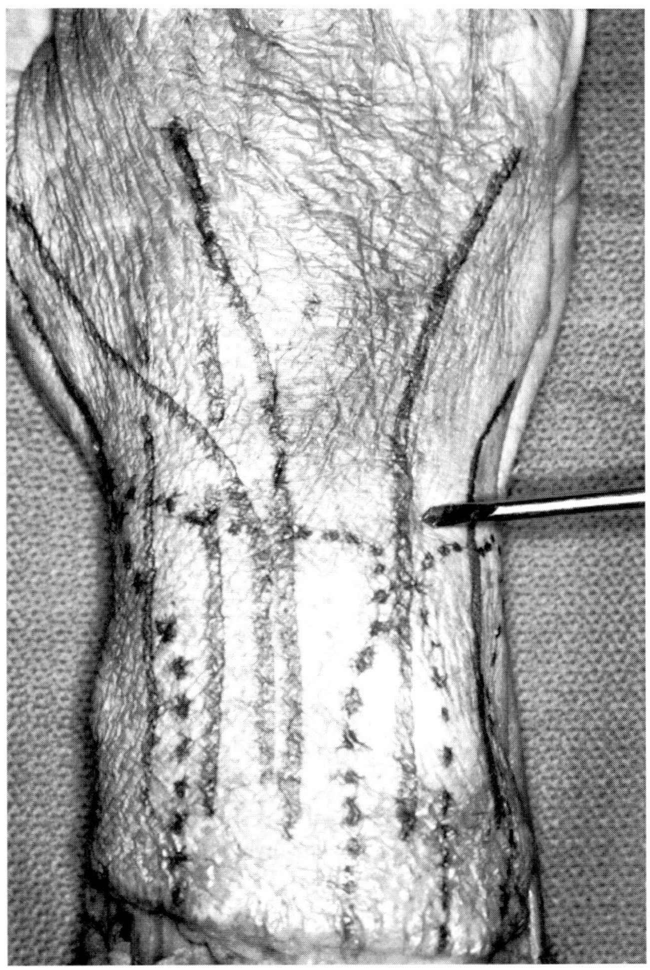

C H A P T E R 9

Chronic Wrist Pain

Terry L. Whipple, MD

The wrist joint, because it contains 8 carpal bones, 17 articulations, 23 ligaments, and a triangular fibrocartilage, all within a two-inch space, challenges the clinician with an array of potential diagnoses. For example, ulnar wrist pain has 44 separate entities and multiple permutations.[1] Wrist arthroscopy allows direct visualization of cartilage surfaces and the synovium and visually directed palpation of the ligaments. Given this ability, wrist arthroscopy is the best, and in some cases the only, technique for the diagnosis of certain chondral lesions, extrinsic ligament tears, and peripheral triangular fibrocartilage.

Chronic, obscure wrist pain is defined as wrist pain that has been present longer than 3 months without definitive diagnosis and that is unresponsive to conservative measures. Obvious carpal instability and fractures should be excluded. The clinical evaluation requires an orderly sequential approach (Outline 1). Step 1 involves a careful history regarding the onset of the problem and mechanism of injury. If the pain is work related, the history should include a thorough description of job activities. Pain should be characterized relative to its location, intensity, duration, radiation, and aggravating or relieving factors. Symptoms that are worse when the wrist is loaded and pain that is associated with clicking or catching suggest a mechanical source of the problem.

Step 2 involves inspection for swelling or masses, palpation for points of maximum tenderness, and a careful analysis of range of motion comparing the injured wrist with the uninjured side. Step 3 in the physical examination is the use of provocative maneuvers (Table 1). Here the examiner tries to recreate the conditions that reproduce the pain in the patient. Catches, clicks, clunks, and crepitus are recorded and looked for in both wrists. These noises are significant if they are unilateral and if they reproduce the patient's symptoms. Step 4 requires grip strength testing using a Jamar dynamometer. Valid grip strength testing should show a bell-shaped curve going from the small intrinsic grip through the combined intrinsic/extrinsic grip and falling with the larger extrinsic grip. Significant wrist pain results in grip strength weakness with a valid, but lower, bell-shaped curve. Patients with exaggerated symptoms or secondary gain usually produce inconsistent responses. Finally, in step 5, a trial injection of local anaesthetic to assess the

Outline 1
A stepwise approach to the clinical examination of the painful wrist

Step 1	History
	Onset, mechanism of injury, characterization of pain
Step 2	Inspection
	Palpation area maximal tenderness, ROM
Step 3	Provocative maneuvers
Step 4	Grip strength
Step 5	Trial injection and retest

Table 1
Provocative wrist maneuvers

Name of Test	Tests	Procedure
The radial stress test (Watson test, scaphoid shift)	Scapholunate stability volarly	Grasp wrist from radial side. Place thumb volarly against scaphoid tubercle and fingers on Lister's tubercle. Use opposite hand to control wrist position. Start in ulnar deviation and slight extension. Move the wrist radially and towards flexion with constant thumb pressure on the scaphoid. Normally, as the wrist radially deviates and flexes, the scaphoid palmar flexes. The examiner's thumb opposes this motion and causes a subluxation stress. With rigid ligaments, the scaphoid pushes the examiner's thumb out of the way and rotates/flexes normally. With ligament laxity, the scaphoid shifts up onto the dorsal rim of the radius. When thumb pressure is withdrawn, the scaphoid returns to its normal position with a "clunk". A positive test is one that elicits a click or a clunk that is greater than the other side and that reproduces the patient's symptoms.
The Shear Test	Pisotriquetral problems	Fingers dorsal to triquetrum, thumb rocks or pushes the pisiform into the triquetrum. A positive test produces grinding and pain.
The Shuck Test	Lunatotriquetral stability	Fingers dorsal to lunate while thumb is on the pisotriquetral joint, then, radial and ulnar deviation of the wrist, both actively and passively. A positive test produces pain at the lunotriquetral articulation.
Lunatotriquetral Ballottement Test	Lunatotriquetral stability	Fix lunate with thumb and index of one hand, while other hand displaces the triquetrum and pisiform both volarly and dorsally. Pain indicates instability or inflammation at the lunotriquetral joint.
Piano-key Test	Distal radioulnar joint stability	Hold distal ulna between index and thumb and test the volar-dorsal translation of the distal ulna at different rotatory positions. Look for excessive mobility compared with opposite wrist.
Triangular Fibrocartilage Load Test	TFC injury	Hold wrist in ulnar deviation, apply axial load. Passive manipulation of carpus against the ulna and rotation will produce painful crepitus.

affects on the pain and the retesting of the provocative maneuvers gives the examiner further information. After completion of the history and physical examination, the examiner may have a definitive clinical diagnosis and, therefore, need no further studies. In other cases, the examiner may suspect the clinical diagnosis but need further studies to confirm that hypothesis. Finally, the diagnosis may still be elusive.

Imaging

Following the five-step clinical examination, any number of imaging techniques are available.[2] As part of our diagnosis of chronic wrist pain, the standard four-view series of the wrist should be augmented by provocative positions and special views. Plain films can include provocative views. If ligament instability or ulnar abutment is suspected, a clenched fist view in pronation and supination and a clenched fist view in radial and ulnar deviation may help to reveal a dynamic scapholunate shift or positive ulnar variance. Special positions, such as carpal tunnel views and pisotriquetral views, can also be useful. In certain instances, comparison views of the normal wrist may help show subtle abnormalities. Video fluoroscopy can be helpful if carpal instability, especially of the midcarpal joint, is suspected.

Wrist arthrography[2] remains the gold standard for diagnosis of ligament injury. The accuracy of the technique can be improved by the use of the pain marker, fluoroscopic observation and/or fast sequence filming of the injection, post-exercise filming, and digital subtraction. Palmer has shown the advantage of triple injection arthrography in making the diagnosis of intrinsic ligament tears and peripheral triangular fibrocartilage tears. The disadvantages of this technique are that it is invasive, painful, involves irradiation, and, most importantly, it does not confirm the mechanical significance of the entity observed. For example, it is not uncommon to have a person with a tear of the triangular fibrocartilage on the right wrist diagnosed arthrographically, and, when a comparison arthrogram is done of the opposite wrist, a similar but asymptomatic tear is identified.

Magnetic resonance imaging[3] with the use of dedicated wrist coils is becoming an increasingly helpful study. It is the ideal technique to study osteonecrosis of the lunate. It is accurate in defining pathologic fluid in the wrist and the presence of small ganglia. It is as accurate as arthrography in identifying defects in the central portion of the triangular fibrocartilage. It is less sensitive in detecting intrinsic ligament tears. In our series, it was 80% accurate in detecting scapholunate tears but only 50% accurate in identifying defects of the lunatotriquetral intrinsic ligament. New enhancement techniques may improve this efficiency and also allow visualization of the volar extrinsic ligaments. Finally, a triple-phase bone scan may be used as a screening test.

Table 2
Results of arthroscopic diagnosis of 68 wrists with chronic wrist pain

Condition Identified	No. of Wrists
Chondromalacia	
Radiocarpal joint	9
Midcarpal joint	21
Triangular fibrocartilage tears	
Central	1
Peripheral	15
Ligament tears	
Scapholunate	2
Lunatotriquetral	5
Ulnar extrinsic	1
Radial extrinsic	1
Synovitis (rheumatoid arthritis)	1

While this scan is not specific for any entity, it is extremely sensitive to the presence of synovitis, arthritis, occult fracture, and the presence of more diffuse entities such as reflex sympathetic dystrophy. It is, therefore, used as a validation study.

Unlike the studies above, wrist arthroscopy allows direct visualization of joint anatomy. It is performed under regional or general anesthesia, which provides the examiner with another opportunity to palpate the wrist and perform the provocative maneuvers. Diagnostic arthroscopy requires a careful step-by-step viewing sequence to visualize and probe all structures. A minimum of three portals is necessary. Generally, we use the 3-4 portal and ulnar portal for the radiocarpal joint and a radial portal for the midcarpal joint. When there is a type II lunate[4] with a large hamate facet, an ulnar midcarpal portal is often added. Lastly, when indicated, the distal radial ulnar joint can be viewed. The 3-4 viewing portal used for this examination is easily entered about 50% of the time. Presence of synovitis, either local or general, should be noted. Localized inflammation is often a clue to the underlying abnormality. If intrinsic ligament instability is suspected, not only should the intrinsic ligament be inspected and palpated in the radiocarpal joint, but the examiner should evaluate the midcarpal joint. If scapholunate instability is present, there is generally chondromalacia in the scaphoid-trapezoid-trapezium (STT) joint. Conversely, if lunatotriquetral or midcarpal instability is present, there is chondromalacia of the triquetral hamate interface. It is often useful to use joystick Kirschner wires to manipulate the respective carpal bones and evaluate translations of the midcarpal artificial interfaces, which are normally concave, devoid of ligament, and level.

In a recent study that examined 68 wrists with chronic wrist pain and normal imaging studies, the 68 patients in the series had normal radiocarpal arthrography. Of the 68, 37 had normal triple compartment arthrography, and 46 had normal MRI studies. Triple-phase bone scanning was performed in 45 of the patients, and the

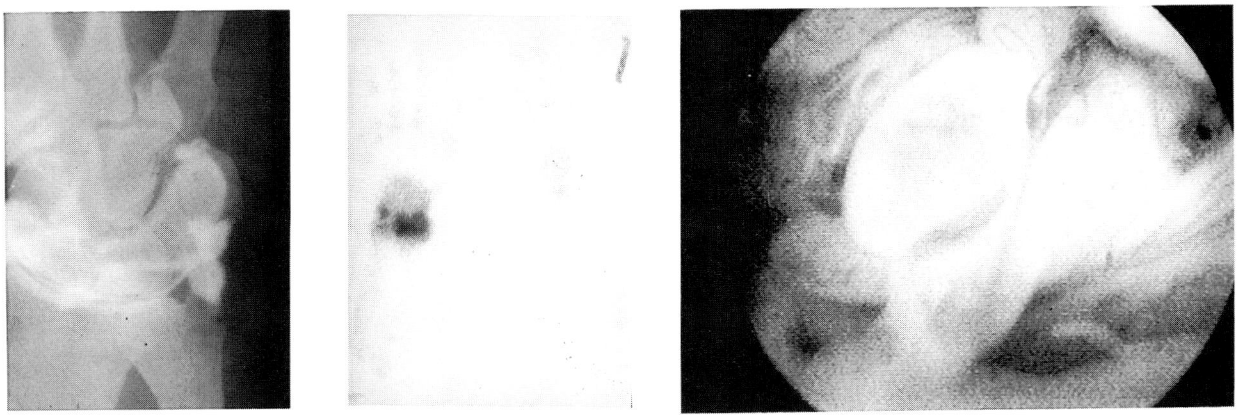

Fig. 1 **Left,** Normal radiocarpal arthrogram and **center**, markedly positive bone scan showing the uptake throughout the wrist. **Right**, Arthroscopic view of inflammatory rheumatoid synovitis.

results were normal in 29 and positive in 16 patients. The arthroscopic diagnoses are listed in Table 2. The diagnoses most commonly missed by the sophisticated imaging techniques were the presence of chondromalacia, particularly when this was present in the midcarpal joint. Peripheral tears of the triangular fibrocartilage, which are obvious at arthroscopy by the laxity of the triangular fibrocartilage, were the second most missed diagnosis. Finally, ulnar extrinsic ligament tears and lunatotriquetral ligament tears were often missed by the imaging techniques.

Thus, without wrist arthroscopy, the diagnosis would have remained unknown in over half of these patients. Arthroscopy was also helpful when there were multiple lesions. Common combinations included perforations of both the scapholunate and lunatotriquetral intrinsic ligaments, tears of the triangular fibrocartilage and the lunatotriquetral ligament, and chondromalacia in the midcarpal joint associated with intrinsic ligament tears.

Case 1

This 19-year-old college student had a 9-month history of insidious swelling and stiffness of right wrist. Physical examination showed generalized wrist soreness with limited wrist motion and mild effusion. Carpal shake test was positive; other provocative tests were negative. Grip strength was significantly decreased on Jamar dynamometer testing. Rheumatologic studies were normal. Plain films were normal and showed no ulnar styloid erosion. Radiocarpal arthrography was normal, but triple-phase bone scanning was markedly positive (Fig. 1, *left* and *center*). At arthroscopy, marked synovitis was noted of the radiocarpal and midcarpal joints. A synovial biopsy confirmed the diagnosis of rheumatoid arthritis (Fig. 1, *right*).

Case 2

A 33-year-old, right-hand dominant carpenter had sustained a high torque twisting injury of his right (dominant) wrist 7 months previously. Ulnar wrist pain, weakness of grip, and ulnar deviation persisted despite conservative care. Physical examination showed maximal tenderness over the lunatotriquetral joint, normal provocative tests, and grip strength reduced by 40% on ulnar deviation only. Plain films, triple compartment arthrography, and magnetic resonance imaging were normal (Fig. 2, *left*). The bone scan was mildly positive over the ulnar aspect of the wrist. The presumptive diagnosis was a partial tear of the lunatotriquetral ligament. At arthroscopy, the lunatotriquetral ligament was intact and the examination of the radiocarpal joint was normal. In the midcarpal joint a Type II lunate[4] was noted; localized midcarpal synovitis and marked chondromalacia were present on the proximal pole of the hamate (Fig. 2, *right*). Arthroscopic chondroplasty was performed. At 2.4 years, the patient is working full duty as a carpenter and is asymptomatic. In this case, wrist arthroscopy not only altered the diagnosis but provided an appropriate therapeutic option.

Extrinsic Ligament Injury

Extrinsic wrist ligaments originate from the radius or ulna and insert on the carpal bones (Fig. 3).[5-7] The extrinsic ligaments often merge with the volar and dorsal aspects of the intrinsic scapholunate and lunatotriquetral ligaments. On the radial side of the joint, they are four in number. The radioscaphocapitate is the first ligament visualized, followed by the broader long radial lunate ligament. Often a small sulcus separates the two ligaments. The radioscapholunate ligament (often referred to as the ligament of Testut), lies beneath the synovial fat pad directly in line with the scapholunate interval. Finally, originating from the lunate facet of the radius and inserting on the lunate, is the short radiolunate ligament. The ulnolunate and ulnotriquetral ligaments originate from the ulna and merge with the peripheral portion of the triangular fibrocartilage. They then reinforce the volar edge of the

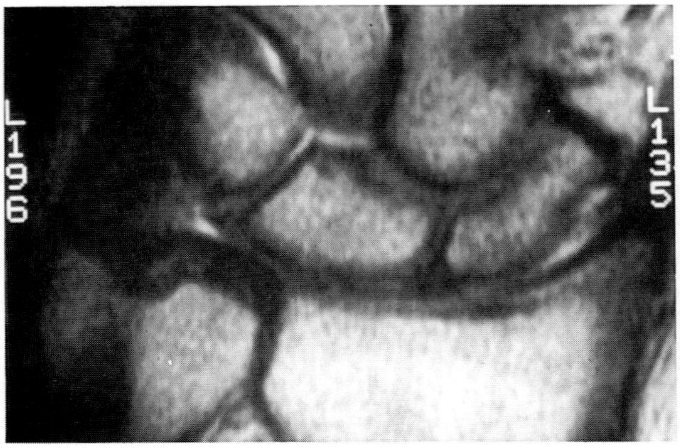

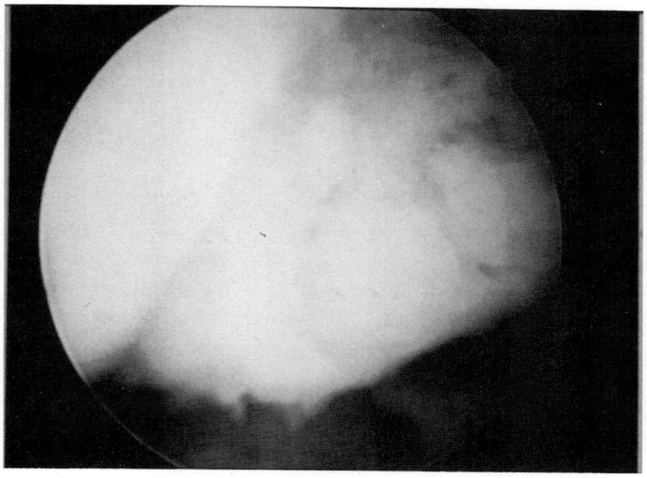

Fig. 2 **Left,** Normal T1 MRI of the wrist. Note the Type II lunate with its hamate facet. **Right**, Arthroscopic view of right midcarpal joint of the capito-hamate interface. Note the significant chondromalacic changes on the proximal pole of the hamate.

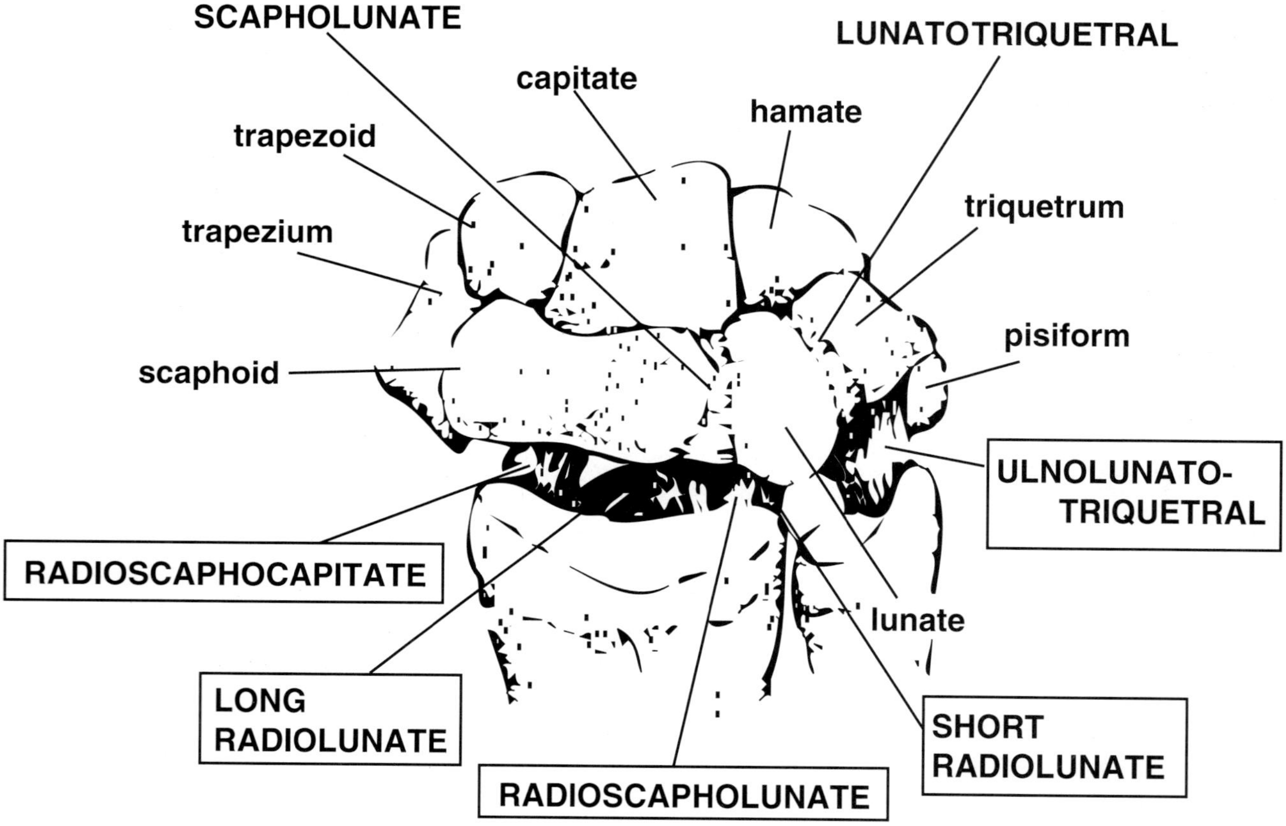

Fig. 3 In this schematic diagram, the five extrinsic radiocarpal ligaments that can be identified arthroscopically are named in the boxes at the lower part of the diagram. The two intrinsic ligaments, the scapholunate and lunotriquetral, are shown at the top.

intrinsic lunatotriquetral ligament. The dorsal extrinsic radiocarpal ligaments and the carpometacarpal extrinsic ligaments cannot generally be visualized arthroscopically.

Extrinsic ligament tears are recognized as part of the injured structures in frank carpal dislocation and static carpal instabilities.[6] Isolated tears of these ligaments were once felt to be rare,[8] but wrist arthroscopy has confirmed that such lesions are more frequent than had been suspected. For example, in a study that involved the arthroscopic evaluation and treatment of intra-articular distal radial fractures, we found a 35% incidence of injury to the radioscaphocapitate ligament, a 40% incidence of injury to the long radiolunate ligament, and a 20% incidence of injury to the short radiolunate ligament.

The clinical diagnosis of an injury to an extrinsic ligament is often difficult. Generally, there is tenderness volarly and dorsally, and pain at the extremes of the motion restrained by that ligament. Provocative tests are not particularly helpful. In ulnar extrinsic ligament damage, a relative supination deformity of the ulnar carpus on the ulna can be seen. A similar type of laxity can be present with peripheral tears of the triangular fibrocartilage and disruption of the extensor carpi ulnaris sheath, and both of these entities should be considered when a carpal supination deformity is noted.

Imaging studies have not been particularly helpful in defining extrinsic ligament tears. Arthrography may be helpful in the acute situation, in which dye may leak through the rent in the volar capsule. Generally, however, in the chronic injury, scar tissue fills the area in and renders the arthrogram normal. Magnetic resonance imaging with special coils can increasingly visualize the volar ligaments. On T2 images, edema may be noted in the volar ligaments as a pathognomonic sign.

Arthroscopy allows direct visualization of the disrupted fibers of a torn extrinsic ligament. In the acute situation, the presence of hemorrhage may fill the ligament interstices. Use of a probe at arthroscopy enables the examiner to palpate the tension in the ligaments directly (Fig 4). In ulnar extrinsic ligament injury, the floor of the ulnar wrist is disrupted and it is generally possible to visualize the pisotriquetral joint directly.

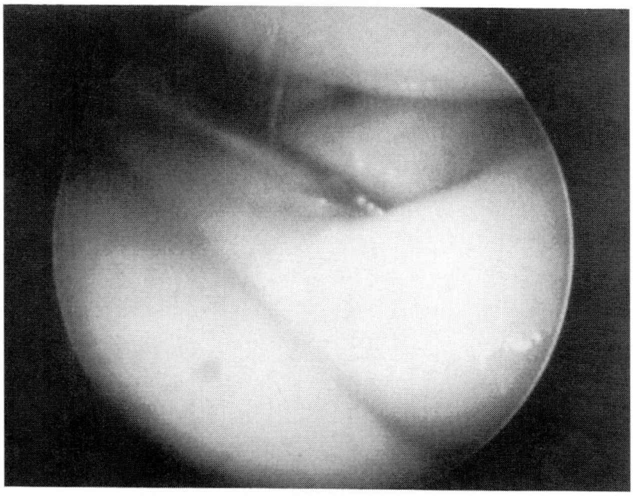

Fig. 4 Radiocarpal arthroscopy of the right wrist showing the probe palpating the interval between the extrinsic radioscaphocapitate ligament and the broader long radiolunate ligament. In the lower left-hand corner is the scaphoid facet of the radius and superiorly the proximal pole of the scaphoid.

Case 3

A 31-year-old left-hand dominant professional golfer had the sudden onset of left ulnar wrist pain with a divot shot. Initial radiographs were normal, and she continued to play. For 6 weeks the pain made her play ineffective. Physical examination showed tenderness in the volar and dorsal aspects of the wrist at the level of the lunato-triquetral joint. There was no hook of hamate tenderness. A shuck test produced pain but no clicking. There was a mild supination deformity not present on the opposite wrist. A Tinel's sign was positive over the ulnar nerve at Guyon's canal, but otherwise the ulnar neurovascular examination was normal. Triple compartment arthrogram showed pisotriquetral filling, which was read as a normal variant (Fig. 5, *top left*). A magnetic resonance image was initially read as showing only increased fluid in the ulnar aspect of the wrist (Fig. 5, *top right*).

At arthroscopy, tears of the extrinsic ulnolunate and ulnotriquetral ligaments were found (Fig. 5, *center left*). The tears allowed direct visualization of the pisotriquetral joint (Fig. 5, *center right* and *bottom left*). No palpable tension was present in the ligaments. Adjacent to the tear, a small osteochondral fracture was noted in the lunate (Fig. 5, *bottom right*). Treatment involved arthroscopic removal of the osteochondral fragment, followed by a volar open approach to the ligament tears with a primary capsular repair and augmentation with a slip of the flexor carpi ulnaris. Following 3 weeks of cast immobilization and 3 months of a therapy program, the patient returned to professional golf.

Central Tear of the Triangular Fibrocartilage

Tears of the triangular fibrocartilage (TFC) are frequently implicated as a cause of ulnar wrist pain.[9,10] Over the last 20 years, a number of studies have extended our knowledge of the anatomy and biomechanics of the triangular fibrocartilage.[11-14] Compared to the peripheral zones of the triangular fibrocartilage, the central zone is thin, cartilaginous, and mechanically weak. Vascular studies[15] have shown it to be relatively avascular with a poor potential for healing. Biomechanically, the TFC bears 20% of the applied load when there is neutral ulnar variance. When there is positive ulnar variance, this load share increases dramatically. Although the triangular fibrocartilage complex is an important stabilizer of the distal radial ulnar joint, studies[14] have confirmed that the central two-thirds can be excised with no change in load bearing or stability. Age-related

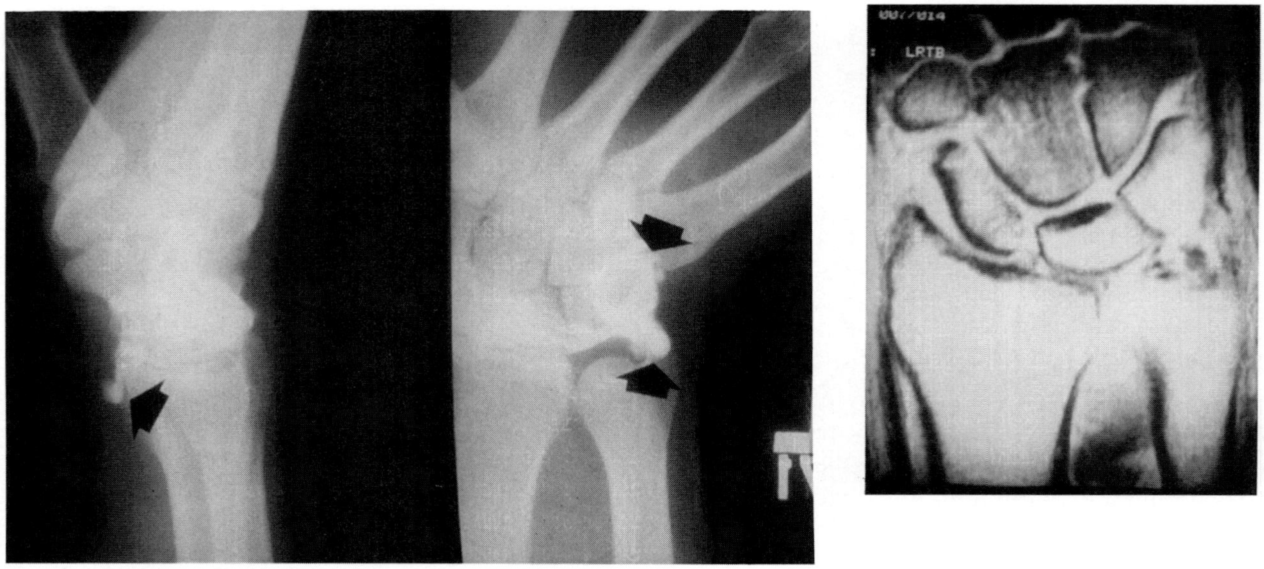

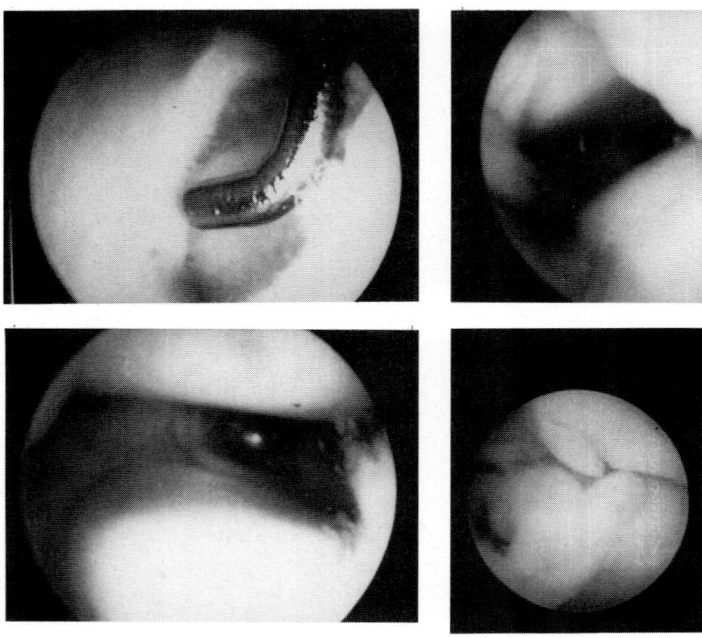

Fig. 5 **Top left,** Radiocarpal arthrogram, left wrist, initially read as normal. It does show pisotriquetral filling which can be a normal variant. **Top right,** Magnetic resonance imaging of the same wrist. Initial reading was increased fluid on the ulnar side of the wrist and a retrospective reading was consistent with edema in the ulnar extrinsic ligaments. **Center left,** Arthroscopic view of the radiocarpal view, left wrist, showing a defect in the ulnar extrinsic ligaments. Probe spans the defect and immediately below the probe is the pisotriquetral joint. **Center right,** On placing the arthroscope closer to the defect at the distal aspect of the tear superiorly and the dark area representing the piso-triquetral joint. **Bottom left,** Final arthroscopic view now looking directly into the piso-triquetral joint, pisiform occupying the lower portion of the picture, triquetrum in the superior portion of the photograph. **Bottom right,** Arthroscopic view of an osteochondral fracture of the ulnar portion of the lunate in this patient with an ulnar extrinsic defect.

perforations of the triangular fibrocartilage occur such that by the fourth or fifth decade more than 40% of wrists have a perforation.[16] Why some tears are symptomatic is controversial. The central portion of the articular disk is devoid of neural fibers. An unstable flap tear, however, may be symptomatic because of the synovitis it causes or because of the tethering effect of the flap on the innervated peripheral zone of the triangular fibrocartilage. Palmer[10] has classified triangular fibrocartilage tears as traumatic or degenerative. Traumatic tears are further subdivided by location: 1A. Central; 1B. Peripheral; 1C. Distal; 1D. Radial. Degenerative tears are frequently associated with positive ulnar variance.

The diagnosis of central tears of the triangular fibrocartilage is usually straightforward.[9] The patient presents with ulnar pain, often with a secondary extensor carpi ulnaris tendinitis. Ulnar deviation, rotation and axial load often create a painful click that reproduces the symptoms (the triangular fibrocartilage compression test). Grip strength is usually reduced by about 20%.

Neutral rotation plain films are helpful in determining ulnar variance. Arthrography is particularly reliable. Radiocarpal injection[17] is 95% accurate for a central tear. Injections of the distal radial ulnar joint are 100% accurate (Fig. 6, *left*). Magnetic resonance imaging[3] is approaching the accuracy of the radiocarpal arthrogram

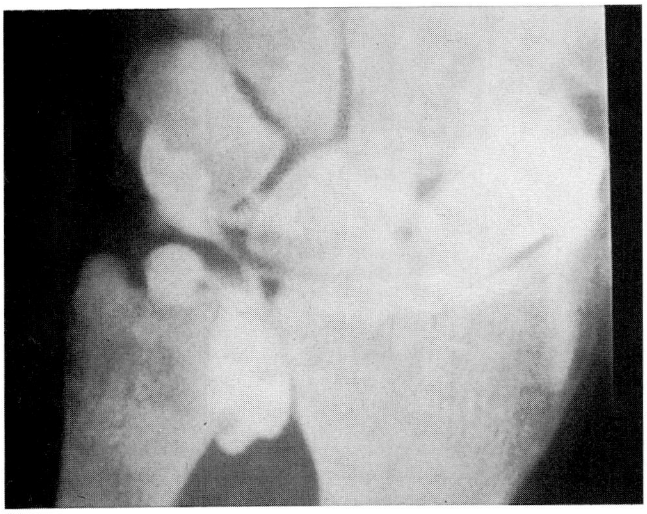

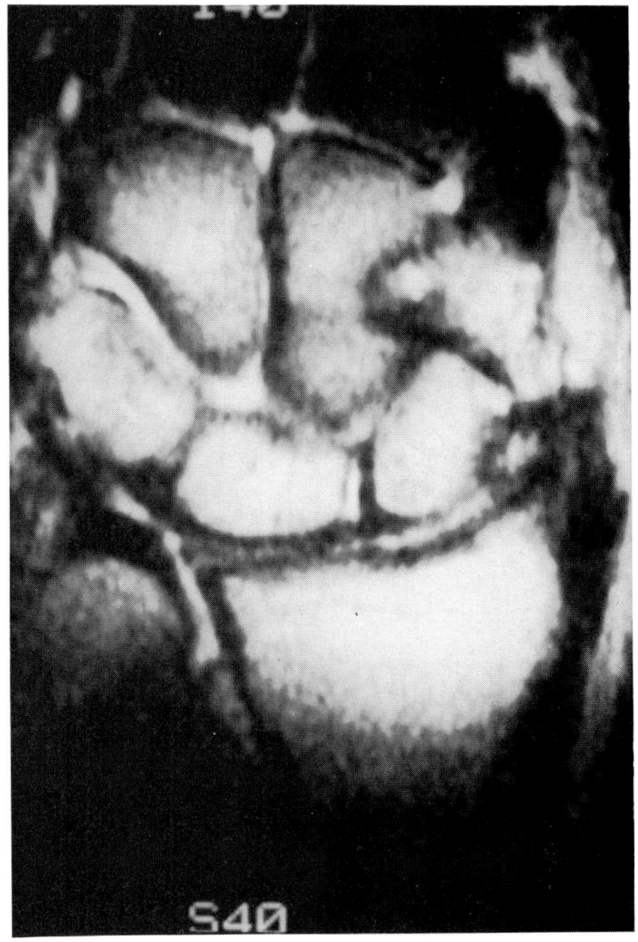

Fig. 6 **Left,** Radiocarpal arthrogram of the patient with a traumatic central triangular fibrocartilage tear. **Right,** Magnetic resonance image of the same person and demonstrating fluid crossing a defect in the triangular fibrocartilage.

(Fig. 6, *right*). Despite this, diagnostic arthroscopy remains the best way to evaluate the size, shape, and stability of the tear. It also allows the examiner to assess the joint reaction to the tear, ie, the amount of synovitis as well as the presence of any chondral or other associated lesions.

Treatment

Many injuries of the triangular fibrocartilage heal or become asymptomatic with time alone. We generally allow 4 months before considering an arthroscopic evaluation. Use of appropriate wrist splints, anti-inflammatories, localized cortisone injection and wrist exercises remain the stalwarts of initial care. If significant symptoms persist, then arthroscopic evaluation and debridement of the central tear are indicated.

Technique

Regional or general anesthetic is used. It is important to examine the anesthetized wrist and perform appropriate provocative maneuvers, in particular to examine the stability of the distal radial ulnar joint and to check for subluxation of the extensor ulnaris tendon. Standard arthroscopic distraction is used, and I favor the use of a wrist tower. The initial viewing portal is the 3-4, and the accessory portal is either the 4-5 or 6R. First, a probe is used to define a tear. A full-radius motorized shaver ranging from 2.0 mm to 3.5 mm is used to clear the synovitis. If an unstable central tear is noted, a banana blade knife is used to excise the unstable portion. A small suction punch is used to smooth and level the edges of the excision. To smooth the ulnar margins of the tear, the viewing portal is usually switched to the ulnar side and the suction punch or shaver brought in radially. After excision it is important to examine the distal ulna for any chondromalacia and to determine the integrity of the lunatotriquetral intrinsic ligament and the ulnar extrinsic ligaments by palpation. If positive ulnar variance, an unstable lunatotriquetral tear, or significant chondromalacia of the distal ulna are present, then simple triangular fibrocartilage debridement is inadequate treatment, and it must be supplemented by such techniques as wafer resection of the distal ulna, leveling procedures of the distal ulna, or stabilization of the lunatotriquetral interval. After completion of the radiocarpal joint examination and debridement, the

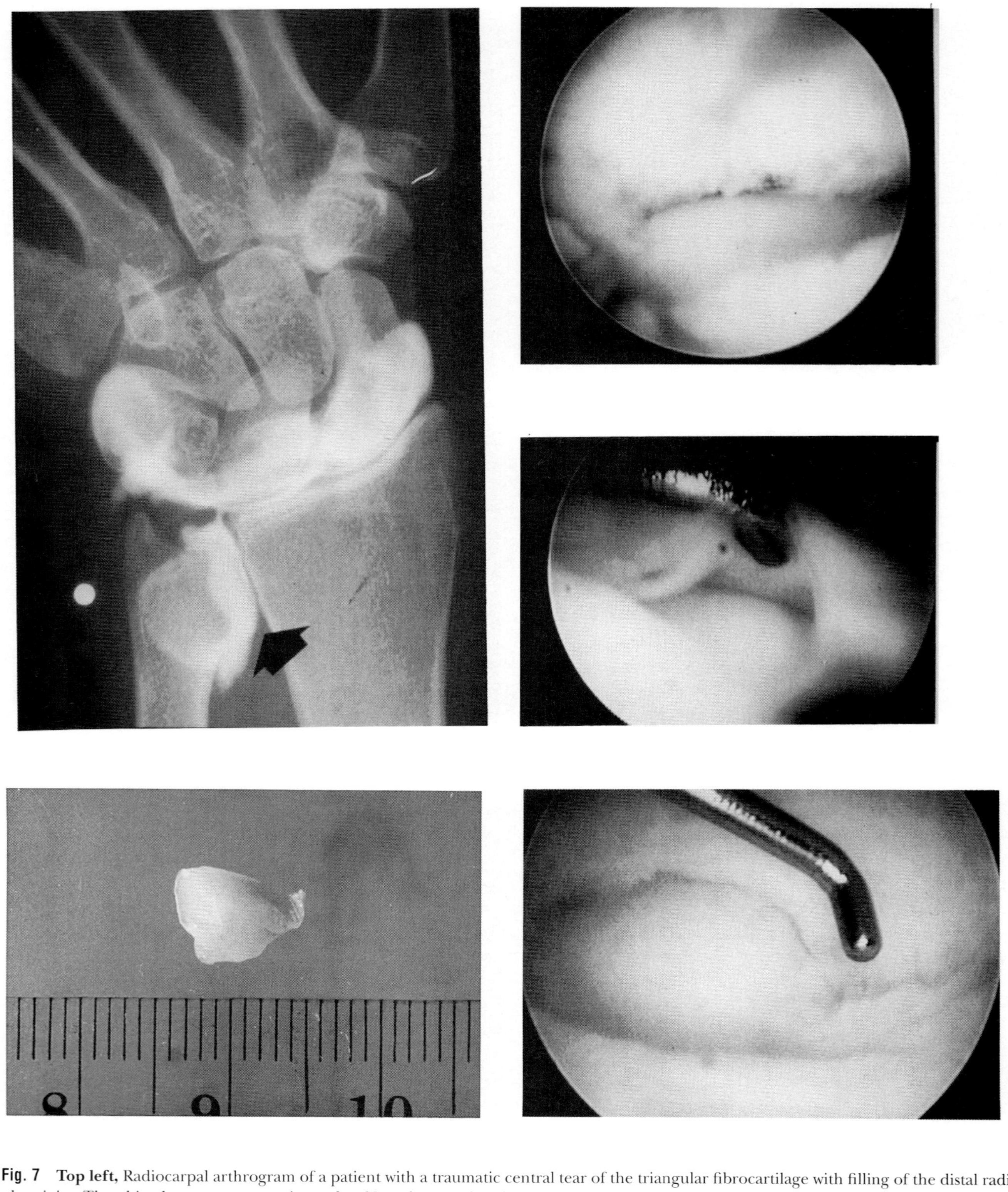

Fig. 7 **Top left,** Radiocarpal arthrogram of a patient with a traumatic central tear of the triangular fibrocartilage with filling of the distal radial ulnar joint. The white dot represents a pain marker. Note the negative ulnar variance. **Top right,** Radiocarpal arthroscopic view of the same patient showing a longitudinal tear of the triangular fibrocartilage. **Center right,** Another view of the triangular fibrocartilage now with the probe in place and revealing the unstable nature of the central tear. Note the normal cartilage surface of the underlying distal ulna. **Bottom left,** Excise unstable central portion of the triangular fibrocartilage. **Bottom right,** Arthroscopic view of the wrist after excision of the unstable central portion. Note the smooth edges of the retained triangular fibrocartilage and the intact peripheral portions.

midcarpal joint is examined. Postoperatively, a splint is used for 1 to 3 weeks for comfort, and graduated strengthening exercises are begun. The patient is allowed to resume vigorous activities at 6 to 8 weeks. There are several pitfalls which should be avoided. Excise only the unstable portion of the tear and be mindful of the volar peripheral attachments, especially the volar and dorsal radioulnar ligaments. The dorsal radioulnar ligament is especially vulnerable when blades or shavers are being passed through the dorsal ulnar portal. Also, avoid using the distal ulna as a cutting board for the triangular fibrocartilage resection.

Case 4

A 28-year-old right-hand dominant physician fell on his outstretched right hand in a football game and later noted ulnar wrist pain associated with a click and difficulty with rotatory activities. Physical examination showed maximum tenderness over the distal radioulnar joint and some tenderness over the extensor carpi ulnaris tendon, but it did not sublux. A triangular fibrocartilage stress test was positive and reproduced his symptoms. A radiocarpal arthrogram showed a tear of the triangular fibrocartilage (Fig. 7). Despite intermittent splinting and a transient response to a cortisone injection, his symptoms persisted.

At arthroscopy, an unstable flap tear of the triangular fibrocartilage was noted. Moderate localized ulnar synovitis of the wrist was present. The underlying cartilage of the distal radial ulnar joint was normal, as were the articular surfaces of the lunate and triquetrum. Extrinsic and intrinsic ligaments were normal. After removing the synovitis with a power shaver, a banana blade and suction punch were used to excise the unstable portion of the tear. The edges of the triangular fibrocartilage were then smoothed. Examination during the procedure confirmed full rotary motion without evidence of instability and elimination of the triangular fibrocartilage click. All portal sites were closed with a single suture and a splint was used for 1 week. At a follow-up of 6 years, the patient remains totally asymptomatic and is participating in all desired activities.

References

1. Taleisnik J: Pain on the ulnar side of the wrist. *Hand Clin* 1987; 3:51-68.
2. Manaster BJ, Mann RJ, Rubenstein S: Wrist pain: Correlation of clinical and plain film findings with arthrographic results. *J Hand Surg* 1989;14A:466-473.
3. Skahen JR III, Palmer AK, Levinsohn EM, et al: Magnetic resonance imaging of the triangular fibrocartilage complex. *J Hand Surg* 1990;15A:552-557.
4. Viegas SF, Wagner K, Patterson R, et al: Medial (hamate) facet of the lunate. *J Hand Surg* 1990;15A:564-571.
5. Berger RA, Kauer JMG, Landsmeer JMF: Radioscapholunate ligament: A gross anatomic and histologic study of fetal and adult wrists. *J Hand Surg* 1991;16A:350-355.
6. Mayfield JK: Wrist ligamentous anatomy and pathogenesis of carpal instability. *Orthop Clin North Am* 1984;15:209-216.
7. Taleisnik J: The ligaments of the wrist. *J Hand Surg* 1976;1:110-118.
8. Mooney JF, Poehling GG: Disruption of the ulnolunate ligament as a cause of chronic ulnar wrist pain. *J Hand Surg* 1991;16A:347-349.
9. Osterman AL: Arthroscopic debridement of triangular fibrocartilage complex tears. *Arthroscopy* 1990;6:120-124.
10. Palmer AK: Triangular fibrocartilage complex lesions: A classification. *J Hand Surg* 1989;14A:594-606.
11. Chidgey LK, Dell PC, Bittar ES, et al: Histologic anatomy of the triangular fibrocartilage *J Hand Surg* 1991;16A:1084-1100.
12. Kauer JMG: The articular disc of the hand. *Acta Anat* 1975;93:590-605.
13. Palmer AK, Werner FW: The triangular fibrocartilage complex of the wrist: Anatomy and function. *J Hand Surg* 1981;6:153-162.
14. Palmer AK, Werner FW, Glisson RR, et al: Partial excision of the triangular fibrocartilage complex. *J Hand Surg* 1988;13A:391-394.
15. Bednar MS, Arnoczky SP, Weiland AJ: The microvasculature of the triangular fibrocartilage complex: Its clinical significance. *J Hand Surg* 1991;16A:1101-1105.
16. Mikic ZD: Age changes in the triangular fibrocartilage of the wrist joint. *J Anat* 1978;126:367-384.
17. Roth JH, Haddad RG: Radiocarpal arthroscopy and arthrography in the diagnosis of ulnar wrist pain. *Arthroscopy* 1986;2:234-243.

CHAPTER 10

Wrist Arthroscopy

Terry L. Whipple, MD
William P. Cooney III, MD
A. Lee Osterman, MD
Steven F. Viegas, MD

Until 1986, wrist arthroscopy was a futile exercise of passing interest to a handful of investigators.[1] Early attempts, which afforded, at best, fleeting glimpses of articular surfaces in the wrist, were of no practical clinical value. In 1986, Whipple and associates reported the use of distraction techniques to provide adequate exposure in the radiocarpal and midcarpal spaces for manipulation of 1.9-mm to 2.7-mm arthroscopes, and described precisely located portals based on anatomic landmarks that would give access to nearly all intra-articular structures and surfaces.[2] The development of small 2- to 3-mm instruments designed specifically for use in the wrist followed shortly thereafter, and soon arthroscopic surgeons and hand surgeons began exploring the wrist visually with predictable clarity and magnification.

In eight short years, wrist arthroscopy has evolved into one of the most reliable and productive means of diagnosing, qualifying, and treating wrist pathology. Although it is a relatively new modality, it is an easily learned skill with ever-increasing indications. This chapter will attempt to define the indications as well as the techniques for diagnostic and operative wrist arthroscopy through the experience of surgeons who have helped to pioneer its applications. This brief review is not intended to be a comprehensive exposition on the subject, but rather should help to place the technique in perspective and within reach for surgeons who see and treat wrist pathology on a frequent basis. The basic tenets of surgical technique will be emphasized, followed by a survey of arthroscopic approaches to specific disorders of the wrist.

Indications

Of course, the most productive and least costly means of evaluating wrist problems are the taking of a thorough history and performance of a skilled physical examination. Even these measures require considerable knowledge of wrist anatomy, mechanics, and mechanisms of injury. The wrist is a complex joint, which provides combined movements in six directions to position the hand for a myriad of tasks. No diagnostic effort for the wrist can be undertaken casually.

Plain radiographs and fluoroscopic examination of the wrist will reveal most bone defects and bony relationships, but they cannot demonstrate soft-tissue lesions. Arthrograms and magnetic resonance images can provide indirect evidence of soft tissue defects in ligaments and tendons. Magnetic resonance imaging (MRI), however, may be too sensitive and not sufficiently specific to be of clinical value for diagnostic purposes. Neither arthrograms nor MRI are reliable means of evaluating synovium or articular cartilage defects.

Visual inspection and palpation are unparalleled means for examination of soft tissues and articular surfaces in the wrist; there is no better alternative. The texture of articular cartilage, the contours and tension of intrinsic and extrinsic ligaments, and the color of synovial villi can all be evaluated by arthroscopic examination, with no significant disruption of the joint capsule, supporting ligaments, retinaculum, blood vessels, or cutaneous nerves. Arthroscopy, therefore, provides the optimal means for internal examination of the soft tissues and articular surfaces of the wrist by minimally invasive techniques.

There are acute, subacute, and chronic wrist problems that may require arthroscopic evaluation. The most common chronic and subacute problems include ligament injuries and certain patterns of carpal instability, articular defects, osteoarthritis, and injuries to the triangular fibrocartilage complex (TFCC). Acute circumstances in which arthroscopic examination may be warranted usually involve injuries in which expedient or timely intervention would provide the best therapeutic results. Intra-articular fractures of the distal radius that cannot be perfectly reduced by closed manipulation are a classic example. Extra-articular distal radius fractures also are associated with a significant incidence of intra-articular soft-tissue injury, such as triangular fibrocartilage tears and intrinsic ligament disruption, and in younger individuals in whom the mechanism of injury is particularly violent, early arthroscopic evaluation might be considered. Scaphoid fractures that are reducible in individuals who cannot tolerate the prospect of long-term cast immobilization can be internally stabilized with arthroscopic assistance to avoid unnecessary division of important supporting ligaments. Likewise, acute injuries to the scapholunate or lunotriquetral ligaments, or to the major extrinsic capsular ligaments of the wrist, may warrant early arthroscopic evaluation to afford the most timely surgical repair. All of these situations will be discussed in the following sections of this chapter.

Surgical Technique

Successful wrist arthroscopy requires appropriate instrumentation and precise attention to recommended surgical technique. Random or forceful insertion of instruments into the joint may jeopardize cutaneous nerves, tendons, the radial artery, and fragile articular cartilage surfaces.

Adequate room for intra-articular instrumentation can only be provided by distracting the carpus; distension of the joint with crystalloid solution will not suffice. Soft nylon finger traps are the gentlest means of capturing the hand for the application of traction. Because these finger traps have a larger surface area than conventional wire finger traps, they distribute the applied forces more evenly on the skin of the fingers. Two finger traps, applied to the index and long fingers, are usually sufficient, but in rheumatoid patients or in circumstances in which the skin may be especially fragile or thin, three or four finger traps should be used, to allow greater distribution of the force.

A TractionTower® (Linvatec, Inc., Largo, Florida), developed for use with the nylon finger traps, provides a convenient and effective means for applying measurable degrees of wrist distraction (Fig. 1). The tower, which can be sterilized, enables the surgeon to position the wrist in varying degrees of flexion, extension, and radial or ulnar deviation as may be necessary during the course of the arthroscopic procedure. This device also maintains the wrist and forearm in a stable position, so that portals are preserved for the exchange of instruments with minimal trauma or struggle.

Installation of a clear, physiologic, crystalloid solution into the joint affords the clearest visibility while protecting the articular tissues from dehydration and desiccation. We prefer to use lactated Ringer's solution, but other solutions are available. Crystalloid irrigant can be introduced through the sheath of the arthroscope with the assistance of a mechanical fluid pump. Pressurized injection increases the risk of fluid extravasation into the subcutaneous tissue, however, and as pressurized distension is unnecessary for surgical exposure, gravity-assisted irrigation has proven adequate without major fluid extravasation in the vast majority of cases. We prefer to use a small atraumatic plastic cannula for joint insufflation (Fig. 2, *left*). The cannula has a small collar, which holds it securely in the joint, and a flexible tip that will not scuff the articular surface as metal cannulas do. This cannula is provided with an irrigation line that contains a small pinch chamber that is used to introduce small boluses of crystalloid when slightly greater pressure is required to clear the visual field of particulate matter or blood (Fig. 2, *right*). Usually elevation of the crystalloid source approximately 1 m above the level of the wrist provides adequate gravity-assisted inflow pressure.

A large variety of small-diameter powered or hand-operated instruments have been designed for feeling, cutting, and grasping tissues in the wrist during arthroscopic procedures (Fig. 3). The ample selection available allows surgeons to choose preferred configurations. Instruments should not exceed 3 mm in diameter, and they should be examined to assure that their surfaces are smooth and pose no risk of inadvertent injury to articular cartilage. Smoother instrument designs are also easier to insert through the subcutaneous tissue and joint capsule. Experienced manufacturers can make these instruments strong, durable, and dependable for years of repeated use.

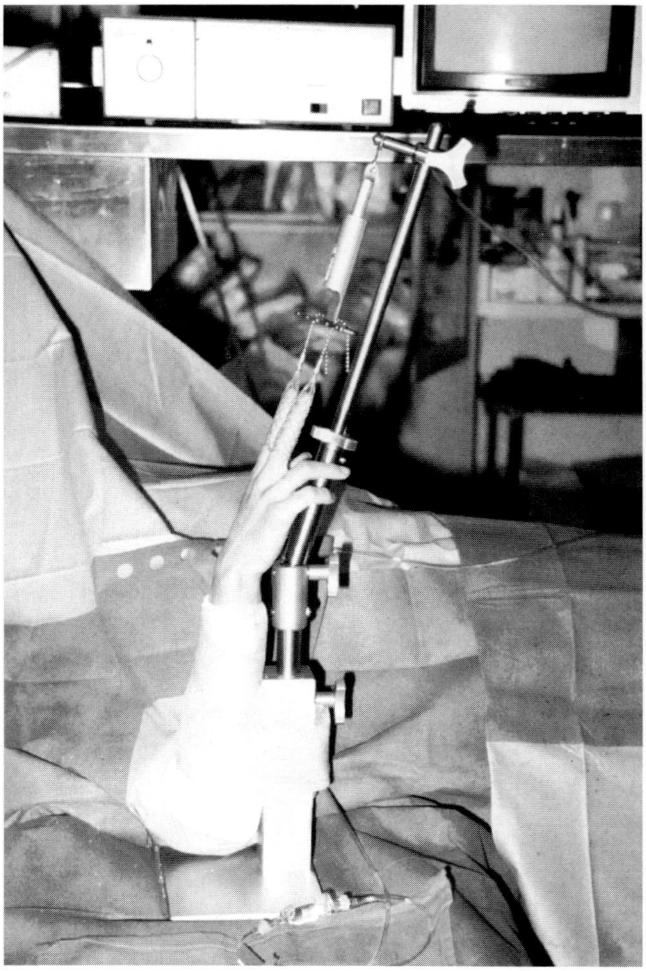

Fig. 1 Wrist distraction is provided through nylon finger traps by means of a TractionTower® (Linvatec, Inc., Largo, FL). With this Tower, the wrist can be positioned in flexion or extension, radial or ulnar deviation, and the extremity remains stable throughout the procedure.

Surgical Landmarks

The location of optimal arthroscopy portals in the wrist depends on accurate identification of certain anatomic landmarks. It is recommended that these landmarks be accurately drawn on the skin in each case. Without this topographical mapping, injury to tendons, articular surfaces, cutaneous nerves, or the radial artery is more likely. After application of 10 to 12 pounds of finger-trap traction, the bony contours of the distal

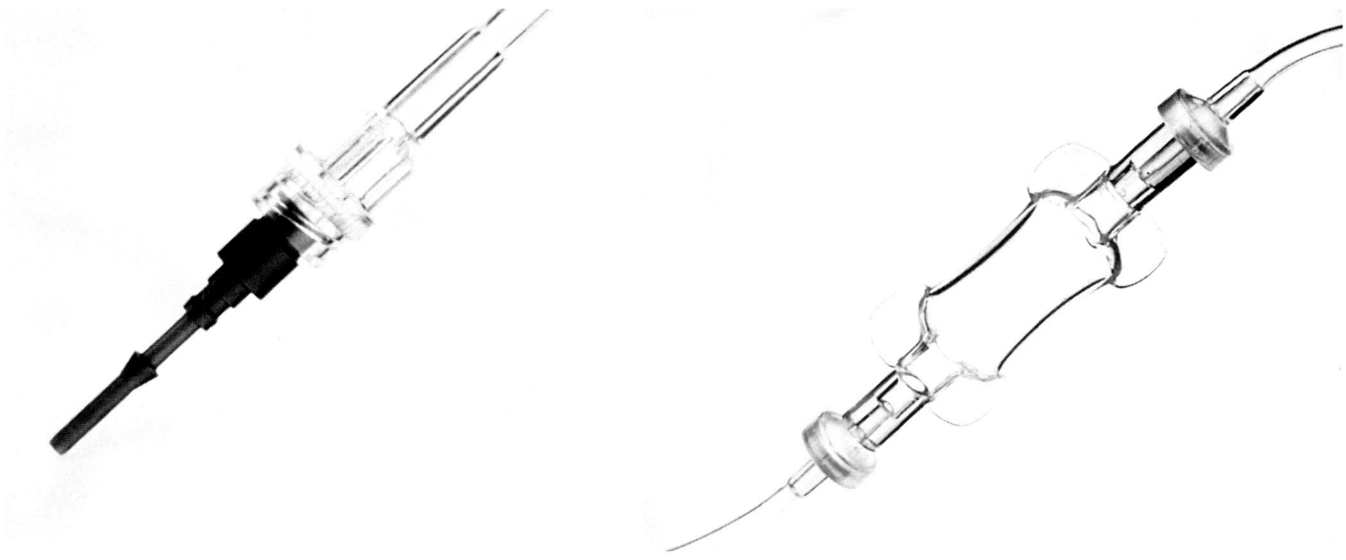

Fig. 2 Irrigation system for small joint arthroscopy (Linvatec, Inc., Largo, FL). **Left,** An atraumatic plastic cannula has a shoulder to maintain its position in the joint, and a Luer lock attachment to the inflow line. **Right,** A 3-cc pinch chamber equipped with one-way flow valves provides inflow assistance to supplement gravity pressure when needed.

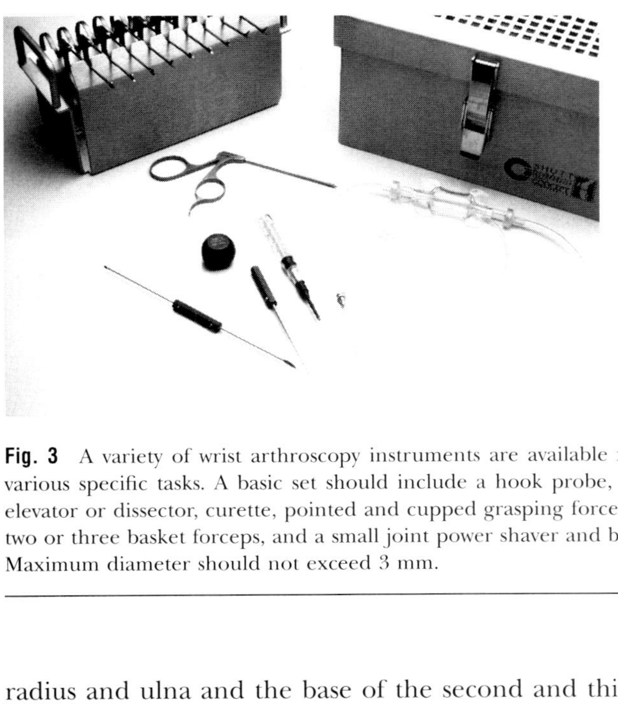

Fig. 3 A variety of wrist arthroscopy instruments are available for various specific tasks. A basic set should include a hook probe, an elevator or dissector, curette, pointed and cupped grasping forceps, two or three basket forceps, and a small joint power shaver and bur. Maximum diameter should not exceed 3 mm.

radius and ulna and the base of the second and third metacarpals can be identified and marked. Similarly, the course of the extensor pollicis longus (EPL) tendon around Lister's tubercle can be identified and drawn, along with the outline of the extensor digitorum communis (EDC) tendon to the index and little fingers. The extensor carpi ulnaris (ECU), and the extensor carpi radialis longus and brevis tendons are easily palpated and should be drawn as well. It is the intersection of these tendons with the bony margins that allows accurate identification and placement of optimal arthroscopy portals. The surgeon will soon appreciate the importance of convenient portal placement to facilitate arthroscopic instrumentation of the wrist with ease and finesse (Fig. 4).

The primary portal for examination of the radiocarpal space is located between the third and fourth extensor compartments just distal to the dorsal margin of the radius (3-4). The inflow cannula is usually placed just ulnar to the ECU tendon, paralleling the proximal slope of the triquetrum (6-U). Here the cannula enters the ulnar side of the joint directly through the prestyloid recess, a normal anatomic aperture in the ulnar wrist capsule. In cases of suspected extensive ulnar pathology, an alternative placement for the inflow cannula on the radial side of the wrist is between the first and second extensor compartments immediately adjacent to the intersection of the extensor carpi radialis longus (ECRL) and the extensor policis longus tendons (1-2). It is important that this portal be established in the dorsal aspect of the anatomic snuffbox to avoid the radial artery, which courses through the volar aspect of the interval between the first and second extensor compartments.

Accessory portals for instrumentation of the radiocarpal space lie between the fourth and fifth extensor compartments (4-5) and just radial to the ECU (6-R). These accessory portals on the dorsal ulnar aspect of the wrist are in close proximity to one another. The 6-R portal is identified as such because palpation of the extensor digiti quinti (EDQ) in the fifth compartment is rarely possible.

Like other instruments for the wrist, the outside diameter of the arthroscope sheath should not exceed 3 mm. Arthroscopes are available in 1.9 mm and 2.7

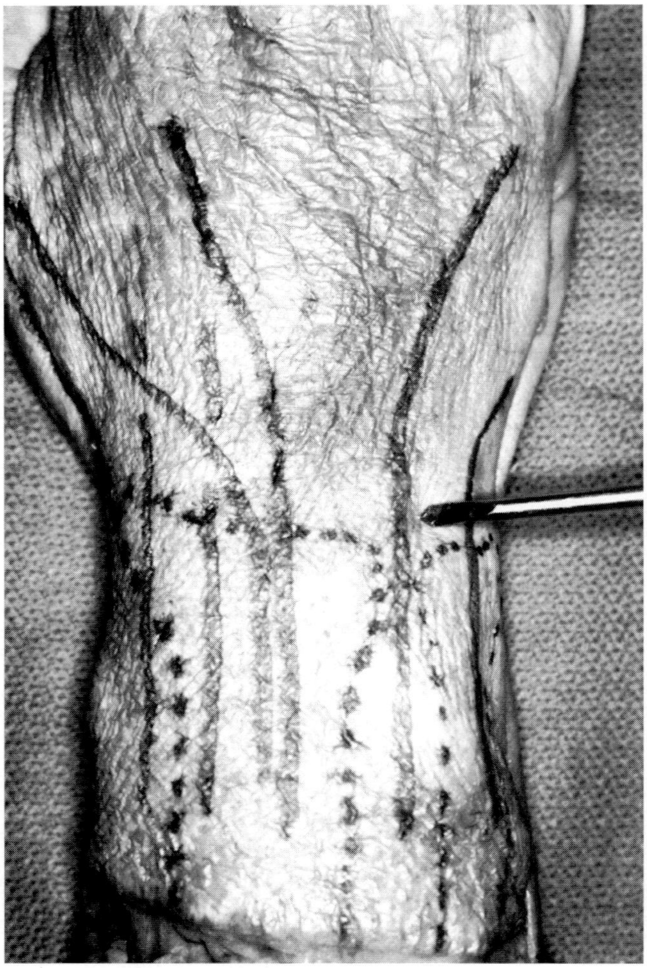

Fig. 4 Right wrist demonstrating topographic landmarks, including outlines of the radius, ulna, and the tendons of the extensor compartments. The pointer indicates the location of the 4-5 portal.

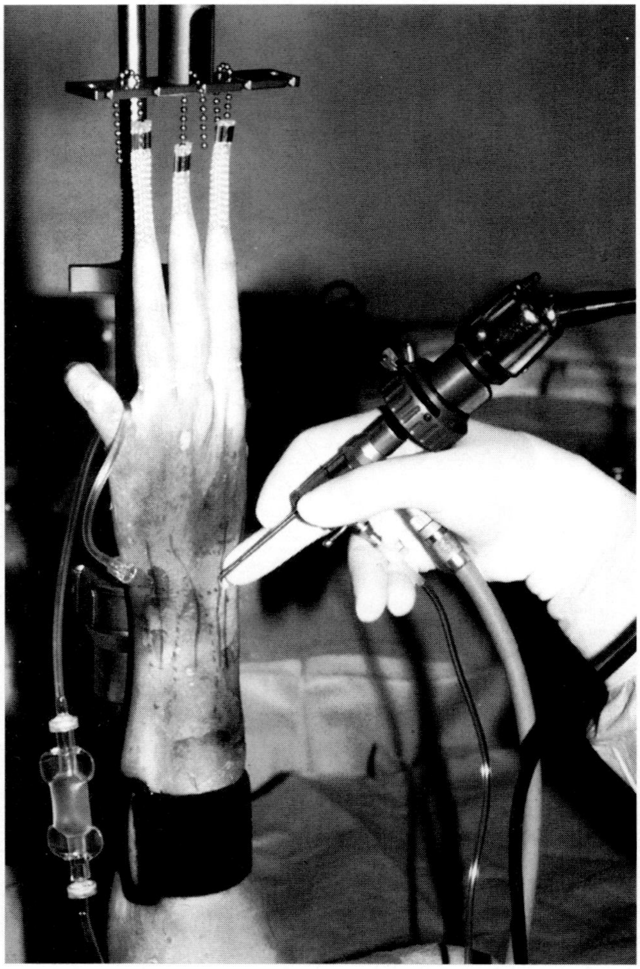

Fig. 5 With the wrist distracted and stable, the arthroscope and camera are cradled in the surgeon's thumb web space. The surgeon's long finger touches the dorsum of the wrist to assist with depth control of the arthroscope. The inflow cannula is placed in the 6-U portal with the inflow line draped over the surgeon's little finger.

mm diameters from most manufacturers. The 2.7-mm arthroscope is stiffer of course, and therefore it is more durable than the 1.9 mm. The 1.9-mm arthroscope may be preferred, however, for the wrists of children or other individuals with small wrists.

Introduction of the arthroscope through the 3-4 portal affords visual access to most of the radiocarpal interval. By cradling the scope and camera in the surgeon's thumb web space, one finger can be extended to touch the dorsum of the patient's wrist, which will allow the surgeon to piston the arthroscope in and out of the joint more easily and with less fatigue (Fig. 5).

The first visual field encountered through the 3-4 portal will be the sagittal ridge of the distal radius articular surface that divides the scaphoid facet from the lunate facet (Fig. 6). Distally, the proximal articular surface of the lunate or the concave horizon of the scapholunate ligament will be seen. By sweeping the arthroscope radially and ulnarward, the examiner will see the proximal articular surface of the scaphoid, the radial joint capsule, and the radial styloid to the radial side; and the triangular fibrocartilage articular disk and the prestyloid recess to the ulnar side. With deeper insertion of the arthroscope, the volar radiocarpal ligaments can be identified and examined.

In most wrists, especially in smaller patients, the arthroscope should be transferred to the 6-R or the 4-5 portal for optimal visual examination of the lunotriquetral ligament, the proximal articular surface of the triquetrum, and the ulnocarpal ligaments (Fig. 7). The advantage of introducing a hook probe to palpate intra-articular structures and surfaces cannot be overstated. With the arthroscope in the 3-4 portal, the 4-5 portal is the most useful placement of the probe. Conversely, when the arthroscope is introduced through the 4-5 or 6-R portals, the probe should be placed in the 3-4 position.

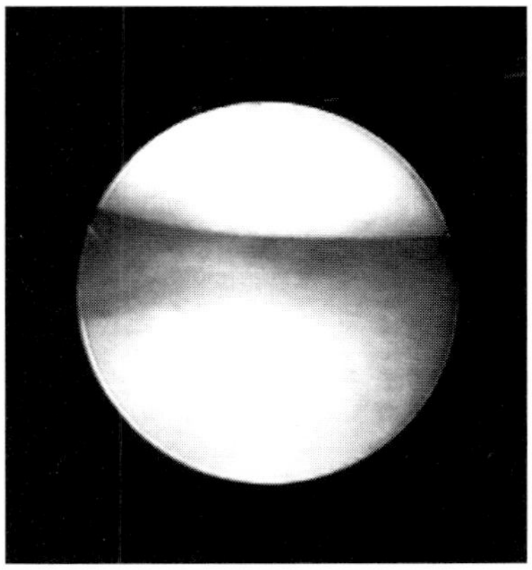

Fig. 6 Arthroscopic view of the right wrist from the 3-4 portal showing articular surface of lunate above, sagittal ridge and lunate facet of the radius below.

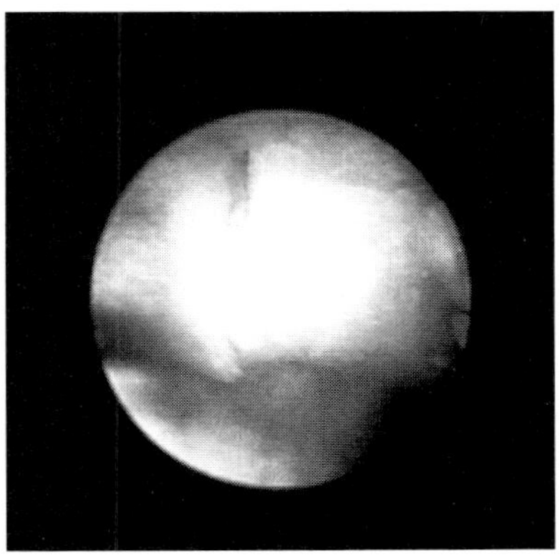

Fig. 7 Arthroscopic view of the right wrist from the 4-5 portal showing a tear in the lunotriquetral ligament above, and the small articular surface of the triquetrum to the right.

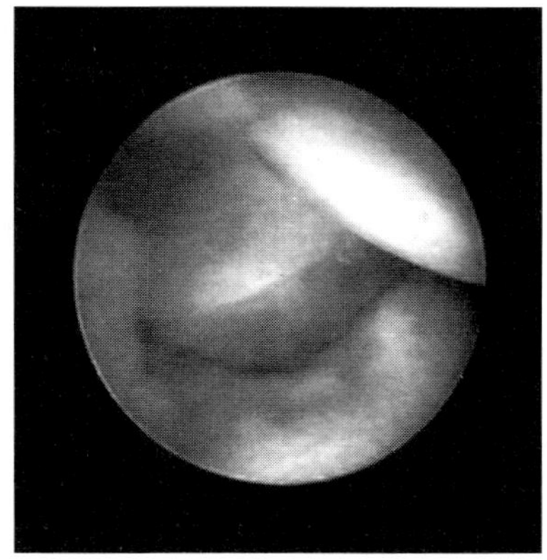

Fig. 8 Arthroscopic view of a bulging dorsal ganglion of the dorsal capsule of the right wrist radiocarpal space, seen from the 6-R portal. The dorsal proximal edge of the lunate is seen above the ganglion and a concave defect in the dorsal margin of the radius is below the ganglion.

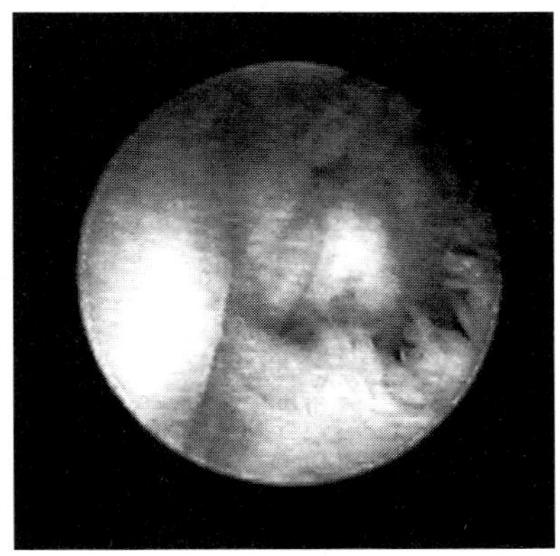

Fig. 9 Arthroscopic view of an opening in the ulnar joint capsule (normal variant) of a right wrist seen from the 6-R portal. This aperture exposes the pisiform on the right articulating with the triquetrum on the left.

Special circumstances may require placement of instruments in the 1-2 portal or 6-R portal. For example, visualization of dorsal ganglia will be gained best by placing the arthroscope in the 6-R or the 1-2 portal (Fig. 8). Frequently, from the 6-R or 4-5 portals, the examiner will identify a second aperture in the ulnar wrist capsule located slightly volar and distal to the prestyloid recess. This aperture exposes the articulation of the pisiform with the triquetrum. In some cases, the pisotriquetral articulation is surrounded by a separate synovial compartment from the radiocarpal space, and this second aperture will not be present. When present, this aperture represents a normal variant, which affords the examiner an opportunity to look for synovial hypertrophy or marginal articular degeneration in the pisotriquetral joint (Fig. 9).

The midcarpal space, which can also be examined arthroscopically, will frequently reveal gross or subtle signs of pathologic change. The primary portal for introduction of the arthroscope in the midcarpal space lies on a line extended proximally from the radial margin of the third metacarpal midway between the base of the metacarpal and the dorsal margin of the radius. A soft spot can be palpated here. Only the skin should be lanced because, in some patients, the extensor digitorum communis to the index finger crosses this portal. When the EDC overlies the ideal radial-midcarpal (RMC) portal, the portal should be placed just radial to the tendon.

In the radial-midcarpal portal, the arthroscope enters between the capitate and the concave surface of the scaphoid. The examiner can sweep the arthroscope radially and distally to visualize the scaphotrapezium-trapezoid (STT) joint or ulnarward to visualize the interval between the scaphoid and lunate (Fig. 10) and

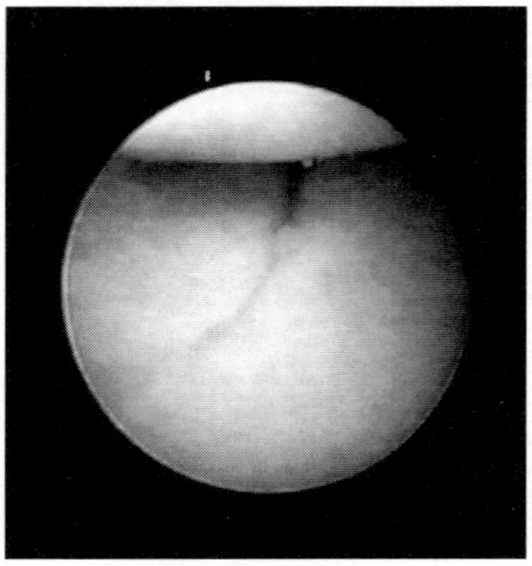

Fig. 10 Arthroscopic view of the midcarpal space, right wrist, from the radial-midcarpal portal (RMC) showing the scapholunate interval below and the head of capitate above.

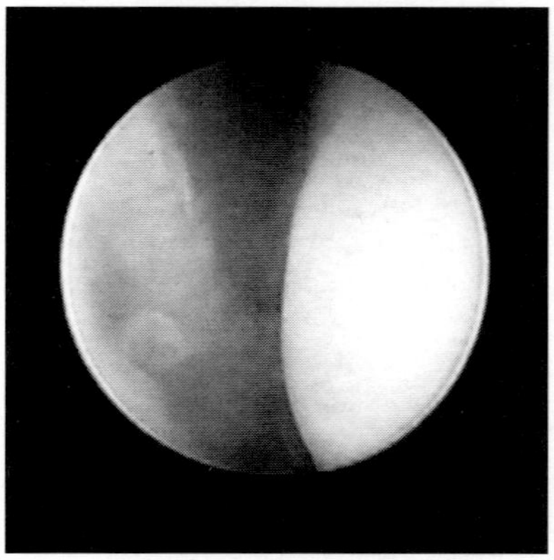

Fig. 11 Arthroscopic view of the right wrist from the proximal distal radioulnar joint (P-DRUJ) portal showing the dorsal edge of the sigmoid notch of the radius to the left and the radial side of the head of the ulna on the right.

the four-corner intersection of the lunate, triquetrum, hamate, and capitate.

An accessory portal for the midcarpal space used primarily for instrumentation, but occasionally for introduction of the arthroscope, is on the ulnar side of the joint. The ulnar-midcarpal (UMC) portal is located on a line extended proximally from the midline of the fourth metacarpal midway between the proximal pole of the triquetrum and the base of the fourth metacarpal with the wrist in neutral position. An additional accessory portal for the STT joint (STT portal) is located just ulnar to the extensor pollicis longus tendon over the STT joint. Placing this portal ulnar to the EPL tendon provides ample protection for the radial artery as it courses toward the first and second metacarpal interval.

Finally, the distal radioulnar joint (DRUJ) can be examined arthroscopically. Occasionally, loose bodies are found in the DRUJ, but more commonly, the concern is for subtle articular changes on the sigmoid notch or the head of the ulna. DRUJ arthrosis shows radiographic changes in advanced stages. When the triangular fibrocartilage complex is intact and the DRUJ is stable to clinical evaluation, early arthritic changes in this joint can only be identified arthroscopically.

The most useful portal for examination of the distal radioulnar joint overlies the axilla of the DRUJ capsule. The forearm should be rotated into supination to relax the dorsal capsule of the distal radioulnar joint. The arthroscope is inserted just proximal to the most prominent radial contour of the head of the ulna. Through this proximal distal radioulnar joint (P-DRUJ) portal one can examine the synovial membrane of the joint proximally, and visualize the articular surface of the sigmoid notch of the radius distally. Through pronation and supination, the articular margin of the ulna can be paraded in front of the arthroscope lens (Fig. 11).

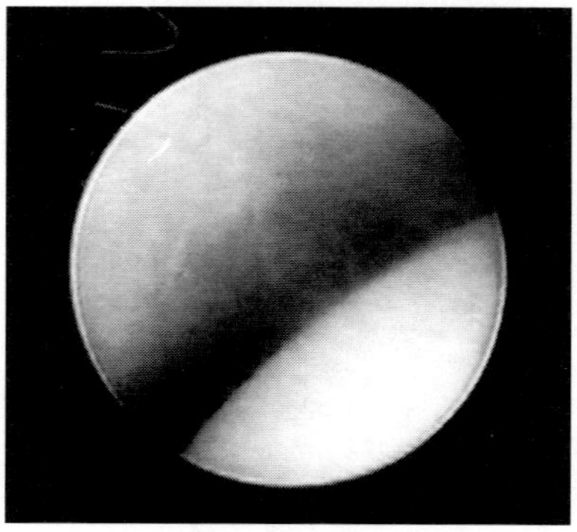

Fig. 12 Arthroscopic view of the right wrist from the proximal distal radioulnar joint (P-DRUJ) portal showing the juncture of the proximal surface of the TFC disk above with the sigmoid notch of the radius on the left. The contour of the seat of the ulna head is seen bottom right.

Except in cases of positive ulnar variance, the arthroscope can be swept gently in a distal direction to visualize the attachment of the triangular fibrocartilage (TFC) to the sigmoid notch of the radius, and to examine the distal articular surface of the seat of the ulna (Fig. 12). Significant pathology is rarely appreciated in this location, because the TFCC is best visualized from the radiocarpal space. However, traumatic partial thickness tears of the triangular fibrocartilage central articular disk have been found in the distal radioulnar joint when the distal surface of the TFC appeared normal.

It should be reemphasized at this point that rigid adherence to surgical technique, precise identification of anatomic landmarks and portal placement, and gentleness in the introduction and exchange of instruments into the wrist are extremely important measures to assure successful and productive arthroscopic examination of the wrist joint.

References

1. Whipple TL (ed): *Arthroscopic Surgery: The Wrist.* Philadelphia, PA, JB Lippincott, 1992.

2. Whipple TL, Marotta JJ, Powell JH III: Techniques of wrist arthroscopy. *Arthroscopy* 1986;2:244-252.

CHAPTER 11

Assessment and Treatment of Common Sites and Causes of Arthrosis in the Wrist

Steven F. Viegas, MD

Direct visualization is the best means to assess the location, pattern, and extent of arthrosis within a joint. Arthroscopy affords us the opportunity to do exactly that in the proximal and midcarpal wrist joints. In fact, it allows better visualization, less invasively, of a greater amount of the joint surface than is possible using the standard open surgical approaches.

The most common location of chondromalacia and/or arthrosis is at the proximal pole of the hamate. This not only has been seen arthroscopically, but it has also been documented in cadaver dissections, in which 28% of 393 cadaver wrists were found to have some degree of exposed subchondral bone at the proximal pole of the hamate (Fig. 1). There was a strong correlation between the presence of arthrosis or chondromalacia at the proximal pole of the hamate and Type II lunate morphology, in which there is a medially located hamate facet on the distal surface of the lunate.[1] The specific type of lunate morphology cannot be reliably identified radiographically and, therefore, pain or tenderness in the location of the ulnar midcarpal joint is a criteria for arthroscopic assessment of the midcarpal joint. However, despite the high incidence of arthrosis and/or chondromalacia at the proximal pole of the hamate, for the most part, this seems to be a relatively silent lesion. In those cases where it is symptomatic, arthroscopic assessment and debridement of the proximal pole of the hamate appears to hold some promise.

In assessing ligament instabilities, such as scapholunate dissociation, treatment planning requires accurate assessment of the articular surfaces both at the proximal and midcarpal joints. Radiographs alone are not adequate to fully assess the condition of the joint surfaces (Fig. 2). In conditions of dorsal intercalary segment instability (DISI) with scapholunate dissociation, degenerative changes will first occur at the articulation between the radial styloid and the scaphoid. If all other surfaces are in reasonable condition, one treatment approach can be to perform an arthroscopic

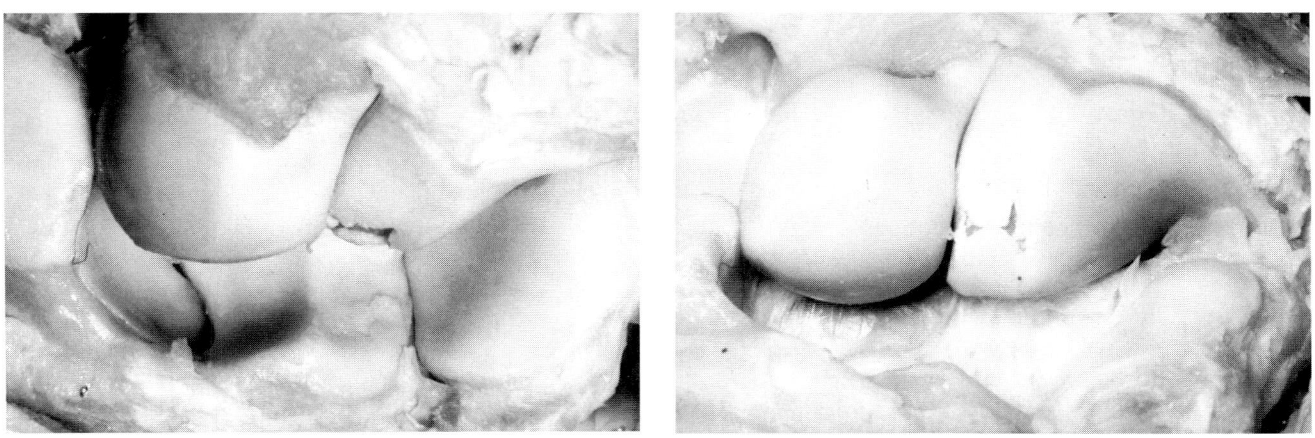

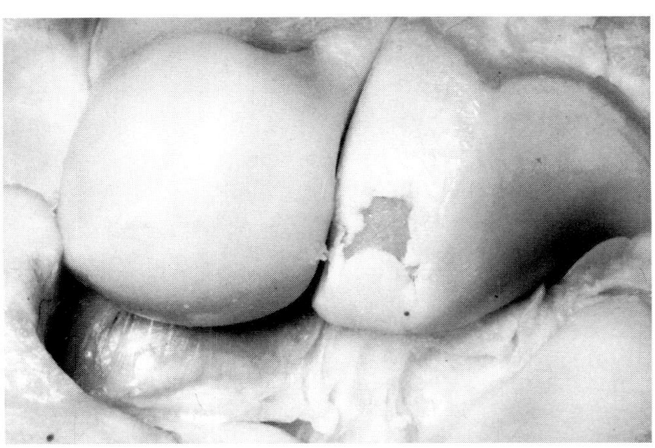

Fig. 1 **Top left,** A photograph of a cadaver dissection of the midcarpal joint of the right wrist in a 71-year-old male demonstrating Type II carpal morphology with a hamate facet with some mild chondromalacia on the lunate and a chondral defect at the proximal pole of the hamate. **Top right,** A photograph of the same dissection viewing the proximal poles of the capitate and hamate with a loose chondral fragment lying in the defect at the proximal pole of the hamate. **Bottom,** A view of the exposed subchondral bone following removal of the loose chondral fragment.

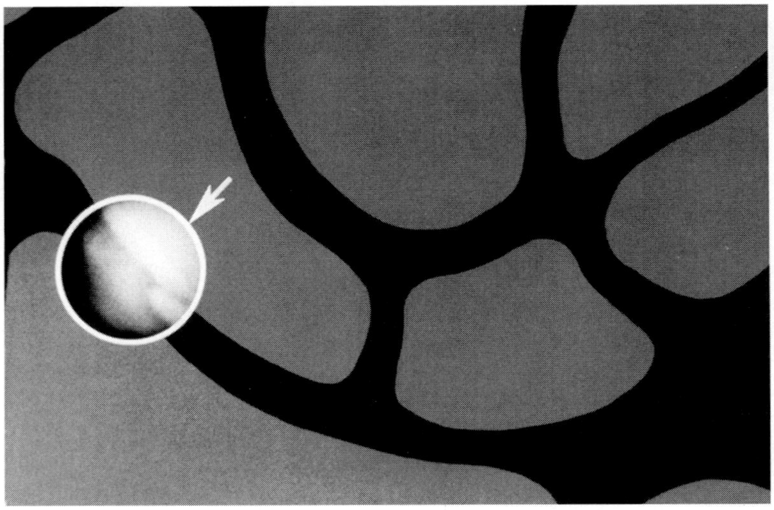

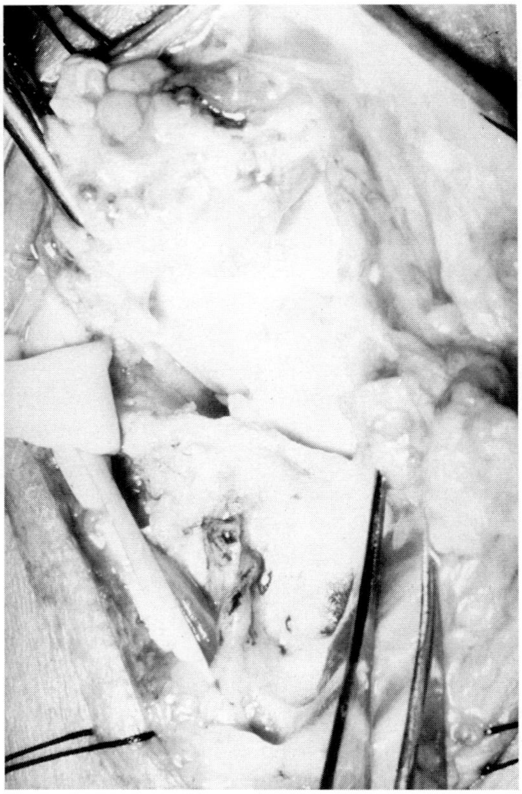

Fig. 2 **Left,** An arthroscopic view of the radial styloid scaphoid joint superimposed on a diagram of the wrist, demonstrating the exposed subchondral bone of the radial styloid and scaphoid with a chondral flap on the scaphoid. **Right,** An exposure of the dorsal radial aspect of the same wrist, again demonstrating the exposed subchondral bone of the scaphoid and radius at the radial styloid scaphoid articulation. (Reproduced with permission from Viegas SF: Lesiones sinoviales y condrales, in *Principios de Artroscopia y Cirurgia Artroscopia.* Iberica, Spain, Springer-Verlag, 1993, pp 324-330.)

radial styloidectomy. Although the underlying instability and cause of the arthrosis has not been addressed, this may offer some improvement and/or temporize an otherwise painful and difficult treatment dilemma. If arthroscopy shows that the changes are more extensive and involve the entire radioscaphoid articulation without changes at the capitolunate joint, one could consider either proximal row carpectomy or open surgical excision of the scaphoid with lunate-triquetrum-capitate-hamate fusion. If arthroscopic examination reveals not only complete involvement of the radioscaphoid articulation but also of the capitolunate joint, it is my opinion that a proximal row carpectomy is not advisable and, alternatively, either an open scaphoid excision with lunate-triquetrum-capitate-hamate fusion or wrist arthrodesis are the remaining surgical treatment options.

Scaphoid nonunion is another wrist lesion that continues to be problematic in its treatment. This problem is particularly substantial if there is associated DISI collapse, radiocarpal degenerative changes, and poor scaphoid bone quality. Studies on the natural history of scaphoid nonunion have detailed the progressive collapse and carpal arthrosis that can develop in chronic, untreated nonunions. Biomechanical studies in simulated scaphoid fractures have demonstrated the transfer of load to the articulation between the distal scaphoid fragment and radial styloid.[2] Mack and associates,[3] Ruby and associates,[4] and Vender and associates[5] all observed that degenerative changes develop in the articulation between the distal scaphoid fragment and the radius, and that the articulations between the proximal scaphoid fragment and the radius and between the radius and the lunate are spared from degenerative changes. Within the first decade from the original scaphoid fracture, they commonly found changes in the quality of bone, including cystic lesions at the site of the scaphoid nonunion. During the second decade, radioscaphoid degenerative changes were evident, followed in the third decade by progressive pain and carpal arthritis.

Arthroscopy affords a means to accurately determine the extent of articular changes when there is some question left by radiographs, CT, or MR studies. In the case of a scaphoid nonunion, wherever feasible, if a reasonable chance of obtaining union and restoring the normal anatomy of the scaphoid is present, this should be the line of treatment. However, despite the spectrum of treatments described for scaphoid nonunion, a number of cases remain resistant to treatment of the nonunion and require a salvage or reconstructive approach. Alternatively, a number of patients delay seeking medical evaluation until carpal deformity and degenerative changes related to the scaphoid nonunion are already evident.

If a scaphoid nonunion exists and the articular surface is in good condition, then certainly bone grafting, with or without fixation to restore the normal scaphoid morphology, is the treatment of choice. My preference in this situation is open reduction, iliac crest bone grafting, and fixation with a Herbert screw. In those individuals who have developed some limited arthrosis between the radial styloid and the distal scaphoid, fixation and bone grafting of the scaphoid, with the addition of a limited radial styloidectomy, is a reasonable option. Alternatively, radial styloid impingement, either from an old scaphoid fracture or degenerative changes, also may be a good candidate for a limited arthroscopic radial styloidectomy. In cases in which degenerative changes have occurred not only in the articulation between the radial styloid and distal scaphoid fragment, but also in the articulation between the proximal scaphoid and the proximal radial aspect of the capitate, excision of the distal portion of the scaphoid and incorporation of the proximal scaphoid into a limited arthrodesis, including the proximal scaphoid, lunate, and capitate, has been shown to be a good treatment option if the quality of the bone in the proximal pole of the scaphoid is reasonably good. An alternative treatment approach could be a scaphocapitate fusion. In this procedure, the proximal and distal poles of the scaphoid are reduced and are aligned with the capitate. Scaphocapitate fusion is combined with a limited radial styloidectomy, where necessary. If the quality of the bone in the proximal pole of the scaphoid is not good, excision of the proximal and distal poles of the scaphoid and an arthrodesis that incorporates the capitate, hamate, lunate, and triquetrum is an alternative. Other alternatives at this stage are a proximal row carpectomy, if the proximal pole of the capitate has a good cartilage surface, or, alternatively, a wrist fusion.

A reasonable and logical approach to these difficult problems is helpful. Arthroscopy can often add important information that will assist in the decision-making process.

References

1. Viegas SF, Patterson RM, Hokanson JA, et al: Wrist anatomy: Incidence, distribution, and correlation of anatomic variations, tears, and arthrosis. *J Hand Surg* 1993;18A:463-475.
2. Viegas SF, Patterson RM, Hillman GR, et al: Simulated scaphoid proximal pole fracture. *J Hand Surg* 1991;16A:495-500.
3. Mack GR, Bosse MJ, Gelberman RH, et al: The natural history of scaphoid non-union. *J Bone Joint Surg* 1984;66A:504-509.
4. Ruby LK, Stinson J, Belsky MR: The natural history of scaphoid non-union: A review of fifty-five cases. *J Bone Joint Surg* 1985; 67A:428-432.
5. Vender MI, Watson HK, Wiener BD, et al: Degenerative change in symptomatic scaphoid non-union. *J Hand Surg* 1987;12A:514-519.

CHAPTER 12

Arthroscopic Assessment of Carpal Instabilities and Ligament Injuries

Steven F. Viegas, MD

Introduction

In 1943, Gilford, Bolton, and Lambrinudi were the first to refer to carpal instability.[1] Linscheid and associates,[2] in 1972, and Dobyns and associates,[3] in 1975, collaborated and published articles on the topic of traumatic instability of the wrist. Their classification, based primarily on the capitolunate angle in the lateral radiograph, provided a way to group and identify different categories of carpal instabilities. These included dorsiflexion instability, palmar flexion instability, ulnar translocation, and dorsal subluxation. These papers originated the terms dorsal intercalated segment instability (DISI), volar intercalated segment instability (VISI), ulnar translocation, and dorsal subluxation. It is arguably this body of work that launched the ever-increasing number of presentations and publications on carpal instabilities.

In 1980, Taleisnik[4] suggested that the classification system be expanded to include static and dynamic forms of instability. More recently, Dobyns and associates,[5] in 1987, and Cooney and associates,[6] in 1990, had proposed to further expand and adapt their classification to include the terms carpal instability dissociative, or CID, and carpal instability nondissociative, or CIND, lesions. This classification, which is based on whether or not there is a disruption within or between the carpal bones of the proximal and/or distal row, complements their earlier approach, which dealt only with the capitate, lunate, and radius alignment.

Dorsal Intercalated Segment Instability

DISI deformity is certainly the most commonly recognized and, presumably, the most commonly occurring of the carpal instability patterns. It occurs when there is disruption of the scapholunate interosseous ligament complex.

Cadaveric dissections help elucidate the incidence of tears of the wrist ligament complex and help characterize the anatomy. In previous dissections on 393 wrists, the scapholunate interosseous ligament was disrupted 28% of the time. Moreover, in those specimens in which both wrists could be dissected, the scapholunate interosseous ligament in the contralateral wrist was also found to be disrupted 66% of the time.[7] Berger and associates[8] recently delineated differences in the dorsal portion of the scapholunate interosseous ligament. They found these differences to be histologically and mechanically the most substantial, followed by those in the volar portion. The least substantial and more membranous portion was that of the proximal aspect of the scapholunate interosseous ligament. It is, therefore, quite possible that there can be a disruption in this proximal membranous portion of the scapholunate interosseous ligament that would result in a positive arthrogram and may, in fact, be the cause of some wrist pain, but that would not result in DISI.

Arthroscopic examination of a wrist in which there may be scapholunate disruption can assist in better detailing the pathology, as well as assessing the degree of carpal instability, if present. Even before arthroscopy, an examination under anesthesia or regional block can afford a more accurate clinical assessment of any scaphoid instability. Arthroscopic examination of the proximal wrist joint through the 3-4 portal can identify the integrity, or lack of integrity, of the radioscaphocapitate, radiolunate, scapholunate interosseous, lunotriquetral interosseous, and ulnocarpal ligaments. The integrity of the radioscapholunate ligament, or ligament of Testut, can also be assessed. Although it is not a true ligament, its assessment can sometimes offer additional information regarding the extent of trauma and/or disruption that may have occurred. During the arthroscopic examination of the proximal wrist joint, the wrist can be brought through a limited range of motion and/or the scaphoid stress test can be performed while the scaphoid and lunate are under arthroscopic observation. Additionally, a probe can be used to assess the anatomic and mechanical integrity of the various portions of the scapholunate interosseous ligament. Chondral lesions resulting from acute trauma or, in chronic cases, any chondromalacia or exposed subchondral bone can be identified and documented. The appropriateness of the various treatment options depends on the existence and extent of chondral pathology.

If there is only a disruption within the membranous proximal portion of the scapholunate interosseous ligament complex, I recommend simple debridement of the disrupted portion of the ligament. When disruption of the dorsal component of the scapholunate interosseous ligament has resulted in significant scapholunate diastasis and instability without significant chondral changes and this condition is diagnosed in the acute phase of the injury, some surgeons perform arthroscopic reduction and pinning of the scapholunate joint. In this case, reduction of the scapholunate joint is maintained, and percutaneous pin fixation of the scapholunate joint is performed under direct arthroscopic visualization through the midcarpal joint. It is rare that patients either present or are referred to our medical center acutely. My usual approach, therefore, is to assess, diagnose, and document the extent of the ligament disruption and chondral damage and, if appropriate for ligament repair and reconstruction, proceed at that point with an open reduction and ligament reconstruction.[9]

Other types of pathology that have been demonstrated to result indirectly in a DISI deformity are scaphoid fracture, malunion or nonunion, and malunion of the distal radius. All these forms of apparent carpal instability generally result from the bone deformity and usually do not involve ligament disruption, although ligament disruption cannot automatically be excluded.

Volar Intercalated Segment Instability

Although there is a relative paucity of cases in the literature of what could be classified as volar intercalated segment instability, this entity is increasingly identified in patients and in the literature. A number of different lesions have been reported to result in VISI deformity. Garth and associates[10] described laxity of the capitotriquetral ligament that resulted in failure of the triquetral hamate joint. Trumble and associates[11] also listed triquetral hamate disruption, as well as capitate and lunate laxity, as causes of VISI deformity. Gibson[12] and Hankin and associates[13] have published case reports in which they attribute a VISI deformity to injury of the scaphotrapezial ligament. All these VISI deformities would be categorized as CIND lesions. The etiology most commonly attributed to the development of a VISI deformity was linked to lunate triquetrum laxity. Recent studies by Viegas and associates[14] have identified the importance of the dorsal capsule and dorsal radiocarpal ligament complex in the development of a static VISI instability. Lunotriquetral disruptions, however, can be a part of the disruption pattern that can result in a VISI instability.

Arthroscopic examination of the proximal wrist joint can help to assess the integrity of the lunotriquetral interosseous ligament complex, as well as the ulnocarpal ligaments. Visualization of these structures from the proximal wrist joint, however, may require visualization through the 6-R or 6-U portals. Additionally, the laxity and diastasis of the lunotriquetral joint can often be assessed by means of midcarpal arthroscopy through the radial midcarpal or ulnar midcarpal portals. The approach used to assess lunotriquetral instability is similar to that used to assess scapholunate stability. Examination under anesthesia is used to assess what I describe as the midcarpal clunk test, which is positive if a static or dynamic VISI instability is present. This midcarpal clunk test is performed by applying a palmarly directed translational force over the dorsum of the capitate. The wrist is in neutral flexion/extension and is brought from a position of radial deviation to a position of ulnar deviation. During this maneuver, if there is sufficient laxity, the capitate subluxes volarly out of the lunate concavity while the wrist is in radial deviation. As the wrist is brought into ulnar deviation, the lunate is forced into a more neutral and slightly extended posture. The capitate remains transiently perched at the volar lip of the lunate and then abruptly shifts or "clunks" dorsally to seat suddenly in a reduced position in the lunate articulation (Fig. 1). This maneuver can also be performed, to a limited extent, while viewing the midcarpal joint from the radial midcarpal or ulnar midcarpal portal. Here, too, when assessing whether or not there is a lunotriquetral interosseous ligament complex disruption, it is important to remember that previous studies by Viegas and associates[7] have shown the lunotriquetral interosseous ligament to be disrupted in 36% of 393 cadaver wrists dissected. Additionally, in those cadavers in which both wrists could be dissected, if there was a lunotriquetral interosseous ligament disruption on one side, there was a 53% incidence of disruption of the lunotriquetral interosseous ligament on the contralateral side. Here again, through visual inspection and probing, the integrity of the lunotriquetral interosseous ligament and, where possible, the dorsal radiocarpal capsule and dorsal radiolunotriquetral ligament should be assessed, and any chondral lesions identified.

Berger and associates[8] have again studied the various components of the lunotriquetral interosseous ligament and found that the most substantial portion of this complex, both histologically and mechanically, is its volar component. The dorsal component is next, and the least substantial portion again is the proximal membranous portion of this complex. If arthroscopy shows the proximal membranous portion of the lunotriquetral interosseous ligament complex to be disrupted, and this disruption is the likely cause of symptoms, a local debridement of the disrupted portion of the membranous portion of the ligament is advised. Here, too, if the disruption and instability are more significant, some surgeons approach these injuries with arthroscopically assisted reduction and percutaneous pin fixation. My approach, however, is to approach the injury through an open procedure and, depending on the patient's wishes, either attempt a ligament reconstruction and repair or, alternatively, proceed to a lunate-triquetrum-capitate-hamate fusion. It is particularly important in the VISI instabilities to examine the contralateral wrist. It is not uncommon to identify physiologic laxity and a physiologic midcarpal clunk in the contralateral wrist. Although this does not preclude the option of ligament repair and reconstruction, it does raise the concern of subsequent stretching or compromise of the ligament repair. In these individu-

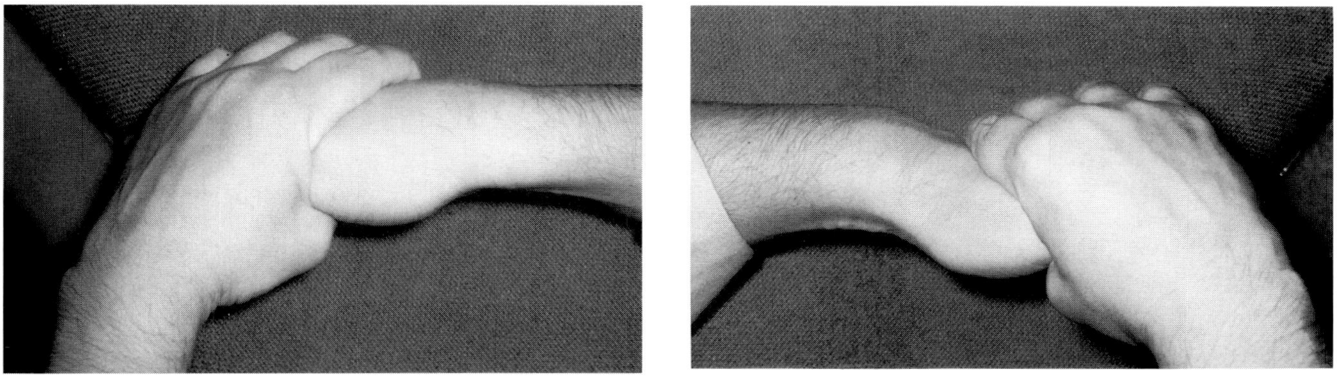

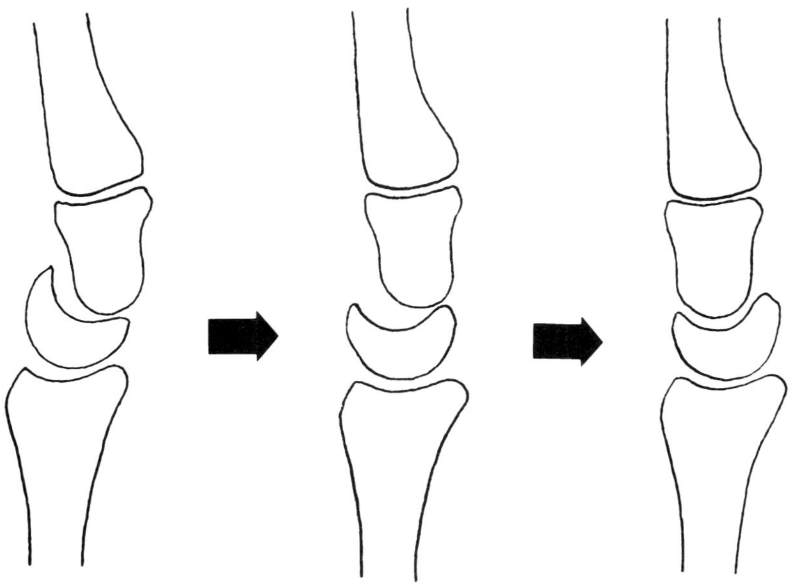

Fig. 1 The examination for a mid-carpal clunk is performed by (**top left**) exerting a palmarly directed translational force over the dorsal aspect of the distal carpal row with the wrist in neutral flexion/extension and slight radial deviation. The hand can be seen to be volarly translated in relation to the forearm. While maintaining the palmarly directed translational force, (**top right**) the wrist is deviated in an ulnar direction which will result in a sudden clunk, as the wrist relocates into a more anatomic position. (**Bottom**) Demonstrates a diagrammatic representation of the third metacarpal, capitate, lunate, and radius in the VISI alignment. When the palmar translational force is exerted over the dorsal aspect of the capitate as the wrist is deviated in an ulnar direction, the scaphoid and then lunate are forced into a more neutral position. Transiently, the capitate remains perched on the volar lip of the lunate and then suddenly relocates into the distal lunate articulation.

als, one might give stronger consideration to a limited arthrodesis.

Arthroscopic examination of wrist injuries affords us the ability to better identify and detail the various ligament disruptions. It has demonstrated a greater incidence of ligament disruptions with concomitant distal radius fractures than had previously been identified. Arthroscopic examination of wrist injuries is a valuable tool that offers an excellent way of assessing the extent and import of a number of ligament disruptions.

References

1. Gilford WW, Bolton RH, Lambrinudi C: The mechanism of the wrist joint with special reference to fractures of the scaphoid. *Guy's Hosp Rep* 1943;92:52-59.
2. Linscheid RL, Dobyns JH, Beabout JW, et al: Traumatic instability of the wrist: Diagnosis, classification, and pathomechanics. *J Bone Joint Surg* 1972;54A:1612-1632.
3. Dobyns JH, Linscheid RL, Chao EYS, et al: Traumatic instability of the wrist, in Evans EB (ed): *American Academy of Orthopaedic Surgeons Instructional Course Lectures XXIV*. St. Louis, MO, CV Mosby, 1975, pp 182-199.
4. Taleisnik J: Post-traumatic carpal instability. *Clin Orthop* 1980; 149:73-82.
5. Dobyns JH, Linscheid RL, Macksoud WS, et al: Carpal instability, nondissociative. Presented at the 54th Annual Meeting of the American Academy of Orthopaedic Surgeons, San Francisco, CA, January 1987.
6. Cooney WP, Dobyns JH, Linscheid RL: Arthroscopy of the wrist: Anatomy and classification of carpal instability. *Arthroscopy* 1990;6:133-140.
7. Viegas SF, Patterson RM, Hokanson JA, et al: Wrist anatomy: Incidence, distribution, and correlation of anatomic variations, tears, and arthrosis. *J Hand Surg* 1993;18A:463-475.
8. Berger RA, Imaeda T, Berglund L, et al: The anatomic, constraint and material properties of the scapholunate interosseous ligament: A preliminary study, in Schuind F, An KN, Cooney WP III, et al (eds): *Advances in the Biomechanics of the Hand and Wrist*. New York, NY, Plenum Press, 1994, pp 9-16.
9. Viegas SF: Ligamentous repair following acute scapholunate dissociation, in Gelberman RH (ed): *Master Techniques in Orthopaedics: The Wrist*. New York, NY, Raven Press, 1994, pp 135-146.

10. Garth WP Jr, Hofammann DY, Rooks MD: Volar intercalated segment instability secondary to medial carpal ligament laxity. *Clin Orthop* 1985;201:94-105.
11. Trumble TE, Bour CJ, Smith RJ, et al: Kinematics of the ulnar carpus related to the volar intercalated segment instability pattern. *J Hand Surg* 1990;15A:384-392.
12. Gibson PH: Scaphoid-trapezium-trapezoid dislocation. *Hand* 1983;15:267-269.
13. Hankin FM, Amadio PC, Wojtys EM, et al: Carpal instability with volar flexion of the proximal row associated with injury to the scaphotrapezial ligament: Report of two cases. *J Hand Surg* 1988;13B:298-302.
14. Viegas SF, Patterson RM, Peterson PD, et al: Ulnar-sided perilunate instability: An anatomic and biomechanic study. *J Hand Surg* 1990;15A:268-278.

CHAPTER 13

Endoscopic Carpal Tunnel Release: Chow Dual-Portal Technique

Daniel J. Nagle, MD

James C. Y. Chow, MD, published his dual-portal technique in 1989[1] and reported his clinical results in 1990.[2] Since then other endoscopic techniques have been reported.[3,4,5] Endoscopic carpal tunnel release (ECTR) was developed for many of the same reasons that prompted the development of other endoscopic techniques, such as laparoscopic cholecystectomy and arthroscopy. The rationale for its development was that a minimal incision approach to carpal tunnel release would hopefully reduce postoperative pain and, possibly, allow an earlier return of function of the involved hand.

Viegas and associates[6] compared ECTR with open carpal tunnel release in regard to postoperative widening of the carpal arch. They concluded that the carpal arch widens less after ECTR. Nagle and Yue[7] reported similar results in 1992.

Indications

The indications for endoscopic and open carpal tunnel release are similar. There are, however, certain patients for whom ECTR may not be helpful. This group includes patients who have undergone previous carpal tunnel release. Although some surgeons have successfully used ECTR in such patients, its outcome is not predictable. A fused wrist constitutes a contraindication for ECTR. The inability to extend the wrist on the hand-holder precludes the safe placement of the cannula. Also, if one suspects the presence of proliferative tenosynovitis, open carpal tunnel release is preferable. Of course, any suspicion of the presence of a mass within the carpal tunnel would be an indication for an open carpal tunnel release rather than an ECTR.

Anesthesia

The anesthetic used is a matter of personal preference. James Chow, MD, feels very strongly that local anesthesia should be used because it allows instant feedback from the patient if the median or ulnar nerve is touched. Local anesthesia also allows the surgeon to assess the neurovascular status of the patient immediately after completion of the carpal tunnel release, while the patient's hand is still prepped. If signs of a nerve, tendon, or arterial injury are noted, immediate exploration can be carried out. It should be understood that the local anesthetic is supplemented with intravenous fentanyl and midazolam just before the cannula is passed into the carpal tunnel. Local anesthesia is particularly well-suited to performing bilateral ECTR in one sitting.

Intravenous regional anesthesia (Bier block) can also be used. It does not allow the instant feedback of local anesthesia, but once the tourniquet is released, the patient's neurologic status returns quickly to preoperative levels, which makes it possible to perform a complete neuromuscular examination before breaking the sterile field. The Bier block eliminates the need to give fentanyl and midazolam in the doses needed with pure local anesthesia, because, with the Bier block, the patient does not feel the cannula pass into the carpal tunnel. Axillary block and general anesthesia have also been used, but they do not allow the patient feedback that is possible with the local techniques.

Technique

The dual-portal ECTR, as described by Chow and modified by others, uses a proximal portal that is established just proximal to the wrist flexion crease in the midline of the forearm at the ulnar border of the palmaris brevis, and a distal portal which is established just distal to the distal edge of the transverse carpal ligament along the long axis of the ring finger. The volar antebrachial fascia is carefully entered and a curved dissector is passed into the carpal tunnel, taking care to hug the hook of the hamate. A "washboard" sensation is felt as the tip of the dissector passes over the ridges in the dorsal surface of the transverse carpal ligament (TCL). If this "washboard" sensation is not felt, the dissector is either palmar to the TCL or is in Guyon's canal. The distal edge of the TCL is palpated with the curved dissector and the position of the distal edge of the TCL is marked on the overlying palmar skin. The curved dissector is removed and the slotted cannula/obturator is placed into the carpal tunnel. The operator's hand is placed on the palmar aspect of the hand between the thenar and hypothenar eminences and the cannula system is lifted (the *lift* test). The examiner's palpating fingers should not be able to feel the cannula. If the cannula is palpable it is either palmar to the TCL or is in Guyon's canal and must be removed and repositioned. Once the cannula is safely placed, taking care to stay close to the hook of the hamate and keeping the cannula system parallel to the long axis of the arm, the wrist and fingers are extended and the hand is placed on the hand-holder. The tip of the cannula system is palpated just distal to the distal edge of the TCL (Fig. 1). The cannula system is then passed through the distal portal while the superficial

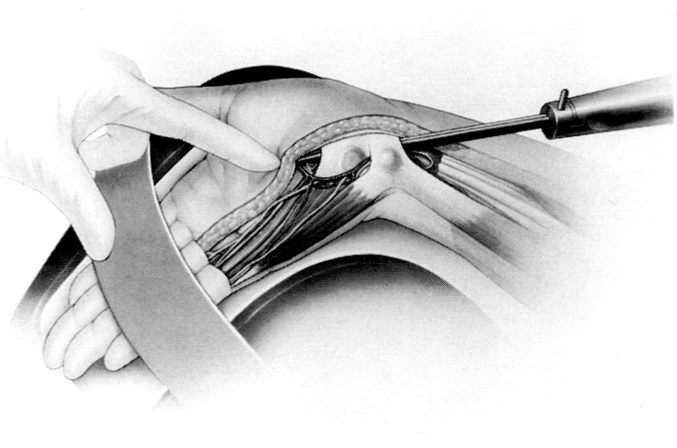

Fig. 1 The cannula system is placed in the carpal tunnel against the hook of the hamate. The tip of the obturator is palpated 3 to 5 mm distal to the distal edge of the TCL, passing palmar to the superficial palmar arch, ulnar to the third common digital nerve, and radial to the fourth common digital nerve. (Reproduced with permission from Smith & Nephew Dyonics, Inc, Andover, MA.)

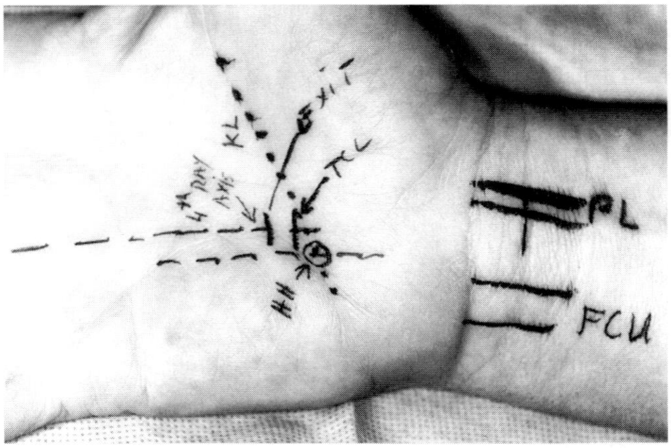

Fig. 2 The portals and surface anatomy. Note the proximal portal just at the ulnar border of the palmaris longus approximately 1 cm proximal to the wrist crease. The distal portal must lie just distal to the TCL along the long axis of the fourth ray. (HH, hook of the hamate; TCL, transverse carpal ligament; PL, palmaris longus; FCU, flexor carpi ulnaris.)

palmar arch is pushed dorsally with the palmar arch depressor. The distal portal is established approximately 4 to 5 mm distal to the distal edge of the TCL along the long axis of the ring finger. This effectively allows the cannula system to pass between the common digital nerves of the third and fourth web spaces, distal and palmar to the superficial palmar arch, and palmar to the communicating branch of the sensory branch between the median and ulnar nerves.[8] Once the cannula system passes out through this distal portal, the system is fixed in position (Fig. 2). The elastic band is placed across the fingers to hold the hand in position. The assistant extends the patient's thumb, thus placing tension on the TCL.

The endoscope is then passed into the proximal end of the cannula. A 30° 4 mm scope is used. Oftentimes a layer of synovial-like tissue lining the dorsal aspect of the TCL must be cleared. A "nerve hook" or commercially available rasps can be used for this. It is of paramount importance that the surgeon *clearly* identifies the TCL and that there are *no* intervening soft tissues! The TCL has a very characteristic feel and morphology. Its transverse fibers are visible and palpable (the washboard feeling). Proximally the TCL is white, while distally it is yellowish. The distal edge of the TCL should be clearly identifiable. Just distal to the distal edge of the TCL a fat pad will be noted to fall into the cannula system.

The cannula system, when placed as described, is *extrabursal*, that is, it lies palmar to the flexor tendon bursa. The median nerve is also extrabursal and can occasionally be seen in the cannula system (Fig. 3). If this is the case, the cannula system can be rotated radially 350°. This will push the median nerve away

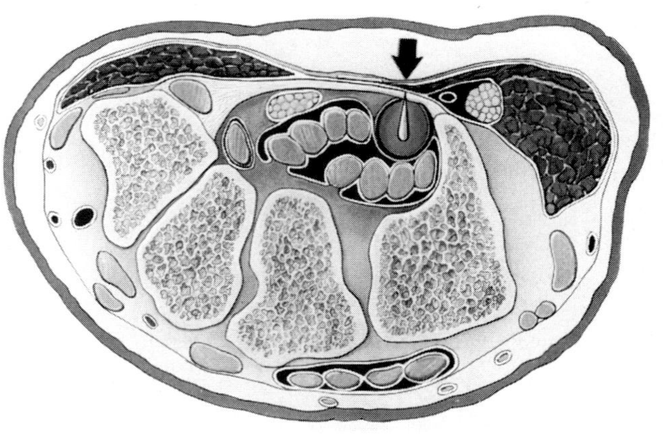

Fig. 3 The extrabursal technique places the cannula palmar to the flexor tendon bursa. (Reproduced with permission from Smith & Nephew Dyonics, Inc, Andover, MA.)

from the cannula. If this action does not clear the cannula system, the cannula/obturator should be removed and reinserted. If clear visualization of the TCL still cannot be achieved, an open carpal tunnel release should be carried out.

Once the surgeon is absolutely certain there is no obstruction and that there are no intervening structures, such as the median nerve, flexor tendon, or superficial palmar arch, the probe blade is inserted. This blade, which resembles a meniscotome, is designed to cut forward and is blunt except at its axilla. The probe blade is passed into the cannula system under direct vision and then withdrawn from proximal to distal until it slips palmarly and its axilla engages the

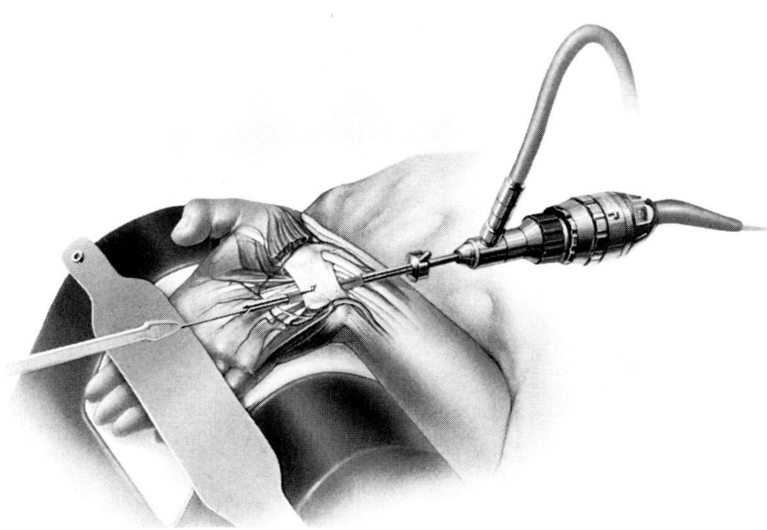

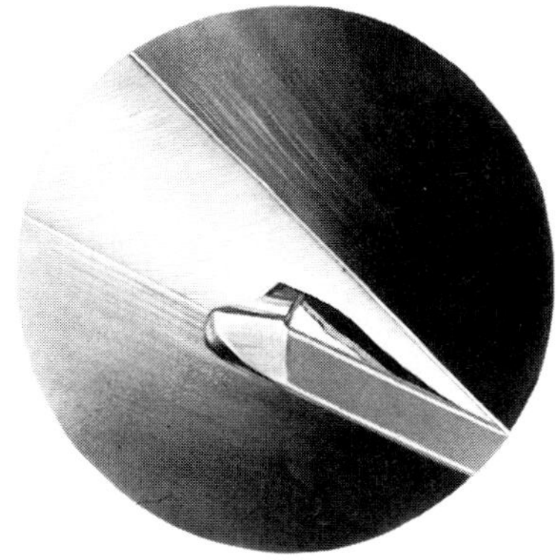

Fig. 4 **Left,** the probe blade pushes safely away from the superficial palmar arch during the first distal cut. **Right,** Interior view of the probe blade. (Reproduced with permission from Smith & Nephew Dyonics, Inc, Andover, MA.)

distal edge of the TCL. This maneuver allows the surgeon to retract any structures that may have been in the area of the distal edge of the TCL, such as a communicating branch of the median and ulnar nerves or the superficial palmar arch. The probe blade is then advanced from distal to proximal for 1 cm to cut the distal edge of the TCL (Fig. 4). This blade is then removed, and the triangular blade is inserted approximately 1.5 cm proximal to the distal edge of the TCL. It is used to make an incision into the TCL, an incision large enough to accept the retrograde blade and deep enough to penetrate the full thickness of the TCL (Fig. 5). The triangular blade is then removed, and the retrograde blade is passed into the cannula system and into the defect created by the triangular blade. The retrograde blade is then used to cut the rest of the distal edge of the TCL from proximal to distal (Fig. 6). This technique is safe as long as the surgeon has full control of the retrograde blade. The surgeon should hold the handle of the retrograde knife in his or her palm with the small and ring fingers. The shank of the blade is held between the long finger and the thumb while the index finger controls the cut by pushing off the cannula or palm. The initial cut, that is, the cut with the probe blade, cuts the distal edge of the TCL and creates a safety zone into which the retrograde blade can be drawn. The probe blade is usually not sharp enough to completely cut the distal edge of the TCL, which can be as thick as 7 to 10 mm. The triangular blade should not be used to cut the distal edge of the TCL, because it has

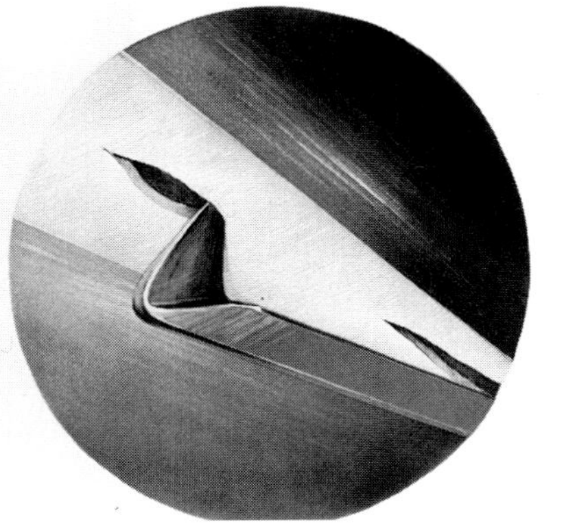

Fig. 5 The second cut, made with the triangular blade, is just large and deep enough to allow the retrograde (hook knife) to fully engage the full thickness of the TCL. (Reproduced with permission from Smith & Nephew Dyonics, Inc, Andover, MA.)

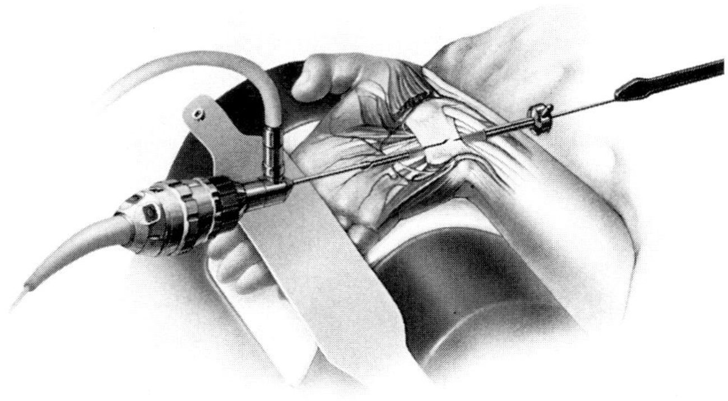

Fig. 6 The final cut is made with the retrograde blade pulling away from the superficial palmar arch. (Reproduced with permission from Smith & Nephew Dyonics, Inc, Andover, MA.)

a tendency to cut too deeply and cause more bleeding as it enters the palmar fascia and fat.

Once the distal edge of the TCL is released, the retrograde blade is placed proximally and the scope distally and the proximal edge of the TCL is released under direct vision from distal to proximal. Occasionally there are attachments between the palmar fascia and the TCL that must be released. This can be done accurately using the triangular blade.

Once the release is complete, the proximal subfascial fat should cascade into the cannula system. In the rest of the cannula system, one should see the palmar fascia. The cut edges of the TCL will retract out of the field of view in such a way that the cannula system must be rotated to see them. If this is not the case, the TCL has not been completely released and further release is needed. Once a complete release has been performed, the obturator is reinserted into the cannula and the cannula system is removed.

The incisions are closed with a subcuticular stitch at the wrist and a simple stitch at the palm, and a bulky dressing is applied. No splint is needed. The patient's circulation, sensation, and motor function are then tested, and the patient is discharged from the operating room. Follow-up is as for any carpal tunnel release.

Results of ECTR

With each passing month, more and more papers are being published regarding ECTR. The results of a multicenter prospective study of ECTR was presented to the American Society for Surgery of the Hand in Phoenix, Arizona in 1992.[9] This study reviewed 640 cases carried out by eight surgeons. Approximately 30% of the cases were worker's compensation and 70% were non-worker's compensation. Two ECTR techniques were used. Early in the study the original technique as described by Dr. Chow was used. Approximately 17% of the cases were treated using the original Chow transbursal technique. This is called a transbursal technique because of the fact the cannula system actually entered and exited the flexor tendon bursa. The remaining 83% of the cases were carried out using the modified Chow technique or extrabursal technique, in which the bursa is not entered. This is the technique that is described above. The authors noted the rate of conversion from endoscopic to open carpal tunnel release was 1.3% for the modified Chow (extrabursal) technique and 7.8% for the transbursal or original Chow technique. The study also reported perioperative complications that included 14 neurapraxias, all of which resolved. There was one superficial palmar arch lacerated and the flexor digitorum sublimis of the ring and small fingers were lacerated in one patient. There was one hematoma and four incomplete releases. Late complications included three reflex sympathetic dystrophies. These statistics translate to a complication rate of 2.2% for the modified Chow technique and 11% for the Chow technique, which led to the conclusion that the transbursal or original Chow technique was associated with a higher complication rate. It was also concluded that there is a steep learning curve with this procedure, and that appropriate training is essential.

Nagle and associates[10] have recently published a study of 278 cases carried out by two surgeons and reviewed prospectively. The worker's compensation and non-worker's compensation ratios were about the same as in the multicenter study cited above. However, all cases were treated using the extrabursal technique, and the conversion rate was 0.7%. There were five neurapraxias, all of which resolved, and there were no tendon, artery, or nerve lacerations, hematomas, or incomplete releases. There was one reflex sympathetic dystrophy, and three stitch abscesses at the proximal portal. This translated to a complication rate of 3.2%, including the three superficial stitch infections. Without the stitch infections, the complication rate was 2.2%.

Other authors have reported their results, including Okutsu and associates,[11] who reviewed 51 ECTRs in 1989 and reported no nerve or arterial injuries. More recently, Okutsu and associates[12] reported the results of 39 ECTRs, in which they note no complications and resolution of all sensory disturbances within an average of 20 weeks. In 1991, Resnick and Miller[5] reported results of a study that compared the transbursal and extrabursal approaches. The only complications noted were with the transbursal approach and consisted of one partial median nerve laceration and six ulnar neurapraxias. Brown and associates[4] reported on their results comparing the single-portal approach (149 cases) to a dual-portal approach (152 cases). They noted the average cessation of preoperative symptoms was approximately 15 days with either technique and the average return-to-work time was between 15 and 17 days. The complication rate was 6% for the single-portal procedure and 5% for the dual-portal. There were no iatrogenic vascular or nerve injuries in either series. However, they did note five patients with "transient paresthesias" with the two-portal technique prior to the use of "customized" instruments. One case of reflex sympathetic dystrophy was noted with each technique. Two cases had to be converted to an open carpal tunnel release using the single-portal approach and they concluded the single-portal approach is more difficult than the dual-portal approach.

In 1994, Malek and associates[13] presented to the American Academy of Orthopaedic Surgeons the results of a questionnaire that was sent to participants in the Chow Endoscopic Carpal Tunnel Release Courses. The questionnaire queried the surgeons as to their results using the dual-portal ECTR technique. Data were collected on 10,624 cases, of which 30% were carried out

Table 1
Complications seen in 10,624 dual-portal ECTRs

Technique	Number	Nerve Injuries	Tendon Injuries
Transbursal	3,186	102 (3.2%)	15 (0.5%)
Extrabursal	7,438	52 (0.7%)	0 (0.0%)

with the original transbursal approach and 70% with the extrabursal approach. The complication rate was 4.8% for the original Chow approach and 1.2% for the extrabursal approach. Complications, however, were serious and included median, ulnar, and digital nerve lacerations and tendon and artery injuries (Table 1).

Results of Open Carpal Tunnel Release

Nearly 3,000 articles have been written on carpal tunnel syndrome since 1964. Among those articles, several have dealt with the complications associated with open carpal tunnel release. Phalen,[14] who reported on 212 cases in 1966, noted one superficial infection and one reflex sympathetic dystrophy. In 1977, Ariyan and Watson[15] reported on 429 cases, with a 1.4% complication rate (one infection, one hematoma, and four recurrences). MacDonald and associates[16] reported in 1978 on 186 cases in which they reported an 18% complication rate, and in 1979 Lichtman and associates[17] reported on 100 cases, with a 7% complication rate. It should be noted that in many of these reports, particularly in the MacDonald study, the complications existed prior to the referral to the team that performed the release. MacDonald reported a 6% incidence of injury to the palmar cutaneous branch of the median nerve; Lichtman reported a 2% incidence. Lichtman points out that these were neurapraxias, which resolved. In MacDonald's series, there was a 1% incidence of injury to the superficial palmar arch and a 6.5% incidence of neurapraxia. MacDonald reported a 2.1% incidence of reflex sympathetic dystrophy; Lichtman reported a 5% incidence. In MacDonald's series, there was a 2% incidence of hypertrophic scars, a 0.5% incidence of tendon adhesions, and a 2% incidence of bowstringing. Deep infection appears to be a rare occurrence after open carpal tunnel release, with Hanssen and associates[18] reporting a 0.4% incidence.

Recurrence of carpal tunnel syndrome symptoms after a successful open carpal tunnel release has not been critically reviewed by many authors. Ariyan and Watson,[15] in one of the few reports of this phenomenon, noted a 0.9% rate of recurrence.

Brown and associates[19] reported on a prospective randomized multicenter study that compared endoscopic and open carpal tunnel release. The endoscopic technique used was the dual-portal extrabursal approach. There were 85 open carpal tunnel releases and 84 ECTRs. They reported no complications using the open carpal tunnel release, but four complications using the ECTR. These included a partial laceration of the superficial palmar arch, a digital nerve neurapraxia, an ulnar nerve neurapraxia, and one hematoma. These researchers stated that the relief of pain and paresthesias was similar with both techniques. Eighty-four percent of the patients who had open carpal tunnel release and 89% of the patients with ECTR were satisfied. The return of sensation and motor strength was the same in both groups. The open carpal tunnel release patients complained of more scar tenderness, and the median return-to-work time for these patients was 28 days as opposed to 14 for ECTR.

Nancollas reported the results of a retrospective review of 60 open carpal tunnel releases with a 5-year follow-up.[20] At 5 years, he noted that 30% of the patients reported their results as being poor to fair. Fifty-seven percent noted the return of some of their preoperative symptoms beginning at 2 years after their surgery.

Worker's Compensation

Several studies have reported on the difference in return-to-work times between worker's compensation cases and non-worker's compensation cases. Indeed, the multicenter study[9] cited earlier as well as that of Nagle and associates[10] reported that the average time before return to work was between 57 and 65 days for worker's compensation cases as opposed to 21 to 22 days for non-worker's compensation cases. Both these studies went on to assess whether or not there was a difference between the worker's compensation and non-worker's compensation groups according to the work classification. These studies concluded that, regardless of the type of work performed, on average the worker's compensation patients return to work later than non-worker's compensation patients. Further corroborating this trend are the results reported by Chow,[21] in which at 4 weeks, 63% of the worker's compensation patients were back to work as opposed to 90% of the non-worker's compensation patients.

Feinstein[22] noted that non-worker's compensation patients returned to work an average of 17 days after their ECTR as opposed to 34 days for worker's compensation patients. Kerr and associates[23] have recently noted the time to return to work was no different for worker's compensation cases, whether they were done endoscopically or by open technique.

Nancollas also noted that, with open carpal tunnel release, 42% of the worker's compensation patients had a slower initial improvement.[20] His statistics show the average time to return to work for a worker's compensation patient after an open carpal tunnel release was 8.4 months as opposed to 1.7 months for non-worker's compensation cases.

It is clear from this review of the currently available literature that the return-to-work issue remains unresolved. Some studies have suggested ECTR in fact does lead to an earlier return to work, while others have suggested it does not, at least in regard to worker's compensation cases. All the studies agree that in patients not influenced by secondary gain, ECTR does, in fact, allow an earlier return to normal activities. It is naive to suppose a surgical technique will accelerate the slow postoperative recovery noted in worker's compensation patients.

Conclusions

These studies demonstrate that ECTR is not a procedure to be taken lightly. It is a demanding surgical exercise that requires exacting knowledge of the anatomy of the hand, and it is not something that should be carried out by the surgeon who does an occasional carpal tunnel release. For those who do not meet these criteria, open carpal tunnel release remains the procedure of choice. However, in the hands of surgeons who are well trained and who are aware of the anatomy of the hand, ECTR allows them to provide their patients with a safe, predictable solution to their carpal tunnel syndrome that will allow them a rapid return to normal activities.

Further studies will be required to see how well ECTR holds up to the test of time. Long-term studies are currently underway by many authors and should be available in the not-too-distant future.

References

1. Chow JC: Endoscopic release of the carpal ligament: A new technique for carpal tunnel syndrome. *Arthroscopy* 1989;5:19-24.
2. Chow JC: Endoscopic release of the carpal ligament for carpal tunnel syndrome: 22-month clinical result. *Arthroscopy* 1990;6:288-296.
3. Menon J: Endoscopic carpal tunnel release: Preliminary report. *Arthroscopy* 1994;10:31-38.
4. Brown MG, Keyser B, Rothenberg ES: Endoscopic carpal tunnel release. *J Hand Surg* 1992;17A:1009-1011.
5. Resnick CT, Miller BW: Endoscopic carpal tunnel release using the subligamentous two-portal technique. *Contemp Orthop* 1991;22:269-277.
6. Viegas SF, Pollard A, Kaminski K: Carpal arch alteration and released clinical status after ECTR. *J Hand Surg* 1992;17A:1012-1016.
7. Nagle DJ, Yue J: Changes in the carpal tunnel arch after endoscopic carpal tunnel release: A preliminary report. Presented at the Fifth International Congress of Hand Surgery. Paris, France, May 25-28, 1992.
8. Meals RA, Shaner M: Variations in digital sensory patterns: A study of the ulnar nerve-median nerve palmar communicating branch. *J Hand Surg* 1983;8A:411-414.
9. Nagle DJ, Fischer T, Harris GD, et al: A multi-center prospective review of 640 endoscopic carpal tunnel releases using the Chow technique. Presented at the 47th Annual Meeting of the American Society for Surgery of the Hand, Phoenix, Arizona, November 10-11, 1992.
10. Nagle D, Harris G, Foley M: Prospective review of 278 endoscopic carpal tunnel releases using the modified Chow technique. *Arthroscopy* 1994;10:259-265.
11. Okutsu I, Ninomiya S, Takatori Y, et al: Endoscopic management of carpal tunnel syndrome. *Arthroscopy* 1989;5:11-18.
12. Okutsu I, Ninomiya S, Takatori Y, et al: Results of endoscopic management of carpal tunnel syndrome. *Orthop Rev* 1993;22:81-87.
13. Malek MM, Chow JCY, Berch D: Complications of endoscopic carpal tunnel release: Analysis of 10,624 cases. Presented at the 61st Annual Meeting of the American Academy of Orthopaedic Surgeons, New Orleans, LA, February 1994.
14. Phalen GS: The carpal-tunnel syndrome: Seventeen years' experience in diagnosis and treatment of six hundred fifty-four hands. *J Bone Joint Surg* 1966;48A:211-228.
15. Ariyan S, Watson HK: The palmar approach for the visualization and release of the carpal tunnel: An analysis of 429 cases. *Plast Reconstr Surg* 1977;60:539-547.
16. MacDonald RI, Lichtman DM, Hanlon JJ, et al: Complications of surgical release for carpal tunnel syndrome. *J Hand Surg* 1978;3A:70-76.
17. Lichtman DM, Florio RL, Mack GR: Carpal tunnel release under local anesthesia: Evaluation of the outpatient procedure. *J Hand Surg* 1979;4A:544-546.
18. Hanssen AD, Amadio PC, DeSilva SP, et al: Deep postoperative wound infection after carpal tunnel release. *J Hand Surg* 1989;14A:869-873.
19. Brown RA, Gelberman RH, Seiler JG III, et al: Carpal tunnel release: A prospective, randomized assessment of open and endoscopic methods. *J Bone Joint Surg* 1993;75A:1265-1275.
20. Cotton P: Symptoms may return after carpal tunnel surgery. *JAMA* 1991;265:1922-1925.
21. Chow JC: The Chow technique of endoscopic release of the carpal ligament for carpal tunnel syndrome: Four years of clinical results. *Arthroscopy* 1993;9:301-314.
22. Feinstein PA: Endoscopic carpal tunnel release in a community-based series. *J Hand Surg* 1993;18A:451-454.
23. Kerr CD, Gittins ME, Sybert DR: Endoscopic versus open carpal tunnel release: Clinical results. *Arthroscopy* 1994;10:266-269.

CHAPTER 14

Endoscopic Carpal Tunnel Release: Single Portal Agee Technique

David H. Palmer, MD

Introduction

The first single portal endoscopic carpal tunnel release was described in 1989 by Okutsu and associates.[1] Most endoscopic carpal tunnel releases in the United States, however, are currently being performed using the two-portal technique and instrumentation designed by Dr. James Chow,[2] or the single-portal method and instrumentation developed by Dr. John Agee.[3] Other single-portal techniques have also subsequently been described.[4] This chapter on carpal tunnel release focuses on the technique and results obtained using the Agee single-portal method.

Rationale for Endoscopic Carpal Tunnel Release

Because endoscopic carpal tunnel release leaves the overlying skin, the subcutaneous fat, and the palmar fascia and its attachments to the thenar and hypothenar musculature intact, its proponents maintain that their patients have less scar tenderness, quicker recovery of strength, and earlier return to activities of daily living and work. Studies by Okutsu and associates[5] and Brown and associates[6] showed that carpal tunnel compartment pressure measurements after endoscopic release were reduced to levels similar to those obtained in normal controls and after open release. Peimer and associates[7] demonstrated an increase in volume of the carpal tunnel as measured by magnetic resonance imaging (MRI) after endoscopic release to values comparable with those after open release. Gelberman and associates[8] and Mackinnon and associates[9] have shown that internal neurolysis is not necessary in primary carpal tunnel syndrome and fails to improve the results of open carpal tunnel decompression.

Indications for Endoscopic Carpal Tunnel Release

Patients with typical signs and symptoms of idiopathic carpal tunnel syndrome who have failed conservative treatment are candidates for the endoscopic procedure. There is a steep learning curve associated with this technique, which requires an intimate knowledge of hand anatomy, the proper use and positioning of instrumentation, and the ability to differentiate under video monitoring between the transverse carpal ligament and nerve or synovial tissue. Therefore, it is mandatory for any surgeon performing this procedure to attend a BioSkills course offering hands-on cadaver experience to master the technique. It is also a good idea to augment one's surgical skills by scrubbing-in with a colleague who has had prior experience with endoscopic carpal tunnel release. For surgeons who perform carpal tunnel release only occasionally, it is best to continue to use open methods. There are several contraindications to endoscopic carpal tunnel release: The procedure is not advised for patients with prior surgery in or around the carpal tunnel. Those patients who have posttraumatic carpal tunnel syndrome or inflammatory arthropathy and who may require an associated tenosynovectomy are not good candidates for the endoscopic procedure. Patients with limited wrist extension present difficulty with device insertion, and any patient with altered carpal anatomy or a suspected space-occupying lesion within the carpal canal should be approached by an open technique. To insure optimal visualization of the transverse carpal ligament, all video and fiberoptic equipment must be in excellent working order.

Instrumentation

The Agee device consists of a trigger assembly handpiece and 2.7-mm endoscope, which attach to any standard video camera and light source. The disposable blade assembly, when trigger-activated, extends 3.5 mm under the direct view of the endoscope through the viewing portal. Other instruments include a synovial elevator and hamate pathfinders. In the room set-up, an assistant is positioned opposite the surgeon. If ambidextrous, the surgeon is usually positioned on the axillary side of the patient, but a right-hand dominant surgeon may, for a left-hand case, work from the cephalic side of the patient. The video monitor is placed off the end of the table so the surgeon has a clear view of both the monitor and operating field.

Initially the procedure is best performed under general or axillary block anesthesia. Once the technique is mastered, 1% local Xylocaine can be infiltrated subcutaneously transversely on the volar side of the wrist, with care taken to avoid injecting any fluid directly within the carpal canal, which can cause difficulties in visualization. An IV regional block should be avoided for the same reason. If necessary, local anesthesia may be augmented with IV sedation or a distal forearm block as described by Wilson.[10]

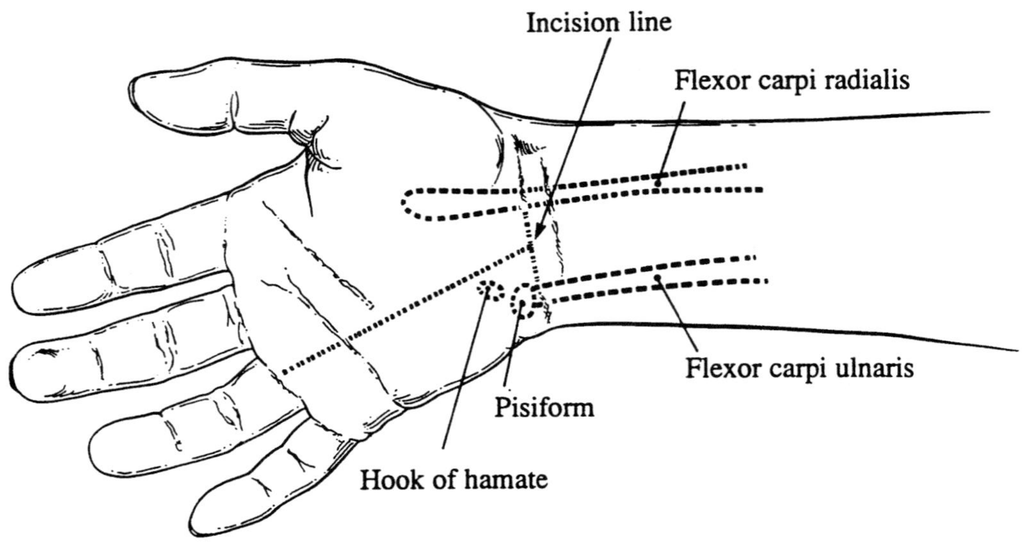

Fig. 1 Important superficial orientation landmarks. (Reproduced with permission from 3M Health Care: *The Agee Surgical Technique and User's Guide*. St. Paul, MN, 3M, 1992, pp 1-15.)

Anatomic Landmarks

Important palpable surface landmarks are the volar flexor tendons (palmaris longus, flexor carpi ulnaris, and flexor carpi radialis), the pisiform, and the hook of the hamate (Fig. 1). It is important to draw an orientation line from the midpoint of the portal incision down the long axis of the ring finger. Rotman and Manske,[11] working with cadaver dissections, measured the narrow tolerances of the carpal tunnel between the Agee device and the median nerve, its branches, the ulnar nerve, and superficial palmar arch. The safe region of blade elevation is located in line with the ring finger axis and is defined by a triangular zone formed by the distal margin of the transverse carpal ligament, the ulnar border of the median nerve and its branches, and the superficial palmar arch (Fig. 2).

Agee Technique

A 1.5- to 2-cm incision is made at a proximal wrist flexor crease transversely between the flexor carpi radialis and flexor carpi ulnaris tendons or just ulnar to the palmaris longus tendon. The subcutaneous tissue is spread bluntly to the antebrachial fascia and a 1-cm, distally based, U-shaped flap is made in the fascia to enter the carpal canal. This flap is elevated and the synovium removed from the dorsal surface of the transverse carpal ligament with a synovial elevator. This step ensures an adequate view of the transverse fibers of the ligament and its distal margin and also establishes the initial path down the ring finger axis. A small hamate pathfinder is placed down the carpal canal hugging the hook of the hamate and defining the distal margin of the ligament by palpation (Fig. 2).

The Agee blade assembly is then introduced down the carpal canal in line with the ring finger axis. It is passed proximally and distally to define the distal margin of the transverse carpal ligament and to ensure that no intervening vital structures are in view. The blade is then elevated at the ligament's distal margin and the entire assembly withdrawn, applying an upward pressure to keep the viewing portal snug against the ligament surface while hugging the radial border of the hook of the hamate (Fig. 3). The blade is then retracted and the assembly reinserted to check for adequacy of release. On occasion, a secondary pass is necessary to transect additional fibers. When completely released, the ligament spreads to create a trapezoidal defect that allows the blade assembly to fit between the cut edges (Fig. 4). Adequacy of the release can also be determined by tilting the viewing portal to visualize the cut edges of the ligament or by placing a retractor at the portal to view directly or palpate with a probe the transected ligament fibers.

The antebrachial fascia is then released proximally another 1.5 to 2 cm under direct view using a tenotomy scissors.

The portal is closed with an intracuticular suture, and a light compression dressing is applied. Activities of daily living are encouraged immediately, but the patient should avoid power gripping, pushing, or pulling for two weeks.

Indications for conversion to an open procedure, which in our experience occurs 3% to 4% of the time,

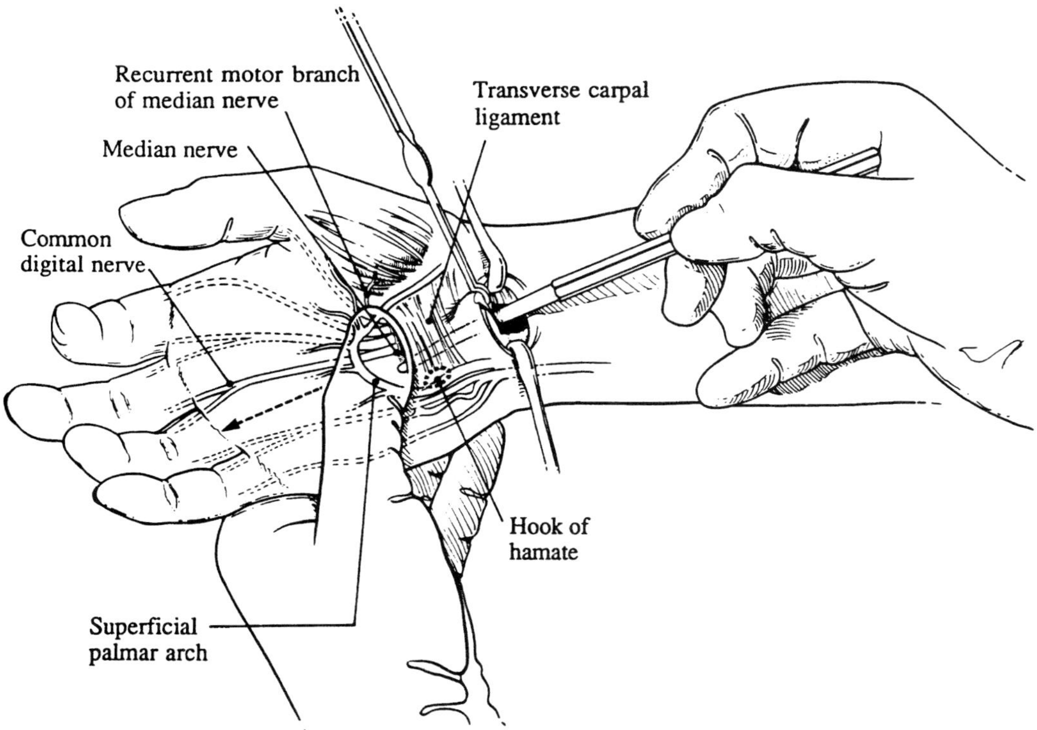

Fig. 2 The triangular safe zone formed by the distal margin of the TCL, ulnar border of the median nerve, and superficial palmar arch. Palpating the distal margin of the carpal tunnel with the hamate finder. (Reproduced with permission from 3M Health Care: *The Agee Surgical Technique and User's Guide*. St. Paul, MN, 3M, 1992, pp 1-15.)

include resistance to the device insertion, possibly indicating an anatomic abnormality within the carpal canal; failure to adequately clear synovium precluding a clear view of the transverse carpal ligament; and poor visualization caused by repeated fogging of the endoscope or by the presence of fluid in the carpal canal. The patient should be forewarned of the possibility that it may be necessary to do the procedure by standard open methods.

Study Results

Two prospective studies have compared the Agee method of endoscopic carpal tunnel release with that of standard open release. Both the multicenter study by Agee and associates[3] and a subsequent single-center study by Palmer and associates[12] showed the endoscopic release and the open release to be equally effective in relieving symptoms of paresthesias and nocturnal pain. In addition, the Palmer study showed that patients treated endoscopically had less perceived weakness and pain with activities of daily living than did those patients treated by open release. More objective testing revealed no difference in sensation and motor (abductor pollicis brevis) test results between the Agee

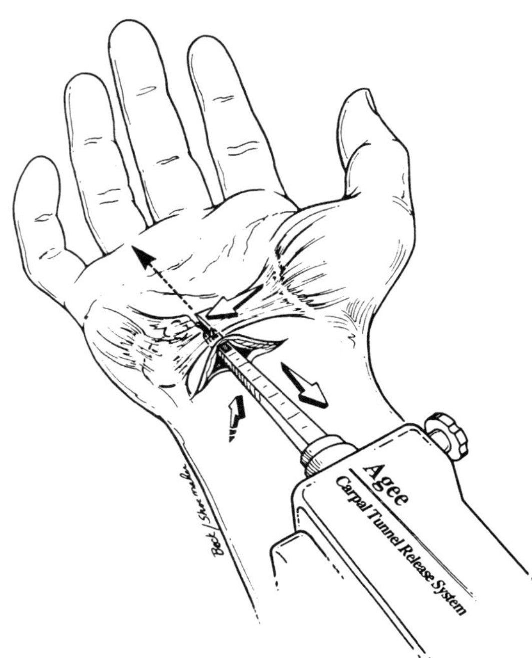

Fig. 3 Incising the transverse carpal ligament with the Agee device. (Reproduced with permission from 3M Health Care: *The Agee Surgical Technique and User's Guide*. St. Paul, MN, 3M, 1992, pp 1-15.)

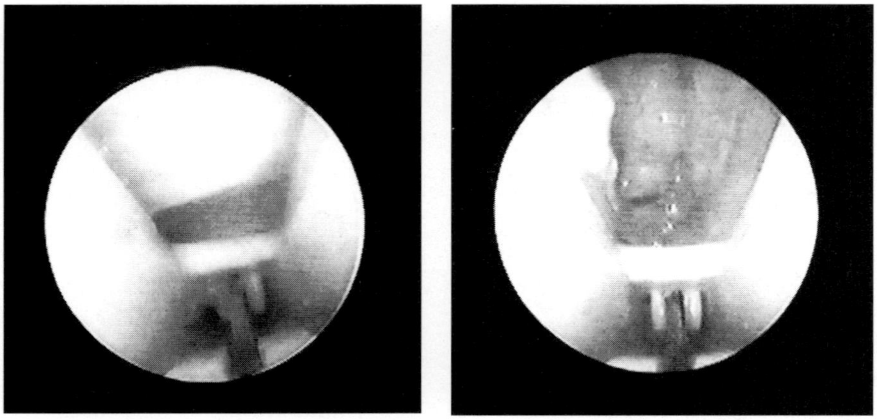

Fig. 4 Endoscopic view of the distal margin of the transverse carpal ligament before **(left)** and after **(right)** release. (Reproduced with permission from 3M Health Care: *The Agee Surgical Technique and User's Guide.* St. Paul, MN, 3M, 1992, pp 1-15.)

device and open controls in either study. Both evaluations, however, demonstrated that patients treated endoscopically had quicker recovery of grip and lateral pinch strength compared to the open group. In addition, patients who underwent open surgery had significantly more palmar scar tenderness in both studies.

In the Agee study, the overall median time for patients to return to work was 25 days for the endoscopic patients, and 46.5 days for those treated by the open method. In the Palmer study,[12] the corresponding times to return to work were 20.7 days and 44.1 days, again favoring the endoscopic group. Patients receiving workers' compensation required significantly longer periods of time to return to work in both studies (Table 1).

Complications

While there are advantages to performing a carpal tunnel release endoscopically, there remains concern over inadvertent injury to important neurovascular structures within the carpal canal. Most of the published and anecdotal reported injuries associated with this device occurred before it was redesigned to permit direct visualization of the blade's point of entry at the distal margin of the transverse carpal ligament. Of the 82 endoscopic procedures performed in the Agee study,[3] two patients had transient ulnar neurapraxias and two patients required an open release for unresolved symptoms. One of the latter two was noted to have an incomplete release. In the Palmer study,[12] 90 Agee endoscopic procedures were performed. Of these, two were converted to an open procedure at the time of surgery and two required a subsequent procedure. One of these patients had an open carpal tunnel release and another had a pronator tunnel release. Ten percent of the endoscopic group had transient ulnar neurapraxias, but this figure was also similar in the open group.

Table 1
Median return-to-work time (in days)

Study	Group	Overall	Workers' Compensation	Non-Workers' Compensation
Agee et al[3]	Endoscopic	25*	71	6.5*
	Open	46.5	78	45.5
Palmer et al[12]	Endoscopic	20.7*	29.2*	10.8*
	Open	44.1	56.1	26.8

*Significant difference between endoscopic and open ($p < 0.01$)

Feinstein,[13] in a retrospective review of 61 procedures performed with the original design, reported one median nerve laceration and one reoperation for unresolved symptoms. Brown and associates[14] reported on 149 procedures. Two of these patients were converted to an open operation, two had recurrences with incomplete releases, and one developed a reflex sympathetic dystrophy.

Limited information is currently available on complication rates associated with use of the point-of-entry blade. The manufacturer has gathered data on 1,049 Agee endoscopic procedures from 63 centers using the newer design.[15] Reported complications at the 4-week follow-up period include a 2.5% rate of conversion to an open procedure due to aberrant anatomy or poor visualization, one patient with a palmar cutaneous median nerve branch injury and another patient with loss of sensation on the radial side of the ring finger. Three patients had transient ulnar nerve paresthesias and three had resolving median nerve paresthesias. One patient developed a reflex sympathetic dystrophy and one a superficial infection for an overall complication rate of 1.1%. Even though this complication rate compares favorably with those reported for open carpal tunnel release,[16-18] there remains a need for a large, independent, multi-center review of complications encountered in both single-portal and two-portal techniques of endoscopic carpal tunnel release.

References

1. Okutsu I, Ninomiya S, Takatori Y, et al: Endoscopic management of carpal tunnel syndrome. *Arthroscopy* 1989;5:11-18.
2. Chow JC: Endoscopic release of the carpal ligament: A new technique for carpal tunnel syndrome. *Arthroscopy* 1989;5:19-24.
3. Agee JM, McCarroll HR Jr, Tortosa RD, et al: Endoscopic release of the carpal tunnel: A randomized prospective multicenter study. *J Hand Surg* 1992;17A:987-995.
4. Menon J: Endoscopic carpal tunnel release: Preliminary report. *Arthroscopy* 1994;10:31-38.
5. Okutsu I, Ninomiya S, Hamanaka I, et al: Measurement of pressure in the carpal canal before and after endoscopic management of carpal tunnel syndrome. *J Bone Joint Surg* 1989; 71A:679-683.
6. Brown RA, Gelberman RH, Seiler JG III, et al: Carpal tunnel release: A prospective, randomized assessment of open and endoscopic methods. *J Bone Joint Surg* 1993;75A:1265-1275.
7. Peimer C, Ablove R, Diao E, et al: Morphologic changes after endoscopic and two-portal subcutaneous carpal tunnel release. *J Hand Surg*, in press.
8. Gelberman RH, Pfeffer GB, Galbraith RT, et al: Results of treatment of severe carpal tunnel syndrome without internal neurolysis of the median nerve. *J Bone Joint Surg* 1987;69A:896-903.
9. Mackinnon SE, McCabe S, Murray JF, et al: Internal neurolysis fails to improve the results of primary carpal tunnel decompression. *J Hand Surg* 1991;16A:211-218.
10. Wilson KM: Distal forearm regional block anesthesia for carpal tunnel release. *J Hand Surg* 1993;18A:438-440.
11. Rotman MB, Manske PR: Anatomic relationships of an endoscopic carpal tunnel device to surrounding structures. *J Hand Surg* 1993;18A:442-450.
12. Palmer DH, Paulson JC, Lane-Larsen CL, et al: Endoscopic carpal tunnel release: A comparison of two techniques with open release. *Arthroscopy* 1993;9:498-508.
13. Feinstein PA: Endoscopic carpal tunnel release in a community-based series. *J Hand Surg* 1993;18A:451-454.
14. Brown MG, Keyser B, Rothenberg ES: Endoscopic carpal tunnel release. *J Hand Surg* 1992;17A:1009-1011.
15. Agee JM, Peimer C, Walsh B, et al: Endoscopic carpal tunnel release: A prospective study of complications and surgical experience. *J Hand Surg*, in press.
16. Kulick MI, Gordillo G, Javidi T, et al: Long-term analysis of patients having surgical treatment for carpal tunnel syndrome. *J Hand Surg* 1986;11A:59-66.
17. Kuschner SH, Brien WW, Johnson D, et al: Complications associated with carpal tunnel release. *Orthop Rev* 1991;20:346-352.
18. MacDonald RI, Lichtman DM, Hanlon JJ, et al: Complications of surgical release for carpal tunnel syndrome. *J Hand Surg* 1978; 3A:70-76.

CHAPTER 15

Social and Economic Costs of Carpal Tunnel Surgery

David H. Palmer, MD
Lawrence P. Hanrahan, PhD, MS

Introduction

Any attempt to assess the economic impact of carpal tunnel surgery depends on its incidence. Estimates of the number of carpal tunnel surgeries performed each year in the United States have varied widely. In 1988, a national survey of 400 hand surgeons estimated that more than 100,000 such procedures were performed in the United States annually.[1] In the same year, the National Center for Health Statistics survey of 44,000 workers estimated that 1.89 million U.S. workers were afflicted with carpal tunnel syndrome.[2] Other surveys have reported that up to 50% of occupationally related carpal tunnel syndrome will be surgically treated.[3]

When evaluating surveillance data one needs to be aware of the population denominator being surveyed. In general, there is a paucity of data on both the total population and the working population as a whole in the United States. A relatively large amount of information is collected, however, at the state level on workers whose injuries are covered by the workers' compensation system. These figures generally include both surgical and nonsurgical cases. Industry-specific evaluations are helpful in defining incidence rates only for that particular industry or work site. Also, many studies report on upper extremity cumulative trauma disorders in general, rather than on carpal tunnel syndrome specifically. Prior national data collection efforts have demonstrated shortcomings, including lack of specific coding, employer incentives to under-report, limited collection of demographic data, and lack of work site verification.[4,5]

The 1991 Bureau of Labor Statistics annual survey of private industry estimated that there were 6.3 million job-related injuries in the United States. The incidence of injury has remained relatively constant since 1980 at about 8.4 injuries per 100 full-time workers (Fig. 1).[6] These data are in marked contrast to statistics on occupational illnesses, which reveal a 300% increase in the incidence of cumulative trauma disorders since 1986 (Fig. 2).[6] Carpal tunnel syndrome is a sub-set of this population.

There are several reasons for the rising incidence of carpal tunnel syndrome, including job automation requiring a single task to be performed many times an hour, an increased public awareness of carpal tunnel syndrome generally, and a work force awareness of it as an occupational disorder. Several state court decisions have broadened the legal definition of carpal tunnel syndrome to include it as an occupationally related disease.[7] This rising incidence of cumulative trauma and repetitive stress injuries has prompted Dr. Christopher Browne to label it "the new industrial epidemic".[8]

The increasing incidence of cumulative trauma disorders is one of the reasons why workers' compensation rates have increased so rapidly in many states. The National Council on Compensation Insurance reports that medical costs have increased at an average rate of 14% per year, and indemnity costs, which include wage compensation reimbursement and permanent partial disability awards, have increased at a rate of 11%.[9] The same organization estimates the average carpal tunnel cost per claim, including lost productivity time, to be $29,000.[10] Liberty Mutual Insurance Company reports that upper extremity cumulative trauma disorder costs have quadrupled since 1987 and now comprise 3% of all workers' compensation claims and 3.5% of total cost.[10] Occasional cases of carpal tunnel syndrome under litigation can cost in excess of $100,000.[11]

Carpal Tunnel Syndrome Incidence Studies

One of the first studies on the incidence of carpal tunnel syndrome to evaluate surgical and nonsurgical cases was conducted for the community of Rochester, Minnesota, during the years 1961 through 1980.[12] This study revealed an age-adjusted incidence of 105 cases per 100,000 population with a ratio of almost 8:1 of females over males. The incidence gradually increased from 88 to 125 per 100,000 population over the course of this study.

Washington state workers' compensation data on carpal tunnel syndrome revealed a lower female-to-male ratio and an overall incidence somewhat higher, at 175 per 100,000 full-time employees.[13] Here, too, the incidence rate increased gradually from 1985 through 1990. The incidence of disabling carpal tunnel syndrome claims in Oregon from 1987 through 1991 was 91 per 100,000 workers. The percentage of carpal tunnel cases increased from 1.9% to 3.7% of total claims during this time, with claims costs reaching nearly $10,000 per case.[14]

In 1987, the Sentinel Event Notification System for Occupation Risk was established to perform surveillance of selected occupational conditions, including carpal tunnel syndrome.[15] This cooperative state/federal program is funded by the National Institute for Occupational Safety and Health. The organizational components include an interactive transmission of data from health care providers to surveillance centers

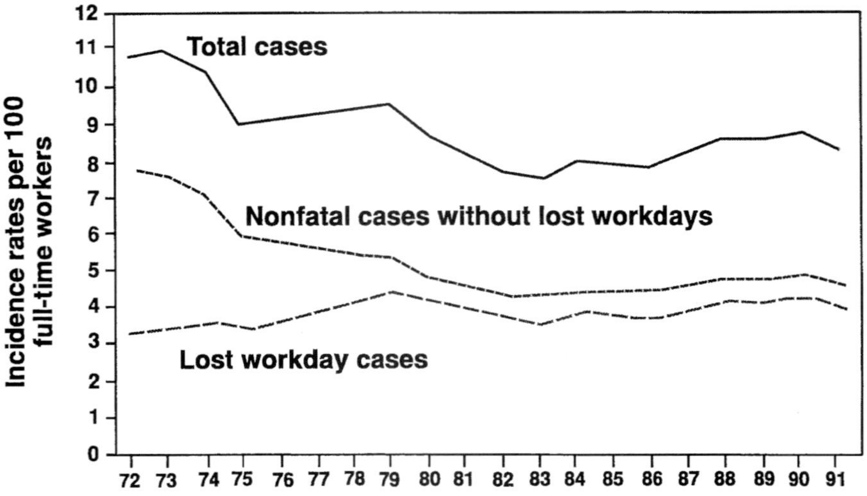

Fig. 1 Occupational injury and illness incidence rates, private industry, 1972-1991. (Reproduced from the Department of Labor: *Occupational Injuries and Illnesses in the U.S. by Industry*. Washington, DC, Bureau of Labor Statistics, 1993, pp 1-84.)

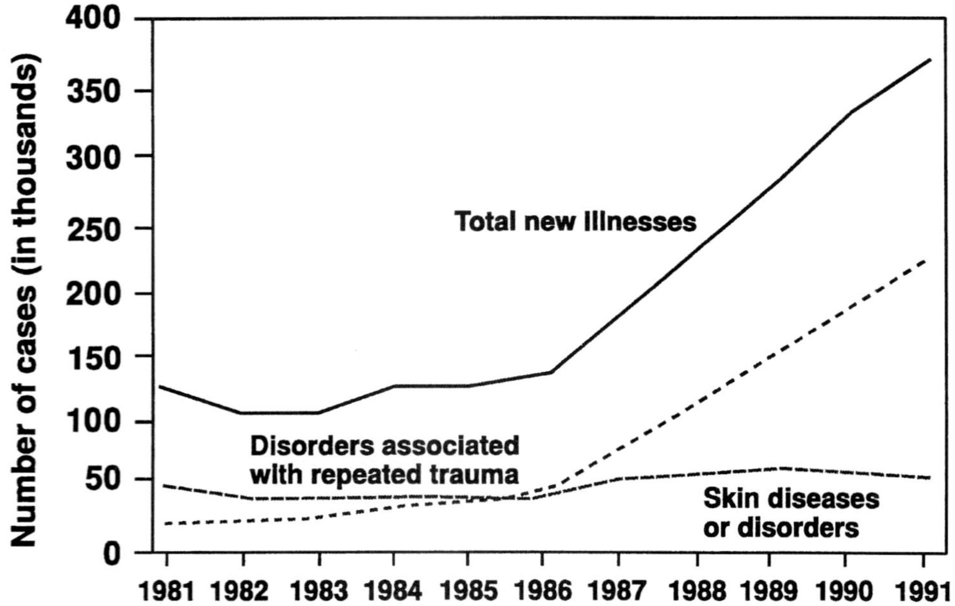

Fig. 2 Number of new occupational illnesses, private industry, 1981-1991. (Reproduced from the Department of Labor: *Occupational Injuries and Illnesses in the U.S. by Industry*. Washington, DC, Bureau of Labor Statistics, 1993, pp 1-84.)

where the data are analyzed with the ultimate goals of identifying workers at risk and initiating specific recommendations to reduce work place hazards.

Under this program, the most comprehensive data relative to the incidence of carpal tunnel surgery have recently been compiled by the Wisconsin Division of Health.[3] Wisconsin initiated mandatory reporting of all surgical cases under procedural codes 04.43 (ICD 9-CM) or 64721 (CPT-4). This covered all free-standing ambulatory and hospital outpatient surgeries in the state. During the time period from July 1990 through March 1993 there were almost 25,000 surgical cases involving almost 20,000 patients. Of these, 26.1% were workers' compensation patients. The overall incidence was 148 per 100,000 population. The surgical incidence for females peaked in the 45- to 55-year-old group whereas that for males gradually rose in incidence to almost equaling females in the over 65-year-old age group (Fig. 3). The workers' compensation case rate peaked in the prime working ages of 35 to 55 for both sexes (Fig. 4).

Return to Work Studies

Accurate estimates of productivity and wage loss reimbursement costs depend on return to work data. There have been three published series comparing open and endoscopic carpal tunnel release relative to return to work. Dr. Agee and associates[16] reported in 1992 an overall difference of 22 days earlier return to work by the endoscopically treated patients. For patients not covered by workers' compensation, there was a difference of 29 days. Dr. Browne and associates[17] compared a dual portal endoscopic technique with open carpal tunnel release and showed an improvement in return to work of 14 days earlier by the endoscopic group. The Palmer and associates[18] study of Minnesota patients in 1993 showed an overall improvement of 23 days earlier return to work with a single portal technique over the open procedure. There was a 27-day improvement in the workers' compensation group and a 16-day improvement in the group not covered by workers' compensation. As a whole, the latter group also returned to work statistically sooner than the workers' compensation patients.

A follow-up survey by telephone and written questionnaire on this patient population was recently completed by one of the authors (DHP) to evaluate the direct and indirect costs of carpal tunnel surgery. Data were collected on salaries, wage loss reimbursement, permanent partial disability awards and patient satisfaction. Of patients in the original study, 68% were contacted. The time of follow-up was a mean of 2.2 years after their procedure.

Economic Analysis

Wisconsin and Minnesota are contiguous midwestern states with similar population numbers and demographics. In this analysis, the Wisconsin surveillance study was used as the prime incidence data base, and statistics from the Minnesota study on patient costs

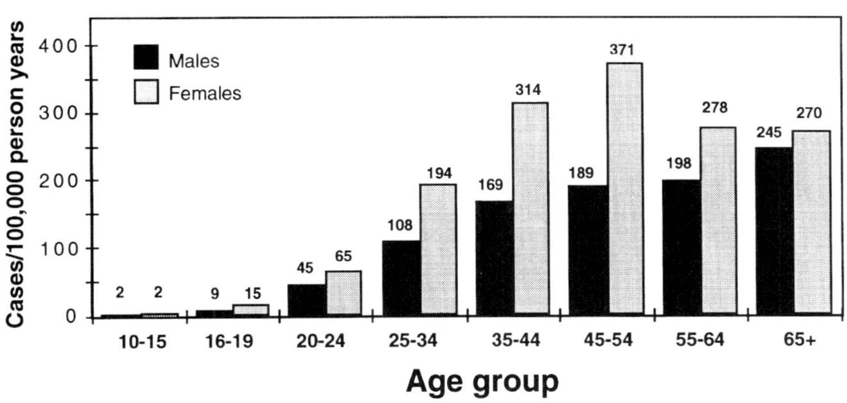

Fig. 3 Wisconsin carpal tunnel syndrome surgery incidence case rate, July 1990 to March 1993. (Reproduced with permission from Hanrahan L, Higgins D, Anderson H, et al: Wisconsin occupational carpal tunnel syndrome surveillance: The incidence of surgically treated cases. *Wis Med J* 1993;12:685-689.)

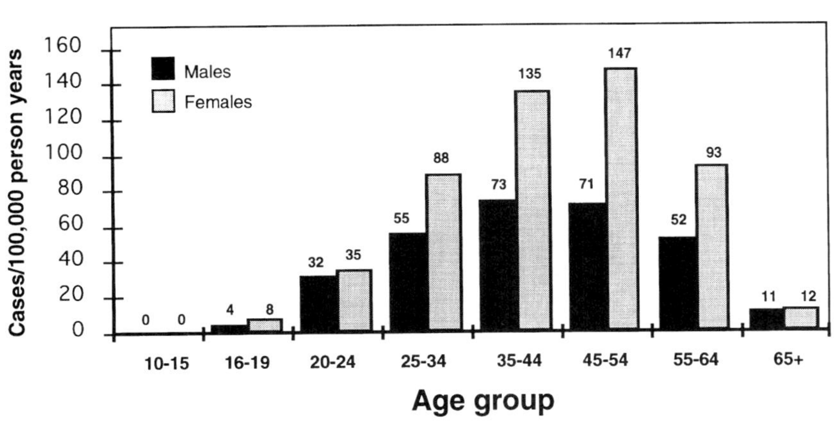

Fig. 4 Wisconsin carpal tunnel syndrome surgery incidence workers' compensation case rate, July 1990 to March 1993. (Reproduced with permission from Hanrahan L, Higgins D, Anderson H, et al: Wisconsin occupational carpal tunnel syndrome surveillance: The incidence of surgically treated cases. *Wis Med J* 1993;12:685-689.)

Table 1
Wisconsin surveillance study groups according to work status

		No. Cases/Year	Percent
Group I	Medicare (over 65)*	1,808	19.9
Group II	Other nonworkers	2,800	30.8
Group III	Workers not covered by Workers' Compensation	2,108	23.2
Group IV	Workers covered by Workers' Compensation	2,372	26.1
Total		9,088	100.0

*Excluding cases covered by Workers' Compensation

Table 2
Economic costs—open carpal tunnel surgery

	Per Case	Wisconsin (Millions)	U.S. (Millions)
Group I	1,804	3.26	166.4
Group II	1,804	5.05	257.6
Group III	3,353	7.06	360.4
Group IV	9,644	22.89	1,167.8
Total		38.26	1,952.2

Table 3
Economic costs—endoscopic carpal tunnel surgery

	Per Case	Wisconsin (Millions)	U.S. (Millions)
Group I	2,136	3.86	196.9
Group II	2,136	5.98	305.1
Group III	2,782	5.86	298.8
Group IV	6,963	16.52	842.8
Total		32.22	1,643.6

and return to work were used to arrive at an estimate of the economic cost of carpal tunnel surgery in Wisconsin.

The Wisconsin surgical survey population was divided into four groups depending on work status (Table 1). Group I is the over age 65 Medicare group, excluding cases covered by workers' compensation. Group II are patients not employed excluding Medicare patients. Group III are those workers not covered by workers' compensation. Group IV are those patients covered by workers' compensation. During the time period covered by the survey there were 9,088 surgeries performed per year in Wisconsin. According to the 1990 U.S. Census Report,[19] the Wisconsin population is 1.96% of the U.S. population. Even though Wisconsin may not be precisely representative of the United States as a whole, it is still possible to use this data to estimate that approximately 463,673 carpal tunnel procedures are performed in the United States annually.

Direct costs of carpal tunnel surgery include physician reimbursement costs, which average $641 for patients not covered by workers' compensation and $889 for those covered under workers' compensation. Facility fees were $1,163 per case in the Wisconsin survey.[20] Other medical costs, which are harder to quantify and were not part of this analysis, include the cost of preoperative treatment, physical therapy, and electrophysiologic testing. Direct costs affect all patients in all groups.

Indirect economic costs include the loss of productivity (which affects Groups III and IV), wage loss reimbursement (Groups III and IV), and permanent impairment awards (Group IV). According to the Bureau of Labor Statistics, the average worker loses $399 per week in productivity costs when out of work.[21] In our follow-up survey, wage loss reimbursement costs averaged $21 per week from private disability for patients not covered by workers' compensation and $383 per week for workers' compensation cases. Permanent partial disability awards averaged $1,383. Other potential indirect costs relating to carpal tunnel surgery, including attorney fees, cost to industry to retrain or hire replacement workers, administration costs, and others, are not part of this analysis.

In our center, endoscopic carpal tunnel release increased the direct costs by $332 per case due to the cost of endoscopic equipment.[18] However, for patients treated endoscopically, the cost of lost productivity decreased by the effect of 3.85 weeks earlier return to work in the workers' compensation group and 2.30 weeks in the group not covered. Wage loss reimbursement also decreased by the effect of 3.85 weeks per case in the workers' compensation group.

Cost estimates for each of the Wisconsin surgical groups can be calculated from this data. The estimated cost for the population of Wisconsin is in excess of $38 million for open carpal tunnel surgery and for the United States nearly $2 billion annually (Table 2). Although costs for patients having endoscopic carpal tunnel surgery increased in Groups I and II, the overall estimated cost for the total population decreased by $6 million for the state of Wisconsin and by approximately $300 million for the nation (Table 3). These figures represent about 16% of total costs.

Although the number of endoscopic carpal tunnel releases being performed in the United States is not currently known, due to more accurate coding requirements we now have reliable figures from the Health Care Financing Administration for the Medicare population. HCFA reports there were 75,321 carpal tunnel procedures performed in 1992 and of these, 3,168, or 4% of the total, were performed endoscopically (personal communication, HCFA, October 22, 1993). This represents an incidence of 233 surgical cases per 100,000 of the covered Medicare population.

Discussion

From the follow-up survey, non-workers' compensation patients were generally satisfied with the results of their procedure, whether performed open or endoscopically, with an overall satisfaction rating of 8.2 on a 0 to 10 scale (Fig. 5). Workers' compensation patients were much less satisfied. To paraphrase Henry Sigerist's statement in 1958, it is apparent that even though occupational carpal tunnel syndrome, particularly those cases covered under workers' compensation, may be biologically similar to nonoccupational carpal tunnel syndrome, the disorder is vastly different socially, psychologically, and economically.[22]

The cost figures presented here are likely to underestimate the actual costs of carpal tunnel treatment for several reasons. The dollar amounts do not reflect cases treated without surgery; nor do they include costs relating to pre- or postoperative treatment or diagnostic testing. Other indirect costs to industry, exclusive of productivity losses, wage loss reimbursement, and permanent impairment awards, are also not represented. Other states have reported higher medical and indemnity costs for carpal tunnel surgery, and data from Minnesota and Wisconsin may not be representative of the rest of the country.[14,23]

The higher incidence in Wisconsin of surgically treated cases of carpal tunnel syndrome (compared to the Rochester data, which includes both surgical and nonsurgical cases) may indicate a higher percentage of patients being treated surgically in Wisconsin or more likely a true increase in incidence since 1980, when the Rochester study was completed. Washington state experienced an even higher rate of occupational carpal tunnel syndrome, and these rates include nonsurgical cases as well.[13] The Wisconsin data also exhibit good distributional agreement with an earlier study from Canada.[24]

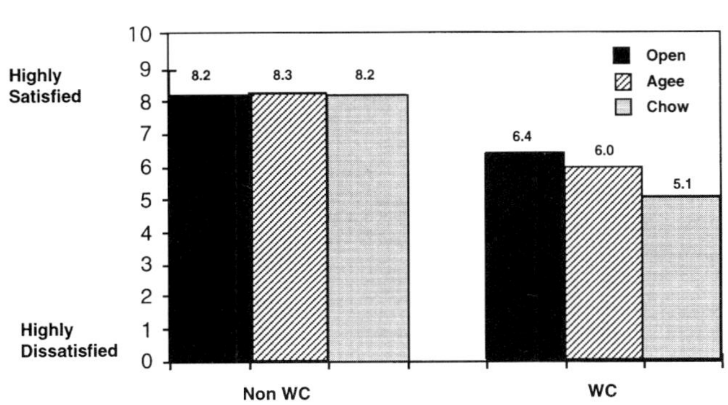

Fig. 5 Results of a carpal tunnel release patient satisfaction survey.

The ultimate purpose of gathering surveillance data is to identify hazards and establish preventive programs to reduce the incidence of occupational carpal tunnel syndrome. Prevention of this disorder is possible in the work place.[25] The state of Oregon, using a number of preventive measures, reduced its lost work day incidence rate by over 21% and total case rate by 18% from 1988 through 1991.[14] Zurn Industries, using ergonomic training sessions and work-site modifications, experienced a 30% reduction in cumulative trauma disorder claims in 1992.[9] Surveillance of carpal tunnel syndrome should play a vital role in the collection of occupational data, its analysis, dissemination of health-care information, and initiation of work-site modifications in those populations at risk.

Summary

In conclusion, we estimate the incidence of carpal tunnel surgery to be between 400,000 and 500,000 cases annually in the United States, with economic costs in excess of $2 billion per year. The costs incurred in workers' compensation cases are almost three times those of other workers and five times those of nonworkers. Despite an increase in medical costs for endoscopic carpal tunnel release, the procedure has a potential to decrease overall costs by lowering productivity and wage reimbursement losses. With better surveillance and data collection systems, workers at risk can be identified and the incidence of occupational carpal tunnel syndrome reduced through appropriate work-site intervention.

References

1. Schenck RR: Keep in touch with pain. *Safety Health* 1988;12:39-42.
2. Park CH, Wagener DK, Winn DM, et al (eds): *Health Conditions Among the Currently Employed: United States, 1988.* National Center for Health Statistics, Hyattsville, MD, Department of Health and Human Services (Publication No. 93-1514), 1993.
3. Hanrahan LP, Higgins D, Anderson H, et al: Project SENSOR: Wisconsin surveillance of occupational carpal tunnel syndrome. *Wis Med J* 1991;90:80-83.
4. McNeely EM: Who's counting anyway? The problem with occupational safety and health statistics. *J Occup Med* 1991;33:1071-1075.
5. Hanrahan LP, Moll MB: Injury surveillance. *Am J Pub Health* 1989;79(suppl):38-45.
6. Bureau of Labor Statistics: *Occupational Injuries and Illnesses in the United States by Industry, 1991.* Washington, DC, BLS Release, Department of Labor 1993;5:1-3.
7. Hadler NM: Is carpal tunnel syndrome an injury that qualifies for workers compensation insurance? *NCCI Digest* 1987;2:49-58.
8. Browne CD, Nolan BM, Faithfull DK: Occupational repetition strain injuries: Guidelines for diagnosis and management. *Med J Aust* 1984;140:329-332.
9. National Council on Compensation Insurance: *Workers' Compensation: Business at Risk. 1993 Issues Report.* Boca Raton, FL, National Council on Compensation Insurance, 1993.

10. Tallying the true costs of on-the-job cumulative trauma disorders. *CTD News* 1993;2:1-4.
11. St. Paul Fire and Marine Insurance Co: *Upper Extremity Cumulative Trauma Disorders, Oct 1989 to Oct 1990.* St. Paul, MN, Loss Central Services, 1992.
12. Stevens JC, Sun S, Beard CM, et al: Carpal tunnel syndrome in Rochester, Minnesota, 1960-1980. *Neurology* 1988;38:134-138.
13. Franklin GM, Haug J, Heyer N, et al: Occupational carpal tunnel syndrome in Washington State, 1984-1988. *Am J Pub Health* 1991; 81:741-746.
14. *Carpal Tunnel Syndrome in Oregon, 1987-1991.* Salem, OR, Oregon Department of Insurance and Finance, September 1992.
15. Baker EL: Sentinel Event Notification System for Occupational Risks (SENSOR): The concept. *Am J Pub Health* 1989;79 (suppl):18-20.
16. Agee JM, McCarroll HR Jr, Tortosa RD, et al: Endoscopic release of the carpal tunnel: A randomized prospective multicenter study. *J Hand Surg* 1992;17A:987-995.
17. Brown RA, Gelberman RH, Seiler JG III, et al: Carpal tunnel release: A prospective, randomized assessment of open and endoscopic methods. *J Bone Joint Surg* 1993;75A:1265-1275.
18. Palmer DH, Paulson JC, Lane-Larsen CL, et al: Endoscopic carpal tunnel release: A comparison of two techniques with open release. *Arthroscopy* 1993;9:498-508.
19. Population trends and congressional apportionment, in *1990 Census Profile.* Washington, DC, U.S. Department of Commerce, 1990.
20. Hanrahan L, Higgins D, Anderson H, et al: Wisconsin occupational carpal tunnel syndrome surveillance: The incidence of surgically treated cases. *Wis Med J* 1993;12:685-689.
21. Brown RA, Gelberman RH, Seiler JG III, et al: Carpal tunnel release: A prospective randomized assessment of open and endoscopic methods. *J Bone Joint Surg* 1993;75A:1265-1275.
22. Falk LA: Medical sociology: The contributions of Dr. Henry E. Sigerist. *J Hist Med Allied Sci* 1958;143:214-228.
23. Detailed claim information for 1991 purchased insurance indemnity claims with incurred losses of $5,000 or more. *The Research Review* 1994;2:1-6.
24. Liss GM, Armstrong C, Kusiak RA, et al: Use of provincial health insurance plan billing data to estimate carpal tunnel syndrome morbidity and surgery rates. *Am J Ind Med* 1992;22:395-409.
25. Silverstein BA, Fine LJ, Armstrong TJ: Carpal tunnel syndrome: Causes and a prevention strategy. *Semin Occup Med* 1986;1:213-221.

Elbow

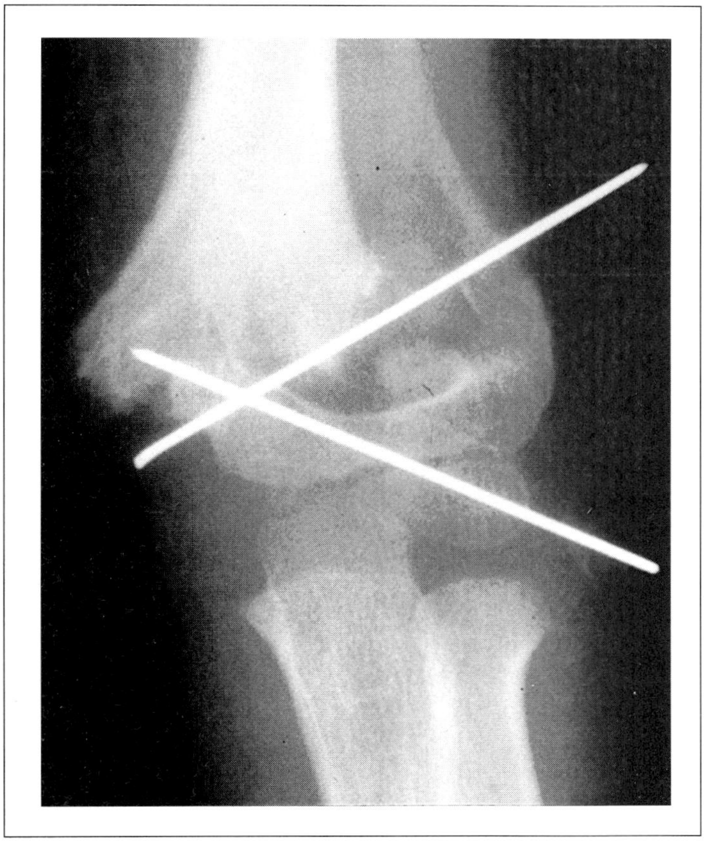

Current Concepts in the Treatment of Fractures of the Radial Head, the Olecranon, and the Coronoid

Bernard F. Morrey, MD

Fractures of the radial head and the olecranon are two of the most common fractures of the elbow; together, they account for more than half of the fractures that occur at that site. An isolated fracture of the coronoid process is a rare and infrequently reported injury. Although most elbow fractures are treated readily with existing techniques, the unpredictable and sometimes sinister behavior of these seemingly innocuous fractures is well known. Thus, it is appropriate to consider some of the more current concepts with regard to their treatment.

Fractures of the Radial Head

Classification

The well-recognized Mason classification is particularly useful in the treatment of radial head fractures.[1] However, it is critical to realize that its true utility is limited to fractures without an associated injury. From a practical standpoint, therefore, it is appropriate first to consider fractures of the radial head as either simple or complex.

Simple fractures, by definition, are fractures without an associated injury. They are best analyzed and treated according to the Mason classification as Type I, undisplaced; Type II, displaced, with involvement of more than 30% of the head; and Type III, comminuted.

Complex fractures are associated with another fracture or with a ligamentous injury. The associated fracture typically is of the proximal part of the ulna and occasionally is of the distal part of the humerus, particularly the capitellum. Ligamentous injury occurs more commonly and can involve either the medial or the lateral collateral ligament as the result of an elbow dislocation. Although this complex popularly has been referred to as a Mason Type-IV fracture, it was described by Johnston,[2] not Mason, and in my system it is considered as a complex injury rather than as an extension of the Mason classification. An injury of the distal radioulnar joint commonly is referred to as the Essex-Lopresti injury.[3,4] The isolated injury of a collateral ligament and the Essex-Lopresti injury each occur with a frequency of less than 5%; only 20 such injuries were treated at the Mayo Clinic over a 35-year period.[4]

Treatment

Simple Fractures There is little question that the undisplaced (Type-I) fracture, because of its excellent prognosis and lack of concurrent soft-tissue or osseous injury, should be treated nonsurgically. Treatment should consist of early motion, usually within several days or as early as pain allows. I prefer to aspirate a painful, tense hemarthrosis and to inject the joint with a local anesthetic with epinephrine.

In a previous study,[5] early motion was associated with a 90% chance of a good result; however, complications still can occur, the most common and serious of which is nonunion. Although its exact prevalence is difficult to estimate, nonunion has followed about 5% of the Mason Type-I injuries in my experience. Other complications include the loss of elbow extension, mild loss of forearm rotation, and occasional aching with use.

The treatment of a symptomatic nonunion is radial head resection. I have not found it helpful or prudent to remove only the fracture fragment, because doing so tends to cause the residual radial head to subluxate. Other authors, however, have reported that this technique is effective.[6,7] If a partial resection is carried out, careful inspection of the radiohumeral relationship throughout pronation and supination is necessary to assure the surgeon that there is no tendency for the radial head to subluxate.

The treatment of the displaced (Type-II) fracture of the radial head is controversial.[5,7-9] Currently, decisions regarding treatment tend to be made on the basis of an examination of the elbow after the administration of a local anesthetic block. If at least 20° to 140° of flexion and 70° of forearm rotation in both directions can be obtained, it is appropriate to treat this fracture nonsurgically. I typically immobilize the elbow and wrist for 2 to 3 weeks and then allow and encourage an active range of motion. Thus, with the exception of the somewhat longer period of rest and protection, the treatment is similar to that of the Type-I fracture. Failure to achieve a satisfactory range of motion after the administration of the local anesthetic block is an indication for surgical treatment, especially in younger adults.

Immediate, complete radial-head resection no longer is thought to be an acceptable treatment of a Type-II fracture. The results of acute resection of the fracture fragment are unpredictable, as was noted previously. Therefore, open reduction and internal fixation should be offered to patients who have an inadequate range of motion when examined after the administration of the local anesthetic block (Fig. 1).[10-12] A Kocher approach should be used (Fig. 2). The capsular incision should not be placed too far posteriorly or directed too

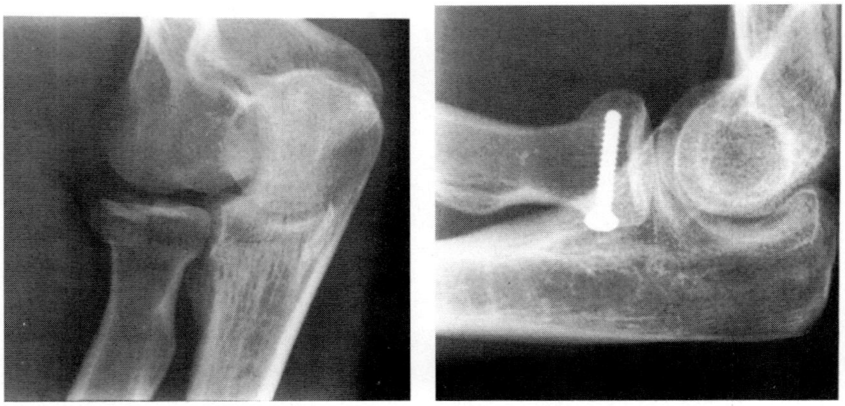

Fig. 1 **Left,** A Type-II radial-head fracture. **Right,** After open reduction and internal fixation with the most standard technique using an AO mini-screw.

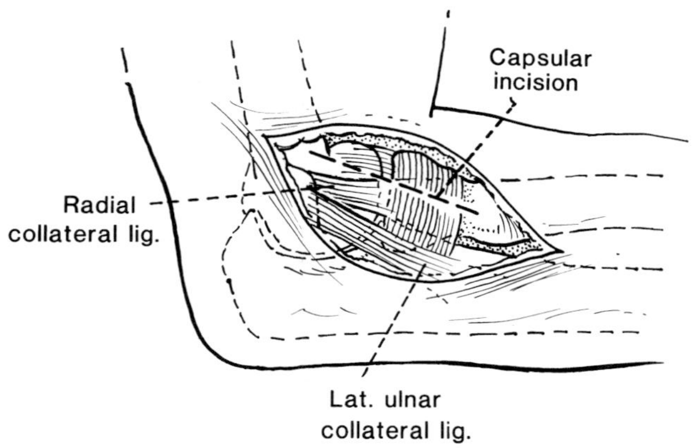

Fig. 2 The exposure of the fracture through the Kocher interval, in which the capsular incision is made anterior to the inferior aspect of the radial humeral capsular ligamentous complex. This approach avoids injury to the fibers that stabilize the ulna to the humerus. (Reproduced with permission from the Mayo Foundation.)

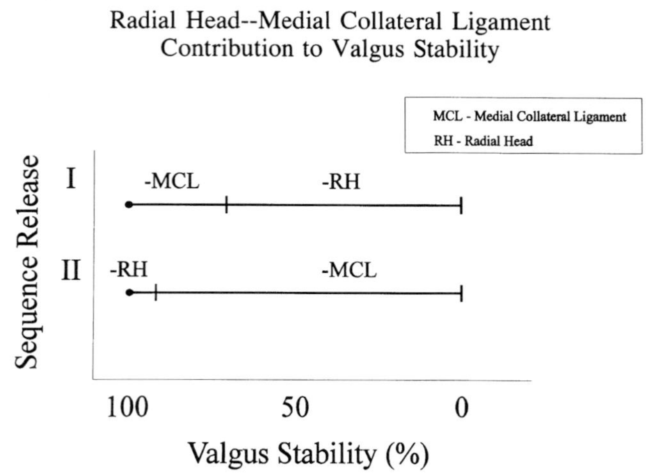

Fig. 3 The relationship of valgus stability to the presence of the radial head and the medial collateral ligament. When the medial collateral ligament is intact, the radial head is less important. When the medial collateral ligament is compromised, valgus stability is provided by the competency of the radiohumeral joint.

obliquely because of the risk of injuring the posterior fibers of the lateral collateral ligament complex. These fibers are called the lateral ulnar collateral ligament, and their disruption can result in late instability of the elbow. I prefer to use one or two AO cortical mini-screws to fix the fragment. Herbert screws also are effective fixation devices but are more expensive. I avoid the use of smooth pins. Placement of the screw can be difficult when the fragment lies in the sigmoid notch. When this rare event occurs, I insert a lag screw into this segment if it is of adequate size for secure fixation. The radiohumeral joint can be explored through a more distal capsular incision if direct access to the fragment is required.

Delayed radial-head excision may be a useful alternative to immediate open reduction and fixation when the patient is seen late or has residual symptoms after initial nonsurgical management. This method has been reported only rarely in the literature.[6] In the experience of Broberg and myself,[13] however, it led to a reduction of pain in 76% and to an improvement in elbow function in 81% of 21 patients for whom nonsurgical management had failed.

There continues to be relative agreement that a comminuted (Type-III) fracture of the radial head is best treated with complete excision within 48 hours after the injury. This method is preferred to simple removal of the displaced fragments.[5,6,8] Biomechanical studies have revealed that the elbow is stable to valgus stress if the medial collateral ligament has been preserved (Fig. 3);[14] the stabilizing effect of the radial head comes into play only when this ligament has been disrupted. Early excision is more critical for Type-III fractures than for Type-II injuries because late excision for Type-III fractures has been less successful than that for the persistently symptomatic elbow after a Type-II injury.[15] Furthermore, while internal fixation has been described for Type-III fractures,[16] it is a difficult procedure to perform, and I do not recommend it for these injuries. In my experience, approximately 10% of comminuted fractures of the radial head have occurred in association with an elbow dislocation; this combination of injuries constitutes one of the most difficult management problems.[15,17]

Complex Fractures Approximately 10% of patients who have a radial head fracture have an elbow dislocation, and conversely, about 10% of patients who have an elbow dislocation have a fracture of the radial head.[5] Little has been published with regard to the outcome of elbow fracture-dislocations. My approach is based largely on an analysis of the Mayo experience.[15] Type-I fractures associated with an elbow dislocation are protected in a splint for 10 to 14 days. I then encourage intensive active motion, because late instability rarely occurs after this injury.[15] Type-II radial-head fractures are treated with open reduction and internal fixation. In fact, this fracture-dislocation with a single displaced fragment is the ideal indication for open reduction and internal fixation of the radial head (Fig. 4).[11,12] The nonarticulating portion of the radial head is the most common portion to be fractured because it lacks strong subchondral osseous support. This anatomic feature is advantageous during fixation of the fragment because a single AO mini-screw can be inserted through the fragment and into the remainder of the radial head.[5] Even if the screw head is slightly prominent, it rarely engages the ulna. As was demonstrated previously,[15] comminuted (Type-III) fractures with elbow dislocation are best treated with early, complete excision of the radial head and immobilization for less than 3 weeks. An active range of motion then is allowed and encouraged.

Occasionally, marked valgus displacement of the elbow causes compression of the radial head and an isolated injury of the medial collateral ligament. This injury presents as a radial neck fracture, and the radiograph shows only a tilt of the radial head (Fig. 5, *left*). Unless carefully sought, the injury of the medial collateral ligament may be undetected. In this setting, my treatment of choice is reduction and fixation of the radial neck fracture with an AO mini-plate (Fig. 5, *right*). This method stabilizes the lateral column and allows the medial collateral ligament to heal.

In the treatment of fracture-dislocations of the elbow, I have never repaired the medial collateral ligament in an attempt to render it more stable and to allow a more rapid and functional rehabilitation. Although Josefsson and associates[18] recommended such an approach for the treatment of pure elbow dislocations, they did not show it to be superior to the nonsurgical treatment of that particular injury. Furthermore, those authors did not address the issue of fracture-dislocation of the elbow in their study.[18]

In some patients who have a combined radial-head fracture and elbow dislocation (Fig. 6, *left*), the ulnohumeral joint may tend to subluxate even after the radial head fracture has been fixed. In this setting, I prefer to use a distraction device rather than to perform a ligament repair. The device consists of a pin

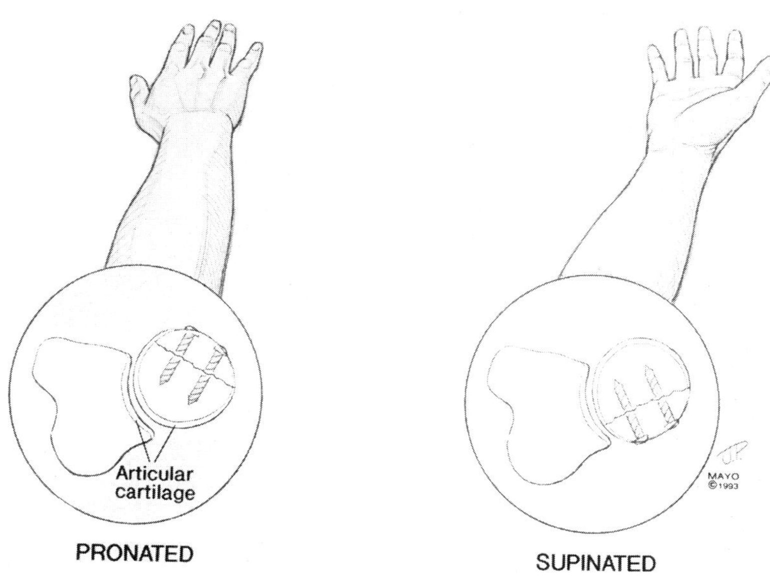

Fig. 4 Pronation and supination after reduction and internal fixation of the radial head. Most fractures of the radial head involve the nonarticulating margin; thus, fixation with screws should not cause problems with pronation and supination. (Reproduced with permission from the Mayo Foundation.)

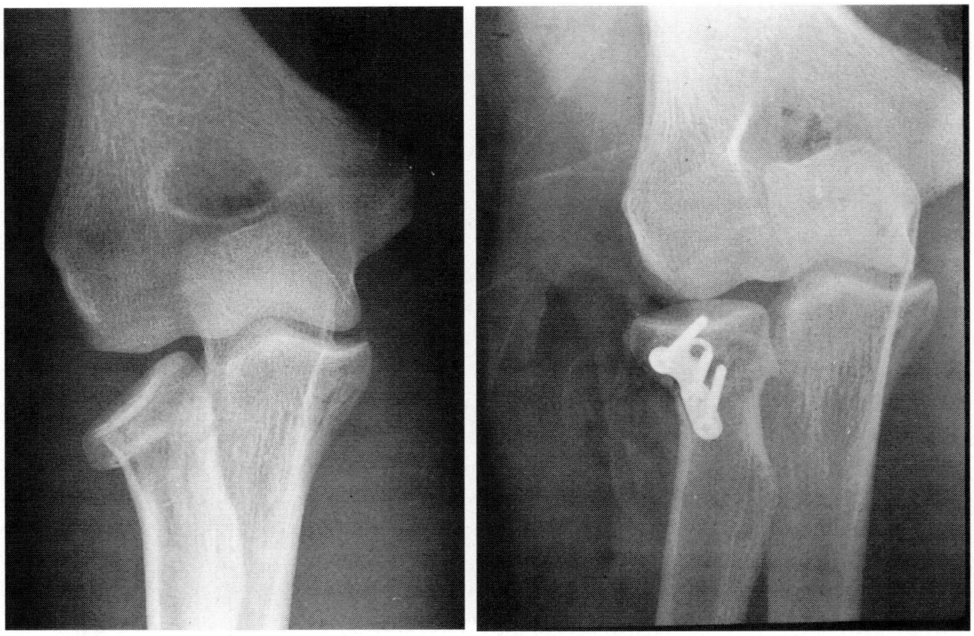

Fig. 5 **Left,** Radial neck fracture with a concurrent medial collateral ligament disruption. **Right,** After treatment with reduction and fixation with an AO mini-plate.

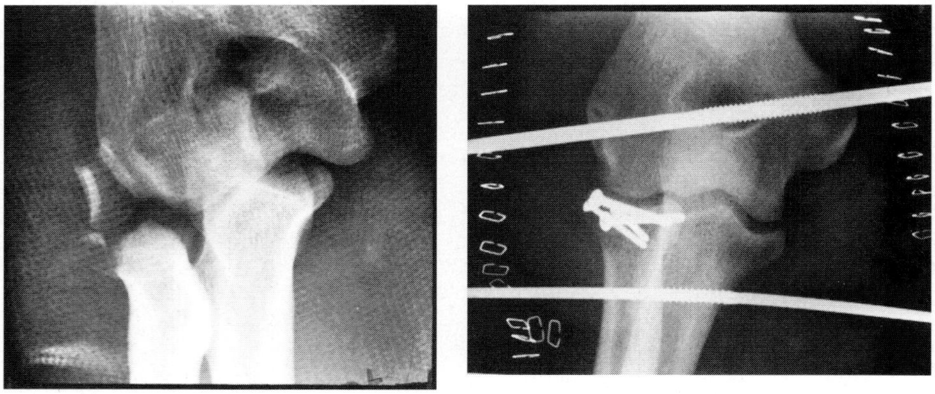

Fig. 6 **Left,** Severe fracture-dislocation of the elbow involving the radial head and the medial and lateral collateral ligaments. **Right,** The radial head was reduced and fixed and the elbow stabilized with the dynamic joint distractor.

placed across the distal part of the humerus and two pins placed in the ulna.[5] The construct, which rotates about the humeral pin, allows normal motion and maintains elbow joint stability. Forces on the radial head are neutralized or the radial head is protected by the distraction provided by the external fixation device, and varus-valgus stress is resisted by the frame (Fig. 6, *right*). Although other devices may be equally effective, I have no experience with them.

Clearly, the detection of this combined injury is the first step in its treatment.[3,4] In my experience, approximately 5% of radial head fractures were complicated by distal ligamentous disruption. Thus, physicians must have a high index of suspicion and exercise constant vigilance to avoid missing this injury, because it is very difficult to treat when not properly treated initially. My observations of the consequences of this injury occurring several months after the event suggest a spectrum of severity or instability of the wrist. I believe that an attempt to elicit tenderness over the distal radioulnar joint is the most sensitive test to suggest, if not to diagnose, this injury. The lateral radiograph of a pronated wrist is confirmatory if it shows the ulna to be dorsally subluxated.

When a radial head fracture is combined with an acute distal radioulnar disruption, the treatment begins with stabilization of the radial head with use of open reduction and internal fixation. Full supination of the forearm then usually results in reduction of the radioulnar joint. If adequate reduction is obtained, this position of supination is maintained in a cast or splint for 3 weeks. Crossed pins may be considered for stabilization of the distal radioulnar joint, but I have not used them. Surgical repair of the triangular fibrocartilage or other soft-tissue attachments of the wrist is controversial.[3,4] At the Mayo Clinic, the hand surgeons have been willing to explore and to repair the torn structures when an adequate closed reduction could not be achieved.

If the injury is not found when it is acute, the patient may have severe wrist symptoms as well as radial migration and subluxation, usually of 5 to 6 mm, as a result of the ligamentous deficiency.[19] The value of any specific treatment of this complication has not been documented in the literature.[4] I prefer an ulnar resection with the amount of ulna removed being based on the amount of radial shortening that has occurred.

Prostheses

Because of the compelling and ever-lengthening list of complications associated with silicone,[20,21] the use of this implant material has been all but abandoned in the United States. Thus, some consideration again is being given to the use of a metal implant for the treatment of a severely comminuted radial-head fracture. Carr and Howard[22] described the use of a metal radial-head implant in the 1950s, Edwards and Rostrup[23] reported the use of a similar implant in the 1960s, and Harrington and Tountas[24] reported satisfactory results with the use of a metal replacement device for the treatment of unstable radial-head fractures in the early 1980s. More recently, Knight and associates[25] reported the cases of 21 patients in whom a fracture-dislocation of the elbow had been treated with a Vitallium radial-head implant; at a mean of 4 years, minimum problems with dislocation or with prosthetic failure had been encountered, although the implant had loosened in two patients. The metal implant appears to be a potentially viable solution when radial head resection is indicated and the joint is unstable.

Prognosis

Overall, the prognosis for an uncomplicated radial-head fracture is considered quite good, with at least a 90% probability of a satisfactory result.[1,6] In my experience, 80% of 22 patients who had an elbow or ulnohumeral dislocation had a satisfactory result. In a previous report,[4] four of five patients who had a radial head fracture with an associated distal radioulnar joint disruption had a satisfactory result if diagnosed correctly.

Fractures of the Olecranon

Fractures of the olecranon generally are considered to be rather straightforward with regard to treatment and prognosis.

Classification

Colton[26] apparently was the first author to classify these fractures systematically. The AO Group recently provided a comprehensive and thorough classification system that is based on concepts that are universally applied to fractures of all joints.[27] In my practice, I have not found either of these classification systems to be particularly useful. To treat a fracture of the olecranon, the orthopaedic surgeon must determine whether the fracture is stable or unstable, comminuted or noncomminuted, and displaced or undisplaced.[28] The Mayo classification was the result of a logical consideration of these variables (Fig. 7).

Mayo Classification

Type I: Undisplaced Fractures In an undisplaced fracture, it matters little whether a single fragment or several fragments are present; thus, noncomminuted (Type-IA) and comminuted (Type-IB) fractures may be considered to be essentially the same lesion.

Type II: Displaced, Stable Fractures In this pattern, the fracture fragments are displaced more than 3 mm, but the collateral ligaments are intact and the forearm is stable in relation to the humerus. The fracture may be either noncomminuted (Type IIA) or comminuted (Type IIB).

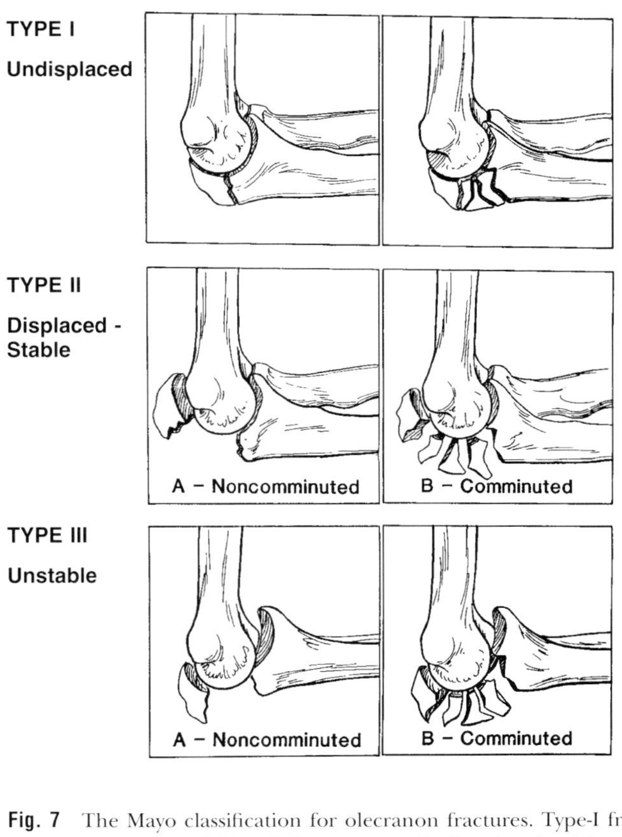

Fig. 7 The Mayo classification for olecranon fractures. Type-I fractures are undisplaced; Type-II fractures are displaced and stable; and Type-III fractures are displaced, with the forearm unstable in relation to the humerus. (Reproduced with permission from Morrey BF: Fracture of the radial head, in Morrey BF (ed): *The Elbow and Its Disorders*, ed 2. Philadelphia, PA, WB Saunders, 1993, p 408.)

Type III: Displaced, Unstable Fractures The Type-III fracture is one in which the fracture fragments are displaced and the forearm is unstable in relation to the humerus. This injury is really a fracture dislocation. It also may be either noncomminuted (Type IIIA) or comminuted (Type IIIB). Clearly, the comminuted, unstable fracture is the most difficult to treat and, of all of the fractures of the olecranon, it has the poorest prognosis.

A review of 100 olecranon fractures that were treated consecutively at the Mayo Clinic revealed 12 Type-I, 82 Type-II, and six Type-III fractures.

Treatment

The value of the Mayo classification system is that it provides a basis for treatment. Several treatment options (tension-band wiring, screw fixation, plate fixation, and resection and distraction) all have merit, depending on the fracture type (Fig. 8).

Type I: Undisplaced Fractures The Type-I injury is treated symptomatically with immobilization for comfort for about one week. Motion then is allowed as tolerated.

Under the very uncommon circumstance in which the patient cannot chance a nonunion or displacement, open reduction and internal fixation might be considered. This method of treatment provides absolute stability to a fracture fragment that is displaced 2 to 3 mm, and thus it allows immediate motion with confidence. Typically, however, such treatment is not necessary.

Type II: Displaced, Stable Fractures The noncomminuted, displaced, stable (Type-IIA) fracture is the classic injury pattern (Fig. 9, *left*). It is the most common type of olecranon fracture, and it can be treated effectively with tension-band wiring (Fig. 9, *right*).[28-35] I prefer to use a 6.5-mm AO cancellous-bone screw, because it has less of a tendency to back out and therefore does not need to be removed.[36] There is evidence that this method of fixation creates a stable construct.[37] If the security of fixation is in question, a figure-of-eight tension-band wire may be added to the screw.

The treatment of a comminuted but stable (Type-IIB) fracture depends on the age of the patient. When the patient is 60 years of age or older, the comminuted fragments are removed and the triceps is advanced (Fig. 10).[38,39] Care should be taken to reattach the triceps tendon as closely as possible to the articular surface of the ulna. Use of this technique virtually ensures that a second operation will not be necessary, and the functional result of this method is comparable with that of fixation.[39] In patients who are younger than 60 years of age, I employ a 3.5-mm AO dynamic-compression plate contoured to fix the comminuted fragments after they have been reduced anatomically (Fig. 11). The advantage of this technique is that it stabilizes and neutralizes the forces across the coronoid fracture from the tip of the olecranon to the shaft (Fig. 12). The distance between the coronoid process and the olecranon should not be compromised by compressing the comminuted fragments. The disadvantage of the technique is that the edge of the plate is prominent

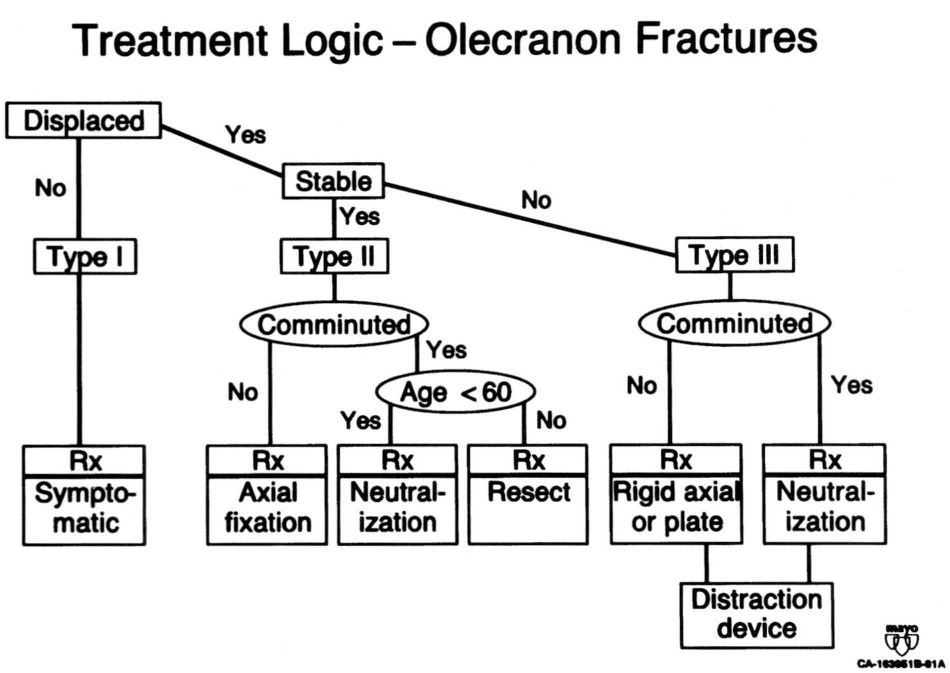

Fig. 8 Recommended treatment for olecranon fractures as based on the elements of the Mayo classification. (Reproduced with permission from the Mayo Foundation.)

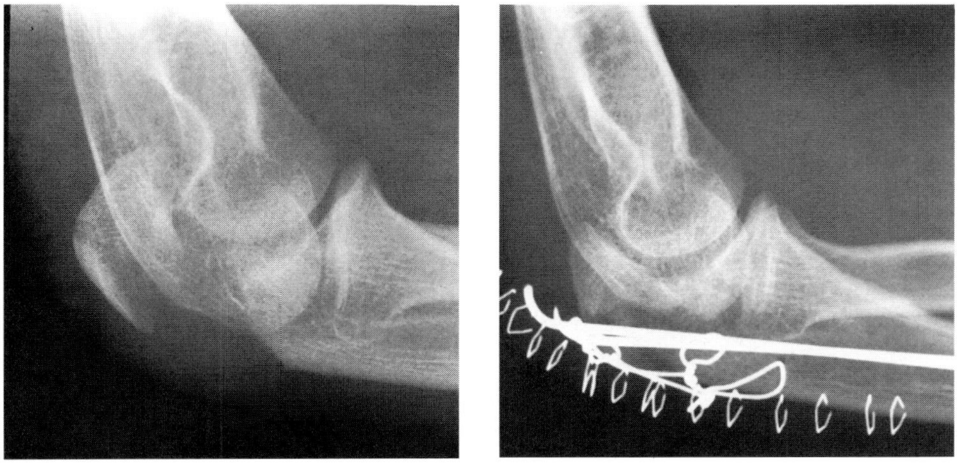

Fig. 9 **Left,** A noncomminuted, displaced, stable (Type-IIA) fracture of the olecranon. **Right,** After treatment with the AO tension-band technique. The prominence of the Kirschner wire is a common problem associated with this technique.

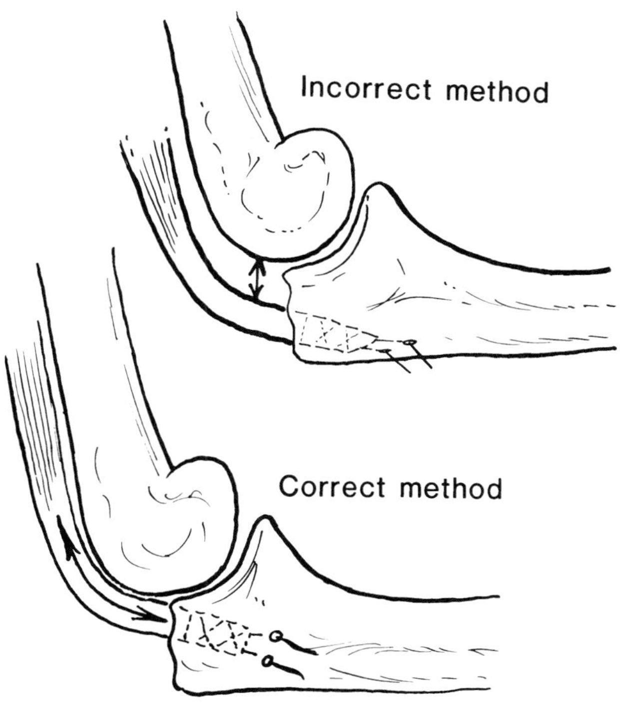

Fig. 10 Treatment of a comminuted, displaced, stable (Type-IIB) fracture of the olecranon with resection of comminuted fragments and advancement of the triceps—the treatment of choice for patients who are 60 years of age or older. The triceps should be advanced close to the articular surface to provide a stable and smooth articulation. (Reproduced with permission from the Mayo Foundation.)

under the skin at the site of the olecranon, which necessitates the removal of the plate later. Mild comminution may be treated with a tension-band wire,[40] although care must be taken to stabilize the intercalary fragments and to avoid compressing the olecranon around the coronoid process. Screw fixation is not used, however, for these displaced fractures.

Type III: Unstable, Displaced Fractures Although all Type-III fractures are extremely difficult to treat, the lack of comminution of a Type-IIIA fracture should make it possible to stabilize the olecranon to the shaft of the ulna with use of screws and a neutralization plate. Either the AO plate or specially designed plates may be used, but rigid fixation of the fracture, to provide stability to the displaced forearm, is essential. I add a distraction device to neutralize the force on the fracture; the device that I use, which is described later, allows motion while it decreases the stresses across the fracture site. I have found the distraction device to be more useful than simple external fixation that provides rigidity but does not allow motion.[41]

The comminuted, unstable, displaced (Type-IIIB) fracture is unquestionably the most difficult type to treat. The comminution threatens the adequacy of plate fixation alone. In this setting, the distraction device is particularly helpful, if not essential. The olecranon fracture should be reduced and rigidly fixed, and the distraction device can be added to further neutralize the force on the system, provide stability to the construct, and allow some controlled elbow motion immediately after fixation is accomplished (Fig. 13). The distraction device (DJD; Howmedica, Rutherford, NJ) consists of a pin that is threaded through the axis of rotation of the humerus—that is, it enters through the lateral epicondyle, crosses the trochlea, and emerges at the inferior aspect of the medial epicondyle. The ulnar pins are placed across the ulna distal to the ulnar fixation device. The technique of application of the device has been described elsewhere.[5] The ulnar nerve must be exposed sufficiently to protect it when the device is being applied. Postoperatively, motion is allowed in a continuous-passive-motion machine with the distraction device in place. Active assisted motion then is encouraged. The fixator is maintained for approximately 4 weeks and then is removed with the patient

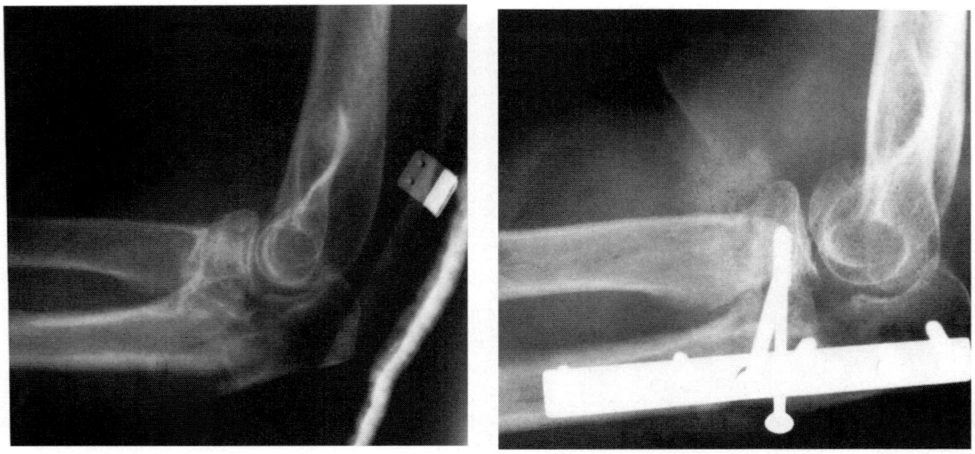

Fig. 11 **Left,** Type-IIB olecranon fracture. **Right,** After treatment with a dynamic compression neutralization plate.

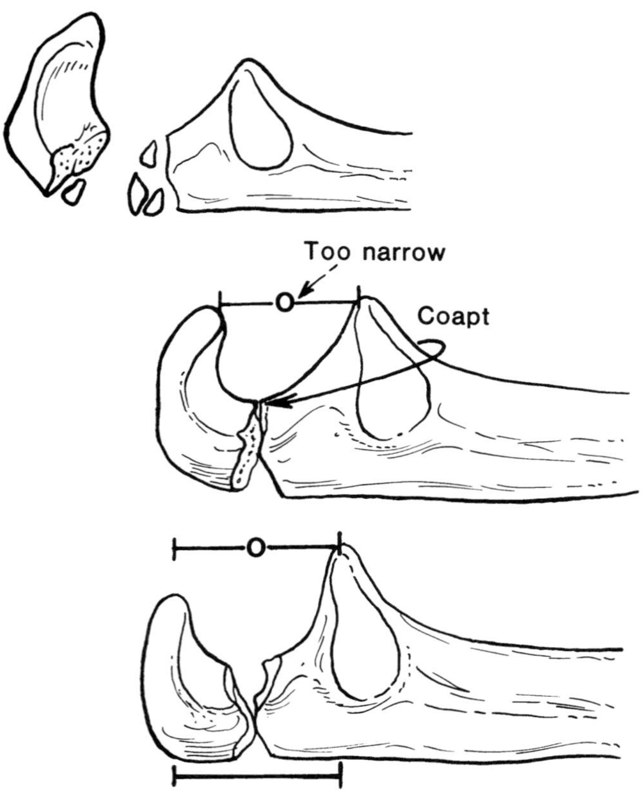

Fig. 12 Treatment of a comminuted, displaced, stable (Type-IIB) fracture of the olecranon in a patient who is younger than 60 years of age. Care should be taken not to compress the comminuted segments, because to do so will narrow the distance between the coronoid process and the olecranon and predispose to early osteoarthrosis. (Reproduced with permission from the Mayo Foundation.)

under general anesthesia. I then rely heavily on splints both to protect the collateral ligaments and to restore motion. Adjustable splints are worn by the patient at night to restore flexion or extension, depending on which motion is most needed. During the day, an adjustable splint is applied to restore motion in the opposite direction.[5]

The results of the treatment of an uncomplicated olecranon fracture have been quite good. In several series, the union rate has been more than 95%;[29,30,32,36] however, the complication rate has been extremely high, if a reoperation to remove the hardware is considered to be a complication.[28,33,42,43] With the exclusion of hardware removal, ulnar nerve paresthesia and nonunion are the two most common complications.[42] It is typical for a patient to lose 10° to 15° of extension. Unless severe soft-tissue injury has occurred, the loss of more than 10° of flexion is uncommon. Ectopic bone is seen occasionally, but usually only when there is a major soft-tissue component to the injury or a closed head injury, or when multiple surgical procedures have been performed within the first 3 to 5 days.

Fractures of the Coronoid Process

Very little has been written with regard to fractures of the coronoid process, and most published studies have been isolated case reports.[44,45] The classification system of Regan and myself[46] is useful as a guide for prognosis and treatment (Fig. 14).

A Type-I fracture is a small chip fracture that has no clinical importance except to suggest the possibility of an elbow dislocation. The fracture is treated symptomatically, because the soft-tissue element (the elbow dislocation) is the more serious part of the injury pattern.

A Type-II fracture involves about 50% of the coronoid process. It may or may not be associated with an unstable ulnohumeral joint. If the ulnohumeral joint is unstable, the fracture should be fixed. Alternatively, the elbow may be stabilized with the distraction device without fixation of the fragment. Early motion can and should be encouraged when either technique is used.

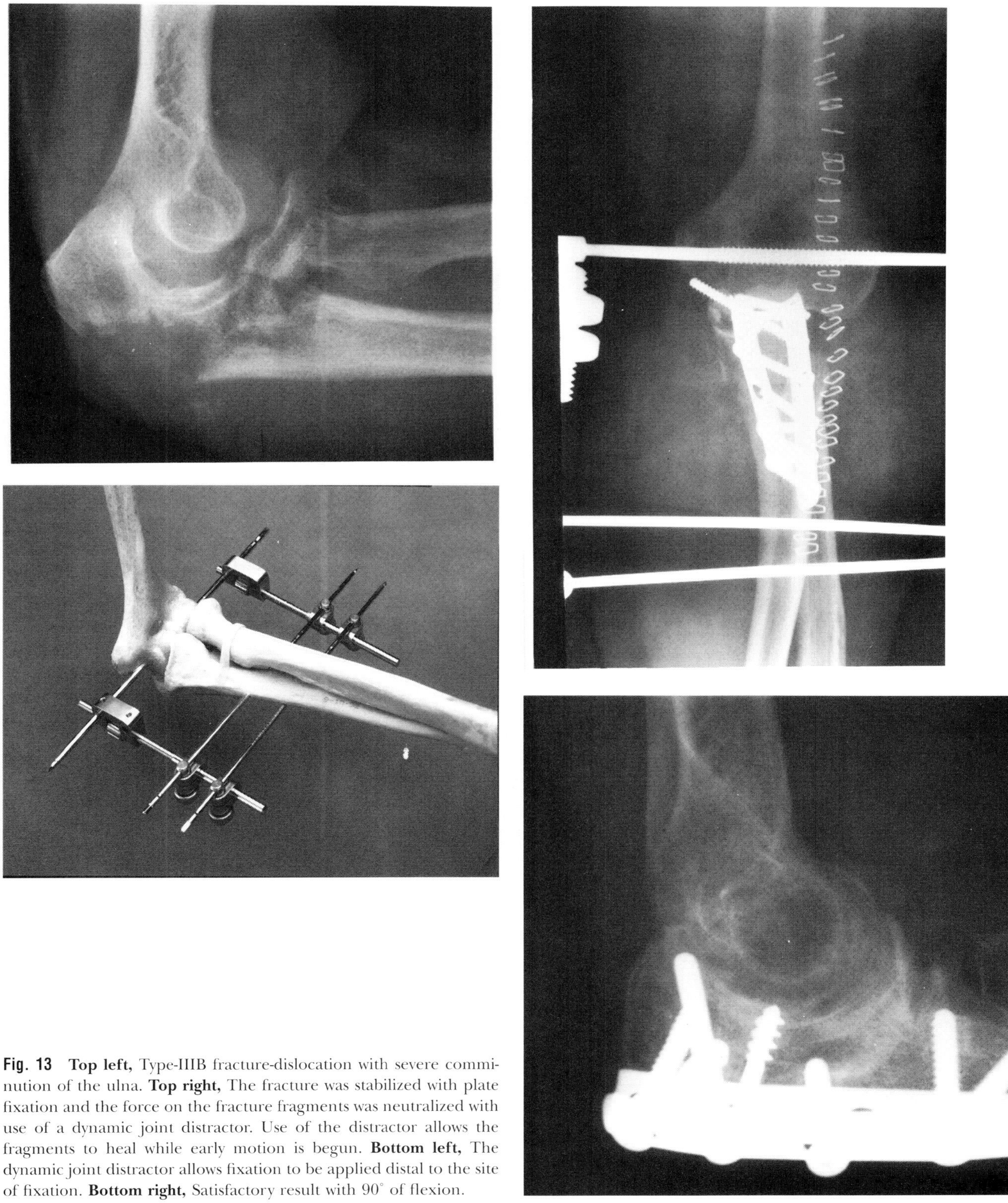

Fig. 13 **Top left,** Type-IIIB fracture-dislocation with severe comminution of the ulna. **Top right,** The fracture was stabilized with plate fixation and the force on the fracture fragments was neutralized with use of a dynamic joint distractor. Use of the distractor allows the fragments to heal while early motion is begun. **Bottom left,** The dynamic joint distractor allows fixation to be applied distal to the site of fixation. **Bottom right,** Satisfactory result with 90° of flexion.

A Type-III fracture is one in which the entire coronoid process has been fractured. If it is not badly comminuted, I recommend open reduction and internal fixation. Fracture fixation is supplemented with the distraction device to reduce pressure or to neutralize the force on the segment that has been fixed and thus allow the fracture to unite without deforming forces. When confronted with a severely comminuted Type-III fracture (fortunately a rare circumstance), I do not resect the fragments. The fragments may be stabilized

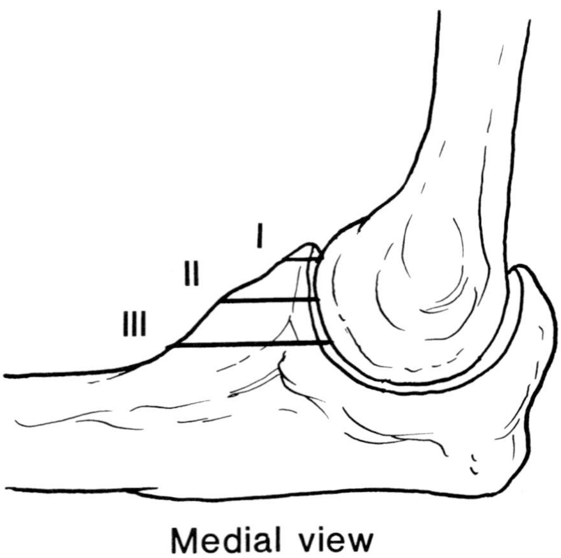

Fig. 14 The classification of coronoid fractures, which correlates with the prognosis.

with number-5 nonabsorbable suture placed through holes in the ulna to approximate them. The distraction device, which then is applied, is the only option of which I am aware that stabilizes the joint and allows early motion. It is particularly helpful with this type of fracture (Fig. 13). In my experience with 35 patients, a satisfactory result was obtained for approximately 90% of those who had a Type-I fracture, for 67% of those who had a Type-II fracture, and for only 25% of those who had a Type-III fracture.[46]

Final Comment

I have found in my practice that, although it has been variably reported in the literature,[15] one of the most important features of elbow injuries is that immobilization for more than 3 to 4 weeks after virtually any traumatic event is associated with an unsatisfactory result. Thus, the rationale for treatment of any of these fractures first must be to stabilize the injury in any way possible (reduction and fixation of fractures and repair of ligaments). The attainment of early motion is the next most decisive prognostic factor. Once the repair has been accomplished, protected early motion should be instituted to minimize the risk of late elbow stiffness. The distraction external fixator helps to achieve these goals in the treatment of the uncommon severe unstable fracture.

References

1. Mason ML: Some observations on fractures of the head of the radius with a review of one hundred cases. *Br J Surg* 1954;42:123-132.
2. Johnston GW: A follow-up of one hundred cases of fracture of the head of the radius with a review of the literature. *Ulster Med J* 1962;31:51-63.
3. Edwards GS Jr, Jupiter JB: Radial head fractures with acute distal radioulnar dislocation: Essex-Lopresti revisited. *Clin Orthop* 1988; 234:61-69.
4. Trousdale RT, Amadio PC, Cooney WP, et al: Radio-ulnar dissociation: A review of twenty cases. *J Bone Joint Surg* 1992;74A:1486-1497.
5. Morrey BF: Fracture of the radial head, in Morrey BF (ed): *The Elbow and Its Disorders*, ed 2. Philadelphia, PA, WB Saunders, 1993, pp 383-404.
6. Arner O, Ekengren K, von Schreeb T: Fractures of the head and neck of the radius: A clinical and roentgenographic study of 310 cases. *Acta Chir Scand* 1957;112:115-134.
7. Wexner SD, Goodwin C, Parkes JC II, et al: Treatment of fractures of the radial head by partial excision. *Orthop Rev* 1985;14:229-232.
8. Goldberg I, Peylan J, Yosipovitch Z: Late results of excision of the radial head for an isolated closed fracture. *J Bone Joint Surg* 1986;68A:675-679.
9. Khalfayan EE, Culp RW, Alexander AH: Mason type II radial head fractures: Operative versus nonoperative treatment. *J Orthop Trauma* 1992;6:283-289.
10. Bunker TD, Newman JH: The Herbert differential pitch bone screw in displaced radial head fractures. *Injury* 1985;16:621-624.
11. King GJ, Evans DC, Kellam JF: Open reduction and internal fixation of radial head fractures. *J Orthop Trauma* 1991;5:21-28.
12. Perry CR, Tessier JE: Open reduction and internal fixation of radial head fractures associated with olecranon fracture or dislocation. *J Orthop Trauma* 1987;1:36-42.
13. Broberg MA, Morrey BF: Results of delayed excision of the radial head after fracture. *J Bone Joint Surg* 1986;68A:669-674.
14. Morrey BF, Tanaka S, An K-N: Valgus stability of the elbow: A definition of primary and secondary constraints. *Clin Orthop* 1991;265:187-195.
15. Broberg MA, Morrey BF: Results of treatment of fracture-dislocations of the elbow. *Clin Orthop* 1987;216:109-119.
16. Sanders RA, French HG: Open reduction and internal fixation of comminuted radial head fractures. *Am J Sports Med* 1986;14:130-135.
17. Desault PJ: *A Treatise on Fractures, Luxations, and Other Affections of the Bones*, ed 2. Edited by X. Bichat, translated by C. Caldwell. Philadelphia, PA, Kimber and Conrad, 1811, p 165.
18. Josefsson PO, Gentz CF, Johnell O, et al: Surgical versus non-surgical treatment of ligamentous injuries following dislocation of the elbow joint: A prospective randomized study. *J Bone Joint Surg* 1987;69A:605-608.
19. Morrey BF, Chao EY, Hui FC: Biomechanical study of the elbow following excision of the radial head. *J Bone Joint Surg* 1979; 61A:63-68.
20. Carter PR, Benton LJ, Dysert PA: Silicone rubber carpal implants: A study of the incidence of late osseous complications. *J Hand Surg* 1986;11A:639-644.
21. Morrey BF, Askew L, Chao EY: Silastic prosthetic replacement for the radial head. *J Bone Joint Surg* 1981;63A:454-458.
22. Carr CR, Howard JW: Metallic cap replacement of radial head following fracture. *West J Surg Obstet Gynecol* 1951;59:539-546.
23. Edwards GE, Rostrup O: Radial head prosthesis in the management of radial head fractures. *Can J Surg* 1960;3:153-155.

24. Harrington IJ, Tountas AA: Replacement of the radial head in the treatment of unstable elbow fractures. *Injury* 1981;12:405-412.
25. Knight DJ, Rymaszewski LA, Amis AA, et al: Primary replacement of the fractured radial head with a metal prosthesis. *J Bone Joint Surg* 1993;75B:572-576.
26. Colton CL: Fractures of the olecranon in adults: Classification and management. *Injury* 1973;5:121-129.
27. Müller ME, Allgöwer M, Schneider R, et al: *Manual of Internal Fixation: Techniques Recommended by the AO Group*, ed 2. Berlin, Springer-Verlag, 1979.
28. Cabanela ME, Morrey BF: Fractures of the proximal ulna and olecranon, in Morrey BF (ed): *The Elbow and Its Disorders*, ed 2. Philadelphia, PA, WB Saunders, 1993, pp 405-428.
29. Holdsworth BJ, Mossad MM: Elbow function following tension band fixation of displaced fractures of the olecranon. *Injury* 1984;16:182-187.
30. Horne JG, Tanzer TL: Olecranon fractures: A review of 100 cases. *J Trauma* 1981;21:469-472.
31. Larsen E, Jensen CM: Tension-band wiring of olecranon fractures with nonsliding pins: Report of 20 cases. *Acta Orthop Scand* 1991;62:360-362.
32. Murphy DF, Greene WB, Dameron TB Jr: Displaced olecranon fractures in adults: Clinical evaluation. *Clin Orthop* 1987;224:215-223.
33. Rowland SA, Burkhart SS: Tension band wiring of olecranon fractures: A modification of the AO technique. *Clin Orthop* 1992;277:238-242.
34. van der Horst CM, Keeman JN: Treatment of olecranon fractures. *Neth J Surg* 1983;35:27-29.
35. Wolfgang G, Burke F, Bush D, et al: Surgical treatment of displaced olecranon fractures by tension band wiring technique. *Clin Orthop* 1987;224:192-204.
36. Johnson RP, Roetker A, Schwab JP: Olecranon fractures treated with AO screw and tension bands. *Orthopedics* 1986;9:66-68.
37. Horner SR, Sadasivan KK, Lipka JM, et al: Analysis of mechanical factors affecting fixation of olecranon fractures. *Orthopedics* 1989;12:1469-1472.
38. Aldredge GN Jr, Gregory CF: Triceps advancement in olecranon fractures. *J Bone Joint Surg* 1969;51A:816.
39. Gartsman GM, Sculco TP, Otis JC: Operative treatment of olecranon fractures: Excision or open reduction with internal fixation. *J Bone Joint Surg* 1981;63A:718-721.
40. Weseley MS, Barenfeld PA, Eisenstein AL: The use of the Zuelzer hook plate in fixation of olecranon fractures. *J Bone Joint Surg* 1976;58A:859-863.
41. Burghele N, Serban N: Fractures of the olecranon: Treatment by external fixation. *Ital J Orthop Traumatol* 1982;8:159-161.
42. Helm RH, Hornby R, Miller SW: The complications of surgical treatment of displaced fractures of the olecranon. *Injury* 1987;18:48-50.
43. Kiviluoto O, Santavirta S: Fractures of the olecranon: Analysis of 37 consecutive cases. *Acta Orthop Scand* 1978;49:28-31.
44. Hanks GA, Kottmeier SA: Isolated fracture of the coronoid process of the ulna: A case report and review of the literature. *J Orthop Trauma* 1990;4:193-196.
45. Selesnick FH, Dolitsky B, Haskell SS: Fracture of the coronoid process requiring open reduction with internal fixation: A case report. *J Bone Joint Surg* 1984;66A:1304-1306.
46. Regan W, Morrey B: Fractures of the coronoid process of the ulna. *J Bone Joint Surg* 1989;71A:1348-1354.

CHAPTER 17

Complex Fractures of the Distal Part of the Humerus and Associated Complications

Jesse B. Jupiter, MD

Injuries involving the distal end of the humerus represent a constellation of complex articular fractures. Recommendations for treatment have ranged from essentially no treatment to operative reduction and stable internal fixation.[1-11] In the past decade, there has been widespread acceptance of operative treatment of articular fractures of the distal end of the humerus. The publication of favorable results with the use of these methods has led to an increase in the application of the techniques for fixation of small fractures to distal humeral fractures, including those associated with polytrauma and the complex comminuted fractures of the elderly. Unfortunately, the rates of complications associated with operative intervention remain disturbingly high. Residual stiffness of the elbow, nonunion, malunion, post-traumatic osteoarthrosis, ulnar neuropathy, and overall functional disability continue to be adverse sequelae of the operative treatment of these challenging fractures.

While substantial advances, such as improved techniques of exposure and methods of fixation of small articular and osseous fragments, have been made, a number of difficulties in the operative treatment of fractures of the distal humerus remain. This should not be surprising, given the intricate anatomy of the elbow, which is composed of three distinct articulations. The proximity of the neurovascular structures, the meager skeletal support of the articular surfaces, and the lack of soft-tissue attachments to the osseous structures all contribute to the unforgiving nature of these fractures and have led many to recommend against operative intervention.[12-18]

Contemporary issues that form the basis of the present paper include methods of fracture classification, the operative exposure, methods of surgical fixation of complex fractures, the problems involved in the achievement of secure fixation in an elderly patient, multiplane articular injuries, and an understanding of and an approach to the management of complications following the operative treatment of fractures of the distal end of the humerus.

Anatomy

A thorough understanding of the surgical anatomy of the distal humerus and its direct correlation to basic fracture patterns is essential before any operation is performed. The distal humerus comprises two osseous columns, one medial and one lateral, which flare out distally to be separated by the olecranon fossa and, more distally, by the trochlea. The lateral column diverges at approximately a 20° angle to the perpendicular of the humeral shaft, while the medial column diverges at a 40° to 45° angle from the longitudinal axis of the humerus. One way to view the distal end of the humerus is as a triangle with the spool-shaped trochlea interposed between the divergent medial and lateral columns.[19] The capitellum is the anterior aspect of the most distal part of the lateral column; the most distal aspect of the medial column is the medial epicondyle, which terminates just proximal to the trochlea. The articulation between the trochlear notch of the olecranon and the trochlea is the most important element of the flexion-extension arc of elbow motion and provides as much as 50% of the intrinsic stability of the elbow.[20] The medial and lateral ridges of the trochlea add to the intrinsic stability of this articulation. Therefore, restoration of the trochlea is of paramount importance during reconstruction of the fractured distal humerus. In particular, care must be taken to avoid narrowing of the width of the trochlea, as doing so may prevent its seating properly within the trochlear notch of the ulna.

Even in patients with underlying osteopenia, the cortical bone at the margins of the medial and lateral columns is adequate for the purchase of bone screws. The surgeon must keep this in mind and, whenever possible, orient the fixation screws to engage the cortical bone of the columns rather than the central portion of the distal end of the humerus (Fig. 1).

The goal in the restoration of the articular and osseous anatomy of the distal humerus is to reconstruct an equilateral triangle consisting of the medial column, the lateral column, and the trochlea. The internal fixation must make each limb sufficiently stable to support postoperative mobilization. Instability of any one of the three limbs will dramatically weaken the entire operative construct.

Classification

With operative treatment of articular fractures of the distal end of the humerus has come a much greater understanding of the nature of the patterns of these fractures. Historical classifications describing T or Y patterns of intercondylar fractures inadequately reflect the variety of fractures seen at operations.[16] When one recognizes that the articular surfaces are supported by the medial and lateral osseous columns, a classification of fractures of the distal end of the humerus that accurately reflects the architecture can be established by the division of the fractures into three major groups: extracapsular; transcolumnar; and intra-articular, in-

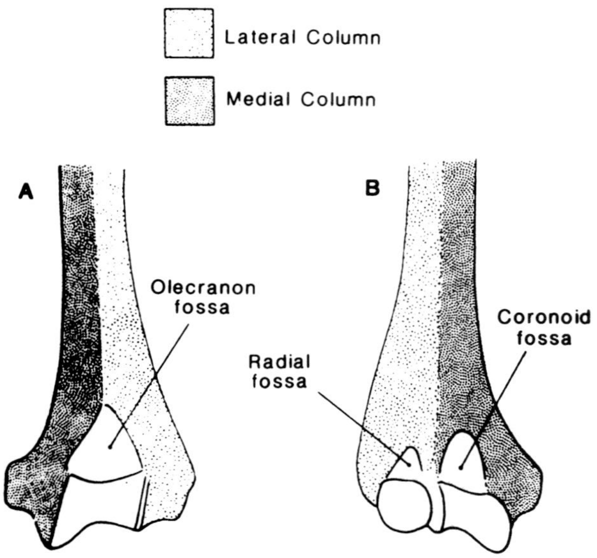

Fig. 1 Illustration of the operative anatomy of the distal end of the humerus, which comprises the articular trochlea supported by two osseous columns. The cortical bone along the margins of these columns is capable of engaging screw purchase even in elderly patients. (Reproduced with permission from Mehne DK, Jupiter JB: Fractures of the distal humerus, in Browner BD, Jupiter JB, Levine AM, et al (eds): *Skeletal Trauma: Fractures, Dislocations, Ligamentous Injuries.* Philadelphia, PA, WB Saunders, 1992, pp 1146-1176.)

Table I
Classification of Fractures of the Distal Part of the Humerus

- I. Intra-articular fractures
  - A. Single-column
    - 1. Medial
      - a. High
      - b. Low
    - 2. Lateral
      - a. High
      - b. Low
  - B. Bicolumnar
    - 1. T pattern
      - a. High
      - b. Low
    - 2. H pattern
    - 3. Lambda pattern
      - a. Medial
      - b. Lateral
  - C. Capitellar
  - D. Trochlear
- II. Extra-articular intracapsular fractures
  - A. Transcolumnar fractures
    - 1. High
      - a. Extension
      - b. Flexion
      - c. Abduction
      - d. Adduction
    - 2. Low
      - a. Extension
      - b. Flexion
- III. Extracapsular fractures
  - A. Medial epicondyle
  - B. Lateral epicondyle

(Reproduced with permission from Jupiter JB, Mehne DK: Fractures of the distal humerus. *Orthopedics,* 1992;15:826.)

cluding single and bicolumnar fractures, fractures involving the capitellum, and those involving the trochlea (Table 1).[21]

Bicolumnar fractures of the distal end of the humerus were classified by Mehne and Matta into six main types (Fig. 2).[19]

High T fracture This is a transverse fracture that divides both columns proximal to or at the proximal limits of the olecranon fossa.

Low T fracture This may be the most common fracture pattern in the elderly and may be among the more difficult to treat. The transverse fracture line crosses the olecranon fossa just proximal to the trochlea, leaving a relatively small amount of bone supporting the articular surfaces.

Y fracture Oblique fracture lines crossing each column join at or about the olecranon fossa to extend distally in a sagittal plane, splitting the trochlea.

H fracture The medial column has a fracture line proximal or distal to the medial epicondyle, and the lateral column is fractured in a T or Y pattern. The trochlea is a free-floating fragment and may be further comminuted.

Medial lambda fracture The most proximal fracture line exits medially, and the lateral fracture line extends distally to the level of the lateral epicondyle.

Lateral lambda fracture The pattern is similar to the H fracture but the lateral column is not involved. While in most intra-articular fractures the trochlea is split in one or two pieces in the sagittal plane, on occasion an additional coronal fracture of the trochlea can occur.[22] In this pattern, the coronoid may serve as a fulcrum to split the trochlea in the coronal plane (Fig. 3).[23]

Another type of fracture of the distal part of the humerus is a shearing injury involving the anterior articular surface of the distal end of the humerus (Fig. 4, left). This fracture pattern also occurs in the coronal plane. The capitellum and the lateral half of the trochlea are separated from the distal end of the humerus. While this pattern may present as an isolated injury or be part of a more complex fracture, its recognition is critical to the successful restoration of the articular surface. In some patients, the characteristic double-arc sign can be seen on the lateral radiograph of the elbow (Fig. 4, right). The double arc is created by the capitellum and trochlea having been displaced as a single unit.

The efforts to define more precisely the patterns of fracture of the distal humerus have culminated in the AO/ASIF classification,[24] which is perhaps the most effective system. In this classification, all fractures involving the metaphysis and articular surfaces of long bones are divided into three main groups: type

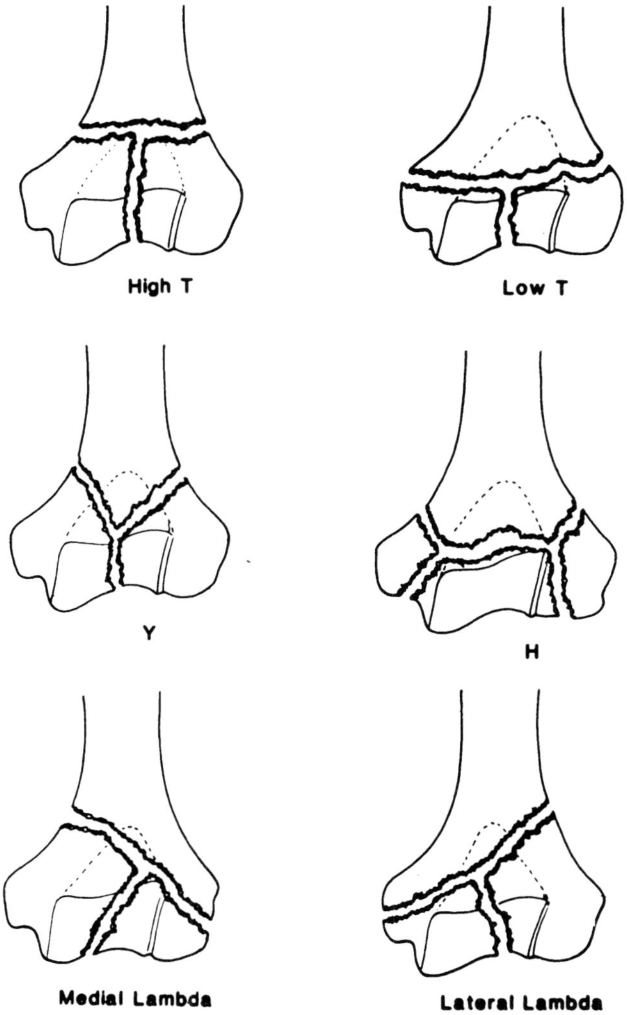

Fig. 2 Illustration showing the system of classification for fractures of the distal end of the humerus proposed by Mehne and Matta, which consists of six basic categories (shown on the anterior aspect of the distal end of the left humerus). (Reproduced with permission from Mehne DK, Jupiter JB: Fractures of the distal humerus, in Browner BD, Jupiter JB, Levine AM, et al (eds): *Skeletal Trauma: Fractures, Dislocations, Ligamentous Injuries*. Philadelphia, PA, WB Saunders, 1992, pp 1146-1176.)

A—extra-articular fractures; type B—partial articular fractures in which a portion of the joint is disrupted, leaving intact a part of the joint attached to the more proximal osseous support; and type C—complete articular fractures in which there is complete disruption between the joint surface and the supporting osseous structures. These three basic types are further divided on the basis of the location and orientation of the major fracture lines and the amount of metaphyseal and articular comminution. In fact, there are twenty-seven different categories in this classification scheme (Fig. 5). I have found this system to be most helpful in the treatment of my patients.

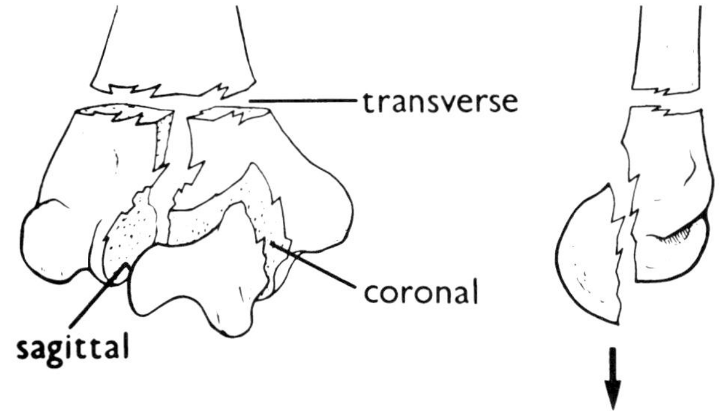

Fig. 3 Illustration of a multiplane fracture, which is characterized by articular fracture lines in both the sagittal and the coronal plane. (Reproduced with permission from Jupiter JB, Barnes KA, Goodman LJ, et al: Multiplane fracture of the distal humerus. *J Orthop Trauma* 1993;7:216-220.)

Surgical Treatment

The operative procedure for more complex fractures can be lengthy, and iliac-crest bone graft may be needed. Therefore, I prefer general endotracheal anesthesia for most patients. The patient is placed in the lateral decubitus position with the injured side up and the involved limb supported on soft bolsters, with the elbow positioned in approximately 90° of flexion. The ipsilateral iliac crest is readily available for bone graft, should it be needed, and it is always prepared and draped. The involved upper limb is draped free, and a sterile tourniquet is applied.

I always use a posterior midline longitudinal incision, modified to incorporate any previous incision. This incision rarely results in any sensitivity of the scar, despite its being located over the posterior part of the elbow.

The next step is to identify and protect the ulnar nerve. Ulnar nerve neuritis is a recognized, adverse sequela of surgical intervention for fractures about the elbow.[21,25,26] The potential for both intraoperative damage and postoperative scarring about the nerve can be reduced by elevating the nerve from the cubital tunnel, proximally to the level of the medial intermuscular septum and distally for approximately 6 cm past its entrance between the two heads of the flexor carpi ulnaris. The fascia over the flexor carpi ulnaris should be split longitudinally, with particular care taken to identify and preserve individual muscle branches to the flexor pronator muscle group. The distal 4 cm of the intermuscular septum should also be resected. Doing so allows the nerve to sit freely in the surrounding soft tissue and avoids the possibility of its becoming tethered in and about the elbow after the operation. One of the complications that has been noted during elbow reconstruction after failed surgical treatment of a com-

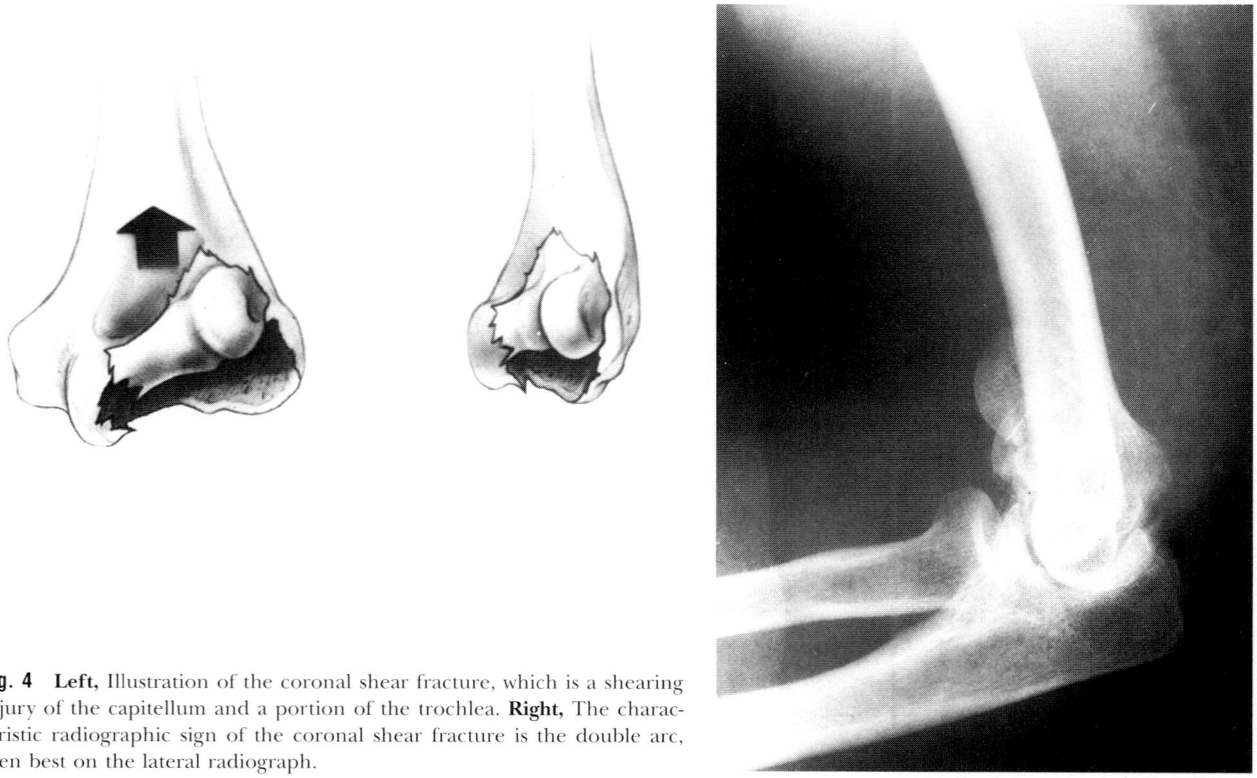

Fig. 4 **Left,** Illustration of the coronal shear fracture, which is a shearing injury of the capitellum and a portion of the trochlea. **Right,** The characteristic radiographic sign of the coronal shear fracture is the double arc, seen best on the lateral radiograph.

plex distal humerus fracture is adherence of the ulnar nerve directly to the medial epicondylar region. This can be avoided by mobilizing the nerve sufficiently so that it lies freely in the subcutaneous tissue in the anteromedial space alongside the distal humerus.

Surgical Approach

An extensile approach is preferable for articular fractures of the distal humerus. Three basic approaches (medial, lateral, and posterior) have been described. While the posterior approach through an olecranon osteotomy is the most widely used, the surgeon should also be familiar with the medial approach, which may prove beneficial when a total elbow arthroplasty is being considered for a complex articular fracture in an elderly patient, and the lateral approach, which may be preferable for a complex lateral column or coronal shear fracture.

Medial approach The medial epicondyle, trochlea, and ulnar nerve are exceptionally well visualized through the medial approach, and it is the best approach for a total elbow arthroplasty. Because the triceps tendon is elevated from medial to lateral, as described by Bryan and Morrey,[21,27] the olecranon is left intact. Care must be taken, however, to reattach the triceps securely to the olecranon during closure. The main disadvantage of this approach is that visualization of lateral column injuries may be more difficult. Additionally, the medial collateral ligament of the elbow may be compromised if the surgeon does not carefully protect (and repair) this important structure during the procedure.

Lateral approach The lateral approach is perhaps the simplest.[27] It, too, features elevation of the triceps from the olecranon and provides excellent exposure of the lateral column, capitellum, and radial head. Fractures of these lateral structures can be well visualized and secured stably through this approach. When this approach is extended distally, care must be taken to identify and protect the posterior interosseous nerve as it passes through the supinator muscle. The lateral approach is not optimum for complex low fractures of both columns of the distal end of the humerus.

Posterior approach The posterior approach through a transolecranon osteotomy provides excellent visualization, particularly of the distal articular fragments. A chevron osteotomy is started with a thin oscillating saw and completed with a thin-bladed osteotome cracking the articular surface of the semilunar notch. The proximal olecranon may then be elevated with the triceps, which provides excellent exposure as far as 7 cm proximal to the joint line before the radial nerve is threatened. The osteotomy is made in the center of the olecranon sulcus because this area of the olecranon has the least amount of articular cartilage. The center can be identified accurately by elevating the anconeus

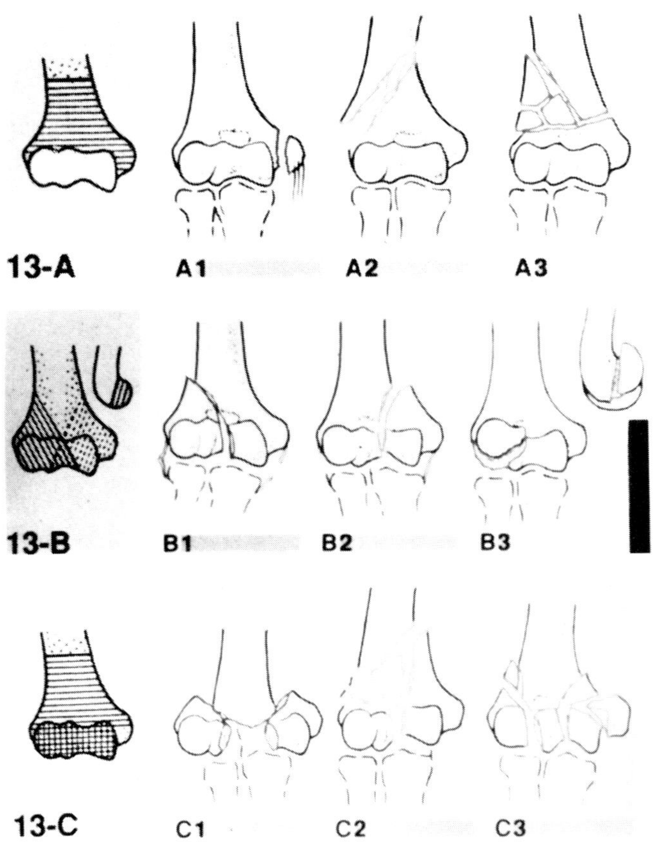

Fig. 5 The AO/ASIF classification divides the fractures into three main groups: Type A, extra-articular; Type B, partial articular; and Type C, complete articular. The three basic types are subdivided on the basis of the location and orientation of the major fracture line or lines. **Top,** The main group, Type A (extra-articular fractures), is divided into Type A1 (apophyseal avulsion), A2 (metaphyseal simple), and A3 (metaphyseal multifragmentary). Type-A1 fractures are further defined as 1 (lateral epicondyle), 2 (medial epicondyle, nonincarcerated), or 3 (medial epicondyle, incarcerated); Type A2, as 1 (oblique downward and inward), 2 (oblique downward and outward), or 3 (transverse); and Type A3, as 1 (with an intact wedge), 2 (with a fragmented wedge), or 3 (complex). **Center,** The main group, Type B (partial articular fractures), is divided into Type B1 (lateral sagittal), B2 (medial sagittal), and B3 (frontal). Type-B1 fractures are further defined as 1 (capitellum), 2 (transtrochlear simple), or 3 (transtrochlear multifragmentary); B2, as 1 (transtrochlear simple, through the medial side [Milch I]), 2 (transtrochlear simple, through the groove), or 3 (transtrochlear multifragmentary); and B3, as 1 (capitellum), 2 (trochlea), or 3 (capitellum and trochlea). **Bottom,** The main group, Type C (complete articular fractures), is divided into Type C1 (articular simple, metaphyseal simple), C2 (articular simple, metaphyseal multifragmentary), and C3 (multifragmentary). Type-C1 fractures are further defined as 1 (with slight displacement), 2 (with marked displacement), or 3 (T-shaped epiphyseal); C2, as 1 (with an intact wedge), 2 (with a fragmented wedge), or 3 (complex); and C3, as 1 (metaphyseal simple), 2 (metaphyseal wedge), or 3 (metaphyseal complex). (Reproduced with permission from Muller ME, Nazarian S, Koch P, et al: *AO Classification of Fractures.* Berlin, Springer-Verlag, 1987.)

muscle from its insertion on the olecranon to directly visualize the articular surface. A sponge is placed from lateral to medial through the joint and is used as countertraction as the osteotomy is created. Although this approach provides excellent visualization, its main disadvantage is that the osteotomy must be securely stabilized at the conclusion of the operative procedure. Nonunion of the olecranon osteotomy has been reported to occur between 2% and 5% of the time.[28-30] In addition, the hardware that is used to fix the osteotomy is often prominent and painful and must be removed later. Finally, this approach is not ideal for total elbow arthroplasty, should that become the treatment of choice.

Fracture Fixation

Once the fracture anatomy has been confirmed, efforts are made to reduce the articular fragments and to restore them anatomically to their origins on the osseous columns. Provisional fixation with smooth 0.045- or 0.062-inch (1.143- or 1.575-mm) Kirschner wires (K-wires) helps to secure the small articular fragments together. The use of an oscillating attachment to the drill is of particular importance at this stage as the specific anatomy of the distal humerus limits the available places in which these provisional K-wires can be positioned. With an oscillating attachment, there is little possibility of injury to the surrounding soft tissues or, in particular, to the ulnar nerve.

Fractures in the Coronal Plane

When a surgeon is faced with a complex articular fracture that involves displacement in the coronal plane, the techniques of definitive fixation are limited. Herbert screws have been useful, as their threads can be buried under the articular surface (Fig. 6). Alternatively, fine-threaded, small K-wires can be buried under the articular surface, but the risk of migration may be somewhat higher.

Fractures in the Sagittal Plane

Articular disruption in the sagittal plane is secured by the placement of one or two 3.5-mm screws across the trochlea. Given the cancellous nature of the bone in this region, these screws should be sufficient to provide a firm hold on the fragments. When there is a central defect or comminution, or both, the surgeon must take great care to avoid overcompressing the fragments and narrowing the trochlea. Narrowing of the trochlea threatens the integrity of the articulation between the trochlea and the trochlear sulcus of the olecranon, which leads to the possibility of instability and posttraumatic osteoarthrosis. Compact cancellous or corticocancellous bone grafts can be used to bridge defects quite effectively (Fig. 7).

With the lambda fracture patterns, the surgeon may find that the definitive fixation is facilitated by restoring one major articular fragment onto the lateral or medial osseous column with screws or with screws and plates.

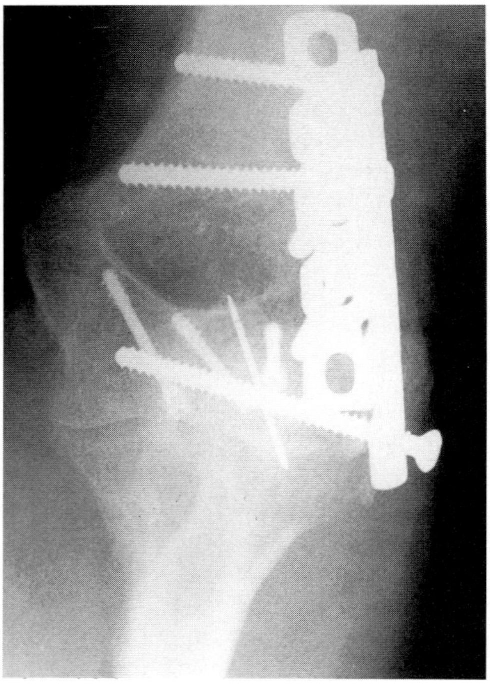

Fig. 6 A coronal shear fracture well secured with Herbert screws, which can be buried beneath the surface of the articular cartilage.

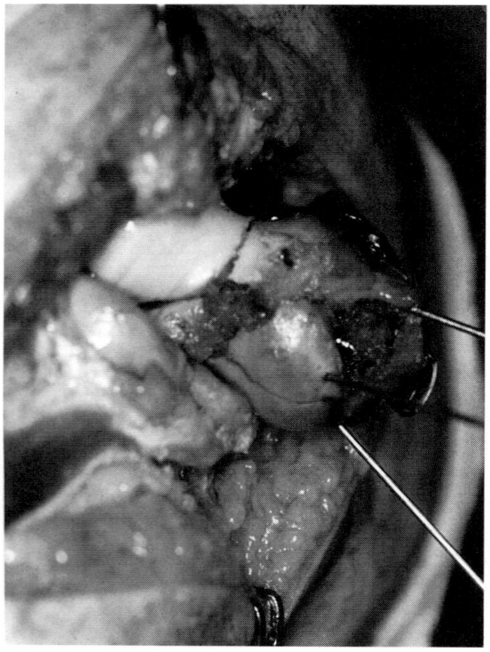

Fig. 7 Comminution and loss of substance of the trochlea; cortico-cancellous bone graft is used to help maintain the anatomic width of the trochlea.

Doing so often facilitates restoration of the remaining articular fragments onto the reconstruction (Fig. 8).

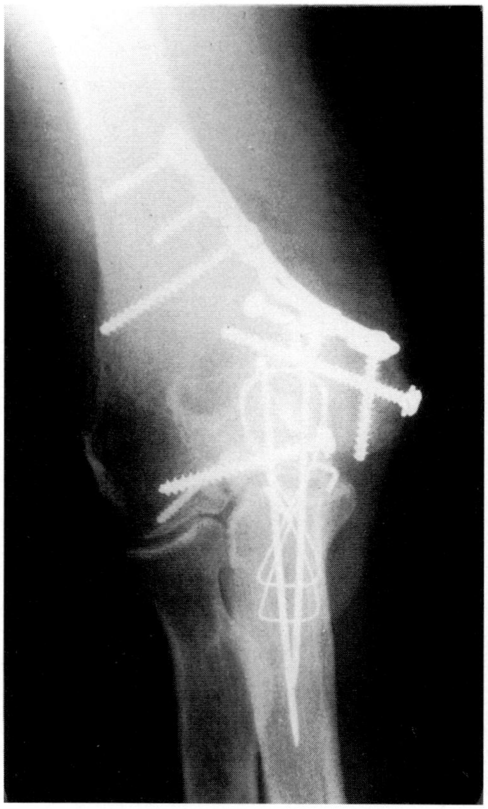

Fig. 8 A complex lambda fracture that had been secured by reassembling the articular fragments onto the intact osseous column of the distal end of the humerus.

The use of strategically placed plates and screws forms the basis of definitive fixation of the articular fragments onto the osseous columns. The overall mechanical strength of the fixation will be enhanced by placement of the plates and their respective screws as close to 90° to each other as possible.[31] For most fractures that extend more proximally, splitting the columns proximal to the olecranon sulcus, plates can be applied along the medial ridge of the medial column and the posterior aspect of the lateral column.

Stable fixation of very distal fractures of the medial side requires special attention to placement of the plates.[32-34] Using 3.5-mm reconstruction plates, I contour the medial plate to bend around and cradle the medial epicondyle. The most distal screws can be directed into the medial epicondyle, diverging from each other at approximately a 90° angle, or a screw can be directed from very distal to proximal into the lateral osseous column proximal to the horizontal fracture line. An additional option, which I have found to be effective in elderly patients, is placement of a third plate directly along the lateral edge of the lateral column. Doing so requires elevation of the origin of the brachioradialis and radial wrist extensors, which should

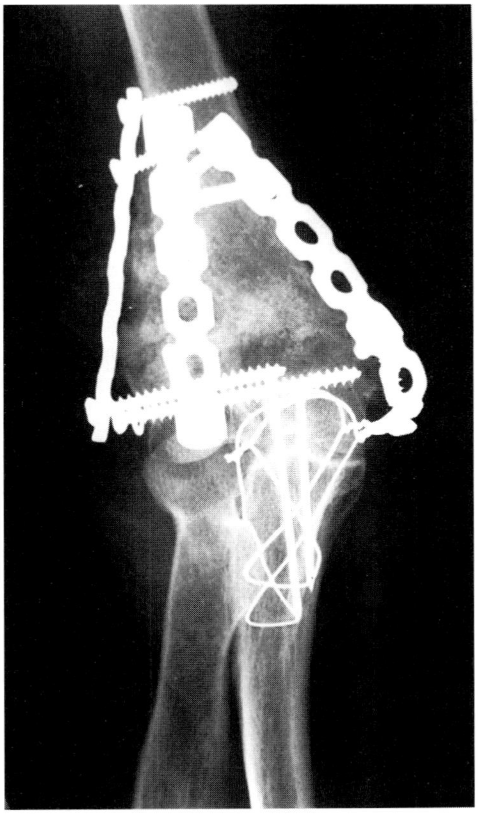

Fig. 9 Fixation of a difficult fracture in an elderly patient; the screw fixation was enhanced by application of a third plate directly along the lateral side of the lateral osseous column (Reproduced with permission of the Mayo Foundation.)

be sutured back into place after the plate has been applied (Fig. 9). Liberal use of autogenous bone graft to fill defects within the architecture of the distal end humerus is important.

Fractures of the distal humerus will become more common as the general population ages. Because the elderly will remain healthier and will lead more active lives, it will be even more important to restore function to their injured joints. Tailoring of the internal fixation to the specific architecture of the fracture will become even more crucial in this patient population. Liberal use of bone graft to fill defects in the osteopenic bone will also be needed more often.

Polymethylmethacrylate has been used effectively to enhance screw fixation in the treatment of fractures, although I do not know of any reports of the effectiveness of this technique for fractures of the distal humerus. Screws that are not fixed securely should be identified and removed, and their location should be marked. The methylmethacrylate is mixed and, while still in liquid phase, poured into a 12-ml syringe with a straight tip. The tip is then placed into the screw-hole, and enough cement to just fill the hole is injected. Extravasation of cement, particularly near the fracture lines, should be carefully avoided. The screws are then sequentially reinserted and allowed to remain in place until the cement begins to become firm, at which point each screw should be advanced a final one or two turns. Excess cement should be removed after it has hardened completely.[35]

Once the fixation hardware is in place, the elbow should be put through a full range of motion to assess visually the stability of the internal fixation. In the event that motion is observed at a fracture line, additional fixation should be provided. Tenuous fixation should be supplemented with cancellous bone graft to enhance and speed healing. Simple placement of the limb in a cast in anticipation that the cast will provide the necessary stability has unfortunately proved, all too often, to be unpredictable and unsatisfactory.[33]

The olecranon osteotomy is secured with two oblique 0.045-inch (1.143-mm) smooth K-wires and a tension-band wire. The proximal ends of the K-wires must be carefully bent and impacted into the bone to prevent migration. If these pins back out, elbow extension may be limited. A tension wire is placed through a drill-hole in the ulna distal to the osteotomy and passed under the K-wires and triceps proximally to create a tension band. The tightening loops of the wire should also be bent carefully around the shaft of the ulna to avoid irritation of the skin.

Postoperative Management

It has become evident from my experience, as well as that of others,[19,21,28-30] that early controlled motion is needed to obtain a functional arc of motion after the surgical treatment of these complex fractures. Union of the fracture without a functional arc of motion is not a successful outcome. It is crucial that the surgeon take an active interest in the supervision as well as the maintenance of the rehabilitation program.

In the early postoperative period—within 24 to 48 hours, depending on the status of the wound—a lightweight, removable thermoplastic splint is made for the patient to use as a resting splint. Because full extension of the elbow is often difficult to obtain, I have found that allowing the patient to rest with the elbow in extension during the first week facilitates the recovery of elbow extension.

Motion exercises are initiated, with the patient lying supine and flexing the involved shoulder to bring the elbow overhead. With the uninjured arm supporting the involved forearm, gravity is used to assist elbow flexion. The approach that is instituted for elbow extension is similar, except that the patient sits upright and the forearm is gently assisted into extension. Patients who have had a posterior surgical approach, especially when the triceps tendon has been elevated, are cautioned to avoid active extension of the elbow for the initial 6 postoperative weeks and to avoid resisted extension for an additional month after that time.

The patient should be encouraged to discontinue use of the splint by 7 to 14 days postoperatively. Doing so will ensure that the patient continues to mobilize the elbow and reincorporates the upper extremity into activities of daily living. Muscle-strengthening and endurance exercises are instituted by 8 to 12 weeks postoperatively, when the surgeon is certain that osseous union has occurred. It is important that the patient either returns for regular office visits or is visited by a nurse, so that compliance with the rehabilitation program is ensured throughout the postoperative period. This step has proved to be of particular importance for elderly patients. I have not found continuous passive motion to be efficacious in the postoperative management of these fractures and have not incorporated it into the protocols that I use.

Once fracture union has been confirmed, the use of a turnbuckle splint can help the patient to regain motion when stiffness of the elbow is a problem. The use of a turnbuckle splint for as long as 6 months after the injury can produce clinical improvement.[20,36]

Complications

Inadequate or unstable fixation, a failure to reposition the articular fragments anatomically, prolonged postoperative immobilization, or the development of soft-tissue complications will result in substantial disability for the patient. Nonunion, malunion, ulnar neuropathy, and heterotopic ossification are all complications that require further discussion.

Nonunion and Malunion

Nonunion or malunion of a fracture of the distal end of the humerus can be disabling because of associated pain or loss of motion. Loss of motion of the elbow may be due to articular deformity, intra-articular or extra-articular adhesions, or pain at the nonunion site.[32,37-41] Ulnar neuropathy may also be associated with a nonunion or malunion, as will be discussed. Surgical procedures aimed at achieving union or correction of deformity are technically demanding, given the distorted anatomy, the limited and osteoporotic bone stock, and the often extensive periarticular fibrosis. Alternatives to surgical reconstruction have included functional bracing, distraction arthroplasty,[36] allograft replacement,[42] and total elbow arthroplasty.[36,42] These latter reconstructive alternatives have their own substantial limitations and are not satisfactory options for young or active individuals.[43,44]

The goals of the management of a malunion or a nonunion must be functional restoration of motion as well as secure osseous union and appropriate alignment. I have found that the surgical approach to these problems is, in effect, a blend of previously described reconstructive procedures.[36,45] The tactics involve mobilization and neurolysis of the ulnar nerve if necessary, extensile exposure through a transolecranon or a triceps-elevation approach, resection of areas of periarticular fibrosis (both posteriorly and anteriorly), and realignment and stable fixation of the distorted osseous architecture. The contouring and placement of the plates and screws mirror the techniques described for the low intra-articular T or transcolumnar fractures. I have found the fixation to be successful, even in the face of distorted anatomy or poor bone stock, or both. In particular, the use of three plates in osteoporotic bone has proved to be extremely helpful.[33]

In two reported series, the functional arc of motion averaged 100° after the successful reconstruction of complex nonunions or intra-articular malunions of fractures of the distal part of the humerus.[33,34] In addition, elbow stability was restored, alleviating the preoperative pain and limitation of function, in each patient. Furthermore, there was no evidence, on late follow-up, of post-traumatic osteoarthrosis (Fig. 10). These results are equal to those reported after total elbow arthroplasty for complex nonunions of the distal part of the humerus,[38] and there is the added benefit that the patient's intrinsic architecture is restored while the use of an implant is avoided.

Ulnar Neuropathy

Complications involving the ulnar nerve have been reported in a number of series of operatively treated intra-articular fractures of the distal humerus.[30,37,38,46,47] Surgical manipulation of the nerve, inadequate release of the fascia over the flexor carpi ulnaris, and postoperative immobilization of the elbow all contribute to fibrosis about the nerve. In addition to neuritic pain, both motor and sensory deficits can occur in the hand, creating an extended disability that may have a greater impact on function than the loss of elbow motion.

In my experience, operative neurolysis and mobilization of the nerve for the treatment of ulnar neuropathy following a failed operation on the elbow has been quite successful, even in elderly patients. In a group of 19 patients (20 elbows) who were treated for post-traumatic ulnar neuropathy associated with failure of primary treatment of a periarticular fracture of the elbow, I observed a substantial improvement in the function of the ulnar nerve following its release. The neurolyses were performed an average of 19 months after the primary injury. At an average of 27 months, patient satisfaction averaged 7.8 points on a scale of 10 points. The average Gabel and Amadio score for ulnar-nerve function[48] improved from 3.2 points preoperatively to 6.5 points postoperatively. There were one excellent, 15 good, and two poor results, with both of the poor results being due to failure of the elbow reconstruction rather than to a persistent ulnar-nerve

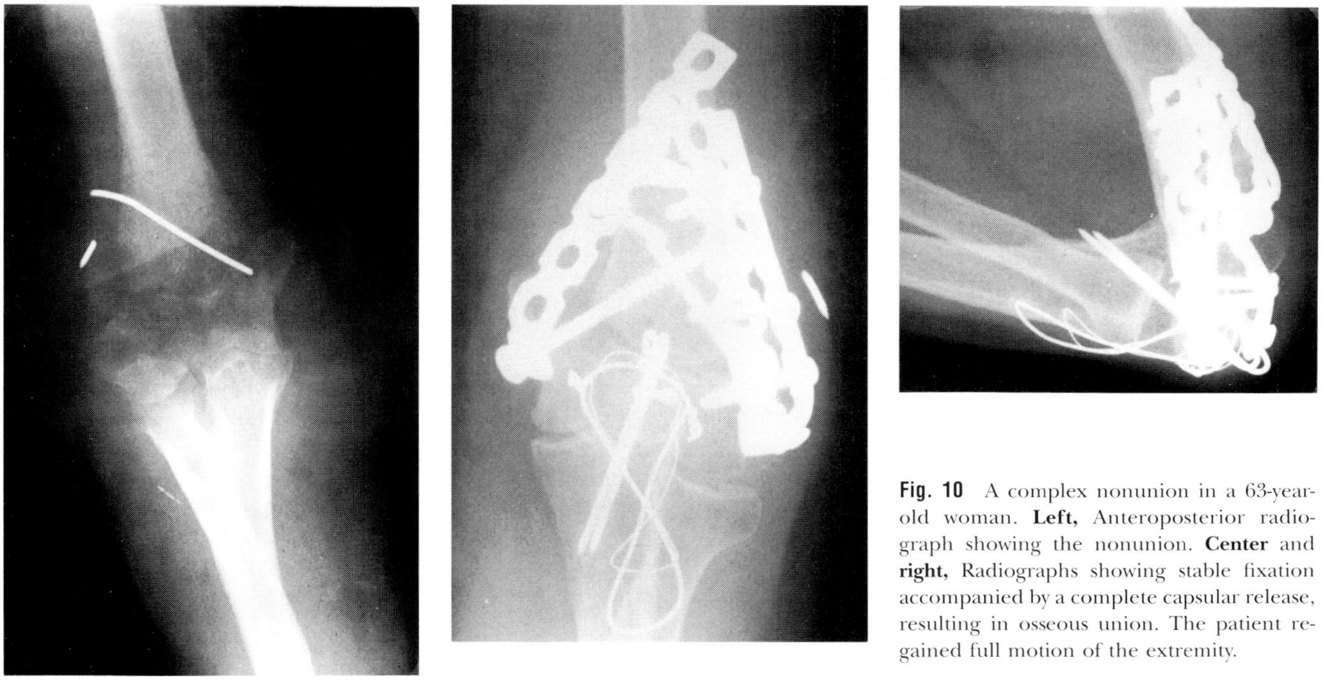

Fig. 10 A complex nonunion in a 63-year-old woman. **Left,** Anteroposterior radiograph showing the nonunion. **Center** and **right,** Radiographs showing stable fixation accompanied by a complete capsular release, resulting in osseous union. The patient regained full motion of the extremity.

problem. Importantly, return of intrinsic muscle strength was observed in all 14 patients who had had intrinsic muscle weakness preoperatively. Twelve recovered grade-V power and two, grade-IV power, as defined by the Medical Research Council.[34] While it is evident that some improvement of these chronic conditions can be gained by neurolysis and mobilization of the ulnar nerve, it is most important that the ulnar nerve is mobilized adequately at the time of the initial operation and that the risk of this potentially disabling complication is thus minimized.

Heterotopic Ossification

Much has been written about heterotopic ossification as a complication of traumatic injuries of the elbow.[2,3,5,9-11] It may be surprising to some that, in the absence of an injury of the central nervous system or the head, heterotopic ossification is uncommon following closed elbow trauma. Thompson and Garcia[11] reviewed the records of 1,314 patients in whom a traumatic injury of the elbow had been treated at New York Orthopaedic Hospital from 1926 to 1964. Overall, they observed a prevalence of heterotopic ossification of only 3% (41 patients). They concluded that the ossification was more likely to be seen following an elbow fracture-dislocation and that the risk could be lessened by atraumatic reduction under adequate anesthesia, early surgical intervention, and the avoidance of passive manipulation to regain elbow motion. In contrast, Garland and O'Hollaren,[3] in a series of 496 patients who had an injury of the central nervous system or the head, observed a 5% prevalence of heterotopic ossification about elbows that had not been injured. This rate increased to 89% when a specific injury of the elbow was identified in these patients.

Part of the confusion regarding heterotopic ossification can be found in its definition. Heterotopic or ectopic bone formation reflects a series of events that result in highly organized bone in and about the elbow joint.[5] This is different from myositis ossificans, in which organized bone forms within skeletal muscle, usually in the brachialis after elbow trauma. These two conditions should be contrasted to heterotopic calcification, in which the collateral ligaments or joint capsule becomes calcified after an injury. In contrast to ossification, calcification tends to be amorphous and without evidence of trabeculation. The lack of specific distinction between these two processes has led to some variation in the reported prevalence of heterotopic bone about the elbow. Mikić and Vukadinović[8] noted periarticular ossification in 34 of 60 patients who had had a radial head excision, whereas Josefsson and associates[4] reported that only one of 52 patients had ectopic ossification following elbow dislocation, although 38 had periarticular calcification.

In addition to head injury, the traumatic conditions that may increase the risk of the development of heterotopic ossification include open fractures or fracture-dislocations, injuries due to high-energy trauma, fractures associated with thermal injury,[49] fractures treated with multiple operative procedures, and failed internal fixation requiring revision surgery within 3 months after the initial injury.[2] Although the timing of the initial operative treatment after the elbow trauma, especially that involving fracture of the radial head, has been suggested by some to have a direct relationship with the development of heterotopic ossification,[4,11] this has not been my experience and I do not know of any prospective studies supporting this anecdotal observation.

Pain, swelling, and warmth about the elbow are the most common symptoms associated with heterotopic ossification. Commonly, a progressive loss of motion is associated with these symptoms. Infection, reflex sympathetic dystrophy, and failure of internal fixation devices are among the conditions that can present with similar symptoms.

Both technetium bone scans and serum alkaline phosphatase levels have been used to detect heterotopic ossification. However, both lack specificity and offer little predictable information.

Treatment

The problem of heterotopic ossification can be addressed from two perspectives: prophylaxis, both at the time of the injury and after surgical resection, and the indications and techniques of surgical excision of existing lesions. Because heterotopic ossification following elbow trauma is not common in the absence of head trauma, prospective studies offer little guidance regarding the prophylactic measures to be taken at the time of the injury. For the most part, the principles of prophylaxis have been formulated in conjunction with total hip arthroplasty or after resection of established heterotopic ossification.[50-55] While orally administered diphosphonates have been used in the past, the clinical results have been disappointing. They have little effect on formation of the osteoid matrix, and calcification of the osteoid appears to occur once the therapy has been discontinued.[55] Furthermore, if the diphosphonates are administered over a long period of time, osteomalacia may ensue; this further limits the attractiveness of these agents as a prophylactic measure.

Nonsteroidal anti-inflammatory agents, particularly indomethacin, have been shown to be effective.[6] These agents have been shown experimentally to inhibit the cyclo-oxygenase needed for the production of prostaglandin E_2,[52] which is thought to be a formative agent in the inflammatory response and a chemical mediator of heterotopic ossification.[56]

A third modality that has been used effectively to prevent heterotopic ossification about the hip is low-dose radiation therapy. Clinical trials in high-risk patients managed with total hip replacement or an acetabular procedure have had encouraging results, even with dosages as low as ten gray in five fractions initiated as early as possible (before the fourth postoperative day).[50,51,54,57] Delay of radiation treatment for more than 72 hours undoubtedly compromises its effectiveness. The clinician must take into account, however, the potential risks of even low-dose radiation, especially for young individuals.[58,59] Furthermore, the theoretical concerns that the radiation could interfere with wound-healing or could delay bone-healing have made its application somewhat controversial for most elbow injuries. I have had no experience with the prophylactic use of radiation after elbow trauma, although the experience at the Mayo Clinic has suggested that it can be applied effectively, and there has been no evidence to date of any associated nonunions, wound problems, or post-irradiation sarcomas.[2]

Surgical excision of heterotopic bone about the elbow should not be considered unless function is substantially impaired. If excision is to be performed, the timing is important. Anecdotal evidence has suggested that excision should not be considered until the bone has matured, as demonstrated by a change in the activity seen on a technetium bone scan. This has not been my experience. After trauma, technetium bone scans may show activity for a considerable period of time, during which a delay in the restoration of elbow mobility can result in capsular or ligamentous contracture and even in degeneration of the articular cartilage. These complications can preclude an effective return of function.

I think that, in the absence of an injury of the head or central nervous system, operative excision of heterotopic bone about the elbow can be considered as early as 6 to 9 months after the injury. While capsular or ligamentous release may be necessary to restore mobility, procedures involving manipulation of the underlying skeleton, such as osteotomies or implant removal, should be avoided, as they may increase the potential for reformation of the heterotopic bone. To some degree, the surgical approach depends on the location of the heterotopic bone as well as on the specific underlying lesion of the elbow. I usually use a medial approach for excision of heterotopic bone after elbow trauma. In some patients, however, the anterolateral approach effectively allows extensile exposure to both the anterior and the posterior part of the elbow. Certainly, when the heterotopic bone lies posteriorly or posteromedially, I use a medial approach. In many situations, it is important to identify and protect the ulnar nerve. This is particularly true after an operation that has included mobilization of the ulnar nerve for the treatment of an elbow fracture or after thermal injury when the ulnar nerve may be compressed.[1,28] Furthermore, if there is bone surrounding the nerve, capsular release and mobilization of the joint may cause local compression of the nerve, resulting in the development of ulnar neuropathy after the heterotopic bone has been removed. In these circumstances, a medial approach allows the surgeon to be sure that the nerve is free of compression when the release of the joint is completed.

After excision, a careful and controlled rehabilitation protocol should be followed. Splints or a continuous-passive-motion machine should be used with caution when the soft-tissue envelope is traumatized. I prefer only a soft dressing postoperatively. With the use of indomethacin as a prophylactic measure in 18 consecutively treated patients, I did not see a recurrence of heterotopic ossification after excision.

The surgical approach to heterotopic ossification in patients with associated head or central nervous system trauma is quite different. Patient selection is of fundamental importance. Garland and associates[60] reported the results of 23 resections of heterotopic ossification about the elbow in patients with head trauma. They noted that patients with minimum cognitive disability, a normal level of alkaline phosphatase, and heterotopic bone that appeared mature on radiographs had improvement in motion and function of the limb with limited complications and a lower rate of recurrence of heterotopic ossification. In contrast, the heterotopic bone recurred in all five elbows in patients who had ongoing, severe, cognitive and physical defects.

References

1. Evans EB: Heterotopic bone formation in thermal burns. *Clin Orthop* 1991;263:94-101.
2. Frassica FJ, Coventry MB, Morrey BF: Ectopic ossification about the elbow, in Morrey BF (ed): *The Elbow and Its Disorders*, ed 2. Philadelphia, PA, WB Saunders, 1993, pp 505-514.
3. Garland DE, O'Hollaren RM: Fractures and dislocations about the elbow in the head-injured adult. *Clin Orthop* 1982;168:38-41.
4. Josefsson PO, Johnell O, Gentz CF: Long-term sequelae of simple dislocation of the elbow. *J Bone Joint Surg* 1984;66A:927-930.
5. Jupiter JB: Heterotopic ossification about the elbow, in Tullos HS (ed): *Instructional Course Lectures XL*. Park Ridge, IL, American Academy of Orthopaedic Surgeons, 1991, pp 41-44.
6. McLaren AC: Prophylaxis with indomethacin for heterotopic bone: After open reduction of fractures of the acetabulum. *J Bone Joint Surg* 1990;72A:245-247.
7. McLaughlin HL: Some fractures with a time limit. *Surg Clin North Am* 1955;35:553-561.
8. Mikić ZD, Vukadinović SM: Late results in fractures of the radial head treated by excision. *Clin Orthop* 1983;181:220-228.
9. Mohan K: Myositis ossificans traumatica of the elbow. *Int Surg* 1972;57:475-478.
10. Roberts PH: Dislocation of the elbow. *Br J Surg* 1969;56:806-815.
11. Thompson HC III, Garcia A: Myositis ossificans: Aftermath of elbow injuries. *Clin Orthop* 1967;50:129-134.
12. Brown RF, Morgan RG: Intercondylar T-shaped fractures of the humerus: Results in ten cases treated by early mobilisation. *J Bone Joint Surg* 1971;53B:425-428.
13. Evans EM: Supracondylar-Y fractures of the humerus. *J Bone Joint Surg* 1953;35B:381-385.
14. Horne G: Supracondylar fractures of the humerus in adults. *J Trauma* 1980;20:71-74.
15. Keon-Cohen BT: Fractures at the elbow. *J Bone Joint Surg* 1966;48A:1623-1639.
16. Reich RS: Treatment of intercondylar fractures of the elbow by means of traction. *J Bone Joint Surg* 1936;18:997-1004.
17. Riseborough EJ, Radin EL: Intercondylar T fractures of the humerus in the adult: A comparison of operative and non-operative treatment in twenty-nine cases. *J Bone Joint Surg* 1969;51A:130-141.
18. Watson-Jones R: *Fractures and Other Bone and Joint Injuries*, ed 2. Baltimore, MD, Williams & Wilkins, 1941.
19. Mehne DK, Jupiter JB: Fractures of the distal humerus, in Browner BD, Jupiter JB, Levine AM, et al (eds): *Skeletal Trauma: Fractures, Dislocations, Ligamentous Injuries*. Philadelphia, PA, WB Saunders, 1992, pp 1146-1176.
20. Morrey BF: Post-traumatic stiffness: Distraction arthroplasty, in Morrey BF (ed): *The Elbow and Its Disorders*, ed 2. Philadelphia, PA, WB Saunders, 1993, pp 476-491.
21. Bryan RS, Morrey BF: Fractures of the distal humerus, in Morrey BF (ed): *The Elbow and Its Disorders*. Philadelphia, PA, WB Saunders, 1985, pp 302-339.
22. Jupiter JB, Barnes KA, Goodman LJ, et al: Multiplane fracture of the distal humerus. *J Orthop Trauma* 1993;7:216-220.
23. Smith FM: The upper extremity of the ulna, in Smith FM (ed): *Surgery of the Elbow*, ed 2. Philadelphia, PA, WB Saunders, 1972, pp 137-165.
24. Muller ME, Nazarian S, Koch P: *AO Classification of Fractures*. Berlin, Germany, Springer-Verlag, 1987.
25. Bryan RS: Fractures about the elbow in adults, in Murray DG (ed): *American Academy of Orthopaedic Surgeons Instructional Course Lectures Volume XXX*. St. Louis, MO, CV Mosby, 1981, pp 200-223.
26. Lecestre P: Les fractures de l'extremite inferieure de l'humerus chez l'adulte. *Rev Chir Orthop* 1980;66(suppl 2):21.
27. Morrey BF: Surgical exposures of the elbow, in Morrey BF (ed): *The Elbow and Its Disorders*. Philadelphia, PA, WB Saunders, 1985, pp 122-146.
28. Aitken GK, Rorabeck CH: Distal humeral fractures in the adult. *Clin Orthop* 1986;207:191-197.
29. Gabel GT, Hanson G, Bennett JB, et al: Intraarticular fractures of the distal humerus in the adult. *Clin Orthop* 1987;216:99-108.
30. Waddell JP, Hatch J, Richards R: Supracondylar fractures of the humerus: Results of surgical treatment. *J Trauma* 1988;28:1615-1621.
31. Helfet DL, Hotchkiss RN: Internal fixation of the distal humerus: A biomechanical comparison of methods. *J Orthop Trauma* 1990;4:260-264.
32. Ackerman G, Jupiter JB: Non-union of fractures of the distal end of the humerus. *J Bone Joint Surg* 1988;70A:75-83.
33. Jupiter JB, Goodman LF: The management of complex distal humerus nonunion in the elderly by elbow capsulectomy, triple plating, and ulnar nerve neurolysis. *J Shoulder Elbow Surg* 1992;1:37-46.
34. McKee M, Jupiter J, Toh CL, et al: Reconstruction after malunion and nonunion of intra-articular fractures of the distal humerus: Methods and results in 13 adults. *J Bone Joint Surg* 1994;76B:614-621.
35. Rosen H: Nonunion and malunion, in Browner BD, Jupiter JB, Levine AM, et al (eds): *Skeletal Trauma: Fractures, Dislocations, Ligamentous Injuries*. Philadelphia, PA, WB Saunders, 1992, pp 501-541.
36. Morrey BF: Post-traumatic contracture of the elbow: Operative treatment, including distraction arthroplasty. *J Bone Joint Surg* 1990;72A:601-618.
37. Bryan RS, Bickel WH: "T" condylar fractures of distal humerus. *J Trauma* 1971;11:830-835.
38. Figgie MP, Inglis AE, Mow CS, et al: Salvage of non-union of supracondylar fracture of the humerus by total elbow arthroplasty. *J Bone Joint Surg* 1989;71A:1058-1065.
39. Mitsunaga MM, Bryan RS, Linscheid RL: Condylar nonunions of the elbow. *J Trauma* 1982;22:787-791.
40. Sanders RA, Sackett JR: Open reduction and internal fixation of delayed union and nonunion of the distal humerus. *J Orthop Trauma* 1990;4:254-259.
41. Sim FH: Nonunion and delayed union of distal humeral fractures, in Morrey BF (ed): *The Elbow and Its Disorders*. Philadelphia, PA, WB Saunders, 1985, pp 340-354.
42. Urbaniak JR, Black KE Jr: Cadaveric elbow allografts: A six-year experience. *Clin Orthop* 1985;197:131-140.

43. Beckenbaugh RD: Resectional arthroplasty and arthrodesis of the elbow, in Evarts CM (ed): *Surgery of the Musculoskeletal System.* New York, NY, Churchill Livingstone, 1983, vol 2, pp 3:265-3:272.
44. Rashkoff E, Burkhalter WE: Arthrodesis of the salvage elbow. *Orthopedics* 1986;9:733-738.
45. Dellon AL: Review of treatment results for ulnar nerve entrapment at the elbow. *J Hand Surg* 1989;14A:688-700.
46. Jupiter JB, Neff U, Holzach P, et al: Intercondylar fractures of the humerus: An operative approach. *J Bone Joint Surg* 1985;67A:226-239.
47. Letsch R, Schmit-Neuerburg KP, Stürmer KM, et al: Intraarticular fractures of the distal humerus: Surgical treatment and results. *Clin Orthop* 1989;241:238-244.
48. Gabel GT, Amadio PC: Reoperation for failed decompression of nerve in the region of the elbow. *J Bone Joint Surg* 1990;72A:213-219.
49. Dias DA: Heterotopic para-articular ossification of the elbow with soft tissue contracture in burns. *Burns* 1982;9:128-134.
50. Ayers DC, Evarts CM, Parkinson JR: The prevention of heterotopic ossification in high-risk patients by low-dose radiation therapy after total hip arthroplasty. *J Bone Joint Surg* 1986; 68A:1423-1430.
51. Coventry MB, Scanlon PW: The use of radiation to discourage ectopic bone: A nine-year study in surgery about the hip. *J Bone Joint Surg* 19881;63A:201-208.
52. Ho SSW, Stern PJ, Bruno LP, et al: Pharmacological inhibition of prostaglandin E_2 in bone and its effect on pathological new bone formation in a rat burn model. *Trans Orthop Res Soc* 1988;13:536.
53. Jowsey J, Coventry MB, Robins PR: Heterotopic ossification: Theoretical consideration, possible etiologic factors, and a clinical review of total hip arthroplasty patients exhibiting this phenomenon, in *The Hip: Proceedings of the Fifth Open Scientific Meeting of The Hip Society.* St. Louis, MO, CV Mosby, 1977, pp 210-221.
54. Sylvester JE, Greenberg P, Selch MT, et al: The use of postoperative irradiation for the prevention of heterotopic bone formation after total hip replacement. *Int J Radiat Oncol Biol Phys* 1988;14:471-476.
55. Thomas BJ, Amstutz HC: Results of the administration of diphosphonate for the prevention of heterotopic ossification after total hip arthroplasty. *J Bone Joint Surg* 1985;67A:400-403.
56. Stern PJ, Bruno LP, Hopson CN: Skeletal deformities after burn injuries: An animal model. *Trans Orthop Res Soc* 1985;10:175.
57. Bosse MJ, Poka A, Reinert CM, et al: Heterotopic ossification as a complication of acetabular fractures: Prophylaxis with low-dose irradiation. *J Bone Joint Surg* 1988;70A:1231-1237.
58. Brady LW: Radiation-induced sarcomas of bone. *Skeletal Radiol* 1979;4:72-78.
59. Kim JH, Chu FC, Woodard HQ, et al: Radiation-induced soft-tissue and bone sarcoma. *Radiology* 1978;129:501-508.
60. Garland DE, Hanscom DA, Keenan MA, et al: Resection of heterotopic ossification in the adult with head trauma. *J Bone Joint Surg* 1985;67A:1261-1269.

CHAPTER 18

Fractures About the Elbow

James H. Beaty, MD
James R. Kasser, MD

Fracture Separation of the Distal Humeral Physis

In children younger than 2 or 3 years of age, an apparent dislocation of the elbow frequently is a fracture-separation of the distal humeral physis (Fig. 1). This injury is difficult to diagnose, because the only ossified structure about the elbow in children of this age is the ossification center of the lateral humeral condyle. In addition, the radius, proximal olecranon, and lateral condyle move medially or laterally as a single unit, giving the appearance of an elbow dislocation.[1-6] When this entity was first recognized, it occasionally was diagnosed by arthrography or magnetic resonance imaging; however, an increased awareness of the injury has made it easier to recognize on plain radiographs.[5,6]

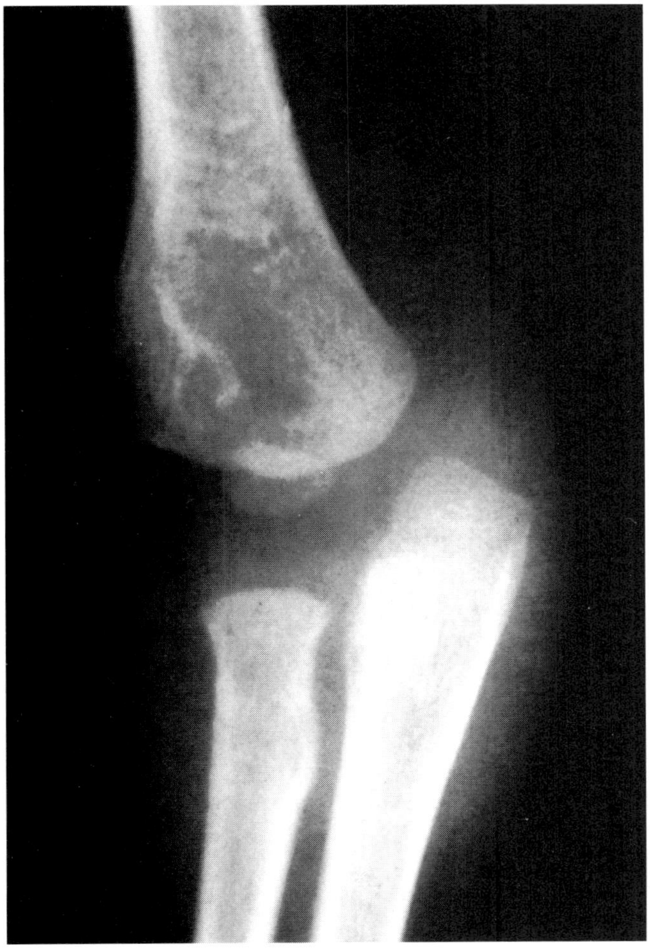

Fig. 1 Transepiphyseal fracture-separation of the distal humeral physis in a 2-year-old child. Ulna, radius, and lateral condyle are displaced medially as a single unit.

At one time, closed reduction and splinting were recommended for this injury,[3,7,8] but, more recently, closed or open reduction and percutaneous pinning have become the treatment of choice to avoid the possibility of instability and loss of reduction.

T-Condylar-Supracondylar Fracture

This rare fracture is difficult to diagnose and treat in young children (Fig. 2).[9] If the T-condylar component of the injury is not displaced, the supracondylar fracture can be treated either by splinting or by closed reduction and percutaneous pinning, but displacement of more than 2 to 3 mm requires open reduction and pinning (Fig. 3).[9-11] The fixation used depends on the age of the child. In very young children, pins can be used to fix the two condylar fragments and crossed Kirschner wires (K-wires) can be used for fixation of both condyles to the humeral shaft. In adolescents approaching skeletal maturity, fixation should be the same as in adults, with acetabular reconstruction plates

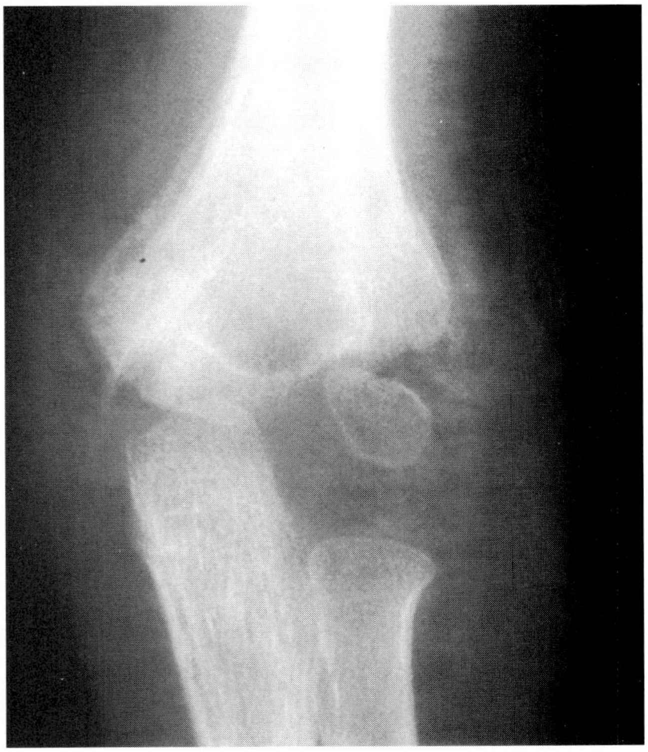

Fig. 2 T-condylar supracondylar fracture in a 4-year-old girl that was initially diagnosed as a supracondylar fracture only. After percutaneous pinning, malunion of the medial condyle and nonunion of the laterally displaced lateral condyle are present.

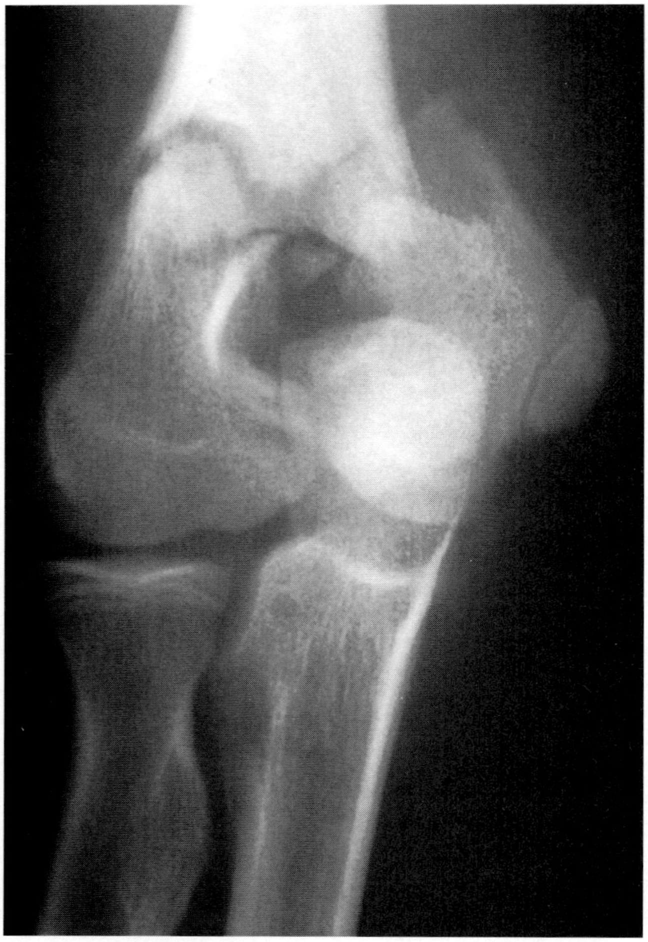

Fig. 3 T-condylar fracture in a 14-year-old boy with mild comminution at the supracondylar level, displacement and rotation of the medial condyle, and 1-cm displacement of the articular surface.

and screw fixation as needed. The triceps-splitting approach may be used, or olecranon osteotomy can be performed for severe comminution or additional exposure. The "pearl" is fixation and early motion to make rehabilitation more effective.[10]

Supracondylar Fracture

Incompletely displaced supracondylar fractures may have the same clinical appearance as fractures of the lateral condylar physis or avulsion of the medial epicondyle. Careful palpation of the bony landmarks about the elbow will pinpoint the area of maximum tenderness and will help in making the diagnosis.

Minimally displaced supracondylar fractures may be difficult to diagnose on plain anteroposterior and lateral radiographs. Signs of a supracondylar fracture on a true lateral view include displacement of the anterior fat pad and posterior displacement of the capitellum relative to the anterior humeral line.[2,7,12] If a supracondylar fracture is suspected but is not visible on routine views, oblique views may be helpful.[7]

Treatment

Generally accepted treatment guidelines are based on the classification of Gartland:[13] type I, nondisplaced; type II, displaced with some cortical contact; and type III, completely displaced. Type I (nondisplaced) fractures are treated with posterior plaster splinting with a collar and a cuff for 2 to 3 weeks. Type II fractures must be evaluated carefully to determine the position of the fracture fragments. If the fragments are in an acceptable alignment on anteroposterior and lateral radiographs, posterior splint immobilization may be appropriate. Excessive angulation, especially in "medial impacted" type II varus injuries, is an indication for closed reduction and percutaneous pinning (Fig. 4). Treatment options for type III injuries include reduction and splinting, skin or skeletal traction, closed reduction and percutaneous pinning, and open reduction. Although each of these options has advantages and disadvantages, the currently recommended treatment for type III injuries is closed reduction and percutaneous pinning, if acceptable closed reduction can be obtained with the patient anesthesized.[14-20] Skeletal traction is used rarely, but it may be helpful in certain situations, for example, when comminution is significant or when reduction and percutaneous pinning are not technically possible.[7,21-23]

Open reduction is indicated for open fractures that require irrigation and debridement and for fractures that cannot be adequately reduced by closed methods. Most fractures with posteromedial or posterolateral displacement of the distal fragment can be reduced through an anterior incision because the soft-tissue dissection has been completed by the fracture itself. After open reduction, fixation can be accomplished with percutaneous medial and lateral crossed K-wires or two lateral wires.

A special problem is the "flexion" supracondylar fracture, which accounts for approximately 2% of all supracondylar fractures.[7,16] If the fracture is in good position, splinting with a collar and cuff for 3 weeks is appropriate. If the fracture is in excessive flexion, reduction and percutaneous pinning are recommended. The difficulty of obtaining a satisfactory closed reduction of these fractures has been noted by several authors,[7,24-26] and open reduction of completely displaced flexion supracondylar fractures frequently is required (Fig. 5).

Pearls

Techniques for closed reduction and percutaneous pinning have been well-described in the literature, but some technical points should be considered.

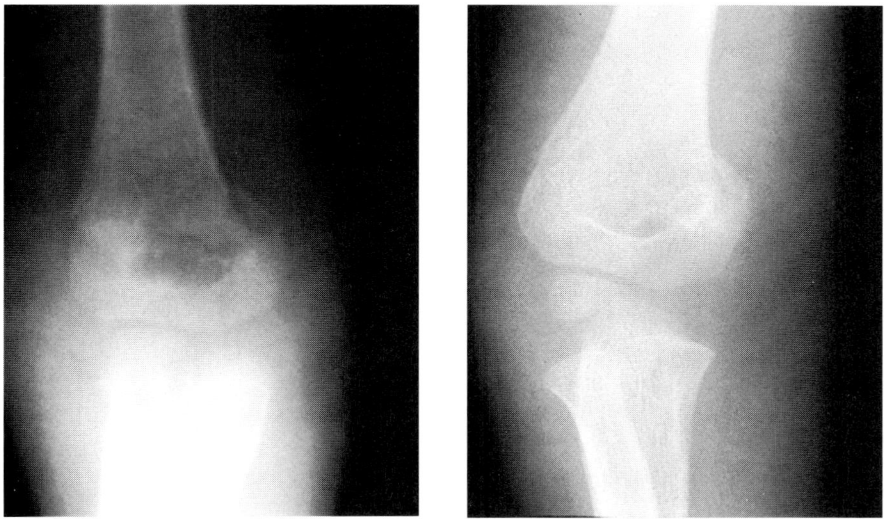

Fig. 4 **Left,** Type II "medially-impacted" supracondylar fracture of the right elbow in a 6-year-old child. **Right,** Three days after injury, medial collapse into varus alignment required manipulation and pinning.

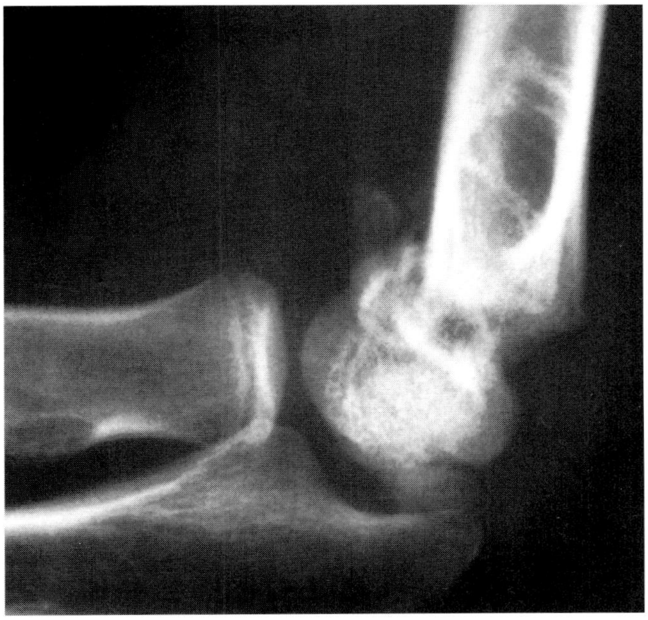

Fig. 5 Flexion supracondylar fracture in a 9-year-old boy. Note anterior displacement and rotation of the distal fragment on the lateral radiograph. Open reduction and internal fixation was required because closed reduction was not acceptable.

General anesthesia should be used, and reduction is done as an emergency procedure, to delay continued edema about the elbow.

Image intensification can be used to evaluate reduction and assist in placement of the pins.[27]

Pin size should be selected carefully. For children younger than 5 or 6 years of age, a 0.062-in smooth K-wire usually is used; for children older than 6 years of age, a 5/64-in wire is appropriate.

The elbow is reduced by longitudinal traction with counter-traction, correction of the medial and lateral displacement, and flexion of the elbow to reduce the extension injury.

After the fracture is reduced, fixation can be obtained with either crossed K-wires (Fig. 6, *left*) or two lateral pins (Fig. 6, *right*). Although crossed wires are more stable mechanically, either technique is acceptable. What is important is that the fracture reduction is stable and in acceptable position before fixation. The more stable the reduction, the more likely two lateral pins will be acceptable. For unstable fractures, crossed medial and lateral K-wires are preferred.

Leaving the wires or pins protruding from the skin and bending them 90° makes removal easier. Removal usually is done as an outpatient procedure approximately 3 weeks after injury. Postoperative immobilization should include a well-padded posterior plaster splint and a collar-and-cuff sling.

Complications

Ulnar Nerve Injury When medial and lateral crossed K-wires are used for fixation, special care must be taken to avoid injury to the ulnar nerve when the medial pin is inserted.[28,29] If necessary, a small 1- to 2-cm incision can be made medially to allow palpation of the medial epicondyle to insure that the medial pin enters at this point. If the pin is distal to the medial epicondyle on image intensification or radiograph, it may pierce the ulnar nerve. For this reason, the ulnar groove should be avoided when the medial wire is inserted.

Brachial Artery Injury Injuries to the brachial artery, although rare, are the most serious complication of supracondylar fractures.[30,31] In a child with a supracondylar humeral fracture, a pink, viable hand with no radial or ulnar pulses must be distinguished from a

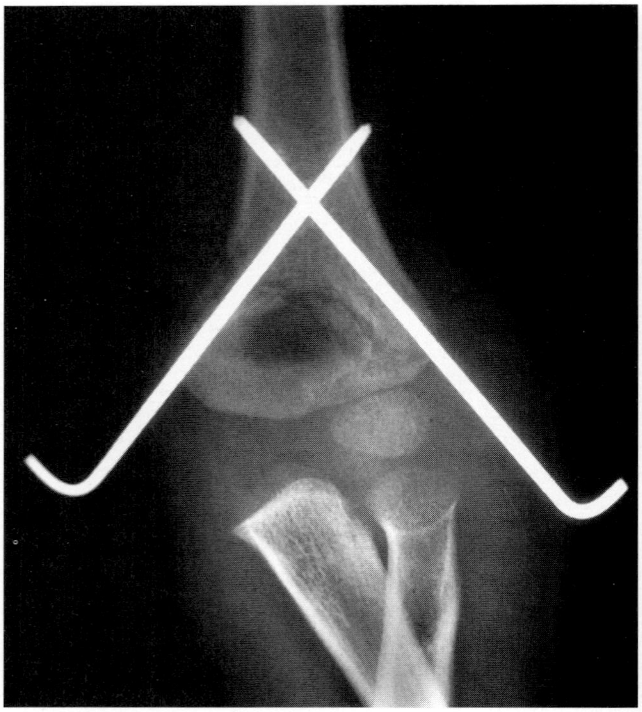

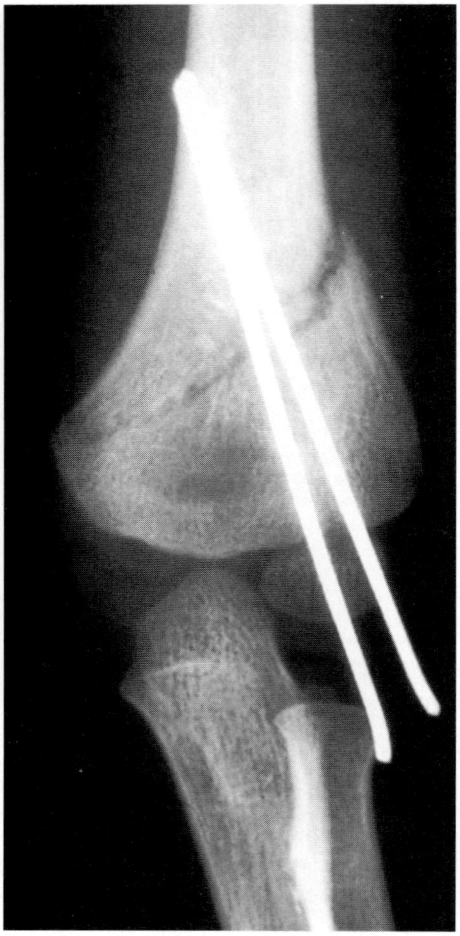

Fig. 6 **Left,** Closed reduction and percutaneous pinning of a type III supracondylar fracture with crossed medial and lateral Kirschner wires. Note good position in medial and lateral columns, slight penetration of the opposite cortex. Pins are bent 90° outside the skin for easier removal. **Right,** Closed reduction and percutaneous pinning with two lateral Kirschner wires. This fracture configuration made placement of a medial pin difficult.

pale, nonviable hand, which is an orthopaedic emergency. Reported injuries to the brachial artery include arterial spasm, laceration, "kinking" by soft tissues, and intimal tear with thrombus formation.

After closed reduction, if pulses are not palpable but the child has a pink, apparently viable hand with good capillary refill and pulses that can be detected by Doppler evaluation, observation is appropriate. If pulses cannot be detected by physical examination or Doppler evaluation, and if the hand appears pale and nonviable, brachial artery exploration is recommended (Fig. 7). In isolated elbow injuries, an arteriogram is not absolutely necessary because the site of the injury is known. If an arteriogram is requested it should be obtained in the operating room rather than in the radiology department to avoid delay in treatment of the arterial injury. Recently, the necessity of obtaining an arteriogram has been questioned when exploration is already planned for a suspected arterial injury.[31]

Findings at arterial exploration include laceration, thrombus formation, and spasm. The pathology dictates treatment, which may range from incision and removal of a thrombus to segmental removal of a portion of the artery and vein grafting. In type III

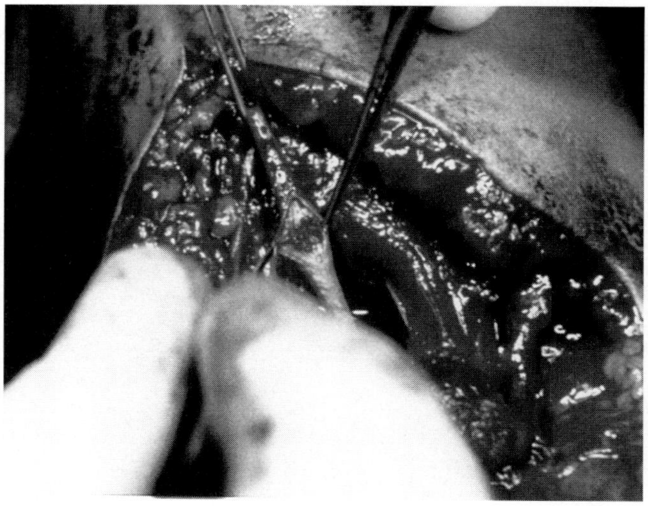

Fig. 7 Arterial exploration identified an intimal tear with thrombus formation in this child with a supracondylar fracture and a nonviable hand (no palpable or Doppler pulse).

fractures with arterial injuries, the fracture should be reduced and percutaneously pinned as quickly as possible to allow extension of the elbow for anterior arterial exploration without fear of instability of the fracture.

Volkmann's Ischemic Contracture and Compartment Syndrome Because of an increasing awareness of the association of compartment syndrome with supracondylar humeral fractures, the incidence of this complication is decreasing. Close observation is recommended for at least 24 hours after treatment of acute fractures. The most important clinical finding is pain with passive motion of the digits, because good capillary refill and even palpable pulses may be present in a child with ischemic forearm musculature or compartment syndrome. If compartment syndrome is suspected, the splint should be removed to allow careful inspection of the elbow and forearm. If the forearm compartment appears normal and pain is immediately relieved, continued observation may be appropriate; however, if compartment syndrome is suspected, compartment pressures may be measured. If pressures are more than 30 mm/Hg, or, more important, if clinical examination suggests compartment syndrome, elbow and forearm fasciotomies are indicated.

Cubitus Varus Cubitus varus has been estimated to occur after approximately 10% of supracondylar humeral fractures.[7,32-34] Although osteonecrosis of the trochlea and growth arrest of the medial aspect of the distal humeral physis rarely have been reported as causes of cubitus varus deformities, most such deformities are caused by malunion of the fracture. Cubitus varus deformities are most frequent after type II impacted varus fractures that heal in varus alignment and after type II or III injuries treated with closed reduction and splinting that displace into a varus position (Fig.

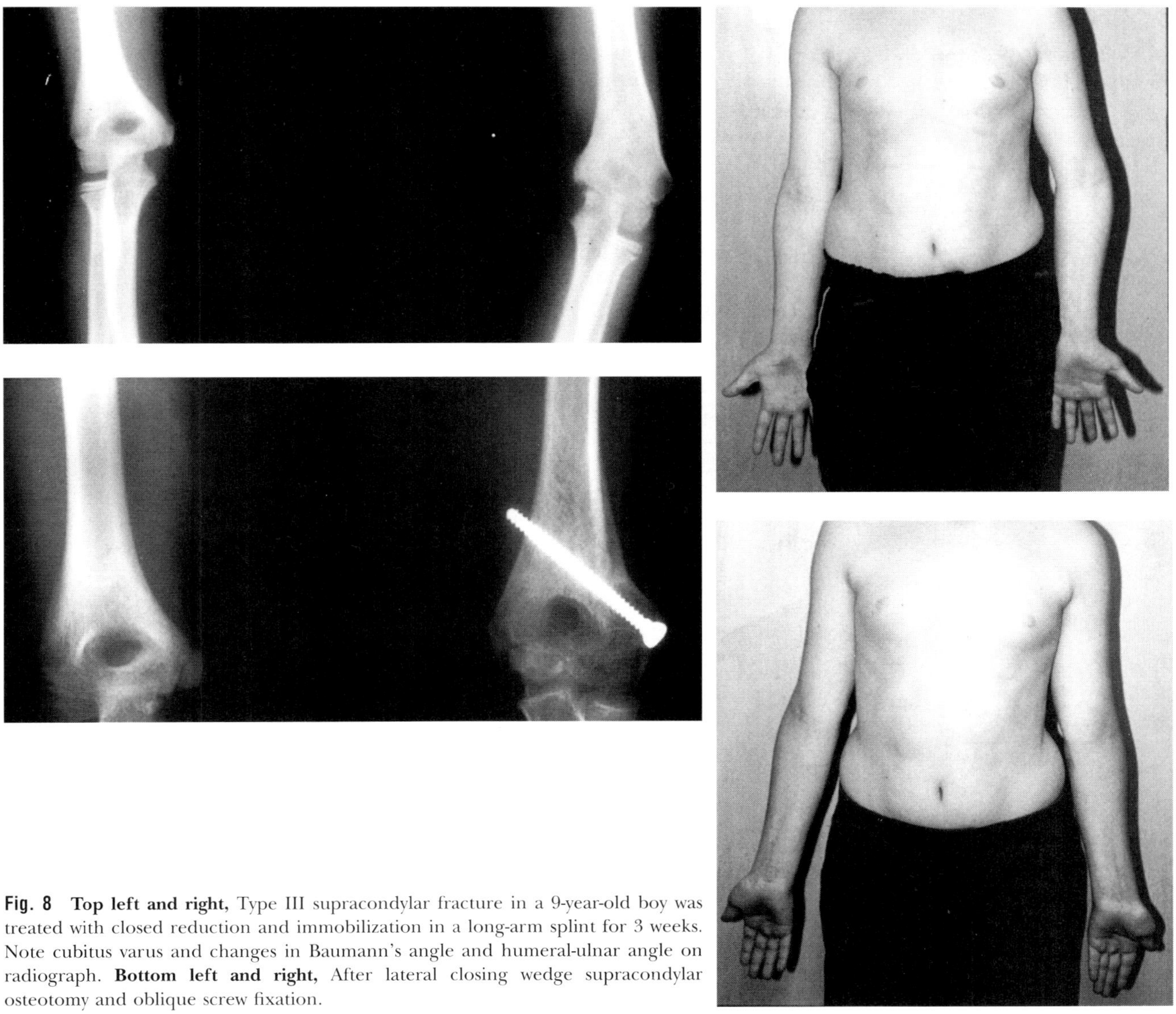

Fig. 8 **Top left and right,** Type III supracondylar fracture in a 9-year-old boy was treated with closed reduction and immobilization in a long-arm splint for 3 weeks. Note cubitus varus and changes in Baumann's angle and humeral-ulnar angle on radiograph. **Bottom left and right,** After lateral closing wedge supracondylar osteotomy and oblique screw fixation.

8). Finally, cubitus varus can occur in fractures that are pinned in varus after closed or open reduction.[26]

Most children with cubitus varus deformities have little functional impairment, but the cosmetic appearance may be unacceptable to the patient or parents. Correction can be obtained with humeral osteotomy, preferably a lateral closing wedge osteotomy of the supracondylar region (Fig. 8, *bottom left*).[32,33,35-37] Care must be taken not to make the osteotomy too far proximally in the diaphyseal bone rather than in the metaphyseal region. As noted by Wilkins,[7] if pins are used for fixation of the osteotomy, the position of the ulnar nerve should be checked with the elbow flexed as well as extended after the pins are inserted. Rigid screw fixation may be used to allow early motion and insure stability of the osteotomy (Fig. 8, *bottom right*).

Late Displacement Occasionally, after closed reduction and splinting or pinning, displacement may occur 7 to 21 days after injury (Fig. 9).[2,7,26,38] If the fracture is in acceptable position, and adequate remodeling can be expected, no treatment is indicated. Even if the fracture position is unacceptable, late open reduction or excessive manipulation may increase the risk of myositis ossificans and is not recommended. Humeral osteotomy can be performed for correction of severe cubitus varus deformity.[31]

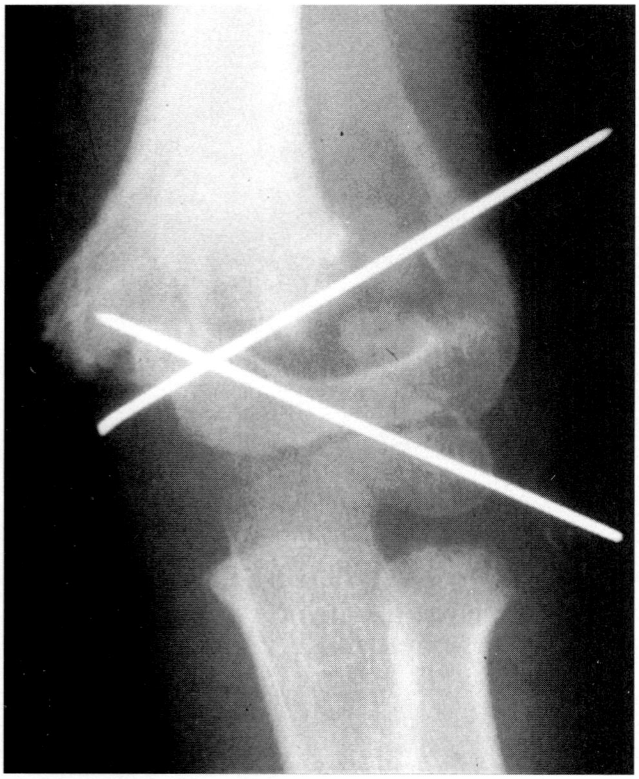

Fig. 9 Late displacement of a type III supracondylar fracture in a 10-year-old girl 2 weeks after closed reduction and percutaneous pinning. Note that the medial pin passes through the fracture site, but the lateral pin is too distal. The fracture displaced laterally 30%, but the carrying angle is acceptable and fracture was allowed to heal in this position.

Myositis Ossificans Myositis ossificans has been reported occasionally in children who have severe soft-tissue injuries or who have participated in an aggressive passive range-of-motion exercise program after fracture treatment. In most children, the bone formation resolves spontaneously over 12 to 24 months. If it impairs function, the heterotopic bone can be excised after it has matured.

Fractures of the Lateral Humeral Condyle

Approximately 15% of fractures about the elbow are fractures of the lateral humeral condyle.[7,39] These fractures may appear to be Salter-Harris type II injuries of the distal humeral physis with lateral metaphyseal fragments. Because the trochlea is not ossified in children younger than 8 years of age, it is also difficult to differentiate this injury from a lateral condylar fracture with extension into the joint.[40-42] Lateral humeral condylar fractures are classified as type I, nondisplaced or displaced less than 2 mm; type II, moderately (2 to 4 mm) displaced; or type III, completely displaced.[41]

The standard treatment of types II and III fractures is open reduction and internal fixation (Fig. 10).[39,43-47] The treatment of type I fractures is more controversial. Several authors have reported late displacement of approximately 10% of type I fractures, with an increased risk of nonunion. Splinting generally is recommended for type I fractures, with close follow-up until union occurs, but some authors recommend percutaneous pinning of nondisplaced or minimally displaced (type I or type II) lateral humeral condylar fractures.[45] If splinting is used, weekly follow-up until radiographic union is essential. Late displacement can be treated as an early nonunion.

Pearls

Open reduction may be performed through a lateral incision, with dissection through the interval between the brachioradialis and triceps muscles.

The soft tissue attached to the posterior aspect of the lateral condyle should be left intact because it is the primary source of blood supply to the condyle.

Clots in the joint should be gently suctioned out and removed with a hemostat, without aggressive debridement of the metaphyseal fragment.

Fracture reduction can be held with a towel clip or bone clamp while the pins are inserted.

In children younger than 5 or 6 years of age, two 0.062-in K-wires are inserted from lateral to medial to penetrate the medial cortex. In children older than 6 years of age, two 5⁄64-in K-wires are used.

The wound is closed in layers and a suction drain is left in place for 24 hours.

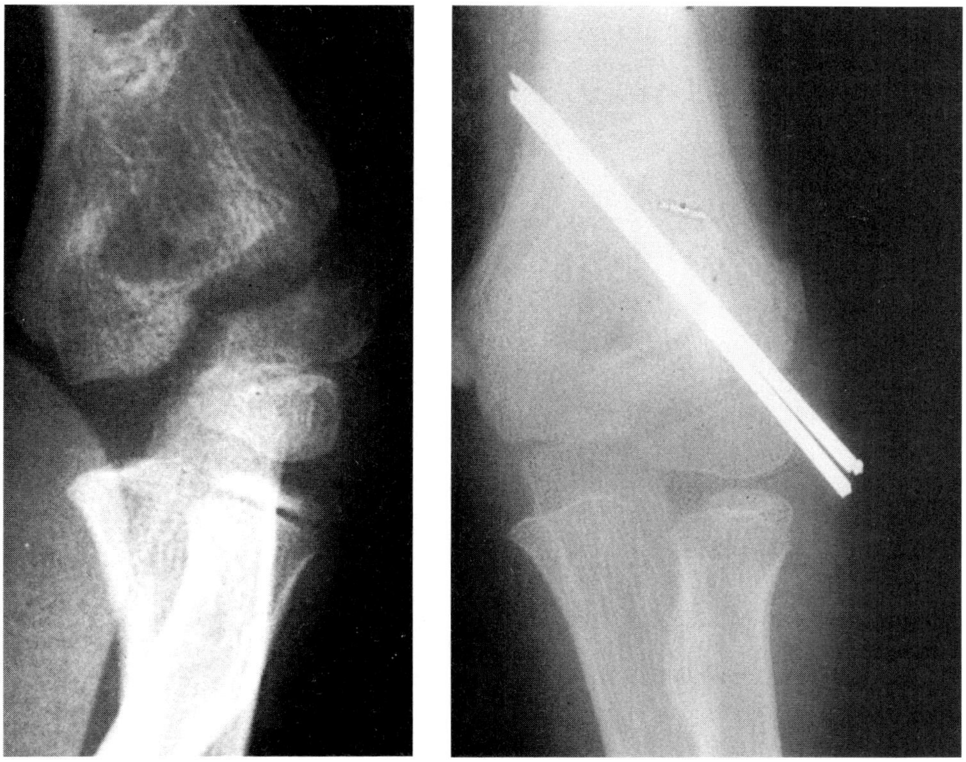

Fig. 10 **Left,** Type III fracture of the lateral condyle with displacement and rotation. **Right,** After open reduction through lateral brachioradialis-triceps interval and fixation with two Kirschner wires.

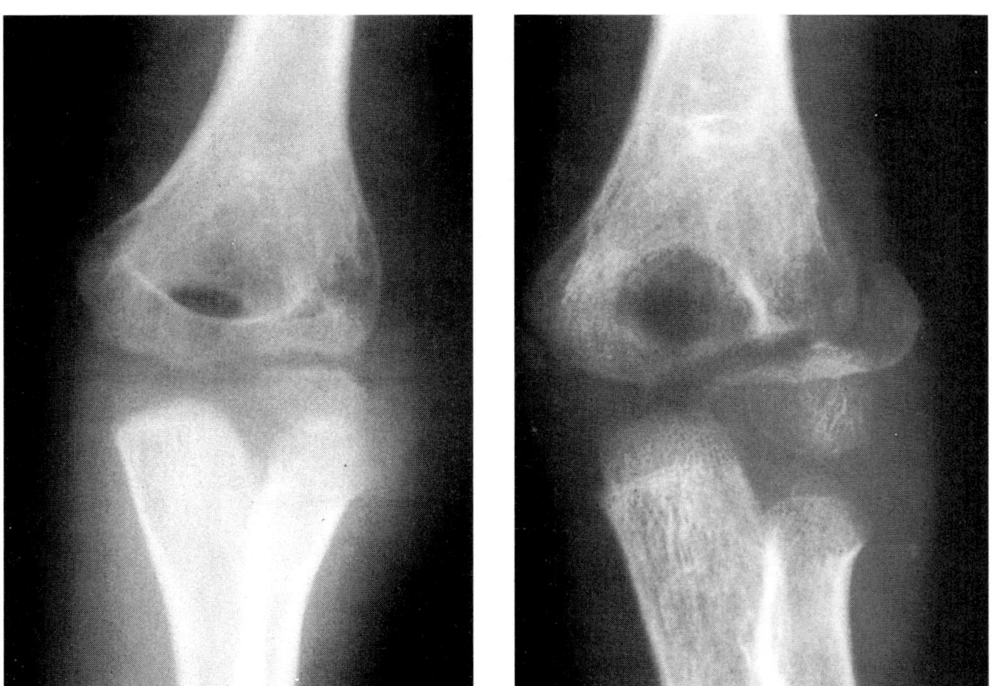

Fig. 11 **Left,** Nondisplaced type I fracture of the lateral condyle in a 6-year-old boy treated with immobilization in a long-arm cast. **Right,** Four weeks after injury, lateral displacement and nonunion of the lateral humeral condyle.

Children with lateral humeral condylar fractures should begin motion early, especially after open reduction and internal fixation, approximately 2 weeks after surgery.

Pins are left buried beneath the skin. They may be removed with the use of local or general anesthesia approximately 3 to 5 weeks after injury when radiographic union is certain.

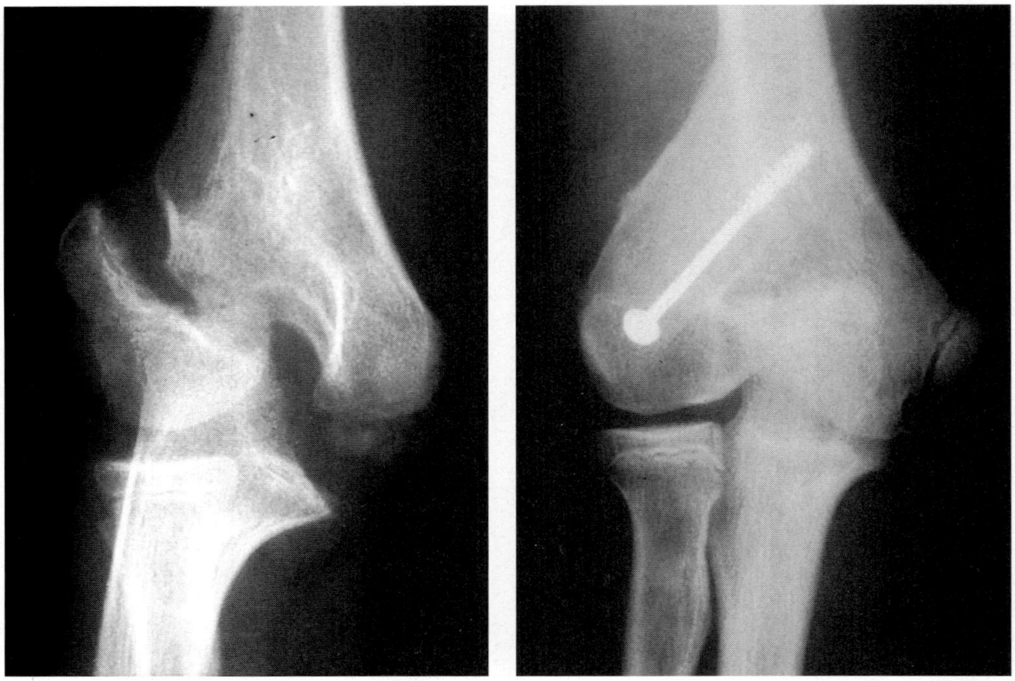

Fig. 12 **Left,** Nonunion of the lateral condyle in a 7-year-old boy. At 5 years of age, he was treated with a sling for what was believed to be an "elbow sprain". Note the large metaphyseal fragment, open physis, and 1-cm joint displacement. **Right,** Postoperative radiograph showing late reconstruction, screw fixation, bone grafting.

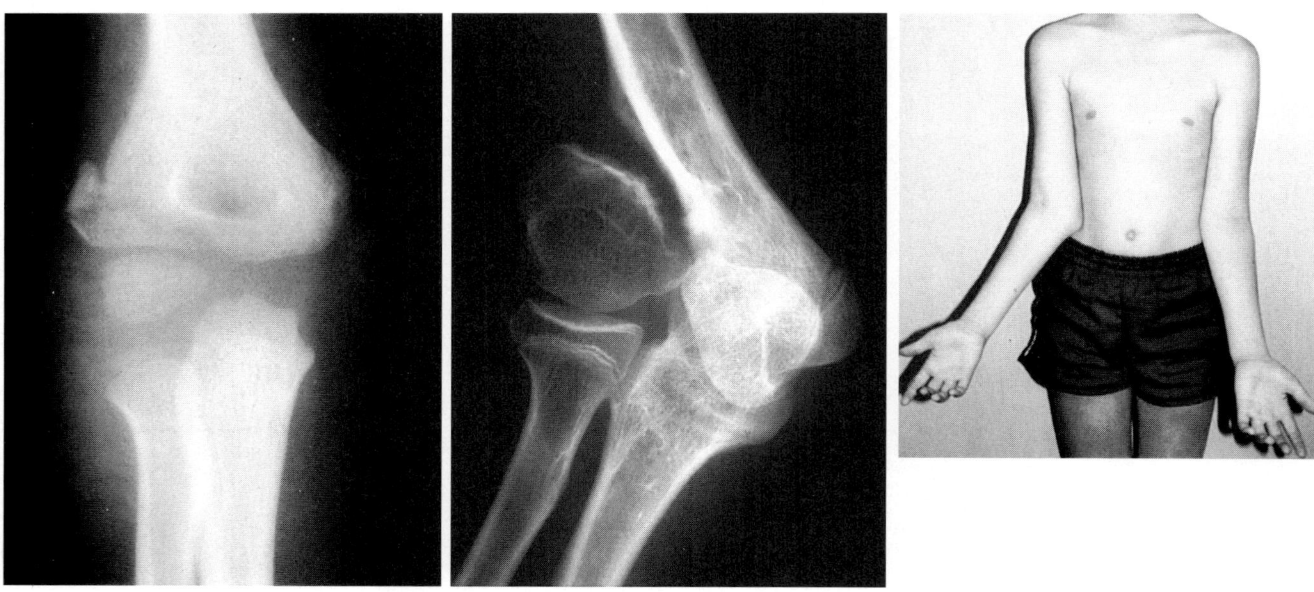

Fig. 13 **Left,** Type II fracture of the lateral condyle in a 6-year-old boy treated with immobilization in a long-arm cast for 3 weeks. **Center,** At age 13 years, lateral condylar fracture is ununited and cubitus varus deformity is 45°. **Right,** Clinical appearance. Tardy ulnar nerve palsy was treated by anterior transposition of the ulnar nerve.

Complications

Nonunion and Cubitus Valgus Deformity Nonunion can occur in fractures with late displacement and in unrecognized, untreated fractures (Fig. 11).[48-51] Treatment of nonunions of lateral condylar fractures depends on the position of the nonunion. Nonunions in good position (within 1 cm of the joint and with a large metaphyseal fragment), in a child with a viable, growing lateral condylar physis, may be treated with late reconstruction, but attention to detail is mandatory. The reconstructive technique is considerably different from that used for open reduction and intra-articular alignment of an acute fracture. A lateral incision is used, but no dissection is made into the articular

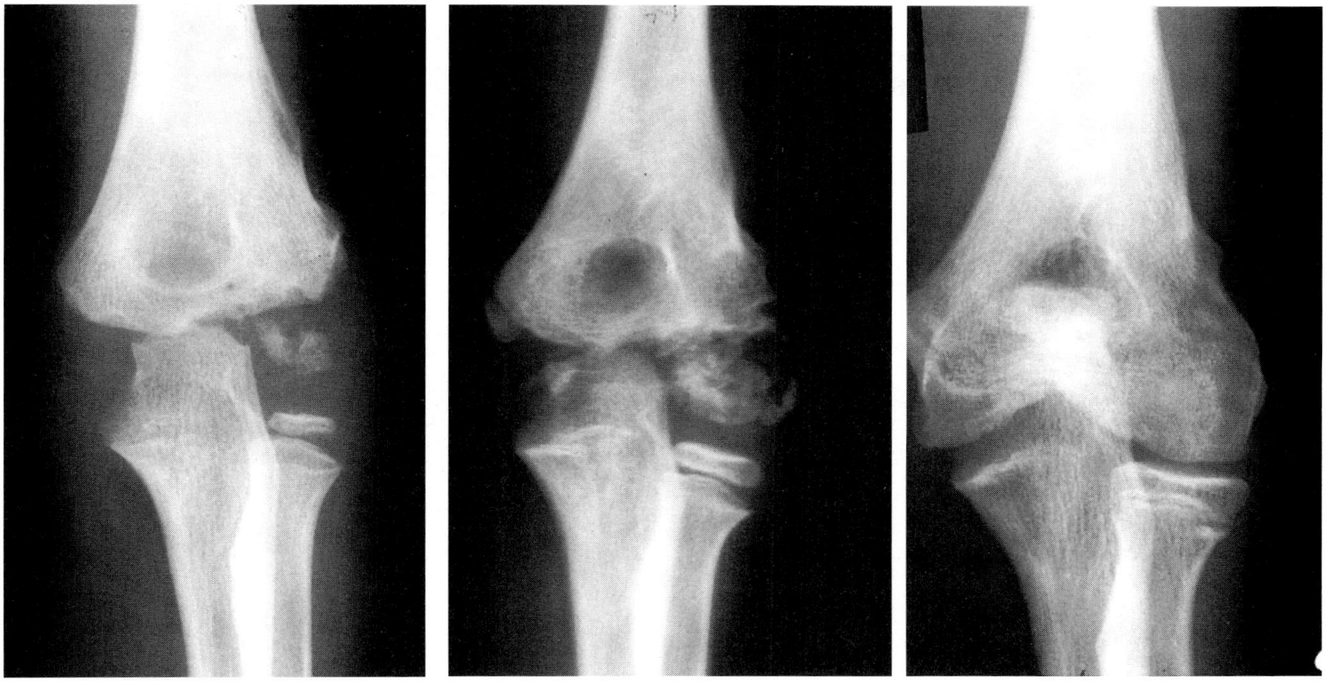

Fig. 14 **Left,** Six months after open reduction and internal fixation of fracture of the lateral condyle in a 7-year-old boy. Note osteonecrosis of the lateral condyle and the irregular metaphysis and physeal region. **Center,** At age 9 years, lateral condyle is beginning to remodel and trochlea is beginning to ossify medially. **Right,** At age 15 years, lateral condyle has reossified and remodeled. "Fishtail" appearance of the distal humerus is caused by central growth arrest. Patient had a good functional result with satisfactory range of motion.

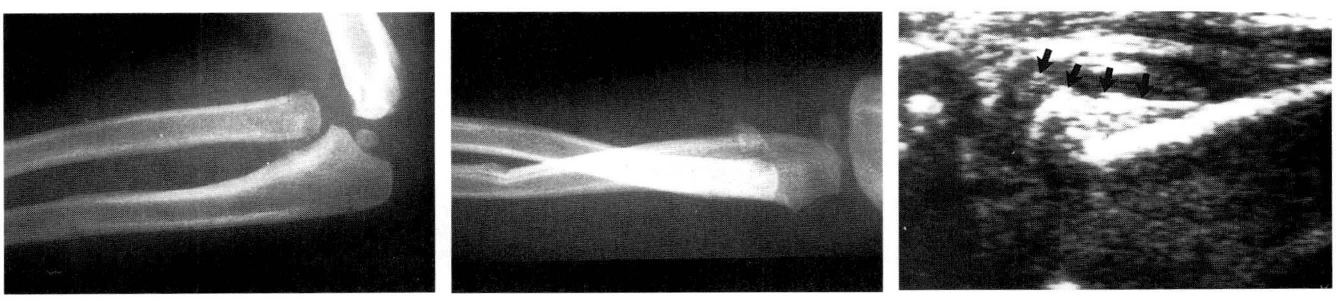

Fig. 15 **Left** and **center,** On plain radiographs, this fracture in an 18-month-old child could be confused with a Monteggia lesion. **Right,** Ultrasound demonstrates normal articulation of the radial head with the capitellum, confirming the diagnosis of radial head fracture without dislocation. Arrows outline periosteum and radial head.

surface of the elbow joint or beyond the fracture. The fibrous tissue is resected at the nonunion, and the lateral condyle is positioned against fresh metaphyseal bone of the lateral distal humerus. A screw is inserted for fixation, and a bone graft is placed along the posterolateral aspect of the fracture (Fig. 12). For nonunions not in good position, or nonunions of long duration, observation is the appropriate treatment. Anterior transposition of the ulnar nerve should be performed if early symptoms of tardy ulnar nerve palsy appear (Fig. 13).

Osteonecrosis Osteonecrosis of the lateral condyle may be caused by the injury itself or by excessive dissection of the soft tissues along the posterior aspect of the condyle.[7] If the fracture unites, the osteonecrosis usually reossifies with time, much like the process in Legg-Perthes disease about the hip (Fig. 14).

Physeal Growth Arrest Growth arrest in the area where the fracture crosses the distal humeral physis is a common radiographic finding after lateral humeral condylar fractures. The "fish-tail" appearance of the

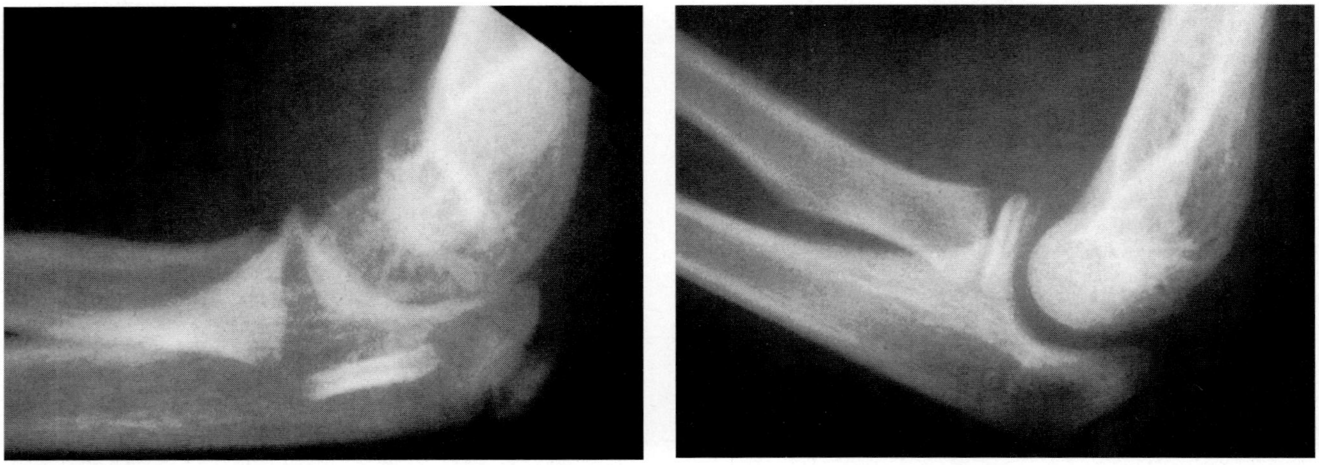

Fig. 16 **Left,** After closed reduction of this posterior elbow dislocation, the radial head was completely displaced. **Right,** After attempted closed reduction, the radial head was inverted 180°, and open reduction was required.

distal humerus on radiographs is interesting, but rarely is it of any clinical consequence.[2,7]

Fractures of the Radial Head

Fractures of the radial head usually occur in the radial neck or metaphysis, at the insertion of the annular ligament. Most frequently, these are Salter-Harris types I and II fractures.

Especially in young children, injuries around the radial head may be difficult to diagnose. Fractures of the cartilaginous epiphysis in young children may mimic Monteggia fracture-dislocations (Fig. 15).[52,53] The radial diaphysis and metaphysis are displaced so that the longitudinal axis of the bone does not cross the capitellum, while the cartilaginous radial head remains located relative to the capitellum. After closed reduction of an elbow dislocation with an associated radial head fracture, ultrasound or MRI may be necessary to determine the location of the radial head. An inverted Salter-Harris type I fracture of the radial head may appear as a subtle malposition after closed reduction (Fig. 16). The diagnosis of this injury is based on apparent physeal widening, an abnormal joint space, and irregular ossification. It is an absolute indication for open reduction and internal fixation.

Most radial head and neck fractures can be treated with closed reduction and, depending on the patient's age, a less-than-perfect reduction (less than 4 mm of translation and 30° to 60° of angulation) is acceptable.[2,7,54,55] Closed reduction of displaced fractures may be attempted by applying direct thumb pressure over the radial head with the forearm in supination. Varying the position of forearm rotation, especially into supination, will make reduction easier, and position should be confirmed by radiographs. Closed reduction of impacted or totally displaced fractures may be impossible because there is no "handle" on the small radial head. A K-wire can be used as a lever for percutaneously manipulating the fracture fragments.

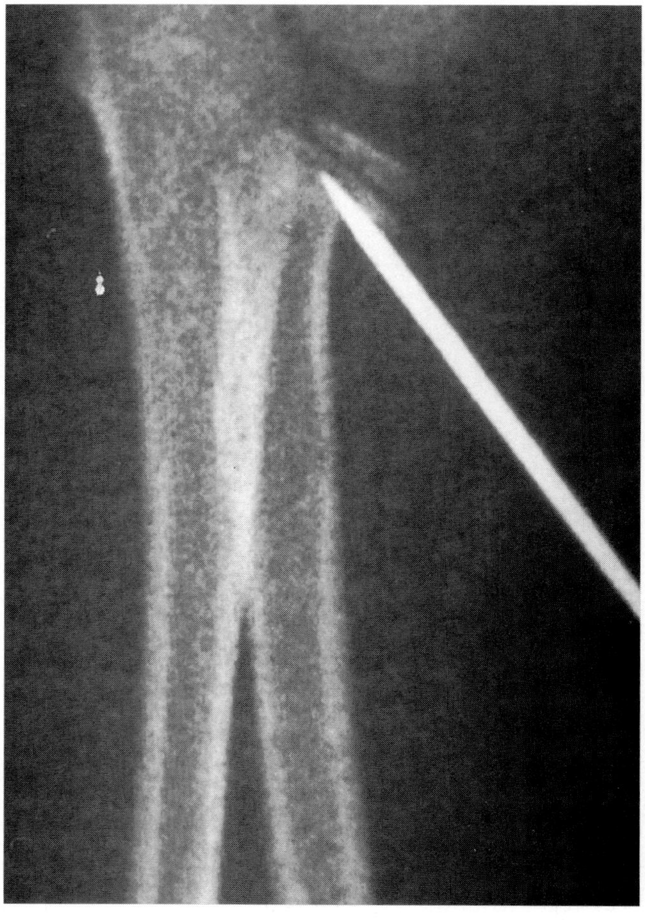

Fig. 17 A K-wire is inserted percutaneously and is used as a "lever" for reduction of the radial head fracture.

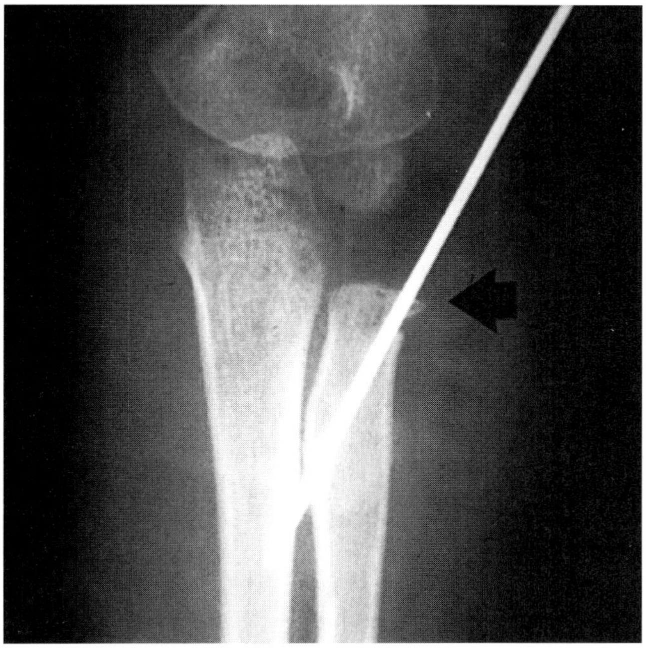

Fig. 18 After open reduction, a single oblique K-wire is sufficient for fixation.

The wire is inserted percutaneously, from distal to proximal (Fig. 17) and is used to gently push the proximal radial fragment under image intensifier control. This may allow acceptable reduction of the radial head without open reduction. Percutaneous internal fixation of the radial head fragment rarely is necessary if this maneuver is successful.

If the displaced radial head fracture cannot be reduced closed or with the percutaneous K-wire technique, open reduction is indicated.[52,56-59] As much of the annular ligament as possible and all of the soft-tissue attachments to the radial head should be preserved. These fractures usually are unstable after reduction and require internal fixation. A single 0.062-in or 5⁄64-in K-wire may be inserted obliquely across the fracture site, beginning at the articular margin of the radial head and crossing through the opposite cortex (Fig. 18); a long-arm cast is used postoperatively. Transcapitellar fixation is unnecessary and is contraindicated because of the risk of pin breakage (Fig. 19). Whether osteonecrosis and loss of motion after severe radial fractures are caused by the extent of the injury or by the open reduction remains controversial. With the lever technique of reduction, we have found that open reduction is rarely necessary. If open reduction is performed, minimal dissection of soft tissues and the use of a single oblique K-wire for fixation keep operative trauma to a minimum. We encourage early pin removal and early motion, by 2 weeks after surgery.

If the radial head is totally displaced from the joint and all soft tissues are detached (Fig. 20), the avascular radial head should be replaced and fixed with an oblique K-wire. Key,[60] in 1946, reported normal growth after replacement of the radial head in one child, but

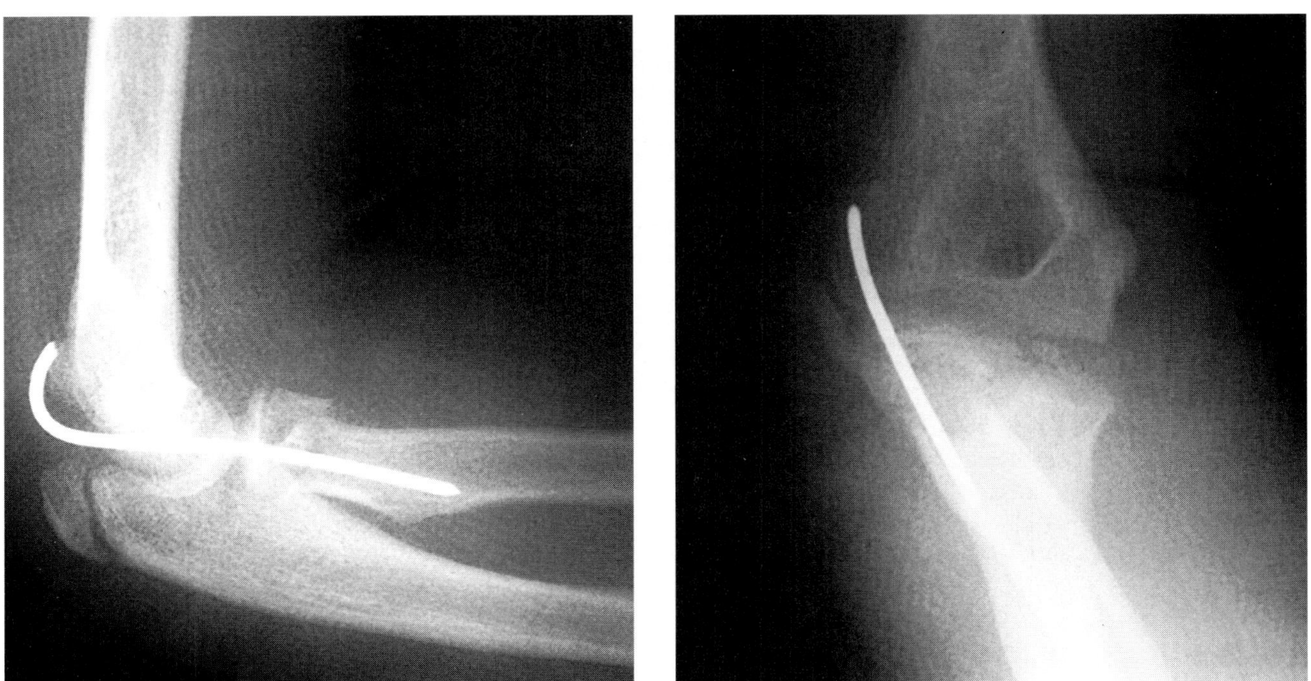

Fig. 19 A transcapitellar wire should be avoided. Note the bent pin in this patient.

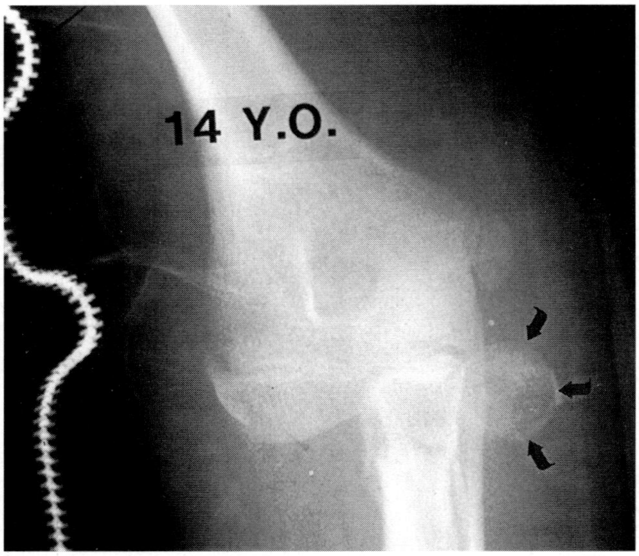

Fig. 20 A radial head that is totally displaced from the radiocapitellar articulation (arrow) should be replaced and internally fixed rather than removed.

this has not been noted by other authors. Posttraumatic resection of the radial head in children has unacceptably high risks of progressive elbow valgus deformity, proximal migration of the radius, and wrist pain. Even if osteonecrosis and growth arrest occur after replacement of the radial head, excision is not indicated. The totally detached radial head is an ideal biologic spacer, with articular cartilage and some potential for healing. Pain caused by radial head deformity may require surgical excision of the radial head, but this should be delayed until skeletal maturity.

Monteggia Fracture-Dislocations

A Monteggia[61] fracture is a combination of radial head dislocation and ulnar fracture.[62,63] These injuries are classified as type 1, extension type with anterior radial head dislocation; type 2, flexion type with posterior radial head dislocation; type 3, with lateral head dislocation; and type 4, with an associated fracture of the radial shaft. Most Monteggia fractures in children are type 1. Missed diagnosis of the radial head dislocation is the most frequent problem with these injuries.[64-66] Often the obvious fracture leads to a diagnosis of "night-stick" fracture or isolated ulnar shaft fracture. Radial head dislocation should be suspected with all proximal or midshaft ulnar fractures. "Mild" radiocapitellar malalignment should not be accepted and is an indication for examination with the patient anesthesized. On all radiographs, the long axis of the radius must transect the capitellum. The radiocapitellar articulation should be carefully scrutinized on anteroposterior, lateral, and oblique views before the diagnosis of isolated ulnar fracture is made.

Treatment

The key to treatment of Monteggia injuries is maintenance of ulnar length and alignment. The radial head usually can be reduced easily if the ulna is aligned and "out to length." Closed reduction of the ulnar fracture may be sufficient if the fracture configuration is stable and anatomically aligned.[67] After reduction of the type 1 Monteggia fracture, the arm is immobilized with the elbow in 110° of flexion and 120° of supination.

If the ulnar fracture is unstable, with shortening and angulation, closed reduction is never satisfactory, and fixation with an intramedullary rod or a plate-and-screw device is mandatory. Because of the remodeling potential of children, acceptance of "reasonable" ulnar alignment may be tempting. However, progressive ulnar shortening and angulation can occur insidiously, followed by radial head dislocation (Fig. 21). Intramedullary fixation of the ulna is simple and can be done with closed technique by inserting a single appropriately sized K-wire through the olecranon apophysis under fluoroscopic guidance. Intramedullary fixation of very oblique unstable ulnar fractures may not prevent shortening and radial head dislocation (Fig. 22), and use of a four-hole 3.5 mm AO plate with interfragmentary screw fixation (Fig. 23) is preferable.

Complications

Compartment Syndrome Although not as frequent as after supracondylar fractures, compartment syndrome may rarely occur after Monteggia fractures. If compartment syndrome or vascular compromise is questionable, internal fixation of the ulnar fracture makes management easier. If the cast must be bivalved or removed, internal fixation decreases the need for tight external support. Although the elbow is immobilized in 120° of flexion after most type 1 Monteggia fractures, if impending compartment syndrome or vascular insufficiency is suspected, the elbow should be extended less than 90°. Management of the compartment syndrome or vascular compromise obviously takes priority over management of the radial head dislocation. A second closed manipulation of the radial head may be necessary after the vascular problems are resolved. Determining the range of stability of the radial head at the time of closed reduction is helpful in determining the length of immobilization or in managing postoperative complications.

Nerve injuries Nerve injuries also may occur with Monteggia fractures.[2,7,68,69] Most commonly, the posterior interosseous nerve, which crosses anterior to the radial head, is injured. If the nerve is not functioning at initial examination, but anatomic reduction can be obtained, exploration of the nerve is not indicated. If closed reduction cannot be obtained, the radial head probably has button-holed through the anterior capsule and

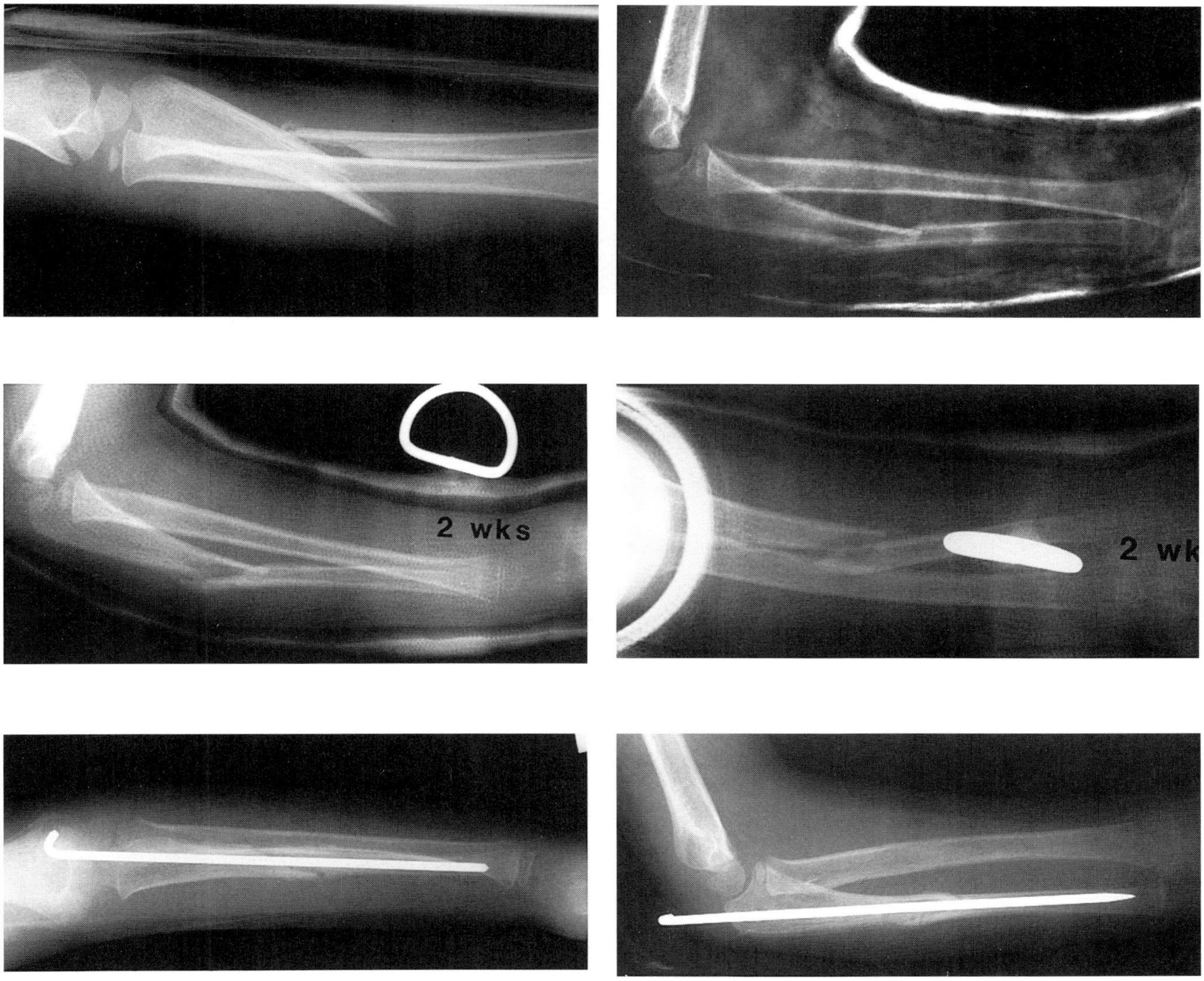

Fig. 21 **Top,** In this Monteggia injury, closed reduction obtained good radial head alignment, but marginal alignment of the ulna. **Center,** At 2 weeks, the ulna has shortened and angulated further and the radial head has subluxed. **Bottom,** After open reduction and internal fixation of the ulnar and a second closed reduction of the radial head.

torn the annular ligament; the posterior interosseous nerve may be trapped under the radial head. If open reduction is required, the posterior interosseous nerve should be carefully identified and relocated to its normal anatomic position.

Untreated Dislocations The annular ligament usually can be repaired primarily, but untreated radial dislocations often require reconstruction of the annular ligament, using a portion of the triceps (Bell-Tawse[70] procedure).

Late reconstruction of untreated radial head dislocations is somewhat controversial.[64,65,71,72] Kasser and associates have attempted reconstruction in seven patients over the past 15 years, some of whom were totally asymptomatic. Reconstruction usually consisted of ulnar osteotomy and lengthening, open reduction of the radial head, and reconstruction of the annular ligament. Results with this protocol have been mixed: two excellent results with near normal motion but diminished strength, three good results with persistent lack of motion, and two poor results with nerve injuries at the time of surgery. Although late reconstruction seems appropriate for symptomatic chronic Monteggia injuries, its usefulness for asymptomatic patients with almost full motion is questionable because of the frequency of nerve injuries and loss of motion after reconstruction.

Fractures of the Medial Condyle

Fractures of the medial condyle are rare in children.[7,73,74] Because the trochlea does not begin to ossify until about the age of 8 years, this injury may be missed in young children, or it may be confused with an isolated fracture of the medial epicondyle (Fig. 24).[75]

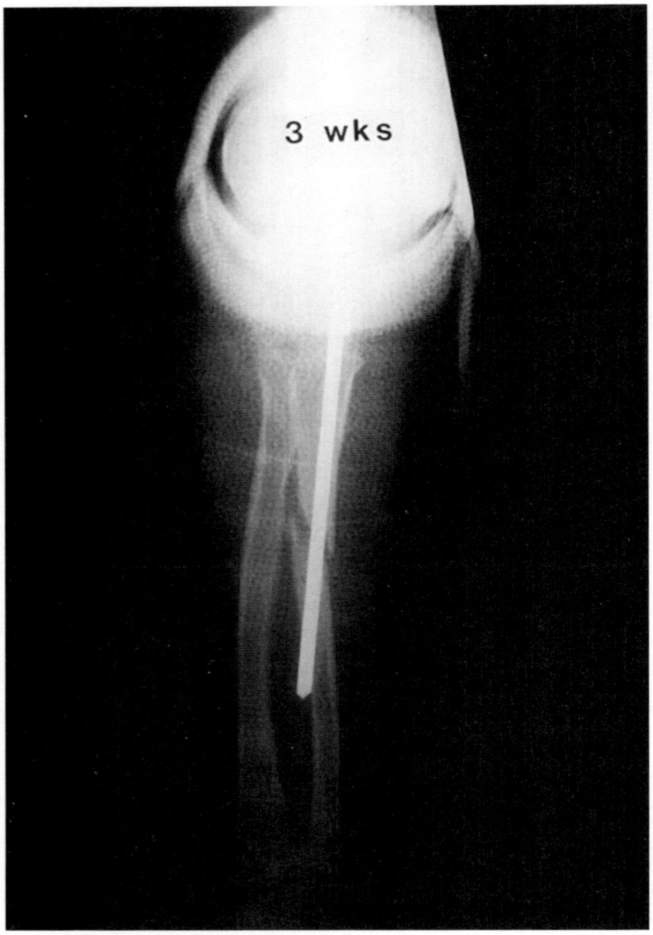

Fig. 22 Despite intramedullary rod fixation of the ulna, shortening and recurrent radial head dislocation may occur in very unstable oblique ulnar fractures.

Medial epicondyle avulsions usually are mild injuries with minimal elbow instability, unless they are associated with an elbow dislocation. If a child has marked medial swelling, ecchymosis, and instability, isolated fracture of the medial epicondyle is less likely, and arthrography or MRI should be performed to determine the diagnosis. Use of arthrography or MRI is especially important in very young children with a suspected intra-articular injury but no radiographic evidence of fracture.

Treatment of medial condylar fractures follows the general principles of treatment of all intra-articular fractures in children. For displaced fractures in young children, open reduction and internal fixation of the fragment are indicated. A medial approach is used, with protection of the ulnar and median nerves and the brachial artery. Care must be taken not to injure the physis or the blood supply to the trochlea. Aggressive dissection should be avoided around the perichondral ring and posterior to the trochlea. K-wire fixation usually is sufficient in the young child.

In adolescents, what appears to be an isolated medial or lateral condylar fracture may be a T-condylar injury that requires open reduction through a posterior approach and rigid internal fixation (Fig. 25). Because 80% of the growth of the humerus occurs proximally, transepiphyseal screws cause little growth inhibition in older children and adolescents.

A long-term problem after medial condylar fractures is osteonecrosis of the trochlea.[73,74,76] Malunion may occur, but accurate diagnosis and treatment minimize the risk of this complication.

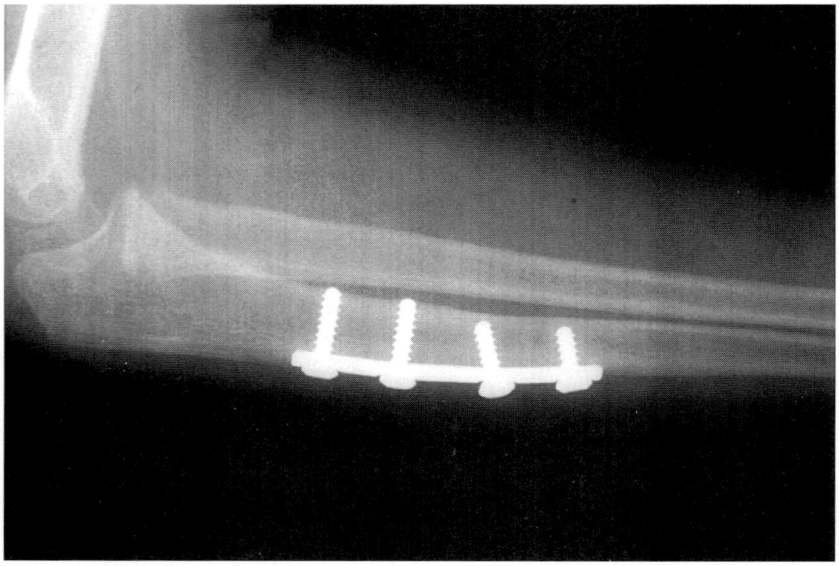

Fig. 23 A small 3.5-mm AO plate with four screws can be used for unstable Monteggia fractures.

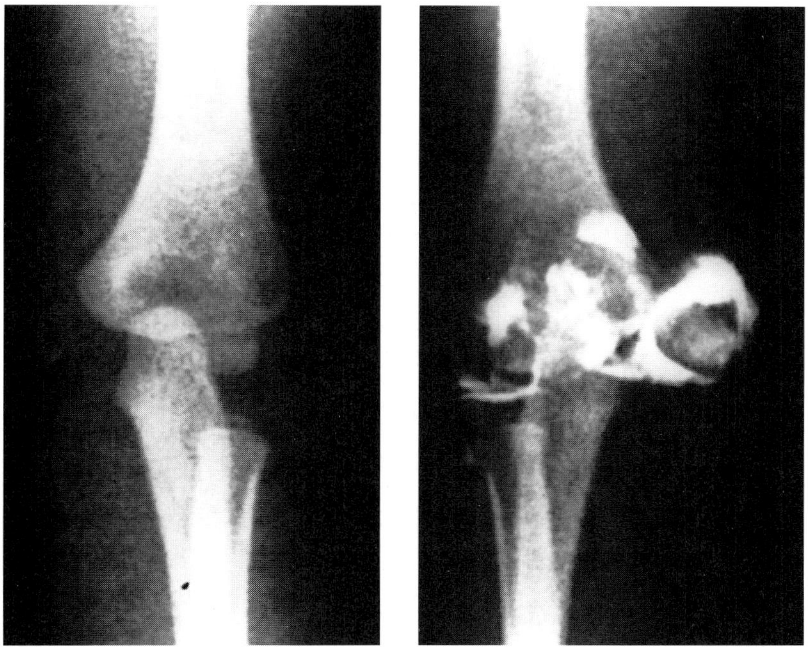

Fig. 24 **Left,** On radiograph this fracture appears to be a small displaced fracture of the medial epicondyle. **Right,** Arthrogram shows fracture of the medial condyle.

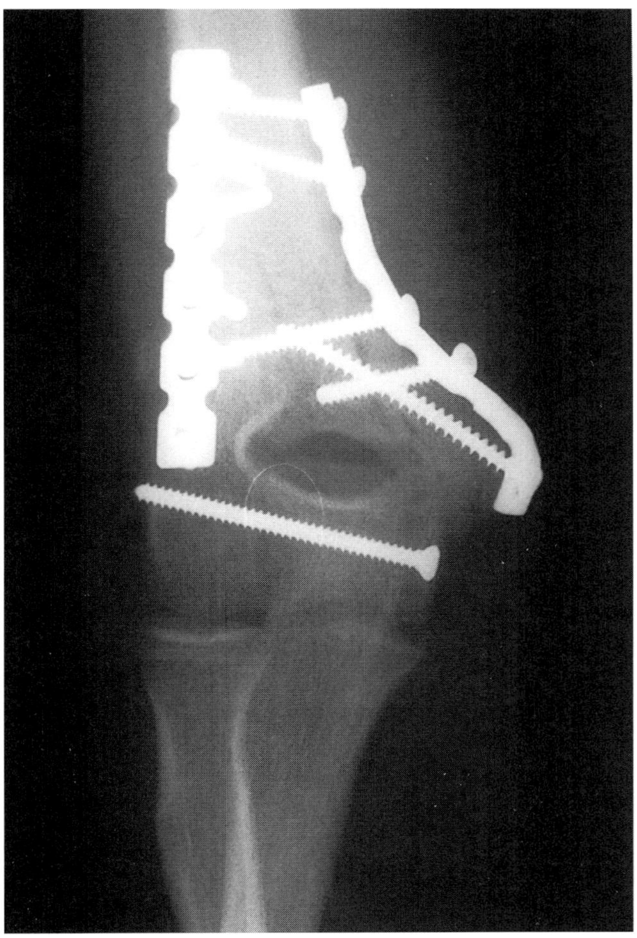

Fig. 25 An intercondylar lag screw and a neutralization plate can be used on fractures of the medial and lateral columns for rigid fixation.

References

1. Barrett WP, Almquist EA, Staheli LT: Fracture separation of the distal humeral physis in the newborn. *J Pediatr Orthop* 1984;4:617-619.
2. Canale ST: Fractures and dislocations, in Canale ST, Beaty JH (eds): *Operative Pediatric Orthopaedics.* St. Louis, MO, Mosby Year Book, 1991, pp 837-1032.
3. DeLee JC, Wilkins KE, Rogers LF, et al: Fracture-separation of the distal humeral epiphysis. *J Bone Joint Surg* 1980;62A:46-51.
4. Holda ME, Manoli A II, LaMont RI: Epiphyseal separation of the distal end of the humeral with medial displacement. *J Bone Joint Surg* 1980;62A:52-57.
5. Kaplan SS, Reckling FW: Fracture separation of the lower humeral epiphysis with medial displacement: Review of the literature and report of a case. *J Bone Joint Surg* 1971;53A:1105-1108.
6. Mizuno K, Hirohata K, Kashiwagi D: Fracture-separation of the distal humeral epiphysis in young children. *J Bone Joint Surg* 1979;61A:570-573.
7. Wilkins KE: Fractures and dislocations of the elbow region, in Rockwood CA Jr, Wilkins KE, King RE (eds): *Fractures in Children,* ed 3. Philadelphia, PA, JB Lippincott, 1991, pp 509-828.
8. Yoo CI, Suh JT, Suh KT, et al: Avascular necrosis after fracture-separation of the distal end of the humerus in children. *Orthopedics* 1992;15:959-963.
9. Beghin JL, Bucholz RW, Wenger DR: Intercondylar fractures of the humerus in young children: A report of two cases. *J Bone Joint Surg* 1982;64A:1083-1087.
10. Jarvis JG, D'Astous JL: The pediatric T-supracondylar fracture. *J Pediatr Orthop* 1984; 4:697-699.
11. Peterson HA: Triplane fracture of the distal humeral epiphysis. *J Pediatr Orthop* 1983;3:81-84.
12. Biyani A, Gupta SP, Sharma JC: Determination of medial epicondylar epiphyseal angle for supracondylar humeral fractures in children. *J Pediatr Orthop* 1993;13:94-97.
13. Gartland JJ: Management of supracondylar fractures of the humerus in children. *Surg Gynecol Obstet* 1959;109:145-154.

14. Aronson DD, Prager BI: Supracondylar fractures of the humerus in children: A modified technique for closed pinning. *Clin Orthop* 1987;219:174-184.
15. Boyd DW, Aronson DD: Supracondylar fractures of the humerus: A prospective study of percutaneous pinning. *J Pediatr Orthop* 1992;12:789-794.
16. Kallio PE, Foster BK, Paterson DC: Difficult supracondylar elbow fractures in children: Analysis of percutaneous pinning technique. *J Pediatr Orthop* 1992;12:11-15.
17. Kasser JR: Percutaneous pinning of supracondylar fractures of the humerus, in Eilert RE (ed): *Instructional Course Lectures, Volume XLI.* Rosemont, IL, American Academy of Orthopaedic Surgeons, 1992, pp 385-390.
18. Kurer MH, Regan MW: Completely displaced supracondylar fracture of the humerus in children: A review of 1708 comparable cases. *Clin Orthop* 1990;256:205-214.
19. Mehserle WL, Meehan PL: Treatment of the displaced supracondylar fracture of the humerus (type III) with closed reduction and percutaneous cross-pin fixation. *J Pediatr Orthop* 1991;11:705-711.
20. Pirone AM, Graham HK, Krajbich JI: Management of displaced extension-type supracondylar fractures of the humerus in children. *J Bone Joint Surg* 1988;70A:641-650.
21. Berghausen T, Leslie BM, Ruby LK, et al: The severely displaced pediatric supracondylar fracture of humerus: Treated by skeletal traction with olecranon pin. *Orthop Rev* 1986;15:510-515.
22. Rodriguez-Merchan EC: Supracondylar fractures of the humerus in children: Treatment by overhead skeletal traction. *Orthop Rev* 1992;21:475-482.
23. Millis MB, Singer IJ, Hall JE: Supracondylar fracture of the humerus in children: Further experience with a study in orthopaedic decision-making. *Clin Orthop* 1984;188:90-97.
24. Alburger PD, Weidner PL, Betz RR: Supracondylar fractures of the humerus in children. *J Pediatr Orthop* 1992;12:16-19.
25. Celiker O, Pestilci FI, Tuzuner M: Supracondylar fractures of the humerus in children: Analysis of the results in 142 patients. *J Orthop Trauma* 1990;4:265-269.
26. France J, Strong M: Deformity and function in supracondylar fractures of the humerus in children variously treated by closed reduction and splinting, traction, and percutaneous pinning. *J Pediatr Orthop* 1992;12:494-498.
27. Thometz JG:Techniques for direct radiographic visualization during closed pinning of supracondylar humerus fractures in children. *J Pediatr Orthop* 1990;10:555-558.
28. Culp RW, Osterman AL, Davidson RS, et al: Neural injuries associated with supracondylar fractures of the humerus in children. *J Bone Joint Surg* 1990;72A:1211-1215.
29. Royce RO, Dutkowsky JP, Kasser JR, et al: Neurologic complications after K-wire fixation of supracondylar humerus fractures in children. *J Pediatr Orthop* 1991;11:191-194.
30. Clement DA: Assessment of a treatment plan for managing acute vascular complications associated with supracondylar fractures of the humerus in children. *J Pediatr Orthop* 1990;10:97-100.
31. Shaw BA, Kasser JR, Emans JB, et al: Management of vascular injuries in displaced supracondylar humerus fractures without arteriography. *J Orthop Trauma* 1990;4:25-29.
32. Ippolito E, Moneta MR, D'Arrigo C: Post-traumatic cubitusvarus: Long-term follow-up of corrective humeral supracondylar osteotomy in children. *J Bone Joint Surg* 1990;72A:757-765.
33. Labelle H, Bunnell WP, Duhaime M, et al: Cubitus varus deformity following supracondylar fractures of the humerus in children. *J Pediatr Orthop* 1982;2:539-546.
34. Smith L: Deformity following supracondylar fractures of the humerus. *J Bone Joint Surg* 1960;42A:235-252.
35. DeRosa GP, Graziano GP: A new osteotomy for cubitus varus. *Clin Orthop* 1988;236:160-165.
36. Graham B, Tredwell SJ, Beauchamp RD, et al: Supracondylar osteotomy of the humerus for correction of cubitus varus. *J Pediatr Orthop* 1990;10:228-231.
37. Oppenheim WL, Clader TJ, Smith C, et al: Supracondylar humeral osteotomy for traumatic childhood cubitus varus deformity. *Clin Orthop* 1984;188:34-39.
38. Ippolito E, Caterini R, Scola E: Supracondylar fractures of the humerus in children: Analysis at maturity of fifty-three patients treated conservatively. *J Bone Joint Surg* 1986;68A:333-344.
39. Badelon O, Bensahel H, Mazda K, et al: Lateral humeral condylar fractures in children: A report of 47 cases. *J Pediatr Orthop* 1988;8:31-34.
40. Herring JA, Fitch RD: Lateral condylar fracture of the elbow. *J Pediatr Orthop* 1986;6:724-727.
41. Jakob R, Fowles JV, Rang M, et al: Observations concerning fractures of the lateral humeral condyle in children. *J Bone Joint Surg* 1975; 57B:430-436.
42. Silberstein MJ, Brodeur AE, Graviss ER: Some vagaries of the lateral eipcondyle. *J Bone Joint Surg* 1982;64A:444-448.
43. Wood AB, Beaty JH: Fractures of the lateral human condylar in children. Presented at the 52nd Annual Meeting of the American Academy of Orthopaedic Surgeons, Las Vegas, NV, 1985.
44. Conner AN, Smith MG: Displaced fractures of the lateral humeral condyle in children. *J Bone Joint Surg* 1970;52B:460-464.
45. Foster DE, Sullivan JA, Gross RH: Lateral humeral condylar fractures in children. *J Pediatr Orthop* 1985;5:16-22.
46. Hardacre JA, Nahigian SH, Froimson AI, et al: Fractures of the lateral condyle of the humerus in children. *J Bone Joint Surg* 1971;53A:1083-1095.
47. Jeffery CC: Non-union of the epiphysis of the lateral condyle of the humerus. *J Bone Joint Surg* 1958;40B:396-405.
48. Flynn JC: Nonunion of slightly displaced fractures of the lateral humeral condyle in children: An update. *J Pediatr Orthop* 1989; 9:691-696.
49. Flynn JC, Richards JF Jr: Non-union of minimally displaced fractures of the lateral condyle of the humerus in children. *J Bone Joint Surg* 1971;53A:1096-1101.
50. Zeier FG: Lateral condylar fracture and its many complications: Shall it be truth or consequences? *Orthop Rev* 1981;10:49-55.
51. Roye DP Jr, Bini SA, Infosino A: Late surgical treatment of lateral condylar fractures in children. *J Pediatr Orthop* 1991;11:195-199.
52. Fowles JV, Kassab MT: Observations concerning radial neck fractures in children. *J Pediatr Orthop* 1986;6:51-57.
53. Olney BW, Menelaus MB: Monteggia and equivalent lesions in childhood. *J Pediatr Orthop* 1989; 9:219-223.
54. Goldenberg RR: Closed manipulation for the reduction of fractures of the neck of the radius in children. *J Bone Joint Surg* 1945;27:267-273.
55. Jones ER, Esah M: Displaced fractures of the neck of the radius in children. *J Bone Joint Surg* 1971;53B:429-439.
56. Kaufman B, Rinott MG, Tanzman M: Closed reduction of fractures of the proximal radius in children. *J Bone Joint Surg* 1989; 71B:66-67.
57. Scullion JE, Miller JH: Fracture of the neck of the radius in children: Prognostic factors and recommendations for management. *J Bone Joint Surg* 1985;67B:491.
58. Steinberg EL, Golomb D, Salama R, et al: Radial head and neck fractures in children. *J Pediatr Orthop* 1988;8:35-40.
59. Wedge JH, Robertson DE: Displaced fractures of the neck of the radius in children. *J Bone Joint Surg* 1982;64B:256.
60. Key JA: Survival of the head of the radius in a child after removal and replacement. *J Bone Joint Surg* 1946;28:148-149.
61. Monteggia GB: *Istituzioni Chirurgiche*, ed 2. Milan, Italy, Presso Giuseppe Maspero, 1814.
62. Bado JL: The Monteggia lesion. *Clin Orthop* 1967;50:71-86.

63. Fowles JV, Sliman N, Kassab MT: The Monteggia lesion in children: Fracture of the ulna and dislocation of the radial head. *J Bone Joint Surg* 1983;65A:1276-1282.
64. Freedman L, Luk K, Leong JC: Radial head reduction after a missed Monteggia fracture: Brief report. *J Bone Joint Surg* 1988; 70B:846-847.
65. Hurst LC, Dubrow EN: Surgical treatment of symptomatic chronic radial head dislocation: A neglected Monteggia fracture. *J Pediatr Orthop* 1983;3:227-230.
66. Wright PR: Greenstick fracture of the upper end of the ulna with dislocation of the radio-humeral joint or displacement of the superior radial epiphysis. *J Bone Joint Surg* 1963;45B:727-731.
67. Letts M, Locht R, Wiens J: Monteggia fracture-dislocations in children. *J Bone Joint Surg* 1985;67B:724-727.
68. Holst-Nielsen F, Jensen V: Tardy posterior interosseous nerve palsy as a result of an unreduced radial head dislocation in Monteggia fractures: A report of two cases. *J Hand Surg* 1984; 9A:572-575.
69. Jessing P: Monteggia lesions and their complicating nerve damage. *Acta Orthop Scand* 1975;46:601-609.
70. Bell-Tawse AJS: The treatment of malunited anterior Monteggia fractures in children. *J Bone Joint Surg* 1965;47B:718-723.
71. Hirayama T, Takemitsu Y, Yagihara K, et al: Operation for chronic dislocation of the radial head in children: Reduction byosteotomy of the ulna. *J Bone Joint Surg* 1987;69B:639-642.
72. Kalamchi A: Monteggia fracture-dislocation in children: Late treatment in two cases. *J Bone Joint Surg* 1986;68A:615-619.
73. El Ghawabi MH: Fracture of the medial condyle of the humerus. *J Bone Joint Surg* 1975:57A:677-680.
74. Papavasiliou V, Nenopoulos S, Venturis T: Fractures of the medial condyle of the humerus in childhood. *J Pediatr Orthop* 1987;7:421-423.
75. Fahey JJ, O'Brien ET: Fracture-separation of the medial humeral condyle in a child confused with fracture of the medial epicondyle. *J Bone Joint Surg* 1971;53A:1102-1104.
76. Fowles JV, Kassab MT: Displaced fractures of the medial humeral condyle in children. *J Bone Joint Surg* 1980;62A:1159-1163.

CHAPTER 19

Arthroscopy of the Elbow

Gary G. Poehling, MD
Evan F. Ekman, MD

Although historically it was thought that arthroscopy of the elbow was too dangerous to be of clinical use,[1] an evolution in techniques and equipment, especially over the past decade, has proved it to be an acceptable alternative for the treatment of many lesions about that joint.[2-4] This chapter discusses the arthroscopically pertinent anatomy of the elbow, the operating-room setup, the development of the portals, the operative technique, and the indications for and complications of elbow arthroscopy. After reading this lecture, one should: (1) know the superficial anatomy of the elbow and be able to create standard arthroscopic portals, (2) know the arthroscopic anatomy of the elbow joint, (3) understand common lesions of the elbow and the clinical indications for elbow arthroscopy, (4) understand how to treat specific intra-articular problems of the elbow arthroscopically, and (5) know the complications of elbow arthroscopy and the strategies for avoiding them.

Elbow arthroscopy is a technically demanding operation, and extensive hands-on training and supervised experience are needed to acquire proficiency. Elbow arthroscopy is important in that it provides an opportunity to intervene in the elbow, both diagnostically and therapeutically, without creation of an arthrotomy with its subsequent morbidity, which may include contracture and an increased risk of infection. When performed with appropriate judgment and technique, elbow arthroscopy is an excellent intervention for the correction of many lesions of the elbow, with minimum risk.

Technique

This section discusses the technique of elbow arthroscopy with prone positioning of the patient, although the operating-room setup and the technique are not very different for a supine patient. Naturally, the preferences of the surgeon allow small changes in this technique.

Prone Position

Traditionally, elbow arthroscopy was performed with the patient resting supine on the operating table,[5] until use of the prone position was introduced in 1989.[4] The prone position improves the mobility of the arthroscope within the joint, facilitates manipulation of the joint, provides for a more complete intra-articular inspection (especially in the posterior aspect of the joint), and eliminates the need for an overhead suspension device to support the elbow. After an appropriate level of anesthesia (general endotracheal or axillary block) has been achieved, the patient is placed prone, with chest-rolls under the torso. An arm-board is placed on the operative side of the table and parallel to it. To increase the mobility of the upper extremity intraoperatively, a sandbag is placed under the shoulder. The forearm is then allowed to hang in a dependent position over the arm-board. A tourniquet may be placed around the proximal aspect of the arm to help to control bleeding during the procedure, but we have rarely found this to be necessary when using a mechanical irrigation system.

Operating-Room Setup

With the patient prone and the anesthesia personnel positioned at the head of the table, the surgeon stands directly lateral to the flexed elbow and the assistant stands toward the head of the patient. The ancillary scrubbed personnel stand toward the foot of the patient or behind the surgeon and the assistant. A Mayo stand with the appropriate surgical instrumentation is placed toward the foot of the patient. The video monitor, recorder, light source, camera, fluid bags, and mechanical irrigation system are placed either on a rolling platform on the side of the patient that is not being operated on or on a suspended platform partially above the patient (Fig. 1).

Anatomy of the Elbow and Development of the Portals

Similar to all other aspects of orthopaedic surgery, elbow arthroscopy requires a complete understanding of the regional anatomy. A thorough knowledge of both the superficial neurovascular and the intra-articular structures is essential for the procedure to be safe and effective. It can be helpful to outline the surface

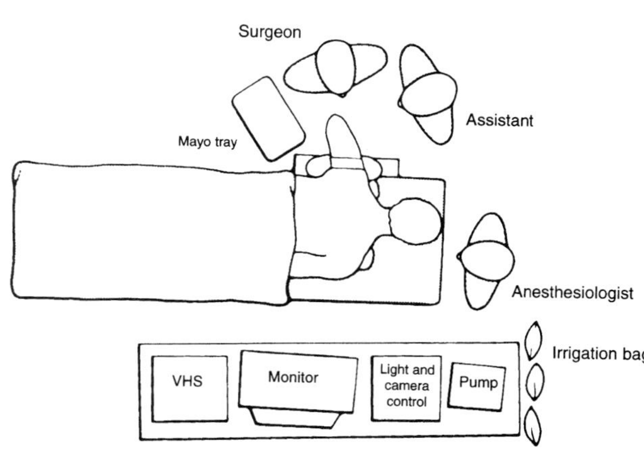

Fig. 1 Operating-room setup for the elbow arthroscopy, with the patient in the prone position. (VHS = video recorder)

landmarks with a sterile marking pen; these structures include the olecranon, the medial and lateral humeral epicondyles, the radial head, and the medial intermuscular septum. To avoid injury to nearby neurovascular structures, it also is helpful to diagram the median, radial, and ulnar nerves and the brachial artery on the skin.

Before creation of the first portal, it is helpful to fill the joint with fluid to distend the capsule and make it easier to enter this relatively small space. Also, egress of fluid from the joint when the portal is made verifies that the cannula is in the joint. To fill the joint with fluid, the boundaries of the anconeus triangle are first identified. The three corners of this triangle are the radial head, the lateral humeral epicondyle, and the tip of the olecranon (Fig. 2). An 18-gauge needle is then placed in the joint through the soft spot bounded by these structures, and 30 to 50 ml of lactated Ringer solution is injected.

Three standard portals are used routinely. A fourth portal is necessary when instruments must be introduced into the posterior aspect of the elbow. All four portals will be described here.

Proximal-Medial Portal This portal is of particular benefit when arthroscopy is performed in a prone patient.[4] The joint is pre-distended with fluid, as already described. The surface location of the proximal-medial portal is 2 cm proximal to the medial epicondyle and just anterior to the intermuscular septum (Fig. 3, *top left*). The medial intermuscular septum is palpated with the surgeon's free hand to locate the proper point of insertion. Failure to identify clearly the intermuscular septum puts the ulnar nerve at risk, especially in an obese patient. A 0.5-cm longitudinal incision is then made through the skin only. A hemostat is used to spread the subcutaneous tissue; this must be done bluntly to protect the medial brachial cutaneous and the medial antebrachial cutaneous nerves. A 4-mm arthroscope sheath is loaded onto a blunt trocar of an appropriate size. The surgeon continues to palpate the medial intermuscular septum, while advancing the trocar anterior to it. The trocar must be kept anterior to the intermuscular septum to protect the ulnar nerve (Fig. 3, *top right*). As the trocar is advanced, care must be taken to maintain contact with the anterior surface of the humerus and to direct the trocar toward the radial head. Use of the anterior surface of the humerus as a constant guiding surface helps to prevent injury to the median nerve and the brachial artery (Fig. 3, *bottom*). The return of fluid through the arthroscope sheath after removal of the trocar ensures that the capsule has been entered. A provisional observation with the telescope at this point, before further development of the portal, helps to orient the system.

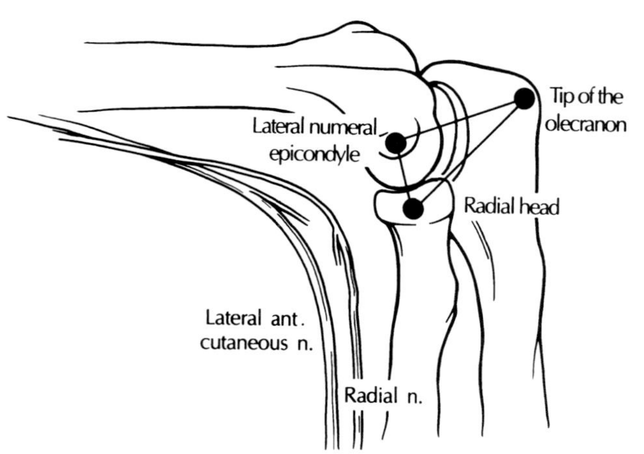

Fig. 2 The anconeus triangle on the lateral aspect of the elbow.

A 4-mm, 30°-angled telescope is excellent for routine elbow arthroscopy, especially in the anterior parts of the joint. From the proximal-medial portal, most of the structures in the anterior aspect of the elbow joint can be visualized, including the radial head, the capitellum, the trochlea, the coronoid process, the medial condyle, and the anterior aspect of the joint capsule (Fig. 4).

Posterolateral Portal The posterolateral portal is created in the anconeus triangle, the same location where the irrigation solution was originally introduced into the joint (Fig. 2). Palpation and outlining of the tip of the olecranon, the radial head, and the lateral humeral epicondyle help to define the corners of the anconeus triangle. The soft spot in the center of this triangle is palpated, and a 0.3-cm vertical skin incision is made. We have found this to be an excellent portal for positioning the pressure monitoring-outflow cannula when performing arthroscopy in the anterior aspect of the joint. If arthroscopy is to be performed in the posterior aspect of the joint, the cannula must be moved from this spot, usually to the anterolateral portal, to free the posterolateral portal for introduction of the telescope or the instrumentation, or both. With the telescope in the posterolateral portal, a view of the olecranon fossa, the tip of the olecranon, and the posterior aspect of the joint capsule is provided (Fig. 5).

Anterolateral Portal The anterolateral portal is essential whenever two portals in the anterior aspect of the joint are required (Fig. 6). As described by Andrews and Carson,[5] the anterolateral portal is created 3 cm distal and 2 cm anterior to the lateral epicondyle with the elbow flexed 90°. This portal is often the first one made when arthroscopy is performed with the patient supine, and in this case the portal is developed in a standard fashion after needle localization of the joint. For the prone patient, the anterolateral portal can be created in an inside-out manner. After the proximal- medial portal has been created and the anterior aspect of the elbow has been inspected arthroscopically, the telescope is removed from the sheath and, with the sheath

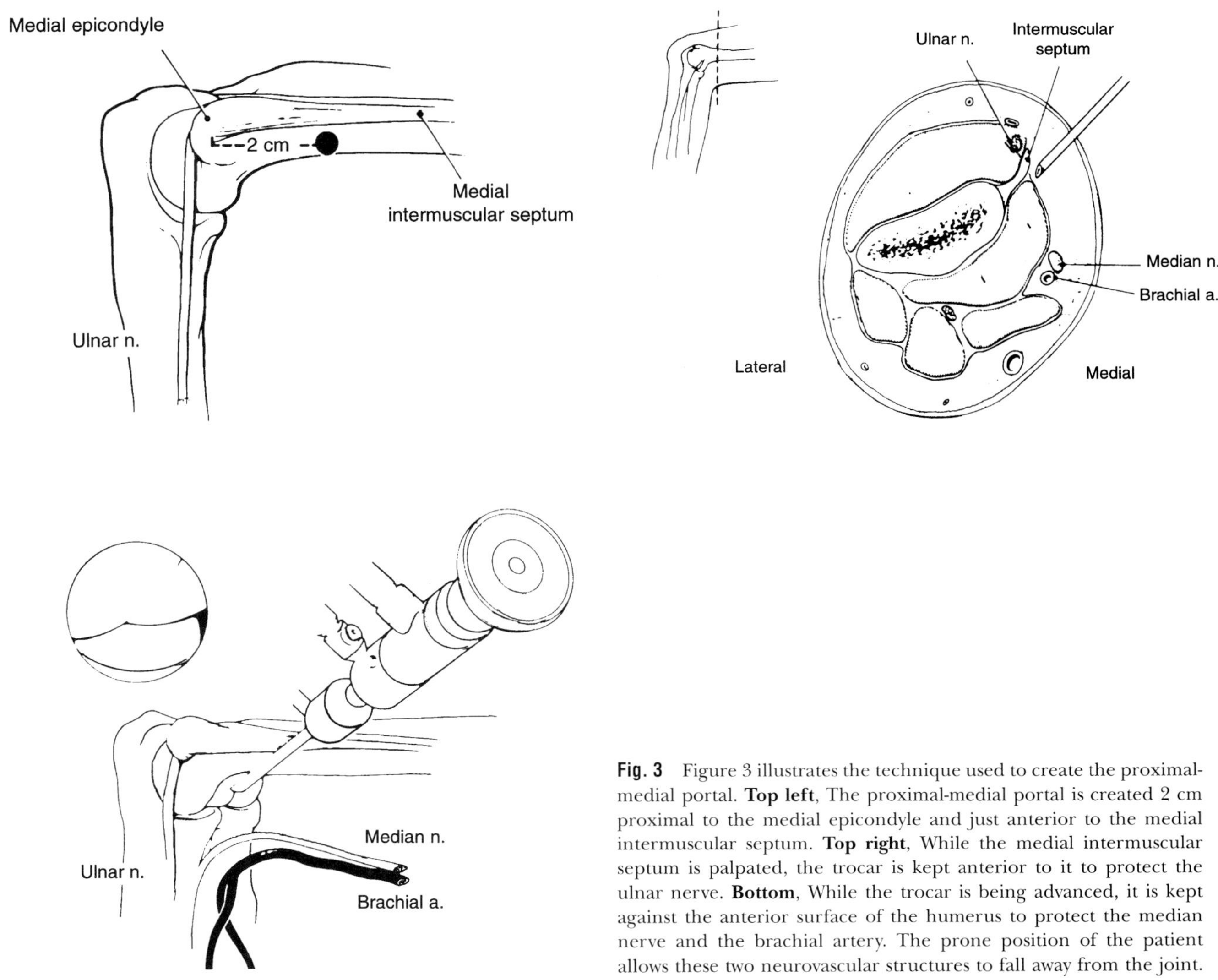

Fig. 3 Figure 3 illustrates the technique used to create the proximal-medial portal. **Top left**, The proximal-medial portal is created 2 cm proximal to the medial epicondyle and just anterior to the medial intermuscular septum. **Top right**, While the medial intermuscular septum is palpated, the trocar is kept anterior to it to protect the ulnar nerve. **Bottom**, While the trocar is being advanced, it is kept against the anterior surface of the humerus to protect the median nerve and the brachial artery. The prone position of the patient allows these two neurovascular structures to fall away from the joint.

still in place and the elbow flexed 90°, a blunt rod is passed through the sheath and directed toward the radial head.[6] In order to protect the posterior interosseous nerve, care must be taken to keep the rod relatively more lateral than anterior to the radial head while it is moved through the capsule. If the elbow is not flexed to 90°, the surgeon will find it difficult to stay lateral to the radial head. The rod is then advanced through the anterolateral portion of the joint capsule and the subcutaneous tissue until it tents the skin. This tenting should occur immediately anterolateral to the radial head and approximately 1 cm distal to the radiocapitellar joint (Fig. 7). A knife can then be used to make a skin incision directly over the tip of the rod. The rod is then advanced through the skin so that a sheath can be placed over it from the anterolateral side and into the joint.

The anterolateral portal is an excellent working portal for instrumentation and manipulation. With the telescope placed in this portal, one can see the lateral portion of the distal aspect of the humerus, the coronoid process of the ulna, and the radial head. The position of the anterolateral portal can be varied slightly to accommodate specific lesions. For example, if performing an excision of the radial head, the surgeon may prefer to make this portal slightly more proximal than described, to create an easier angle for the excision.

Direct Posterior Portal The direct posterior portal is developed when it is necessary to place instrumentation in the posterior aspect of the joint. A 5-mm skin incision is made 1.5 to 2 cm proximal to the tip of the olecranon, directly over the triceps tendon, and a sheath, mounted on a blunt trocar, is advanced through the triceps tendon directly into the olecranon fossa. This should be done while the entry of the sheath into the capsule is observed through the telescope placed in the posterolateral portal. Direct arthroscopic visualization confirms successful positioning of the trocar in the

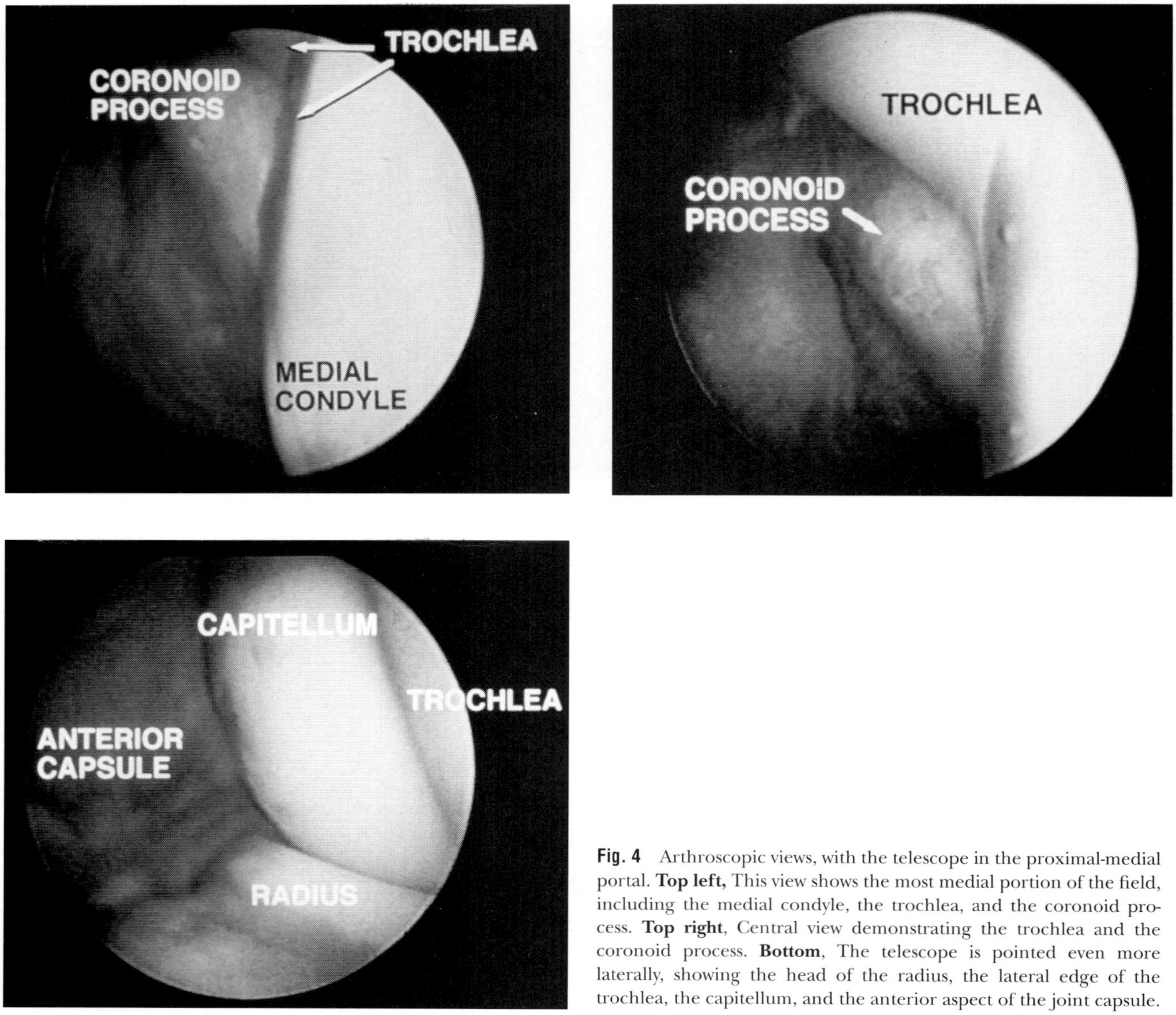

Fig. 4 Arthroscopic views, with the telescope in the proximal-medial portal. **Top left,** This view shows the most medial portion of the field, including the medial condyle, the trochlea, and the coronoid process. **Top right**, Central view demonstrating the trochlea and the coronoid process. **Bottom**, The telescope is pointed even more laterally, showing the head of the radius, the lateral edge of the trochlea, the capitellum, and the anterior aspect of the joint capsule.

olecranon fossa. The direct posterior portal serves primarily as a site for the introduction of instruments into the posterior aspect of the elbow joint; however, the telescope can be placed through this portal, allowing the posterolateral portal to become the working instrument portal. This portal allows visualization of the structures of the posterior aspect of the joint: the olecranon, the olecranon fossa, and the posterior aspect of the capsule. Some surgeons prefer to use a posterior working portal, created at approximately the same level but just lateral to the triceps tendon.

Indications for Arthroscopy of the Elbow

Arthroscopy of the elbow is a relatively new technique, and its indications are still being defined. It can be used for the diagnosis of intra-articular lesions, the removal of loose and foreign bodies, irrigation of the joint, debridement of an infected joint, excision of osteophytes, synovectomy, capsular release, and excision of the radial head. Arthroscopy has also been used in the evaluation and treatment of acute fractures of the elbow.

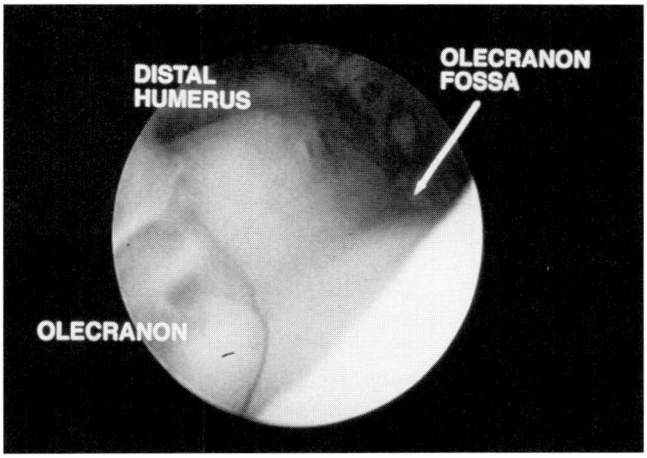

Fig. 5 Arthroscopic view, with the telescope in the posterolateral portal. Both the olecranon and the olecranon fossa can be visualized from this portal.

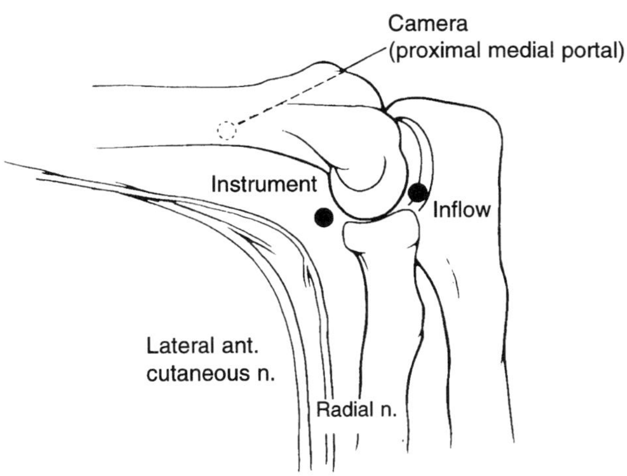

Fig. 6 Illustration of the lateral portals. The inflow portal is in the posterolateral position, which is established in the middle of the anconeus triangle. The instrument portal is in the anterolateral position, immediately anterior to the radial head and near the radiocapitellar joint.

Removal of Loose and Foreign Bodies

A number of authors have reported on the removal of loose bodies with arthroscopy;[7-11] a similar technique has been used for the removal of foreign bodies.[12] Several pathological processes may initiate the formation of a loose body. Regardless of the etiology, one can expect less swelling, locking, and pain, as well as improved motion, if the loose body is removed.

To remove loose bodies from the anterior aspect of the joint, the telescope is positioned in either the proximal-medial portal or the anterolateral portal. A grasping forceps, with or without suction attached, is introduced through the contralateral portal. The pressure monitoring-outflow device remains in the posterolateral portal. To remove loose bodies from the posterior aspect of the joint, the telescope is placed in the posterolateral portal after the pressure monitoring-outflow device has been moved to the anterolateral portal. A grasping instrument can then be inserted through a direct posterior portal.

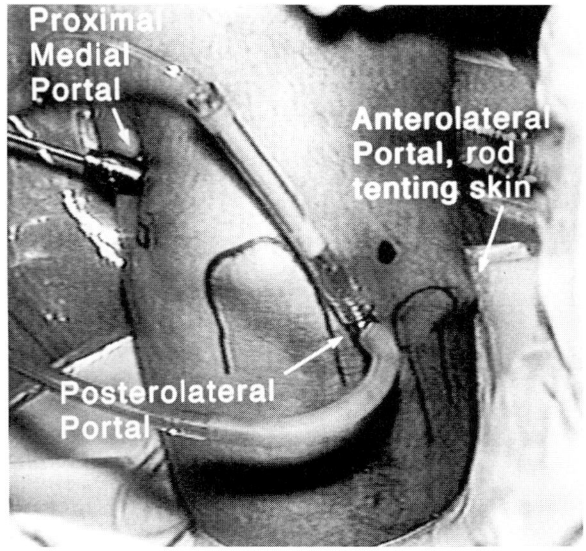

Fig. 7 Clinical photograph of a blunt rod tenting the skin in the anterolateral position. The tenting is a step in the creation of the portal with use of the inside-out technique.

Irrigation of an Infected Joint

If the diagnosis of an infection of the elbow is made or suspected, arthroscopy is an effective way to lavage the joint with minimum invasiveness. Only two portals are needed: the proximal-medial portal and the posterolateral portal. After the joint has been irrigated with a copious amount of fluid, the condition of the underlying bone, cartilage, and synovial tissue can be assessed arthroscopically.

Excision of Osteophytes

The presence of osteophytes, or osseous spurs, is another condition that lends itself to arthroscopic management.[11,13] We have used a variety of burrs to remove osteophytes. Preoperative radiographs can help the surgeon to plan the appropriate margins of the excision. A true lateral radiograph of the elbow is useful for the identification of osteophytes that may limit the range of motion. Also helpful is an intraoperative assessment of the full range of flexion, extension, pronation, and supination after a provisional removal of the osteophyte has been performed. These movements, although simple to execute with the patient in a prone position and the arm free, are quite difficult to do with the patient supine. It must be remembered that arthroscopic excision of osteophytes creates a substantial amount of intra-articular debris, and thorough irrigation of the elbow before the cannula is removed is essential.

Synovectomy

A partial or near-total synovectomy can be performed arthroscopically and often provides considerable relief of pain for a patient with chronic synovitis.[14] Anterior and posterior synovectomy require that the telescope and shaver be moved from portal to portal in both the anterior and the posterior aspects of the joint to obtain the best result. Synovectomy can result in a large amount of blood, and we recommend that the portals be left open postoperatively to allow blood and fluid to drain from the joint. This decreases the prevalence of hemarthrosis and its inherent complications, including an increased risk of infection and postoperative pain.

Capsular Release

Like loose bodies and osteophytes, capsular contracture can also limit elbow motion. Release of the anterior aspect of the capsule, with or without debridement of bone in the olecranon fossa, improves motion of the elbow in all axes.[15] In the anterior aspect of the joint, with use of the distal part of the humerus as a guide, the capsule is released proximally at its insertion onto the humerus. Because the neurovascular structures about the elbow may be closely adherent to the capsule, capsular release is a very risky procedure and should be undertaken only with great care, by a surgeon experienced in elbow arthroscopy.

Excision of the Radial Head

Successful excision of the radial head can be performed arthroscopically. In addition to the entire radial head, as much as 2 to 3 mm of the radial neck can be removed. With the telescope placed in the proximal-medial portal, an arthroscopic burr is placed through the anterolateral portal. After the radial head and a portion of the neck have been removed, the elbow should be supinated and pronated under arthroscopic visualization to ensure that no osseous block remains. To maintain stability at the proximal radioulnar joint, however, the annular ligament must be left intact.

Complications

Complications due to elbow arthroscopy can be minimized if the surgeon has a sound knowledge of the anatomy of the elbow and uses proper equipment and meticulous technique. The most commonly reported complications of this procedure are neurologic. Jones and Savoie[16] reported a case of transection of the posterior interosseous nerve; Cascells,[15] a case of irreparable damage to the ulnar nerve; and Papilion and associates,[17] a case of a compression neuropathy of the radial nerve. Permanent dysfunction of the sensory branch of the radial nerve[18] and transient dysfunction of the median nerve, the radial nerve, and the medial antebrachial cutaneous nerve have also been reported.[3,5] Infection is, of course, a possible complication whenever a joint has been entered; however, with use of meticulous sterile technique and appropriate care of the instruments, this risk is small. One case of aseptic bursitis of the olecranon has been reported.[16] The authors thought that the establishment of two adjacent portals through the olecranon bursa may have caused the problem. Theoretically, the brachial artery is in a position of risk;[3] hence, care must be taken to avoid this structure, particularly when anterior capsular release is attempted. Finally, as with arthroscopic procedures at other sites, the instruments can break. Appropriate care of the telescope and tools and minimum use of force should decrease the prevalence of this complication.

Other measures that decrease the risk of complications include placement of the patient in the prone position, so that gravity can pull the anterior neurovascular structures (the median nerve and the brachial artery) away from the capsule;[4] full distention of the joint and flexion of the elbow to 90° before the creation of a portal; and use of the inside-out technique for the creation of the anterolateral portal. The use of these measures, combined with precise surgical technique, greatly minimizes the risks associated with elbow arthroscopy, making it a safe procedure.

Overview

Arthroscopy of the elbow has come of age. With the advent of new technology, such as smaller instruments and mechanical fluid pumps, and with innovations in technique, the orthopaedic surgeon can treat a variety of lesions of the elbow. We advocate the prone position for the patient because of its simplicity, safety, and effectiveness. Although elbow arthroscopy is now used primarily for the indications outlined in this chapter, we can expect the list of indications to expand. As in all areas of orthopaedics, however, enthusiasm for this technique should not override sound clinical and surgical judgment.

References

1. Burman MS: Arthroscopy or the direct visualization of joints: An experimental cadaver study. *J Bone Joint Surg* 1931;13:669-695.

2. Carson WG Jr: Arthroscopy of the elbow, in Bassett Frank H III (ed): *American Academy of Orthopaedic Surgeons Instructional Course Lectures Volume XXXVII.* St. Louis, MO, CV Mosby, 1988, pp 195-201.
3. Lynch GJ, Meyers JF, Whipple TL, et al: Neurovascular anatomy and elbow arthroscopy: Inherent risks. *Arthroscopy* 1986;2:190-197.
4. Poehling GG, Whipple TL, Sisco L, et al: Elbow arthroscopy: A new technique. *Arthroscopy* 1989;5:222-224.
5. Andrews JR, Carson WG: Arthroscopy of the elbow. *Arthroscopy* 1985;1:97-107.
6. Poehling GG, Ekman EF: Elbow arthroscopy: Introduction and overview, in Poehling G, Koman LA, Pope T, et al (eds): *Arthroscopy of the Wrist and Elbow.* New York, NY, Raven Press, 1994, pp 129-136.
7. Boe S: Arthroscopy of the elbow: Diagnosis and extraction of loose bodies. *Acta Orthop Scand* 1986;57:52-53.
8. O'Driscoll SW: Elbow arthroscopy for loose bodies. *Orthopedics* 1992;15:855-859.
9. Ogilvie-Harris DJ, Schemitsch E: Arthroscopy of the elbow for removal of loose bodies. *Arthroscopy* 1993;9:5-8.
10. Parisien JS: Arthroscopic surgery of the elbow. *Bull Hosp Joint Dis* 1988;48:149-158.
11. Ward WG, Anderson TE: Elbow arthroscopy in a mostly athletic population. *J Hand Surg* 1993;18A:220-224.
12. Cameron SE, Travis MT, Kruse RW: Foreign body arthroscopically retrieved from the elbow. *Arthroscopy* 1993;9:220-221.
13. Woods GW: Elbow arthroscopy. *Clin Sports Med* 1987;6:557-564.
14. Angelo RL: Advances in elbow arthroscopy. *Orthopedics* 1993;16:1037-1046.
15. Cascells SW: Editorial: Neurovascular anatomy and elbow arthroscopy: Inherent risks. *Arthroscopy* 1986;2:190.
16. Jones GS, Savoie FH III: Arthroscopic capsular release of flexion contractures (arthrofibrosis) of the elbow. *Arthroscopy* 1993;9:277-283.
17. Papilion JD, Neff RS, Shall LM: Compression neuropathy of the radial nerve as a complication of elbow arthroscopy: A case report and review of the literature. *Arthroscopy* 1988;4:284-286.
18. Guhl JF: Arthroscopy and arthroscopic surgery of the elbow. *Orthopedics* 1985;8:1290-1296.

Hip

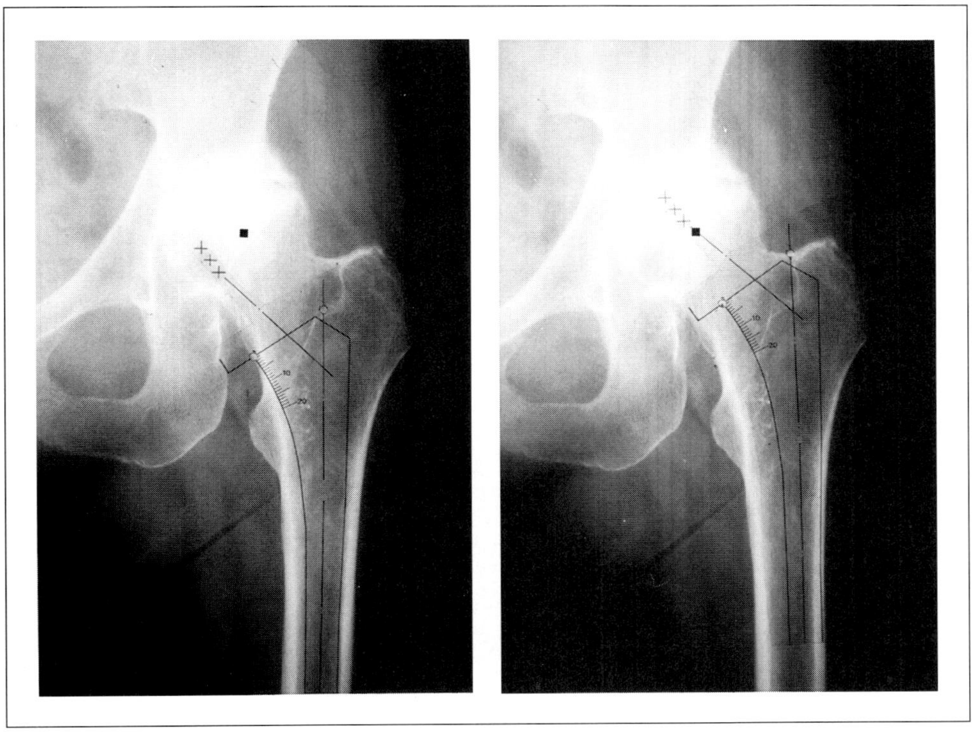

CHAPTER 20

Fractures of the Proximal Part of the Femur

Richard F. Kyle, MD
Miguel E. Cabanela, MD
Thomas A. Russell, MD
Marc F. Swiontkowski, MD
Robert A. Winquist, MD
Joseph D. Zuckerman, MD
Andrew H. Schmidt, MD
Kenneth J. Koval, MD

Prevalence and Prevention

The worldwide prevalence of fractures of the proximal part of the femur is increasing as the average age of the population increases. The actual number of these fractures in the United States doubled from the mid-1960s through the 1980s. Frandsen and Kruse[1] predicted that the number of such fractures will triple that of today by the year 2050. Thus, fractures of the proximal part of the femur are an important cause of morbidity and mortality in all age groups, especially the elderly.

Approximately 250,000 fractures of the proximal part of the femur occur in the United States each year, resulting in annual health-care costs of more than 8.7 billion dollars.[2] Extensive debate continues with regard to the cost-effectiveness of various medical and surgical therapies, including the treatment of fractures of the proximal part of the femur. Using the concept of quality-adjusted life-years, Parker and associates[3] determined that surgical treatment is the most cost-effective approach for displaced intracapsular fractures and all extracapsular fractures. Thus, the proper treatment of fractures of the proximal part of the femur is important not only for the continued health and vitality of the population but also for the health of the economy.

Fractures of the proximal part of the femur occur predominantly as low-energy injuries in elderly patients and as high-energy injuries in younger patients. The high prevalence of these fractures in the elderly is related to numerous factors, including osteoporosis, malnutrition, decreased physical activity, impaired vision, neurologic impairment, poor balance, altered reflexes, and muscular weakness. Firooznia and associates[4] showed, however, that elderly patients who sustained fractures of the proximal part of the femur did not have a higher rate of osteoporosis than age-matched control subjects.

Fractures of the proximal part of the femur in elderly patients are generally the result of a single fall and are more common in women than in men.[5] The absolute rate of fracture is highest for white women, followed by white men, black women, and black men.[6] These rates are thought to reflect a difference in bone density between black and white people. Alffram[7] reported that patients who have intertrochanteric fractures are, as a group, slightly older and have higher rates of morbidity and mortality compared with patients who have fractures of the femoral neck.

Falls are the single most common cause of fractures of the proximal part of the femur, and the prevention of falls is a primary way to control the increasing prevalence of these injuries.[5] Alterations in living conditions to improve lighting and eliminate obstacles that can cause tripping, such as throw rugs, are practical steps that can be taken. The treatment of conditions that cause weakness and imbalance is another way to decrease the prevalence of these fractures.[5]

Pertinent Anatomy

Most of the vascular supply to the femoral head comes from the posterior medial and lateral femoral circumflex arteries that form an extracapsular ring about the femoral neck (Fig. 1). Ascending cervical branches arise from this network and enter the capsule at its insertion. Fractures of the femoral neck have been shown, both by injection techniques and by histologic study, to disrupt this vascular supply to the femoral head.[8-10] Experimental study has shown that, if both the medial circumflex and the lateral epiphyseal vessels have been disrupted, the collateral circulation maintains viability of the femoral head in less than 20% of specimens.[10] However, Claffey[11] showed that displaced fractures of the femoral neck can occur without complete disruption of the medial femoral circumflex or lateral epiphyseal systems. These vessels may only be kinked; therefore, early anatomic reduction and internal fixation of displaced femoral-neck fractures is advocated in order to restore blood flow.

The osseous anatomy of the proximal end of the femur dictates where the internal fixation device should be placed for maximum purchase in the femoral head. Maximum bone density is found in the area where the compression and tension trabeculae coalesce in the center of the head (Fig. 2). Careful evaluation of the trabecular patterns allows the surgeon to estimate the degree of osteoporosis and to gauge the likelihood of success of internal fixation; however, the subjective nature of the grading systems used for this purpose limits their reliability.[12,13]

The ball-and-socket configuration of the hip joint is inherently stable and allows an excellent range of

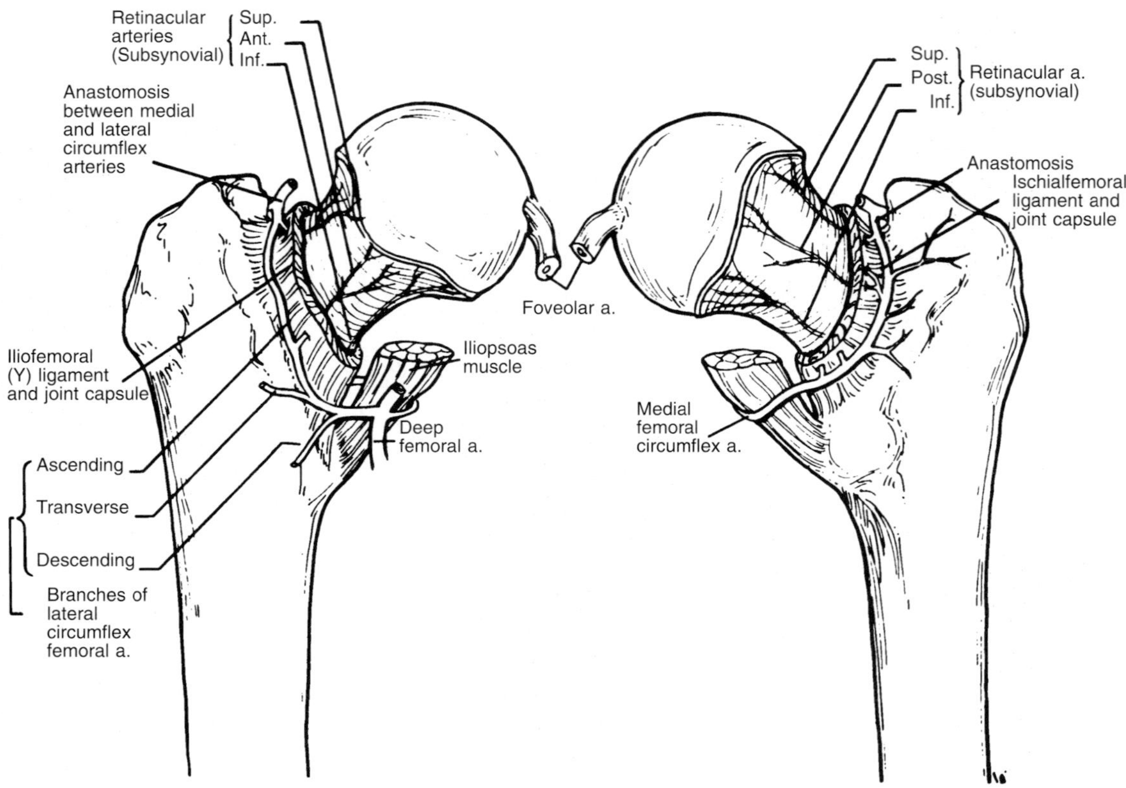

Fig. 1 Drawing showing the blood supply to the proximal end of the femur. The major sources are the lateral and medial circumflex arteries, which traverse the capsule to become the lateral retinacular arteries supplying the femoral head. (Reproduced with permission from Kyle RF: Fractures of the hip, in Gustilo RB, Kyle RF, Templeman DC (eds): *Fractures and Dislocations*. St. Louis, MO, Mosby-Yearbook, 1993, vol 2, p 789.)

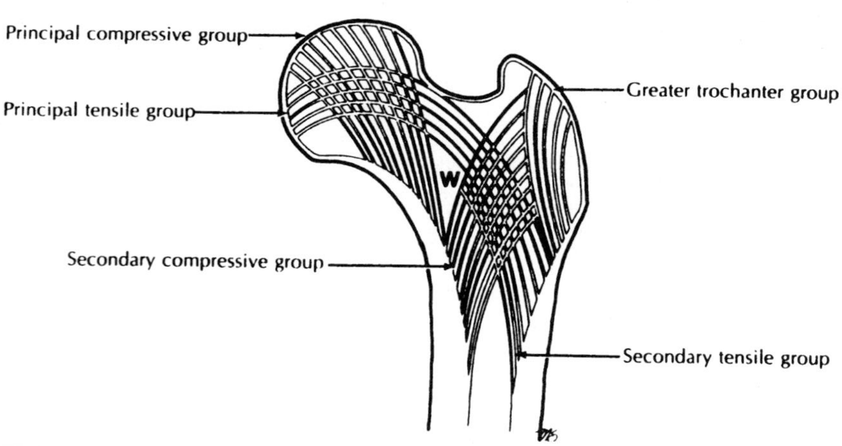

Fig. 2 Drawing showing the internal trabecular pattern of the proximal third of the femur. The primary compressive and tension trabeculae coalesce in the center of the head. W = Ward's triangle. (Reproduced with permission from Rockwood CA Jr, Green DP, Bucholz RW (eds): *Fractures in Adults*, ed 3. Philadelphia, PA, JB Lippincott, 1991, vol 2, p 1488.)

motion in all directions. The two major forces acting on the hip joint are abductor muscle tension and body weight, as defined by the joint-reaction force. In men, the normal joint-reaction force can be as much as four to seven times body weight, and in women, 2.5 to four times body weight.[14,15] Stair-climbing causes peak hip forces of as much as seven times body weight.[16] The mechanics of the hip are such that implants designed for the fixation of fractures or for prosthetic replacement must withstand extremely high loads and bending moments. The activities of a bedridden patient can produce forces on the implant equivalent to those that occur during walking with the use of external supports.[14] Even when the structural integrity of the hip has been restored, the major muscle forces continue to test the stability of the fracture fixation or of the prosthetic replacement. Using instrumented nail-plate implants, Nordin and Frankel[14] showed that only one-fourth of the total load is borne by the fixation device.

Highly sophisticated procedures and techniques can now guide the surgeon to a more accurate placement of internal fixation devices, optimizing impaction and stabilization of the fracture. Image intensification has reduced operating time and has allowed the surgeon the opportunity for immediate evaluation of the reduction and of the placement of the fixation device. This has led to fewer complications and better results in patients who have an intracapsular or extracapsular fracture. New, high-strength stainless-steel and titanium alloys and computer-assisted designs ensure maximum strength of the implant by the reduction of stress-risers and the elimination of weak areas.[17,18] The use of these materials and designs has reduced the frequency of breakage of the implant to less than 1%; failures of the implant that do occur are usually associated with a failure of fracture-healing and are indicative of nonunion.[19] The one fracture pattern that still poses a great problem is the displaced intracapsular fracture with compromised blood supply to the femoral head. This fracture, so aptly named by Speed,[20] remains today the "unsolved fracture."

An improved understanding of fracture patterns, along with advancements in internal fixation, have led to greater expectations of good results and to the need for a more critical review of the results of treatment of these injuries. Many factors conspire to make generalizations about treatment difficult, and comparisons of the results of treatment are nearly impossible. There have been few prospective, randomized comparative studies. Most clinical reviews are incomplete because of poor follow-up. Rapid developments in implant technology make the standardization of surgical procedures an elusive task. Finally, the age and poor health of the patients who sustain these fractures make it difficult to conduct comprehensive, long-term follow-up studies.

Fractures of the Femoral Neck

Clinical Presentation and Classification

Fractures of the femoral neck occur in two distinctly different populations: the elderly and younger adults. In an elderly patient, the fracture usually results from a fall, while in a younger patient, it is generally caused by an accident involving a motor vehicle or by another high-energy pattern of injury. Because of the intracapsular nature of the fracture, an elderly patient is usually stable on initial presentation, unless transport has been delayed or overriding medical problems are present. This is often not true for young adults. Fifty per cent of the time, a younger patient has sustained multiple trauma and may have other serious injuries.[21,22] Twenty per cent of young patients who have a femoral neck fracture also have a fracture of the ipsilateral femoral shaft.[22,23] Because the surgeon focuses on the femoral shaft fracture, the femoral neck fracture may be missed in as many as 40% of these patients.[21]

Clinical Signs of Intracapsular Fractures of the Hip

Clinical signs and symptoms at presentation may be minor in a patient who has an incomplete, impacted, or nondisplaced fracture of the femoral neck. Internal rotation of the limb almost always elicits pain in the region of the hip and groin when a femoral neck fracture is present. In displaced femoral-neck fractures, there is shortening and external rotation of the limb, with the hip usually held in slight abduction. The patient is in severe pain, and any attempt to move the hip causes pain. If a femoral neck fracture is suspected, the patient will be most comfortable with a pillow placed beneath the knee and the hip moderately flexed. This position allows relaxation of the hip capsule and reduces pressure on and pain in the hip joint.

Radiographic Evaluation

Standard anteroposterior and lateral radiographs of the hip are essential for the evaluation of a femoral neck fracture. Any discontinuity in the cortical outline or overlapping of the trabecular pattern of the head and neck should be noted. Displaced femoral-neck fractures are quite obvious; the surgeon should pay particular attention to the lateral radiograph to evaluate the amount of posterior comminution because the greater the degree of comminution, the greater the instability of the fracture. Nondisplaced fractures that cannot be seen on plain radiographs are apparent on a magnetic resonance image immediately and on a bone scan after 3 days. A negative result on the magnetic resonance image assures the surgeon that no fracture of the hip is present.[24]

Garden's classification, which is the most widely accepted classification of femoral neck fractures, primarily describes subcapital fractures.[23,25-28] Types I through IV are based on the degree of displacement evident on an anteroposterior radiograph of the hip (Fig. 3). These grades correspond to both the prognosis for healing and the rate of osteonecrosis. Displaced fractures (types III and IV) are associated with a higher prevalence of osteonecrosis and nonunion than are nondisplaced fractures (types I and II).[25-28]

An alternative classification system, in which the type of femoral neck fracture is based on the angle formed by the fracture line and the horizontal plane, was proposed by Pauwels.[29] Fractures that are more vertical are subject to higher shear stresses and are associated with a correspondingly poorer prognosis, and they are given a higher classification.[29] The closer the fracture line to the horizontal, the less shear force exerted on the fracture or on any device used to fix the fracture.

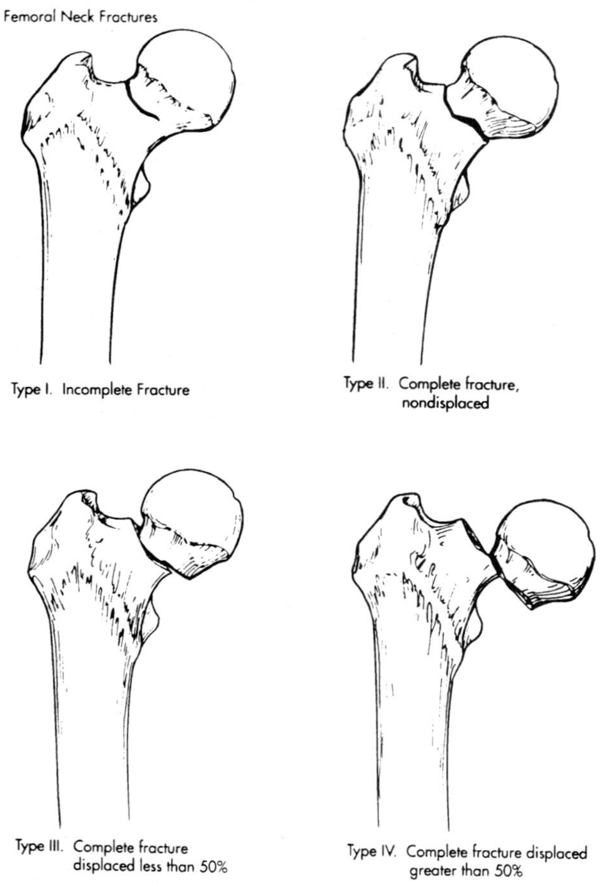

Fig. 3 Drawings showing the classification of Garden[25-28] for fractures of the femoral neck. The rates of both osteonecrosis and nonunion, as well as the method of treatment, are based on the amount of displacement. (Reproduced with permission from Kyle RF: Fractures of the hip, in Gustilo RB, Kyle RF, Templeman DC (eds): *Fractures and Dislocations.* St. Louis, MO, Mosby-Yearbook, 1993, vol 2, p 795.)

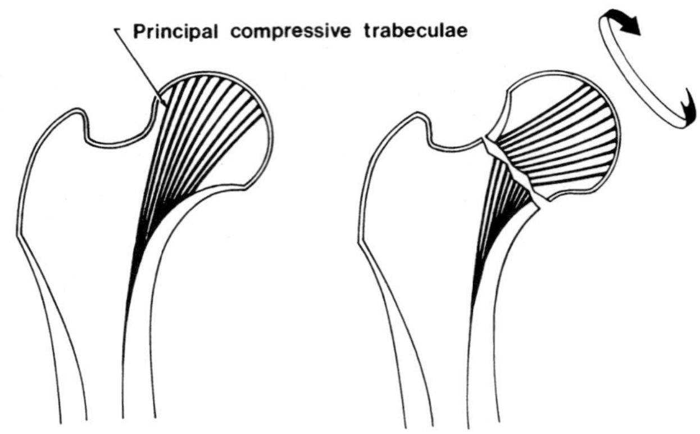

Fig. 4 Rotational malalignment of the femoral head may be determined on the basis of observation of the malalignment of the compressive trabeculae. (Reproduced with permission from Kyle RF: Fractures of the hip, in Gustilo RB, Kyle RF, Templeman DC (eds): *Fractures and Dislocations.* St. Louis, MO, Mosby-Yearbook, 1993, vol 2, p 796.)

The rotation of the femoral head and the amount of comminution of the femoral neck must also be considered when the severity of the fracture is estimated. Neither of the classification systems just described takes into account the rotational alignment of the head or the degree of posterior comminution. Rotational malalignment is difficult to diagnose, but its presence should be suspected when the major compressive trabeculae in the head and neck are not aligned accurately, even if there is overall good alignment of the cortical shells (Fig. 4).

All patients must be evaluated thoroughly and their medical condition must be stabilized before they are taken to the operating room.[30] The optimum timing for internal fixation of femoral neck fractures remains controversial.[31-33] Several authors have reported lower rates of osteonecrosis and nonunion in patients who had reduction and rigid internal fixation of the fracture on an emergent basis.[33-36] In contrast, Barnes and associates,[31] in one of the largest overall series of femoral neck fractures, did not identify a significant increase in the rate of osteonecrosis or nonunion when fixation had been delayed for as long as a week. Swiontkowski and associates[37] showed, in animal studies, that a minimum increase in intracapsular pressure occludes the blood supply to the femoral head. We believe that there is a theoretical advantage, on the basis of the pathophysiology of the fracture, to reduction and stabilization of the fracture as soon as the patient is medically stable.

The treatment of the fracture depends primarily on the age of the patient and the degree of displacement (Fig. 5). A patient who has a nondisplaced or a minimally displaced femoral-neck fracture is at low (0 to 10%) risk for osteonecrosis or nonunion if the displacement of the fracture remains unchanged.[28] Thus, these fractures are best treated with internal fixation to prevent displacement and to decrease the attendant risks of osteonecrosis and nonunion.[38]

A patient who has a displaced femoral-neck fracture is at high risk for both osteonecrosis and nonunion. Several authors, in studies of more than 100 patients, reported an average rate of nonunion of 20% (range, 6% to 40%) and an average rate of osteonecrosis of 25% (range, 10% to 43%).[31,39-47] Arnold and associates,[39] in a study of 1,000 nonpathological fractures, including 670 displaced fractures, reported an overall rate of nonunion of 15%. In the patients who had a displaced fracture, the rate of osteonecrosis was 12%, and in those who had a nondisplaced fracture, it was 7%. Barnes and associates,[31] in a study of 1,503 subcapital fractures, reported that 289 (19%) were ununited and 183 (12%) had late segmental collapse after three years of follow-up. Treatment of displaced femoral-neck fractures is based on the age and the physical demands of the patient. In a younger, healthy, physically active patient,

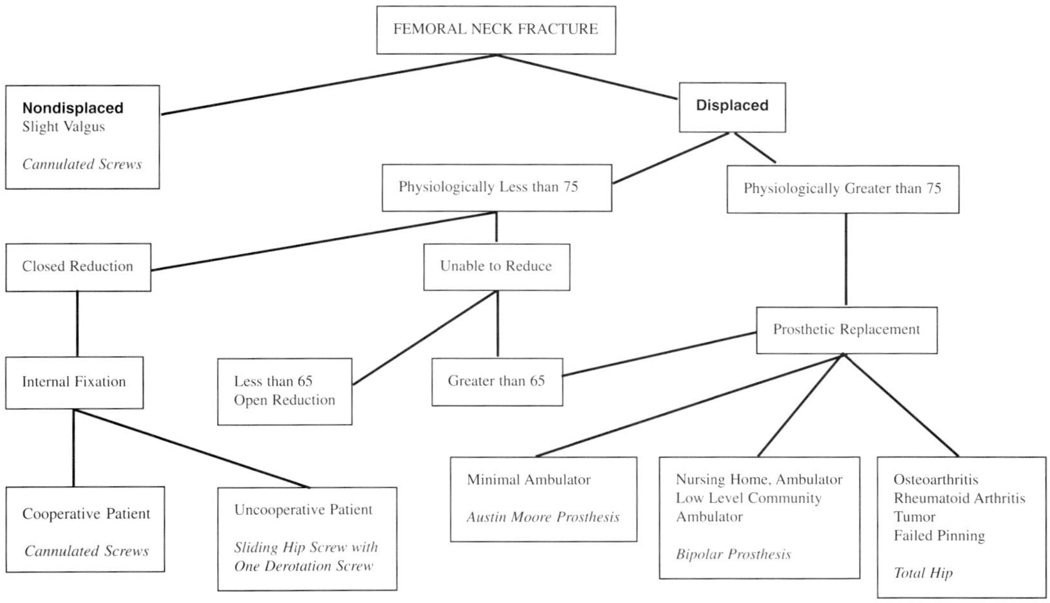

Fig. 5 Flowchart showing the various methods of treatment for fractures of the femoral neck, as determined by the amount of displacement of the fracture, the age of the patient, and whether there is a history of hip disease. (Reproduced with permission from Kyle RF: Fractures of the hip, in Gustilo RB, Kyle RF, Templeman DC (eds): *Fractures and Dislocations*. St. Louis, MO, Mosby-Yearbook, 1993, vol 2, p 800.)

every effort should be made to preserve the femoral head. In an elderly, physically debilitated patient, a second operation can be avoided by the use of primary prosthetic replacement. There is, however, no documentation as to the exact age at which open reduction and internal fixation to preserve the femoral head should be abandoned in favor of prosthetic replacement. In a patient who is physiologically younger than 70 to 75 years old and is capable of withstanding a second operation if the fixation fails, the treatment of choice is open reduction and internal fixation. A patient who is physiologically more than 70 to 75 years old should be considered a candidate for primary prosthetic replacement to avoid a second operation. A person's physiologic age is dependent on concurrent medical problems that result in a change in activities of daily living; it is not always the same as the chronologic age. Prosthetic replacement may also be chosen for a patient who has severe, pre-existing hip disease, such as osteoarthrosis, compounded by a femoral neck fracture.

Various options for prosthetic replacement are available. The choice of the prosthesis depends on the walking requirements of the patient and the degree of associated hip disease. In a patient who cannot walk or transfer from bed to chair, a one-piece hemiprosthesis without cement may be used. This type of prosthesis is best suited for sedentary patients because weight-bearing on the prosthesis is associated with a high prevalence of both pain in the thigh and later acetabular protrusion.[48] In a patient who has moderate functional requirements, such as one who lives in a nursing home or who is restricted to walking about the house, a bipolar prosthesis with cement has been used, with excellent results.[49] A modular hemiprosthesis, with a solid, exchangeable head on the femoral stem, is currently available; however, there have been no long-term comparative studies of its clinical success, to our knowledge. A total hip replacement is the treatment of choice for femoral neck fractures associated with severe osteoarthrosis, rheumatoid arthritis, or cancer.

Treatment of Fractures of the Femoral Neck in Younger Adults

Protzman and Burkhalter[23] reported disastrous results, including very high rates of osteonecrosis and nonunion (19 patients [86%] and 13 patients [59%], respectively), in 22 patients who had a femoral neck fracture and were younger than 55 years of age. In more recent series, however, the rates of osteonecrosis (20% to 30%) and nonunion (15% to 20%) have been found to be the same as those in elderly patients. Swiontkowski and associates,[22] in a study of 27 patients who were younger than 50 years of age, reported no nonunions;

osteonecrosis developed in five patients (19%). In a study by the Orthopaedic Trauma Hospital Association, the rates of osteonecrosis and nonunion in 112 patients who were younger than 55 years of age were consistent with those reported in elderly patients.[21]

Evaluation of Reduction, and Acceptable Guidelines

A poor reduction of a femoral neck fracture prevents reestablishment of the blood supply to the femoral head and decreases the amount of apposition of bone between the proximal and distal fragments, leaving poor mechanical stability after fixation. Garden[27] and others[21,22] have shown that reduction in more than 20° of valgus is associated with a higher rate of osteonecrosis. Any varus deformity after reduction is also associated with increased rates of osteonecrosis and nonunion.[21] Anterior or posterior angulation of more than 10° should not be accepted, particularly in osteoporotic bone; such angulation increases the potential for redisplacement of the fracture because the bone is weak. The surgeon should pay particular attention to the degree of posterior comminution seen on the lateral radiograph. Both Garden[26,28] and Banks[50] have shown that fractures with marked posterior comminution have a higher prevalence of nonunion. When treating fractures with a large amount of posterior comminution, the surgeon should place the superior and posterior screws along the calcar femorale to resist posterior collapse (Fig. 6). In some patients, bone-grafting of the posterior aspect of the femoral neck may be considered.

A displaced fracture that cannot be reduced in a closed fashion in an elderly patient who has high functional requirements and is able to walk about the community (generally, a patient who is younger than 75 years of age and has few medical problems) or in a younger patient should be treated with open reduction and internal fixation. In a more fragile, elderly patient, the surgeon should proceed with prosthetic replacement.

The use of multiple pins, such as Knowles pins, or of screws is a simple and effective technique for fixation of well-reduced femoral-neck fractures. This technique can be done percutaneously with use of a local anes-

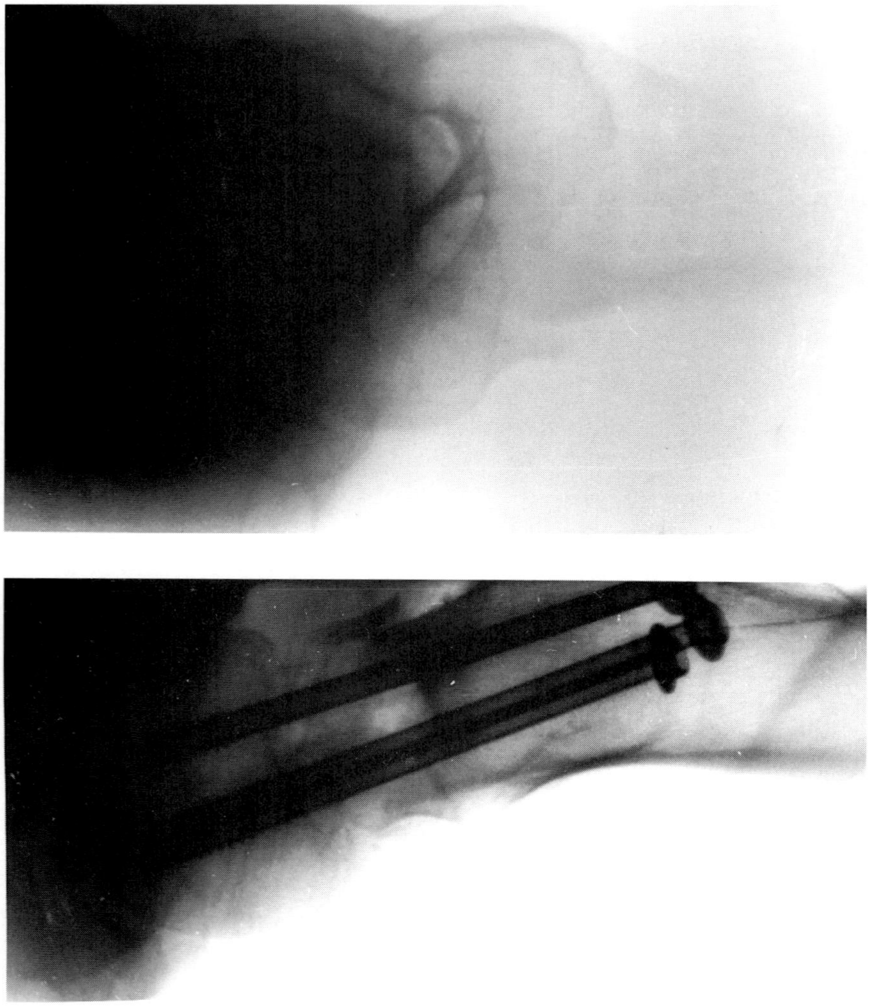

Fig. 6 Lateral radiographs of a fracture of the femoral neck. **Top,** The radiograph shows posterior comminution. **Bottom,** Radiograph made after fixation. The screws have been placed along the posterior cortex to buttress the comminuted region.

thetic, or it can be performed with an open technique with the patient under general or spinal anesthesia. Stability at the site of the fracture is maximized by the placement of three pins in a triangular configuration.[51] Mechanical studies have not proved the effectiveness of the use of more pins. Care must be taken to place the pins or screws at an angle of 130° to 135° in relation to the femoral shaft. If they are positioned at a higher (140° to 145°) angle, the holes will be created in the lateral cortex, at or distal to the level of the lesser trochanter. Holes at this location have been associated with a 20% prevalence of subtrochanteric fracture.[52]

Surgical Technique with the Use of Three Cannulated Screws

A one-eighth-inch (0.32-cm) guide-pin is laid along the anterior aspect of the femoral neck at an angle of 135°, according to the technique of Tronzo.[53] This guide-pin should appear, on image intensification, to lie adjacent to the medial cortex of the femoral neck. A 3.8-mm drill-hole is made in the mid-part of the lateral cortex, parallel to the anterior guide-pin. The position of the drill-bit is checked on the anteroposterior and lateral radiographs. The drill is then removed, and the guide-pin is placed in the drill-hole. Under image intensification, the guide-pin is tapped into place along the medial cortex of the femoral neck and into the head to within 5 mm of the subchondral bone. The guide-pin should lie slightly inferior in the femoral head on the anteroposterior radiograph and in the center of the head on the lateral radiograph. After this guide-pin has been placed, two more guide-pins are inserted with use of image intensification. On the anteroposterior radiograph, these pins lie slightly superior in the femoral head; on the lateral radiograph, one lies slightly anterior and the other, slightly posterior, forming a triangular pattern of guide-pins. Next, the length of the screws to be implanted is determined by direct measurement of the guide-pins, each of which lies within 5 mm of the subchondral bone of the femoral head (Fig. 7). Cannulated screws are then driven over the guide-pins. The inferior screw is placed first, followed by the superior screws. The screws should be tightened simultaneously, to apply uniform compression across the fracture and to avoid tipping of the femoral head into varus angulation. The guide-pins are then removed, and image intensification is used to confirm the proper position of all three screws.

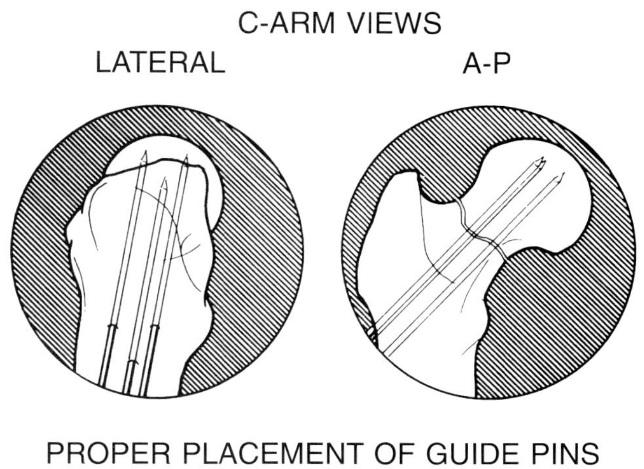

Fig. 7 Diagrams showing the proper placement of the guide-pins. The cannulated screws are driven over one-eighth-inch (0.32-cm) guide-pins to within 5 mm of the subchondral bone. Three screws, placed in a triangular pattern, provide optimum stability. The distal screw lies against the medial cortex, to resist varus forces on the femoral head. The proximal screws are spread out and placed anterior and posterior, to resist displacement and rotation. (Reproduced with permission from Kyle RF: Fractures of the hip, in Gustilo RB, Kyle RF, Templeman DC (eds): *Fractures and Dislocations.* St. Louis, MO, Mosby-Yearbook, 1993, vol 2, p 807.)

Complications

Nonunion Nonunion of femoral neck fractures, which usually becomes apparent within one year, was reported in 34 (11%) of 301 patients in one series,[54] in 39 (33%) of 119 patients in another series,[41] and in none of five patients in a third series.[50] Arnold and associates[39] reported a 15% rate of nonunion in 1,000 patients who had a displaced fracture. This range of occurrence may be explained by differences in the types of fractures and in the methods used for reduction and fixation.[55] Nonunion may or may not be accompanied by osteonecrosis. If nonunion occurs, a magnetic resonance image must be made to evaluate the viability of the femoral head before the options for treatment are considered. In an elderly patient who is able to walk about the community, a nonunion is treated with a total hip replacement; in a younger patient, a Pauwels valgus osteotomy and repeat fixation are used.[56] In a younger patient who has collapse of the femoral head concurrent with a nonunion, a total hip replacement is indicated. Most nonunions have drifted into some varus angulation, and a valgus intertrochanteric osteotomy allows compression loads to occur at the fracture site to promote healing (Fig. 8).[56] Another option for treatment is the use of a posterior muscle-pedicle graft. The success of this treatment is difficult to assess, because the reported series have been so small.[57-59]

Osteonecrosis Overall, the reported rate of osteonecrosis in patients who have had a displaced femoral-neck fracture has ranged from 4% to 40%.[31,35,38,39,41-43,46,47,54] Fielding and associates[43] reported osteonecrosis in 40 (16%) of 256 patients. The wide range in rates may, again, be explained, at least in part, by differences in the types of fracture and in the respective authors' chosen methods of reduction and fixation. Osteonecrosis is usually partial and does not involve the entire femoral head. In many patients, the head does not collapse. If a patient is asymptomatic, no additional treatment is indicated. If the osteonecrotic fragment has collapsed and the patient is

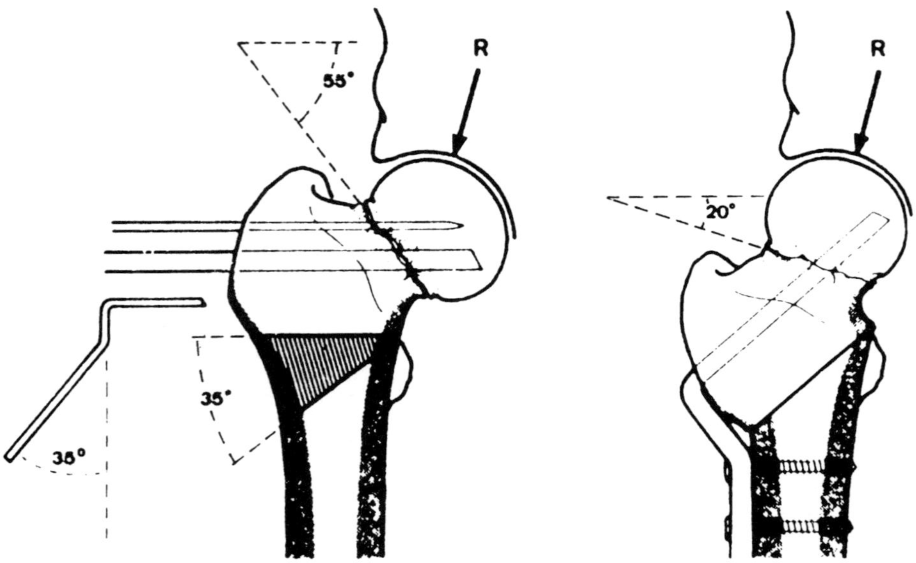

Fig. 8 Schematic drawings showing the technique for a valgus osteotomy of the proximal end of the femur in the treatment of a nonunion of a femoral neck fracture. The osteotomy has changed the vertical orientation of the fracture line from 55° to 20°. (Reproduced with permission from Weber, BG, Cech O: *Pseudoarthrosis.* Bern, Switzerland, Hans Huber, 1976.)

symptomatic but is able to walk about the community, total hip arthroplasty is indicated.

Surgical Technique for Fractures of the Femoral Neck and the Ipsilateral Femoral Shaft

Special considerations may be necessary for a patient who has a fracture of the ipsilateral femoral shaft. The injury of primary importance in this fracture complex is the femoral neck fracture, which must be reduced and stabilized before fixation of the femoral shaft is attempted.

The fracture of the shaft may be treated with intramedullary fixation. The femoral neck should be reduced, and it may be pinned temporarily with three one-eighth-inch (0.32-cm) Kirschner wires, placed anteriorly to avoid interference with the intramedullary nail. The intramedullary nail can then be introduced through the piriformis fossa. The femoral shaft should be over-reamed by 2 mm to facilitate driving of the nail without excessive force, which could displace the femoral neck fracture. After the fracture of the femoral shaft has been reduced and fixed with the nail, the temporary fixation of the neck is removed, and three guide-wires are placed around the intramedullary nail and into the femoral head under image intensification. Cannulated screws are driven over the guide-wires, with use of the technique described earlier. The intramedullary nail must be locked to prevent rotation and shortening at the site of the fracture of the shaft.

Alternatively, a second-generation locking nail (one with two proximal locking screws, which are inserted into the greater trochanter and angled into the femoral head) may be used to stabilize the femoral neck, but proper placement of the locking screws in the femoral head may be difficult, because the screws must be driven through the nail. If there is a problem with placement of the screws through the second-generation nail, additional screws can be used outside of the nail. Swiontkowski and associates,[22] as well as Sanders and associates,[60] described a method in which a nail is inserted, after reaming, retrograde from the medial femoral condyle. This technique requires the use of a very flexible nail, and it may result in valgus deformity at the site of the femoral shaft fracture if it is not performed properly.

An acceptable, and recently more popular, alternative is the routine stabilization and fixation of the femoral neck fracture with multiple pins, followed by plating of the femoral shaft fracture (Fig. 9). This approach allows the surgeon to stabilize the more critical femoral-neck fracture adequately in a standard fashion. The femoral shaft may then be exposed and plated without fear of disruption of the femoral neck fixation. This is the easiest and most reliable way of treating this complex pattern of injury in most patients.

In summary, proper treatment of femoral neck fractures depends on the age of the patient and the degree of displacement of the fracture. A suggested algorithm

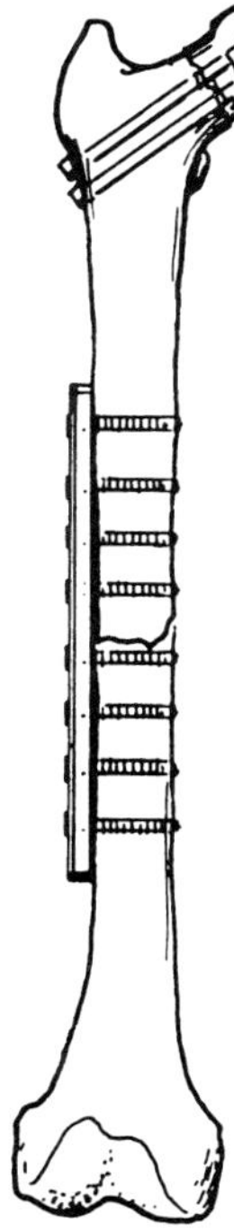

Fig. 9 Multiple-screw fixation of a fracture of the femoral neck and plating of a fracture of the femoral shaft. (Reproduced with permission from Kyle RF: Fractures of the hip, in Gustilo RB, Kyle RF, Templeman DC (eds): *Fractures and Dislocations*. St. Louis, MO, Mosby-Yearbook, 1993, vol 2, p 810.)

for treatment has been developed (Fig. 5). Concomitant injuries and medical problems must also be evaluated. A nondisplaced femoral-neck fracture should be fixed in situ for the best results. A displaced femoral-neck fracture remains, in some ways, the "unsolved fracture."[20] Reduction and fixation should be performed as soon as the patient is medically stable, to restore the blood supply to the femoral head. Anatomic reduction and solid stabilization with multiple-point fixation, with use of pins or cannulated screws, is the best way to prevent osteonecrosis and nonunion. In an elderly patient, a hemiprosthetic replacement is a good option. Total hip replacement should be reserved for a patient who has concomitant hip disease or in whom fixation has failed.

Intertrochanteric Fractures

The treatment of intertrochanteric fractures has advanced greatly in the last few decades. In the 1930s, Jewett[61] introduced the triflanged nail, which allowed the surgeon to achieve immediate stability of the fracture and early mobilization of the patient.[37] However, use of the Jewett nail for the fixation of unstable intertrochanteric fractures has been problematic and loss of fixation has been common. Such a rigid implant does not allow the impaction of comminuted fracture fragments to occur. As a result, there is increased stress on the implant if union does not occur rapidly; the implant will ultimately fatigue and fail, or it will penetrate and cut out of the femoral head (Fig.10).[62-64]

The shortcomings of fixed nail-plate devices were recognized by the mid-1960s, and techniques were developed to recreate medial stability in patients who had an unstable intertrochanteric fracture. These techniques combined the use of rigid devices with various types of osteotomies. Dimon and Hughston[65] advocated a procedure in which the lateral trochanter is osteotomized and the shaft is displaced medially to force the head and neck into the shaft (Fig. 11, *left*). Sarmiento and Williams[66,67] recommended a valgus osteotomy in which a laterally based wedge at the proximal end of the fracture of the shaft is resected and the neck fragment is placed on the medial cortex in a valgus position to create a stable configuration (Fig. 11, *right*).

During the same period, Clawson,[68] as well as Massie,[69] introduced sliding devices that allowed impaction of the fracture fragments. Biomechanical and clinical studies showed that a stable fracture configuration results from reduction of the fracture in an anatomic or slightly valgus position and fixation with a sliding device. This technique has produced results that are equal to or better than those of osteotomies,[65,67,70-72] and it remains the mainstay of treatment today.

In the mid-to-late 1970s, flexible intramedullary devices for the fixation of intertrochanteric fractures were introduced in the form of the Ender nail and the condylocephalic nail. The mechanical advantage of these devices derives from their intramedullary position, which places them closer to the resultant force across the fracture and reduces the bending moment on the device. In addition, the use of distal sites of insertion to decrease operative time and loss of blood, compared with the use of proximal sites, has been reported.[73,74] This surgical technique was made possible by the use of image intensification and was promoted as a closed method for the fixation of intertrochanteric fractures. However, a high prevalence of varus deformity, as well as pain in the knee caused by distal migration of the pins, was reported in association with this procedure (Fig. 12).[55,75] These problems led to a high rate of reoperation for extraction of the pins and correction of deformity. A high rate of failure due to loss of reduction, shortening, and external rotation has resulted both from the use of Ender nails and from the use of condylocephalic nails.[73] Accordingly, most authors have recommended that these devices not be used for the fixation of intertrochanteric fractures.[76]

Second-generation rigid, locking, intramedullary devices, introduced in the 1980s, have also been asso-

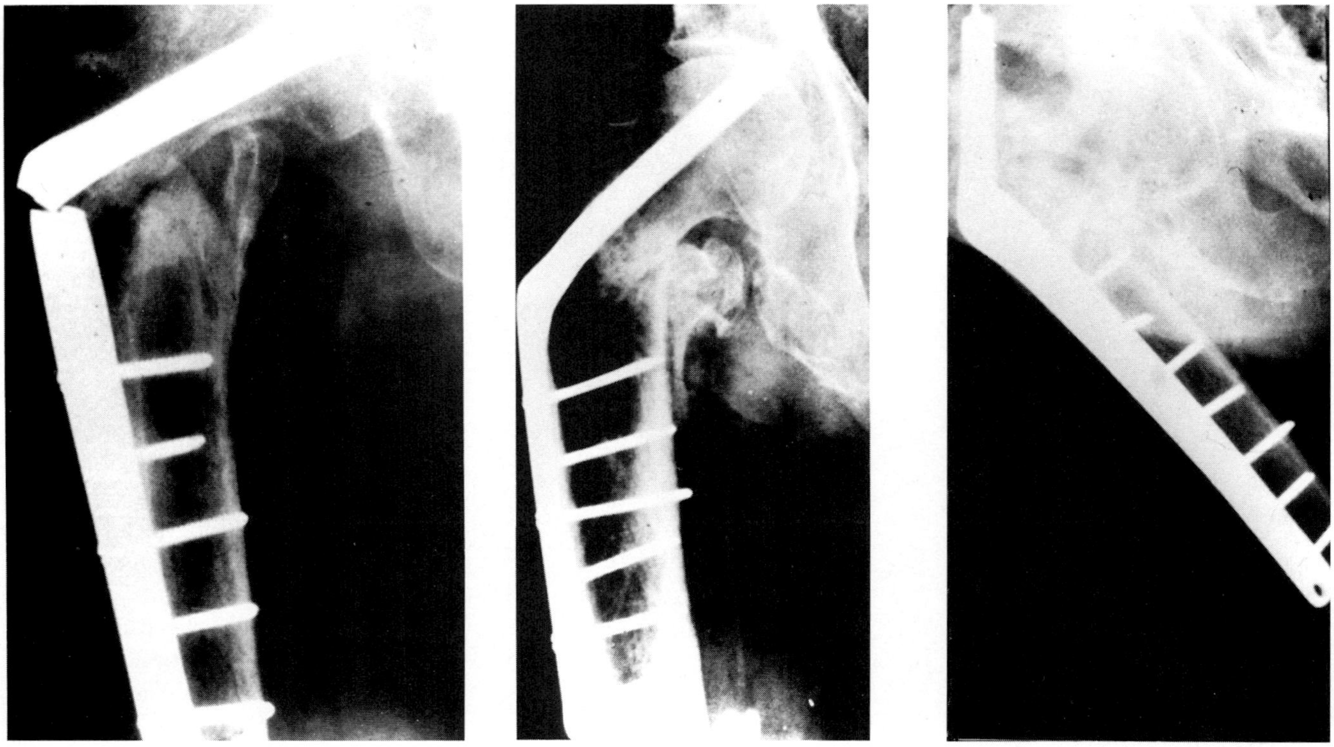

Fig. 10 Radiographs showing various problems with the older, solid fixation devices. The bone has impacted to a stable position, causing the implant to break, **left;** to penetrate the hip joint, **center;** or to cut out of the femoral head, **right.** (Reproduced with permission from Kyle RF: Fractures of the hip, in Gustilo RB, Kyle RF, Templeman DC (eds): *Fractures and Dislocations.* St. Louis, MO, Mosby-Yearbook, 1993, vol 2, p 845.)

ciated with a higher rate of complications than the sliding hip-screw when they have been used for routine intertrochanteric fractures.[17,77] These devices are most useful for the fixation of distal subtrochanteric fractures as well as for selected fractures of the ipsilateral shaft and hip.

Classification

Intertrochanteric fractures may be classified as stable or unstable. In a stable fracture, the posteromedial buttress remains intact or is minimally comminuted. Collapse of the fracture fragments is minimum, and stability is obtained with reduction and re-establishment of medial cortical contact. In an unstable fracture, a large segment of the posteromedial wall has broken free, with comminution posteriorly (Fig. 13), and the outcome may be varus collapse, malunion, or nonunion.[78,79]

The classification of Boyd and Anderson[80] is useful, because it further subdivides stable fractures into those without comminution, those with minimum comminution, and those with a subtrochanteric component. With use of a modification[62] of the classification of Boyd and Anderson, four basic types of intertrochanteric fracture were described in a prospective study of 268 patients (Fig. 14). Type I consists of nondisplaced, stable intertrochanteric fractures without comminution (57 fractures [21%]). Type-II fractures are stable, minimally comminuted, and displaced (97 fractures [36%]); reduction of these fractures leads to a stable construct. Stable fractures heal well with any type of fixation device, because the bone is essentially in a stable configuration after the major fragments have been fixed together. Type-III fractures—the so-called problem fractures—are unstable and have a large posteromedial comminuted area (74 fractures [28%]) (Fig. 15). Type-IV fractures, which have a subtrochanteric component, are also unstable and are relatively rare (40 fractures [15%]) and consist of an intertrochanteric fracture with a subtrochanteric component. A type-IV fracture is the most difficult to fix because of the great forces across the subtrochanteric region of the femur.[62,74]

Clinical Signs

A patient who has a displaced intertrochanteric fracture is typically seen in the emergency room with the affected limb externally rotated and shortened. Because movement of the limb causes severe pain, a forced range of motion should not be attempted. Kenzora and associates[30] showed that medical stabilization of the patient is essential before an operation and that the timing of the operation should be dictated by the patient's medical condition, which must be evaluated very carefully.

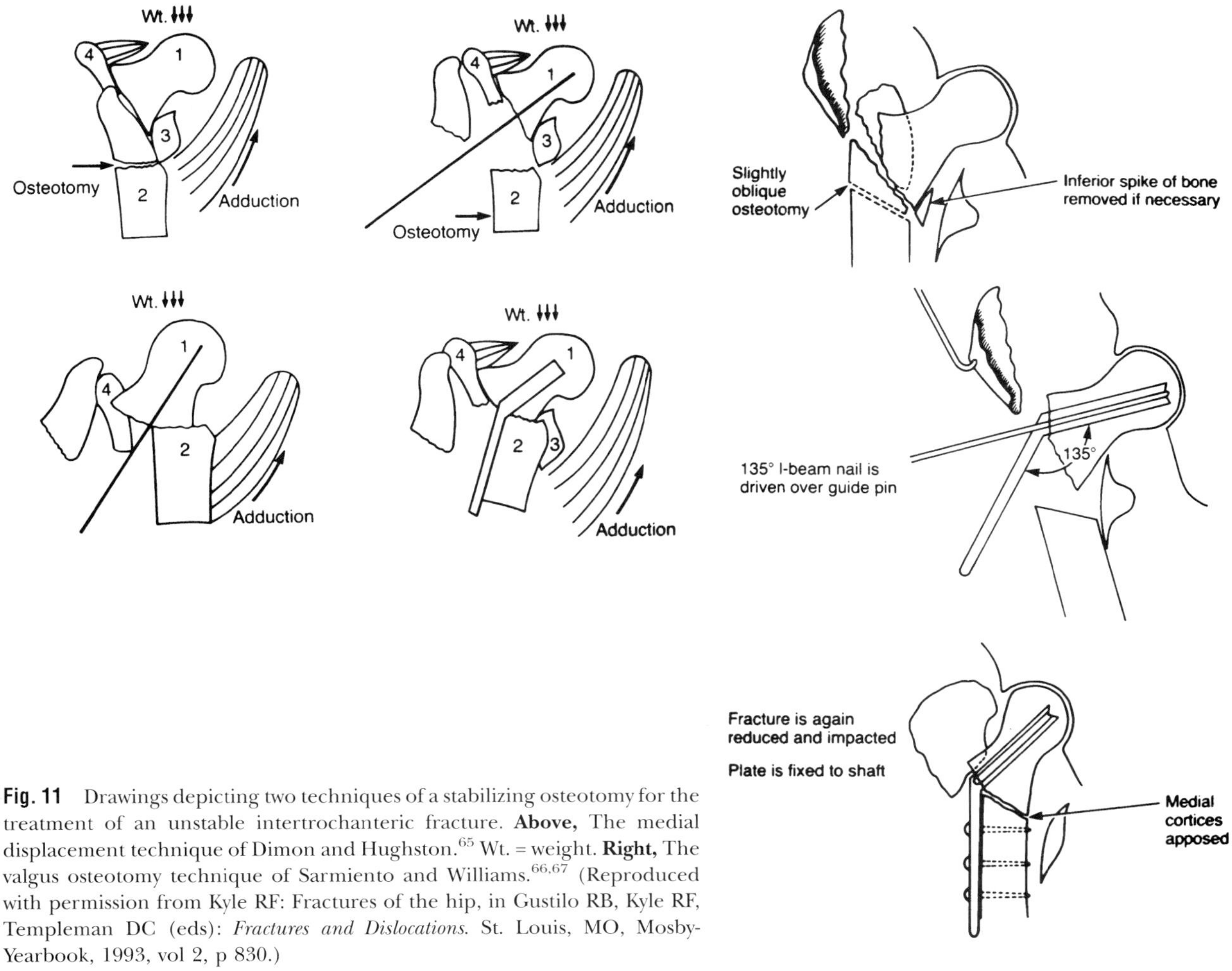

Fig. 11 Drawings depicting two techniques of a stabilizing osteotomy for the treatment of an unstable intertrochanteric fracture. **Above,** The medial displacement technique of Dimon and Hughston.[65] Wt. = weight. **Right,** The valgus osteotomy technique of Sarmiento and Williams.[66,67] (Reproduced with permission from Kyle RF: Fractures of the hip, in Gustilo RB, Kyle RF, Templeman DC (eds): *Fractures and Dislocations.* St. Louis, MO, Mosby-Yearbook, 1993, vol 2, p 830.)

Radiographic Evaluation

Standard anteroposterior and lateral radiographs of the hips are made for evaluation. A fracture between the greater and lesser trochanters can be seen on the anteroposterior radiograph. The larger the fracture of the lesser trochanter, the more unstable the fracture. The surgeon should note the amount of posterior comminution on the lateral radiograph. The greater the degree of posterior comminution, the more unstable the fracture (Fig. 15).

Surgical Technique for Fixation

The most important step in the fixation of an intertrochanteric fracture is the proper placement of the guide-pin in the center of the femoral head (Fig. 16). A small drill-bit should be used to allow rapid repositioning of the guide-hole for accurate placement of the pin. The drill-bit should be advanced at a high angle across the fracture site to the subcapital level of the femoral head. During advancement, the position of the drill-bit should be checked under image intensification on both anteroposterior and lateral radiographs to ensure proper aim toward the center of the head. The drill-bit should lie at the highest angle anatomically possible along the medial cortex of the neck fragment, yet it should be in the center of the femoral head on both anteroposterior and lateral radiographs. After drilling has been accomplished, the drill-bit should be removed and the guide-pin should be passed into the drill-hole, to the level of the subchondral bone. A variable-angle guide is used to determine the exact nail-plate angle required for fixation.

If posterior sag of the fracture occurs, the fracture should be reduced with upward pressure applied to the buttock or femur. Pressure must be reapplied during each passage of the instruments across the fracture to avoid jamming the instruments on the guide-pin.

After insertion of the screw, the plate should be fixed to the lateral aspect of the shaft with at least four cortical-bone screws. In osteoporotic bone, six screws are necessary. Medial fragments may be secured with a lag-screw technique if they can be captured without extensive dissection or periosteal stripping. Biomechanical studies have shown increased stability of the fracture

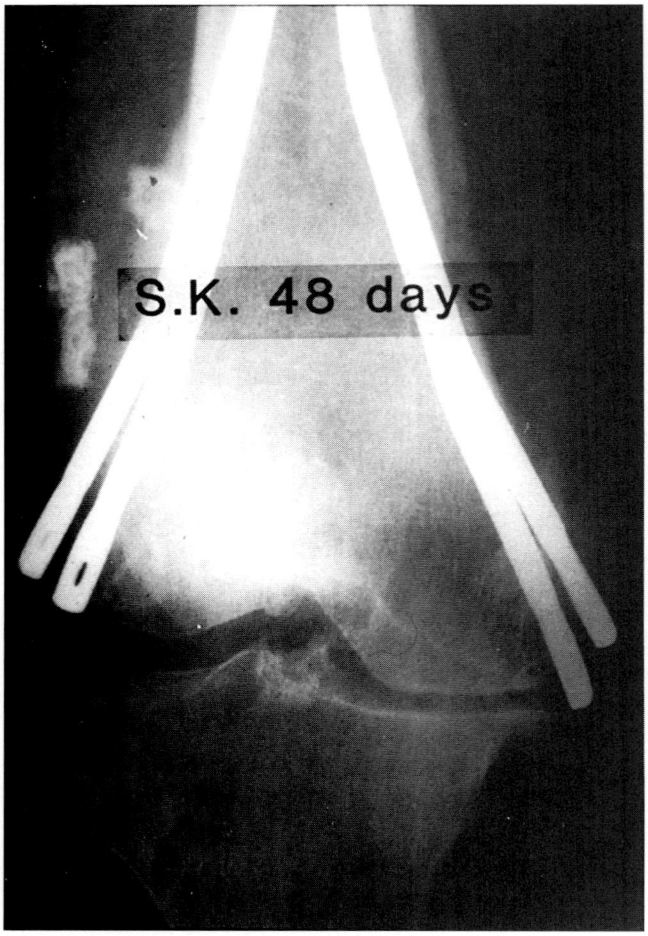

Fig. 12 Radiograph showing migration of Ender nails in an intertrochanteric fracture. Nail migration is associated with high rates of varus deformity and knee pain. (Reproduced with permission from Kyle RF: Fractures of the hip, in Gustilo RB, Kyle RF, Templeman DC (eds): *Fractures and Dislocations*. St. Louis, MO, Mosby-Yearbook, 1993, vol 2, p 831.)

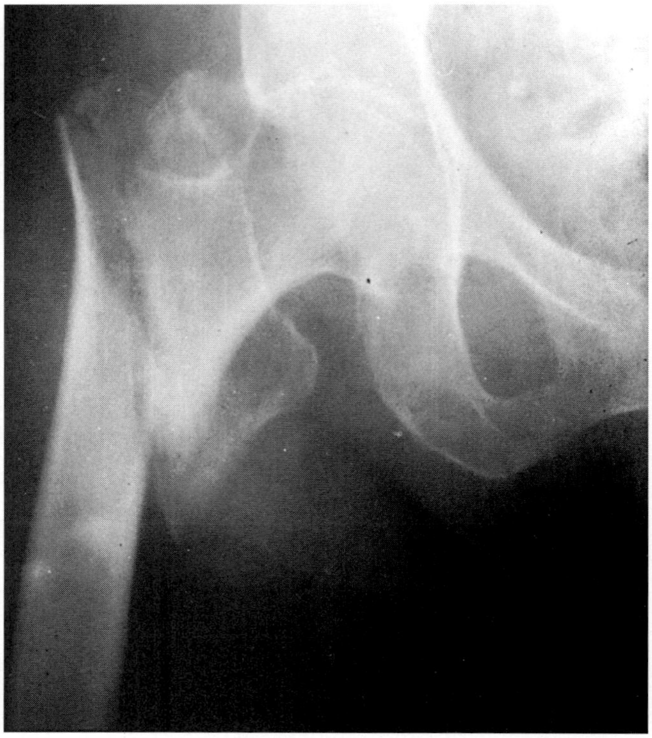

Fig. 13 Radiograph showing a large fragment of the posteromedial wall in an intertrochanteric fracture, which has resulted in instability.

after fixation of large medial fragments.[81] Image intensification should be used during the final seating of the nail or screw to ensure that the implant is well within the femoral head and lying within 5 mm of the subchondral bone. This placement ensures adequate purchase in the femoral head and solid fixation of the femoral head and neck fragment to the shaft fragment.

Successful treatment of intertrochanteric fractures depends on stable osteosynthesis. The ability of the fixation device to obtain firm purchase in the proximal and distal fracture fragments depends on the degree of osteoporosis of the bone, the fracture pattern, and the correct use of the fixation device. The ability of severely osteoporotic bone to bear a substantial segment of the load is impaired even when a collapsible device is used properly. For this reason, many of these fractures must be protected with limited weightbearing postoperatively. The purchase of the cortical-bone screws through the side-plates may also be impaired in osteoporotic bone and may result in the plate pulling away from the femoral shaft. This problem may be corrected by the use of either a longer plate and more screws or supplemental cerclage wiring. A patient who has severe arthritis of the acetabulum can be managed with an arthroplasty; however, primary arthroplasty is difficult and is associated with a high rate of dislocation. In most patients who have an intertrochanteric fracture with associated mild degenerative changes, internal fixation is the procedure of choice. If a patient is symptomatic after the fracture has healed, an arthroplasty can be performed more easily later than when the fracture was fresh.

The value of prophylactic use of antibiotics has been proved.[82] The rates of infection have been reduced from 5% to less than 1% with the use of broad-spectrum antibiotics, begun before the operation and given for at least one day postoperatively.

Biomechanics of Sliding Devices in the Fixation of Fractures of the Hip

To use a sliding device correctly in a patient who has a fracture of the hip, it is essential to understand the mechanics of the device and the forces that it must withstand. In 1935, Pauwels[29] concluded that the forces acting on the hip in single-limb stance are equivalent to approximately three times the body weight, applied at an angle of 159° to the vertical plane. These data were confirmed later by numerous authors.[69,72,83] These

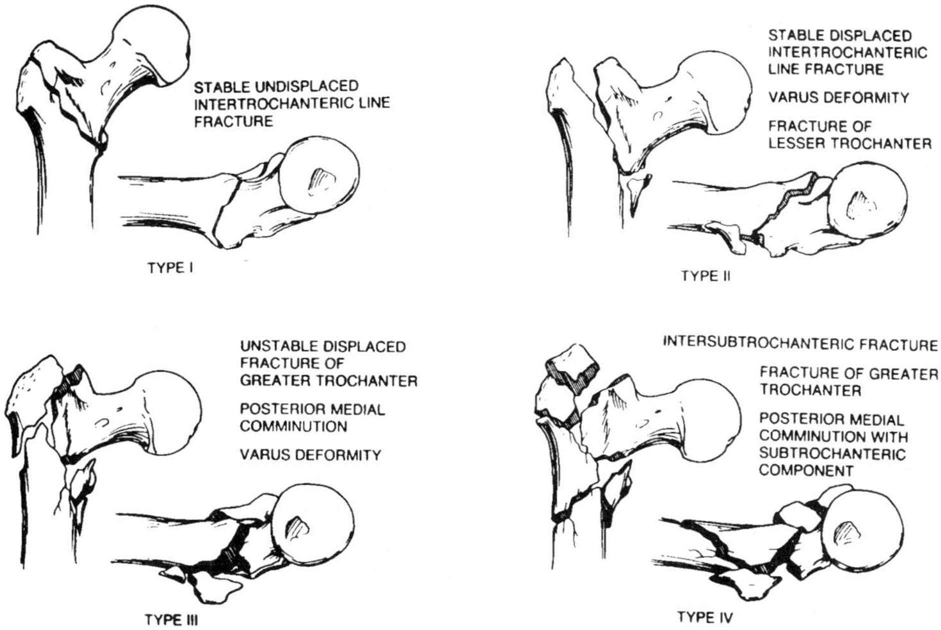

Fig. 14 Classification of intertrochanteric fractures, used at the Hennepin County Medical Center.[62] The classification is based on stability. Types III and IV are unstable and are associated with the highest rates of failure.

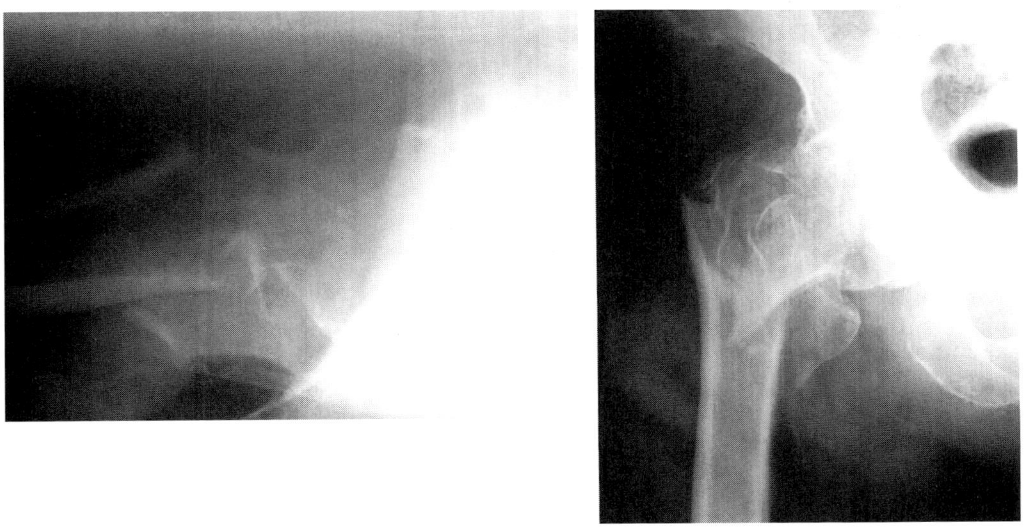

Fig. 15 Radiographs showing a type-III intertrochanteric fracture. **Left,** The lateral radiograph shows posteromedial comminution (arrow), which indicates instability. **Right,** Comminution is not seen on the anteroposterior radiograph.

same forces act on any hip-fixation device that is placed across the fracture site.

A sliding device with a screw-plate angle closest to the combined force vector allows optimum sliding and impaction. The closer the nail-plate angle to the resultant vector of the forces across the hip, the more force available to assist impaction (Fig. 17).[84] A device that is placed at a lower angle has less force working parallel to the sliding axis and more force working perpendicular to the sliding axis. This perpendicular force acts to jam or bend the device, thereby preventing impaction. Technically, however, the surgeon cannot place the sliding device at a high angle in a small hip or in a hip with a varus deformity. Mechanically, it is desirable to place the sliding device at as high an angle as clinically possible while still maintaining the placement of the device in the center of the head. A device that is placed at a lower angle may be used effectively in a stable fracture because controlled collapse is not important for impaction of the fracture and early weightbearing. However, an accurate assessment of the stability of the fracture is sometimes difficult. In these questionable

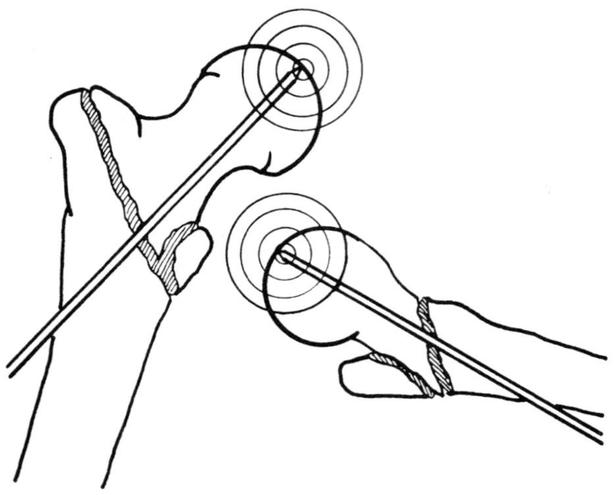

Fig. 16 Placement of the pin in the center of the femoral head on the bull's-eye position is the most important step in the fixation of an intertrochanteric fracture and gives the best bone purchase in the proximal fragment. Malposition may result in cut-out or penetration of the fixation device. (Reproduced with permission from Kyle RF: Fractures of the hip, in Gustilo RB, Kyle RF, Templeman DC (eds): *Fractures and Dislocations.* St. Louis, MO, Mosby-Yearbook, 1993, vol 2, p 839.)

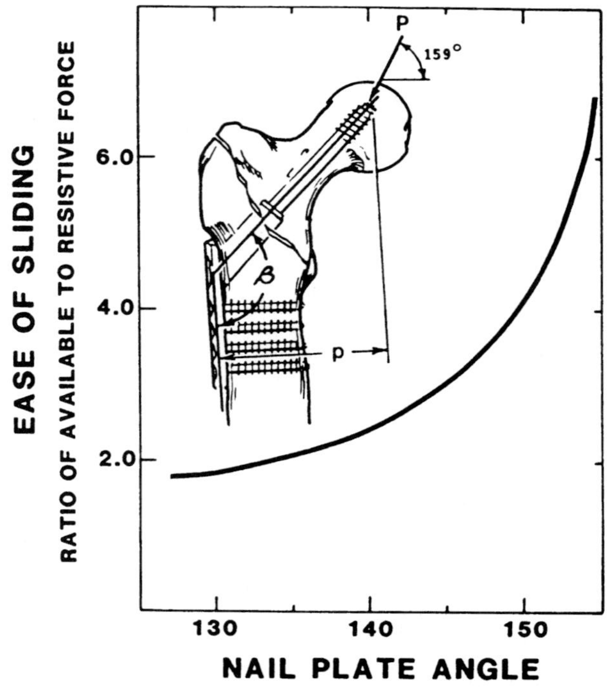

Fig. 17 Graph in which the ease of sliding of the device is plotted against the nail-plate angle. The higher the angle, the greater the ease of sliding. The closer the nail-plate angle to the resultant force across the hip, the more force available to assist impaction of the sliding screw. (Reproduced with permission from Kyle RF: Fractures of the hip, in Gustilo RB, Kyle RF, Templeman DC (eds): *Fractures and Dislocations.* St. Louis, MO, Mosby-Yearbook, 1993, vol 2, p 835.)

situations, placement of the device at a higher angle will allow impaction, regardless of the degree of stability of the fracture.

The ideal position for the nail or screw in the femoral head is apparent from a radiograph of the proximal femur. The point of coalescence of the tension and compression trabeculae results in a dense pattern of cancellous bone in the center of the femoral head. This is where the best purchase in the bone can be obtained for a fixation device. When these trabeculae are absent, the surgeon can expect a higher rate of failure with use of the device. Placement in the center of the femoral head, within 5 mm of the subchondral bone, has resulted in the lowest rate of clinical failure in patients who have an unstable intertrochanteric fracture (Table 1).[18,85] After anatomic reduction, a properly placed sliding device allows spontaneous impaction and medial displacement of all intertrochanteric fractures into a stable configuration (Fig. 18). This allows early mobilization of the patient. If a patient has good fixation, full weightbearing is allowed. If the fixation is unstable, as when the bone is osteoporotic, only partial weightbearing is permitted.

Postoperative Care

The patient is allowed to sit, if doing so is comfortable, on the day after the operation. If solid fixation has been obtained, the patient is allowed to walk between parallel bars, bearing weight on the injured extremity as tolerated, on the second or third postoperative day. Weightbearing is progressed as tolerated. If the bone is osteoporotic or if only poor fixation has been obtained, delayed weightbearing with use of toe-touch only is necessary until callus has formed. If there is a subtrochanteric component to the fracture, weightbearing should be delayed until callus is seen on the radiograph. Radiographs should be made at weekly intervals for the first 2 weeks to ensure that proper impaction of the fragments occurs. Additional radiographs should be made at 4 and 6 weeks after the fracture. The final radiographs should be made 6 months after the fracture.

Low-dose heparin is not effective in the prevention of thromboembolic disease in patients who have a hip fracture.[86] Coumadin (warfarin) is the most effective drug in the prevention of thromboembolic disease, but formation of a hematoma can complicate treatment with anticoagulants if the prothrombin time is not kept within the recommended range of 15 to 18 seconds. Continuous passive motion and intermittent use of a positive-pressure splint may be of value in the prevention of thromboembolic complications, but both require a specialized apparatus, which may interfere with the mobilization of the patient. Stable fixation of the fracture, which allows rapid mobilization of the patient,

Table 1
The relationship between the rate of failure of fixation and the position of the nail in type III fractures[62]

Position of Nail on Antero-posterior and Lateral Radiographs	Position of Nail*	Prevalence[62] No.	Prevalence[62] Percent	Distance of Nail-Tip from Subchondral Bone on AP/Lat. Radiographs (mm)	Failures No.	Failures Percent
2/2	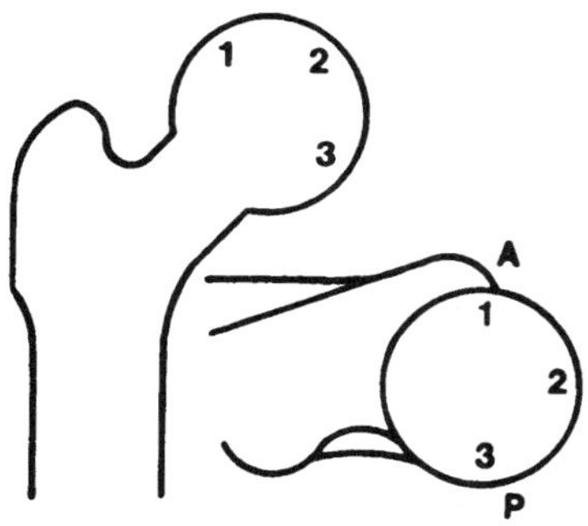	34	46	11/12	0	0
2/3		22	30	14/7	1	5
2/1		4	5	9/5	0	0
1/2		6	8	12/18	2	33
1/3		4	5	14/11	1	25
3/3		4	5	15/16	1	25

*The center position (2) is associated with the lowest rate of failure. A = anterior and P = posterior.
(Adapted with permission from Kyle RF: Fractures of the hip, in Gustilo RB, Kyle RF, Templeman DC (ed): *Fractures and Dislocations.* St. Louis, MO, Mosby-Year Book, 1993, vol 2, p 835.)

is the most effective method for the prevention of thromboembolic disease.

Complications

The complications of fixation of intertrochanteric fractures are minimum, compared with those associated with fixation of other fractures of the hip, if the surgeon uses the appropriate device correctly and pays attention to accepted mechanical principles. The rate of failure with use of a collapsible hip-screw or nail of contemporary materials and design is less than 5%. With prophylactic use of antibiotics, the rate of infection is less than 1%. Osteonecrosis is extremely rare, occurring in less than 1% of patients.[82]

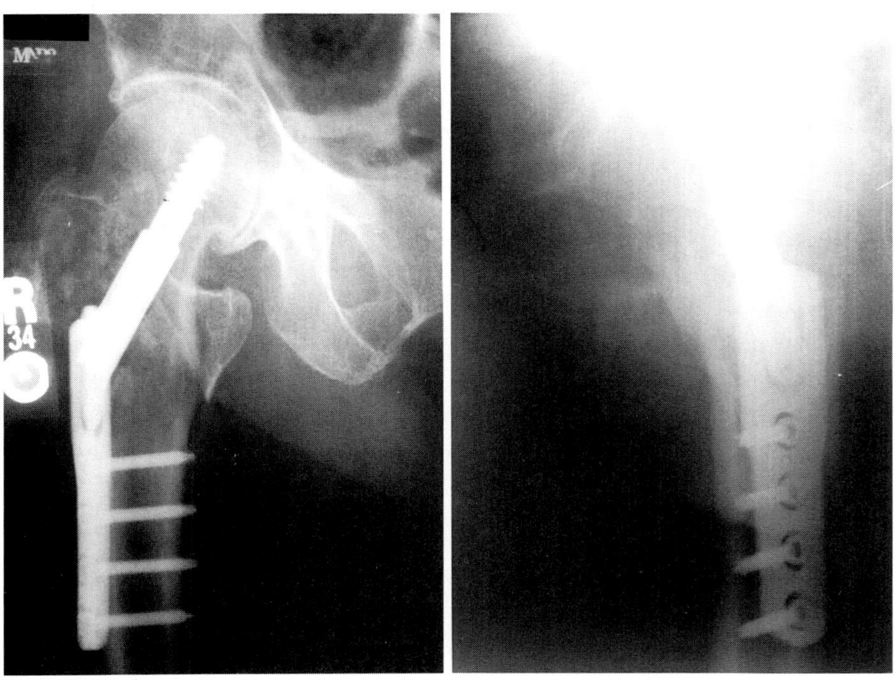

Fig. 18 Anteroposterior, **left**, and lateral, **right**, radiographs showing the proper placement of a sliding device allowing spontaneous impaction and medial displacement of the fracture to a stable position.

The rate of nonunion is less than 10%.[87] If nonunion does occur, the rate of success after simple removal of the device, renailing in a more valgus position, and insertion of a cancellous bone graft has been reported to be 90%,[87] although Boyd and Lipinski[88] found that, of 28 nonunions, 22 (79%) united after surgical treatment.

The most common mode of failure of fixation is the hip-screw cutting out of osteoporotic bone, allowing the fracture to collapse into varus angulation. If little bone is left in the femoral head after this has occurred, a blade-plate can be used to restore stability. The plate provides more surface area to resist cutting out through the femoral head. If the acetabulum has been injured by the protruding nail, a total hip replacement is the treatment of choice.

Type-IV Fractures

A sliding hip-screw or a second-generation locking nail may be used in the treatment of intertrochanteric-subtrochanteric fractures that have a femoral shaft extension. The second-generation locking nail is an excellent form of fixation if the piriformis fossa is intact. When the piriformis fossa is not intact, treatment with a hip-screw with a long side-plate, combined with limited interfragmentary fixation and supplementary bone-grafting, is advisable (Fig. 19). In subtrochanteric fractures that extend quite distally into the shaft and that are combined with an intertrochanteric fracture and involvement of the piriformis fossa, a second-generation intramedullary nail may be the only option; however, the surgeon should anticipate difficulty in its use because the starting point has been destroyed.

Surgical Technique

For type-IV intertrochanteric-subtrochanteric fractures, a one-eighth-inch (0.32-cm) guide-wire is first placed into the proximal neck-and-head fragment, as is done for routine type-I, II, and III fractures. The distal aspect of the shaft is then exposed by dissection of the vastus lateralis from the lateral aspect of the shaft with a periosteal elevator. The posterior sag is reduced by traction and with pressure applied directly under the buttocks or femur at the site of the fracture. The fragments are aligned by traction applied through the soft-tissue attachments with use of the principles of indirect reduction as described by Kinast and associates.[89] The side-plate is then applied to the distal aspect of the shaft and is secured with a Verbrugge bone-clamp. The proximal fragment is well fixed by placement of the hip-screw in the center of the head. The distal fragment is fixed by capture of at least eight cortices with four bone-screws. Large fragments between the proximal and distal segments are stabilized with interfragmentary fixation and placement of bone-screws through the side-plate, if the fragments can be retrieved and fixed without additional periosteal stripping. Anatomic restoration of all comminuted fragments is not necessary. Grafting of the medial defects with autogenous bone should be done to promote early healing if medial comminution is present.

A reverse oblique fracture[53] needs special consideration, because the major fracture line extends from proximal-medial to distal-lateral through the intertrochanteric-subtrochanteric region (Fig. 20). While this type of fracture should be fixed in a manner similar to that used for a type-IV fracture, it may be difficult to reduce, because the adductors and iliopsoas are intact and they pull the distal fragment medially while the proximal fragment is abducted, flexed, and pulled laterally. These fractures should be fixed with a screw-plate placed at a lower angle so that the fixation device does not have to be placed directly along the fracture site. The fracture is reduced with manual traction and is held in place with a bone-clamp. Excessive traction may cause additional displacement; often, the traction must be released and the fragments must be rotated slightly and reduced manually to the side-plate. A longer side-plate is recommended for these fractures because of their distal extension. Some authors, such as Kinast and associates,[89] have advocated the use of a right-angle nail. However, this device places high stresses on the nail-plate junction. A second-generation locking nail may also be used for stabilization.[90] An advantage of the intramedullary position of this device is that it prevents medial displacement of the distal fragments.

Postoperative Treatment

A patient who has a type-IV fracture is allowed to sit the day after the operation. Unlike the protocol for a patient who has a type-I, II, or III fracture, weightbearing is delayed until callus has formed. The patient is then allowed to increase weightbearing gradually as tolerated.

In summary, the treatment of unstable and complex intertrochanteric and intertrochanteric-subtrochanteric fractures has been simplified by the development of newer techniques and devices which, in general, have been highly successful. Solid fixation of the proximal fragment to the distal fragment with use of a sliding device and a side-plate allows bone impaction and the restoration of medial stability, with few complications. Nevertheless, complications can result because intertrochanteric fractures frequently occur in osteoporotic bone and in patients who are quite ill. With a thorough understanding of the biomechanics of these fractures, meticulous attention to surgical technique, and modern medical management, union can be achieved in most patients, with minimum morbidity.

Subtrochanteric Fractures

Subtrochanteric fractures of the femur account for 10% to 15% of all fractures of the hip and are among the most problematic ones to treat. These fractures occur in

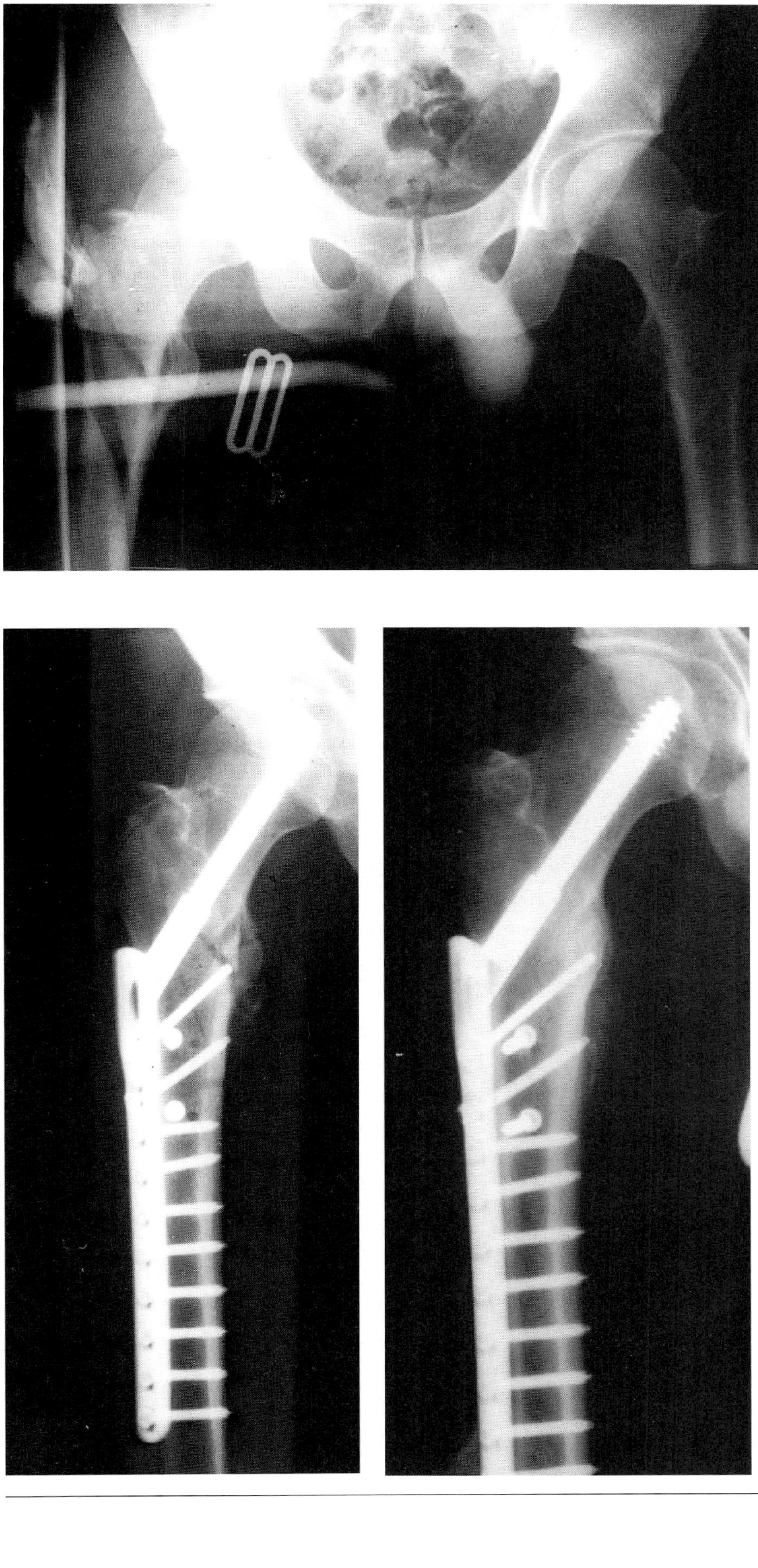

Fig. 19 Radiographs showing a combined intertrochanteric-subtrochanteric fracture of the proximal part of the right femur. **Top,** Radiograph showing involvement of the piriformis fossa. **Bottom left,** Fixation is best accomplished with a sliding hip-screw, as it is very difficult to use an intramedullary nail when the piriformis fossa is fractured. **Bottom right,** Six months postoperatively, the fracture has healed.

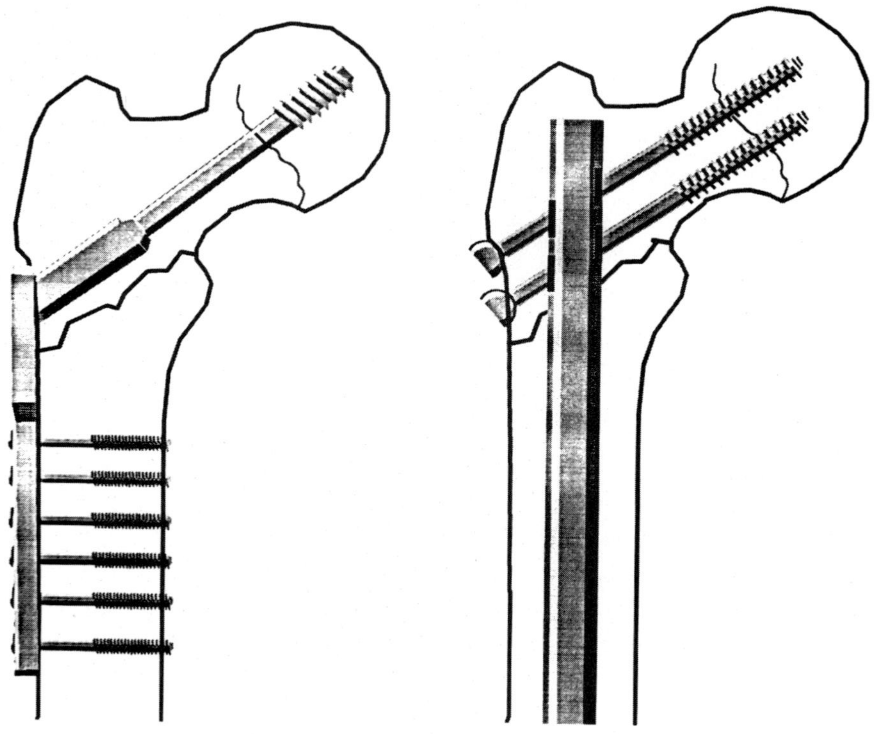

Fig. 20 Schematic drawings of a reverse oblique fracture. These fractures are difficult to reduce and to fix because of the forces that displace the distal fragment medially. **Left,** In this fracture, a low-angle nail has been used. The barrel of the screw is placed through the lateral cortex of the proximal fragment, thus preventing displacement. **Right,** If the piriformis fossa is not involved, a second-generation nail (with two locking screws) may be used to prevent displacement of the distal fragment.

the most highly stressed region of the skeleton. Koch[91] described compressive forces of greater than 1,200 lb/in^2 (8,274,000 Pa) in the medial cortex distal to the lesser trochanter and tensile stresses of 1,000 lb/in^2 (6,895,000 Pa) in the lateral cortex (Fig. 21).[92] Such high stresses predispose internal fixation of these fractures to a high rate of failure and account for the great difficulty in both surgical and nonsurgical treatment.

In 1891, Allis[93] described the difficulty involved in the treatment of these fractures in traction, and the resultant high rates of varus deformity and nonunion. Because of these problems, Lambotte,[94] in 1907, recommended open reduction and internal fixation with a combination of hip-nails and cerclage wiring. Hibbs,[95] in 1902, advocated traction followed by use of a cast. Because of the mechanical problems with early devices, most surgeons, before the 1950s, took the advice of Hibbs and treated these fractures with traction followed by immobilization of the limb in a plaster cast. Most of the fractures healed, but with shortening and varus deformity. In addition, prolonged treatment in bed produced a high rate of medical complications.

After the development of the triflanged nail-plate, internal fixation again became more popular, although complications remained frequent. Fielding and Magliato[96] reported complications in association with 16 (25%) of 64 subtrochanteric fractures that had been consecutively treated with a Jewett nail. The treatment was a failure in ten (40%) of the 25 fractures that were distal to the lesser trochanter.

Küntscher,[97] in 1939, reported on the concept of intramedullary fixation of subtrochanteric fractures with a "Y" nail. However, this double nail, the large triangular metal wedge of which was driven into the head and neck fragment, proved difficult to use, and it did not gain general acceptance.

The first intramedullary device known to be used successfully was developed by Zickel[98-100] in the 1960s (Fig. 22). He reported very low rates of failure in several clinical series: none of five devices failed in a preliminary report; two of 84, in 1976; and three of 184, in 1980. The Zickel nail was a great advance in the treatment of subtrochanteric fractures, and the device was the most effective one used through the early 1980s. However, it could not be inserted with a closed technique, and it did not stabilize the fracture against compressive forces. Shortening of the femur occurred unless cerclage wiring or interfragmentary fixation was used. There were also technical difficulties during insertion, and refracture of the femur occurred occasionally during extraction of the nail.[101,102]

The AO angled blade-plate, introduced in the 1970s, was effective if the medial buttress could be restored and the plate could be used as a tension band. This technique required accurate realignment and stable fixation of all medial fragments.[89,103]

The sliding hip-screw or nail device, popularized by Clawson[68] and by Massie[69] in the 1960s, was used in proximal subtrochanteric-intertrochanteric fractures, but the rate of failure was high in comminuted fractures

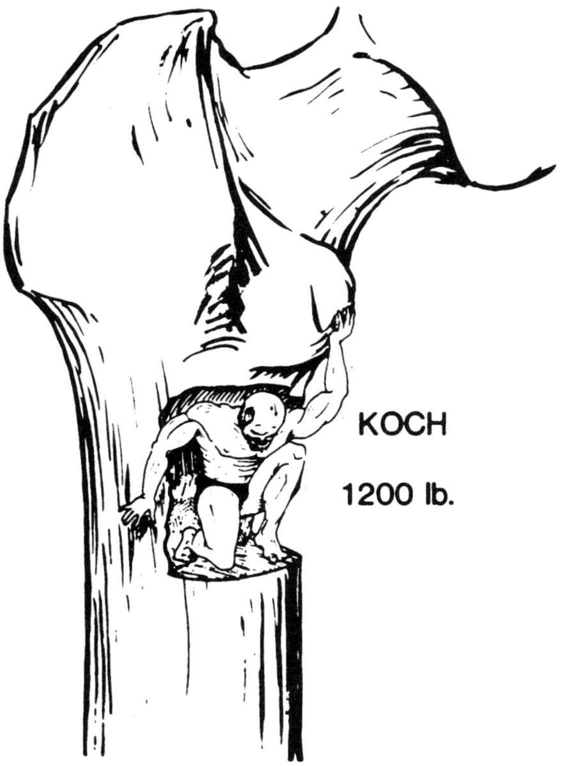

Fig. 21 Compressive forces of more than 1,200 lb/in^2 (8,274,000 pascals)[91] may occur along the medial cortex of the femur, 1 to 3 inches (approximately 2.5 to 7.5 cm) distal to the lesser trochanter. This is the most highly stressed region in the body. (Reproduced with permission from Kyle RF: Fractures of the hip, in Gustilo RB, Kyle RF, Templeman DC (eds): *Fractures and Dislocations.* St. Louis, MO, Mosby-Yearbook, 1993, vol 2, p 814.)

with extension into the femoral shaft.[104] The development of higher-strength metals, such as cold-worked stainless steel and titanium, markedly reduced the rate of failure of these telescoping screw devices. The success of these devices in the treatment of both subtrochanteric and comminuted intertrochanteric-subtrochanteric fractures was improved further by the use of bone-grafting about the highly stressed medial cortex.[89,103] This technique, which is used in conjunction with the method of indirect reduction advocated by Kinast and associates,[89] requires little or no periosteal stripping in the area of comminution, and soft-tissue tension is used to realign the bone fragments.

In the early 1980s, closed treatment of subtrochanteric fractures with an intramedullary nail and locking screws was introduced. More recent advances in both technique and design have made possible the intramedullary fixation of subtrochanteric fractures that extend into the shaft. Although it was believed that locking nails might predispose a fracture to nonunion because they maintain distraction of the fracture fragments, clinically this has not been the case. All known reported series of closed interlocking intramedullary nailing have shown a high rate of union, a low rate of infection, and excellent maintenance of alignment.[90,105-110] The high rate of mechanical failure noted with use of the Jewett nail has not been demonstrated with these newer devices. The rapid rate of healing is attributed to the closed technique, which gives excellent stabilization of the fracture and, through reaming, provides autogenous bone graft to the area of the fracture. With reaming, larger (stronger) nails can be placed in the shaft of the femur. The intramedullary position of the nail, as with the Zickel device, greatly reduces the lever arm at the screw-nail junction, contributing to the decrease in the rate of mechanical failure (Fig. 23). The walls of these nails are thicker than those of standard intramedullary nails, in order to reduce the stress-riser effect of holes placed through them, and the increased thickness enhances their rigidity. For this reason, proper surgical technique is critical to ensure that the wall of the femur is not fractured inadvertently during insertion of the nail.

Mechanism of Injury

The cause of subtrochanteric fractures is related to the age of the patient. In most series, including those that we reviewed at the Hennepin County Medical Center, approximately one-half of the injuries were the result of a high-energy trauma, such as an automobile accident or a fall from a height, usually in young people. The other half were the result of a low-energy fall in elderly patients.[111] A combination of a direct blow on the lateral aspect of the greater trochanter, axial force along the femur, and muscular pull creates various patterns of subtrochanteric fractures. These deforming muscle forces were reported by Froimson,[92] who clearly described the proximal fragment being abducted by the gluteal muscles, flexed by the iliopsoas, and externally rotated by the short external rotators and the distal fragment being displaced medially by the strong pull of the adductors.

Classification

There have been multiple systems of classification of subtrochanteric fractures. Some are complex and others are simple, but few have taken into account the mode of treatment or the prognosis. The classification of Fielding and Magliato[96] describes three types of fractures on the basis of the location of the primary fracture line in relation to the lesser trochanter. In type I, the fracture line is 1 inch (approximately 2.5 cm) distal to the lesser trochanter; in type II, 2 inches (approximately 5 cm) distal; and in type III, 3 inches (approximately 7.5 cm) distal.[96] Zickel,[99] in 1976, described six types of subtrochanteric fractures: four oblique and two transverse. The classification of Seinsheimer[104] included four types, with type I being the most proximal and type IV, the most distal. He further classified each type into subtypes A, B,

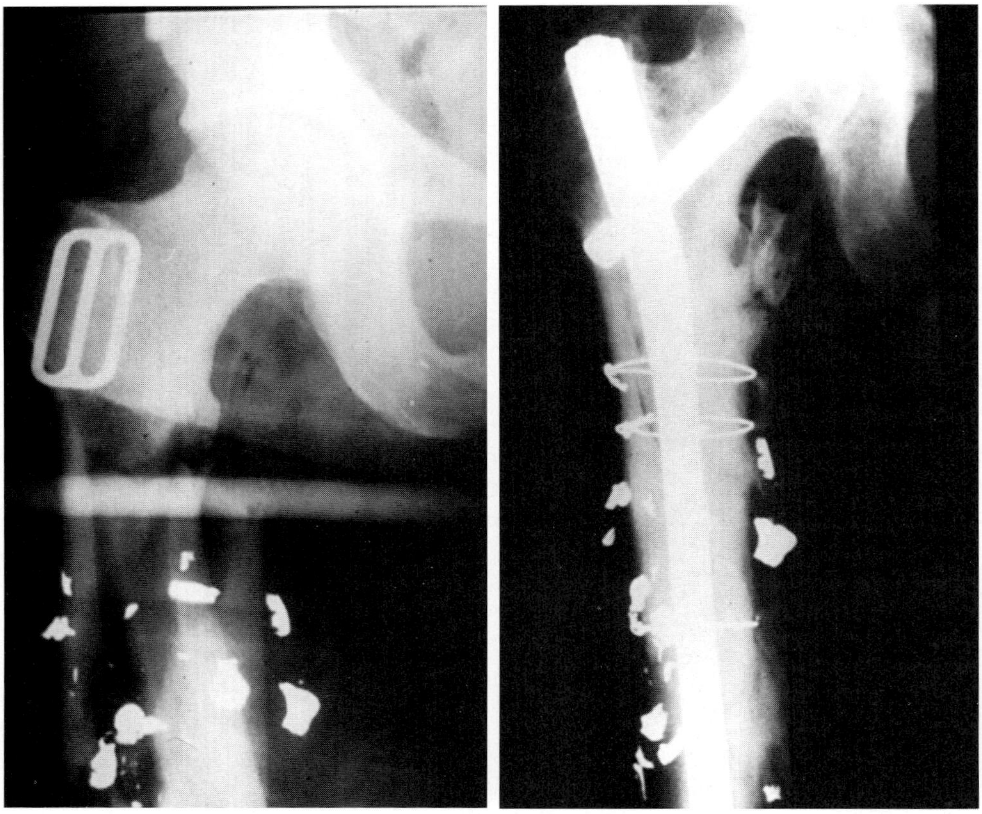

Fig. 22 Subtrochanteric fracture, **left,** fixed with a Zickel nail, **right**. (Reproduced with permission from Kyle RF: Fractures of the hip, in Gustilo RB, Kyle RF, Templeman DC (eds): *Fractures and Dislocations.* St. Louis, MO, Mosby-Yearbook, 1993, vol 2, p 821.)

and C, with subtype A being the most stable and subtype C, the most unstable and comminuted. The AO group developed a classification system that is based on the degree of comminution; however, in their system, the region of the lesser trochanter is always intact.[112]

The classification system currently used by us at the Hennepin County Medical Center is based on the method of treatment, with the fractures divided into two types (Fig. 24). In type I, or high subtrochanteric fractures, the fracture line extends into the lesser trochanter. Because the lesser trochanter is broken off, fixation must be obtained with either a sliding hip-screw or a second-generation locking nail. In type II, or low subtrochanteric fractures, the lesser trochanter remains intact, and the fractures can be treated with a first-generation locking nail (a nail, with a single proximal locking screw, that is positioned retrograde from the greater trochanter to the lesser trochanter). Both types of fracture may be either simple or comminuted, with extension into the shaft.

In a type-I fracture in which the piriformis fossa is fractured, a sliding hip-screw is used because the central entry point for insertion of an intramedullary nail has been lost. In a type-I fracture in which the piriformis fossa is intact, a second-generation locking nail is used because the entry point for the intramedullary nail is undisturbed.

On occasion, in a very distal type-I fracture of the ipsilateral femoral shaft, despite involvement of the piriformis fossa, we use a second-generation locking nail. In a type-II fracture in which the lesser trochanter and the piriformis fossa are intact, we use a first-generation locking nail.

Clinical Signs and Symptoms

On presentation, the affected limb is markedly shortened and externally rotated. In a younger patient who has sustained high-energy trauma, the surgeon must be aware of accompanying injuries to the pelvis, axial spine, and other long bones. Associated pelvic and long-bone fractures were found in 46% of such patients who were evaluated at the Hennepin County Medical Center.[111] The patient must also be evaluated for hemodynamic instability because of the loss of blood due to the high-energy fracture.

After being stabilized in the emergency room, the patient is taken to the radiology suite for evaluation of the bone injuries. The fracture is splinted in Buck traction or in a Thomas splint with a Pearson attachment during transfer. In a patient who has sustained multiple trauma, the fracture should be stabilized on an emergency basis. If the patient has an isolated subtrochanteric fracture, stabilization may be delayed, but it should still be performed within 48 hours after the injury.

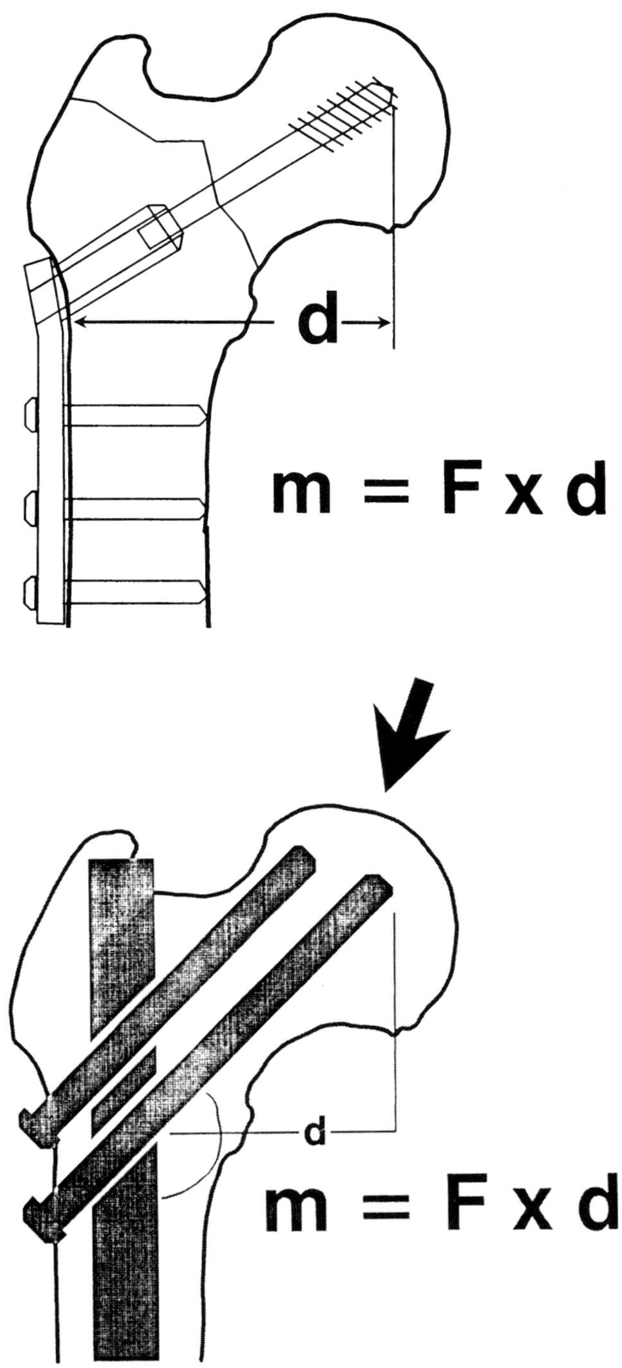

Fig. 23 Diagrams depicting the moment on the nail. An intramedullary position reduces the moment (m) on the angle of the nail by reducing the distance (d) over which the bending force (F) acts.

Surgical Technique for the Use of Locking Intramedullary Nails

The surgeon may elect to perform the intramedullary nailing with the patient in either the supine or the lateral position. The supine position is preferable, because it facilitates radiographic visualization of the hip in both the anteroposterior and the lateral planes and makes positioning of the patient easier. A patient who has sustained multiple trauma should always be placed in the supine position to allow ease of access to the airway as well as to facilitate treatment of the other injuries. The supine position also facilitates reduction of the fracture and obtainment of an acceptable rotational alignment of the femur (Fig. 25). However, with the supine position, it is difficult to gain access to the tip of the greater trochanter for insertion of the intramedullary nail. In these proximal fractures of the femur, the proximal fragment is flexed and abducted, making access to the greater trochanter even more difficult. The lateral position may be used in patients who have an isolated subtrochanteric fracture. Although this position allows easy access to the greater trochanter for insertion of the nail, reduction of the fracture and radiographic visualization of the head- and-neck fragment are more difficult. Good visualization of the proper entry point for an intramedullary nail must be obtained on both the anteroposterior and the lateral radiographs. The point of entry should be in line with the medullary canal on the anteroposterior radiograph and should lie just anterior to the piriformis fossa on the lateral radiograph (Fig. 26).

An incision is made beginning just distal to the flare of the greater trochanter and extending proximally 9 to 10 cm (Fig. 27). The fascia of the gluteus maximus is incised in line with its fibers. The subfascial plane of the gluteus medius is identified, and the piriformis fossa is palpated. This may be difficult in an obese patient, especially if flexion and abduction of the proximal fragment cause the tip of the trochanter to lie against the ilium. Adduction of the limb and positioning of the torso away from the affected extremity can help to expose the tip of the trochanter.

A one-eighth-inch (0.32-cm) guide-wire is inserted into the piriformis fossa, and its correct position is verified with image intensification (Fig. 28). The guide-wire must lie at the base of the femoral neck, just medial to the greater trochanter on the anteroposterior radiograph and just anterior to the piriformis fossa on the lateral radiograph.

After the guide-wire has been positioned correctly and driven into the femur, the proximal end of the femur is opened with use of a .5-inch (1.27-cm) diameter drill-bit. Alternatively, an awl may be used to broach the proximal end of the femur (Fig. 29). A T-handled reamer is then used to ream the proximal part of the medullary canal.

A bulb-tipped guide-wire with a 35° curved tip is then inserted into the medullary canal and passed across the fracture site into the distal fragment. If the passing of the guide-wire proves difficult, pressure on the anterior aspect of the proximal fragment, applied either with the

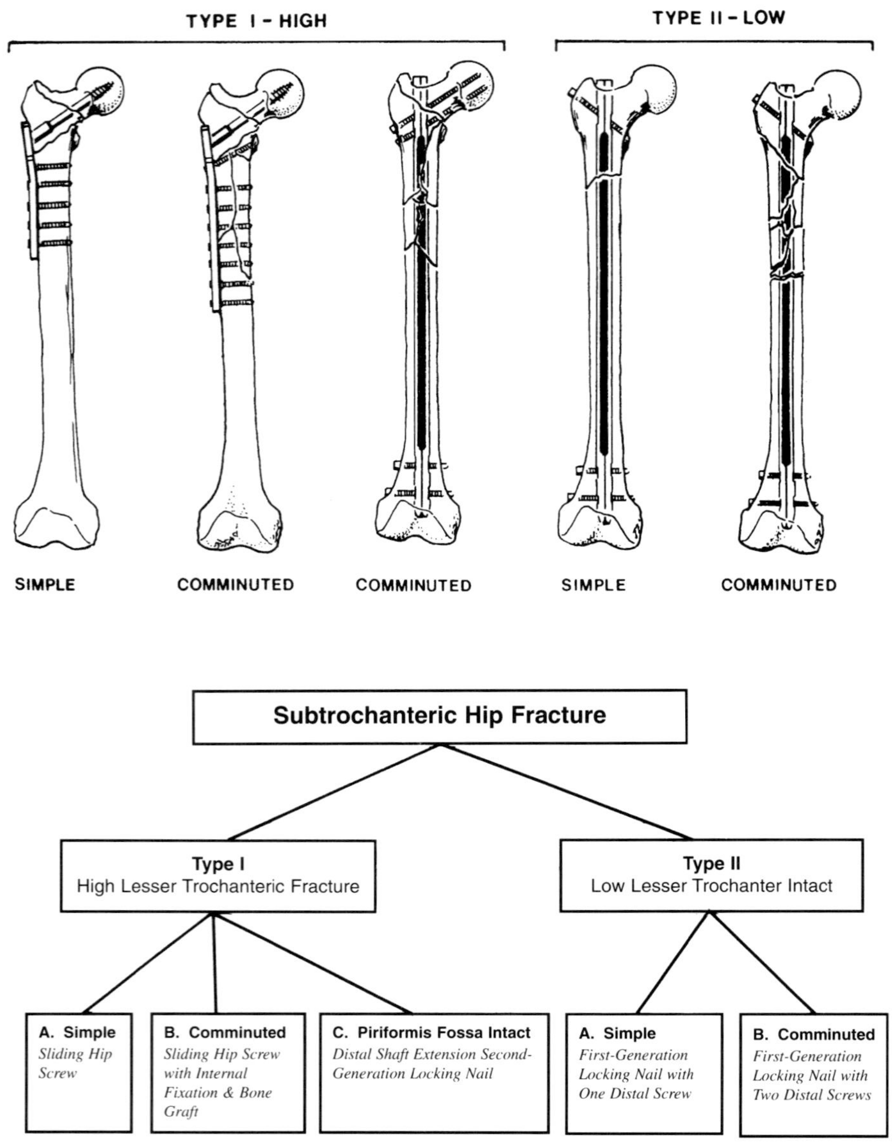

Fig. 24 Classification of subtrochanteric fractures (top), used at the Hennepin County Medical Center, and a flowchart (bottom) showing the various methods of treatment. A type-I simple, high fracture involves the lesser trochanter and is treated with a sliding hip-screw or a second-generation locking nail. In a type-I comminuted fracture that involves the piriformis fossa, the sliding hip-screw is preferred because of the difficulty encountered with insertion of an intramedullary nail. In a type-II simple or comminuted low fracture, a first-generation locking nail (with a single locking screw) is used. (Reproduced with permission from Kyle RF: Fractures of the hip, in Gustilo RB, Kyle RF, Templeman DC (eds): *Fractures and Dislocations.* St. Louis, MO, Mosby-Yearbook, 1993, vol 2, p 819.)

hand or directly with an instrument, may aid in reduction. A small (10 or 11-mm) nail, inserted into the medullary canal, may also be used to manipulate the proximal fragment into alignment with the shaft fragment. Preliminary reaming of the proximal fragment to 12 mm to accommodate the 11-mm guide-nail is necessary. The guide-wire is then passed through the nail and into the distal part of the femur, and the small nail is removed.

The surgeon should not attempt to place the guide-wire with the closed technique for more than 20 to 30 minutes. After such an interval, the fracture site should be opened for placement of the guide-wire.

After the guide-wire has been placed, the femur is reamed according to the surgical technique associated with the particular device being used. Reaming should proceed in 1-mm increments until contact with the cortical wall has been made, and it should then continue in .5-mm increments. If a second-generation locking nail is used, it must be aligned correctly with the anteversion of the femur. The femur should be reamed 1 to 1.5 mm more than the diameter recommended by the manufacturer to allow free rotation of the nail within the femur and easy accommodation for any anteversion encountered.

The reaming nail is then exchanged for a driving wire with use of a plastic exchange tube. The proper length of the intramedullary nail is determined by measuring the length of the guide-wire extending from the femur (Fig. 30) and subtracting this length from the total length. Preoperatively, direct radiographic measurement of the contralateral, intact femur allows the

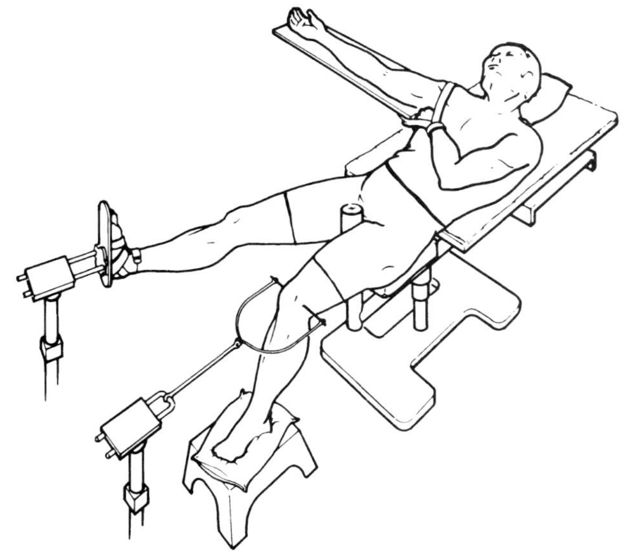

Fig. 25 The patient is positioned on the fracture-table with the hip in adduction and the torso away from the fracture, to aid in exposure of the insertion site. (Figs. 25 through 32 show the surgical technique for the use of locking intramedullary nails.) (Reproduced with permission from Kyle R, Chadwick R Jr: Operative techniques for second-generation interlocking femoral nails. *Op Tech Orthop* 1991;1:288.)

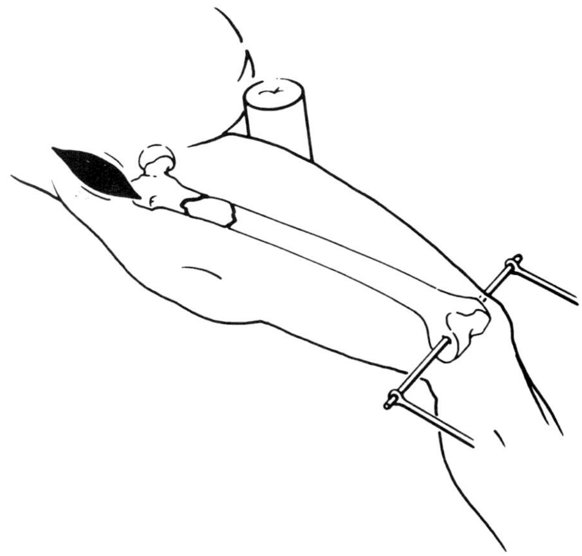

Fig. 27 The skin incision should be in line with the femur and should extend proximally from the greater trochanter. (Reproduced with permission from Kyle R, Chadwick R Jr: Operative techniques for second-generation interlocking femoral nails. *Op Tech Orthop* 1991;1:288.)

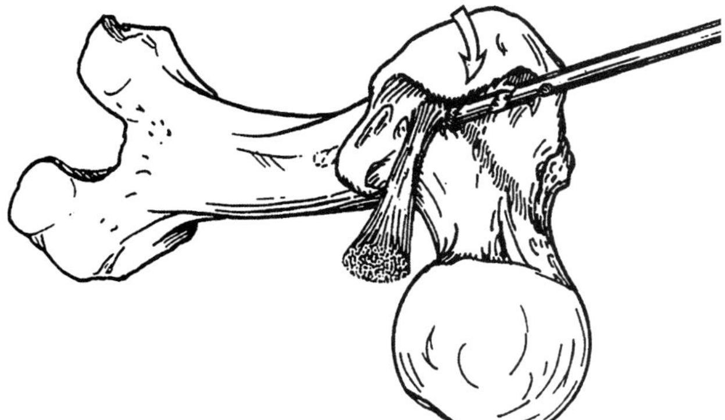

Fig. 26 The intramedullary nail must be inserted precisely: in the piriformis fossa, beneath the flare of the tip of the greater trochanter in the posterior aspect of the femoral neck. (Reproduced with permission from Kyle RF: Fractures of the hip, in Gustilo RB, Kyle RF, Templeman DC (eds): *Fractures and Dislocations.* St. Louis, MO, Mosby-Yearbook, 1993, vol 2, p 815.)

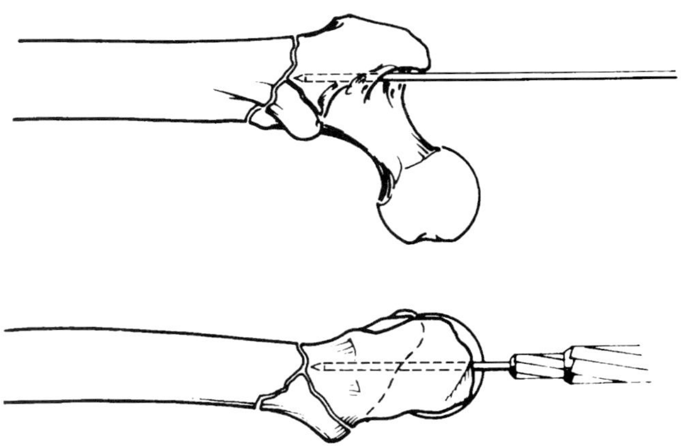

Fig 28 A guide-wire and step-drill are used to create the insertion site. (Reproduced with permission from Kyle R, Chadwick R Jr: Operative techniques for second-generation interlocking femoral nails. *Op Tech Orthop* 1991;1:289.)

surgeon to select a nail of the proper length. This step is particularly useful in the treatment of comminuted fractures.

The nail is inserted over the driving wire, and its proper rotation is estimated by carefully assessing the anteversion as seen on the lateral radiograph of the proximal femur under image intensification. The proximal targeting device is used to insert two screws through the nail into the femoral neck and head. Care must be taken to place the distal screw tightly against the medial cortex to prevent varus deformity as well as to allow room for insertion of the proximal screw (Fig. 31). This may be difficult in a small patient or in a patient who has a varus hip. Careful attention to the amount of ante-

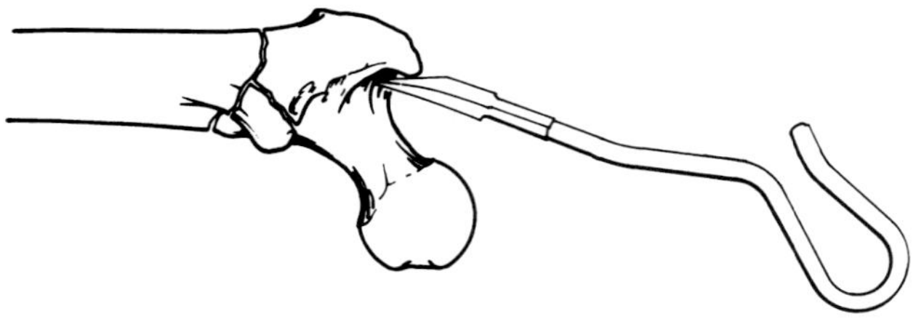

Fig. 29 An alternative method for opening of the femur with use of an awl. (Reproduced with permission from Kyle R, Chadwick R Jr: Operative techniques for second-generation interlocking femoral nails. *Op Tech Orthop* 1991;1:289.)

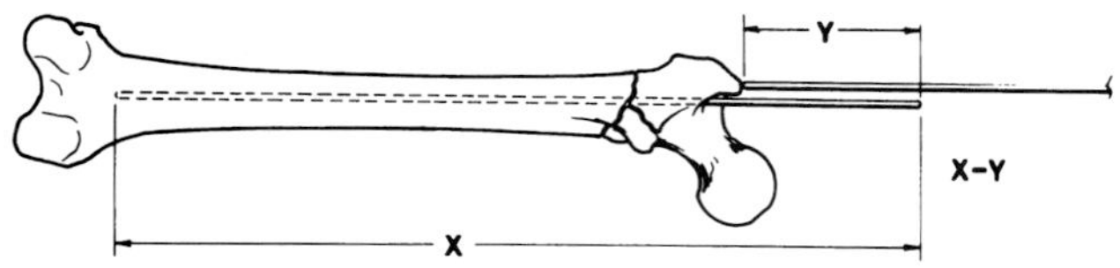

Fig. 30 Method of measurement of the correct size for the intramedullary nail. If the two nails are of identical length, then the length X-Y can be calculated easily. (Reproduced with permission from Kyle R, Chadwick R Jr: Operative techniques for second-generation interlocking femoral nails. *Op Tech Orthop* 1991;1:289.)

version, and the use of guide-wires before insertion of the screws, will help to ensure correct placement of the screws in the femoral head and neck.

Attention is then turned to the distal aspect of the femur and to the placement of locking distal screws to prevent rotational deformity. I have found a modified freehand technique to be the easiest way to insert the distal screws (Fig. 32). After perfectly round distal holes have been visualized under image intensification, a 1-cm incision is made over the lateral aspect of the thigh and a one-eighth-inch (0.32-cm) Kirschner wire, secured to a radiolucent holder, is inserted down to the femur to the center of the proximal hole. The wire is then aligned in both planes under image intensification and is driven through the hole in the nail with a mallet. Proper placement of the Kirschner wire through the proximal hole is verified with image intensification. The wire is then removed, and a hole of proper size is drilled through the nail, following the track made by the wire. A distal locking screw of correct length is inserted. A second screw may be used to provide additional fixation.

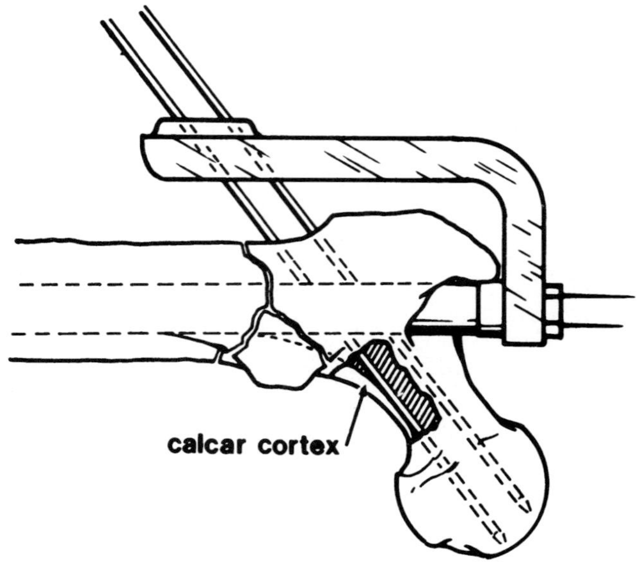

Fig. 31 Placement of the guide-wires for the proximal screws. The guide-wires should lie adjacent to the calcar cortex and in the appropriate amount of anteversion. (Reproduced with permission from Kyle R, Chadwick R Jr: Operative techniques for second-generation interlocking femoral nails. *Op Tech Orthop* 1991;1:290.)

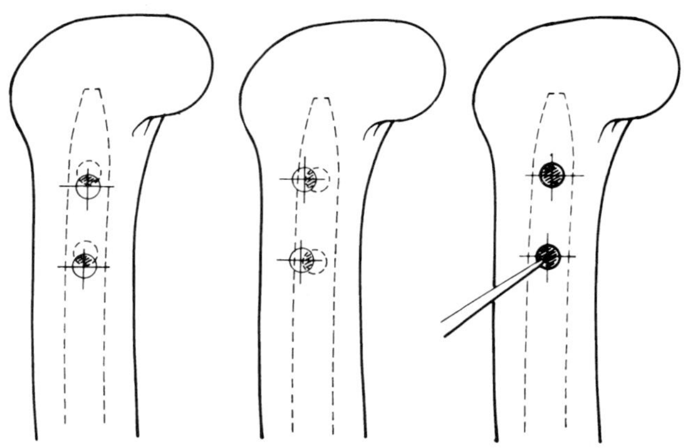

Fig. 32 Freehand technique for distal locking. Care should be taken to align the image so that both holes in the nail are collinear before placement of the Kirschner wire. (Reproduced with permission from Kyle R, Chadwick R Jr: Operative techniques for second-generation interlocking femoral nails. *Op Tech Orthop* 1991;1:290.)

Surgical Technique for the Use of Sliding Hip-Screws

If the piriformis fossa is involved in a proximal (type-I) subtrochanteric-intertrochanteric fracture, a sliding hip-screw should be used. The technique for placement of the screw is the same as that described earlier for the treatment of intertrochanteric-subtrochanteric fractures.

Indirect reduction with minimum periosteal stripping should be used. Bone-grafting of the medial cortex is done if this area is comminuted.

Postoperative Care

Strengthening exercises for the entire lower extremity and range-of-motion exercises are begun immediately. Regardless of the device that is used, the patient is allowed to walk with use of crutches and toe-touching until good formation of callus has been observed on radiographs. After this has occurred, progressive weight-bearing is started. The fracture callus is allowed to mature completely. If complete healing is observed, the fixation device may be removed 15 to 18 months postoperatively in a young and active patient or in one who is symptomatic.

Complications

Varus and Rotational Deformities Rotational deformity is uncommon with use of contemporary methods of treatment of subtrochanteric fractures. When such a deformity occurs and the patient is symptomatic, either an open or a closed derotation osteotomy, with insertion and locking of an intramedullary rod, should be performed. A patient who has a symptomatic varus malunion should be managed with an intertrochanteric valgus osteotomy and fixation with a blade-plate or hip-screw device.

Nonunion Nonunions of the shaft of the femur are treated with repeat reaming and insertion and locking of a larger intramedullary rod. Nonunions in the subtrochanteric region are treated with valgus osteotomy, bone-grafting, and refixation. Osteonecrosis is rare in patients who have a subtrochanteric fracture.

Summary

The orthopaedic surgeon has a multitude of internal fixation devices and techniques available for use in the treatment of subtrochanteric fractures of the proximal femur. The successful use of second-generation locking nails is technically demanding. Close attention to positioning of the patient, reduction of the fracture, placement of the guide-wire, and insertion of the nail and of the proximal and distal locking screws is mandatory. The newer, high-strength hip-screws allow good fixation of a fracture that extends into the piriformis fossa. If medial comminution is present, this technique is best performed in conjunction with indirect reduction and bone-grafting. With proper technique, these devices allow the surgeon to manage predictably a complex subtrochanteric fracture that previously had to be treated with traction or extensive dissection and with (frequently inadequate) internal fixation.

Acknowledgment

The author thanks Laura C. Carroll and Sara J. Campbell for their assistance with the manuscript.

References

1. Frandsen PA, Kruse T: Hip fractures in the county of Funen, Denmark: Implications of demographic aging and changes in incidence rates. *Acta Orthop Scand* 1983;54:681-686.
2. Praemer A, Furner S, Rice DP (eds): *Musculoskeletal Conditions in the United States*. Park Ridge, IL, American Academy of Orthopaedic Surgeons, 1992.
3. Parker MJ, Myles JW, Anand JK, et al: Cost-benefit analysis of hip fracture treatment. *J Bone Joint Surg* 1992;74B:261-264.
4. Firooznia H, Rafii M, Golimbu C, et al: Trabecular mineral content of the spine in women with hip fracture: CT measurement. *Radiology* 1986;159:737-740.
5. Greenspan SL, Myers E, Maitland LA, et al: Fall severity and bone mineral density as risk factors for hip fracture in ambulatory elderly. *JAMA* 1994;271:128-133.
6. Hinton RY, Smith GS: The association of age, race, and sex with the location of proximal femoral fractures in the elderly. *J Bone Joint Surg* 1993;75A:752-759.
7. Alffram P-A: An epidemiologic study of cervical and trochanteric fractures of the femur in an urban population: Analysis of 1,664 cases with special reference to etiologic factors. *Acta Orthop Scand* 1964;65:1-109.
8. Catto M: A histological study of avascular necrosis of the femoral head after transcervical fracture. *J Bone Joint Surg* 1965;47B:749-776.
9. Sevitt S: Avascular necrosis and revascularisation of the femoral head after intracapsular fractures: A combined arteriographic and histological necropsy study. *J Bone Joint Surg* 1964;46B:270-296.
10. Sevitt S, Thompson RG: The distribution and anastomoses of arteries supplying the head and neck of the femur. *J Bone Joint Surg* 1965;47B:560-573.
11. Claffey TJ: Avascular necrosis of the femoral head: An anatomical study. *J Bone Joint Surg* 1960;42B:802-809.
12. Lane JM, Vigorita VJ: Osteoporosis. *J Bone Joint Surg* 1983;65A:274-278.
13. Singh M, Riggs BL, Beabout JW, et al: Femoral trabecular-pattern index for evaluation of spinal osteoporosis. *Ann Intern Med* 1972;77:63-67.
14. Nordin M, Frankel VH: Biomechanics of the hip, in Nordin M, Frankel VH (eds): *Basic Biomechanics of the Musculoskeletal System*, ed 2. Philadelphia, PA, Lea & Febiger, 1989, pp 135-151.
15. Paul JP: Forces at the human hip joint. Chicago, IL, University of Chicago Press, 1967. Thesis.
16. Crowninshield RD, Johnston RC, Andrews JG, et al: A biomechanical investigation of the human hip. *J Biomech* 1978;11:75-85.
17. Bridle SH, Patel AD, Bircher M, et al: Fixation of intertrochanteric fractures of the femur: A randomised prospective comparison of the gamma nail and the dynamic hip screw. *J Bone Joint Surg* 1991;73B:330-334.
18. Davis TR, Sher JL, Horsman A, et al: Intertrochanteric femoral fractures: Mechanical failure after internal fixation. *J Bone Joint Surg* 1990;72B:26-31.
19. Mariani EM, Rand JA: Nonunion of intertrochanteric fractures of the femur following open reduction and internal fixation: Results of second attempts to gain union. *Clin Orthop* 1987;218:81-89.
20. Speed K: The unsolved fracture. *Surg Gynecol Obstet* 1935;60:341-352.
21. Kyle RF: Operative techniques of fixation for femoral neck fractures in young adults. *Tech Orthop* 1986;1:33-38.

22. Swiontkowski MF, Winquist RA, Hansen ST Jr: Fractures of the femoral neck in patients between the ages of twelve and forty-nine years. *J Bone Joint Surg* 1984;66A:837-846.
23. Protzman RR, Burkhalter WE: Femoral-neck fractures in young adults. *J Bone Joint Surg* 1976;58A:689-695.
24. Rizzo PF, Braun JT, Lyden JR, et al: Classification of hip fractures based on MRI: Treatment and follow-up. *Orthop Trans* 1993; 17:467.
25. Garden RS: Low-angle fixation in fractures of the femoral neck. *J Bone Joint Surg* 1961;43B:647-663.
26. Garden RS: Stability and union in subcapital fractures of the femur. *J Bone Joint Surg* 1964;46B:630-647.
27. Garden RS: Malreduction and avascular necrosis in subcapital fractures of the femur. *J Bone Joint Surg* 1971;53B:183-197.
28. Garden RS: Reduction and fixation of subcapital fractures of the femur. *Orthop Clin North Am* 1974;5:683-712.
29. Pauwels F: Der schenkelhalsbruch ein mechanisches problem: Grundlagen des heilungsvorganges. Prognose und kausale therapie. Stuttgart, Ferdinand Enke-Verlag, 1935.
30. Kenzora JE, McCarthy RE, Lowell JD, et al: Hip fracture mortality: Relation to age, treatment, preoperative illness, time of surgery, and complications. *Clin Orthop* 1984;186:45-56.
31. Barnes R, Brown JT, Garden RS, et al: Subcapital fractures of the femur: A prospective review. *J Bone Joint Surg* 1976;58B:2-24.
32. Graham J: Early or delayed weight-bearing after internal fixation of transcervical fracture of the femur: A clinical trial. *J Bone Joint Surg* 1968;50B:562-569.
33. Massie WK: Treatment of femoral neck fractures emphasizing long term follow-up observations on aseptic necrosis. *Clin Orthop* 1973;92:16-62.
34. Brown JT, Abrami G: Transcervical femoral fracture: A review of 195 patients treated by sliding nail-plate fixation. *J Bone Joint Surg* 1964;46B:648-663.
35. Manninger J, Kazar G, Fekete G, et al: Significance of urgent (within 6h) internal fixation in the management of fractures of the neck of the femur. *Injury* 1989;20:101-105.
36. Soto-Hall R, Johnson LH, Johnson RA: Variations in the intra-articular pressure of the hip joint in injury and disease: A probable factor in avascular necrosis. *J Bone Joint Surg* 1964;46A:509-516.
37. Swiontkowski MF, Tepic S, Perren SM, et al: Laser Doppler flowmetry for bone blood flow measurement: Correlation with microsphere estimates and evaluation of the effect of intracapsular pressure on femoral head blood flow. *J Orthop Res* 1986;4:362-371.
38. Holmberg S, Kalén R, Thorngren K-G: Treatment and outcome of femoral neck fractures: An analysis of 2418 patients admitted from their own homes. *Clin Orthop* 1987;218:42-52.
39. Arnold WD, Lyden JP, Minkoff J: Treatment of intracapsular fractures of the femoral neck: With special reference to percutaneous Knowles pinning. *J Bone Joint Surg* 1974;56A:254-262.
40. Barnes R: Editorial: The diagnosis of ischaemia of the capital fragment in femoral neck fractures. *J Bone Joint Surg* 1962; 44B:760-761.
41. Chapman MW, Stehr JH, Eberle CF, et al: Treatment of intracapsular hip fractures by the Deyerle method: A comparative review of one hundred and nineteen cases. *J Bone Joint Surg* 1975;57A:735-744.
42. Christie J, Howie CR, Armour PC: Fixation of displaced subcapital femoral fractures: Compression screw fixation versus double divergent pins. *J Bone Joint Surg* 1988;70B:199-201.
43. Fielding JW, Wilson SA, Ratzan S: A continuing end-result study of displaced intracapsular fractures of the neck of the femur treated with the Pugh nail. *J Bone Joint Surg* 1974;56A:1464-1472.
44. Gerber C, Strehle J, Ganz R: The treatment of fractures of the femoral neck. *Clin Orthop* 1993;292:77-86.
45. Hammer AJ: Nonunion of subcapital femoral neck fractures. *J Orthop Trauma* 1992;6:73-77.
46. Skinner PW, Powles D: Compression screw fixation for displaced subcapital fracture of the femur: Success or failure? *J Bone Joint Surg* 1986;68B:78-82.
47. Swiontkowski MF, Hansen ST Jr: The Deyerle device for fixation of femoral neck fractures: A review of one hundred and twenty-five consecutive cases. *Clin Orthop* 1986;206: 248-252.
48. Beckenbaugh RD, Tressler HA, Johnson EW Jr: Results after hemiarthroplasty of the hip using a cemented femoral prosthesis: A review of 109 cases with an average follow-up of 36 months. *Mayo Clin Proc* 1977;52:349-353.
49. Lausten GS, Vedel P, Nielsen P-M: Fractures of the femoral neck treated with a bipolar endoprosthesis. *Clin Orthop* 1987;218:63-67.
50. Banks HH: Nonunion in fractures of the femoral neck. *Orthop Clin North Am* 1974;5:865-885.
51. Swiontkowski MF, Harrington RM, Keller TS, et al: Torsion and bending analysis of internal fixation techniques for femoral neck fractures: The role of implant design and bone density. *J Orthop Res* 1987;5:433-444.
52. Karr RK, Schwab JP: Subtrochanteric fracture as a complication of proximal femoral pinning. *Clin Orthop* 1985;194:214-217.
53. Tronzo RG: *Surgery of the Hip Joint.* Philadelphia, PA, Lea & Febiger, 1973.
54. Banks HH: Factors influencing the result in fractures of the femoral neck. *J Bone Joint Surg* 1962;44A:931-964.
55. Strathy GM, Johnson EW Jr: Ender's pinning for fractures about the hip. *Mayo Clin Proc* 1984;59:411-414.
56. Marti R K, Schüller HM, Raaymakers ELFB: Intertrochanteric osteotomy for nonunion of the femoral neck. *J Bone Joint Surg* 1989;71B:782-787.
57. Judet R: Traitement des fractures du col du femur par greffe pediculée. *Acta Orthop Scand* 1962;32:421-427.
58. Meyers MH, Harvey JP Jr, Moore TM: Delayed treatment of subcapital and transcervical fractures of the neck of the femur with internal fixation and a muscle pedicle bone graft. *Orthop Clin North Am* 1974;5:743-756.
59. Swiontkowski MF: Current concepts review: Intracapsular fractures of the hip. *J Bone Joint Surg* 1994;76A:129-138.
60. Sanders R, Regazzoni P, Routt M Jr: The treatment of subtrochanteric fractures of the femur using the dynamic condylar screw. *Orthop Trans* 1988;12:683.
61. Jewett EL: One-piece angle nail for trochanteric fractures. *J Bone Joint Surg* 1941;23:803-810.
62. Kyle RF, Gustilo RB, Premer RF: Analysis of six hundred and twenty-two intertrochanteric hip fractures. *J Bone Joint Surg* 1979;61A:216-221.
63. Larsson S, Elloy M, Hansson LI: Stability of osteosynthesis in trochanteric fractures: Comparison of three fixation devices in cadavers. *Acta Orthop Scand* 1988;59:386-390.
64. Steinberg GG, Desai SS, Kornwitz NA, et al: The intertrochanteric hip fracture: A retrospective analysis. *Orthopedics* 1988; 11:265-273.
65. Dimon JH, Hughston JC: Unstable intertrochanteric fractures of the hip. *J Bone Joint Surg* 1967;49A:440-450.
66. Sarmiento A: Intertrochanteric fractures of the femur. 150-degree-angle nail-plate fixation and early rehabilitation: A preliminary report of 100 cases. *J Bone Joint Surg* 1963;45A:706-722.
67. Sarmiento A, Williams EM: The unstable intertrochanteric fracture: treatment with a valgus osteotomy and I-beam nail-plate: A preliminary report of one hundred cases. *J Bone Joint Surg* 1970;52A:1309-1318.
68. Clawson DK: Trochanteric fractures treated by the sliding screw plate fixation method. *J Trauma* 1964;4:737-752.
69. Massie WK: Extracapsular fractures of the hip treated by impaction using a sliding nail-plate fixation. *Clin Orthop* 1962;22:180-202.
70. Chang WS, Zuckerman JD, Kummer FJ, et al: Biomechanical evaluation of anatomic reduction versus medial displacement

osteotomy in unstable intertrochanteric fractures. *Clin Orthop* 1987;225:141-146.
71. Frankel VH: *The Femoral Neck: Function, Fracture Mechanism, Internal Fixation: An Experimental Study*. Springfield, IL, Charles C Thomas, 1960.
72. Rydell NW: Forces acting on the femoral head prosthesis: A study on strain gauge supplied prostheses in living persons. *Acta Orthop Scand* 1966;37(suppl 88):1-132.
73. Aprin H, Kilfoyle RM: Treatment of trochanteric fractures with Ender rods. *J Trauma* 1980;20:32-42.
74. Waddell JP, Czitrom A, Simmons EH: Ender nailing in fractures of the proximal femur. *J Trauma* 1987;27:911-916.
75. Sherk HH, Foster MD: Hip fractures: Condylocephalic rod versus compression screw. *Clin Orthop* 1985;192:255-259.
76. Cobelli NJ, Sadler AH: Ender rod versus compression screw fixation of hip fractures. *Clin Orthop* 1985;201:123-129.
77. Leung KS, So WS, Shen WY, et al: Gamma nails and dynamic hip screws for peritrochanteric fractures: A randomised prospective study in elderly patients. *J Bone Joint Surg* 1992;74B:345-351.
78. Evans EM: The treatment of trochanteric fractures of the femur. *J Bone Joint Surg* 1949;31B:190-203.
79. Evans EM: Trochanteric fractures. A review of 110 cases treated by nail-plate fixation. *J Bone Joint Surg* 1951;33B:192-204.
80. Boyd HB, Anderson LD: Management of unstable trochanteric fractures. *Surg Gynecol Obstet* 1961;112:633-638.
81. Apel DM, Patwardhan A, Pinzur MS, et al: Axial loading studies of unstable intertrochanteric fractures of the femur. *Clin Orthop* 1989;246:156-164.
82. Burnett JW, Gustilo RB, Williams DN, et al: Prophylactic antibiotics in hip fractures: A double-blind, prospective study. *J Bone Joint Surg* 1980;62A:457-462.
83. Inman VT: Functional aspects of the abductor muscles of the hip. *J Bone Joint Surg* 1947;29:607-619.
84. Kyle RF, Wright TM, Burstein AH: Biomechanical analysis of the sliding characteristics of compression hip screws. *J Bone Joint Surg* 1980;62A:1308-1314.
85. Larsson S, Friberg S, Hansson LI: Trochanteric fractures: Influence of reduction and implant position on impaction and complications. *Clin Orthop* 1990;259:130-139.
86. Alho A, Stangeland L, Rottingen J, et al: Prophylaxis of venous thromboembolism by aspirin, warfarin and heparin in patients with hip fracture: A prospective clinical study with cost-benefit analysis. *Ann Chir Gynaecol* 1984;73:225-228.
87. Kyle RF: Intertrochanteric fractures, in Chapman WM, Madison M (eds): *Operative Orthopaedics*. Philadelphia, PA, JB Lippincott, 1988, vol 1, pp 353-359.
88. Boyd HB, Lipinski SW: Nonunion of trochanteric and subtrochanteric fractures. *Surg Gynecol Obstet* 1957;104:463-470.
89. Kinast C, Bolhofner BR, Mast JW, et al: Subtrochanteric fractures of the femur: Results of treatment with the 95-degrees condylar blade-plate. *Clin Orthop* 1989;238:122-130.
90. Wiss DA, Fleming CH, Matta JM, et al: Comminuted and rotationally unstable fractures of the femur treated with an interlocking nail. *Clin Orthop* 1986;212:35-47.
91. Koch JC: The laws of bone architecture. *Am J Anat* 1917;21:177-298.
92. Froimson AI: Treatment of comminuted subtrochanteric fractures of the femur. *Surg Gynecol Obstet* 1970;131:465-472.
93. Allis OH: Fracture in the upper third of the femur exclusive of the neck. *Med News* 1891;59:585-590.
94. Lambotte A (ed): L'intervention opératoire dans les fractures récentes et anciennes, envisagée particulierement au point de vue de l'oste, ó-synthese avec la description de plusieurs techniques nouvelles. Bruxelles, Lamertain, 1907.
95. Hibbs RA: The management of the tendency of the upper fragment to tilt forward in fractures of the upper third of the femur: A question of priority. *NY Med J* 1902;75:239-240.
96. Fielding JW, Magliato HJ: Subtrochanteric fractures. *Surg Gynecol Obstet* 1966;122:555-560.
97. Küntscher G: Dauerbruch und Umbauzone. *Beitr Z Klin Chir* 1939;169:557-572.
98. Zickel RE: A new fixation device for subtrochanteric fractures of the femur: A preliminary report. *Clin Orthop* 1967;54:115-123.
99. Zickel RE: An intramedullary fixation device for the proximal part of the femur: Nine years' experience. *J Bone Joint Surg* 1976;58A:866-872.
100. Zickel RE: Subtrochanteric femoral fractures. *Orthop Clin North Am* 1980;11:555-568.
101. Ovadia DN, Chess JL: Intraoperative and postoperative subtrochanteric fracture of the femur associated with removal of the Zickel nail. *J Bone Joint Surg* 1988;70A:239-243.
102. Yelton C, Low W: Iatrogenic subtrochanteric fracture: A complication of Zickel nails. *J Bone Joint Surg* 1986;68A:1237-1240.
103. Senter B, Kendig R, Savoie FH: Operative stabilization of subtrochanteric fractures of the femur. *J Orthop Trauma* 1990;4:399-405.
104. Seinsheimer F: Subtrochanteric fractures of the femur. *J Bone Joint Surg* 1978;60A:300-306.
105. Brumback RJ, Uwagie-Ero S, Lakatos RP, et al: Intramedullary nailing of femoral shaft fractures: Part II. Fracture-healing with static interlocking fixation. *J Bone Joint Surg* 1988;70A:1453-1462.
106. Tarr RR, Wiss DA: The mechanics and biology of intramedullary fracture fixation. *Clin Orthop* 1986;212:10-17.
107. Thoresen BO, Alho A, Ekeland A, et al: Interlocking intramedullary nailing in femoral shaft fractures: A report of forty-eight cases. *J Bone Joint Surg* 1985;67A:1313-1320.
108. Wile PB, Panjabi MM, Southwick WO: Treatment of subtrochanteric fractures with a high-angle compression hip screw. *Clin Orthop* 1983;175:72-78.
109. Wiss DA, Brien WW, Becker V Jr: Interlocking nailing for the treatment of femoral fractures due to gunshot wounds. *J Bone Joint Surg* 1991;73A:598-606.
110. Wiss DA, Brien WW, Stetson WB: Interlocked nailing for treatment of segmental fractures of the femur. *J Bone Joint Surg* 1990;72A:724-728.
111. Kyle RF: Subtrochanteric and intracapsular hip fracture update. Presented at the 58th Annual Meeting of the American Academy of Orthopaedic Surgeons, Anaheim, California, 1991.
112. Müller ME, Allgöwer M, Schneider R, et al: *Manual of Internal Fixation*, ed 3. Berlin, Springer Verlag, 1991, pp 136-137.

CHAPTER 21

Fractures of the Femur in Children

S. Terry Canale, MD
Vernon T. Tolo, MD

Fractures of the Proximal Part of the Femur

Although fractures of the proximal part of the femur are much more common in adults than in children, complications after such fractures are more frequent and more devastating in children.[1-15] Generally, high-energy trauma is required to produce this fracture in a healthy child. Fractures of the proximal femur in children also differ from those in adults because of the presence of the physis and the vulnerability of the blood vessels that supply the femoral head. The overall rates of complications have been reported in the literature as ranging from 20% to 92%, in series ranging from 11[11] to 132 patients.[12,13] Because of the vulnerability of the vascular supply to the proximal femoral epiphysis, avascular necrosis is a frequent and serious complication of proximal femoral fractures in children. Injury to the physis (premature physeal closure), inadequate reduction, or loss of reduction may cause a limb-length discrepancy or coxa vara. Less frequent complications include delayed union, nonunion, chondrolysis, and infection.

Proximal femoral fractures in children also differ from those in adults because a child can tolerate immobilization much more readily than can an adult. Thus, more options for treatment are available, including traction, use of a spica cast, and bed rest, in addition to surgical treatment. Threaded pins often are used for internal fixation of fractures in adults, and they also may be used through the capital femoral physis in children to secure firm fixation of the femoral neck. However, in infants, doing so may cause premature physeal closure and marked limb-length inequality.

Both the treatment guidelines and the frequency and type of complications are dependent on the type of fracture. Delbet's four-part classification is the most commonly used for proximal femoral fractures in children (Fig. 1).[16] Type I comprises fractures with transepiphyseal separation, with or without dislocation of the femoral head from the acetabulum; type II, transcervical fractures, displaced and non-displaced; type III, cervicotrochanteric fractures, displaced and non-displaced; and type IV, intertrochanteric fractures.[16] Types II and III are the most common fracture patterns; type IV, the next in frequency; and type I, the least common. Ogden,[17] among others, has noted that intracapsular cartilaginous fractures may actually be variants of physeal fractures and may be classified according to the Salter-Harris[18] and the Ogden[19] systems for physeal injuries.

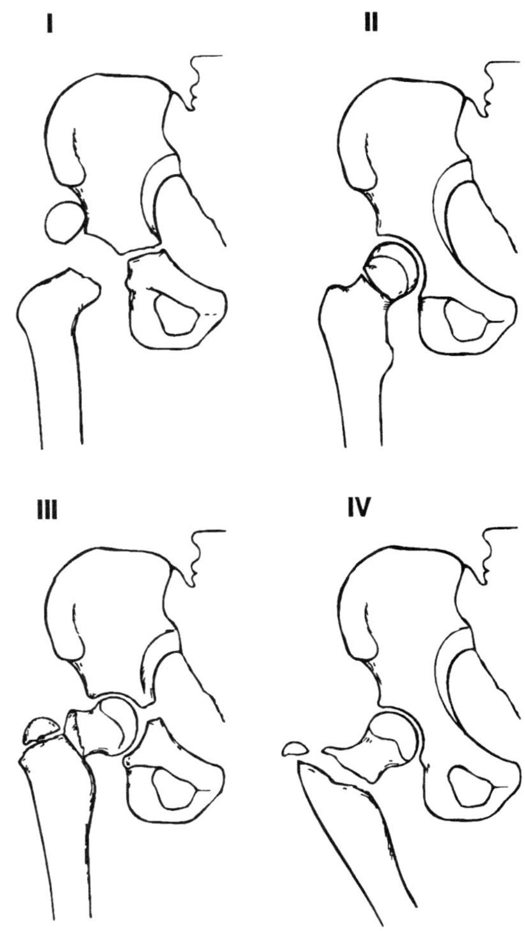

Fig. 1 Classification of hip fractures in children.[16] Type I, transepiphyseal fractures, with or without dislocation of the femoral head from the acetabulum; type II, transcervical fractures; type III, cervicotrochanteric (basicervical) fractures; and type IV, intertrochanteric fractures.

Type-I Fractures (Transepiphyseal Separations)

Although they are the least common fractures of the proximal part of the femur in children, type-I fractures (transepiphyseal separations) were associated with the most complications in the series of Canale and Bourland[1,2] and in most series reported in the literature (20 of 23 type-I fractures in five series were associated with complications).[3,5,6,8,10] Approximately half of the type-I fractures were reported to be associated with dislocation of the capital femoral epiphysis. All five patients with a transepiphyseal separation in the just-mentioned series[2] had dislocation of the femoral head from the acetabulum, and avascular necrosis of the femoral head developed in all five. Forlin and associates[20] suggested that type-I fractures with dislocation from the acetabulum had a better prognosis in children younger than 2.5 years of age than in older children. Ogden[17] reported that the five poor and fair results in his 11 patients with type-I fractures were caused by coxa vara and premature physeal closure; all 11 children were more than two years old.

Severe violence is required to produce a type-I injury in young children,[2,12,13,20] but the injury may result from less trauma in adolescents because it may represent one end of the spectrum of slipped capital femoral epiphysis. The injury often occurs in victims of child abuse.[21]

In infants, in whom the femoral head is not yet ossified, diagnosis of type-I fractures may be difficult. In newborns, an entity called proximal femoral epiphysiolysis, in which the epiphysis separates, occasionally occurs, probably at the time of delivery. Transepiphyseal separation should be suspected in an infant with an apparently shortened extremity that is held flexed, abducted, and externally rotated. In addition to plain radiographs, ultrasonography, arthrography, and magnetic resonance imaging may be needed to make the diagnosis. In older children and adolescents, the diagnosis is more readily apparent on physical examination and plain radiographs, especially when there is a history of severe trauma.

Gentle closed reduction and fixation with smooth pins in younger children and with cannulated screws in adolescents is the appropriate treatment for type-I (transepiphyseal) fractures without dislocation. In children younger than two years of age, closed reduction and application of a spica cast without internal fixation may be adequate if the reduction appears clinically stable. If the femoral head is dislocated from the acetabulum, a single gentle attempt at closed reduction with the child under anesthesia may be made, followed by immediate open reduction and pin or screw fixation if the closed reduction is unsuccessful. Mass and associates[22] and Raju and associates,[23] however, recommended immediate open reduction of transepiphyseal fractures with dislocation of the femoral head to preserve any remaining capsular attachments and to protect any remaining intact blood supply to the femoral head (Fig. 2). Computed tomography is helpful to verify a dislocation presurgically, to determine the direction of the dislocation, and to guide the surgical approach.

Type-II (Transcervical) Fractures

Type-II (transcervical) fractures occur more often than do other proximal femoral fractures in children.[1,6,10,13,14] Most of these fractures are displaced, and the amount of displacement appears to be directly related to the frequency of the development of avascular necrosis. Avascular necrosis occurred after 32 (37%) of 86 proximal femoral fractures and after 17 (52%) of 33 type-II fractures in the series of Canale and Bourland.[1,2] Fracture displacement seems to be responsible for the vascular damage. The maximum amount of displacement probably occurs at the time of the injury.

According to Boitzy,[24] capsular distention by the fracture hematoma and subsequent tamponade of the vessels may increase the prevalence of avascular necrosis; consequently, early evacuation of the hematoma by either aspiration or capsular release may decrease the rate of avascular necrosis. Pförringer and Rosemeyer,[10] in their series of 52 proximal femoral fractures (seven of which were transcervical), reported fewer occurrences of avascular necrosis, premature closure of the

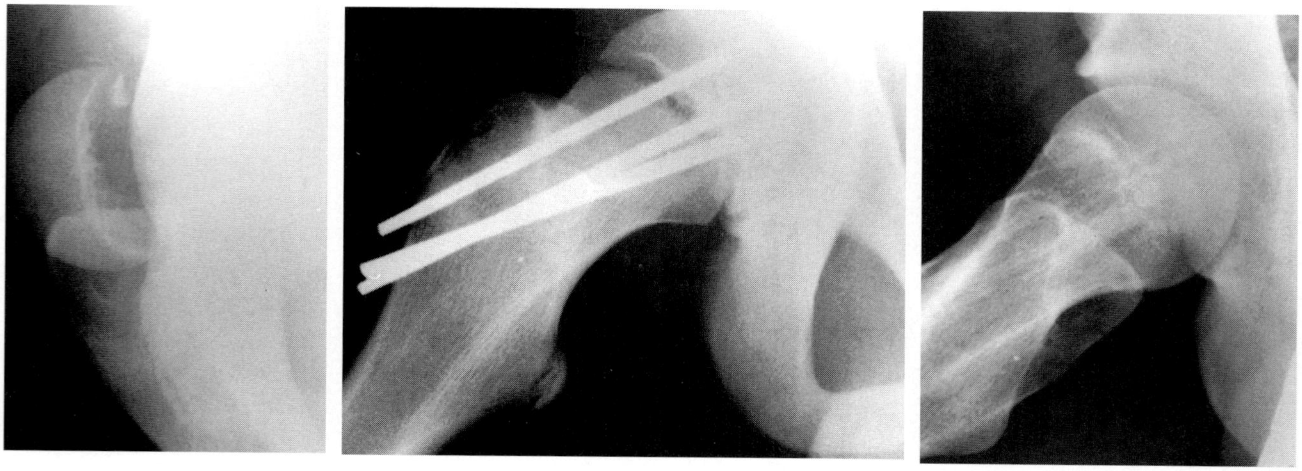

Fig. 2 Transepiphyseal fracture with separation, with the epiphysis dislocated from the acetabulum. **Left**, Before treatment. **Center,** After open reduction and fixation with threaded Kirscher wires. **Right**, At 5-year follow-up, there is no evidence of avascular necrosis.

physis, and nonunion after immediate surgical treatment than after delayed surgery or nonsurgical treatment, regardless of the type of fracture. They recommended decompression of the capsule by fenestration or aspiration for undisplaced fractures treated nonsurgically. Swiontkowski and Winquist[25] recommended immediate open reduction and internal fixation with anterior capsulotomy for evacuation of the intracapsular hematoma for all displaced type-II and type-III fractures. In a review of 29 femoral neck fractures in children managed in seven Swiss (AO) hospitals, however, Gerber and associates[26] found that avascular necrosis developed in nine patients despite early open reduction and internal fixation; seven of the 14 patients with a type-II fracture subsequently had avascular necrosis. Gerber and associates concluded that the occurrence of avascular necrosis was related to the degree of initial fracture displacement and also to the location of the fracture, and that immediate open reduction and internal fixation did not prevent avascular necrosis after displaced type-II and type-III fractures.

We recommend internal fixation for all type-II fractures, because most are unstable. Almost invariably, both displaced and nondisplaced transcervical type-II fractures drift into varus angulation if they are treated only with external fixation or with closed reduction and immobilization in a spica cast. Nonunion also can occur if internal fixation is not used. A gentle closed reduction, similar to that used for femoral neck fractures in adults, should be carried out with longitudinal traction, abduction, and internal rotation, followed by fixation with two cannulated hip-screws (Fig. 3). Percutaneous pinning with Knowles pins can be done with the aid of an image intensifier. In small children, two Knowles pins may suffice, although three can be used. Swiontkowski and Winquist[25] recommended 4.5-mm AO cortical-bone screws, inserted short of the physis, with overdrilling of the near fragment to create a lag effect. Because of problems with noncompliance, a spica cast, with the hip placed in an abducted position, is used for 6 weeks.

Type-III (Cervicotrochanteric) Fractures

Type-III (cervicotrochanteric) fractures are the second most common type of proximal femoral fracture in children and are similar to those occurring at the base of the femoral neck in adults, although avascular necrosis after this fracture is more common in children than in adults.[2,3,5,6,8,10,13,14,27] If the fracture is truly nondisplaced, treatment with an abduction spica cast after 3 to 6 weeks of traction is recommended. If the fracture is displaced, closed reduction and internal fixation should be carried out. Recently, because of several nonunions, we have used a cannulated screw with a side plate for fixation of these fractures in older children. If there is any uncertainty about displacement, the fracture should be treated as if it were displaced. Several fractures in the series of Canale and Bourland[2] were thought to be nondisplaced and were treated with immobilization in a spica cast, only to angulate into an unacceptable varus position in the cast.

Type-IV (Intertrochanteric) Fractures

Type-IV (intertrochanteric) fractures generally result in fewer complications than do the other types of fracture.[2,3,5,6,8,10,13,14,27] Because children have a strong potential for fracture healing in the trochanteric area, union almost always occurs rapidly, usually within 6 to 8 weeks. Initially, skeletal traction can be used to obtain an acceptable reduction. After the fracture alignment appears to be stable, at 2 to 3 weeks (depending on the age of the child), an abduction spica cast is applied and is worn for 6 to 10 weeks. Occasionally, when the fracture cannot be reduced with traction, closed manipulation can be used, followed by application of an

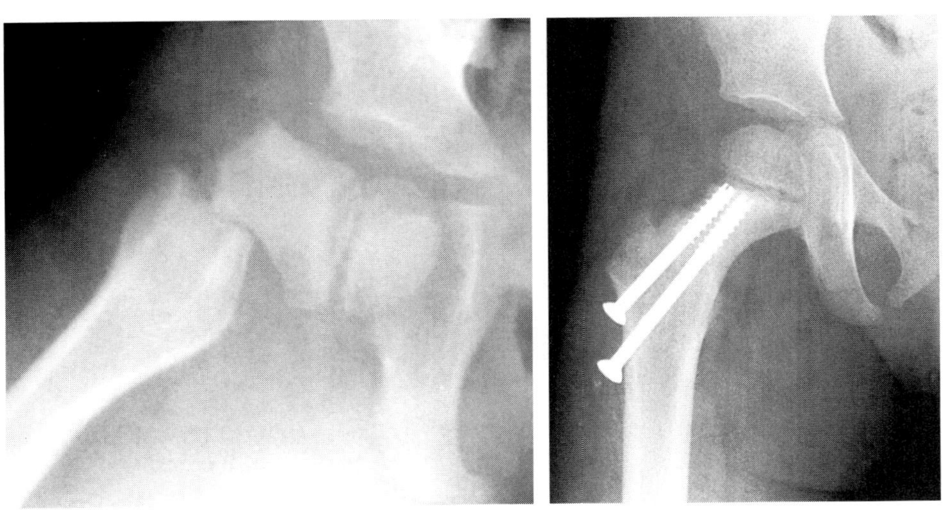

Fig. 3 Displaced type II (distal transcervical) fracture in a 9-year-old boy. **Left**, Before treatment. **Right**, After reduction and fixation with cannulated (4.5-mm) hip-screws.

abduction spica cast or by internal fixation. The type of internal fixation used depends on the age of the child. Because the fracture is some distance from the physis, the internal fixation device should not cross it, especially in young children.

General Considerations of Treatment

When surgical fixation of a fracture of the proximal part of the femur is indicated in a child, several factors must be evaluated before an internal fixation device and an surgical procedure are selected. The most important consideration is the age of the patient.

For fixation of types I, II, and III fractures in very young children (birth to 3 years old), smooth pins may be used; in older children (3 to 8 years old), cannulated 4.0- or 6.5-mm screws can be used. Type-IV (intertrochanteric) fractures can be fixed with pediatric or adult-sized hip-compression screws, depending on the size of the child. Reaming is recommended to avoid displacement when these hip-screws are used. The fixation device should not distract the fracture site or subluxate the femoral head; triflanged nails should not be used.

Several types of cannulated cancellous-bone screws are now available. These screws sometimes are difficult to retrieve because their threads do not cut in reverse. If the fixation device is painful or if the parents wish to have it removed, it should be removed early, 7 to 12 months after the fracture, when union is ensured, or at the first signs of avascular necrosis (Fig. 4). Penetration of the physis by the screws should always be avoided. If the physis must be crossed, smooth pins should be used, especially in younger children.

Complications

Avascular Necrosis The most serious complication of proximal femoral fractures in children is avascular necrosis. Avascular necrosis occurred in 26 (43%) of 61 fractures in a previous series[2] and in six (24%) of 25 fractures in a later series.[1] In the earlier series,[2] avascular necrosis occurred in all five type-I fractures, in 14 of 27 type-II fractures, in six of 22 type-III fractures, and in one of seven type-IV fractures; 25 of the 26 fractures that were followed by the development of avascular necrosis were displaced. Two recent studies confirmed a similar frequency of this complication after proximal femoral fractures in children. Forlin and associates[20] reported avascular necrosis in 14 of 16 children with displaced femoral neck fractures. Davison and Weinstein[3] reported avascular necrosis in nine of 19 children with proximal femoral fractures, seven of whom required surgical treatment.

Ratliff[12] described three types of avascular necrosis: type I, whole head involvement; type II, partial head involvement; and type III, an area of avascular necrosis extending from the fracture line to the physis (Fig. 5).

The first physical symptoms of avascular necrosis are pain and limitation of motion as a result of synovitis. Radiographic signs may be seen as early as 6 weeks after the fracture. A lack of development of the capital epiphysis or osteoporosis of the femoral head with widening of the cartilage space is seen first, followed by fragmentation and gross deformity of the femoral head. Before radiographic signs are evident, radioisotope scanning with a pin-hole collimator may show decreased uptake in the involved femoral head compared with that in the contralateral femoral head.[28] Ogden[19] recommended bone-scanning at 3 to 4 months after the fracture and again at 1 year if avascular necrosis is suspected. Avascular necrosis usually develops within the first year after the injury. The use of magnetic resonance imaging for early detection of avascular necrosis of the femoral head in adults has

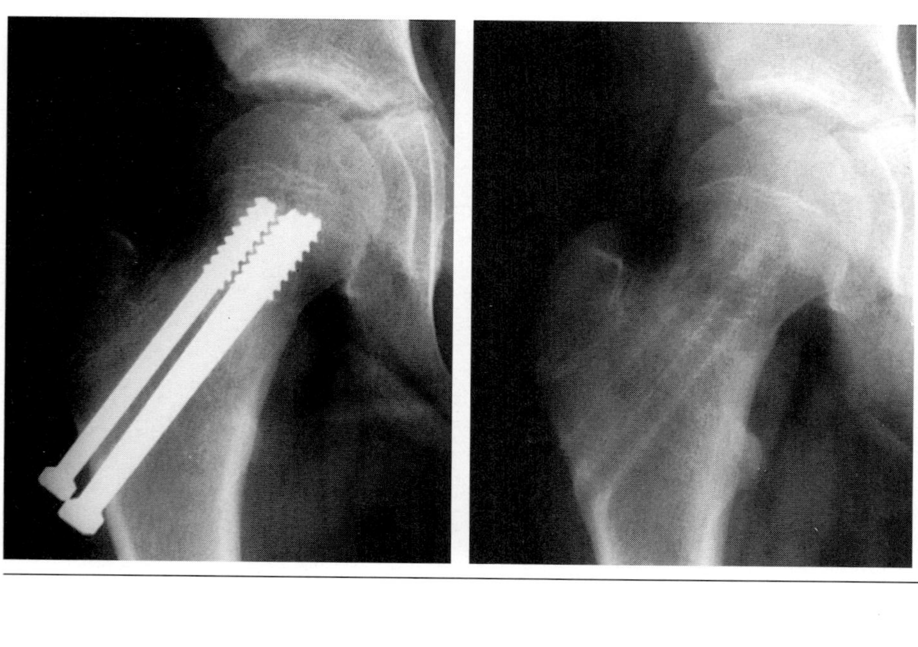

Fig. 4 Type II (transcervical) fracture. **Left**, After closed reduction and internal fixation with cannulated screws, placed to avoid penetration of the physis. **Right**, One year after removal of the screws, there is no evidence of avascular necrosis.

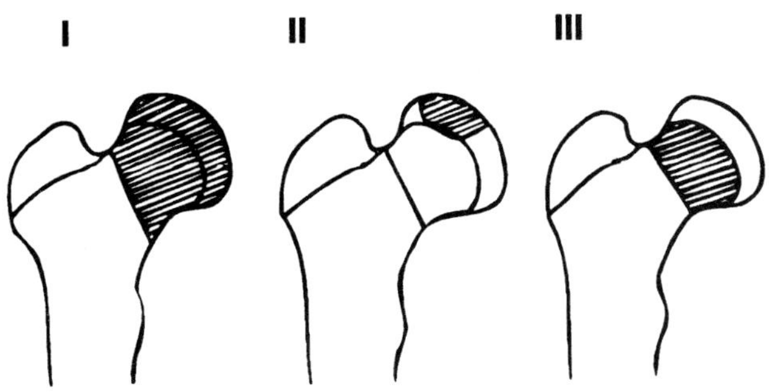

Fig. 5 The three types of avascular necrosis described by Ratliff.[12] Type I, total head involvement; type II, segmental involvement; and type III, involvement from the fracture line to the physis. (Reproduced with permission from Ratliff AHC: Fracture of the neck of the femur in children. *J Bone Joint Surg* 1962;44B:531.)

been reported,[29] but similar use in children has not been well defined.

Treatment recommendations for avascular necrosis have included bed rest, avoidance of weightbearing, and surgical procedures, including soft-tissue releases about the hip for flexion and adduction contractures, osteotomy, arthrodesis, and arthroplasty, but no treatment method has been proved effective.[30,31] For children younger than ten years of age with type-I or II avascular necrosis, removal of the fixation device, followed by the use of an abduction containment orthosis for 12 months, may produce acceptable results (Fig. 6).

Coxa Vara Coxa vara has been reported to occur less often in patients in whom internal fixation was used.[1,2,5,10,12,13] In a previous series,[13] it was found that if the neck-shaft angle was more than 120° in a young child with coxa vara, remodeling usually occurred to some degree, and even if it did not, the mild coxa vara caused little disability. However, if the neck-shaft angle was between 100° and 110°, the coxa vara deformity did not remodel but persisted. Severe coxa vara causes a shortened extremity and an abductor lurch, as well as later degenerative joint changes. Subtrochanteric valgus osteotomy is indicated for a persistent serious coxa vara deformity (Fig. 7). A closing-wedge osteotomy just distal to the greater trochanter, with use of the Campbell screw or another pediatric lag screw with a side plate for internal fixation, is preferred. Although nonunion of the osteotomy is rare, a spica cast is generally used for 6 to 12 weeks postsurgically, depending on the age of the child.

Nonunion Nonunion of these fractures in children is an infrequent complication.[1,2,5,6,8,10] We attribute the low prevalence of nonunion (7%) in a previous series[2] to the use of internal fixation. Surgical treatment for nonunion should be undertaken as soon as possible. A valgus subtrochanteric osteotomy, as recommended by Ratliff,[13] can be used to make the nonunion line more horizontal and to allow compressive vertical forces to aid in union (Fig. 8). This osteotomy can be augmented with bone grafts. Internal fixation is routinely placed across the nonunion site, and a spica cast is worn for 12 weeks.

Recently, one of us (STC) treated a nonunion of a type-II (transcervical) fracture that was associated with an infection in an older child (Fig. 9). Initially, the fracture was internally fixed with an adult-sized hip-compression screw. After the operation, a low-grade infection was treated with antibiotics. The patient was temporarily lost to follow-up after discharge from the hospital. When he returned for examination, 7 months after the fracture, the nonunion appeared to be healing and the hip joint was progressing to early spontaneous fusion. High-concentration antibiotic therapy was instituted, and after union and spontaneous fusion, the hardware was removed. The infection had not recurred at the time of writing, but the position of the fused hip was less than satisfactory. A subtrochanteric osteotomy is planned to realign the lower extremity.

Premature Physeal Closure Premature physeal closure has been reported to occur in 23% of children with proximal femoral fractures (129 of 552 patients in ten series).[1,2,4,5,8-13] In one series,[2] 18 children who had Knowles pins crossing the physis had premature physeal closure. Pförringer and Rosemeyer,[10] however, found no association between premature physeal closure and the type of treatment in their patients. Because the capital femoral epiphysis contributes only 13% of the growth of the entire lower extremity and normally closes earlier than most of the other physes of the lower extremity, shortening usually is less than 2 cm, except when the fracture occurs in a very young child.[25] In the series of children who had Knowles pins,[2] the limb-length discrepancy was more than 2 cm only in patients who also had avascular necrosis. Nevertheless, it is advisable to avoid penetration of the physis if possible, especially in young children, by the use of the newer, more rigid fixation devices (Fig. 4). Limb-length inequality should be determined with scanograms and should be carefully recorded so that epiphysiodesis in the contralateral extremity can be done to prevent a serious discrepancy.

Fractures of the Femoral Shaft and the Distal Part of the Femur

Diaphyseal Fractures

In growing children, most femoral fractures occur in the diaphysis, and almost all unite relatively rapidly, regardless of the type or location of the fracture or the treatment method. The classic method of treatment has been the use of skin or femoral pin traction to obtain fracture alignment, followed by the application of a

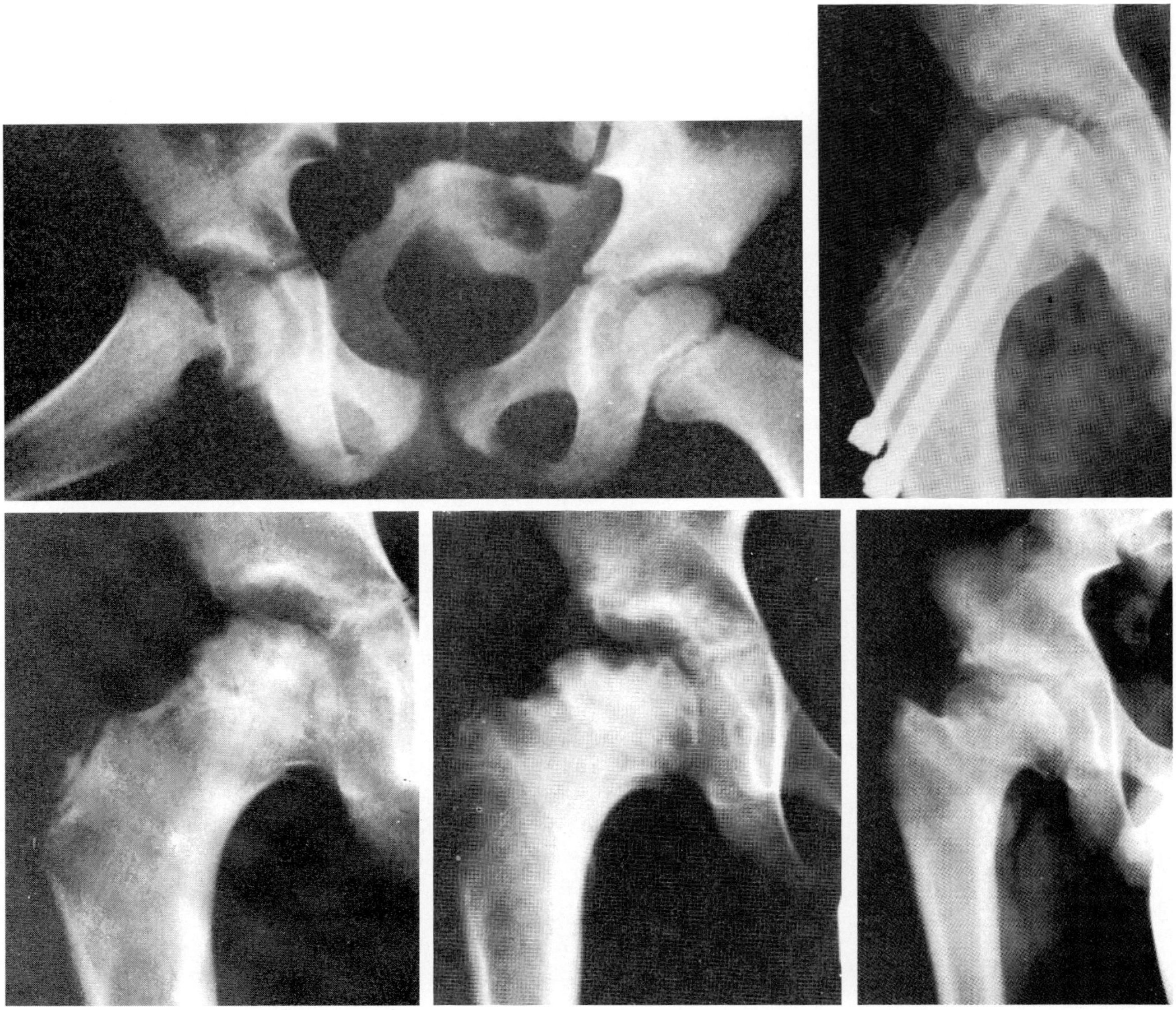

Fig. 6 Type I (transepiphyseal) fracture in a six-year-old child. **Top left**, Before treatment. **Top right**, After closed reduction and pin fixation. **Bottom left**, One year after the fracture, the pins have been removed and avascular necrosis has developed. **Bottom center**, Anteroposterior radiograph made during treatment in abduction. **Bottom right**, Four years after treatment, the femoral neck is short because of premature physeal closure, but the head is reasonably well shaped and the clinical result is acceptable.

hip-spica cast. Although satisfactory results can be obtained with this treatment method, equally good results can be obtained with other methods, without the 2 to 3 weeks of hospitalization required with the traction method.

Treatment of femoral shaft fractures generally is age dependent and must be individualized for each patient. Surgical treatment of femoral shaft fractures is seldom considered for patients younger than 5 years of age, in whom early reduction and immobilization in a spica cast often are possible without lengthy hospitalization. However, in older children and adolescents, surgical treatment should be considered to avoid complications such as delayed union, malunion, rotational deformity, refracture, knee stiffness, limb-length discrepancy, and psychosocial problems.[32]

Treatment in the 5- to 10-Year Age Group

In children from 5 to 10 years old, the primary surgical options for femoral shaft fractures are external fixation, plate-and-screw fixation, and retrograde intramedullary nailing. Antegrade nailing should be avoided in this age group because of the risk of injury to the greater trochanteric apophysis.

Excellent results have been reported after the use of external fixation of femoral shaft fractures in this age group.[33-37] Evanoff and associates[35] reported union, without loss of joint motion, of all 25 femoral fractures

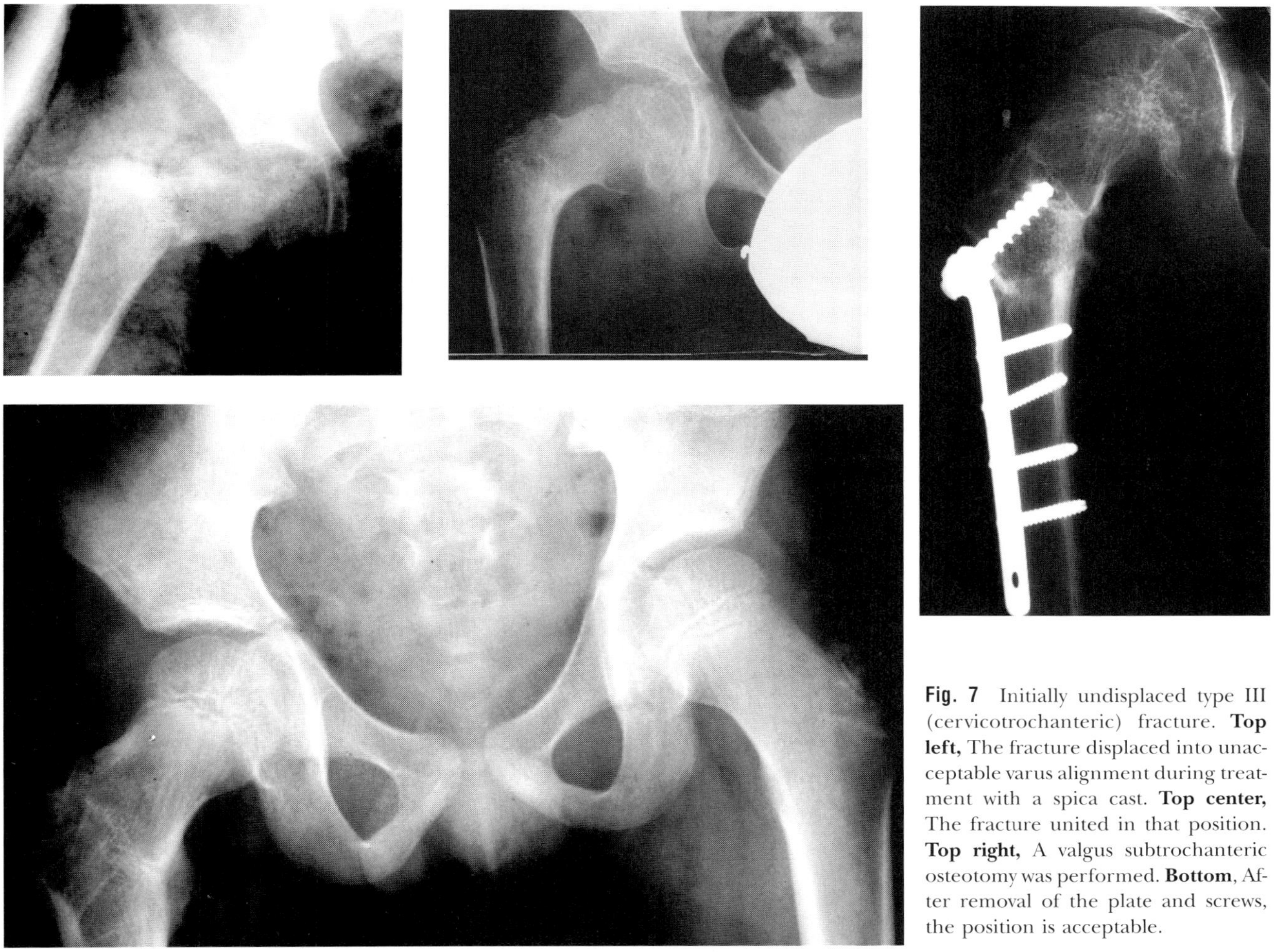

Fig. 7 Initially undisplaced type III (cervicotrochanteric) fracture. **Top left,** The fracture displaced into unacceptable varus alignment during treatment with a spica cast. **Top center,** The fracture united in that position. **Top right,** A valgus subtrochanteric osteotomy was performed. **Bottom,** After removal of the plate and screws, the position is acceptable.

in head-injured or multiply injured children between the ages of 2 years and 4 months and 15 years and 6 months (average age, 8 years and 5 months). Because of the results of this study, one of those authors (Strong) has used external fixation for more than 80 femoral shaft fractures in children without head injuries or multiple injuries and has recommended it for all fractures of the femur in children between the ages of 3 and 13 years. Aronson and Tursky[34] used primary external fixation with early weightbearing for 44 femoral fractures in children. An average of 5.8 mm of femoral overgrowth occurred in six of 16 patients with documented follow-up. As a result, the authors recommended external fixation for isolated femoral fractures in children between the ages of 4 and 12 years.

Generally, a unilateral external fixation frame is used and is applied with the patient under general anesthesia. Numerous devices are available, but some frames are easier to apply than others. Devices with articulations between the upper and lower ends allow more leeway in pin placement because they permit fracture manipulation and reduction after pin placement, but often they are more expensive. If a solid lateral frame is used, the pins must be placed after the fracture has been reduced, and the pin sites should be pre-drilled to achieve optimum purchase of the pins. With a nonarticulated device, two parallel pins are placed proximally and distally in the metaphyseal areas with the fracture reduced. With some nonarticulated frames, extra pins can then be placed adjacent to the fracture to improve reduction and to control the position of the fracture. Pins should be placed no closer than 1 cm to the proximal and distal physes to avoid the risk of premature physeal closure.

The primary difficulty with the use of external fixation is the evaluation of rotation between the proximal and distal fragments. Often, the distal fragment is internally rotated, making it difficult to judge the amount of external rotation of the proximal fragment. In general, the more proximal the fracture, the more externally rotated the proximal fragment. Precise restoration of limb length is not necessary in growing children; fixation in bayonet apposition is satisfactory

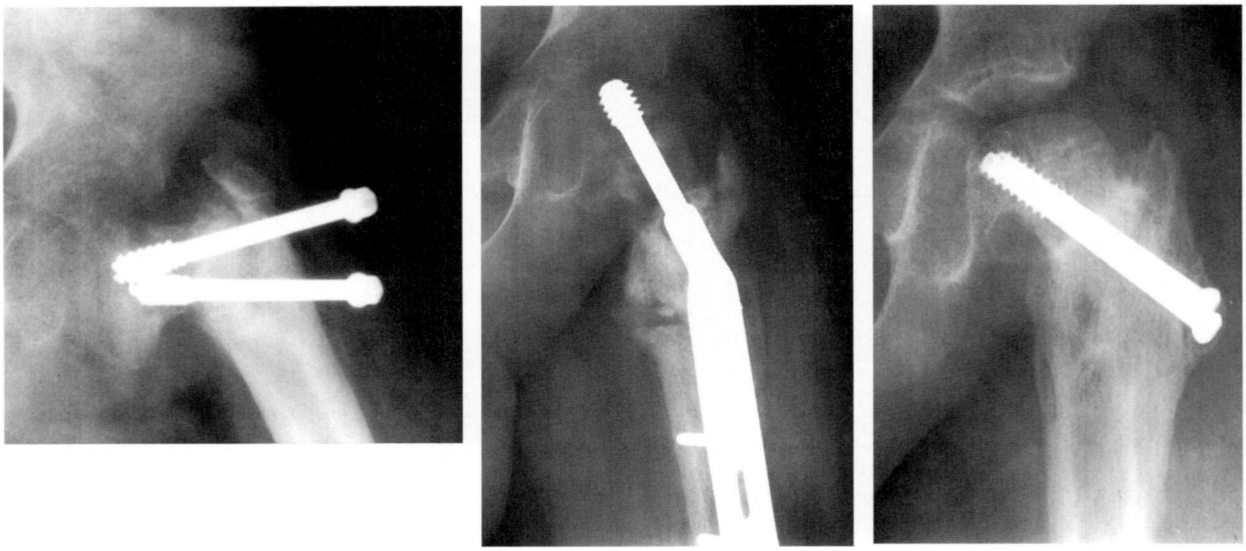

Fig. 8 Displaced type III fracture. **Left**, After treatment with closed reduction and internal fixation, there is definite evidence of a nonunion, with backing out of the points and a severe coxa vara deformity. **Center**, After valgus subtrochanteric osteotomy and internal fixation with a screw, side-plate, and bone-grafting. **Right**, A persistent nonunion necessitated a second bone-grafting procedure and internal fixation with cannulated screws before union was obtained.

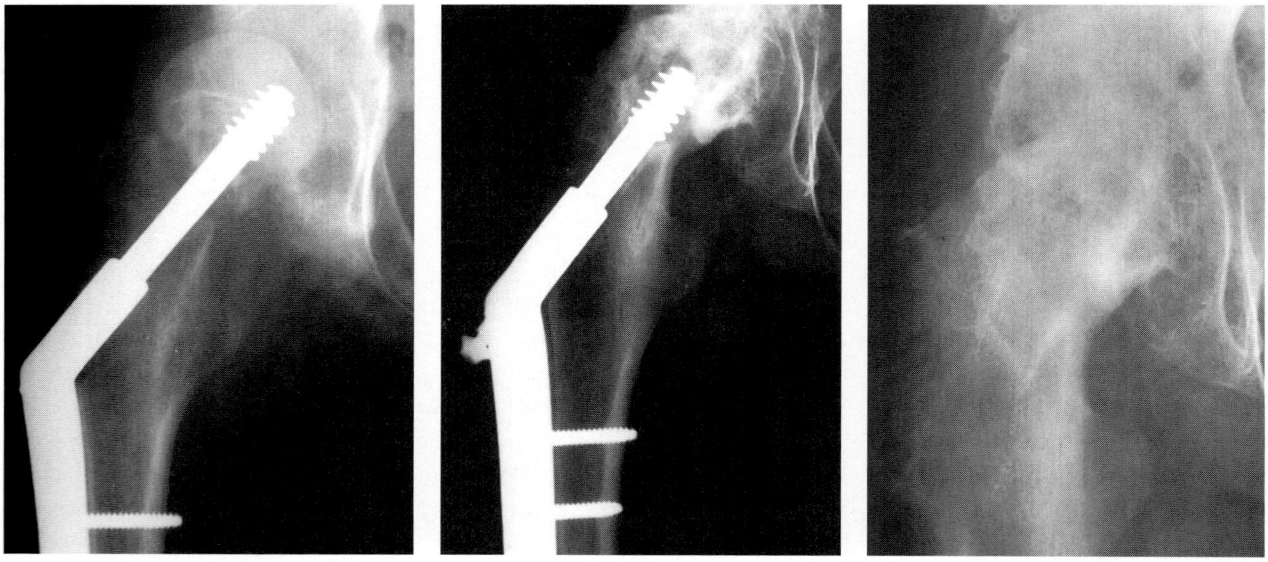

Fig. 9 Displaced type II (transcervical fracture). **Left**, After treatment with internal fixation, there is evidence of an early nonunion. **Center**, Seven months later, there is evidence of infection, union of the fracture, and early fusion of the hip joint. **Right,** One year after spontaneous fusion of the hip and union of the fracture, the fixation device was removed to control the infection.

and will allow for the expected femoral overgrowth of approximately 1 cm after union (Fig. 10).

Skin tension on the pins should be avoided, and daily pin care must be performed. Despite these efforts, pin-tract infections occur in some children. Oral antibiotic therapy is sufficient for most of these infections, but if drainage and local infection persist, pin removal is indicated to prevent osteomyelitis.

Refracture after removal of the external fixator has been reported and may be caused by premature removal of the frame, the use of a very rigid frame, or fracture through a pin tract.[38] To minimize the risk of refracture, we recommend leaving the external fixator in place until abundant bridging callus is seen radiographically. The fixator usually is left in place for 5 to 6 weeks in children younger than 8 years of age, for 6 to

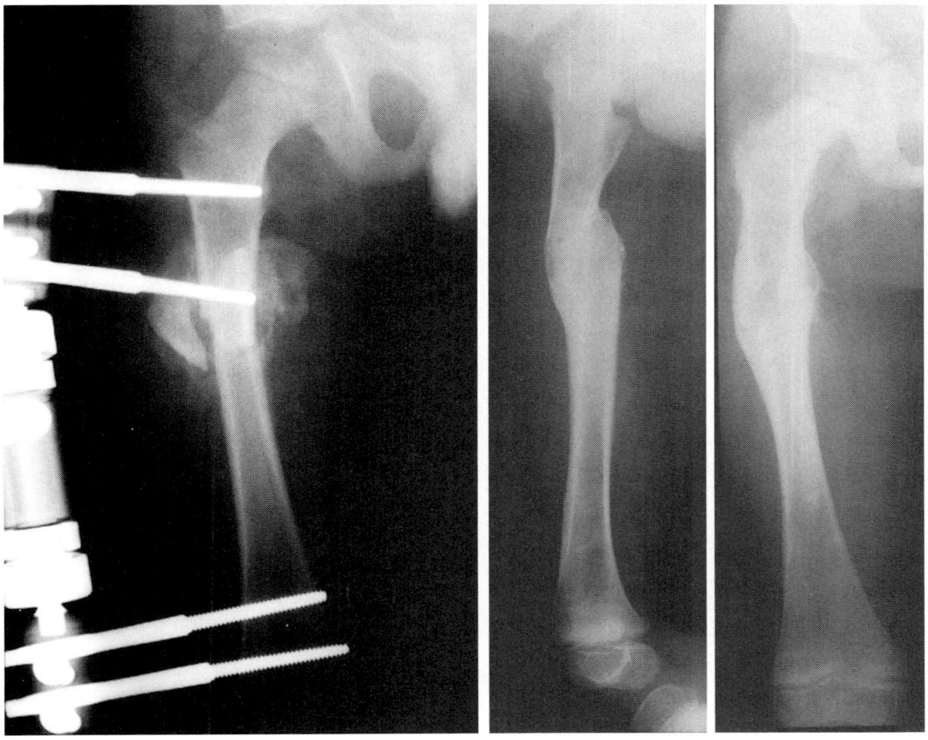

Fig. 10 Femoral shaft fracture in an eight-year-old child. **Left**, The fracture was treated with external fixation. Bayonet apposition allows for expected femoral overgrowth. **Center** and **right**, The healed femoral fracture.

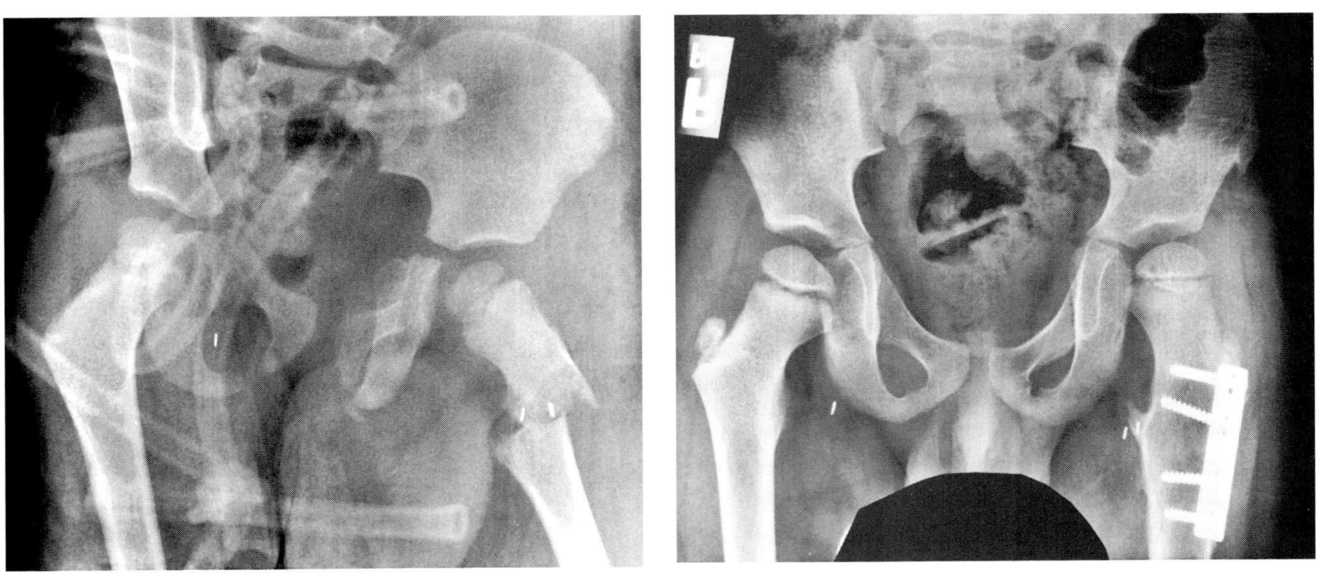

Fig. 11 Proximal femoral fracture in a 5-year-old boy with a severe head injury. **Left**, Before treatment. **Right**, The fracture healed after fixation with a plate and screws. Note the valgus deformity.

8 weeks in those between the ages of 8 and 12 years, and for 8 to 12 weeks in adolescents.

Another surgical option for femoral shaft fractures in 5 to 10-year-old children is plate fixation. In the past, open reduction and plate fixation of femoral fractures in this age group was reported to result in femoral overgrowth and limb-length discrepancy,[39] but these complications have been less frequent in more recent reports (Fig. 11).[40,41] The second surgical procedure required for plate removal may further stimulate growth and increase the limb-length discrepancy. Ziv and Rang[42] reported a deep infection in three of five head-injured children between the ages of 6 and 12 years in whom the femoral fracture had been treated with a

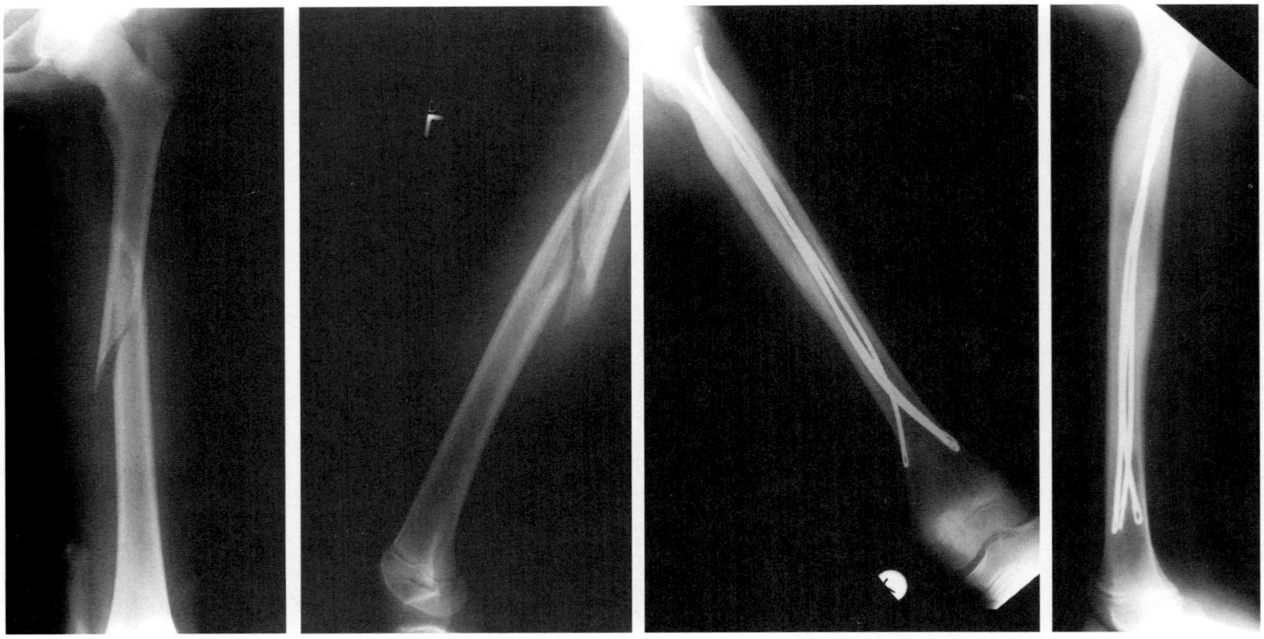

Fig. 12 Femoral shaft fracture in an 8-year-old boy. **Left** and **left center**, Before treatment. **Right center** and **right**, After fixation with retrograde flexible intramedullary nails. (Courtesy of Dr. George S. Bassett.)

plate; these authors discouraged the use of a plate in this age group. Ward and associates[41] reported the use of an AO compression plate for the treatment of femoral fractures in 25 children and adolescents (average age, 11 years). Union was obtained within 11 weeks in 23 patients (92%), no infections occurred, and limb-length discrepancy was not a clinical problem. Kregor and associates[40] reported healing at an average of 8 weeks for 15 femoral fractures in 12 patients with head injuries or multiple injuries. Overgrowth of the injured femur averaged 0.9 cm in their series. Both Ward and associates[41] and Kregor and associates[40] recommended plate fixation for femoral shaft fractures in children with severe head injuries or multiple injuries. Although anatomic reduction is easily obtained with plate fixation, we prefer other methods in growing children. Plate fixation occasionally may be used for fractures in the subtrochanteric area and may aid in the management of head-injured or multiply injured children, but the surgeon should realize that a severe limb-length discrepancy may result from the use of plates.

Good results have been reported in the 5- to 10-year age group with the use of intramedullary nailing (flexible Ender-type nails) by Heinrich and associates,[43] Fein and associates,[44] Kissel and Miller,[45] and Mann and associates[46] (Fig. 12). Ligier and associates[47] reported good results with elastic stable intramedullary nailing of 123 femoral shaft fractures in children with an average age of 10 years. They reported no nonunions or delayed unions, one infection, and minimum limb-length discrepancy. Most advocates of this technique have recommended it for children between the ages of 6 and 10 years for whom traction is not feasible because of head injury or multiple trauma.

The nails are placed from the distal femoral metaphysis and are directed proximally under fluoroscopic guidance into the proximal fragment; the tips of the nails are positioned in the proximal femoral metaphysis or the femoral neck.[44] At least two nails should be used. In many patients, the fixation is stable enough that postsurgical immobilization in a cast is not necessary, but a brace may be used for postsurgical protection, especially after fixation of comminuted fractures. The nails can and should be removed easily through a small incision after union has occurred.

Treatment in Children Who Are Older Than Ten Years of Age

The options for surgical treatment of femoral shaft fractures in this age group include external fixation, plate fixation, and retrograde and antegrade intramedullary nailing. Growth disturbance of the greater trochanteric apophysis is much less of a problem in these older children. Before the age of 9 years, injury to the greater trochanteric apophysis may cause valgus deformity of the proximal part of the femur, but after the age of 10 years, the cessation of apophyseal growth has little effect on the development of the proximal part of the femur. Anatomic alignment of the fracture is more important in this age group because the expected overgrowth and remodeling are less than in younger children.

The advantages and disadvantages of external fixation of femoral shaft fractures in this age group are essentially the same as in younger children, especially if the physes are still open. If the physes are closed, the distal pin can be placed closer to the end of the femur. Anatomic reduction is recommended because little or no femoral overgrowth can be expected.[34] Probe and associates[38] reported refracture through the original fracture site in two adolescents in whom the femoral shaft fracture had been treated with external fixation. Probe and associates believed that prolonged rigid or static fixation impairs sufficient callus formation and healing.

Compression-plate fixation of femoral fractures is feasible in this age group, but plate application often requires extensive exposure, and spiral or butterfly fracture components require the use of a long plate. To avoid postsurgical immobilization in a cast, which is less well tolerated by older children than by younger ones, use of a broad (4.5-mm) AO dynamic compression plate is often necessary to achieve adequate stability. Crutch-assisted walking with limited weightbearing is recommended for several weeks to months after the operation. If an adolescent plans to return to sports activities, plate removal is recommended after fracture union to avoid the persistence of a stress riser that may cause refracture. Partial weightbearing with crutches is required for 4 to 6 weeks after plate removal.

Strengthening of the quadriceps and hamstring muscles is necessary after both operations, which further delays return to full activity.[48] Nonunion and delayed union also are more frequent after open reduction and plate fixation than after other methods of fixation.

In children older than 10 years of age, both retrograde[44-46] and antegrade[49,50] intramedullary nailing should be considered (Fig. 13). Closed antegrade insertion of an intramedullary nail in younger children may cause premature growth arrest of the greater trochanteric apophysis and thinning of the base of the femoral neck.[51,52] Apophyseal growth arrest in children younger than 9 years of age causes valgus deformity of the proximal part of the femur because of the continued growth of the proximal femoral physis. If the operation itself or prolonged retention of the nail causes arrest of appositional bone growth at the base of the femoral neck, this portion of the neck becomes thinned, increasing the risk of fracture (Fig. 14).

Beaty and associates[49] recently reported the results of closed intramedullary nailing of 31 femoral shaft fractures in 30 patients aged 10 to 15 years. All fractures united, and the average limb-length discrepancy was 0.5 cm. Two patients had overgrowth of more than 2.5 cm; none had an angular or rotational malunion. All nails were removed at an average of 14 months after the injury; no refracture or femoral neck fracture occurred after removal.

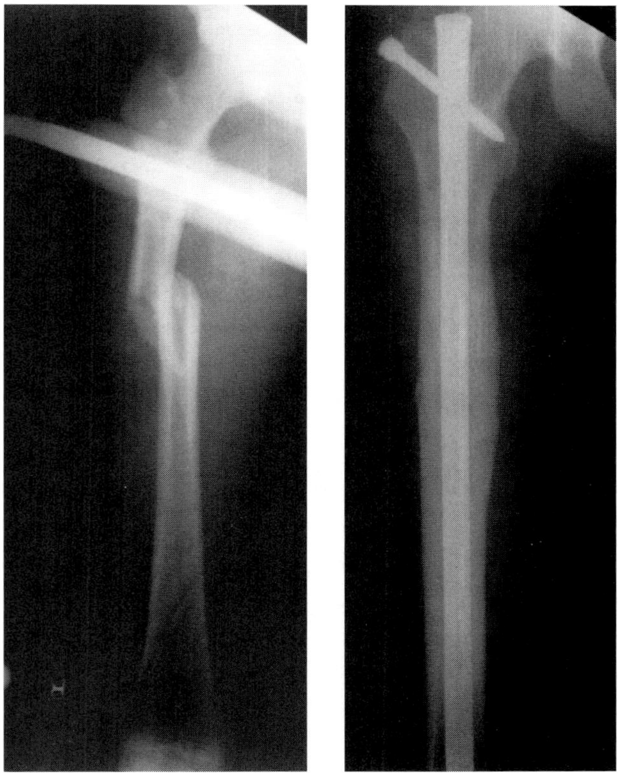

Fig. 13 Femoral shaft fracture in a 13-year-old boy. **Left,** Before treatment. **Right,** The fracture healed after antegrade intramedullary rod fixation.

Chung[53] demonstrated, with injection studies, that the primary vascular supply to the femoral head in pre-adolescents is through the lateral femoral circumflex artery, which courses adjacent to the hip-joint capsule on the posterior part of the neck. Because this artery is at risk for injury during insertion of an intramedullary nail in children, the entry point should be anterior to the piriformis fossa, directly at the superior tip of the greater trochanter. Careful direct observation of this area and fluoroscopic confirmation of the position of the awl and reamer are necessary for safe insertion. Once the initial starting point has been determined, the rest of the surgical technique is similar to that used in skeletally mature patients, with several modifications: (1) the nail must stop short of the distal femoral physis; (2) dissection should be limited to the piriformis fossa and should not be extended proximally on the neck of the femur; (3) the proximal end of the nail should be left 1 cm above the surrounding bone to make removal easier; and (4) the nail should be removed 9 to 18 months after there is radiographic evidence of fracture union so that the femur does not grow over the end of the nail.

If an intramedullary nail designed for adults is used and is stopped short of the distal femoral physis, the distal screw-holes will be more proximal than is opti-

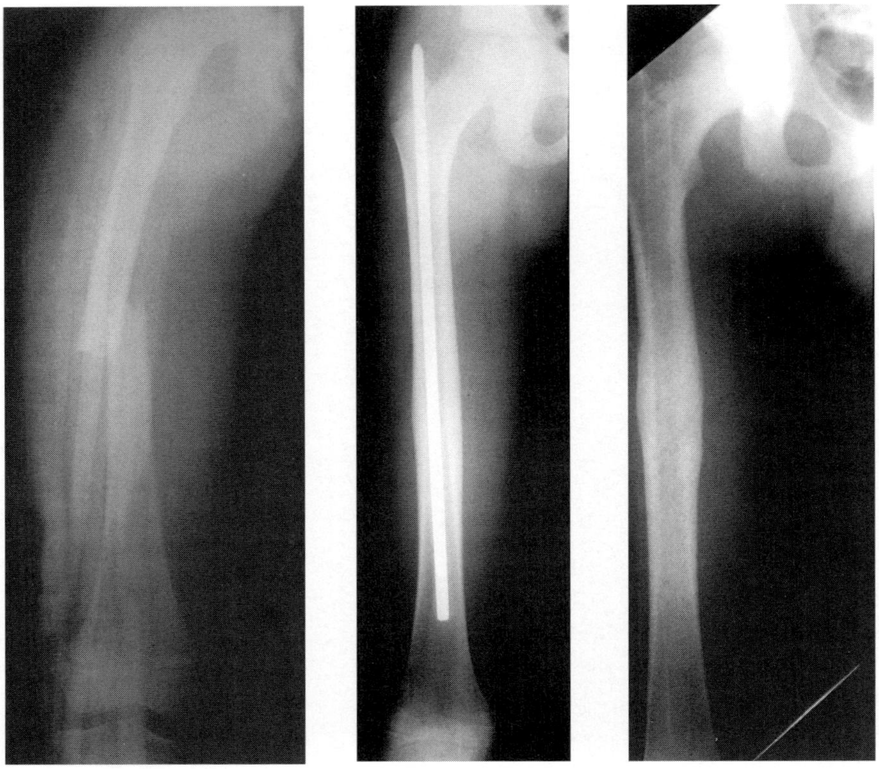

Fig. 14 Femoral shaft fracture in an 8-year-old boy. **Left**, Before treatment. **Center,** The fracture healed after fixation with a self-broaching intramedullary nail without reaming. **Right**, After removal of the nail, there is thinning at the base of the femoral neck, caused by arrested appositional growth.

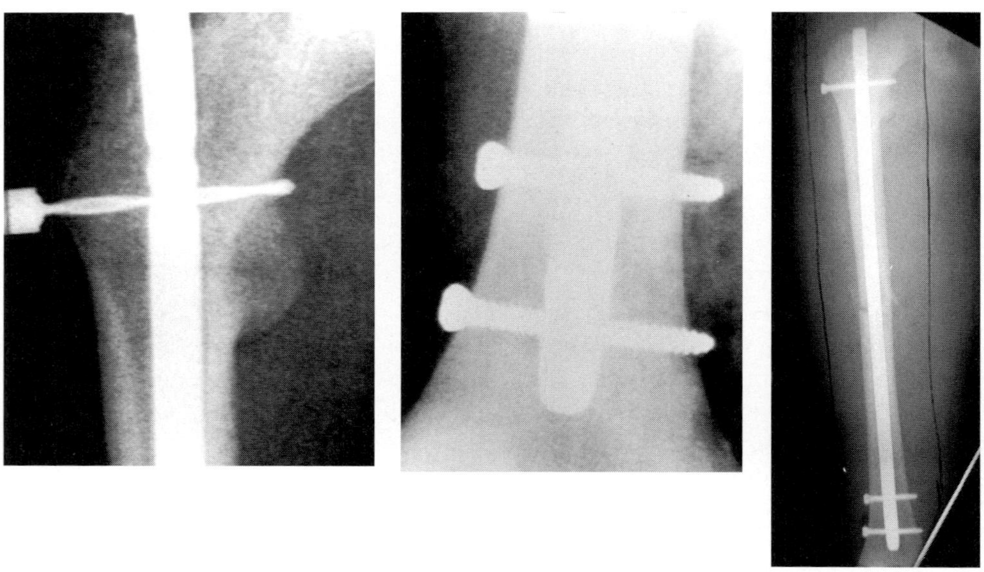

Fig. 15 The technique of proximal transverse screw fixation for children, developed to avoid injury of the trochanteric apophysis. **Left**, The drill-bit is inserted through the proximal locking drill-hole of an 8-mm pediatric intramedullary nail. **Center**, The distal locking screw-holes are placed more distally than in adults so that the nail can be driven down only to the physis and proper position of the distal locking screws can still be achieved. **Right**, After distal and proximal locking has been completed.

mum. An 8-mm nail that has more distally placed holes for the distal locking screws and has a transverse hole for the proximal locking screw designed to avoid the region of the greater trochanteric apophysis has been developed for use in children (Fig. 15).

Potentially, the most damaging complication of antegrade intramedullary nailing of femoral fractures in this age group is avascular necrosis of the femoral head, although this complication was reported by Beaty and associates[49] in only one (3%) of 31 fractures. This one

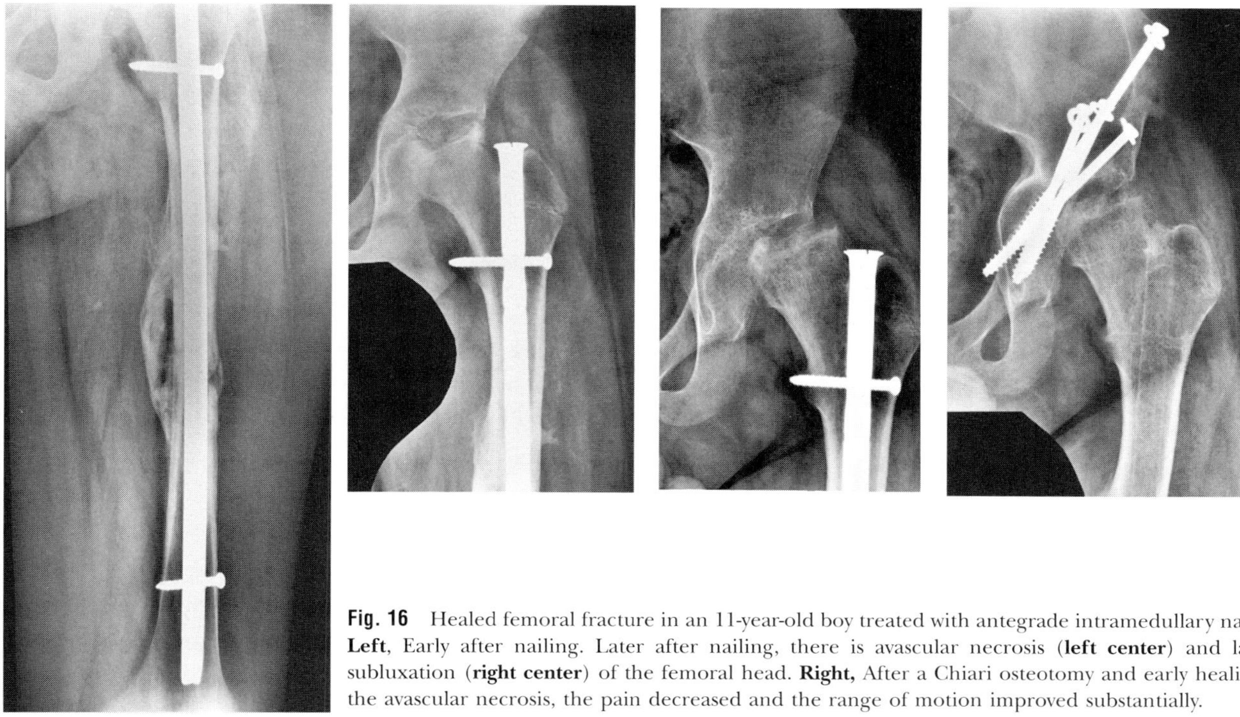

Fig. 16 Healed femoral fracture in an 11-year-old boy treated with antegrade intramedullary nailing. **Left**, Early after nailing. Later after nailing, there is avascular necrosis (**left center**) and lateral subluxation (**right center**) of the femoral head. **Right,** After a Chiari osteotomy and early healing of the avascular necrosis, the pain decreased and the range of motion improved substantially.

occurrence was not seen on radiographs until 15 months after the injury, and the authors were unable to determine if it had been caused by an unrecognized hip injury, by injury to the blood supply of the femoral head and neck during insertion of the nail, or by dissection during removal of the nail. They recommended that dissection be limited to the base of the femoral neck and into the junction of the piriformis fossa and the greater trochanter and that it not extend into the posterior aspect of the capsule of the midportion of the femoral neck. Dissection can be further decreased by removing the posterior third of the tip of the greater trochanter and inserting the nail at the junction of the piriformis fossa with the base of the greater trochanter.

Avascular necrosis of the femoral head in older children and adolescents generally does not heal without treatment, and this complication can limit hip function into adulthood. If only a small segment of the weightbearing portion of the femoral head is involved, limited weightbearing with crutches is the initial treatment, often for several months, as the radiographic changes are monitored. After the extent of avascular necrosis appears to have stabilized, more definitive treatment may be considered. If the medial aspect of the femoral head is unaffected and can be brought to the weightbearing area by adduction of the hip, a proximal valgus femoral osteotomy should be considered. If a larger portion of the femoral head is involved or if the hip is subluxated, a Chiari pelvic osteotomy can be used to provide coverage of the femoral head (Fig. 16).

Less serious, but more frequent, complications of femoral shaft fractures include rotational malunion and delayed union. If healing is delayed, removal of the distal locking screw and continued weightbearing usually will result in fracture healing. Rotational malalignment results either from malreduction or from rotation of the distal fragment around the nail postsurgically when no distal locking screw has been used. If there is any concern about rotational stability at the time of reduction, distal interlocking nailing should be performed.

Supracondylar Femoral Fractures

Supracondylar fractures of the femur often are difficult to control with traditional traction techniques. Because of the pull of the gastrocnemius muscles that originate from the distal part of the femur, the distal fragment angulates posteriorly. Often, this angulation cannot be corrected with longitudinal traction with use of a single traction pin in the distal part of the femur. Flexion of the knee may improve the posterior angulation but also makes it impossible to monitor the frontal plane alignment of the fracture. Because of these difficulties, supracondylar femoral fractures usually require either the placement of a second skeletal traction pin through the distal fragment or open reduction and internal fixation of the fracture. The second, more proximal traction pin adds an anteriorly directed force to the longitudinal force applied by the first pin. This combination eliminates the posterior angulation of the distal fragment, avoids excessive knee flexion, and thus allows evaluation of the varus-valgus alignment. Care must be taken to avoid the physis when the traction pins are inserted into the distal part of the femur.

In some patients, surgical treatment may be preferable to the two-pin traction technique. External fixation can be used, especially in patients with multiple injuries, but maintenance of a safe distance (1 to 2 cm) between the distal femoral physis and the distal pins of the fixation device often is difficult. Alternatively, in younger children, the fracture may be reduced through a limited incision and held with crossed percutaneous Steinmann pins (Fig. 17). Immobilization in a spica or above-the-knee cast is necessary when this type of fixation is used. In older children and adolescents, open reduction and compression-plate fixation can be used to eliminate the need for a postsurgical cast.

Distal Femoral Physeal Fractures

Although Salter-Harris types I and II fractures[18] rarely result in growth disturbances in other long bones, fractures through the distal femoral physis have been reported to cause angular deformity or limb-length discrepancy. Lombardo and Harvey[54] reported a limb-length discrepancy of more than 1 cm in 13 (46%) of 28 patients and angular deformity in 11 (33%) of 33 patients. Riseborough and associates[55] reported a limb-length discrepancy of more than 2.4 cm in 19 (29%) and angular deformity in 17 (26%) of 66 patients. Anatomic reduction of these fractures is especially important to decrease the risk of growth arrest of the distal femoral physis, the physis that contributes most of the length of the growing femur.

Closed reduction of types I and II fractures may be attempted, but anatomic reduction often is difficult, or extreme flexion or extension of the knee is necessary to maintain reduction. If anatomic reduction is obtained by closed means, percutaneous pins or screws can be used for fixation (Fig. 18) and to allow application of a cast with the knee in a slightly flexed position. If closed reduction is unacceptable, limited open reduction with a Steinmann pin or screw fixation is carried out. If the metaphyseal fragment in a type-II fracture is large enough, a 4.5- or 7.0-mm cannulated screw can be used for fixation (Fig. 19). Immobilization in a cast is required for 3 to 4 weeks after either pin or screw fixation.

Displaced Salter-Harris types III and IV fractures[18] require open reduction and internal fixation to realign the articular surfaces and to minimize the risk of physeal growth arrest. Reduction of type-III fractures can be maintained by one or two cannulated screws placed into the epiphysis. In the treatment of type-IV fractures, cannulated screws can be placed in either the epiphysis or the metaphysis, depending on the size of the metaphyseal fragment. Threaded screws or pins should not be placed across the physis because they may damage it.

Follow-up for at least 1 to 2 years is essential for growing children with distal femoral physeal fractures, because these injuries often cause permanent, severe damage to the physis.[54-56] If the entire physis has been damaged by the fracture, approximately 8 to 9 mm of

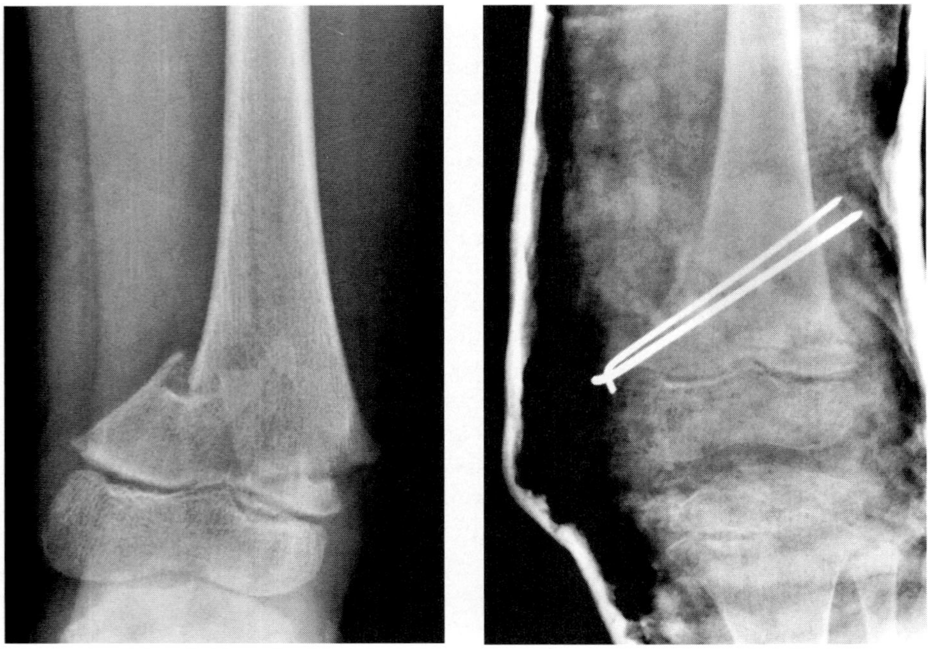

Fig. 17 Supracondylar femoral fracture in a 9-year-old boy. **Left**, Before treatment. **Right**, After anatomic reduction, the limited internal fixation was protected in a spica cast. The fracture healed without deformity.

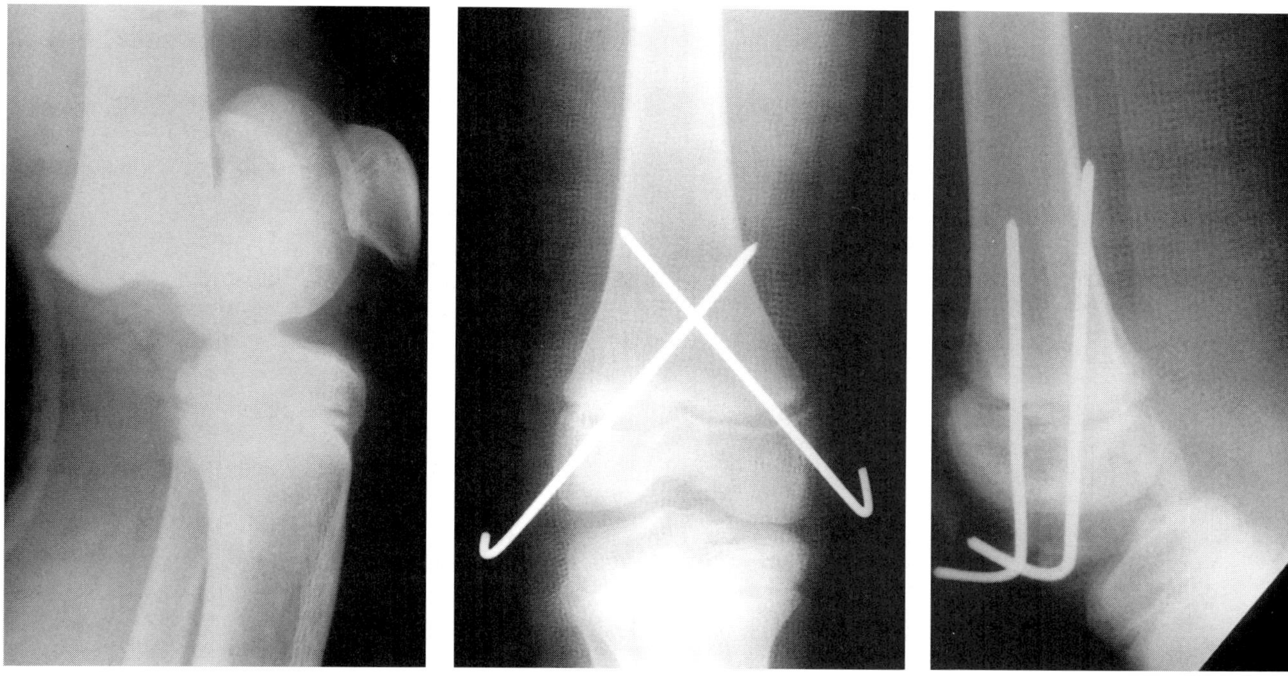

Fig. 18 Extension-type Salter-Harris type I fracture[18] of the distal femoral physis. **Left**, Before treatment. **Center** and **right**, After closed reduction and percutaneous pin fixation.

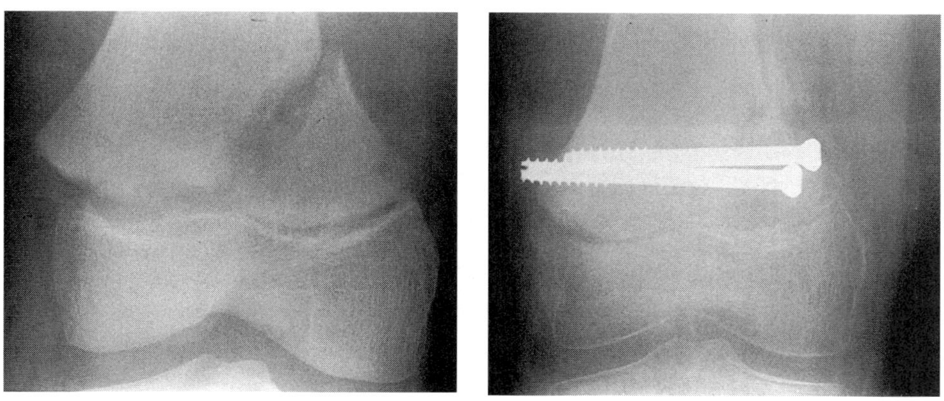

Fig. 19 Posteriorly displaced Salter-Harris type II fracture[18] with a metaphyseal spike. **Left**, Before operative treatment. **Right**, After closed reduction and percutaneous fixation with cannulated screws.

shortening can be expected to occur each year until skeletal maturity has been reached. It should be anticipated that limb-length-equalization procedures will be necessary to correct such discrepancies. If only a portion of the physis has been damaged, angular deformity will occur (Fig. 20). Careful evaluation, including imaging studies such as tomography or magnetic resonance imaging, is necessary to determine if surgical resection of the osseous physeal bridge, with interposition of fat or methylmethacrylate, can be used to reestablish longitudinal growth. If more than 5° of varus or valgus deformity is present, a distal femoral osteotomy should be performed at the time of resection of the osseous bar.

Unrecognized physeal compression or crush injuries, most commonly to the distal femoral or proximal tibial physis, may occur at the time of the femoral shaft fracture. The diagnosis of such physeal injuries usually cannot be made until a resultant growth disturbance becomes evident. The family of the patient should be warned of the possibility of growth disturbance, and the patient should be followed to skeletal maturity to detect any angular deformity or limb-length discrepancy.

Femoral Fractures Associated with Fractures of the Pelvis or Tibia

Ipsilateral femoral and tibial fractures (so-called floating-knee injuries) present special problems in man-

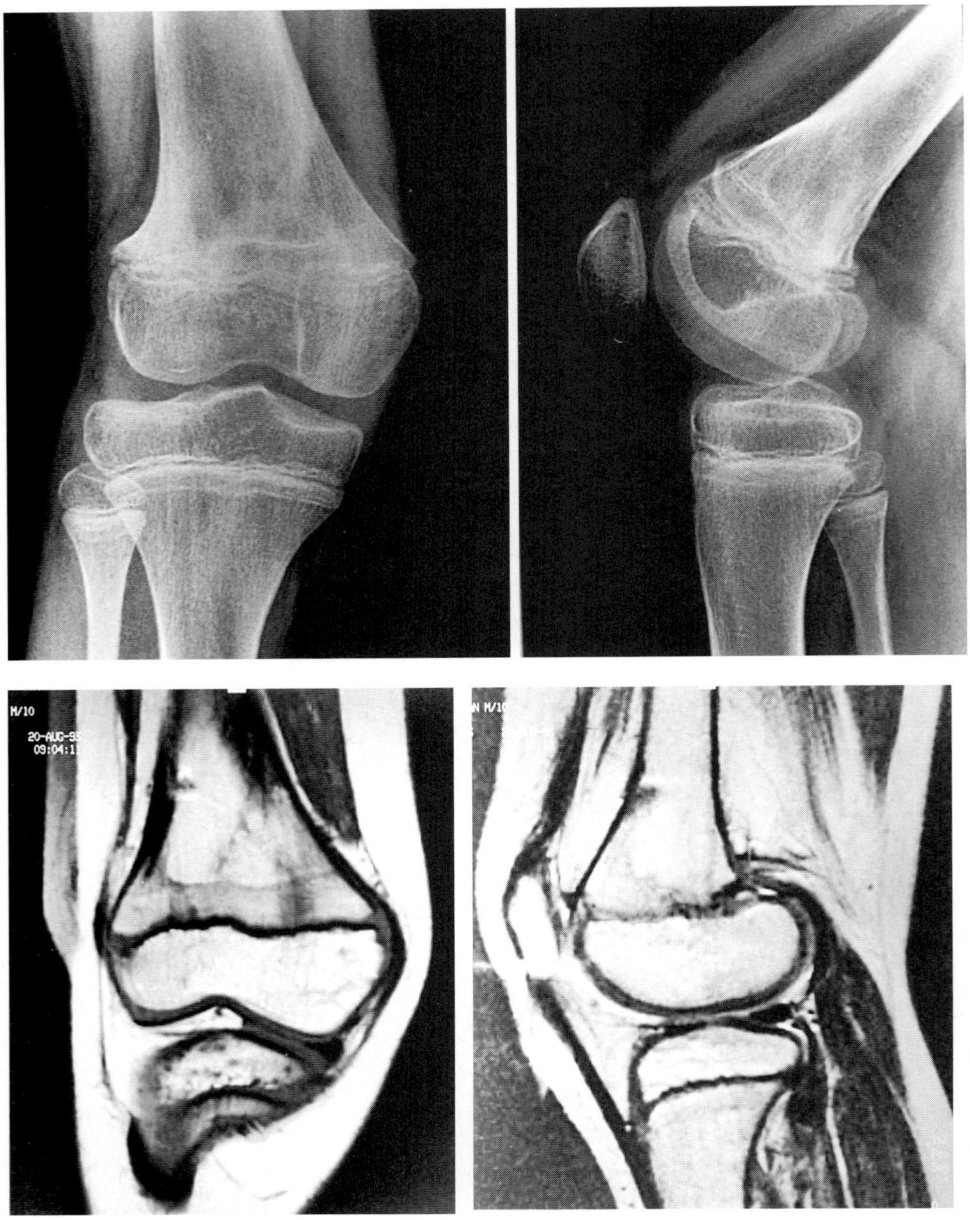

Fig. 20 **Top**, A healed Salter-Harris type I fracture[18] of the distal part of the femur in an 11-year-old boy. Absence of growth arrest lines laterally and posteriorly suggests physeal damage. **Bottom,** Magnetic resonance images demonstrate lateral and posterior physeal damage.

agement (Fig. 21). In 15 children who were younger than 10 years of age, Bohn and Durbin[56] reported that six had an average overgrowth of the lower extremity of 1.8 cm, a consequence of this injury pattern. Older children with these fractures, especially those with distal femoral or proximal tibial physeal injuries, often have knee injuries as well.[57,58] A variety of treatment options are available for floating-knee injuries, but external fixation appears to be the most appropriate. The fixators can be placed separately at each fracture site or they can be linked to immobilize the knee. Spanning the knee joint with external fixation seldom causes permanent knee stiffness in children unless the knee joint itself has been injured. Moderate bone loss in the tibia sometimes can be treated with fixation of the tibia in a shortened position (1 to 2 cm) and reduction of the femoral fracture to length. In young children, this technique may allow healing without bone grafting, and overgrowth of both bones often corrects any limb-length discrepancy. Alternatively, external fixation can be used for the tibial fracture while skeletal traction holds the femoral fracture in alignment until sufficient callus has formed to allow immobilization in a cast. Intramedullary fixation of the tibia should not be used in skeletally immature patients because of the possibility of damage to the tibial physes.

For ipsilateral femoral fractures and vertical shear pelvic fractures, femoral pin skeletal traction is the appropriate treatment, especially in children younger than 10 years of age. Because vertical shear pelvic

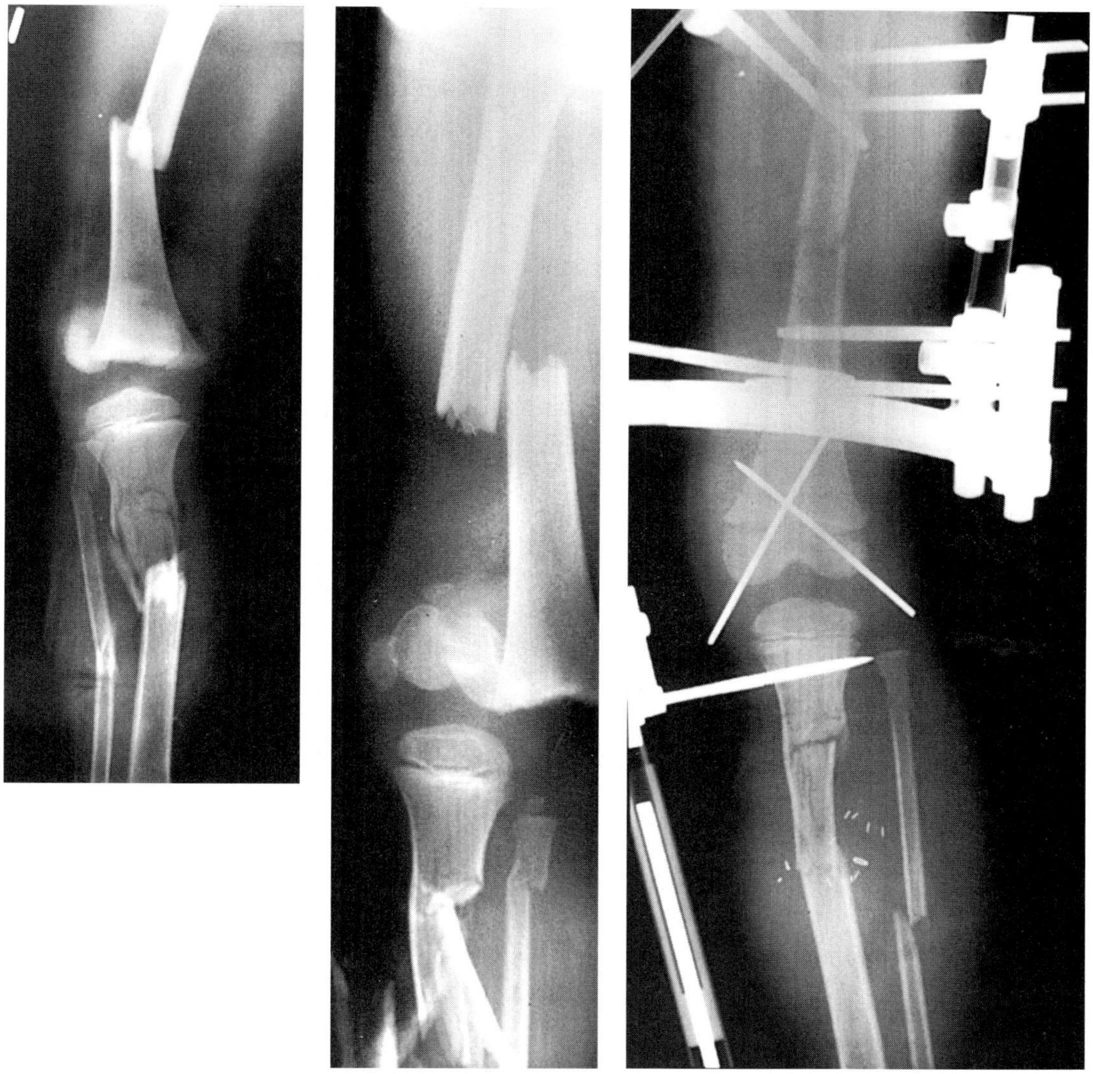

Fig. 21 **Left** and **center**, a severe floating-knee injury with a mid-shaft fracture of the femur, a Salter-Harris type II fracture of the distal femoral physis, and a comminuted fracture of the tibial shaft. **Right**, After internal fixation of the distal femoral physeal fracture with crossed pins and external fixation of the fractures of the femoral and tibial shafts.

fractures heal well in this age group, any limb-length discrepancy of as much as 1 cm resulting from persistent superior displacement will be corrected by femoral overgrowth within 2 years of the injury.

Pathological Fractures of the Femur

Femoral fractures caused by benign or malignant lesions are relatively uncommon in children. Femoral fractures through benign lesions, such as unicameral bone cysts or large fibrous lesions, usually heal with traction and immobilization in a cast, during which time the lesion may ossify enough to avoid surgical excision. For this reason, surgical treatment of acute pathological fractures is rarely indicated.

The treatment of femoral fractures through a malignant lesion depends on the pathology of the lesion and the degree of fracture displacement. A severely displaced fracture through a malignant lesion such as an osteosarcoma usually requires amputation; limb-salvage procedures are not indicated, because displacement of the fracture has usually seeded the soft tissue. Limb-salvage procedures can be considered for non-displaced fractures through malignant lesions. Metastatic disease is a rare cause of femoral fractures in children. In selected patients, after local tumor removal, intramedullary rod fixation can provide stability to the femur during medical treatment of the malignancy (Fig. 22).

Overview

In summary, hip fractures in children, although less frequent than in adults, seem to have a worse prognosis, and parents should be warned of the possibility of

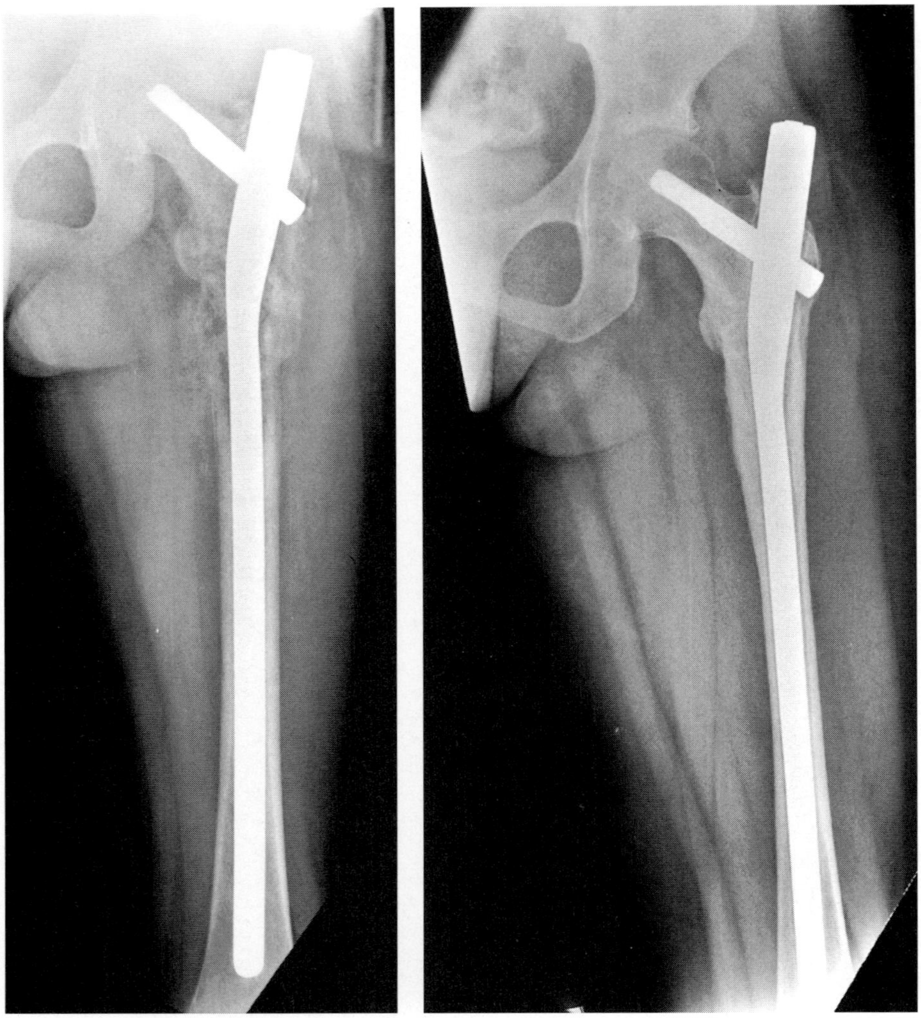

Fig. 22 Pathological femoral fracture caused by a metastatic neuroblastoma in a 12-year-old girl. **Left**, The fracture was treated with Zickel-nail fixation. **Right**, After a bone-marrow transplant and healing of the fracture.

these poor results. Internal fixation should be used for most type-I, for type-II, and for displaced type-III fractures, and the fixation should avoid the physis whenever possible, especially in young children. The theoretical benefits of immediate capsular evacuation, open reduction, and internal fixation have not been proved. Large cannulated screws that produce rigid fixation and avoid distraction should be used, and postsurgical immobilization in a spica cast may be necessary for young, noncompliant children. Avascular necrosis is responsible for most poor results after proximal femoral fractures in children. It occurs most often after displaced fractures. In older children, it can have devastating consequences, while younger children seem to have some potential for reconstitution and remodeling of the avascular head. Nonunion and coxa vara can be avoided with the use of rigid internal fixation. Premature physeal closure usually does not cause severe shortening unless it is associated with avascular necrosis or it occurs in a very young child.

Most femoral shaft fractures in children can be treated nonsurgically, with early reduction and application of a cast or with a few weeks of traction followed by use of a cast, and most heal without difficulty. Surgical treatment, however, is becoming more common in children who are older than 5 years of age, and it may consist of external fixation, application of a compression plate, or intramedullary nailing. Specific anatomic features of the growing femur must be considered if surgical treatment is undertaken.

References

1. Canale ST: Fractures of the hip in children and adolescents. *Orthop Clin North Am* 1990;21:341-352.
2. Canale ST, Bourland WL: Fracture of the neck and intertrochanteric region of the femur in children. *J Bone Joint Surg* 1977; 59A:431-443.
3. Davison BL, Weinstein SL: Hip fractures in children: A long-term follow-up study. *J Pediatr Orthop* 1992;12:355-358.

4. Forlin E, Guille JT, Kumar SJ, et al: Complications associated with fracture of the neck of the femur in children. *J Pediatr Orthop* 1992;12:503-509.
5. Heiser JM, Oppenheim WL: Fractures of the hip in children: A review of forty cases. *Clin Orthop* 1980;149:177-184.
6. Ingram AJ, Bachynski B: Fractures of the hip in children: Treatment and results. *J Bone Joint Surg* 1953;35A:867-887.
7. Kay SP, Hall JE: Fracture of the femoral neck in children and its complications. *Clin Orthop* 1971;80:53-71.
8. Lam SF: Fractures of the neck of the femur in children. *J Bone Joint Surg* 1971;53A:1165-1179.
9. Leung PC, Lam SF: Long-term follow-up of children with femoral neck fractures. *J Bone Joint Surg* 1986;68B: 537-540.
10. Pförringer W, Rosemeyer B: Fractures of the hip in children and adolescents. *Acta Orthop Scand* 1980;51:91-108.
11. Quinlan WR, Brady PG, Regan BF: Fracture of the neck of the femur in childhood. *Injury* 1980;11:242-247.
12. Ratliff AH: Fractures of the neck of the femur in children. *J Bone Joint Surg* 1962;44B:528-542.
13. Ratliff AHC: Complications after fractures of the femoral neck in children and their treatment. *J Bone Joint Surg* 1970;52B:175.
14. Ratliff AH: Fractures of the neck of the femur in children. *Orthop Clin North Am* 1974;5:903-924.
15. Swiontkowski MF: Complications of hip fractures in children. *Complicat Orthop* 1989;4:58-62.
16. Colonna PC: Fracture of the neck of the femur in children. *Am J Surg* 1929;6:793-797.
17. Ogden JA: Hip development and vascularity: Relationship to chondro-osseous trauma in the growing child, in Salvati EA (ed): *The Hip: Proceedings of the Ninth Open Scientific Meeting of The Hip Society.* St. Louis, MO, CV Mosby, 1981, pp 139-187.
18. Salter RB, Harris WR: Injuries involving the epiphyseal plate. *J Bone Joint Surg* 1963;45A:587-622.
19. Ogden JA: *Skeletal Injury in the Child,* ed 2. Philadelphia, PA, WB Saunders, 1990.
20. Forlin E, Guille JT, Kumar SJ, et al: Transepiphyseal fractures of the neck of the femur in very young children. *J Pediatr Orthop* 1992;12:164-168.
21. Gaudinez RF, Heinrich SD: Transphyseal fracture of the capital femoral epiphysis. *Orthopedics* 1989;12:1599-1602.
22. Mass DP, Spiegel PG, Laros GS: Dislocation of the hip with traumatic separation of the capital femoral epiphysis: Report of a case with successful outcome. *Clin Orthop* 1980;146:184-187.
23. Raju KK, Tepler M, Dharapak C, et al: Transepiphyseal fracture of the hips in children. *Orthop Rev* 1984;13:65-77.
24. Boitzy A: Fractures of the proximal femur, in Weber BG, Brunner C, Frueler F (eds): *Treatment of Fractures in Children and Adolescents.* Berlin, Springer-Verlag, 1980, pp 254-267.
25. Swiontkowski MF, Winquist RA: Displaced hip fractures in children and adolescents. *J Trauma* 1986;26:384-388.
26. Gerber C, Lehmann A, Ganz R: Femoral neck fractures in children: Experience in 7 Swiss AO hospitals. *Orthop Trans* 1985; 9:474.
27. Ovesen O, Arreskov J, Bellstrøm T: Hip fractures in children: A long-term follow-up of 17 cases. *Orthopedics* 1987;12:361-367.
28. Herring JA, McCarthy RE: Fracture dislocation of the capital femoral epiphysis. *J Pediatr Orthop* 1986;6:112-114.
29. Kokubo T, Takatori Y, Ninomiya S, et al: Magnetic resonance imaging and scintigraphy of avascular necrosis of the femoral head: Prediction of subsequent segmental collapse. *Clin Orthop* 1992;277:54-60.
30. Morrissy R: Hip fractures in children. *Clin Orthop* 1980;152:202-210.
31. Morrissy RT: Fractured hip in childhood, in Murray JA (ed): *American Academy of Orthopaedic Surgeons Instructional Course Lectures Volume XXXIII.* St. Louis, MO, CV Mosby, 1984, pp 229-241.
32. Reeves RB, Ballard RI, Hughes JL: Internal fixation versus traction and casting of adolescent femoral shaft fractures. *J Pediatr Orthop* 1990;10:592-595.
33. Alonso J, Geissler W, Hughes JL: External fixation of femoral fractures: Indications and limitations. *Clin Orthop* 1989;241:83-88.
34. Aronson J, Tursky EA: External fixation of femur fractures in children. *J Pediat Orthop* 1992;12:157-163.
35. Evanoff M, Strong ML, MacIntosh R: External fixation maintained until fracture consolidation in the skeletally immature. *J Pediatr Orthop* 1993;13:98-101.
36. Gregory RJ, Cubison TC, Pinder IM, et al: External fixation of lower limb fractures in children. *J Trauma* 1992;33:691-693.
37. Tolo VT: External skeletal fixation in children's fractures. *J Pediatr Orthop* 1983;3:435-442.
38. Probe R, Lindsey RW, Hadley NA, et al: Refracture of adolescent femoral shaft fractures: A complication of external fixation. A report of two cases. *J Pediatr Orthop* 1993;13:102-105.
39. Viljanto J, Linna MI, Kiviluoto H, et al: Indications and results of surgical treatment of femoral shaft fractures in children. *Acta Chir Scand* 1975;141:366-369.
40. Kregor PJ, Song KM, Routt MLC Jr, et al: Plate fixation of femoral shaft fractures in multiply injured children. *J Bone Joint Surg* 1993;75A:1774-1780.
41. Ward WT, Levy J, Kaye A: Compression plating for child and adolescent femur fractures. *J Pediatr Orthop* 1992;12: 626-632.
42. Ziv I, Rang M: Treatment of femoral fracture in the child with head injury. *J Bone Joint Surg* 1983;65B:276-278.
43. Heinrich SD, Drvaric D, Darr K, et al: Stabilization of pediatric diaphyseal femur fractures with flexible intramedullary nails (a technique paper). *J Orthop Trauma* 1992;6:452-459.
44. Fein LH, Pankovich AM, Spero CM, et al: Closed flexible intramedullary nailing of adolescent femoral shaft fractures. *J Orthop Trauma* 1989;3:133-141.
45. Kissel EU, Miller ME: Closed Ender nailing of femur fractures in older children. *J Trauma* 1989;29:1585-1588.
46. Mann DC, Weddington J, Davenport K: Closed Ender nailing of femoral shaft fractures in adolescents. *J Pediatr Orthop* 1986;6:651-655.
47. Ligier JN, Metaizeau JP, Prévot J, et al: Elastic stable intramedullary nailing of femoral shaft fractures in children. *J Bone Joint Surg* 1988;70B:74-77.
48. Hennrikus WL, Kasser JR, Rand F, et al: The function of the quadriceps muscle after a fracture of the femur in patients who are less than seventeen years old. *J Bone Joint Surg* 1993;75A:508-513.
49. Beaty JH, Austin SM, Warner WC, et al: Interlocking intramedullary nailing of femoral-shaft fractures in adolescents: Preliminary results and complications. *J Pediatr Orthop* 1994;14:178-183.
50. Herndon WA, Mahnken RF, Yngve DA, et al: Management of femoral shaft fractures in the adolescent. *J Pediatr Orthop* 1989; 9:29-32.
51. Raney EM, Ogden JA, Grogan DP: Premature greater trochanteric epiphysiodesis secondary to intramedullary femoral rodding. *J Pediatr Orthop* 1993;13:516-520.
52. Ziv I, Blackburn N, Rang, M: Femoral intramedullary nailing in the growing child. *J Trauma* 1984;24:432-434.
53. Chung SM: The arterial supply of the developing proximal end of the human femur. *J Bone Joint Surg* 1976;58A:961-970.
54. Lombardo SJ, Harvey JP Jr: Fractures of the distal femoral epiphyses: Factors influencing prognosis. A review of thirty-four cases. *J Bone Joint Surg* 1977;59A:742-751.
55. Riseborough EJ, Barrett IR, Shapiro F: Growth disturbances following distal femoral physeal fracture-separations. *J Bone Joint Surg* 1983;65A:885-893.
56. Bohn WW, Durbin RA: Ipsilateral fractures of the femur and tibia in children and adolescents. *J Bone Joint Surg* 1991;73A:429-439.
57. Bertin KC, Goble EM: Ligament injuries associated with physeal fractures about the knee. *Clin Orthop* 1983;177:188-195.
58. Roberts JM: Fractures and separations of the knee, in Rockwood CA Jr, Wilkins EK, King RE (eds): *Fractures in Children,* ed 3. Philadelphia, PA, JB Lippincott, 1991, vol 3, pp 1165-1233.

Primary Arthroplasty of the Hip in Patients Younger Than 21 Years of Age

John H. Wedge, MD, FRCS(C),
Daniel J. Cummiskey, MD

Thirty years of successful experience with the use of replacement arthroplasty for the treatment of osteoarthrosis of the hip in the elderly has led to an expansion of its indications to younger patients. This broadening of the indications for total hip arthroplasty has permitted us to improve dramatically the quality of life for that small subset of young patients who are unresponsive to other forms of management and who otherwise would be relegated to a life of pain and immobility.

With this increasing application of total hip arthroplasty has come the recognition of its limitations. The literature outlining the results of primary hip arthroplasty in young adults was recently reviewed by Callaghan.[1] This chapter addresses the use of primary hip arthroplasty for a group of younger patients, arbitrarily defined as being younger than 21 years of age. We have separated this population from that of young adults because of the differences between the two groups in terms of the indications for and the biologic responses to arthroplasty.

First, bone maturation does not cease with physeal closure; it continues past the age of 20 years. Peak bone mass is not reached until the third decade of life.[2] Diaphyseal diameter increases throughout life because of continued appositional growth and endosteal resorption. Second, the rate of bone turnover is more rapid in younger patients, which greatly enhances the potential for remodeling, especially in the femur. Third, compliance with instructions to restrict activity is poor in this age group. After a period of severe disability, the newfound functional ability and relief of pain are too much to resist, even for the most compliant of patients. Finally, these younger patients who are candidates for arthroplasty often have poor bone stock as a result of disease, such as juvenile rheumatoid arthritis, or of drug therapy for a malignant lesion.

There are no indications for total hip arthroplasty in young patients who have unilateral disease unless another joint is involved or life expectancy is limited. Arthrodesis is still the procedure of choice for the management of young individuals of both sexes who have unilateral end-stage hip disease when there are no other limitations to activity and when the spine and ipsilateral knee are normal.

Of the various options for the treatment of hip disease in this age group, replacement arthroplasty may be the most shortsighted. The choice of arthroplasty should be based on the expectation that there will be relief of symptoms for approximately one decade and an almost certain return to disability thereafter. The undoubted early success of arthroplasty should not diminish caution.

Alternatives to Arthroplasty

There is little doubt that the initial investment of time and the morbidity encountered usually are greater for osteotomy, arthrodesis, and vascularized grafting of the femoral head than for arthroplasty. In discussions with the patient, the physician should avoid the tendency to explain therapeutic outcomes in terms of the immediate results only, when, in fact, alternative procedures may provide adequate relief and "buy time" whereas total hip replacement may create the need for early revision.

Soft-tissue release of the hip in patients who have juvenile rheumatoid arthritis often has been successful for the relief of pain and the correction of deformity, even in the presence of moderately advanced damage to the joint surface.[3] The use of vascularized grafts for the treatment of early osteonecrosis may prevent femoral head collapse.[4] An osteotomy for the treatment of congenital dysplasia may prevent or delay the onset of disabling secondary arthritis. All of these procedures provide prolonged excellent function and do not necessarily compromise the result of a later arthroplasty.[5] Hip arthrodesis often is the best choice for the treatment of unilateral post-traumatic osteonecrosis.

Indications for Arthroplasty

The long-term results of total hip arthroplasty are not as favorable for young patients as they are for patients who are more than 60 years old.[6-14] Success with arthroplasty in the patient who is younger than 21 is more likely to be achieved by close adherence to restricted indications.

Patients who have advanced hip disease associated with systemic or polyarticular juvenile rheumatoid arthritis can be benefited by arthroplasty when there are other severe limitations of the level of activity (Fig. 1).[13,15-17] Even in patients who are to be managed with bilateral hip and knee arthroplasty, the extra-articular disease and the involvement of the foot and ankle prevent a level of activity great enough to cause excessive prosthetic wear.

Often advanced steroid-induced bilateral osteonecrosis seen with hemopoietic malignant disease (Fig. 2) and after organ transplantation (Figs. 3 and 4) is an appropriate indication for arthroplasty. The sustained requirement for high-dose steroids by these patients

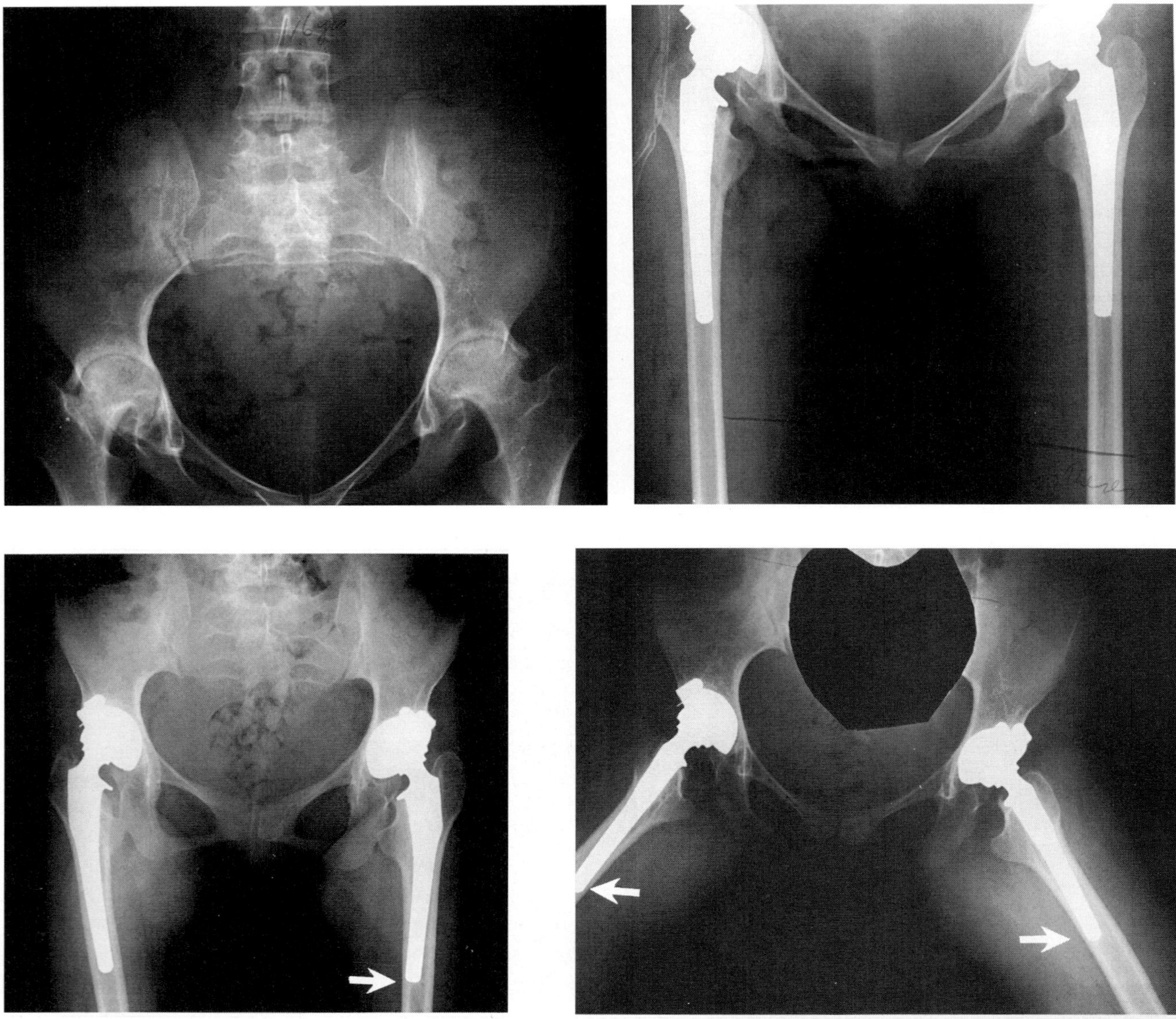

Fig. 1 Radiographs of a 16-year-old girl who had juvenile rheumatoid arthritis. **Top left,** Preoperative anteroposterior radiograph. **Top right,** Early postoperative radiograph. Note the positions of the stems with respect to the femoral cortices. **Bottom left,** Radiograph made 15 months postoperatively, showing medial migration of the tip of the left stem (arrow). **Bottom right,** Lateral radiograph showing bilateral posterior migration of the tip of the stem (arrows). There were no signs of loosening; this suggested that the position was related to remodeling of bone.

makes more biologic procedures, such as osteotomy and bone-grafting (vascularized or strut), less appealing even in the early stages of osteonecrosis. However, bilateral osteonecrosis occurring after the short-term use of steroid therapy for the treatment of an acute condition, such as asthma or an allergic reaction, is more appropriately treated with an osteotomy or grafting because the situation is self-limiting, life expectancy is normal, and there may be no involvement of other joints.

Patients who have a severe form of multiple epiphyseal dysplasia (Fig. 5),[18] spondyloepiphyseal dysplasia, or one of the storage diseases such as the mucopolysaccharidoses and mucolipidoses often are seen with advanced deformities. Osteotomy may fail to preserve joint function, even with seemingly adequate correction of the deformity, because of the involvement of articular cartilage in the disease process. Hip arthroplasty may be the only option to maintain the ability to walk in these individuals.

Less common indications for arthroplasty in carefully selected patients who are younger than 21 years of age include sickle-cell disease and hemophilia. It is important that the patient be assessed in light of the total clinical picture, including the home, school, and work environment.

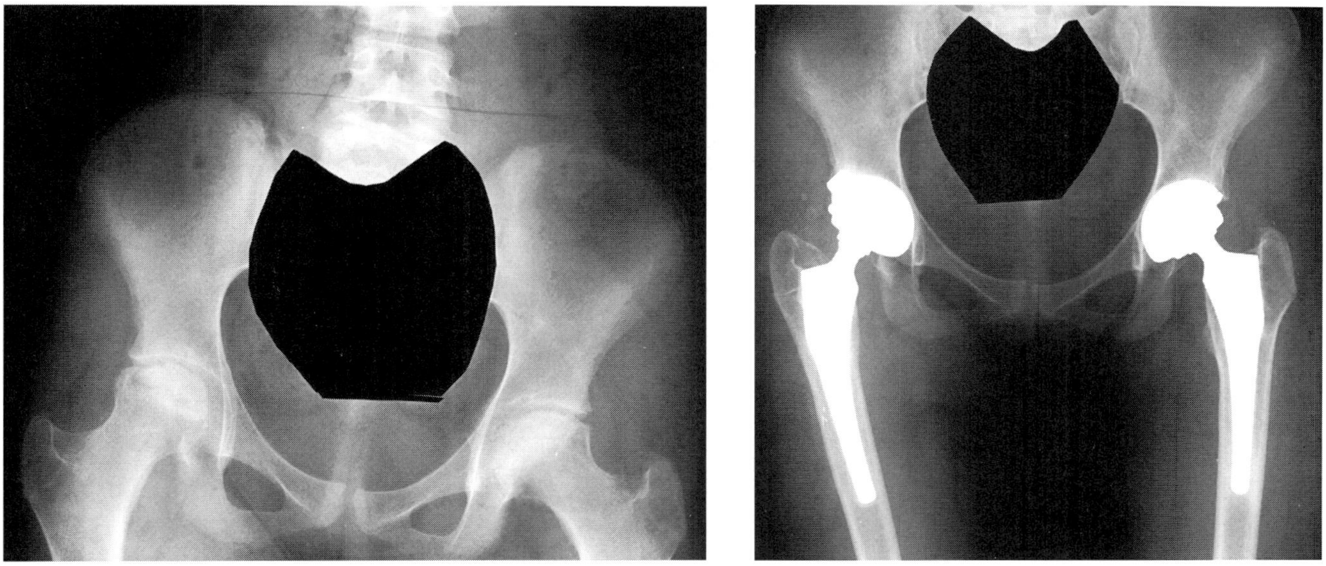

Fig. 2 Radiographs of a 13-year-old who had bilateral osteonecrosis secondary to steroid therapy for leukemia. She also had bilateral osteonecrosis of the lateral femoral condyle and talus. **Left,** Preoperative anteroposterior radiograph. **Right,** Anteroposterior radiograph made four years postoperatively.

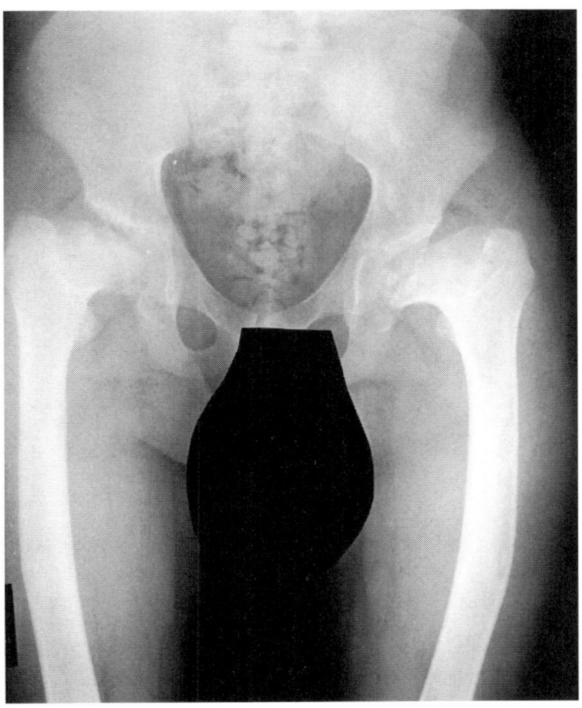

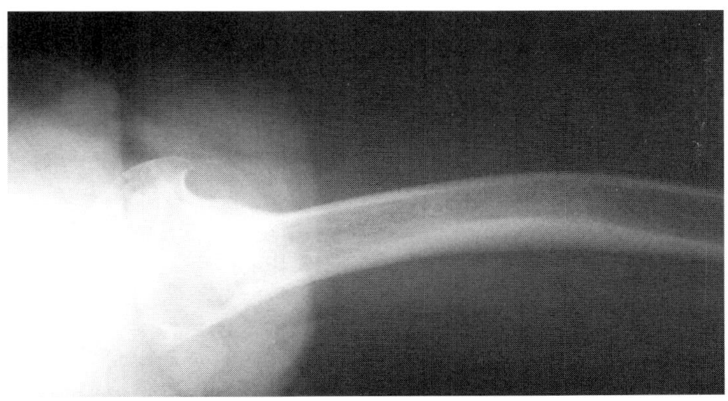

Fig. 3 Radiographs of a 15-year-old boy who had bilateral osteonecrois and metabolic bone disease secondary to renal osteodystrophy. **Left,** Preoperative anteroposterior radiograph. **Right,** Preoperative lateral radiograph demonstrating the extent of the deformity of the left femur.

Problems Specific to Hip Arthroplasty in the Patient Who Is Younger Than 21 Years of Age

The diseases for which hip replacement is indicated for a young patient are different from those that lead to the need for an arthroplasty in an adult. These conditions arise while the skeleton is still developing, and they result in unique anatomic and pathologic variations that must be recognized and planned for before the arthroplasty.

An absolute reduction in the size of the acetabulum and femoral head can markedly restrict the choice of

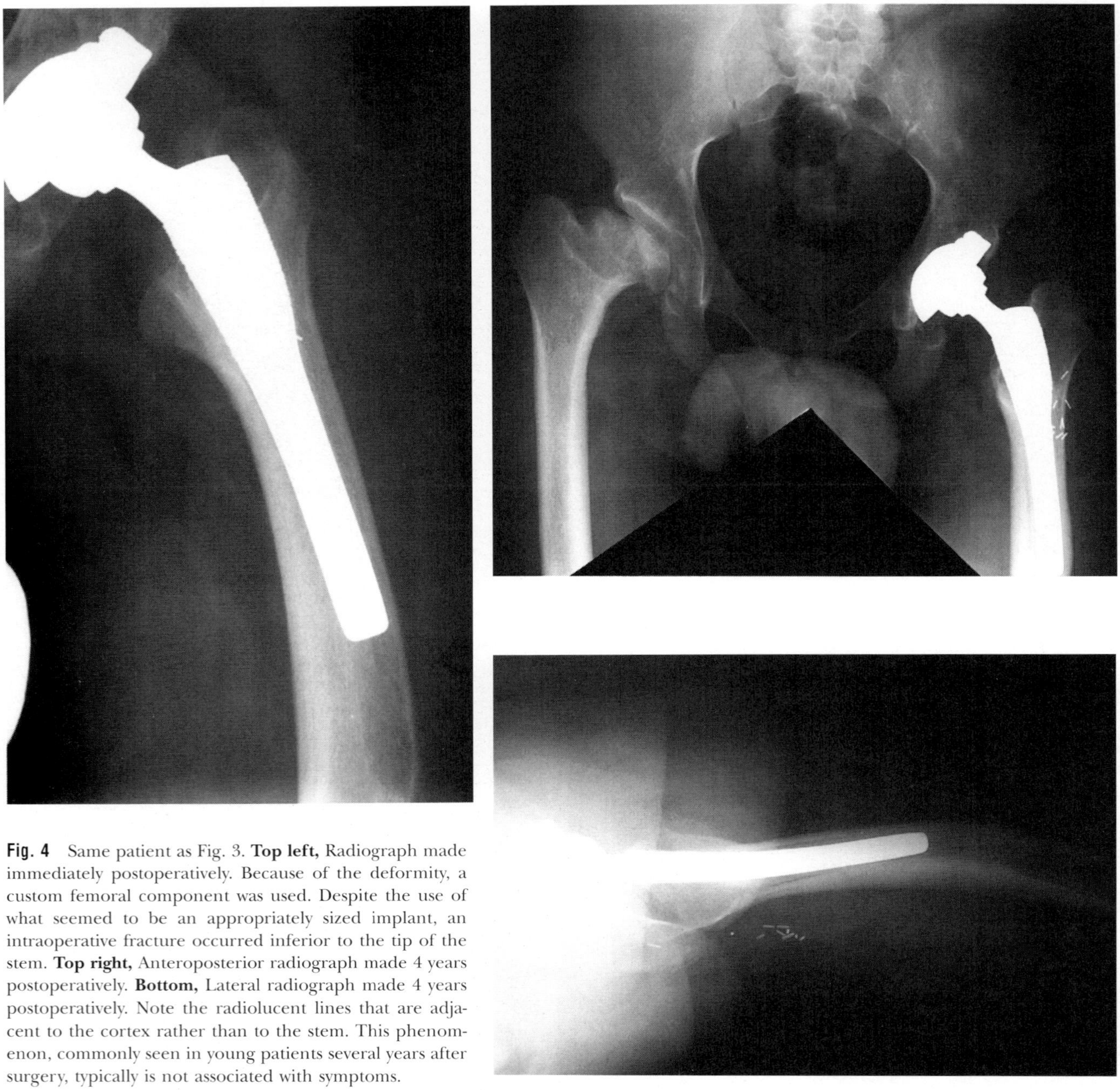

Fig. 4 Same patient as Fig. 3. **Top left,** Radiograph made immediately postoperatively. Because of the deformity, a custom femoral component was used. Despite the use of what seemed to be an appropriately sized implant, an intraoperative fracture occurred inferior to the tip of the stem. **Top right,** Anteroposterior radiograph made 4 years postoperatively. **Bottom,** Lateral radiograph made 4 years postoperatively. Note the radiolucent lines that are adjacent to the cortex rather than to the stem. This phenomenon, commonly seen in young patients several years after surgery, typically is not associated with symptoms.

acetabular and femoral head components. A small acetabulum may require a cemented all-polyethylene cup to provide sufficient thickness and to ensure durability. We use a femoral head that is 26 or 28 mm in diameter, although we are prepared to use one that is 22 mm in diameter if necessary to provide at least an 8-mm-thick polyethylene cup.

There may be a mismatch between the femoral metaphysis and diaphysis.[19] The femoral metaphysis frequently is relatively larger than the diaphysis in these young patients. Standard femoral components that fit the diaphysis may not fill the metaphysis adequately in the young patient. A modular system, custom components, or cement may be needed to obtain optimum fit and a stable implant (Figs. 3 and 4).

The anteroposterior diameter of the medullary canal of the femur may be greater than the mediolateral diameter.[15] This phenomenon must be recognized in order to avoid the use of a standard stem designed to be inserted without cement, which may not fill the anteroposterior dimension of the canal and therefore may result in instability of the prosthesis in the canal. The

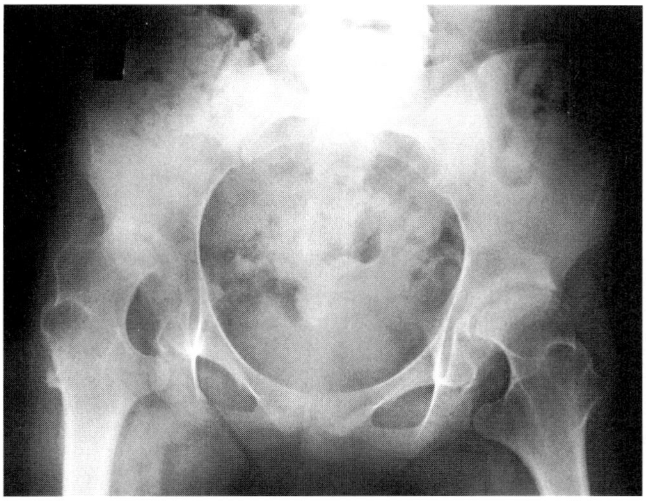

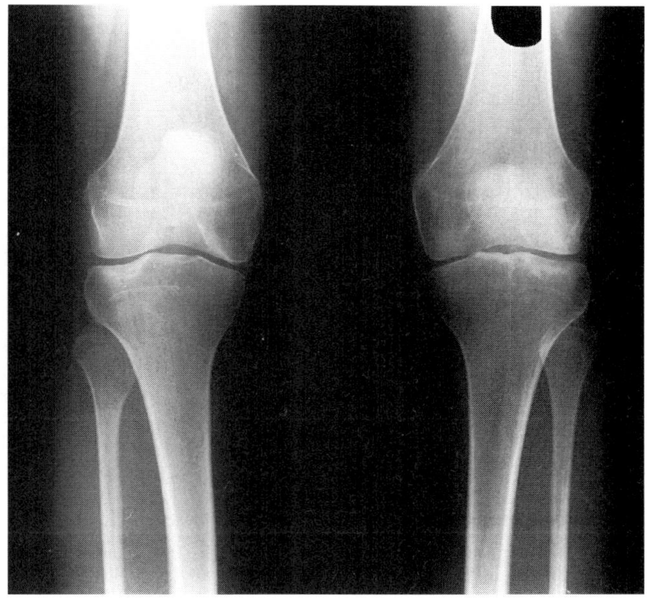

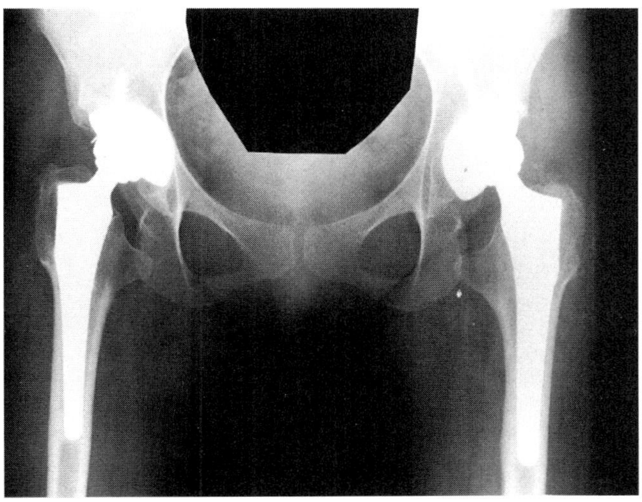

Fig. 5 Radiographs of a 13-year-old girl who had multiple epiphyseal dysplasia. **Top left,** Preoperative anteroposterior radiograph. **Top right,** Preoperative radiograph demonstrating severe deformity of the knee joints that limited activity after the hip arthroplasty. Arthroplasty in young patients should be restricted to those who have the severe form of this disease. **Bottom,** Anteroposterior radiograph made almost 1 year following surgery, demonstrating stable implants.

use of templates on conventional radiographs may be misleading, even when correction for magnification has been done. Computed tomography is helpful in the identification and treatment of this problem. We use porous-coated rather than hydroxyapatite-coated femoral components.

Marked anteversion of the femur may be encountered. The use of standard techniques in the presence of anteversion increases the risk of postoperative dislocation. Preoperative computed tomographic scans can be used to estimate the degree of anteversion and to determine the need for an osteotomy or the use of modular components.

When the disease process was present early in childhood, soft-tissue contractures may be more severe than those in an older patient. Adductor, external rotator, and iliopsoas tenotomies or recessions may be necessary at the time of the arthroplasty.

Young patients who need a hip replacement usually have severe osteoporosis as the result of inactivity and medication.[13] The cortices of the femoral neck and greater trochanter often are eggshell thin while the diaphyseal cortex is relatively thick. Insertion of an implant that provides adequate proximal fill may increase the risk of an intraoperative fracture (Figs. 3 and 4).

Depending on the underlying disease and on the amount of growth remaining, bone turnover may be high, and greater remodeling may occur than is seen in the adult. It is important that the stem be well centralized in order to minimize cortical erosion by the implant (Fig. 1).

We recently have followed the trend toward the use of porous-coated implants designed to be inserted without cement in the young adult, and since the mid-1980s we have not used cement in patients who are younger than 21. There have been situations in which, in retrospect, we probably should have cemented the femoral component in place, and we always are prepared to do so if necessary. It is important to have a wide range of implant sizes available and to recognize when a custom implant is needed.

Complications

The complications of total hip arthroplasty in young patients are similar to those in adults, but more rapid loosening, accelerated wear, and the inability to achieve adequate fixation are expected to occur more frequently. As there always is underlying systemic disease, careful medical management in the perioperative period is essential if respiratory, circulatory, renal, and gastrointestinal complications are to be prevented or recognized promptly when they occur.

Results

It is difficult, if not impossible, to quantify the results of hip arthroplasty in a heterogeneous patient population, a large proportion of which has a limited life expectancy. Moreover, the status of the underlying disease may be more critical to the overall well-being of these patients than the hip function. The results should be viewed in the context of the lack of other options for the maintenance of mobility and the relief of pain. Furthermore, a wide range of implants, both standard and custom, often are used in non-standard ways. Thus, the situation is quite different from that in studies involving a single design of implant designed to be inserted with or without cement for the treatment of a single disease such as osteoarthrosis in an adult population. For a detailed discussion of the results of total hip arthroplasty in young patients, the reader is referred to the article by Callaghan.[1]

The one absolute criterion for the measurement of results in the patient younger than 21 years of age should be that failure of the arthroplasty must leave the patient no worse off than if the operation had not been done. According to this stringent criterion, our own results have been almost universally satisfactory in terms of function and of pain relief. Major complications have been avoided by an awareness of the specific features, identified in this chapter, of the diseased hip in patients younger than 21.

In summary, the outcome of hip arthroplasty in the patient younger than 21 years of age is dependent largely on patient selection, recognition of the problems that may be encountered in this population, and close attention to specific technical considerations at the time of the operation. The best results are obtained for patients who are lighter, are less active because of other physical limitations, have a limited life expectancy, and are compliant with instructions to restrict activity.

References

1. Callaghan JJ: Results of primary total hip arthroplasty in young patients. *J Bone Joint Surg* 1993;75A:1728-1734.
2. Mazess RB: On aging bone loss. *Clin Orthop* 1982;165:239-252.
3. Moreno-Alvarez MJ, Espada G, Maldonado-Cocco JA, et al: Long-term follow-up of hip and knee soft tissue release in juvenile chronic arthritis. *J Rheumatol* 1992;19:1608-1610.
4. Yoo MC, Chung DW, Hahn CS: Free vascularized fibula grafting for the treatment of osteonecrosis of the femoral head. *Clin Orthop* 1992;277:128-138.
5. Kilgus DJ, Amstutz HC, Wolgin MA, et al: Joint replacement for ankylosed hips. *J Bone Joint Surg* 1990;72A:45-54.
6. Chandler HP, Reineck FT, Wixson RL, et al: Total hip replacement in patients younger than thirty years old: A five-year follow-up study. *J Bone Joint Surg* 1981;63A:1426-1434.
7. Collis DK: Cemented total hip replacement in patients who are less than fifty years old. *J Bone Joint Surg* 1984;66A:353-359.
8. Collis DK: Long-term (twelve to eighteen-year) follow-up of cemented total hip replacements in patients who were less than fifty years old: A follow-up note. *J Bone Joint Surg* 1991;73A:593-597.
9. Cornell CN, Ranawat CS: Survivorship analysis of total hip replacements: Results in a series of active patients who were less than fifty-five years old. *J Bone Joint Surg* 1986;68A:1430-1434.
10. Dorr LD, Takei GK, Conaty JP: Total hip arthroplasties in patients less than forty-five years old. *J Bone Joint Surg* 1983;65A:474-479.
11. Gustilo RB, Burnham WH: Long-term results of total hip arthroplasty in young patients, in *The Hip: Proceedings of the Tenth Open Scientific Meeting of the Hip Society*. St. Louis, MO, CV Mosby, 1982, pp 27-33.
12. Harris WH, Penenberg BL: Further follow-up on socket fixation using a metal-backed acetabular component for total hip replacement: A minimum ten-year follow-up study. *J Bone Joint Surg* 1987;69A:1140-1143.
13. Learmonth ID, Heywood AW, Kaye J, et al: Radiological loosening after cemented hip replacement for juvenile chronic arthritis. *J Bone Joint Surg* 1989;71B:209-212.
14. Mattingly DA, Hopson CN, Kahn A III, et al: Aseptic loosening in metal-backed acetabular components for total hip replacement: A minimum five-year follow-up. *J Bone Joint Surg* 1985;67A:387-391.
15. Cage DJN, Granberry WM, Tullos HS: Long-term results of total arthroplasty in adolescents with debilitating polyarthropathy. *Clin Orthop* 1992;283:156-162.
16. Scott RD: Total hip and knee arthroplasty in juvenile rheumatoid arthritis. *Clin Orthop* 1990;259:83-91.
17. Witt JD, Swann M, Ansell BM: Total hip replacement for juvenile chronic arthritis. *J Bone Joint Surg* 1991;73B:770-773.
18. Treble NJ, Jensen FO, Bankier A, et al: Development of the hip in multiple epiphyseal dysplasia: Natural history and susceptibility to premature osteoarthritis. *J Bone Joint Surg* 1990;72B:1061-1064.
19. Forwood MR, Burr DB: Physical activity and bone mass: Exercise in futility? *Bone Miner* 1993;21:89-112.

CHAPTER 23

Complex Primary Total Hip Arthroplasty: The Difficult Femur

Robert Poss, MD

General Considerations

When preparing to perform total hip replacement in an abnormal proximal femur, the surgeon must give careful consideration in the preoperative planning to the exposure, the equipment needed, and the type of prosthesis that must be available.[1] Exposure of the proximal femur by either vastus lateralis retraction and/or trochanteric osteotomy greatly facilitates the orientation of the proximal femoral canal. The availability of a C-arm to confirm the (presumably) intramedullary position of reamers and broaches is also helpful. Where there has been previous hardware or intramedullary fixation, power burrs are necessary to broach the sclerotic intertrochanteric cancellous bone. Power burrs are also useful in actually shaping a sclerotic intertrochanteric bed to receive the proximal part of the femoral prosthesis. The broaches usually used to prepare the proximal femur in primary total hip arthroplasty (THA) may fracture the femur if they are hand driven through the sclerotic track. When metallic plates or screws traverse the canal, appropriate power equipment that is capable of cutting metal is required.

Custom or long-stem prostheses may be necessary either to fit abnormal proximal shapes or to bypass by three diameters the stress risers created by the hardware removal.

Removing Old Hardware

I routinely remove proximal femoral blade plates following osteotomy at approximately 2 years following surgery. I find that the proximal femur subsequently remodels extensively, and that both the osteopenic lateral femoral cortex that was under the plate and the intertrochanteric dimensions are restored to a great degree. Additionally, patients are often relieved of greater trochanteric discomfort caused by the prominent plate and experience some improvement in abductor function, possibly from the now unobstructed function of the iliotibial band.

When performing total hip arthroplasty in a proximal femur with retained hardware, the question arises whether hardware removal should be accomplished at the time of conversion of total hip replacement or in two stages. Obviously, one-stage removal is more efficient, but, in certain instances, two-stage removal should be considered. A very difficult hardware removal requires extensive exposure and prolonged operating time. Also, it can be difficult to control the flow of cement through screw holes or plate tracks, and, in certain instances, intraoperative fracture may occur through osteopenic bone when manipulating a femur during total hip replacement.

When infection is suspected despite a negative preoperative workup (eg, aspiration, nuclear scans), a two-stage conversion, in which the first stage is removal of hardware, will allow multiple tissue biopsies for cultures[2] and will also allow healing of screw holes or plate tracks. With the exception of these special instances, one-stage removal and conversion to total hip replacement is usually satisfactory (Figs. 1 and 2).

Old Intertrochanteric Osteotomy

If hardware has been remotely removed, sufficient remodeling will have occurred in previous varus or valgus osteotomy to allow insertion of a standard prosthesis. The problem with old varus osteotomy may be that the greater trochanter obscures easy access to the intramedullary canal (Fig. 3). In such instances a greater trochanteric osteotomy may be required. Old valgus osteotomy usually does not present any serious problems in broaching the true canal and placing a prosthesis (Fig. 4). The combination of varus or valgus with flexion or extension may present formidable problems in placing a standard prosthesis because of abnormal angulation in the sagittal plane. Even in these instances, a standard prosthesis usually can be inserted, but it is essential in preoperative planning to determine whether one can successfully bypass the abnormally angulated intertrochanteric region. With extreme angulation, it may be necessary to reosteotomize the femur or consider the use of a custom implant.

Old Subtrochanteric Osteotomy

Because of the relatively distal location of this osteotomy, reosteotomy is almost always required to allow prosthetic insertion (Fig. 5). Once the femur has been reosteotomized, a somewhat longer femoral stem will provide stable intramedullary fixation.[3] Rotational stability can be enhanced by the use of a three-holed or four-holed unicortical plate. One should be very careful in assessing the final anteversion of the femoral component, because many of the landmarks of rotational control are obscured by the previous or the present procedure.

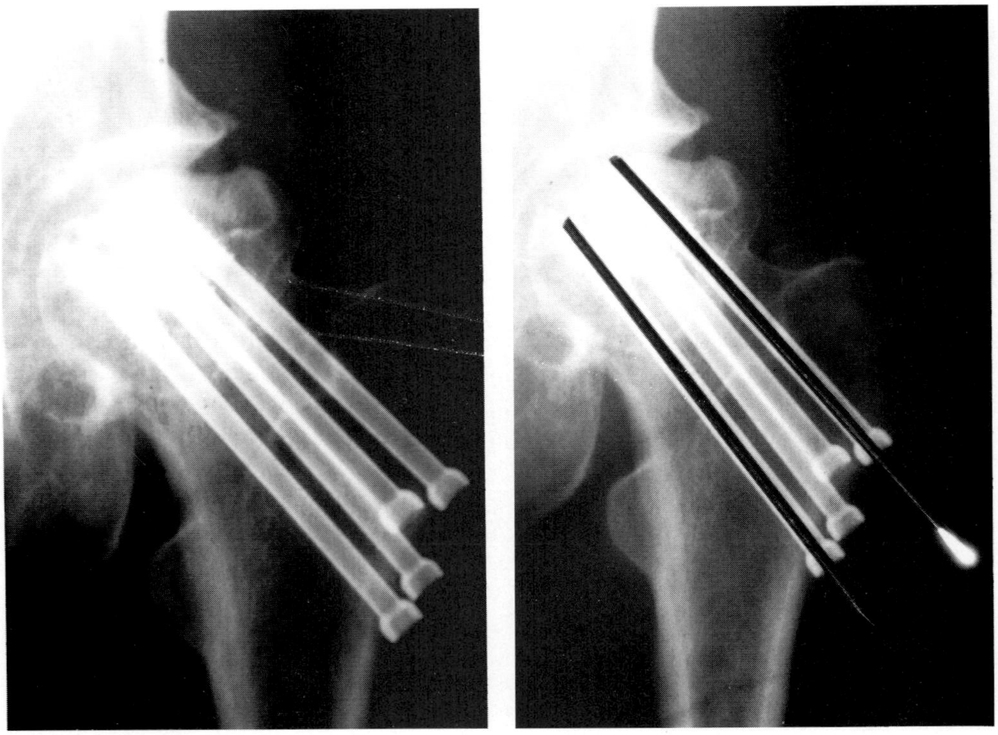

Fig. 1 This patient had undergone previous internal fixation for femoral neck fracture with cannulated screws. The four screw heads were not easily identified during initial exploration, and so the procedure was facilitated by proceeding with hip dislocation and finding the screw heads by retrograde insertion of Steinmann pins through the cannulated screws. This not only saved operating time, but also minimized bone removal from the lateral femoral cortex. This technique is also useful when there are fixed solid screws or threaded Steinmann pins that have been previously inserted into the neck and head. After hip dislocation, the head and neck can be osteotomized and removed, thus exposing the pins for either retrograde or direct removal.

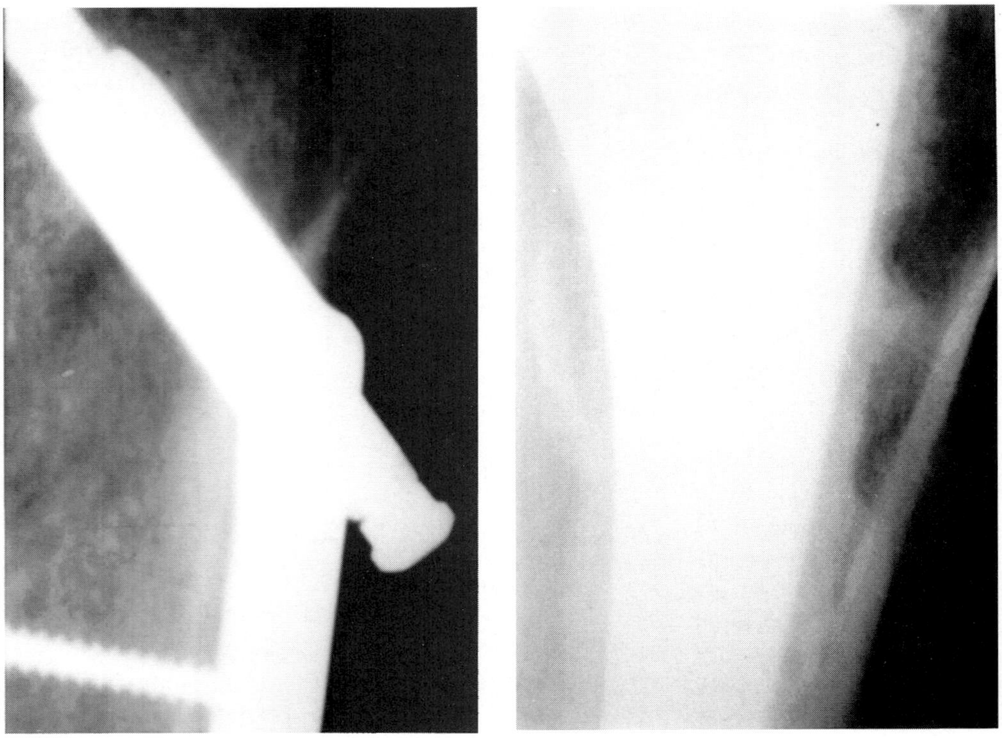

Fig. 2 When large fixation devices are removed from the lateral cortex, a bone plug should be inserted into the defect to enhance cement pressurization and prevent extravasation.

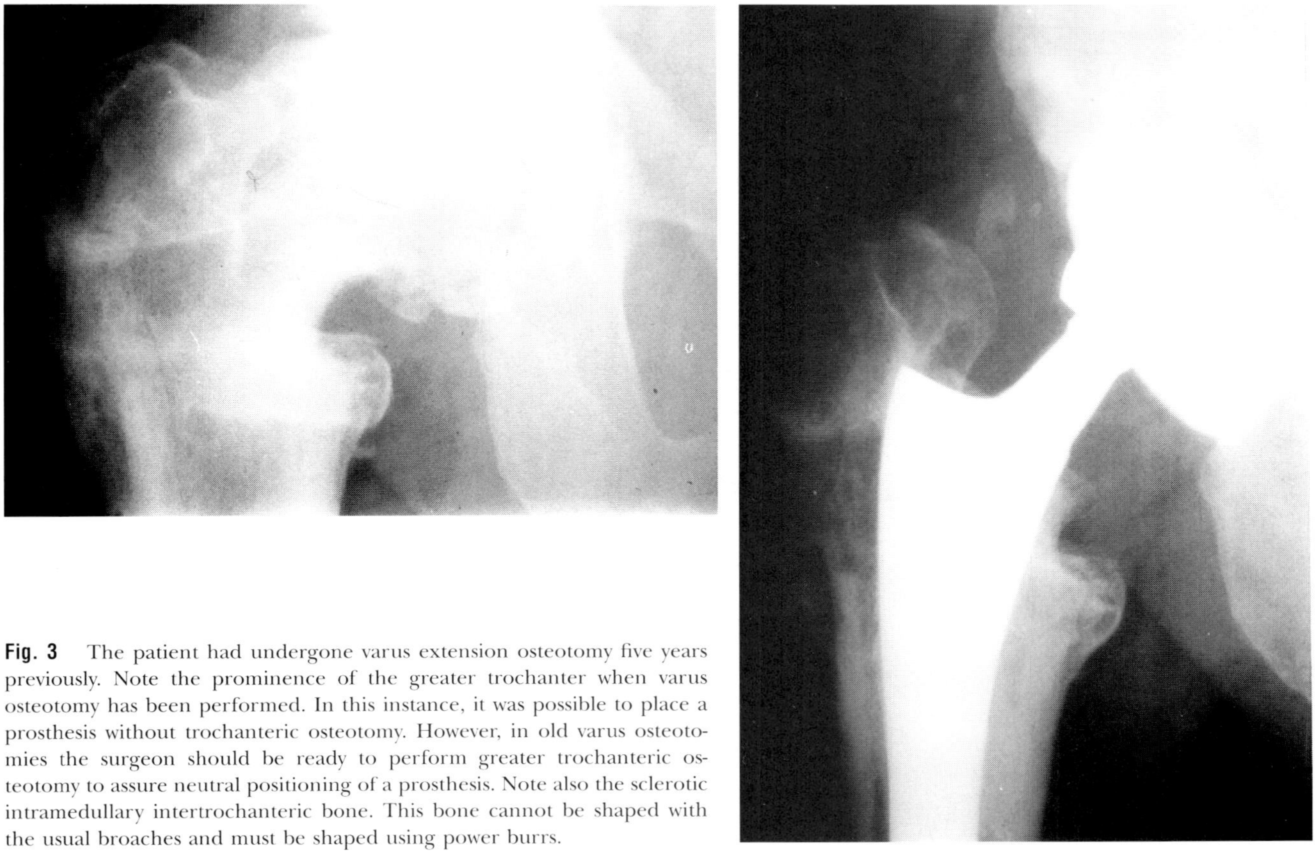

Fig. 3 The patient had undergone varus extension osteotomy five years previously. Note the prominence of the greater trochanter when varus osteotomy has been performed. In this instance, it was possible to place a prosthesis without trochanteric osteotomy. However, in old varus osteotomies the surgeon should be ready to perform greater trochanteric osteotomy to assure neutral positioning of a prosthesis. Note also the sclerotic intramedullary intertrochanteric bone. This bone cannot be shaped with the usual broaches and must be shaped using power burrs.

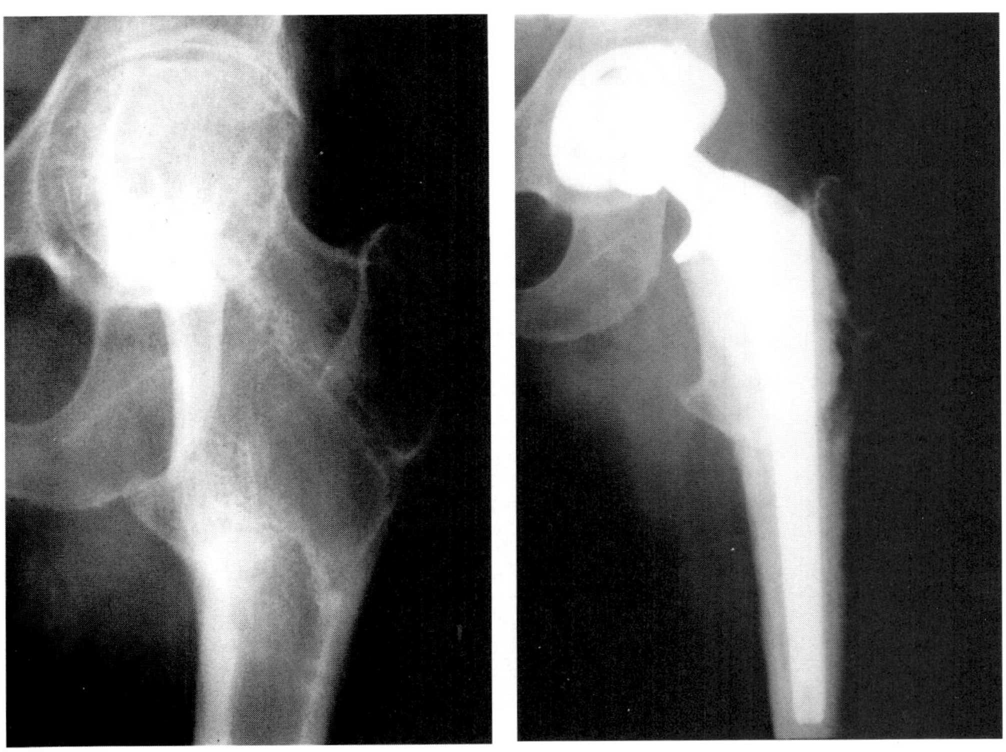

Fig. 4 In patients with old valgus osteotomies, the greater trochanter is usually well lateralized and does not compromise access to the femoral canal.

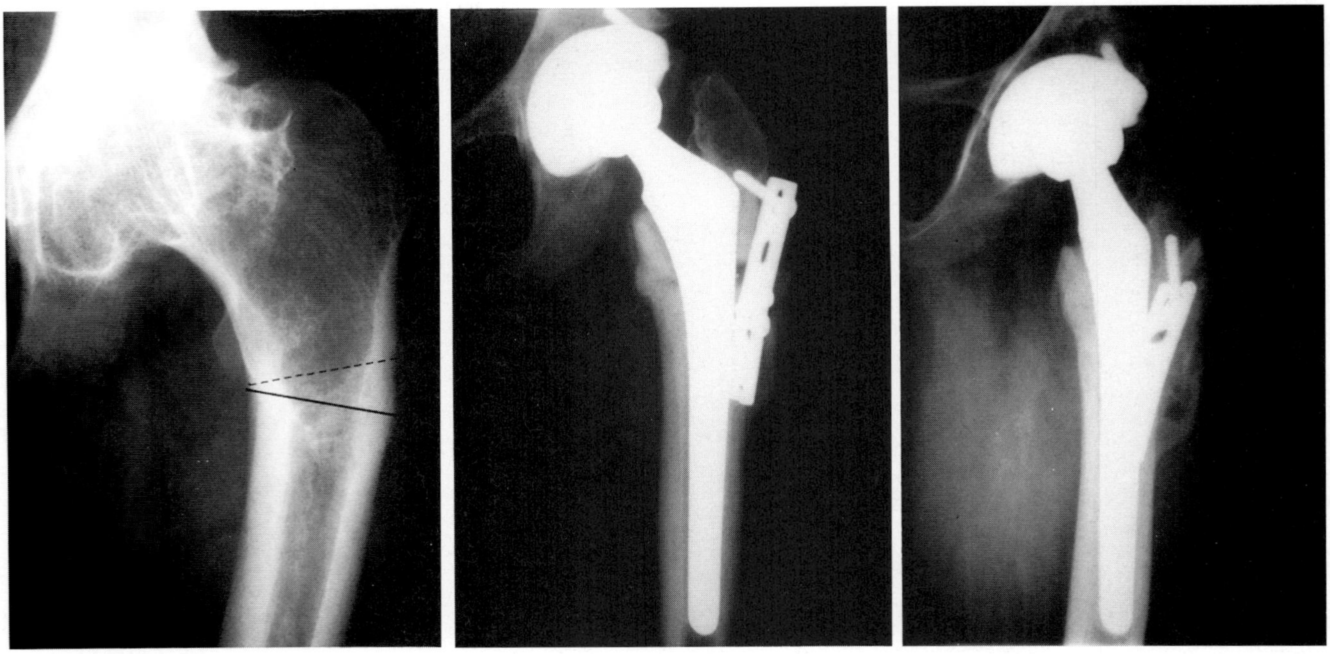

Fig. 5 In previous subtrochanteric osteotomies, the angulation is sufficiently distal so as to preclude the use of a standard prosthesis in most instances. Possible solutions are a custom prosthesis or reosteotomy at the subtrochanteric level and use of a prosthesis sufficiently long and with sufficient rotational stability distally to achieve secure fixation. Rotational stability can be enhanced by the use of a unicortical plate that bridges the osteotomy site.

The Problem of Offset

One of the most frequent problems we face in the planning of primary THA is not in femurs with abnormal femoral anatomy, but in femurs that vary within the limits of normal. We are confronted by the dilemma of trying to achieve conflicting goals: the need to restore optimal abductor mechanics, equal leg lengths, and sufficient soft-tissue stability to render the prosthesis stable. Because the normal proximal femur varies greatly in neck-shaft angle (from approximately 125° to 145°), a standard prosthesis with a fixed neck-shaft angle (usually about 135°) will not satisfy all of these needs in many patients.

In a standard prosthesis with a 135° neck-shaft angle, use of longer modular head/neck combinations will cause a gain of 1 mm in length for every millimeter in offset (Fig. 6). Therefore, if this "standard" 135° prosthesis is used in a femur that has more natural offset (approximately 130°), the distance from the greater trochanter to the center of rotation is decreased (thus increasing the joint-reaction force), which requires the use of longer neck lengths to maintain sufficient tissue tension. This "trade-off" increases the likelihood of lengthening the extremity. In a more valgus hip, this treatment may increase the offset more than the patient's natural offset, producing asymmetry of the two sides.

One solution to this dilemma is to use a standard prosthesis of 135° and reproduce the anatomy of a more varus hip by performing a low neck osteotomy, or in a more valgus hip, by performing a high neck

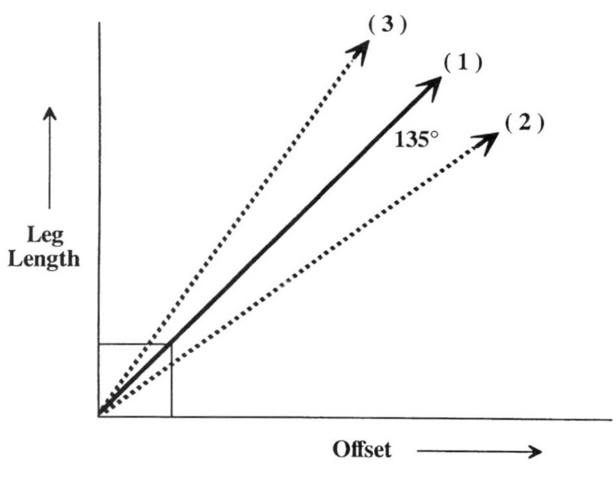

Fig. 6 A prosthesis that has a neck-shaft angle of 135° will produce 1 mm of increased leg length for every millimeter of increased offset. If this prosthesis is used in a hip with more natural varus, it is likely that, to achieve sufficient soft-tissue stability, increased leg length will be produced. A better solution is to use a prosthesis that has a more varus neck-shaft angle. In this instance, soft-tissue stability can be achieved without the concomitant equal increase in leg length.

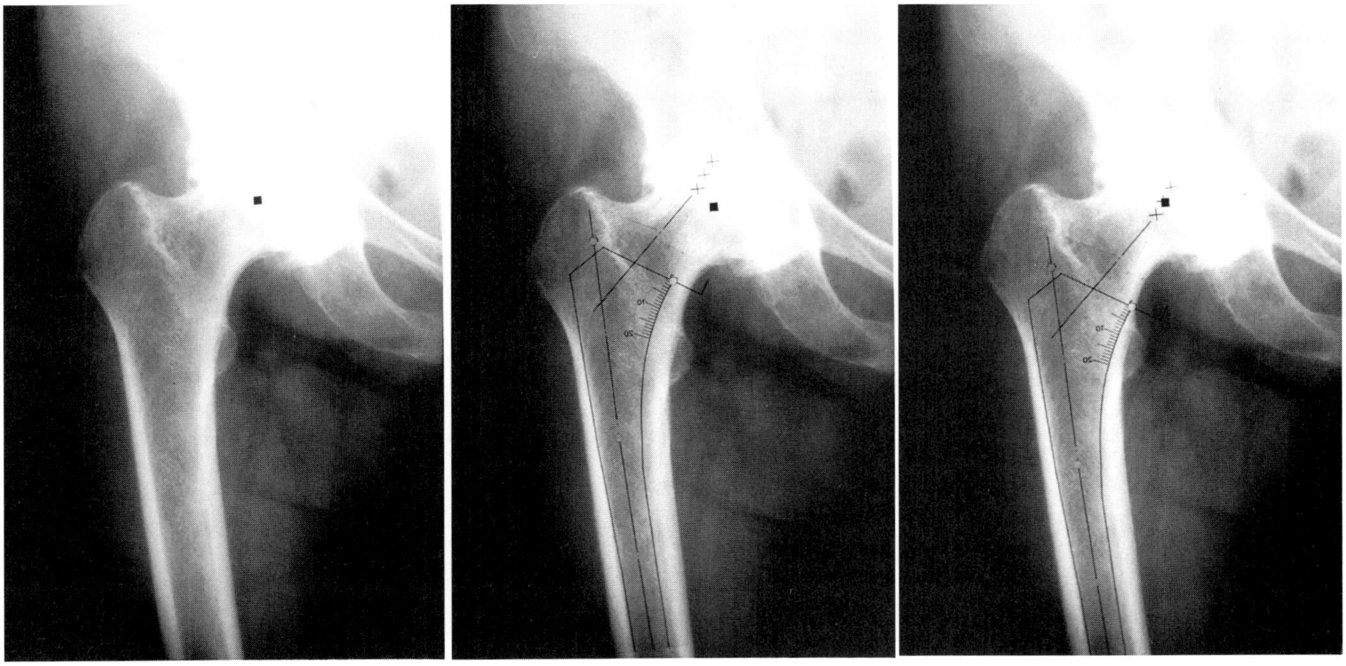

Fig. 7 In the preoperative planning for total hip replacement in this varus hip, a standard prosthesis with a neck-shaft angle of 135° can restore the patient's hip center of rotation by a very low neck osteotomy. Actually achieving this goal at surgery, however, may pose technical difficulties.

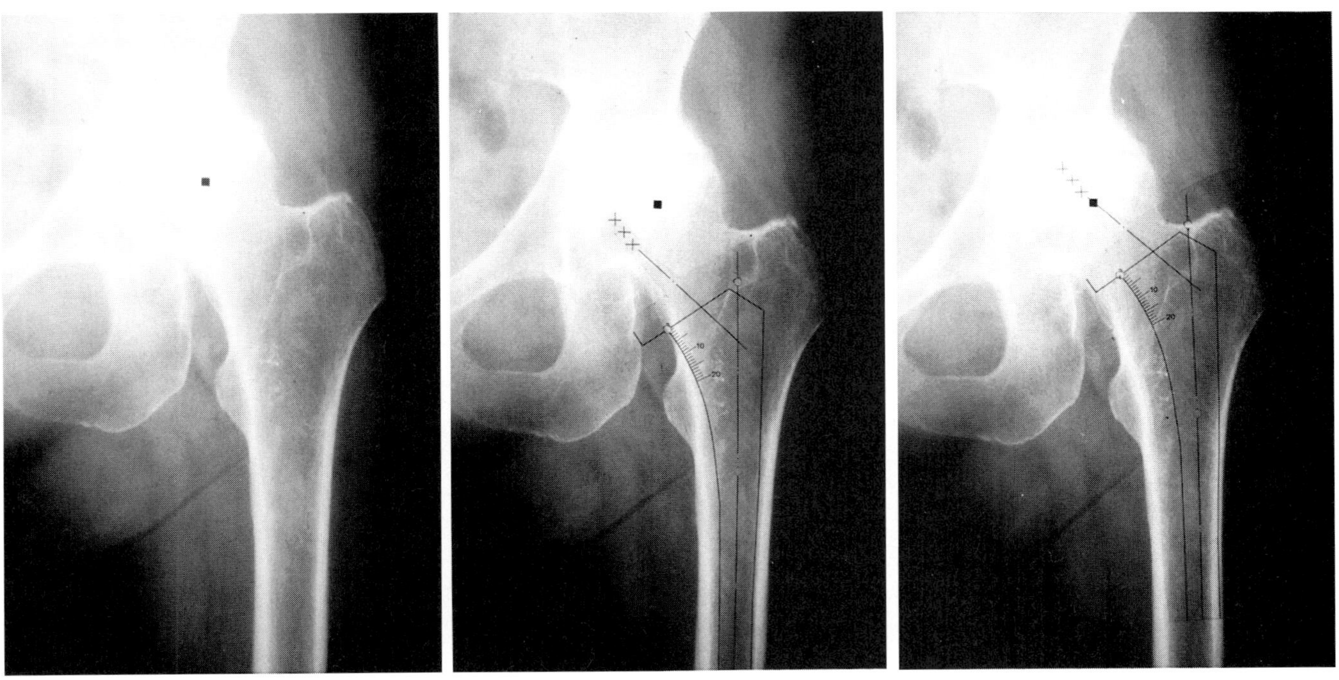

Fig. 8 In a patient with a valgus hip, a high neck osteotomy can achieve restoration of the hip center of rotation. However, a number of technical difficulties can be encountered in trying to achieve proper hip mechanics by these techniques.

osteotomy (Figs. 7 and 8). This approach will satisfy templating requirements in preoperative planning, but this attempted solution may be impossible to achieve in actual practice. Will a prosthesis that is templated to fit the canal also fit at the level of these high or low neck cuts? Will the shortest neck be too long with a high neck cut? Will the longest modular head still leave the soft tissues too lax in a low neck cut? One possible

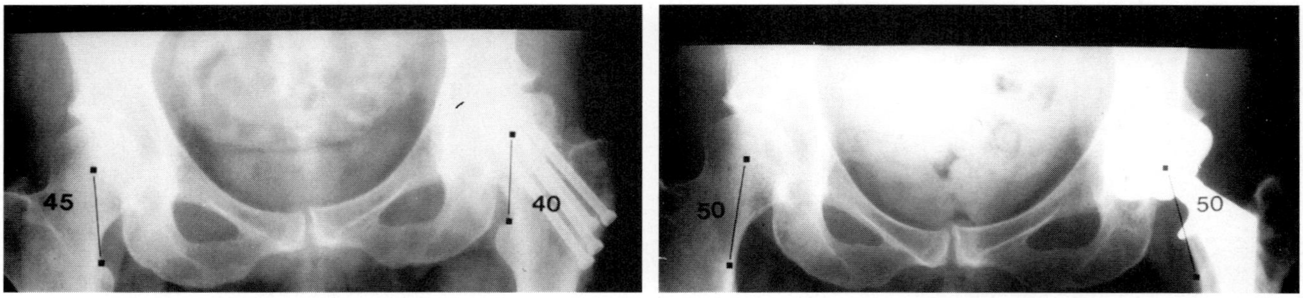

Fig. 9 One of the goals of preoperative planning is to restore equal leg lengths and the proper relationship between the tip of the greater trochanter and the center of rotation of the hip. **Left,** On the preoperative AP pelvis, a magnified ruler is used to measure the distance between the proximal border of the lesser trochanter and the center of rotation of the hip on both the normal and involved sides. In this instance, the patient is found to be 5 mm short on the operative side. **Right,** Intraoperatively, the proximal border of the lesser trochanter is an excellent landmark to confirm the preoperative measurement and is invariably found to reproduce the radiograph measurement preoperatively. The distance from the lesser trochanter to the neck osteotomy can be planned preoperatively. Selection of a prosthesis with appropriate offset will restore the patient's normal trochanter to center-of-rotation relationships.

solution to excessive soft-tissue laxity is to perform a trochanteric osteotomy and advancement.[4] An even better solution is to choose a prosthesis that approximates the patient's anatomic offset.

The best safeguard against these types of intraoperative problems is proper preoperative planning.[1] The apparent lengths should be determined on clinical examination. I prefer to determine this measurement by using blocks under the shorter extremity when the patient is standing. Discrepancies caused by abnormalities in areas other than the hip joint (eg, fixed pelvic obliquity, posttraumatic malalignment and/or shortening of the femur or tibia) can be assessed by this method.

On the preoperative radiographs of the pelvis, one can measure the length discrepancy attributable to the difference between the affected and the contralateral hip. These radiographic measurements can then be confirmed intraoperatively (Fig. 9). An excellent intraoperative and radiographic landmark is the superior border of the lesser trochanter. Its distance to the center of rotation of the femoral head can be measured using magnified templates or rulers on radiographs preoperatively, and it can be confirmed intraoperatively by direct measurement. By selecting a prosthesis that reproduces the patient's offset, one can preselect the length of modular head that will be used and measure the site of neck resection proximal to the lesser trochanter. We have found that intraoperatively, we can reproduce the same lesser-trochanter to center-of-rotation measurements predicted by preoperative planning, achieve satisfactory soft-tissue stabilization, and consistently restore equalization of leg length.

References

1. Müller ME: Lessons of 30 years of total hip arthroplasty. *Clin Orthop* 1992;274:12-21.
2. Barrack RL, Harris WH: The value of aspiration of the hip joint before revision total hip arthroplasty. *J Bone Joint Surg* 1993;75A:66-76.
3. Holtgrewe JL, Hungerford DS: Primary and revision total hip replacement without cement and with associated femoral osteotomy. *J Bone Joint Surg* 1989;71A:1487-1495.
4. Fackler CD, Poss R: Dislocation in total hip arthroplasties. *Clin Orthop* 1980;151:169-178.

Heterotopic Ossification Following Total Hip Arthroplasty

David G. Lewallen, MD

Heterotopic ossification, a commonly observed complication of total hip arthroplasty, occurs in anywhere from 20% to 90% of hip arthroplasties performed.[1-3] Fortunately, fewer than 10% of patients are observed to have a major amount of bone formation and only a small fraction of these are significantly symptomatic. Heterotopic ossification does have the potential to cause major disability and significant symptoms resulting in the need for reoperation in a small subgroup of patients in whom it occurs.

The risk of developing an amount of heterotopic ossification sufficient to produce symptoms varies considerably between groups of patients and appears to be related in part to identifiable risk factors. However, the exact etiology of the new bone formation is not well understood. In 1977, Jowsey, Coventry, and Robins[4] wrote that it is likely that "bone induction is caused by short range diffusion of inductive substances . . . from an epithelial cell . . . to adjacent mesenchymal cells." Since 1977 a great deal of work has been completed on the cellular events that lead to new bone formation, and it seems clear that the development of heterotopic ossification is the end result of a complex cascade of cellular events analogous to those that occur during fracture healing. A variety of growth factors have been implicated in the initiation of new bone formation, and it is reasonable to assume that these same substances play a role in the development of heterotopic ossification. The details of the underlying cellular events, however, are still not completely understood.

Radiographically, the new bone formed within the soft tissues as a result of heterotopic ossification becomes visible by 3 to 6 weeks following surgery. It may be difficult to determine the extent of involvement before 3 months, and, frequently, ongoing radiographic maturation continues for as long as a year (Fig. 1). Bone scan activity in the area of the newly formed bone indicates the amount of continuing activity occurring biologically in the area of heterotopic ossification. This area may continue to show localized increased uptake for many months following surgery, occasionally still showing increased uptake indicative of elevated blood flow to bone and increased new bone formation at the 1-year mark.

Risk Factors for Heterotopic Ossification

A number of significant risk factors have been identified for the development of heterotopic ossification following total hip arthroplasty (THA). Previous heterotopic ossification in the same hip or the opposite hip following arthroplasty definitely increases the risk of heterotopic bone formation following any proposed additional hip surgery and should be an indication for prophylaxis. Patients who have formed heterotopic bone following a prior total hip arthroplasty have a 60% to 100% incidence of heterotopic bone formation when total hip arthroplasty is carried out on the contralateral hip.[5,6] The severity of heterotopic ossification formation tends to be similar in amount or grade to that observed following the first hip replacement.[7] In osteoarthritic patients, hypertrophic changes and osteophyte formation have been shown to be associated with an increased incidence of heterotopic bone formation compared to those with more atrophic changes.[8] Active ankylosing spondylitis has been cited as a risk factor. It has been believed that disease activity may be important in the relative risk of this problem contributing to heterotopic ossification following arthroplasty. However, Sundaram and Murphy[9] were unable to show a correlation between a high erythrocyte sedimentation rate and the incidence or extent of heterotopic bone formation in a group of ankylosing spondylitis patients undergoing arthroplasty. Up to 60% of patients with ankylosing spondylitis have been observed to form heterotopic bone following surgery, and 39% of those patients who did not receive prophylaxis demonstrated grade III to IV ossification.[10] But, in another series, clinically important heterotopic ossification was observed in 11% of ankylosing spondylitis patients undergoing THA. All patients in this series had a preoperative history of prior surgery, postoperative infection, or complete ankylosis.[11]

Both diffuse idiopathic skeletal hyperostosis (DISH syndrome) and spinal hyperostosis (Forstier's disease) have been cited as factors increasing the risk of heterotopic ossification following surgery. Fahrer and associates[12] showed a more than twofold increase in heterotopic ossification formation in patients with the DISH syndrome. However, other authors have been unable to substantiate an increased risk of heterotopic ossification in patients with DISH.[13] Blasingame and associates[14] documented an incidence of 38% to 50% grade III to IV heterotopic bone formation in patients with spinal hyperostosis where prophylaxis was not employed.

In men, the incidence of heterotopic ossification formation is twice that of women, and it has been postulated that this may be related to the increased bulk of the abductor musculature and perhaps to the increased soft tissue trauma required for surgical exposure in those individuals.

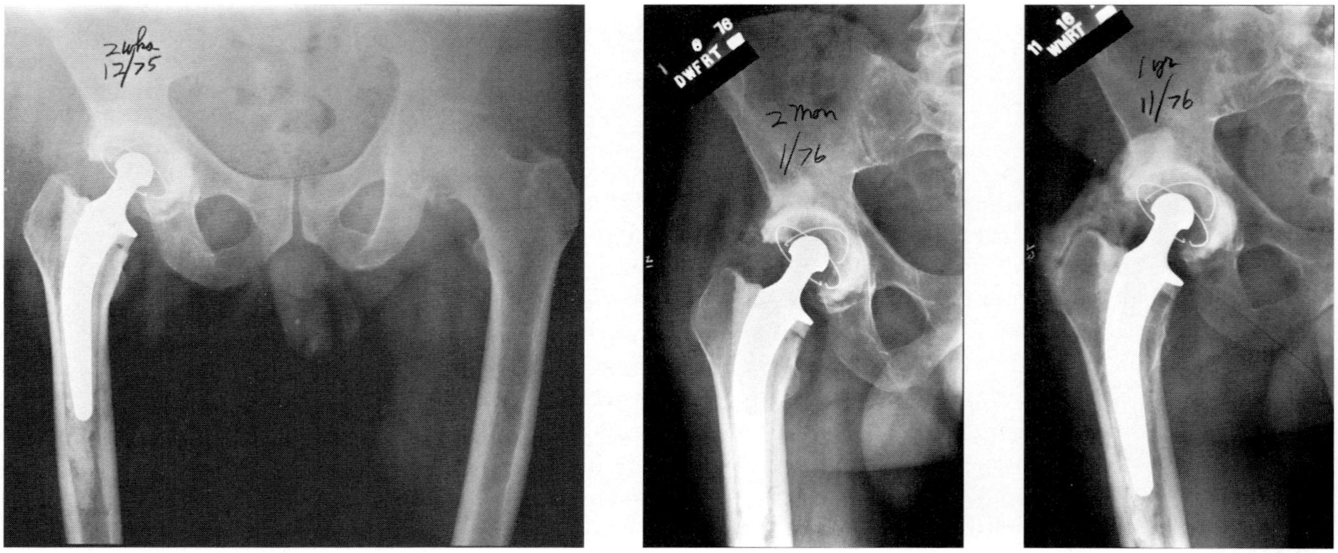

Fig. 1 **Left**, Radiograph 2 weeks following cemented total hip arthroplasty. **Center**, At 2 months following surgery there is radiographic evidence of heterotopic bone formation between the superior lateral margin of the acetabular component and the tip of the trochanter. **Right**, Mature heterotopic ossification is shown at 1 year after surgery, just before surgical excision to restore range of motion and relieve pain.

Some of the most dramatic instances of heterotopic ossification around the hip occur in patients with spine or head injuries. This represents one of the few clinical situations where heterotopic ossification may occur spontaneously about the hip in the absence of surgery or injury. While it is unusual for arthroplasty candidates to have an associated serious injury of the central nervous system, it is possible that this clinical situation might arise. An example might be the polytraumatized patient with head injury who sustained an associated severe femoral head fracture dislocation that requires arthroplasty for reconstruction. Given the high risk of heterotopic bone formation that would otherwise exist, this type of patient is definitely a candidate for prophylaxis.

The type of femoral component fixation used also appears to affect the incidence of heterotopic ossification. Maloney and associates[15] reported a significant increase in incidence and severity of heterotopic bone in a group of osteoarthritis patients who received uncemented stems, compared with a similar group who received a hybrid total hip arthroplasty, in which the stems were cemented.

Potential risk factors that have been less definitely established by the literature include early reoperation of an arthroplasty through the still organizing hematoma around the hip, limited hip motion prior to arthroplasty, trochanteric osteotomy,[16,17] and recent fracture, including intraoperative fractures. In addition, at the time of bone grafting in the area of the acetabulum or proximal femur it seems reasonable to avoid unnecessary spillage of graft into the surrounding soft tissues, because this, too, could conceivably trigger new bone formation in the surrounding muscle envelope.

Classification

The most widely used classification scheme for heterotopic ossification is the one reported by Brooker and associates,[18] which consists of four classes. Class I represents isolated islands of bone. Class II includes bone spurs, with a gap of 1 cm or more between the areas of bone formation. Class III represents near complete bridging with a gap less than 1 cm in size, and Class IV is apparent ankylosis.[18] An alternative system has been recommended by Morrey with grade I involvement measuring 5 mm or less, grade II being cases where ossification represents less than 50% of the area between the trochanter and the pelvis laterally, grade III greater than 50%, and grade IV apparent ankylosis.[17]

It would appear that grading of heterotopic bone formation would be similar in these two systems, except in those instances where patients were either extremely small or very large in terms of body size, in which case percent measurement may be more desirable. It is also possible that multifocal bone formation might be difficult to classify using the Brooker system.

Clinical Presentation

The vast majority of patients with heterotopic ossification detectable by radiography have only limited bone formation present, and these small amounts of heterotopic bone fail to produce any significant symptoms for them. Those with more extensive bone formation may have pain, restricted range of motion, or both.

In some instances, these complaints may be of sufficient severity to require excision of the heterotopic bone.

In addition, case examples exist of individuals whose problems with recurrent dislocation of the hip were felt to be related in part to impingement of heterotopic bone resulting in levering of the femoral component out of the acetabular cup. Impingement along the rim of the acetabulum can cause dislocation and can also cause direct polyethylene damage. Questions have also been raised about a relationship between component loosening and heterotopic bone formation, but the exact interrelationship has not been clearly defined.

Prevention of Heterotopic Bone Formation

There has been considerable interest in prophylaxis against heterotopic ossification, and a variety of potential treatments have been explored. These measures can be grouped into three main categories: surgical technique, low dose radiation, and medication.

Surgical Technique

Careful surgical technique and gentle handling of the soft tissues to avoid excessive muscle stripping and damage seems reasonable, because the degree of trauma to the surrounding musculature and extent of surgical exposure does seem to correlate with the propensity for new bone formation following hip surgery.[19-21] While trochanteric osteotomy has also been implicated as one factor potentially increasing the risk of heterotopic bone when compared with the posterior approach, this effect may not be as great as was previously believed.[16,17] Wound drainage to avoid localized hematoma formation within the area of the gluteus medius and hip joint would seem reasonable. Lavage of the wound using a water pik has been recommended by some as a means of clearing the soft tissues of bony debris from the reaming and bone preparation required for the surgery, but the benefit of this has not been clearly documented. Other measures occasionally employed include sealing the rim of bleeding bone around the acetabulum following excision of osteophytes using bone wax, but this practice, along with many of the above methods, is difficult to document objectively as clearly beneficial.

Low Dose Radiation

Coventry and Scanlon[22] first reported the benefits of low-dose radiation in reducing formation of heterotopic bone or its recurrence following excision. They initially recommended 2,000 rads in 10 fractions, and they were able to show that the treatment was ineffective if radiation was begun after heterotopic bone had become visible on radiograph. In their series of 48 hips so treated they were able to avoid massive bone formation of the grade III to IV variety in all patients who began treatment early (within days) of their arthroplasty.

Because application of 2,000 rads in ten fractions can be difficult to schedule in the postoperative period, numerous authors have investigated lower doses and increasingly fewer treatment fractions. Ayers and associates[23] documented the efficacy of 1,000 rads given in five fractions, as compared with 2,000 rads in ten fractions. Pellegrini and associates[24] were unable to demonstrate any difference in 800 centigray given as a single dose when compared with 1,000 centigray in five fractions, the latter being comparable to the 1,000 rads in five fractions referred to by Ayers (1 centigray = 1 rad). Healy and associates[25] showed that a 700 centigray treatment on postoperative day 1 prevents formation of grade III or IV heterotopic ossification, while Hedley and associates[26] examined the efficacy of 600 rads given as a single dose up to day 3. Recent information suggests that the threshold for effectiveness in radiation treatment is somewhere around 600 to 700 centigray.[26]

Pellegrini and associates[27] recently reported a prospective randomized study of 86 hips, which compared preoperative radiotherapy given 4 hours before the hip replacement with a single 800 centigray dose given 72 hours postoperatively. No difference was observed between the patients treated pre- and postoperatively, and there was no grade III or IV heterotopic ossification at all in the group preoperatively treated. This study not only documents the efficacy of preoperative treatment, but also has significant implications regarding the osteoprogenitor cells responsible for formation of heterotopic bone, suggesting that those cells are derived locally and do not come from circulating cell populations, which would be outside the port of treatment in a preoperative program. Low-dose radiation in the era of porous ingrowth implants has required construction of custom lead shielding to prevent irradiation of bone ingrowth areas, which might otherwise be adversely affected.[28,29]

Medications

Early efforts at suppression of heterotopic bone formation following hip arthroplasty centered on the use of diphosphonates. Diphosphonates, by inhibiting the growth of hydroxyapatite crystals, delay the appearance of new bone on radiograph. However, they do not prevent osteoid formation. It has been shown by Thomas and Amstutz[30] that the osteoid calcifies after the drug is stopped, which explains why this drug has been clinically ineffective in preventing symptomatic heterotopic ossification. Thus, the use of diphosphonates is no longer recommended for prophylaxis against heterotopic bone formation.

More promising has been work using nonsteroidal anti-inflammatory drugs (NSAIDs). Numerous authors have demonstrated the efficacy of Indomethacin in the prevention of heterotopic bone formation.[31-37] Indomethacin, the most extensively studied nonsteroidal medication in this clinical setting, has been documented to be effective in suppressing the formation of heterotopic bone in the period following arthroplasty. In a prospective, double-blind, randomized study by Schmidt and associates,[35] there were no cases of grade III or IV heterotopic bone in patients treated with this drug. Incidence in placebo patients was 18%. In this same study, 85% of patients treated with Indomethacin demonstrated no heterotopic ossification formation at all, while only 25% of the placebo group were free of heterotopic bone formation. Doses of Indomethacin shown to be effective range from 25 mg administered thrice daily for 6 weeks duration down to the same dosage continued for only 2 weeks. The fact that sequential authors have been able to demonstrate the continued efficacy of Indomethacin with shorter and shorter treatment courses is helpful, because a high incidence of gastrointestinal (GI) problems is associated with this medication. In one study, 37% of patients treated with Indomethacin for a 6-week course were unable to complete the recommended treatment program because of adverse GI side effects.[31] A number of other nonsteroidal anti-inflammatories, including aspirin, ibuprofen, naproxen, and diclofenac, have been investigated and found to be at least partially effective in the prevention of heterotopic bone formation.[32,34,36,38-40]

Radiation versus NSAIDs

Clinically, the decision whether to use radiation treatment or nonsteroidal anti- inflammatories for prophylaxis against heterotopic ossification can be difficult, although there are clinical situations that clearly seem to lend themselves to one form of treatment versus the other. Concern exists about using Indomethacin or other NSAIDs in individuals undergoing porous ingrowth arthroplasty because of the systemic effects of those medicines and the documented adverse effect that they have on bone formation during fracture healing.[41] Presumably, the biology at the interface between the porous or hydroxyapatite coated implant is similar to the response seen during fracture healing and thus the concern about their use in young patients undergoing implantation of the devices requiring biological fixation. McMahon and associates[33] have shown satisfactory results short-term using Indomethacin in patients receiving ingrowth components. However, because effective custom shielding of ingrowth components during low-dose radiation is now possible, it has been our practice to favor radiation treatment, except for women of childbearing age, for whom the relative risks might be argued to shift back in favor of the use of NSAIDs.

In those patients undergoing implantation of cemented components, Indomethacin would seem a reasonable choice, particularly because it has now been shown to be effective over a 2- to 3-week course of treatment. One complicating factor, however, is the routine use of Coumadin or low-molecular weight Heparin for deep venous thrombosis prophylaxis in this patient population. This, along with the possibility that many of these often elderly patients may be intolerant to Indomethacin and other nonsteroidals or may have a history of frank peptic ulcer disease, can make NSAID use less attractive. Some of these patients are also best treated by radiation therapy.

Because both methodologies have been shown to be effective by numerous investigators, a choice can be made by the surgeon on an individual basis for the particular patient in question. Decision making, based on the patient's medical history and clinical circumstances, involves weighing the relative advantages and disadvantages of the two competing methods.

Excision of Heterotopic Ossification

Heterotopic bone may require excision if grade III to IV ossification has occurred and has produced significant symptoms of pain and restriction of motion. In addition, patients who are undergoing revision of their arthroplasty for other reasons and who have significant heterotopic bone present should also undergo excision at the time of surgery. For patients who do not have other indications for repeat surgery on their hip, the amount of pain present is the factor that dictates whether isolated excision is attempted. Postoperatively, all such patients should undergo prophylaxis against reformation of heterotopic bone as outlined above.

The decision about when to perform excision of heterotopic ossification may be guided by the use of bone scans. Once bone scan activity begins to fall off significantly, which indicates that the local process about the hip is quiescent and the heterotopic bone is mature, excision can be safely carried out with less chance of heterotopic bone reforming. Usually, excision of this sort can be planned for at 1 year following the original surgery, but on occasion it will have to be deferred longer or, alternatively, may be carried out earlier if the process has reached maturity by that time.

Success of heterotopic ossification excision has tended to be judged by radiographic criteria. However, a recent study by Cobb and associates[42] examined the functional outcome of patients following excision of heterotopic bone. These authors presented 53 cases of isolated heterotopic ossification excision following formation associated with hip arthroplasty. Patients were examined at a mean of 3.5 years following excision, and radiographic follow-up was available at an average of 7.8 years on this patient group. While excision significantly increased the range of motion (by a mean of 33° flexion), it is noteworthy that there was little correlation between final Brooker grade and final range of motion measured clinically. Most importantly, pain relief was unreliable, even when reformation of heterotopic bone was effectively prevented by prophylaxis using either radiation or nonsteroidals, both of which were employed separately in this series. These results further support the importance of prevention of significant heterotopic bone initially following total hip arthroplasty in those patients who are at increased risk. It also suggests that some caution be used in the selection of patients for isolated excision of heterotopic bone following total hip arthroplasty, because, despite dependable improvements in motion and ability to reliably prevent reformation of the heterotopic bone, relief of pain cannot be assured.

Summary

Although heterotopic ossification following total hip arthroplasty is frequently observed radiographically, it fortunately is much less commonly of clinical importance. There are, however, a group of patients that develop significant heterotopic bone formation, which can be symptomatic and, in some cases, can require repeat surgery.

Careful surgical technique seems indicated in all patients undergoing total hip arthroplasty to try to reduce the incidence of this problem. Patients who are recognized to be at risk should be treated with prophylaxis. These include patients with active ankylosing spondylitis, skeletal hyperostosis, and prior heterotopic bone formation. Both low-dose radiation and nonsteroidal anti-inflammatories have been shown to be effective. The choice between these two modalities depends on the patient's individual circumstances, the availability of radiotherapy support (including custom shielding for ingrowth components), and the presence of areas of bone grafting and any osteotomies or fractures. Nonsteroidal anti-inflammatories, particularly Indomethacin, are a very acceptable form of prophylaxis and may be preferred in certain patients, including young women of childbearing age. Radiation is preferred in those patients with known GI intolerance to these medications or with a prior history of peptic ulcer disease. Excision of heterotopic bone, if symptomatic, should not be performed before 6 to 12 months and then only once it is clear that the process is mature. Bone scans can be helpful in assessing the maturity of heterotopic bone and can guide the timing of excision. Prophylaxis should be carried out in all patients following excision of heterotopic bone. Although prophylaxis can effectively prevent reformation of heterotopic ossification, it does not necessarily completely relieve the pain symptoms that prompted the patient to seek further treatment.

References

1. Charnley J: The long-term results of low-friction arthroplasty of the hip performed as a primary intervention. *J Bone Joint Surg* 1972;54B:61-76.
2. Frassica FJ, Frassica DA, Coventry MB: Ectopic bone, in Morrey BF (ed): *Joint Replacement Arthroplasty.* New York, NY, Churchill-Livingstone, 1991, pp 867-876.
3. Rosendahl S, Christoffersen JK, Nørgaard M: Para-articular ossification following hip replacement: 70 arthroplasties ad modum Moore using McFarland's approach. *Acta Orthop Scand* 1977;48:400-404.
4. Jowsey J, Coventry MB, Robins PR: Heterotopic ossification: Theoretical consideration, possible etiologic factors, and a clinical review of total hip arthroplasty patients exhibiting this phenomenon, in *The Hip: Proceedings of the Fifth Open Scientific Meeting of the Hip Society.* St. Louis, MO, CV Mosby, 1977, vol 51, pp 210-221.
5. DeLee J, Ferrari A, Charnley J: Ectopic bone formation following low friction arthroplasty of the hip. *Clin Orthop* 1976;121:53-59.
6. Kromann-Andersen C, Sørensen TS, Hougaard K, et al: Ectopic bone formation following Charnley hip arthroplasty. *Acta Orthop Scand* 1980;51:633-638.
7. Ritter MA, Vaughan RB: Ectopic ossification after total hip arthroplasty: Predisposing factors, frequency, and effect on results. *J Bone Joint Surg* 1977;59A:345-351.
8. Goel A, Sharp DJ: Heterotopic bone formation after hip replacement: The influence of the type of osteoarthritis. *J Bone Joint Surg* 1991;73B:255-257.
9. Sundaram NA, Murphy JCM: Heterotopic bone formation following total hip arthroplasty in ankylosing spondylitis. *Clin Orthop* 1986;207:223-226.
10. Bisla RS, Ranawat CS, Inglis AE: Total hip replacement in patients with ankylosing spondylitis with involvement of the hip. *J Bone Joint Surg* 1976;58A:233-238.
11. Kilgus DJ, Namba RS, Gorek JE, et al: Total hip replacement for patients who have ankylosing spondylitis: The importance of the formation of heterotopic bone and of the durability of fixation of cemented components. *J Bone Joint Surg* 1990;72A:834-839.
12. Fahrer H, Koch P, Ballmer P, et al: Ectopic ossification following total hip arthroplasty: Is diffuse idiopathic skeletal hyperostosis a risk factor? *Br J Rheum* 1988;27:187-190.
13. Bundrick JJ, Cook DE, Resnik CS: Heterotopic bone formation in patients with DISH following total hip replacement. *Radiology* 1985;155:595-597.
14. Blasingame JP, Resnick D, Coutts RD, et al: Extensive spinal osteophytosis as a risk factor for heterotopic bone formation after total hip arthroplasty. *Clin Orthop* 1981;161:191-197.
15. Maloney WJ, Krushell RJ, Jasty M, et al: Incidence of heterotopic ossification after total hip replacement: Effect of the type of fixation of the femoral component. *J Bone Joint Surg* 1991;73A:191-193.
16. Errico TJ, Fetto JF, Waugh TR: Heterotopic ossification: Incidence and relation to trochanteric osteotomy in 100 total hip arthroplasties. *Clin Orthop* 1984;190:138-141.
17. Morrey BF, Adams RA, Cabanela ME: Comparison of heterotopic bone after anterolateral, transtrochanteric, and posterior approaches for total hip arthroplasty. *Clin Orthop* 1984;188:160-167.
18. Brooker AF, Bowerman JW, Robinson RA, et al: Ectopic ossification following total hip replacement: Incidence and a method of classification. *J Bone Joint Surg* 1973;55A:1629-1632.
19. Ahrengart L: Periarticular heterotopic ossification after total hip arthroplasty: Risk factors and consequences. *Clin Orthop* 1991; 263:49-53.
20. Bosse MJ, Poka A, Reinert CM, et al: Heterotopic ossification as a complication of acetabular fracture: Prophylaxis with low-dose irradiation. *J Bone Joint Surg* 1988;70A:1231-1237.
21. Kaempffe FA, Bone LB, Border JR: Open reduction and internal fixation of acetabular fractures: Heterotopic ossification and other complications of treatment. *J Orthop Trauma* 1991;5:439-445.
22. Coventry MB, Scanlon PW: The use of radiation to discourage ectopic bone: A nine-year study in surgery about the hip. *J Bone Joint Surg* 1981;63A:201-208.

23. Ayers DC, Evarts CM, Parkinson JR: The prevention of heterotopic ossification in high-risk patients by low-dose radiation therapy after total hip arthroplasty. *J Bone Joint Surg* 1986; 68A:1423-1430.
24. Pellegrini VD Jr, Konski AA, Gastel JA, et al: Prevention of heterotopic ossification with irradiation after total hip arthroplasty: Radiation therapy with a single dose of eight hundred centigray administered to a limited field. *J Bone Joint Surg* 1992;74A:186-200.
25. Healy WL, Lo TC, Covall DJ, et al: Single-dose radiation therapy for prevention of heterotopic ossification after total hip arthroplasty. *J Arthroplasty* 1990;5:369-375.
26. Hedley AK, Mead LP, Hendren DH: The prevention of heterotopic bone formation following total hip arthroplasty using 600 rad in a single dose. *J Arthroplasty* 1989;4:319-325.
27. Pellegrini VD Jr, Gregoritch SJ, Rubin P: Preoperative radiation therapy for prevention of heterotopic ossification following total hip arthroplasty. Presented at the 61st Annual Meeting of the American Academy of Orthopaedic Surgeons, New Orleans, LA, Feb 28, 1994.
28. Blount LH, Thomas BJ, Tran L, et al: Postoperative irradiation for the prevention of heterotopic bone: Analysis of different dose schedules and shielding considerations. *Int J Radiat Oncol Biol Phys* 1990;19:577-581.
29. Jasty M, Schutzer S, Tepper J, et al: Radiation-blocking shields to localize periarticular radiation precisely for prevention of heterotopic bone formation around uncemented total hip arthroplasties. *Clin Orthop* 1990;257:138-145.
30. Thomas BJ, Amstutz HC: Results of the administration of diphosphonate for the prevention of heterotopic ossification after total hip arthroplasty. *J Bone Joint Surg* 1985;67A:400-403.
31. Cella JP, Salvati EA, Sculco TP: Indomethacin for the prevention of heterotopic ossification following total hip arthroplasty: Effectiveness, contraindication, and adverse effects. *J Arthroplasty* 1988;3:229-234.
32. Kjaersgaard-Andersen P, Ritter MA: Short-term treatment with nonsteroidal anti-inflammatory medications to prevent heterotopic bone formation after total hip arthroplasty: A preliminary report. *Clin Orthop* 1992;279:157-162.
33. McMahon JS, Waddell JP, Morton J: Effect of short-course indomethacin on heterotopic bone formation after uncemented total hip arthroplasty. *J Arthroplasty* 1991;6:259-264.
34. Ritter MA, Gioe TJ: The effect of indomethacin on para-articular ectopic ossification following total hip arthroplasty. *Clin Orthop* 1982;167:113-117.
35. Schmidt SA, Kjaersgaard-Andersen P, Pedersen NW, et al: The use of indomethacin to prevent the formation of heterotopic bone after total hip replacement: A randomized, double-blind clinical trial. *J Bone Joint Surg* 1988;70A:834-838.
36. Sodemann B, Persson PE, Nilsson OS: Prevention of periarticular heterotopic ossification following total hip arthroplasty: Clinical experience with indomethacin and ibuprofen. *Acta Orthop Trauma Surg* 1988;107:329-333.
37. Tozun R, Pinar H, Yesiller E, et al: Indomethacin for prevention of heterotopic ossification after total hip arthroplasty. *J Arthroplasty* 1992;7:57-61.
38. Freiberg AA, Cantor R, Freiberg RA: The use of aspirin to prevent heterotopic ossification after total hip arthroplasty: A preliminary report. *Clin Orthop* 1991;267:93-96.
39. Gebuhr P, Soelberg M, Orsnes T, et al: Naproxen prevention of heterotopic ossification after hip arthroplasty: A prospective control study of 55 patients. *Acta Orthop Scand* 1991;62:226-229.
40. Wahlstrom O, Risto O, Djerf K, et al: Heterotopic bone formation prevented by diclofenac: Prospective study of 100 hip arthroplasties. *Acta Orthop Scand* 1991;62:419-421.
41. Allen HL, Wase A, Bear WT: Indomethacin and aspirin: Effect of nonsteroidal anti-inflammatory agents on the rate of fracture repair in the rat. *Acta Orthop Scand* 1980;51:595-600.
42. Cobb TK, Berry DJ, Morrey BF, et al: Functional outcome of excision of heterotopic ossification after total hip arthroplasty. Presented at the 61st Annual Meeting of the American Academy of Orthopaedic Surgeons, New Orleans, LA, Feb 28, 1994.

CHAPTER 25

Fractures of the Femur After Hip Replacement

Clive P. Duncan, MD, FRCSC
Bassam A. Masri, MD

In the early days of total hip arthroplasty, fractures following hip replacement were a rare occurrence.[1,2] With more and more patients receiving total hip replacements, it is now no longer unusual to encounter and treat a patient with a femoral fracture at or below a total hip replacement stem. These fractures can occur during the intraoperative or postoperative periods. The treatment of such fractures can be complex and is one of the major challenges facing the reconstructive orthopaedic surgeon. With this problem becoming more prevalent, the prevention of such fractures is now increasingly important. A thorough understanding of the biomechanical principles and risk factors is crucial for effective prophylaxis. Intraoperative and postoperative femoral periprosthetic fractures will be discussed in this chapter, with emphasis on prevention and treatment. A new classification system for postoperative periprosthetic fractures will be presented.

Epidemiology of Periprosthetic Femoral Fractures

Incidence

Intraoperative Fractures Recently, the incidence of intraoperative fractures during the course of total hip arthroplasty has increased, especially with the advent of cementless arthroplasty. Prior to the advent of press-fit or porous-coated total hip arthroplasty, the incidence of intraoperative femoral fractures during total hip arthroplasty was about 0.1% to 1%.[3-5] Revision surgery is associated with a higher incidence.[6] Christensen and associates[6] reported an intraoperative fracture in 6.3% of revision hip arthroplasties. With the increased bulk and force of insertion of cementless implants, there has been a significant rise in the incidence of intraoperative fractures. Fracture rates between 3% and 17.6%[7-9] have been reported. Because of the need for a tight press-fit at the isthmus for predictable bone ingrowth,[10] older cementless designs used an undersized femoral broach in order to ensure a good fit for the femoral component. With the use of such a broach, there is an increased risk of intraoperative fracture during insertion of the femoral component.[9] Inadequate reaming of the medullary canal can also cause the metaphyseal portion of the prosthesis to act as a wedge and split the proximal femur. Careful attention to technical detail during cementless total hip arthroplasty by templating, careful preparation of the bone bed with graduated reamers and broaches of increasing size, and hoop stress protection by the application of cerclage wires or bone holders will help decrease the risk of intraoperative fracture.[9]

Postoperative Fractures Fractures of the femur following total hip replacement are becoming an increasingly important problem. In a review of 2,360 cases, Garcia-Cimbrelo and associates[11] encountered 37 postoperative femoral fractures (1.57%). Kavanagh[3] estimated the risk of postoperative femoral fracture to be less than 1% after primary arthroplasty and as high as 4.2% following revision surgery. In a review of 1,442 total hip replacements, Löwenhielm and associates[12] found the accumulated risk of postoperative fracture over the 15 years following a total hip replacement to be 25.3 per 1,000. Based on these figures, one may estimate the risk of postoperative periprosthetic fracture at 1.5% to 4%.

Risk Fractures for Periprosthetic Femoral Fractures

The incidence of intraoperative fractures during total hip arthroplasty is higher in patients with rheumatoid arthritis than it is in those who have osteoarthritis.[13,14] This increased incidence is probably due to the osteopenia seen in individuals who have rheumatoid arthritis. Severe osteoporosis may also be associated with a higher risk of intraoperative fracture. Other conditions that increase bone fragility, such as osteomalacia, Paget's disease, osteopetrosis, and osteogenesis imperfecta also increase the risk of intraoperative fracture. Complex deformities of the proximal femur, particularly when associated with a narrow medullary canal, as seen in degenerative joint disease following developmental dislocation of the hip[15] may also increase the risk of intraoperative fractures. Revision surgery is associated with a higher risk of intraoperative fracture than primary hip replacement surgery.[6,15] Scott and associates[15] found that 12 of 16 intraoperative proximal femoral fractures were associated with secondary surgery. These fractures occurred during hip dislocation, cement extraction, or reaming through old cement.[6,15]

Cortical perforation during total hip replacement has been described as a major risk factor for periprosthetic fractures.[16-22] Talab and associates[16] reviewed the early total hip arthroplasty experience, and noted that the incidence of cortical perforation during the course of total hip arthroplasty varied between 0.4% and 4%. They also concluded that with increasing experience with total hip replacement, this complication became less frequent. Early on, cortical penetration was not recognized as a definite risk factor for periprosthetic fracture. With later studies, it has become apparent that cortical penetration and extruded cement, when not treated properly, can be a significant risk factor for a periprosthetic fracture.[16-20] Talab and associates[16] had 14 perforations in 500 total hip replacements. Most of these occurred during second procedures or revision arthroplasties. Perforation was rare in primary hip replacement. In four of these patients, the hip replacement was complicated by a periprosthetic fracture between 3 and 36 months postoperatively. In a review of fractures adjacent to long-stem femoral components, cortical defects were noted in six of seven patients suffering such fractures.[18] Eschenroeder and Krackow[19] described the new entity of femoral stress fracture in association with a cortical perforation and extruded cement. This entity is seen in a patient who is doing well following a total hip replacement complicated by a cortical perforation and extruded cement. There is a sudden onset of pain that would make the surgeon suspect a diagnosis of loosening or infection. A bone scan shows focal increased uptake at the site of perforation. The authors recommend excision of the extruded cement to the level of the endosteal cortex, with bone grafting of the lesion. Sydney and Mallory[23] described the technique of controlled cortical perforation for cement excision in the course of revision of cemented femoral components. In this technique, multiple perforations are made in the cortex of the femur, to allow improved illumination of the femoral canal, better inspection of the cement mantle, and irrigation of the canal. In a review of 219 revision arthroplasties in which this technique was used, nine periprosthetic fractures were encountered. In eight of these fractures, major trauma was responsible for the fractures. The authors concluded that technique is safe and does not significantly increase the risk of fracture. Clearly, however, with a risk of fracture in the region of 4%, this technique should only be used with good indication. The main differences between this technique and accidental perforation is that with this technique, the perforations are on the anterior femoral cortex, whereas with accidental perforation, the defect is usually on the lateral femoral cortex, which is the tension side of the femur. Moreover, controlled perforations are always bypassed by the femoral stem, whereas accidental perforations, if not recognized at surgery, are not always bypassed by the femoral stem.

The risk factors for cortical perforation include female sex, osteoporosis, previous fracture, or previous hip surgery.[24] Narrow femoral canals, as seen in congenital dislocation of the hip or juvenile rheumatoid arthritis, or preexisting areas of weak femur may also predispose to cortical perforation. In such cases, great care must be taken while removing the old cement mantle in case of revision surgery or during canal reaming. In the patient at risk, a longer incision is recommended, as well as a trochanteric osteotomy for improved exposure. If the perforation is recognized at surgery, it should be bypassed with a long-stem femoral component, and the extruded cement should be removed.

Other risk factors for postoperative fractures following total hip replacement include loosening of the prosthesis with cortical bone loss or stress risers within the cortex, such as old screw holes, the ends of plates, or impingement of a loose stem against the lateral femoral cortex.[22] Localized osteolysis has also been shown to be associated with periprosthetic femoral fractures.[25] As the incidence of osteolysis secondary to particulate matter increases, this will become an increasingly important risk factor, and the early identification and treatment of such lesions will be important for fracture prevention.

Loosening of the prosthesis is associated with a higher risk of postoperative fracture. Bethea and associates[22] noted that 75% of patients with postoperative periprosthetic fractures had underlying loosening of the implant. The risk factors for intraoperative and postoperative periprosthetic femoral fractures are summarized in Table 1.

Classification of Periprosthetic Femoral Fractures

Intraoperative Fractures

The most commonly used classification of intraoperative periprosthetic fractures is that of Johansson and associates.[4] This is the same classification as that described for postoperative periprosthetic fractures. There are three fracture types in this classification. Type I fractures are entirely proximal to the tip of the prosthesis. Type II fractures are located around the tip of the stem, and commonly extend below it, and type III fractures are entirely distal to the tip of the stem. In the study by Johansson and associates,[4] the commonest fracture pattern was type II, followed by types I and III. In cementless arthroplasty, the commonest fracture pattern is type I followed by type II and type III.[26] Types II and III were more common in revision surgery. Stuchin[7] described a similar classification system for intraoperative fractures with cementless total hip re-

Table 1
Risk factors for intraoperative and postoperative fractures of the femur in total hip arthroplasty.

Intraoperative Fracture	Postoperative Fracture
Rheumatoid arthritis	Weakened femur
Cementless arthroplasty	Stress risers: screw holes, end of plate, stem tip impingement, etc.
Metabolic bone disease	Cortical perforation
Paget's disease	Osteolysis
Osteogenesis imperfecta	Extruded cement
Complex deformities of the proximal femur	Loose implant
Revision or secondary surgery	

placement. Types I and II are the same as those of Johansson. Type III fractures are those that are related to a femoral stress riser, and type IV fractures are the ones that are not otherwise classifiable. Mallory and associates[26] described a classification system for intraoperative fractures seen with cementless total hip arthroplasty. Type I fractures are proximal to the lesser trochanter. Type II fractures extend distal to the lesser trochanter, but end more than 4 cm proximal to the tip of the stem. Type III fractures extend more distally than type II fractures. In a review of 56 cases using this classification,[26] 80% of intraoperative fractures during cementless total hip replacement were type I, 16% were type II, and only 4% were type III. Type I and II fractures were not associated with any adverse consequences, and the number of type III fractures was not large enough for a statistical analysis. Schwartz and associates[9] described a classification system that attempted to predict the stability of the fracture. They described the location of the fracture as being either proximal or distal (near the tip of the stem). Proximal fractures were described as complete or incomplete, and distal fractures were classified as incomplete-minimally displaced, incomplete-displaced, or complete. Most intraoperative fractures were incomplete and minimally displaced.[9] The different classification systems are summarized in Table 2.

Postoperative Fractures

The Johansson classification is the most commonly used classification for postoperative periprosthetic femoral fractures.[4] This classification is the same as that used for intraoperative fractures. Bethea and associates[22] described the following classification system. Type A fractures were those below the tip of the implant. Type B fractures were spiral fractures around the femoral component. Comminuted fractures around the stem were designated type C. Cooke and Newman[27] modified the Bethea classification. In their classification, type I fractures were comminuted fractures around the stem, type II fractures were oblique or spiral fractures around the stem, type III fractures were transverse fractures below the tip of the prosthesis, and type IV fractures were spiral or oblique fractures below the tip of the stem. Roffman and Mendes[28] suggested a simple classification that divided fractures into two groups. In one group, the stability of the bone-implant interface is maintained, and in the other group, the stability of the bone-implant interface is not maintained. These various classifications for postoperative periprosthetic femoral fractures are summarized in Table 3.

Treatment of Periprosthetic Femoral Fractures

Intraoperative Fractures

Not all intraoperative fractures during total hip arthroplasty are recognized at surgery. For those fractures that are, the treatment depends on the fracture location and configuration. For fractures that are well above the tip of the planned prosthesis, internal fixation with cerclage wire or cable and a standard-length femoral prosthesis should suffice. Postoperative mobilization would be based on the stability of the fracture and its fixation. Ali Khan and O'Driscoll[5] reported good results with this treatment. If the fracture is close to the tip of the prosthetic stem, it should be bypassed with a long-stem component, and additional cerclage wire or cable fixation may be considered. Fractures that are not recognized at the time of surgery are usually stable and can be treated conservatively with activity restriction, minimal weightbearing, or a hip spica in precarious cases.

Cortical perforations that are recognized at surgery should be bypassed with a longer stem[16] in order to decrease the risk of postoperative fracture. The distal-most extent of the stem should be two diameters below the level of the cortical perforation.[29] This is based on in vitro work[29] on canine femora in which the strength of a femur with a cortical perforation was only 44% that of the intact femur. Bypassing the defect by two diameters raised the strength of the femur to 84% of the contralateral femur. If the perforation is not recognized at surgery, the patient may be treated with activity restriction until the defect is filled in with new bone. In

Table 2
Classification of intraoperative periprosthetic femoral fractures

Johansson[4]	Type I proximal to the tip	Type II around the tip	Type III distal to the tip	
Stuchin[7]	Type I proximal to the tip	Type II around the tip	Type III related to a stress riser	Type IV not otherwise classifiable
Mallory[26]	Type I proximal to lesser trochanter	Type II distal to the lesser trochanter but no closer than 4 cm to the tip of the stem	Type III more distal than type II	
Schwartz[9]	Proximal		Distal	
	complete	incomplete	incomplete and undisplaced	incomplete and displaced

Table 3
Classification of postoperative periprosthetic femoral fractures

Johansson[4]	Type I proximal to the tip	Type II around the tip	Type III distal to the tip	
Bethea[22]	A below the tip	B around the stem	C comminuted	
Cooke & Newman[27]	Type 1 comminuted	Type 2 oblique or spiral around the stem	Type 3 transverse below the tip	Type 4 oblique below the tip
Roffman & Mendes[28]	Stable prosthesis	Loose prosthesis		

the investigation of persisting postoperative pain in the presence of a cortical perforation, the possibility of a stress fracture should be entertained. If a stress fracture is present, reoperation for the removal of bone cement and bone grafting should be considered.[17,19]

Postoperative Fractures

There is little agreement in the literature with respect to the optimum treatment of these difficult fractures. Various treatment modalities have been described and advocated, but the optimum treatment for each fracture depends on numerous factors, and not all methods are appropriate for all fractures. Treatment options include (a) nonsurgical management with traction or a hip spica, (b) revision total hip arthroplasty with a long-stem femoral component and cerclage fixation, (c) revision arthroplasty with proximal femoral prosthetic or allograft replacement, and (d) open reduction and internal fixation (ORIF) using plates, screws, and cerclage bands or cables. In addition to the above traditional methods, there has been recent interest in the use of cortical onlay allografts fixed with cables for the internal fixation of periprosthetic fractures. The choice of treatment methods depends on the nature of the fracture, the stability of the implant, the quality of bone stock, the age of the patient, and the experience of the surgeon.

Nonsurgical Treatment Several authors have recommended nonsurgical treatment for some periprosthetic femoral fractures. McElfresh and Coventry[21] suggested that nonsurgical treatment should be the treatment of choice unless the bone ends cannot be maintained in direct opposition in traction or in a hip spica. Scott and associates[15] reviewed postoperative periprosthetic fractures, but their sample was too small for them to make any strict recommendations. They suggested, however, that conservative treatment is effective, and the risk of surgical intervention may not be justified. Johansson and associates[4] suggested that fractures proximal to the tip of the prosthetic stem be treated conservatively, and, if symptomatic loosening results, a revision replacement may be performed following fracture healing. In our opinion, conservative treatment is not as innocuous as has been suggested. Bed rest in the elderly patient is associated with many risks, such as atelectasis, pneumonia, and thromboembolic disease. Other complications include skin ulceration, knee stiffness, and malunion. A malunited femur may make revision replacement more difficult (Fig. 1), and a loose femoral stem will commonly require revision surgery regardless of the fracture. The results outlined by the above authors, when examined critically, show that it is very difficult to come to any firm conclusions because of the small numbers in these series. Also, because of the early and long-term risks associated with nonsurgical management, as well as the cost of prolonged hospitalization, surgical management is preferable in most cases.

Revision Total Hip Arthroplasty Postoperative periprosthetic femoral fractures are often associated with loosening of the femoral stem. This loosening may or may not have been symptomatic prior to fracture. In one series of postoperative periprosthetic femoral fractures, Bethea and associates[22] reported that 75% of these fractures were associated with prosthetic loosening. In such cases (Fig. 2), we recommend revision total hip arthroplasty with a long-stem prosthesis, especially in the older patient. Other authors have recommended

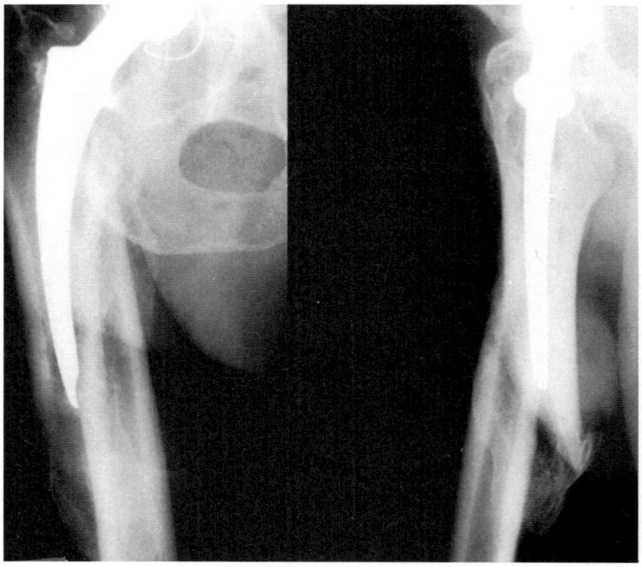

Fig. 1 Conservative treatment of this fracture resulted in the fracture healing with the tip of the stem outside the femur. Reconstruction following malunion of the fracture was more difficult than it would have been at the time of the fracture.

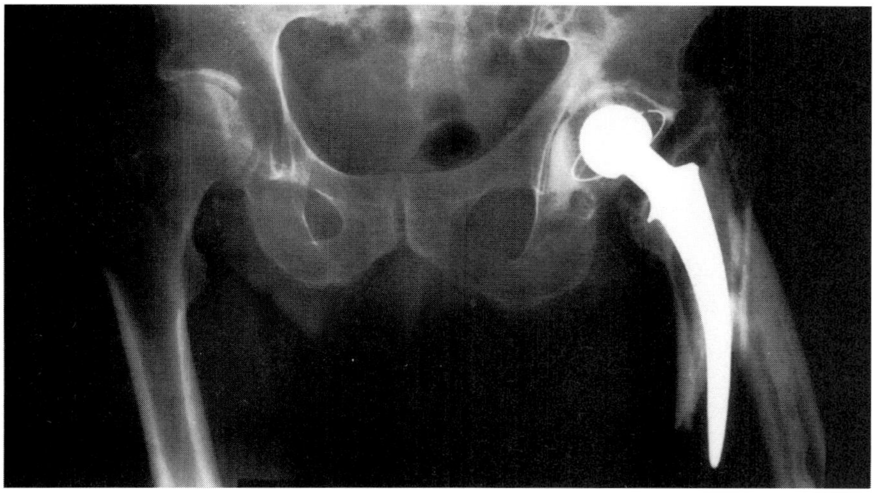

Fig. 2 Because of loosening of the stem, this fracture is best treated by intramedullary stabilization using a long-stem femoral component. This method of treatment uses a single surgical procedure to address both the problems of fracture and of loosening.

such treatment and reported good results, but their series were small and poorly controlled.[3,13,22,30] In cases with adequate bone stock, our preferred method is a cemented long-stem femoral prosthesis, especially in the older patient. The fracture should be reduced and fixed in an intramedullary fashion with the long-stem prosthesis. In addition to the prosthetic stem, supplementary cerclage cables or wires may be required for added stability. To avoid delayed union and nonunion, cement must not be allowed to extrude into the fracture site. Bone grafting of these fractures has been recommended by some authors.[3,22] Although there is no convincing evidence that bone grafting is always indicated, it may be used at the surgeon's discretion, depending on bone quality, soft-tissue preservation, and fracture comminution. In cases in which the bone stock and fracture comminution are such that reconstruction of the femur is impossible (Figs. 3 and 4), revision arthroplasty, using a proximal femoral replacement, must be considered. In the younger patient, we use a proximal femoral allograft replacement, with a step-cut osteotomy at the bone-allograft junction. A long-stem femoral component is cemented into the allograft and press-fitted into the femur distally. It may be necessary to stabilize the bone-allograft junction with supplementary cerclage cables, and morselized bone graft should be added in order to optimize the union rate. All extruded cement at the bone-allograft junction should be carefully removed in order to enhance the union rate. The patient's own femur is retained as a bivalved vascularized autograft around the bone-allograft junction. Nonunion at the bone-allograft junction is an important cause of morbidity following this procedure, and the above techniques help to minimize the risk of this complication. In the elderly patient with a limited life expectancy, we use a prosthetic proximal femoral replacement (Fig. 4), thus avoiding the potential morbidity associated with the longer and more complex procedure of proximal femoral allograft replacement, as well as the more protracted postoperative recovery. The most common complication that we have observed following prosthetic

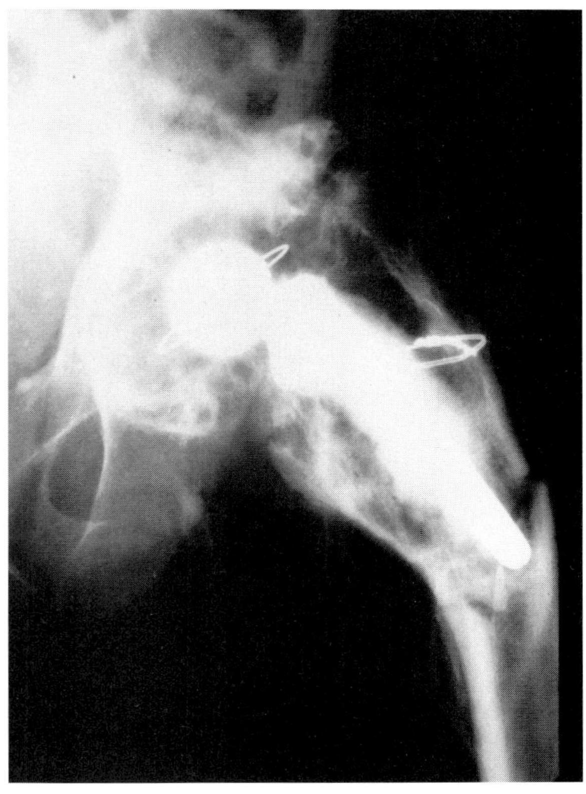

Fig. 3 Bone stock in the proximal femur is so poor that a conventional reconstruction with ORIF and revision THR is impossible. This patient was served well with a proximal femoral allograft replacement.

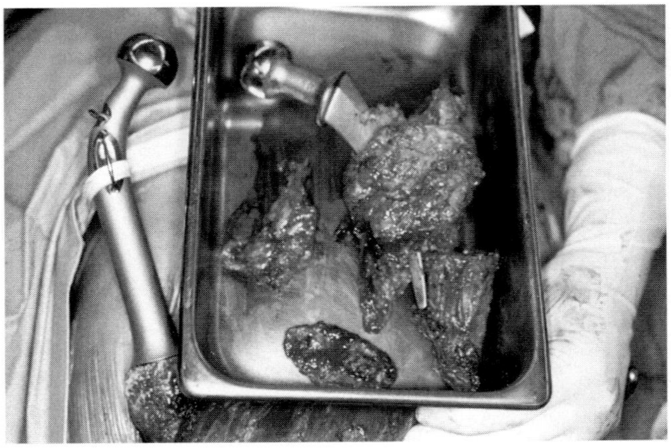

Fig. 4 A prosthetic femoral replacement was used to make up for the poor bone stock in the proximal femur of this elderly patient. The advantages of such treatment include lower cost, immediate mobilization, and lower morbidity.

proximal femoral replacement is dislocation, unless a cup is used that will "capture" the femoral head. When this technique is used, therefore, the surgeon should consider the use of a snap-fit acetabular cup or a bipolar cup in order to minimize the risk of postoperative dislocation.

Open Reduction and Internal Fixation One of the first reports of open reduction and internal fixation of periprosthetic femoral fracture used a combination of intramedullary Rush rods and cerclage wire for the fixation of mid-shaft periprosthetic fractures in the presence of cementless hemiarthroplasty prostheses.[1] These authors also recommended prophylactic bone grafting. Intramedullary nailing was also used by Olerud,[2] who used a long-stem Charnley femoral component wedged into a Küntscher intramedullary femoral nail for the provisional stabilization of a periprosthetic femoral fracture. Following fracture healing, this temporary device was removed and a definitive long-stem revision arthroplasty was performed. Others have recommended condylocephalic Ender nailing in the treatment of proximal femoral fracture below noncemented femoral implants.[31]

Other techniques of open reduction and internal fixation include cerclage fixation using stainless steel wires, multifilament cables, or wide bands such as the stainless steel Parham bands[32] and nylon Partridge bands.[33] In one biomechanical study,[34] Parham bands and swage-lock titanium cables were shown to exhibit the strongest fixation potential. Gauge-18 stainless steel wires followed, and the use of a square knot enhanced the strength of fixation. Nylon bands were less effective. Clinical studies have shown that cerclage fixation alone does not achieve rigid fixation, and such treatment should be supplemented with other methods of rigid internal fixation.[11]

With the increasing popularity of AO/ASIF techniques in the treatment of long bone fractures, such principles were applied to periprosthetic femoral fractures.[35,36] In a review of nine cases treated with open reduction and internal fixation using a standard dynamic compression plate, Stern and associates[35] reported good results with no implant failure and no nonunions. When this technique is used, it is desirable not to violate the cement mantle in the solid femoral component. In those fractures below the tip of the stem (Johanssen type III), it is often possible to achieve rigid internal fixation without violating the integrity of the cement mantle (Fig. 5). To achieve rigid internal fixation in more proximal fractures, the proximal screws must be inserted into the cement mantle around the femoral stem (Fig. 6). Because of the theoretical disadvantage of inserting screws in the cement mantle around a solid femoral component, and because of the current use of canal-filling cementless femoral components, other devices that do not require screws for proximal fixation have been developed. Such devices use proximal cerclage systems to anchor the plate to the femur, while allowing distal fixation with standard screws. The first such device was introduced by Ogden and Rendall[37] and is currently known as the Ogden plate. This plate allows fixation with screws distally, and with Parham bands proximally. Results of treatment of periprosthetic femoral fractures with this plate have been encouraging. Ogden and Rendall[37] reported on ten periprosthetic fractures treated with this plate. All fractures healed. Similarly, Wang and associates[13] reported a 100% union

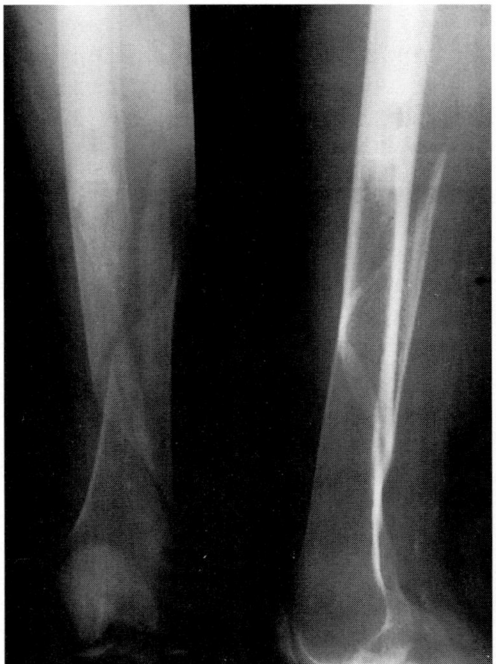

Fig. 5 This distal femoral fracture was treated effectively with ORIF without disturbing the femoral component.

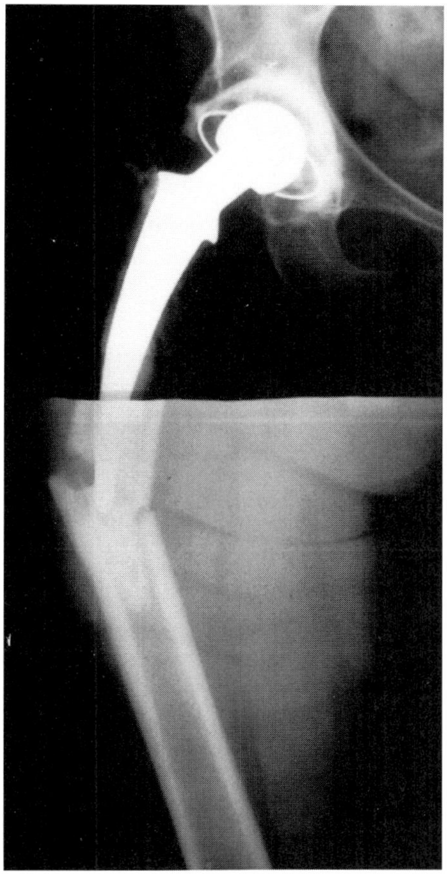

Fig. 6 Because the femoral stem was well fixed, ORIF was chosen to treat the fracture. The proximity of the fracture to the femoral component made it necessary for the screws to penetrate the cement mantle.

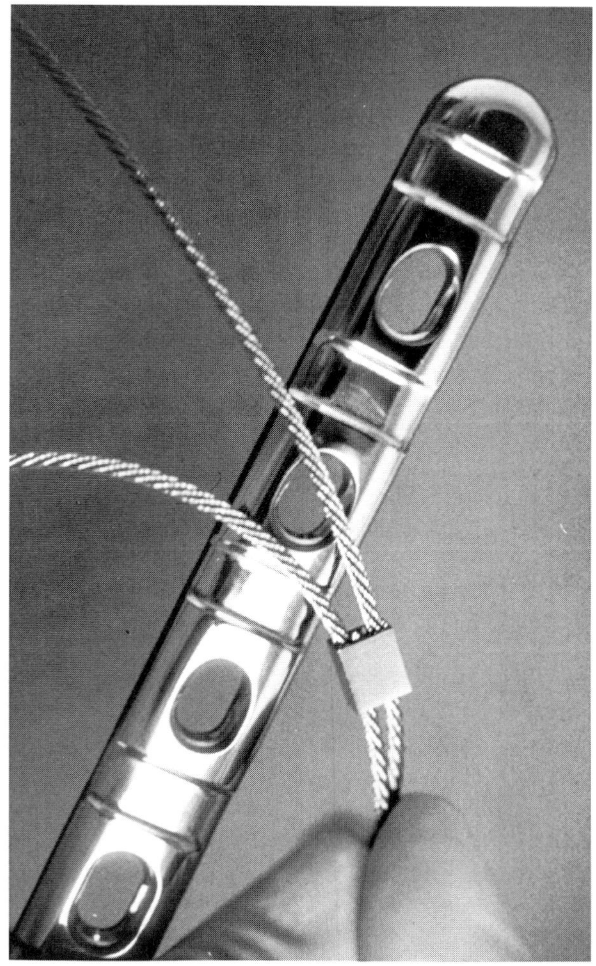

Fig. 7 The Dall-Miles plate (Howmedica Inc., Rutherford, NJ).

rate in six patients treated with the Ogden plate. Zenni and associates[38] reported excellent or good results in 17 of 19 patients treated with this plate. Sixteen fractures healed within 3.5 months, two fractures resulted in delayed union, and one resulted in nonunion. Montijo and associates[39] also reported a 100% union rate in seven fractures treated with the Ogden plate. More recently, the Dall-Miles plate (Howmedica Inc, Rutherford, NJ) has been introduced, although clinical experience had been limited. This is a stainless steel plate with slots between the screw holes (Fig. 7). These slots accept 2.0 mm stainless steel cables that may be crimped into these slots. With this device, a combination of screws and cables may be used anywhere within the plate, which makes it more versatile than the Ogden plate. Pierson and associates[40] had no nonunions when 12 periprosthetic fractures were treated with a new plate-clamp device (Plamp). This device is not yet in widespread use.

Rüedi and Lüscher[41] strongly recommended routine bone grafting of femoral shaft fractures treated by internal fixation, even in the absence of ipsilateral hip replacement. When a total hip replacement is present adjacent to a fracture of the femoral shaft, the intramedullary blood supply is by necessity already compromised. ORIF interferes with the extra-osseous blood supply. Because of this decreased blood supply, we recommend routine bone grafting of all periprosthetic femoral shaft fractures treated with ORIF. Other authors have also recommended routine bone grafting of such fractures.[3,30,36]

Open reduction and internal fixation may be difficult in osteoporotic bone. The poor bone quality may not allow adequate screw purchase and, thus, may not allow rigid fixation. One well-recognized technique that is used for ORIF in pathologic bone is cement supplementation. In periprosthetic fractures with poor bone quality, the medullary canal may be cleaned of debris and then filled with bone cement. Screws are then inserted through the cement mantle for improved fixation. The use of this technique allowed rigid fixation of nine periprosthetic femoral fractures with good results and no failure of fixation.[35] In addition to screw fixation, the use of supplemental cerclage cable fixation throughout the length of the plate, as is possible with the Dall-Miles plate (Howmedica Inc, Rutherford, NJ), may allow more rigid fixation.

In summary, the treatment of choice in unstable periprosthetic femoral fractures when the femoral prosthesis is stable is open reduction and internal fixation with bone grafting. Any of a variety of implants may be used, as long as rigid fixation is achieved.

Bicortical Onlay Allograft Fixation Another technique used in the treatment of periprosthetic femoral fractures is ORIF using two cortical onlay allografts that are applied to the lateral and medial sides of the femur and fixed to it with cerclage cables (Fig. 8). The two onlay allografts act as internal bone plates, thus eliminating the need for plate and screw fixation. This technique is particularly useful in the osteoporotic femur because it eliminates the screw holes as potential stress risers, and because it has the potential to achieve more rigid fixation when good screw purchase is difficult to obtain. The use of bone as an internal plate also minimizes the stress-shielding effect[42] seen when a stainless steel plate is used. In a finite element biomechanical analysis of the bone-plate technique using a single strut, Mihalko and associates[42] showed that there was some stress shielding of the femur, however, this was less than the stress shielding observed with the Ogden plates.[42] Moreover, the authors also found that, in order to improve the fixation with this technique, more wires must be added at the distal end of the proximal and distal fracture fragments, because maximum load transfer occurs at these sites. This technique, using a single cortical strut and Gauge-18 wires, was at least as effective as the Ogden plate. Another advantage of the use of the bicortical onlay allograft technique for the treatment of periprosthetic femoral fractures is the ability of the bone graft to incorporate and strengthen the native femur.[43] On theoretical grounds, it is apparent that the bicortical onlay allograft technique with multifilament cerclage cables is an effective technique, but, as it is a relatively new technique, clinical experience has been limited.

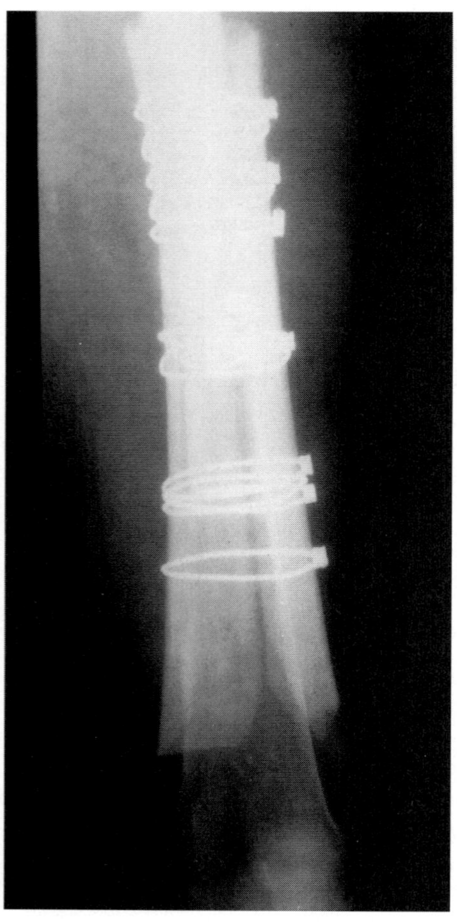

Fig. 8 The bicortical onlay allograft technique is an effective means of achieving rigid fixation of periprosthetic femoral fractures.

Prevention of Periprosthetic Femoral Fractures

As has already been emphasized, periprosthetic femoral fractures are becoming an increasingly important clinical problem, with significant morbidity. It is important to be able to prevent such fractures. Most intraoperative fractures occur during hip dislocation, femoral reaming, cement removal, or final insertion of the prosthesis.[6,9,21] Therefore, it is important to have adequate exposure before any attempt is made to dislocate the hip. In difficult cases, a trochanteric osteotomy may greatly enhance the exposure and help prevent an intraoperative fracture. In one series, 50% of all intraoperative fractures during revision total hip arthroplasty occurred at the time of dislocation.[6] This high incidence was due to inadequate soft-tissue release.

Care should be taken during the preparation of the medullary canal of the femur, especially with cementless arthroplasty. Reaming with flexible, rigid, or conical reamers must be done carefully. Eccentric reaming with rigid reamers may predispose to fracture. If a femoral canal is prepared using a flexible reamer in preparation for the insertion of a straight cementless femoral component, high points may be left because of the normal curvature of the femur.[9] Insertion of a snug prosthesis can cause a wedging effect, and a fracture may occur.[9] Moreover, if the femur is not reamed far enough, the tip of the prosthesis will encounter a tighter medullary canal and can cause a fracture. If undersized broaches are used, the final implant, which has a slightly larger dimension, may fracture the femur as it is being inserted. For this reason, Schwartz and associates[9] have recommended that undersized broaches not be used. Fitzgerald and associates[8] recommended over-reaming the cortex to reduce the risk of intraoperative fractures during cementless total hip arthroplasty.

If the surgeon has concerns regarding the strength of the femur and its ability to withstand the stresses of reaming or insertion of a cementless implant, the hoop stress resistance may be increased by applying cerclage fixation or a bone clamp prophylactically. Herzwurm and associates[44] showed that the use of a single 2.0-mm cerclage cable increased the proximal femoral microstrain at fracture from 962 to 4179. This was highly significant. Incavo and associates[45] also showed that cerclage wiring increases the energy required for crack propagation. Therefore, prior to the insertion of a total hip femoral prosthesis, particularly if a porous-coated prosthesis is used, the surgeon must ensure that there are no cracks in the proximal femur. If such a crack is noted, a cerclage wire or cable should be applied in order to prevent crack propagation,[45] which could transform an inconsequential fracture to a clinically significant fracture that could affect the stability of the implant.[8]

In addition to the preparation of the femoral canal and the insertion of the prosthesis, cement removal may predispose to an intraoperative fracture. Great care should be taken while removing cement from the femur. The cement mantle should be split radially at multiple levels before any attempt is made to separate the cement mantle from bone. The cement column should be well visualized. If there is difficulty seeing the cement mantle, a cortical window with no sharp corners should be made. The prosthetic stem should bypass this window by at least two cortical diameters in order to prevent a postoperative fracture.

Authors' Preferred Method

The literature to date supports many methods in the treatment of periprosthetic femoral fractures. The choice of the most appropriate treatment depends on a number of factors, including the location of the fracture, the stability of the fracture and implant, the quality of bone stock, the age of the patient, and the experience of the surgeon. Our treatment algorithm is summarized in Figure 9. If the fracture is stable and the prosthesis is stable, the fracture may be treated nonsurgically. If the fracture is unstable, the treatment should depend on the stability of the prosthesis. If the prosthesis is loose and the bone stock is adequate, a long-stem revision is preferred. If bone stock is inadequate due to extensive osteolysis or severe comminution, the proximal femur is replaced with a prosthetic proximal femoral replacement in the aged patient, or with an allograft proximal femoral replacement in the physiologically young patient. If a prosthetic proximal femoral replacement prosthesis is chosen, serious consideration should be given to the use of bipolar femoral head or a snap-fit acetabular cup, because of the increased risk of postoperative dislocation with these prostheses. If the prosthesis is not loose, ORIF is our preferred treatment. If bone stock is adequate, particularly in distal fractures, plate fixation is preferred, unless this fixation violates the cement mantle of the femoral stem. In such cases, as well as in cases with poor bone stock and those with a canal-filling cementless

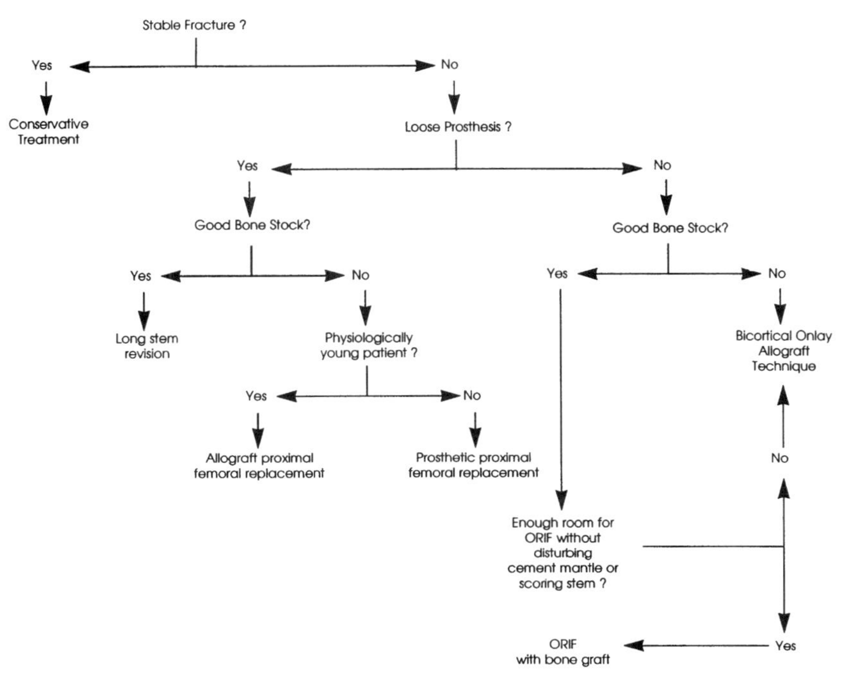

Fig. 9 Our proposed algorithm for the treatment of periprosthetic femoral fractures.

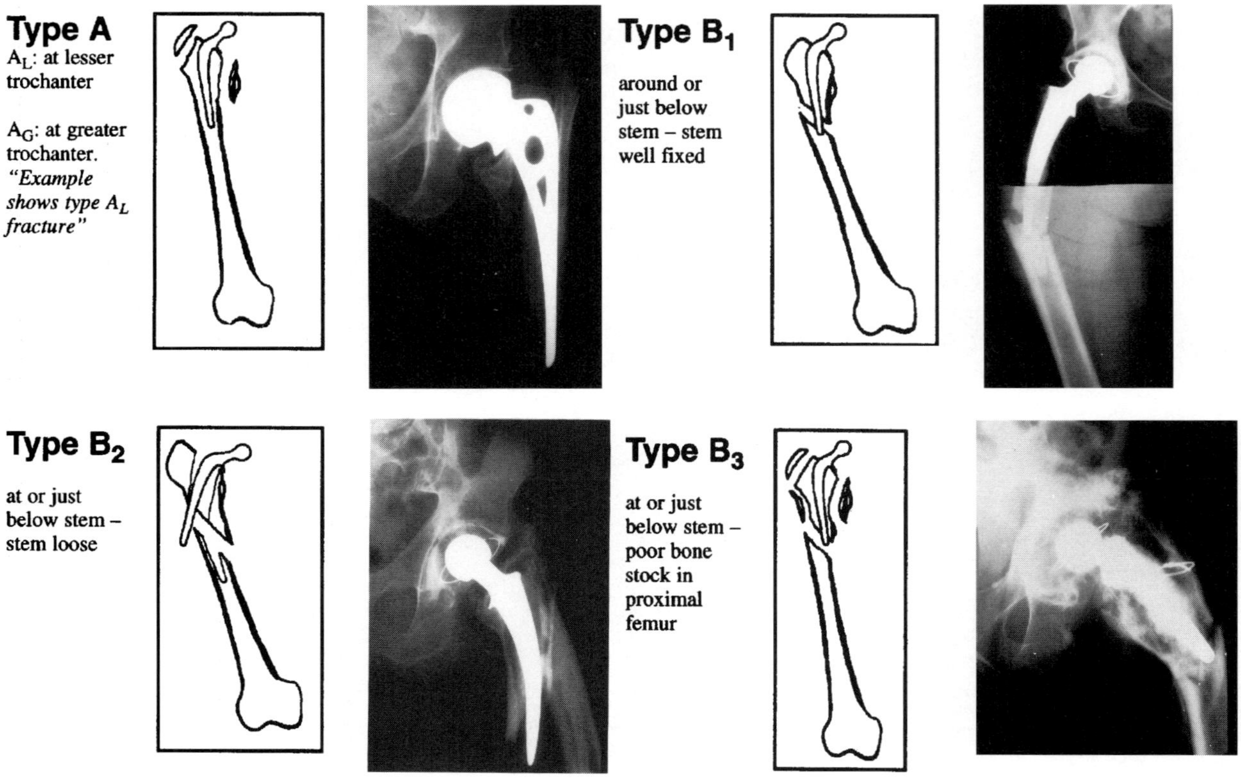

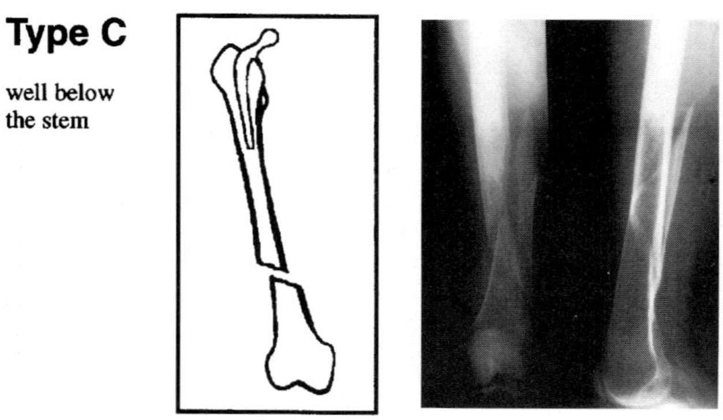

Table 4
Our proposed classification of fractures of the femur following total hip arthroplasty

Type	Location	Subtype
A	Trochanteric Region	A_G: Greater Trochanter
		A_L: Lesser Trochanter
B	Around or just distal to the stem	B_1: Prosthesis Stable
		B_2: Prosthesis Unstable
		B_3: Bone Stock Inadequate
C	Well below the stem	

Fig. 10 The classification system used by the authors for fractures of the femur following total hip arthroplasty.

stem, the bicortical onlay allograft technique is preferred. At present, we have no experience with the plate/cable combinations such as the Ogden or Dall-Miles plates.

The current classification systems for postoperative periprosthetic femoral fractures (Table 3) do not aid the surgeon in choosing the most appropriate treatment. For this reason, we developed a new classification system (Table 4, Fig. 10), which we believe is of more value in guiding the surgeon to the most appropriate treatment for these fractures. The factors that our classification system takes into consideration include the location of the fracture, the fixation of the stem, and the quality of the bone, all of which are important in deciding on the optimal management of the fracture. There are three major types in our classification, depending on the location of the fracture. Type A fractures involve the trochanteric region. Type B fractures are around the stem of the femoral component, or extend slightly distal to it. Type C fractures are so distal to the stem that the presence of the femoral component may be ignored, and the fracture can be treated by conventional methods. Type A fractures are subclassified as follows: Type A_G fractures involve the greater trochanter, and type A_L fractures involve the lesser trochanter. Type B fractures are subclassified based on the stability of the implant and the quality of bone stock. In type B_1 fractures, the implant is stable, whereas in type B_2 fractures, the implant is unstable or loose. Type B_3 fractures are those in which the stem is loose and the bone stock around the femoral component is inadequate. Bone stock may be inadequate because of severe osteopenia, osteolysis, or fracture comminution.

In a review of a series of 75 consecutive periprosthetic femoral fractures treated at Vancouver Hospital and Health Science Centre between February 1985 and February 1994, 4% of fractures were type A, 86.7% were type B, and 9.3% were type C. Among type B fractures, 18.5% were type B_1, 44.6% were type B_2, and 36.9% were type B_3. It is the frequency of types B_2 and B_3 fractures over the years that stimulated the senior author to develop this new classification system, in order to emphasize the significance of the quality of the prosthesis-bone interface and bone stock in the therapeutic decision-making process. With the high proportion of fractures with an unstable prosthesis or poor bone stock, conservative management, in the majority of cases, is contraindicated, and surgery remains the appropriate treatment for the majority of patients with periprosthetic femoral fractures. Using our classification system, type A fractures may be treated either conservatively or surgically, depending on the stability of the fracture. Type B_1 fractures are best treated using ORIF or the bicortical onlay allograft technique. Type B_2 fractures are best treated using long-stem revision total hip arthroplasty. Type B_3 fractures usually require complex reconstruction. Type C fractures are best treated using ORIF.

In summary, fractures of the femur following total hip arthroplasty continue to be among the most demanding problems that face the reconstructive orthopaedic surgeon. The past two decades have seen a gradual shift towards early surgical intervention, with improved results.

References

1. Parrish TF, Jones JR: Fracture of the femur following prosthetic arthroplasty of the hip: Report of nine cases. *J Bone Joint Surg* 1964;46A:241-248.
2. Olerud S: Reconstruction of a fractured femur following total hip replacement: Report of a case. *J Bone Joint Surg* 1979;61A:937-938.
3. Kavanagh BF: Femoral fractures associated with total hip arthroplasty. *Orthop Clin North Am* 1992;23:249-257.
4. Johansson JE, McBroom R, Barrington TW, et al: Fracture of the ipsilateral femur in patients with total hip replacement. *J Bone and Joint Surg* 1981;63A:1435-1442.
5. Ali Khan MA, O'Driscoll M: Fractures of the femur during total hip replacement and their management. *J Bone Joint Surg* 1977;59B:36-41.
6. Christensen CM, Seger BM, Schultz RB: Management of intraoperative femur fractures associated with revision hip arthroplasty. *Clin Orthop* 1989;248:177-180.
7. Stuchin SA: Femoral shaft fracture in porous and press-fit total hip arthroplasty. *Orthop Rev* 1990;19:153-159.
8. Fitzgerald RH Jr, Brindley GW, Kavanagh BF: The uncemented total hip arthroplasty: Intraoperative femoral fractures. *Clin Orthop* 1988;235:61-66.
9. Schwartz JT Jr, Mayer JG, Engh CA: Femoral fracture during non-cemented total hip arthroplasty. *J Bone Joint Surg* 1989; 71A:1135-1142.
10. Engh CA, Bobyn JD, Glassman AH: Porous-coated hip replacement: The factors governing bone ingrowth, stress shielding, and clinical results. *J Bone Joint Surg* 1987;69B:45-55.
11. Garcia-Cimbrelo E, Munuera L, Gil-Garay E: Femoral shaft fractures after cemented total hip arthroplasty. *Int Orthop* 1992;16:97-100.
12. Löwenhielm G, Hansson LI, Kärrholm J: Fracture of the lower extremity after total hip replacement. *Arch Orthop Trauma Surg* 1989;108:141-143.
13. Wang G-J, Miller TO, Stamp WG: Femoral fracture following hip arthroplasty: Brief note on treatment. *J Bone Joint Surg* 1985; 67A:956-958.
14. Poss R, Ewald FC, Thomas WH, et al: Complications of total hip-replacement arthroplasty in patient with rheumatoid arthritis. *J Bone Joint Surg* 1976;58A:1130-1133.
15. Scott RD, Turner RH, Leitzes SM, et al: Femoral fractures in conjunction with total hip replacement. *J Bone Joint Surg* 1975; 57A:494-501.
16. Talab YA, States JD, Evarts CM: Femoral shaft perforation: A complication of total hip reconstruction. *Clin Orthop* 1979; 141:158-165.
17. Fredin H: Late fracture of the femur following perforation during total hip arthroplasty: A report of two cases. *Acta Orthop Scand* 1988;59:331-332.
18. Missakian ML, Rand JA: Fractures of the femoral shaft adjacent to long stem femoral components of total hip arthroplasty: Report of seven cases. *Orthopedics* 1993;16:149-152.
19. Eschenroeder HC Jr, Krackow KA: Late onset femoral stress fracture associated with extruded cement following hip arthroplasty: A case report. *Clin Orthop* 1988;236:210-213.
20. Scher MA: Fractures of the femoral shaft following total hip replacement. *J Bone Joint Surg* 1981;63B:472.
21. McElfresh EC, Coventry MB: Femoral and pelvic fractures after total hip arthroplasty. *J Bone Joint Surg* 1974;56A:483-492.
22. Bethea JS III, DeAndrade JR, Fleming LL, et al: Proximal femoral fractures following total hip arthroplasty. *Clin Orthop* 1982;170:95-106.
23. Sydney SV, Mallory TH: Controlled perforation: A safe method of cement removal from the femoral canal. *Clin Orthop* 1990;253:168-172.
24. Pellicci PM, Inglis AE, Salvati EA; Perforation of the femoral shaft during total hip replacement: Report of twelve cases. *J Bone Joint Surg* 1980;62A:234-240.
25. Pazzaglia U, Byers PD: Fractured femoral shaft through an osteolytic lesion resulting from the reaction to a prosthesis: A case report. *J Bone Joint Surg* 1984;66B:337-339.
26. Mallory TH, Kraus TJ, Vaughn BK: Intraoperative femoral fractures associated with cementless total hip arthroplasty. *Orthopedics* 1989;12:231-239.
27. Cooke PH, Newman JH: Fractures of the femur in relation to cemented hip prostheses. *J Bone Joint Surg* 1988;70B:386-389.

28. Roffman M, Mendes DG: Fracture of the femur after total hip arthroplasty. *Orthopedics* 1989;12:1067-1070.
29. Larson JE, Chao EYS, Fitzgerald RH: Bypassing femoral cortical defects with cemented intramedullary stems. *J Orthop Res* 1991; 9:414-421.
30. Berman AT, Levenberg RJ: Femur fractures associated with total hip arthroplasty. *Orthopedics* 1992;15:751-753.
31. Pankovich AM, Tarabishy I, Barmada R: Fractures below non-cemented femoral implants: Treatment with Ender nailing. *J Bone Joint Surg* 1981;63A:1024-1025.
32. Parham FW: Circular constriction in the treatment of fractures of the long bones. *Surg Gynecol Obstet* 1916;23:541-544.
33. Partridge AJ, Evans PE: The treatment of fractures of the shaft of the femur using nylon cerclage. *J Bone Joint Surg* 1982;64B:210-214.
34. Shaw JA, Daubert HB: Compression capability of cerclage fixation systems: A biomechanical study. *Orthopedics* 1988;11:1169-1174.
35. Stern RE, Harwin SF, Kulick RG; Management of ipsilateral femoral shaft fractures following hip arthroplasty. *Orthop Rev* 1991;20:779-784.
36. Levenberg R, Iorio R, Gingrich K, et al: Femur fractures associated with total hip arthroplasty. *Orthopedics* 1990;13:1188-1189.
37. Ogden WS, Rendall J: Fractures beneath hip prostheses: A special indication for Parham bands and plating. *Orthop Trans* 1978;2:70.
38. Zenni EJ Jr, Pomeroy DL, Caudle RJ: Ogden plate and other fixations for fractures complicating femoral endoprostheses. *Clin Orthop* 1988;231:83-90.
39. Montijo H, Ebert FR, Lennox DA: Treatment of proximal femur fractures associated with total hip arthroplasty. *J Arthroplasty* 1989; 4:115-123.
40. Pierson JL, Burstein AH, Cornell CN, et al: Plamp: A plate-clamp device for the treatment of peri-prosthetic fractures. Presented at the fifty-ninth annual meeting of the American Academy of Orthopaedic Surgeons, Washington, DC, 1992.
41. Rüedi TP, Lüscher JN: Results after internal fixation of comminuted fractures of the femoral shaft with DC plates. *Clin Orthop* 1979;138:74-76.
42. Mihalko WM, Beaudoin AJ, Cardea JA, et al: Finite-element modeling of femoral shaft fracture fixation techniques post total hip arthroplasty. *J Biomech* 1992;25:469-476.
43. Emerson RH Jr, Malinin TI, Cuellar AD, et al: Cortical strut allografts in the reconstruction of the femur in revision total hip arthroplasty: A basic science and clinical study. *Clin Orthop* 1992;285:35-44.
44. Herzwurm PJ, Walsh J, Pettine KA, et al: Prophylactic cerclage: A method of preventing femur fracture in uncemented total hip arthroplasty. *Orthopedics* 1992;15:143-146.
45. Incavo SJ, DiFazio F, Wilder D, et al: Longitudinal crack propagation in bone around femoral prosthesis. *Clin Orthop* 1991; 272:175-180.

CHAPTER 26

The Role of Antibiotic-Loaded Cement in the Treatment of an Infection After a Hip Replacement

Clive P. Duncan, MD, FRCSC
Bassam A. Masri, MD

Since the mid-1960s, total hip replacement has become one of the most popular and successful procedures performed by orthopaedists. However, devastating consequences may result if an infection occurs. Numerous treatment methods have been proposed. The results of attempts to retain an implant, in case of infection, have been unpredictable. Müller[1] described a small series of five patients in whom a deep infection occurred within 3 weeks after the operation and who were managed with a thorough debridement, retention of the implant, and intravenous administration of antibiotics; there was only one failure. Steinbrink[2] noted that an early infection (occurring within 3 weeks after the operation) may be treated with extensive debridement and suction-irrigation followed by systemic antibiotic therapy for 7 days. This was based on previous work by Mella-Schmidt and Steinbrink,[3] in which such an approach was successful for the treatment of 35 (45%) of 77 infections at the site of a total hip or knee replacement (64 hips and 13 knees). With better technique and earlier diagnosis, the authors were able to improve this salvage rate to 19 (56%) of 34 between 1984 and 1987 and to 31 (66%) of 47 when good suction-drainage was established. The same outcome also may apply to acute hematogenous infections that are treated within a few days after the onset of the infection, regardless of the length of time after the initial procedure. In a large review of 3,215 total hip arthroplasties,[4] only eight of 42 implants that were surrounded by a deep infection were salvaged with debridement, irrigation, and administration of antibiotics. Most of the implants that could be salvaged were those around which the infection had occurred within 3 months after the index arthroplasty. In the patients who had an acute hematogenous infection, only one of seven implants was salvaged. The distinction between an acute infection and a chronic infection with an acute flare is ill defined, and no large series is available to identify any marked differences between infections caused by a bacteremic insult and those associated with an acute exacerbation of a chronic low-grade infection.[5]

It is well accepted that a chronic infection following the insertion of a total hip prosthesis is not likely to resolve without the removal of the implant. In a series of patients who had a chronic infection at the site of a total hip replacement, Murray[5] reported a salvage rate of only eight (25%) of 32 implants when debridement, irrigation, and placement of suction tubes were used. Between 1972 and 1982, Goulet and associates[6] managed 19 patients using prolonged antibiotic therapy with or without debridement and irrigation. At a minimum 2-year follow-up, nine patients were considered free of infection. Another two patients were able to retain the prosthesis, although they clearly were worse clinically as a result of the infection. The remaining eight patients were considered treatment failures. In summary, retention of the prosthesis is successful in only a minority of patients; in the rest, removal of the prosthesis and cement is necessary to resolve the infection.

The symptomatic and functional outcome following excision arthroplasty, however, often is not very good. While for many years excision arthroplasty was the most commonly used method of treatment, the results often left something to be desired. In a series of 30 pseudarthroses created for the treatment of an infection at the site of a total hip arthroplasty,[7] six hips continued to drain, two patients had worsening pain, and most patients had marked shortening of the extremity and poor hip function, especially difficulty with walking that necessitated the use of walking aids. Bittar and Petty[8] stressed the poor functional outcome of Girdlestone arthroplasty when used to treat an infection at the site of a total hip arthroplasty. In a review of 33 Girdlestone arthroplasties followed for 3 to 13 years (mean, 6 years), only 14 (42%) of the patients were satisfied with the functional outcome.[9] Bosquet and associates[10] reported similarly poor long-term results. Because of these obvious shortcomings, there was a need for a reasonable alternative, focusing on reconstruction instead of resection. The milestone work by Buchholz and Engelbrecht[11] in the development and use of antibiotic-loaded cement has made revision arthroplasty a feasible alternative.

History of Antibiotic-Loaded Bone Cement

Infection was a common complication during the early days of total hip replacement. With improved surgical technique, and particularly with the introduction of the ultra-clean operating room,[12-14] Charnley was able to reduce the infection rate to as low as three (0.3%) of 1,039 after excluding three exceptional cases because of a positive intraoperative culture. Without any exclusions, the lowest infection rate would have been six (0.6%) of 1,039. Concurrently, Buchholz and Engelbrecht,[11] working at the Endo-Klinik in Hamburg, introduced the concept of antibiotic-loaded cement by impregnating Palacos bone cement (Smith and Nephew Richards, Memphis, Tennessee) with gentamicin. With its use, Buchholz and associates[15] were able to reduce the infection rate from a range of 5.9% to 6.3% (29 of 489 in 1968 to 42 of 665 in 1969) to a range of 0.9% to 2.4% (four of 431 in 1973 to eight of 333 in 1975). Since that time, numerous studies regarding the basic science and clinical applications of antibiotic-loaded bone cement have been published. The success of antibiotic-loaded cement in the prevention of infection at the site of a total hip replacement has led to its use in the treatment of other musculoskeletal infections, such as those at the site of a fracture[16] or a total knee replacement.[17] More recently, a biodegradable antibiotic-carrying cement also has been developed.[18]

Basic Science of Antibiotic-Loaded Bone Cement

The rational use of antibiotic-loaded bone cement requires some understanding of the basic properties of this composite material. The properties of antibiotic-loaded bone cement have been thoroughly investigated since the 1970s. It is now known, through in vitro[19-30] and in vivo[19-23,30-33] studies, that many commonly used antibiotics are released from bone cement in such a way that the local antibiotic levels vastly exceed the minimum inhibitory concentrations needed to treat most susceptible pathogens, and that these levels are much higher than those achieved with parenteral therapy.[32] We have been able to measure tobramycin levels as high as 232 mg/l in the drainage fluid of a patient who had been managed with tobramycin-loaded cement, and vancomycin levels as high as 54 mg/l in the drainage fluid of a patient who had been managed with vancomycin-loaded cement. These levels are therapeutic. Different antibiotics have different elution characteristics. For example, within the first few hours, tobramycin elutes in much higher concentrations than does vancomycin (Fig. 1). The elution rate of both antibiotics decays with time, but the elution rate of tobramycin decays much faster than that of vancomycin. Small concentrations of both antibiotics have been detected as long as 6 months after implantation in our patients. In an in vitro assay, clindamycin was found to elute from cement for as long as 56 days.[25] In rabbits, antibiotic-loaded cement pellets can elute antibiotics for as long as 37 days.[22] It also has been shown that antibiotics in bone cement implanted within the medullary cavity of a cadaveric femur elute from the cement and permeate through the dead cortical bone.[23] This finding has obvious therapeutic implications for patients who have a severe infection at the site of a total hip arthroplasty, with osteomyelitis and devascularized bone.

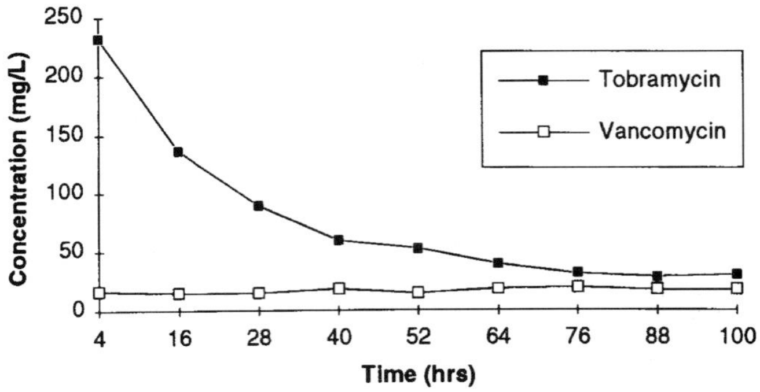

Fig. 1 In vivo elution of tobramycin and vancomycin from bone cement.

A laboratory investigation by Kendall and associates[34] suggested that bacteria can survive on antibiotic-loaded cement containing tobramycin or vancomycin. However, in a further study by the same investigators,[35] antibiotic cement that contained a combination of tobramycin and vancomycin revealed no bacterial growth and no bioadherence when retrieved from humans at the second stage of a total joint revision.

The safety of this antibiotic delivery system also has been clearly established. In our patients who had been managed with antibiotic-loaded bone cement because of an infection at the site of a hip or knee arthroplasty, we never have been able to measure tobramycin or vancomycin serum levels higher than 3 mg/l, despite the addition of as much as 3.6 g of powdered tobramycin per 40 g of bone cement. This level of safety also has been demonstrated in the rabbit model,[22] in the dog model,[26,31] in sheep,[20] and in other studies in humans.[23,30,33]

Baker and Greenham,[20] through in vivo and in vitro studies using scanning electron microscopy, described the mechanism of elution of antibiotics from bone cement. The release of antibiotics occurs only from the surface, from voids and cracks in the bone cement. They concluded that an increase in the concentration of antibiotics within the cement would improve the elution characteristics of the antibiotics. This idea was confirmed in human studies by Wahlig and associates,[33] who showed that when the concentration of gentamicin was doubled, from 0.5 g per 40 g of cement to 1.0 g per 40 g of cement, the concentration of gentamicin in wound secretions was doubled. Baker and Greenham[20] also concluded that a bone cement with greater porosity would be expected to allow more antibiotic release than one with less porosity. It is not surprising, then, that Palacos bone cement, with greater porosity than other cements, has the most rapid elution characteristics.[23,26,30,31,36] Baker and Greenham also noted that methods of cement preparation that are designed to minimize porosity (such as vacuum mixing or centrifugation) could have a deleterious effect on elution characteristics.

The change in the mechanical strength of antibiotic-loaded bone cement compared with that of plain cement also has been investigated.[37-40] In some studies, the addition of small amounts of antibiotics in powder form did not seem to substantially weaken the cement,[38,39] whereas the addition of antibiotics dissolved in liquid markedly weakened the bone cement.[40] Other studies have shown that the addition of any amount of antibiotic powder can cause some weakening of the cement.[37] The degree of weakening depends on the amount of antibiotic added to the cement. Lautenschlager and associates[39] showed that the addition of more than 4.5 g of gentamicin sulphate can substantially weaken bone cement, to the point that its compressive strength is decreased to below the minimum standards set by the American Society for Testing and Materials.

Results of Clinical Studies Using Antibiotic-Loaded Bone Cement

Infection Prophylaxis

The first application of antibiotic-loaded bone cement was in the prophylaxis of infection at the site of a cemented total hip arthroplasty. The data of Buchholz and associates[15] are the most comprehensive to date. At St. Georg Hospital in Hamburg, the infection rate among 1,154 hip replacements in which plain cement had been used was between 5.9% and 6.3% for 1968 and 1969. With the addition of 0.5 g of gentamicin to each 40 g of Palacos bone cement, the infection rate was reduced to between 0.9% and 2.4% in 1,655 hip replacements performed between 1972 and 1975. Systemic antibiotics were used only in exceptional circumstances. Murray[5] reported that the infection rate at the site of primary and revision total hip arthroplasties was eleven (1%) of 1,112 when erythromycin was used in the bone cement, compared with three (0.4%) of 786 when a combination of erythromycin and colistin was used. These data are difficult to interpret because it was a retrospective non-randomized review and because systemic antibiotics also were used.

In a prospective randomized trial, Josefsson and associates[41] compared use of gentamicin-loaded cement alone (0.5 g/40 g) with a variety of parenteral antibiotic protocols. At the 2-year follow-up, there were three deep infections in 821 hips that had been treated with gentamicin-loaded cement, whereas there were 13 deep infections in 812 hips of patients who had received systemic antibiotics. The pattern of superficial infection, however, was quite different. The patients who had been managed with gentamicin-loaded cement had 71 superficial infections, compared with 49 infections in the patients who had received systemic antibiotics. The authors concluded that the high local concentration of antibiotics obtained in the periprosthetic space with antibiotic-loaded cement minimized the risk of deep infection. However, the lack of systemic absorption of antibiotics when antibiotic-loaded cement was used alone, without systemic antibiotics, led to a higher rate of superficial infection.

In another prospective randomized trial,[42] the long-term effect of gentamicin-loaded cement was studied in 1,688 hips. At a 5-year follow-up, there were seven deep infections in the hips of patients managed with gentamicin-loaded cement compared with 16 deep infections in the hips of patients who had been given systemic antibiotics. Furthermore, the rates of aseptic loosening were not noticeably different: 205 (29%) of 698 hips in the patients who had received systemic antibiotics and 171 (24%) of 711 hips in the patients who had received gentamicin-loaded cement. This was an important finding because of the concern that the addition of antibiotics weakens cement.

There are negative aspects to the routine use of antibiotic-loaded cement. In a review of 246 infections at the site of total hip replacements that were done between 1976 and 1987, Hope and associates[43] reported that 91 infections were caused by coagulase-negative staphylococci. Of the 91 infections, 27 were caused by two or more strains of this organism. It was found that in 30 (88%) of 34 patients in whom the primary arthroplasty contained gentamicin-loaded bone cement, at least one of the infecting strains of Staphylococcus was resistant to gentamicin. In contrast, only nine (16%) of 57 patients whose index arthroplasty was not performed with gentamicin-loaded cement had an infection that was caused by gentamicin-resistant coagulase-negative staphylococci. Because of this tendency toward the emergence of resistant strains when antibiotic-loaded bone cement is used, the prophylactic use of antibiotic cement should be approached with caution, and it should be used only when the anticipated benefits outweigh the potential risks.

In summary, there is some evidence that antibiotic-loaded cement is effective in the prevention of deep infection about the hip. The rate of superficial infection, however, is higher when antibiotic-loaded cement is used by itself. The emergence of resistant organisms in subsequent infections should be considered as a potential problem when antibiotic-loaded cement is used prophylactically. When small amounts of antibiotics (0.5 g/40 g of cement) are used, there is no evidence of increased risk of aseptic loosening.[44,45] Our current practice, therefore, is not to use antibiotic-loaded bone cement in straightforward total hip arthroplasties.

Therapeutic Use

Placement of a prosthetic device in an infected wound contradicts all classic orthopaedic teaching, but in the early 1970s reports of reimplantation of total hip prostheses in the presence of infection began to appear. One of the first citations in the English-language literature regarding the reimplantation of a total hip prosthesis in the presence of infection was in a review by Patterson and Brown[46] of the McKee-Farrar total hip arthroplasty. Three prostheses were reimplanted without the use of antibiotic-loaded bone cement. An infection recurred in two of the hips. Since then, there have been many reports of reimplantation of a prosthesis in the treatment of infection at the site of a total hip arthroplasty.[34,47-61] Despite some early negative reports,[55] exchange arthroplasty has become the standard of care in most instances. Obviously, there are exceptions in which the traditional approach of excision arthroplasty is more appropriate, but these are becoming less and less frequent.

Numerous techniques have been used to reimplant a new hip prosthesis in the presence of infection. A one-stage exchange[2,43,48-50,59,61] may be performed, in which the surgeon implants a new prosthesis after the removal of all foreign material. This new prosthesis is secured in place with plain or antibiotic-loaded cement. Alternatively, a two-stage exchange arthroplasty[47,51,52,54,57-59,62-65] may be done, in which all infected tissue and foreign material is removed at the first stage and, after a period of weeks or years, a second prosthesis is implanted, with or without antibiotic-loaded cement. In a modification of this technique, antibiotic-loaded cement spacers may be inserted after the excision arthroplasty.[47,51,52,54,59,65]

The pioneering work of Buchholz[66] at the Endo-Klinik in Hamburg produced a salvage rate, by 1978, of 484 (71%) of 684 infections about a total hip arthroplasty with use of a one-stage exchange technique with antibiotic-loaded Palacos bone cement.[66] Systemic antibiotics were not used except when they were needed for the treatment of another infection.[66] In a multicenter study from Sweden, Carlsson and associates[49] attempted to reproduce the results of Buchholz. Seventy-seven hips were treated either with single-stage exchange arthroplasty (59 hips) or with two-stage exchange arthroplasty (18 hips). In all procedures, antibiotic-loaded Palacos bone cement was used. Of the 77 hips, 60 had a good result; eight remained infected; and nine, despite the lack of obvious evidence of infection, continued to be painful. The authors called these hips "doubtful." For the sake of discussion, they will be considered failures of treatment, so the overall success rate was 60 (78%) of 77 hips, slightly higher than the success rate of Buchholz. It is noteworthy that Carlsson and associates[49] gave systemic antibiotics for 6 months, whereas Buchholz rarely used systemic antibiotics.[66] It also is interesting that the success rates of the single-stage and two-stage exchange procedures were identical (78%). Carlsson and associates[49] concluded that they were unable to detect a difference between the single and the two-stage exchange arthroplasties and recommended the use of the single-stage exchange in the presence of infection, because of its efficiency and simplicity.

In a larger series with longer follow-up, Buchholz and associates[48] reported on their first 10 years of experience with single-stage exchange arthroplasty using antibiotic-loaded Palacos cement. After a one-stage exchange, they were able to salvage 448 (77%) of 583 implants around which an infection had occurred. Following subsequent one-stage exchanges for initial failures, the ultimate success rate was improved to 522 (90%) of 583. The factors that were associated with failure included infection caused by gram-negative organisms or Group-D streptococci and inadequate doses of antibiotics in the cement. Although it seems that this is a reasonable success rate, the failures were serious: there was a 2% mortality rate and a 2% rate of hip disarticulation, and 3% of the patients eventually had a Girdlestone procedure.

Salvati and associates[58] reviewed the literature and compared the results obtained with or without antibiotic-loaded bone cement, as well as the results of one-stage compared with two-stage exchange arthroplasties. Thirty-five (88%) of 40 hips had a successful two-stage procedure with antibiotic-impregnated cement and 169 (84%) of 202 hips had a successful two-stage procedure without antibiotic-impregnated cement. Six hundred and fifty-nine (78%) of 840 hips had a successful one-stage exchange with antibiotic-impregnated cement and 57 (52%) of 110 hips had a successful one-stage procedure without antibiotic-impregnated cement.

Hope and associates[43] reported that nine (13%) of 72 hips had a recurrence of infection after use of the single-stage exchange method and suggested a very selective role for that procedure. Furthermore, Elson and associates[62] reported a failure in 30 (12%) of 243 hips with the one-stage exchange method, compared with three (3%) of 86 hips with the two-stage method. On the basis of this information, it seems that the two-stage exchange method is more effective than the one-stage method, despite its obvious disadvantages.

On the basis of the results of some more recent studies, one may question the need for antibiotic-loaded bone cement.[60,64] In the study by McDonald and associates,[64] 71 (87%) of 82 hips had a successful two-stage exchange arthroplasty without the use of antibiotic-loaded bone cement. There was a high correlation between the presence of retained cement at the time of the initial excision and the rate of recurrence of infection. Also, reimplantation performed within 1 year after the resection arthroplasty was associated with a much higher rate of recurrence (seven [27%] of 26 hips) than reimplantation performed more than 1 year after the resection (four [7%] of 56 hips). The presence of a virulent organism (gram-negative rods and Group-D streptococci) combined with less than 28 days of systemic antibiotic therapy after the resection also worsened the prognosis. Therefore, for a two-stage exchange arthroplasty without antibiotic-loaded bone cement to be successful, it seems that prolonged antibiotic therapy postoperatively and a long period (more than 1 year) of poor hip function must be tolerated. In contrast, Wroblewski[61] reported a successful outcome for 93 (91%) of 102 patients who had been managed with a one-stage exchange arthroplasty with use of antibiotic-loaded cement because of an infection.

Taking into account these and other studies,[50] it is clear that the use of antibiotic-loaded bone cement can improve the salvage rate after an infection at the site of a total hip arthroplasty, regardless of the treatment philosophy that is adopted. Despite the lack of properly controlled randomized prospective trials, it is our impression that the two-stage exchange arthroplasty with use of antibiotic-loaded bone cement is superior. As previously discussed, the use of less than 2 g of antibiotic powder does not seem to weaken the bone cement to any degree,[38,40] and the addition of 0.5 g of gentamicin to bone cement does not appear to lead to increased radiographic signs of loosening when compared with the use of plain bone cement.[44,45]

Hovelius and Josefsson[54] described a variant of the two-stage exchange arthroplasty in which the dead space created at the time of a resection arthroplasty is filled with antibiotic-loaded cement beads. The medullary canal of the femur also is packed with the beads. Much greater amounts of antibiotics can be incorporated in the cement because one does not need to be concerned about changing the biomechanical properties of the cement when it is used simply as a spacer and a drug-delivery system. In a 2- to 9-year follow-up study of two-stage treatment of infection at the site of a total hip arthroplasty,[59] the success rate was improved from 11 of 17 to 11 of 13 with the use of antibiotic-impregnated beads.

The superiority of the two-stage exchange arthroplasty for the treatment of an infection at the site of a total hip arthroplasty does not come without a price. The delayed reimplantation procedures are technically more difficult because of scar formation, shortening, disuse osteoporosis, and distorted anatomy.[2] The patient is uncomfortable, discouraged, and often confined to the hospital with limited mobility and activity during the interval between the two procedures. To avoid these problems, antibiotic-loaded temporary spacers have been developed. Abendschein[47] presented a case report in which a crude spacer made from antibiotic-loaded bone cement was used to fill the gap created by the removal of an implant around which an infection had occurred. An expansile modular prosthesis that is coated with antibiotic-loaded bone cement also has been described[65] for use as a temporary spacer.

Since 1987, we have used a temporary antibiotic-loaded facsimile of a hip prosthesis. Initially, we used a bent intramedullary nail, coated with highly antibiotic-loaded bone cement, as an endoskeleton. A hand-made acetabulum and femoral head were fabricated from the same bone cement. Although this construct maintained the length of the limb and prevented substantial scar formation while eluting high levels of antibiotics into the periprosthetic space, motion and weight-bearing were limited. In 1989, we introduced the Prosthesis of Antibiotic Loaded Acrylic Cement (PROSTALAC) into clinical trials (Fig. 2). This facsimile of a total hip prosthesis has a very thin polyethylene acetabular cup that is loosely cemented, with a large amount of antibiotic-loaded bone cement, into the acetabular fossa (Fig. 3). The femoral component is a modular stainless-steel endoskeleton (Fig. 4) that is coated with antibiotic-loaded bone cement (Fig. 5). This prosthesis is assembled in the operating room and, after hardening of the bone cement, it is inserted into the femur as a press-fit prosthesis. The PROSTALAC system is very versatile. In addition to its modularity, the stem is available in different lengths to compensate for bone loss. There also is a snap-fit acetabular component to compensate for potential instability in patients who are at risk for postoperative dislocation.

In 1993, we reported on the first 15 patients who had been managed with this device because of problems of unique complexity and who had had a minimum follow-up of 2 years.[67] The infection was eradicated in all patients. Two patients had had a reoperation: one because of nonunion at the host-allograft junction after the second stage, and the other because of a loose Lord acetabular component, again after the second stage. The use of this functional facsimile of the hip and proximal part of the femur maintained the length of the extremity and allowed mobilization of the patients out of bed and out of the hospital. The second stage was simplified. In addition to the control of infection, the PROSTALAC system offered other valuable advantages. With earlier mobilization out of bed and out of the hospital, rehabilitation was accelerated and discharge from the hospital between stages became feasible, even when the patient had substantial loss of bone stock. Our total experience to date includes 86 hips, with a minimum follow-up of 2 years for 46. In this larger series, the procedure has failed because of definite or suspected failure to control the infection in three hips (6.5%). This rate of success is comparable with the best results reported in the literature to date, and it indicates that there is no obvious risk or disadvantage to the use of a temporary facsimile of the hip joint, if the results are compared with those obtained

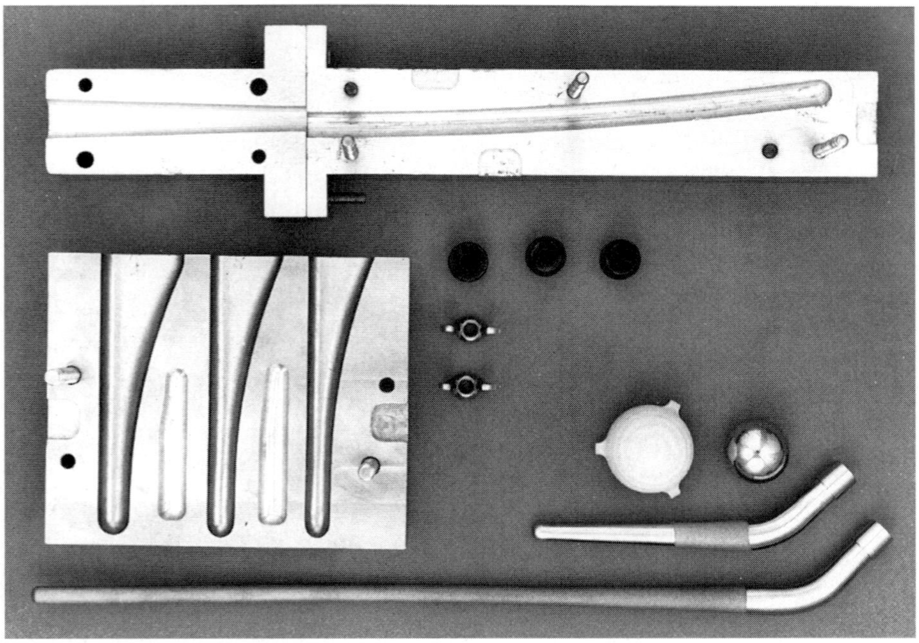

Fig. 2 The PROSTALAC hip system consists of a series of molds used to manufacture a temporary custom-made antibiotic-loaded hip prosthesis that can be used as a spacer after the removal of an infected total hip replacement. The prosthesis consists of a thin polyethylene shell that is coated with a large amount of antibiotic-loaded cement to be used as an acetabular component. The femoral component consists of a stainless-steel endoskeleton that is coated with antibiotic-loaded cement. Stability is ensured by use of the appropriate neck length.

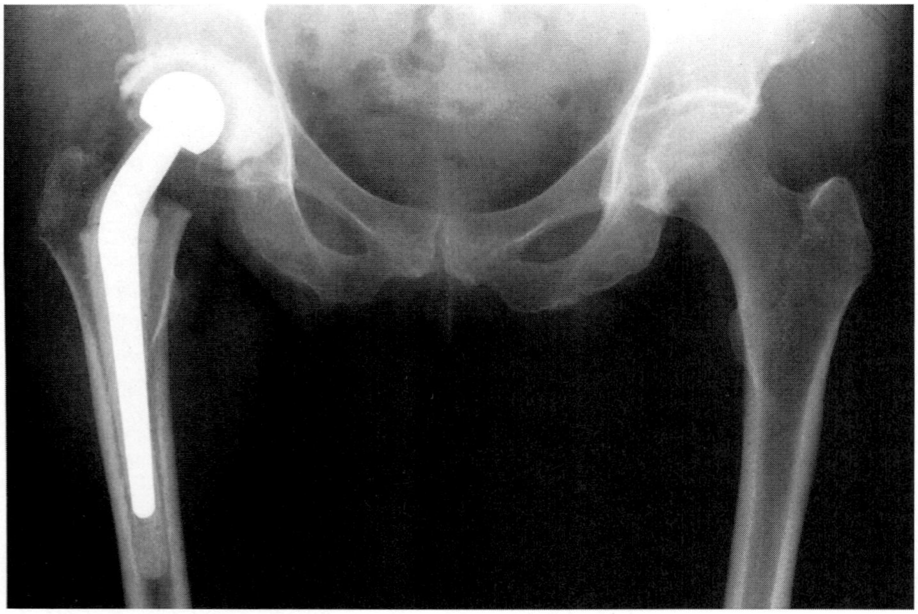

Fig. 3 PROSTALAC hip in situ after the removal of an implant because of an infection.

after a temporary excision arthroplasty or with the use of an antibiotic depot in some other form.

Conclusions

It is clear that properly conducted scientific studies are lacking, and interpretation of the literature obviously is affected by the bias of the individual surgeon. It is difficult to compare different studies performed by different investigators, on different patient populations, for different infections, under different conditions, with many uncontrolled variables. Despite these limitations, it is our interpretation of the literature that the use of antibiotic-loaded bone cement is superior to the use of plain bone cement in the treatment of an infection at the site of a total hip arthroplasty. It is also our conclusion that two-stage exchange arthroplasty is safer than one-stage exchange in the treatment of such

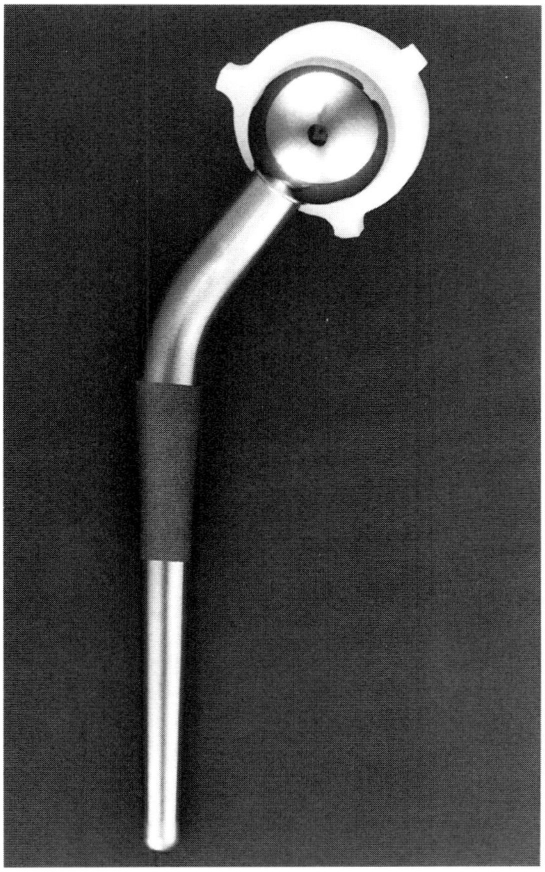

Fig. 4 The endoskeleton used to reinforce the PROSTALAC femoral stem. The surface of this endoskeleton, with the exception of the femoral head, is completely coated with antibiotic-loaded bone cement, minimizing the amount of exposed metal.

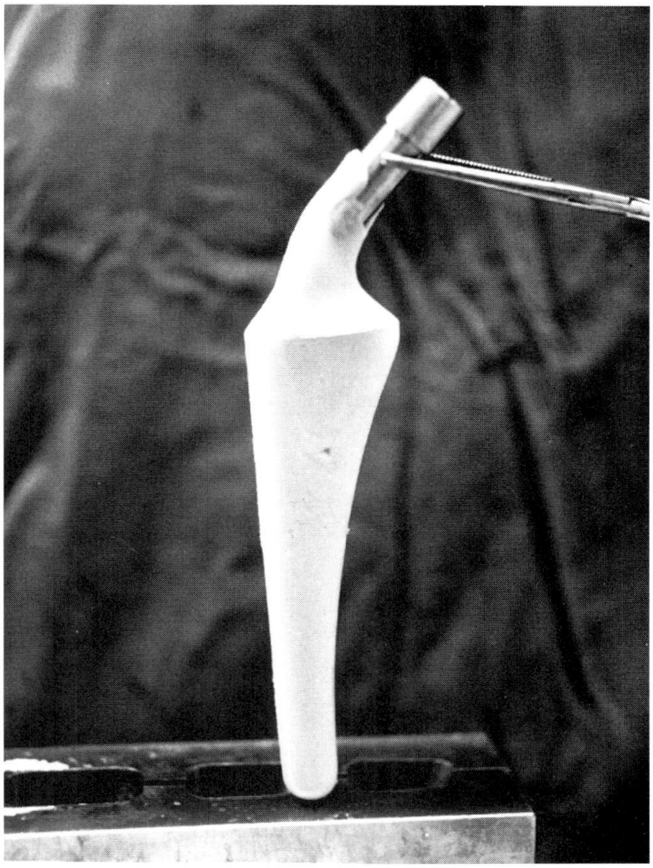

Fig. 5 The finished PROSTALAC femoral component before insertion.

an infection. We favor the use of an antibiotic depot, be it antibiotic-loaded beads, a crude facsimile, or preferably a PROSTALAC prosthesis. The two-stage method allows the use of much higher concentrations of antibiotics in the temporary depot than is otherwise possible. This method allows the use of insertion of components without cement at the time of the revision arthroplasty in a younger patient, and it allows the surgeon a second opportunity to remove any inadvertently retained bone cement, which is associated with a higher rate of failure.[64] There is also less risk associated with the use of an allograft in the final reconstruction when a two-stage approach is used.[36,51,52]

One important consideration when the results of one-stage and two-stage exchange arthroplasties are compared is that Palacos cement has been used in most single-stage exchange arthroplasties, because of its superior elution characteristics.[2,21,23,26,43] However, the higher porosity that is responsible for its improved elution characteristics makes it less amenable to modern cementing techniques[68] and may produce a deleterious effect on the mechanics and long-term durability of the hip reconstruction. It is our practice to use Palacos cement loaded with antibiotics (2.4 to 3.6 g of tobramycin and 1 to 2 g of vancomycin per 40 g of cement) for the temporary spacer; however, when the final components are implanted, Simplex-P bone cement (Howmedica, Rutherford, New Jersey) loaded with antibiotics (0.6 to 1.2 g of tobramycin and 0.5 to 1.0 g of vancomycin per 40 g of cement) is used because of its superior handling characteristics.

Despite the advantages of our modified two-stage exchange method, we still employ the one-stage exchange arthroplasty technique in certain circumstances, as outlined by Miley and associates.[69] The one-stage exchange is particularly well suited for the elderly individual who is unable to tolerate two major surgical procedures and who does not have any contraindications for the use of this technique.[15,48-50,53,55,58-60] These contraindications include severe infection with poorly vascularized and necrotic tissue, persistent draining sinuses, multiple previous operations on the hip, inadequate debridement with retention of old bone cement, sepsis, bone-stock deficiency, and radiographic evidence of osteomyelitis. One-stage exchange also is contraindicated in patients who have a polymicrobial infection; an infection caused by a particularly virulent organism, such as Group-D streptococci or gram-negative organisms (especially Pseudomonas); or a fungal or mycobacterial infection. Single-stage exchange also is contraindicated when preoperative cultures are negative, as often occurs in patients who have been managed with oral or parenteral administration of antibiotics before having a diagnostic hip-aspiration biopsy.

With the discouraging results and poor acceptance of excision arthroplasty by patients, the current treatment of an infection at the site of a total hip replacement has evolved toward exchange arthroplasty. The results of such treatment have been encouraging. Indeed, when we consider that the prevalence of infection in the modern operative setting is 1% or less, and that with modern principles of treatment, at least 90% of infections at the site of a total hip arthroplasty are eradicated, it should be safe to assume that only 0.1% of our patients will have a persistent infection after a total hip replacement. This is quite a remarkable achievement, considering the high rate of infection in the early days of total hip arthroplasty. This dramatic reduction of morbidity is due mainly to our careful attention to the principles of prophylaxis and treatment that have been developed over the past two decades. The advent of antibiotic-loaded bone cement[70] has been a major contributor to this dramatic reduction in morbidity.

References

1. Müller ME: Preservation of septic total hip replacement versus Girdlestone operation, in Harris WH (ed): *The Hip: Proceedings of the Second Open Scientific Meeting of The Hip Society*. St. Louis, MO, CV Mosby, 1974, pp 308-318.
2. Steinbrink K: The case for revision arthroplasty using antibiotic-loaded acrylic cement. *Clin Orthop* 1990;261:19-22.
3. Mella-Schmidt C, Steinbrink K: Stellenwert der spül-saug-drainage bei der behandlung des fruhinfekts von gelenkimplantaten. *Chirurg* 1989;60:791-794.
4. Fitzgerald RH Jr, Nolan DR, Ilstrup DM, et al: Deep wound sepsis following total hip arthroplasty. *J Bone Joint Surg* 1977;59A:847-855.
5. Murray WR: Use of antibiotic-containing bone cement. *Clin Orthop* 1984;190:89-95.
6. Goulet JA, Pellicci PM, Brause BD, et al: Prolonged suppression of infection in total hip arthroplasty. *J Arthroplasty* 1988;3:109-116.
7. Clegg J: The results of the pseudarthrosis after removal of an infected total hip prosthesis. *J Bone Joint Surg* 1977;59B:298-301.
8. Bittar ES, Petty W: Girdlestone arthroplasty for infected total hip arthroplasty. *Clin Orthop* 1982;170:83-87.
9. Bourne RB, Hunter GA, Rorabeck CH, et al: A six-year follow-up of infected total hip replacements managed by Girdlestone's arthroplasty. *J Bone Joint Surg* 1984;66B:340-343.
10. Bosquet MMJ, Duncan CP, Mulier JC, et al: Girdlestone excision arthroplasty of the hip: A review of 49 patients. *Orthop Trans* 1982;6:336.
11. Buchholz HW, Engelbrecht H: Über die depotwirkung einiger antibiotica bei vermischung mit dem kunstharz Palacos. *Chirurg* 1970;41:511-515.
12. Charnley J: A clean-air operating enclosure. *Br J Surg* 1964;51:202-205.
13. Charnley J: Postoperative infection after total hip replacement with special reference to air contamination in the operating room. *Clin Orthop* 1972;87:167-187.
14. Charnley J: *Low Friction Arthroplasty of the Hip: Theory and Practice.* Berlin, Springer-Verlag, 1979.
15. Buchholz HW, Elson RA, Heinert K: Antibiotic-loaded acrylic cement: Current concepts. *Clin Orthop* 1984;190:96-108.
16. McNally MA, Small JO, Tofighi HG, et al: Two-stage management of chronic osteomyelitis of the long bones: The Belfast technique. *J Bone Joint Surg* 1993;75B:375-380.
17. Wilde AH, Ruth JT: Two-stage reimplantation in infected total knee arthroplasty. *Clin Orthop* 1988;236:23-35.
18. Gerhart TN, Roux RD, Horowitz G, et al: Antibiotic release from an experimental biodegradable bone cement. *J Orthop Res* 1988;6:585-592.
19. Adams K, Couch L, Cierny G, et al: In vitro and in vivo evaluation of antibiotic diffusion from antibiotic-impregnated polymethylmethacrylate beads. *Clin Orthop* 1992;278:244-252.
20. Baker AS, Greenham LW: Release of gentamicin from acrylic bone cement: Elution and diffusion studies. *J Bone Joint Surg* 1988;70A:1551-1557.
21. Bayston R, Milner RD: The sustained release of antimicrobial drugs from bone cement: An appraisal of laboratory investigations and their significance. *J Bone Joint Surg* 1982;64B:460-464.
22. Chapman MW, Hadley WK: The effect of polymethylmethacrylate and antibiotic combinations on bacterial viability: An in vitro and preliminary in vivo study. *J Bone Joint Surg* 1976;58A:76-81.
23. Elson RA, Jephcott AE, McGechie DB, et al: Antibiotic-loaded acrylic cement. *J Bone Joint Surg* 1977;59B:200-205.
24. Goodell JA, Flick AB, Hebert JC, et al: Preparation and release characteristics of tobramycin-impregnated polymethylmethacrylate beads. *Am J Hosp Pharm* 1986;43:1454-1461.
25. Hill J, Klenerman L, Trustey S, et al: Diffusion of antibiotics from acrylic bone-cement in vitro. *J Bone Joint Surg* 1977;59B:197-199.
26. Hoff SF, Fitzgerald RH Jr, Kelly PJ: The depot administration of penicillin G and gentamicin in acrylic bone cement. *J Bone Joint Surg* 1981;63A:798-804.
27. Kirkpatrick DK, Trachtenberg LS, Mangino PD, et al: In vitro characteristics of tobramycin-PMMA beads: Compressive strength and leaching. *Orthopedics* 1985;8:1130-1133.
28. Kuechle DK, Landon GC, Musher DM, et al: Elution of vancomycin, daptomycin, and amikacin from acrylic bone cement. *Clin Orthop* 1991;264:302-308.
29. Lawson, KJ, Marks KE, Brems J, et al: Vancomycin vs tobramycin elution from polymethylmethacrylate: An in vitro study. *Orthopedics* 1990;13:521-524.
30. Wahlig H, Dingeldein E: Antibiotics and bone cement: Experimental and clinical long-term observations. *Acta Orthop Scand* 1980;51:49-56.
31. Marks KE, Nelson CL, Lautenschlager EP: Antibiotic-impregnated acrylic bone cement. *J Bone Joint Surg* 1976;58A:358-364.
32. Salvati EA, Chekofsky KM, Brause BD, et al: Reimplantation in infection: A 12-year experience. *Clin Orthop* 1982;170:62-75.
33. Wahlig H, Dingeldein E, Buchholz HW, et al: Pharmacokinetic study of gentamicin-loaded cement in total hip replacements: Comparative effects of varying dosage. *J Bone Joint Surg* 1984;66B:175-179.
34. Kendall R, Duncan CP, Smith J, et al: Persistence of bacteria on antibiotic loaded acrylic depots: A reason for caution. Unpublished data.

35. Kendall R, Duncan CP, Beauchamp CP : Bacterial growth on antibiotic-loaded acrylic cement: A prospective in-vivo retrieval study. Unpublished data.
36. Berry DJ, Chandler HP, Reilly DT: The use of bone allografts in two-stage reconstruction after failure of hip replacements due to infection. *J Bone Joint Surg* 1991;73A:1460-1468.
37. Bargar WL, Martin RB, deJesus R, et al: The addition of tobramycin to contrast bone cement: Effect on flexural strength. *J Arthroplasty* 1986;1:165-168.
38. Davies JP, O'Connor DO, Burke DW, et al: Influence of antibiotic impregnation on the fatigue life of Simplex P and Palacos R acrylic bone cements, with and without centrifugation. *J Biomed Mater Res* 1989;23:379-397.
39. Lautenschlager EP, Jacobs JJ, Marshall GW, et al: Mechanical properties of bone cements containing large doses of antibiotic powders. *J Biomed Mater Res* 1976;10:929-938.
40. Lautenschlager EP, Marshall GW, Marks KE, et al: Mechanical strength of acrylic bone cements impregnated with antibiotics. *J Biomed Mater Res* 1976;10:837-845.
41. Josefsson G, Lindberg L, Wiklander B: Systemic antibiotics and gentamicin-containing bone cement in the prophylaxis of postoperative infections in total hip arthroplasty. *Clin Orthop* 1981;159:194-200.
42. Josefsson G, Gudmundsson G, Kolmert L, et al: Prophylaxis with systemic antibiotics versus gentamicin bone cement in total hip arthroplasty: A five-year survey of 1688 hips. *Clin Orthop* 1990;253:173-178.
43. Hope PG, Kristinsson KG, Norman P, et al: Deep infection of cemented total hip arthroplasties caused by coagulase-negative staphylococci. *J Bone Joint Surg* 1989;71B:851-855.
44. Carlsson ÅS, Egund N, Gentz C-F, et al: Radiographic loosening after revision with gentamicin-containing cement for deep infection in total hip arthroplasties. *Clin Orthop* 1985;194:271-279.
45. Elson RA: Exchange arthroplasty for infection: Perspectives from the United Kingdom. *Orthop Clin North Am* 1993;24:761-767.
46. Patterson FP, Brown CS: The McKee-Farrar total hip replacement: Preliminary results and complications of 368 operations performed in five general hospitals. *J Bone Joint Surg* 1972;54A:257-275.
47. Abendschein W: Salvage of infected total hip replacement: Use of antibiotic/PMMA spacer. *Orthopedics* 1992;15:228-229.
48. Buchholz HW, Elson RA, Engelbrecht E, et al: Management of deep infection of total hip replacement. *J Bone Joint Surg* 1981;63B:342-353.
49. Carlsson ÅS, Josefsson G, Lindberg L: Revision with gentamicin-impregnated cement for deep infections in total hip arthroplasties. *J Bone Joint Surg* 1978;60A:1059-1064.
50. Cherney DL, Amstutz HC: Total hip replacement in the previously septic hip. *J Bone Joint Surg* 1983;65A:1256-1265.
51. Duncan CP, Beauchamp CP: The antibiotic loaded hip replacement: A valuable tool in the management of the complex infected total hip arthroplasty. *J Bone Joint Surg* 1991;73B(suppl 2):115.
52. Duncan CP, Beauchamp CP: Total hip replacement for the management of chronic hip infection. *J Bone Joint Surg* 1992; 74B(suppl 3):275.
53. Goodman SB, Schurman DJ: Outcome of infected total hip arthroplasty: An inclusive, consecutive series. *J Arthroplasty* 1988;3:97-102.
54. Hovelius L, Josefsson G: An alternative method for exchange operation of infected arthroplasty. *Acta Orthop Scand* 1979;50:93-96.
55. Hunter G, Dandy D: The natural history of the patient with an infected total hip replacement. *J Bone Joint Surg* 1977;59B:293-297.
56. James ET, Hunter GA, Cameron HU: Total hip revision arthroplasty: Does sepsis influence the results? *Clin Orthop* 1982;170:88-94.
57. Nasser S: Prevention and treatment of sepsis in total hip replacement surgery. *Orthop Clin North Am* 1992;23:265-277.
58. Salvati EA, Callaghan JJ, Brause BD, et al: Reimplantation in infection: Elution of gentamicin from cement and beads. *Clin Orthop* 1986;207:83-93.
59. Sanzén L, Carlsson ÅS, Josefsson G, et al: Revision operations on infected total hip arthroplasties: Two- to nine-year follow-up study. *Clin Orthop* 1988;229:165-172.
60. Wilson MG, Dorr LD: Reimplantation of infected total hip arthroplasties in the absence of antibiotic cement. *J Arthroplasty* 1989;4:263-269.
61. Wroblewski BM: One-stage revision of infected cemented total hip arthroplasty. *Clin Orthop* 1986;211:103-107.
62. Elson R, Norman P, Scott I, et al: Exchange cemented joint arthroplasties for deep infection. *J Bone Joint Surg* 1992;74B(suppl 3): 295.
63. Evans RP, Nelson CL: Staged reimplantation of a total hip prosthesis after infection with Candida albicans: A report of two cases. *J Bone Joint Surg* 1990;72A:1551-1553.
64. McDonald DJ, Fitzgerald RH Jr, Ilstrup DM: Two-stage reconstruction of a total hip arthroplasty because of infection. *J Bone Joint Surg* 1989;71A:828-834.
65. Zilkens K-W, Casser H-R, Ohnsorge J: Treatment of an old infection in a total hip replacement with an interim spacer prosthesis. *Arch Orthop Trauma Surg* 1990;109:94-96.
66. Buchholz HW: Results of exchange operations for infection, in Elson RA, Caldwell ADS (eds): *Revision Arthroplasty: Proceedings of a Symposium Held at Sheffield University.* Oxford, Medical Education Services, 1979, pp 103-110.
67. Duncan CP, Beauchamp C: A temporary antibiotic-loaded joint replacement system for management of complex infections involving the hip. *Orthop Clin North Am* 1993;24:751-759.
68. Harris WH, McGann WA: Loosening of the femoral component after use of the medullary-plug cementing technique: Follow-up note with a minimum five-year follow-up. *J Bone Joint Surg* 1986;68A:1064-1066.
69. Miley GB, Scheller AD Jr, Turner RH: Medical and surgical treatment of the septic hip with one-stage revision arthroplasty. *Clin Orthop* 1982;170:76-82.
70. Duncan CP, Masri B: Editorial. Antibiotic depots. *J Bone Joint Surg* 1993;75B:349-350.

Foot and Ankle

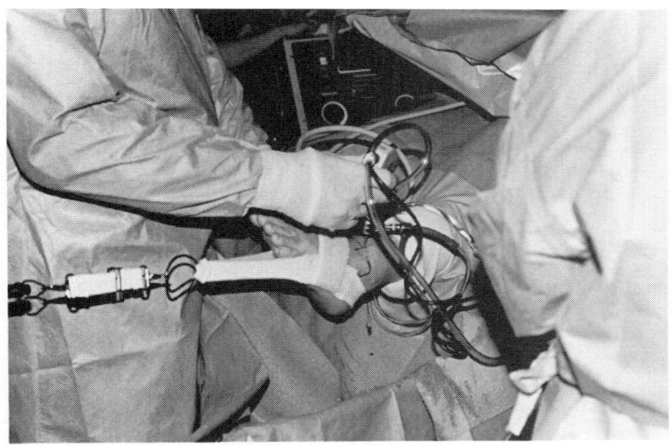

CHAPTER 27

Ankle Fractures in Children

Alvin H. Crawford, MD

Fractures of the distal tibial physis have been reported to be the most common physeal injuries in children.[1] All of the major ligamentous structures about the ankle, except the interosseous ligament, either insert on or originate from the tibial and fibular epiphyses. As a result, when trauma is absorbed through the ankle joint in young children, the physeal structures are more likely to fail than are the ligaments. The physis is involved in more than 50% of tibial fractures and in approximately 75% of fibular fractures.[1]

Ankle injuries commonly are caused by indirect violence, with the fixed foot being forced into eversion, inversion, plantar flexion, external rotation, or dorsiflexion.[2] Fractures also may be caused by direct violence, such as motor vehicle accidents, falls from heights, or contact sports. The type of fracture caused by these forces differs with the age of the child (Fig. 1). Salter-Harris type I through IV injuries usually occur in younger children with open physes; triplane and Tillaux fractures occur in older children in whom the asymmetric physeal closure (from middle to medial side to lateral side) has begun.[3-5]

Diagnosis

Anteroposterior and lateral views should always be taken, and if swelling is severe an oblique view is recommended. All structures around the ankle should be systematically evaluated, including the soft tissues. The normal fat stripe surrounding a bone may be thickened after nondisplaced fracture. The medial and lateral soft tissue usually show increased density and haziness after severe trauma (Fig. 2). Marked swelling ("goose egg") over the lateral aspect of the ankle with an apparently undisplaced Salter-Harris

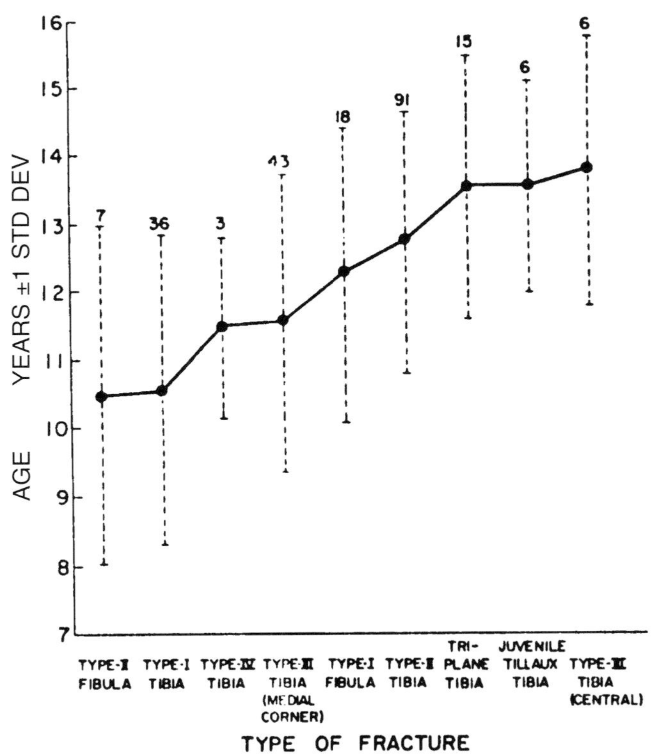

Fig. 1 Type of distal tibial and fibular fractures according to age. (Reproduced with permission from Spiegel PG, Cooperman DR, Laros GS: Epiphyseal fractures of the distal ends of the tibia and fibula: A retrospective study of two hundred and thirty-seven cases in children. *J Bone Joint Surg* 1978;60A:1046-1050.)

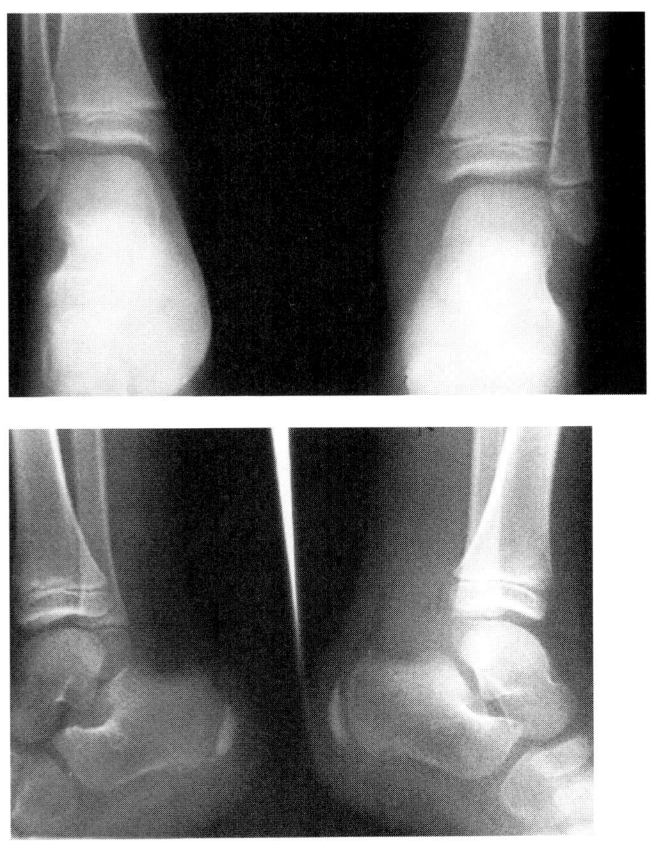

Fig. 2 **Top,** On the anteroposterior view, note the increase in soft tissue density adjacent to the medial malleolus in the injured left ankle compared to the uninjured right ankle. **Bottom,** On the lateral view, the soft tissue density is limited by the fat stripe just anterior to the Achilles tendon shadow, suggesting that an effusion is displacing the posterior soft tissues.

type I fracture of the fibula may indicate that some displacement occurred at the time of injury or that a hematoma is developing. Anteroposterior, lateral, and mortise views should be examined before any type of reduction maneuver.

Treatment

The primary indicators for surgical treatment are open fractures, inability to obtain or maintain closed reduction, displaced physeal or articular fractures, and evidence of massive soft-tissue injury.

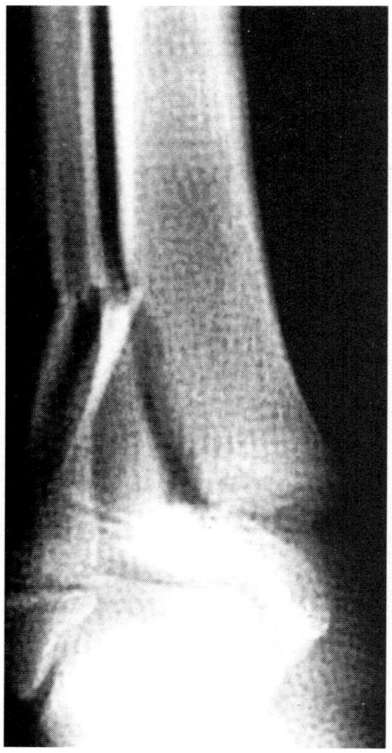

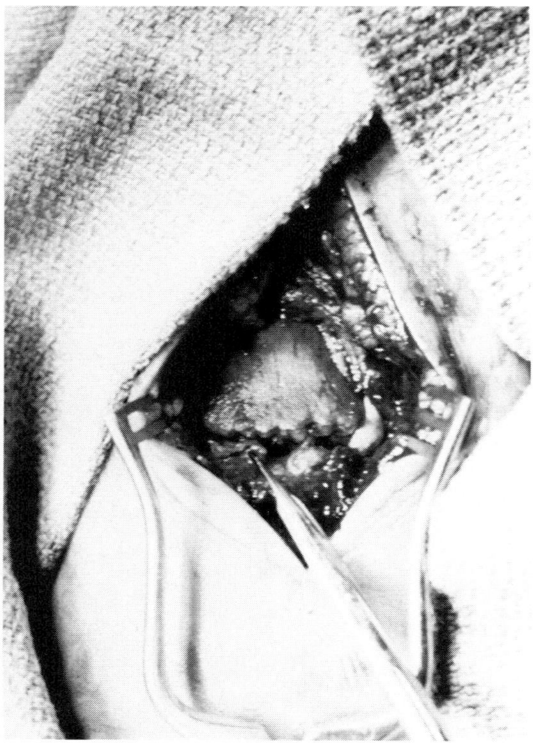

Fig. 3 **Top left,** Multiple attempts failed to obtain anatomic closed reduction of this Salter-Harris type II fracture. **Top right,** At surgery, periosteum was found to be interposed between fragments. **Bottom left,** After removal of the periosteum, anatomic reduction was obtained. **Bottom right,** The fracture healed with no evidence of growth arrest. (Courtesy of Dr. Russell Clark)

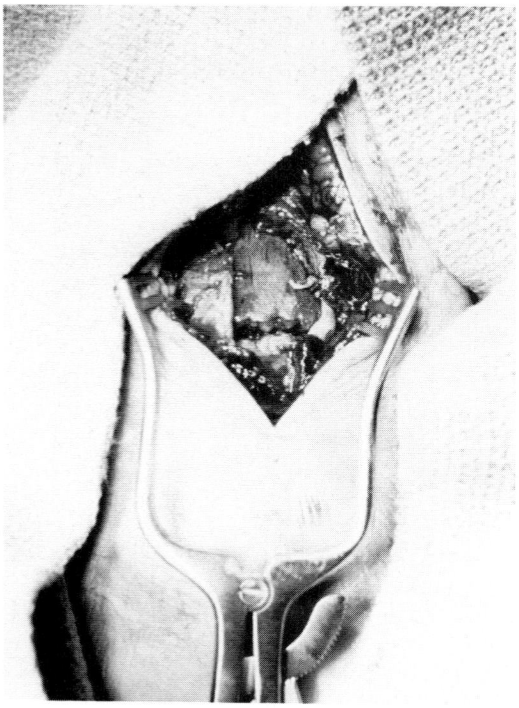

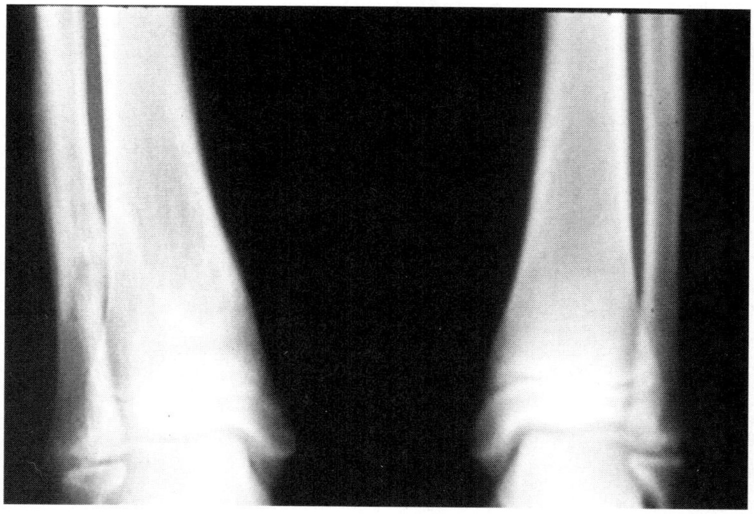

Salter-Harris Types I and II Distal Tibial Epiphyseal Fractures

Salter-Harris types I and II fractures of the distal tibial epiphysis usually can be treated by closed reduction and the application of a bent-knee, long-leg cast. In young children, moderate displacement after closed reduction, especially in the anteroposterior plane, is acceptable, but varus or valgus angulation in older children and adolescents with type I or II fractures will not correct spontaneously.[5-7] If an anatomic reduction can be obtained by closed manipulation, the fracture can be stabilized with percutaneous Steinmann pins, Kirschner wires, or a cannulated screw.

Occasionally, the lateral or posterolateral tibial metaphyseal fragment is caught behind the fibula, making reduction difficult. In severely displaced type II fractures, the periosteum opposite the metaphyseal fragment may be entrapped in the fracture, preventing reduction (Fig. 3). Either of these situations may require open reduction.

Salter-Harris Types III and IV Medial Malleolar Fractures

In young children, faster healing and better remodeling than in older patients usually produces better results with closed reduction of fractures. In ankle fractures, however, this is not always true, especially in types III and IV fractures.[3,8-10] Because of the longer period of growth remaining, the potential for deformity is greater, and accurate reduction is as important in young children as it is in older children and adolescents.

Salter-Harris types III and IV fractures, which must be anatomically reduced to less than 2 mm of displacement, usually require open reduction and internal fixation. The use of tomograms and CT scanning can help determine acceptable displacement. Types III and IV fractures are almost always medial at the plafond. Often a tiny triangular piece of bone is present on the metaphyseal side in type IV fractures. This piece of bone should be removed at open reduction to aid exposure of the physis and perhaps prevent the formation of a bony bar in this area.

For anatomic reduction of types III and IV fractures, adequate exposure of the physis and articular surfaces is mandatory. Soft-tissue dissection can be minimized by placing the incision over the fracture gap, where the periosteum usually is elevated. After the wound has been irrigated, any clots removed, and bony debris curetted, it is usually possible to realign the fracture. Transverse transepiphyseal Kirschner wires or small fragment screws may be used for internal fixation.

Tillaux Fractures

Tillaux fractures occur primarily in older adolescents, after the medial part of the physis has closed but before the lateral part closes.[1,11-13] The fracture line runs through the physis, across the epiphysis, and distally into the joint, creating a Salter-Harris type III or IV fracture. Most juvenile Tillaux fractures can be reduced with gentle internal rotation, but displaced fractures usually

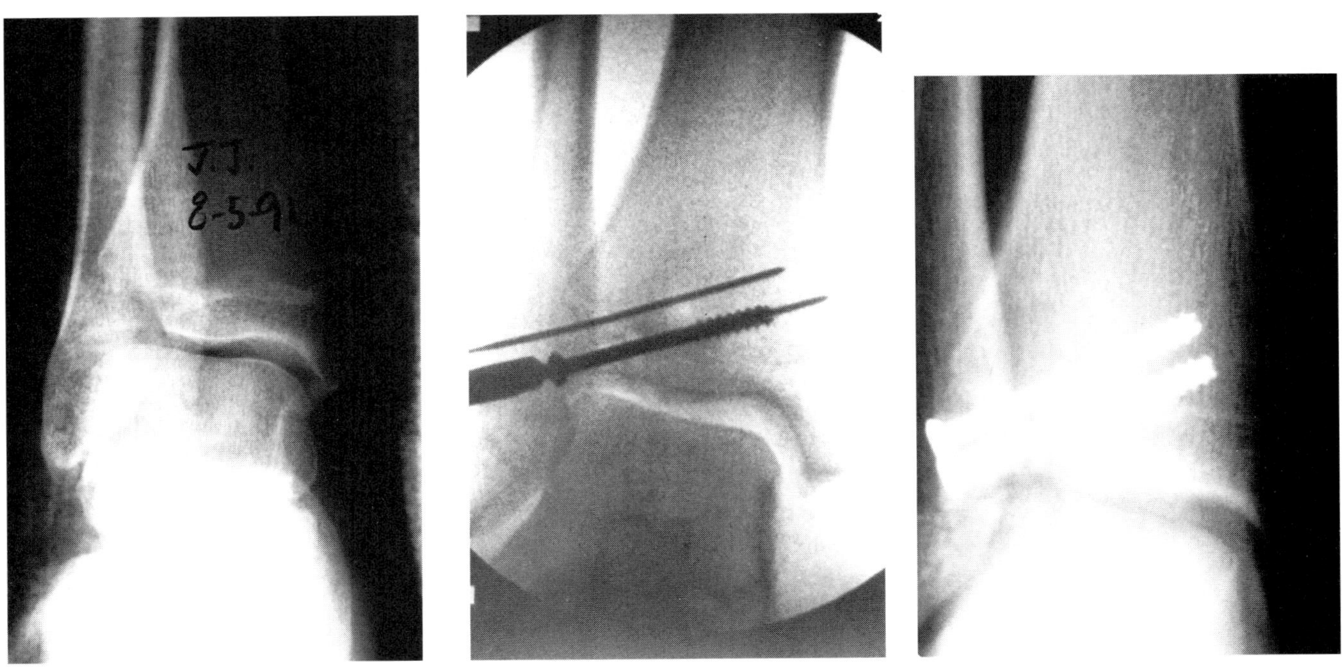

Fig. 4 **Left,** Minimally displaced Tillaux fracture was reduced closed and splint was applied. **Center,** Because reduction was unsatisfactory, indirect reduction was performed with a small guide pin and direct compression of the fragment. Two cannulated screws were then placed obliquely across fracture because skeletal growth was almost complete. **Right,** Eight months after injury, fracture is completely healed.

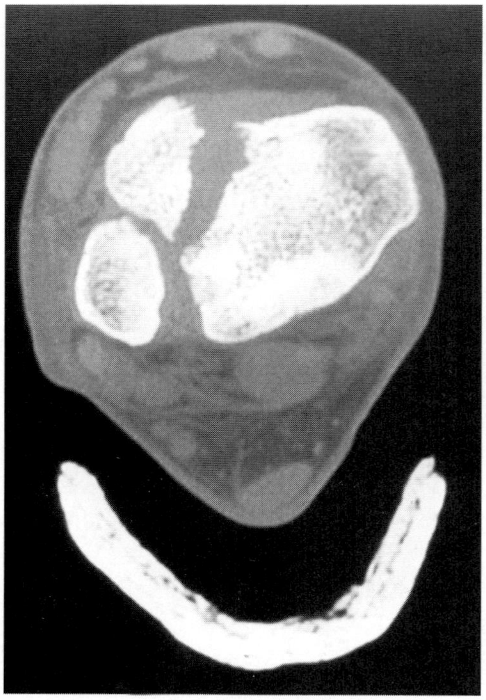

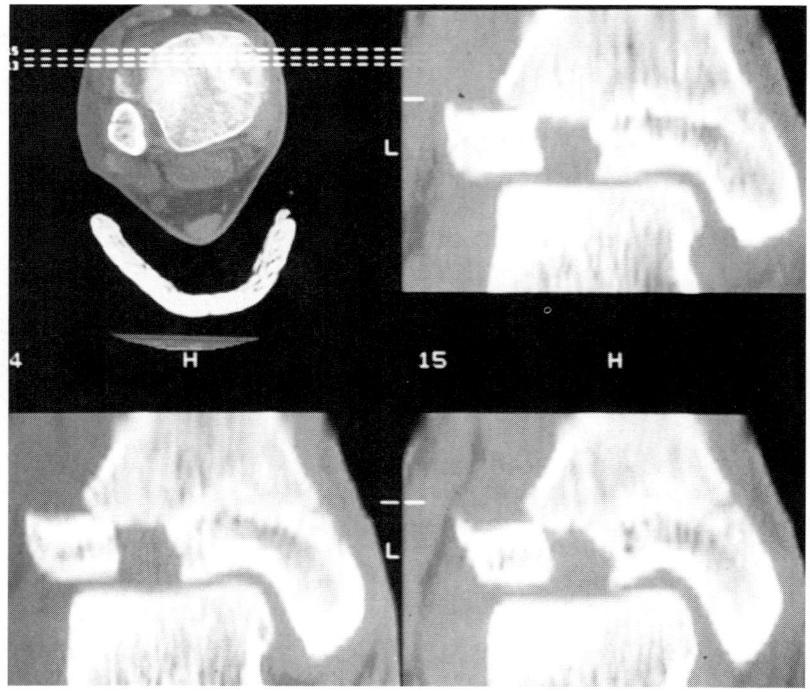

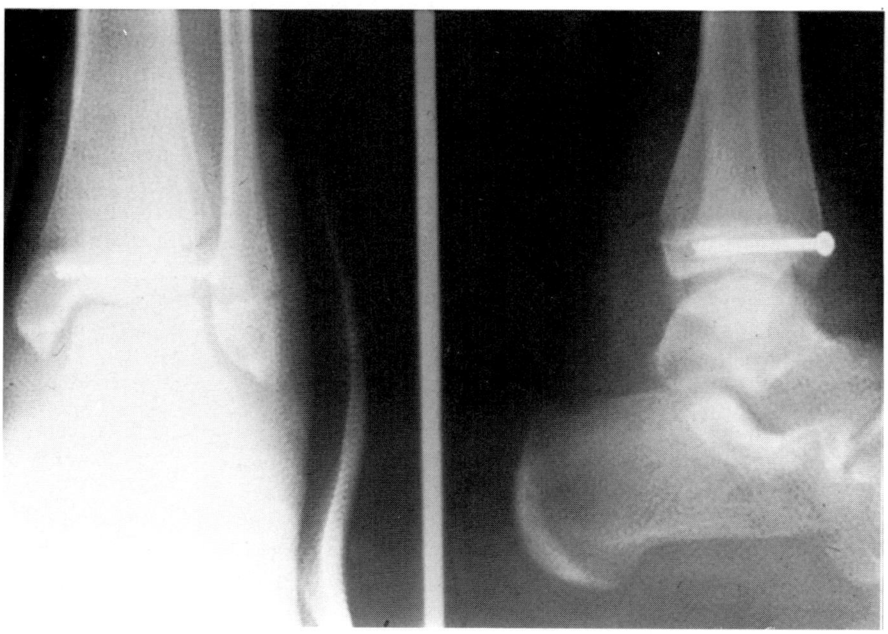

Fig. 5 **Top left,** CT scan of displaced Tillaux fracture. **Top right,** Three-dimensional reconstructed coronal view confirms the amount of displacement. **Bottom,** After indirect reduction and fixation with a cannulated interfragmentary screw placed horizontally because of remaining growth potential.

require open reduction and internal fixation.[14] The fracture fragment pulled off by the anterior tibiofibular ligament is almost always anterior, and osteotomy of the fibula is not necessary for exposure.

For moderately displaced Tillaux fractures, indirect reduction with a Steinmann pin may be attempted (Fig. 4).[15] For indirect reduction, the pin is inserted through the distal fragment and is used as a joy stick to lever the fragment into anatomic alignment. Direct manual compression is applied, and the pin is passed across the fracture. Once anatomic reduction and alignment are obtained, cast immobilization or a cannulated screw placed over the pin can be used to maintain stability. CT scanning is helpful to determine the amount of displacement (Fig. 5).

Triplane Fractures

Triplane fractures consist of three fragments: (1) the anterolateral portion of the distal tibial epiphysis, (2) the remainder of the epiphysis (anteromedial and posterior

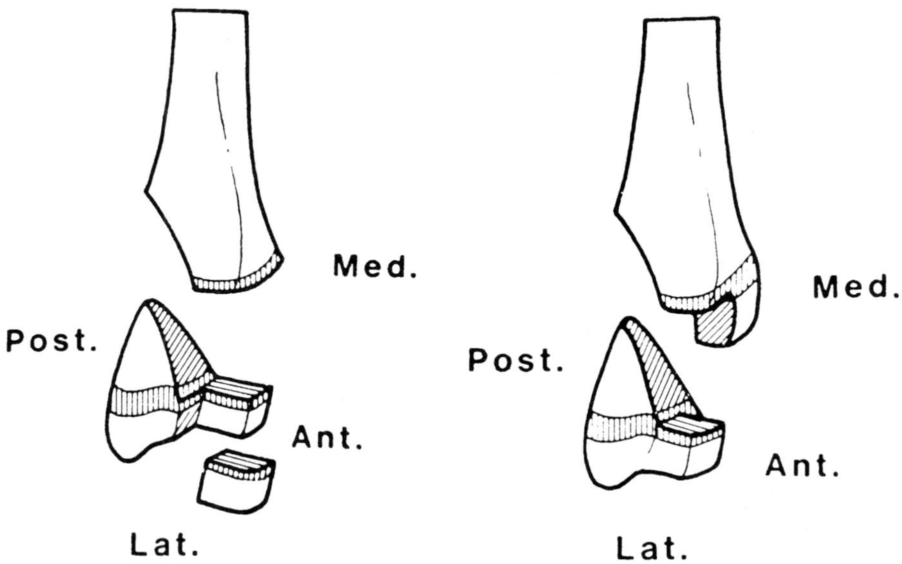

Fig. 6 Triplane fractures. **Left,** Three-part fracture. **Right,** Two-part fracture.

portions) with an attached posterolateral spike of the distal tibial metaphysis, and (3) the remainder of the distal tibial metaphysis and tibial shaft (Fig. 6, *left*). The fracture lines run in three planes: coronal, transverse, and sagittal. Two-part fractures also may result from this fracture pattern (Fig. 6, *right*).[3,4,11,13] Dias and Giegerich[11] found that three-part fractures occurred in younger patients and required surgical treatment more often than did two-part fractures.

Closed reduction may be achieved by internal rotation of the foot. If closed reduction cannot be achieved, indirect reduction techniques may be successful (Fig. 7), but usually open reduction and internal fixation are required. Because of the complex fracture pattern and large fragments, reduction often is difficult and can require extensive dissection. For three-part fractures, open reduction of both the Salter-Harris type II and type III components is necessary. First, the Salter-Harris type III component should be approached laterally. If adequate open reduction can be achieved, the Salter-Harris type II component (medially) may be treated closed; if not, both components require open reduction.

Complications

Using the Salter-Harris classification, Spiegel and associates[5] grouped 183 fractures of the distal tibia and fibula according to the risk of shortening, angular deformity, and joint incongruity (Outline 1). The most frequent and most serious complication after ankle fractures in growing children is premature asymmetrical closure of the physis (Fig. 8).[5-7,10] Medial malleolar fractures with Salter-Harris type III or IV components have the highest risk for this complication.

Outline 1
Classification of distal tibial and fibular fractures according to risk of complications

Low risk group (89) 6.7% complications
- Types I and II fibular fractures
- Type I tibial fractures
- Types III and IV tibial fractures with < 2 mm displacement
- Epiphyseal avulsion injuries

High risk group (28) 32% complications
- Types III and IV tibial fractures with > 2 mm displacement
- Juvenile Tillaux fractures
- Comminuted tibial epiphyseal fractures (type V)

Unpredictable group (66) 16.7% complications
- Type II tibial fractures

(Adapted from Spiegel PG, Cooperman DR, Laros GS: Epiphyseal fractures of the distal ends of the tibia and fibular: A retrospective study of two hundred and thirty-seven cases in children. *J Bone Joint Surg* 1978;60A:1046-1050.)

Severe leg length discrepancy is an infrequent complication of physeal injury at the ankle, because, except with severe compression injuries in very young children, varus deformity is more likely than significant shortening. Approximately 50% of the growth of the tibia is through the distal physis (approximately .25 inch per year). Angulation deformities after physeal injury at the ankle usually are painless varus deformities that do not impair function. Varus angulation after Salter-Harris types III and IV fractures usually is evident within 6 to 18 months of injury.

Residual joint incongruity may cause posttraumatic arthritis, especially after triplane fractures with significant articular disruption. Nonunion and delayed union are rare, as is osteonecrosis.

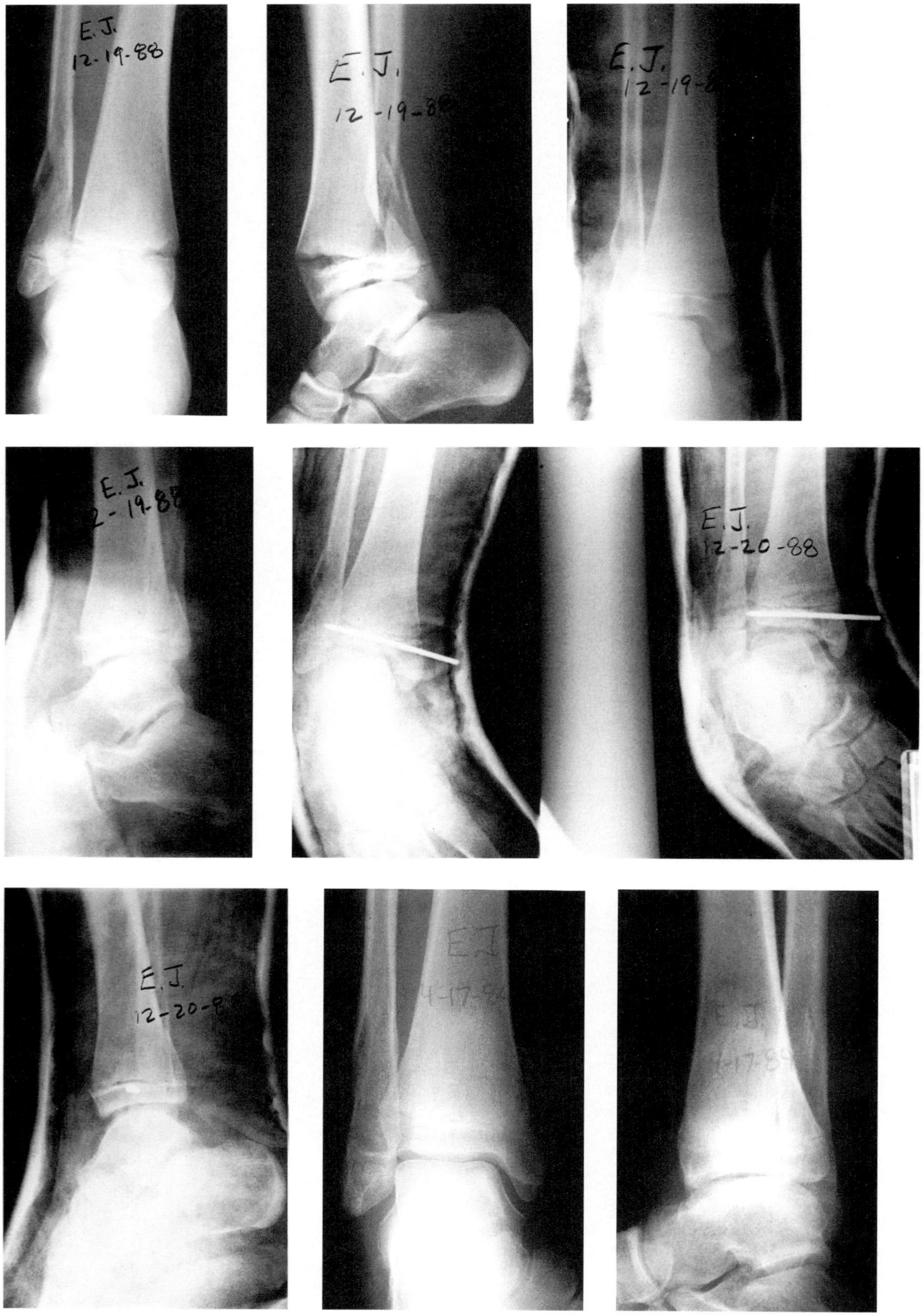

Fig. 7 Two-part triplane fracture. **Top left,** Anteroposterior view shows Salter-Harris type III distal tibial fracture and comminuted nondisplaced fibular fracture. **Top center,** Lateral view shows Salter-Harris type II fracture. **Top right** and **center left,** Closed reduction failed to obtain acceptable reduction. **Center right,** After indirect reduction and percutaneous Steinmann pin fixation. **Bottom left, bottom center,** and **bottom right,** Three months after pin removal, subchondral surface is anatomic. (Reproduced with permission from Crawford AH: Fractures and dislocations of the foot and ankle, in Green DE, Swiontkowski MF (eds): *Skeletal Trauma in Children.* Philadelphia, PA, WB Saunders, 1993.)

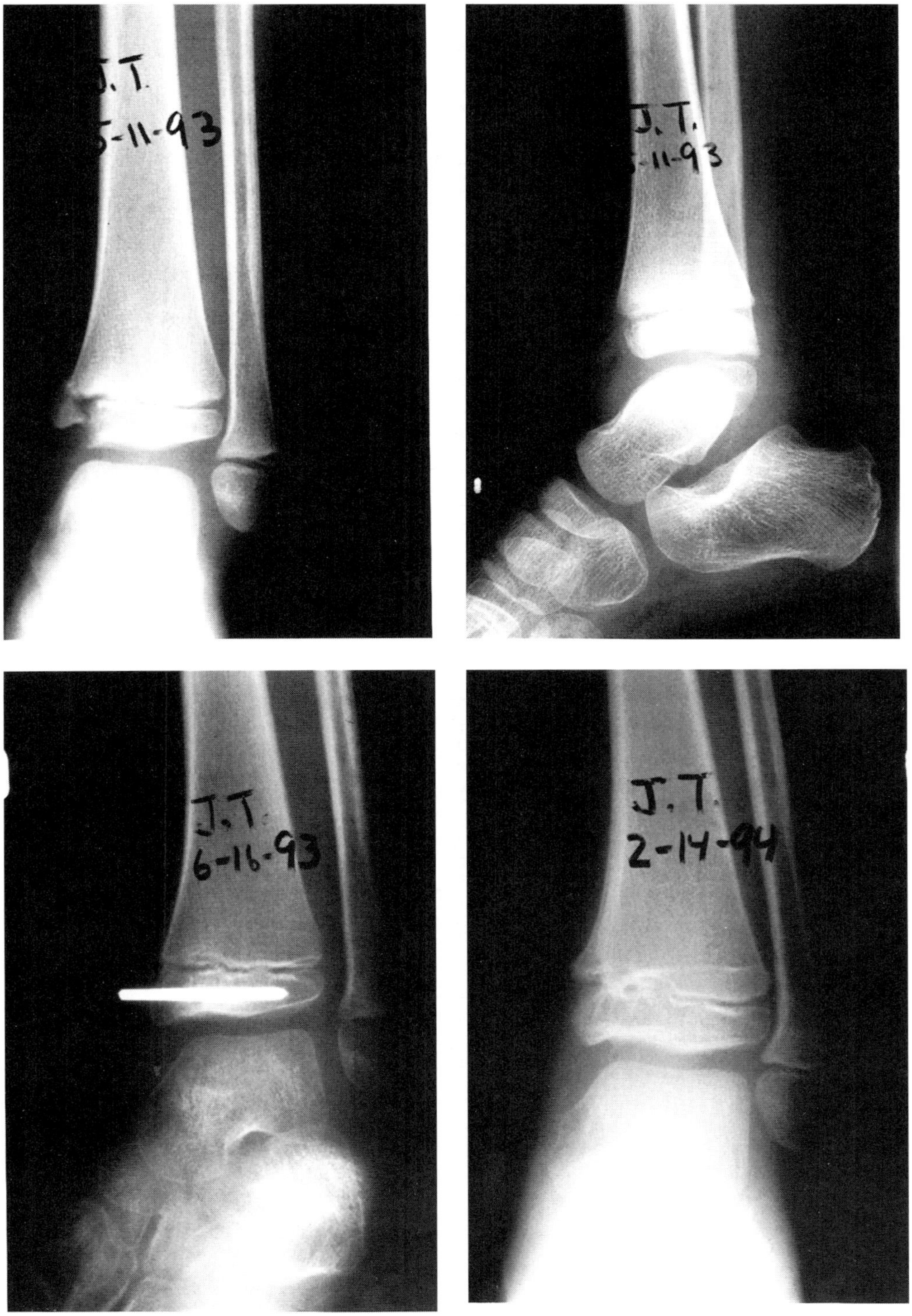

Fig. 8 **Top left** and **right,** Displaced Salter-Harris type IV fracture with small, minimally displaced metaphyseal fragment; note also Salter-Harris type II fracture of distal fibula. **Bottom left,** After open reduction, removal of metaphyseal fragment, and fixation with Steinmann pin. **Bottom right,** Nine months after injury, a physeal bar is developing at the fracture line; note the undulation (Poland's hump) just lateral to the bar and angulation of growth disturbance line. Physeal bar excision was performed.

Pearls and Pitfalls

Pearls

Soft-tissue swelling over the distal fibula after ankle sprain usually indicates injury to the distal fibular physis. This injury rarely results in growth arrest and can be treated with compression and immobilization.

The presence of interosseous ligament calcification after ankle sprain indicates an unrecognized fracture.

In Salter-Harris type II injuries of the distal tibia, the distal fragment may be rotated more than is apparent on radiographs; an oblique view usually will identify any displacement.

Salter-Harris type II fractures of the distal tibial usually can be treated closed; a less-than-perfect reduction is preferable to risking iatrogenic physeal damage from delayed or repeated manipulations. Less than 5° of varus and up to 10° of valgus are acceptable. Angulation into plantar flexion should be avoided.

An epiphyseal fragment gap of more than 2 mm requires anatomic reduction; if adequacy of the reduction is questionable, CT scanning should be used.

Any fixation (wires, pins, screws) should be placed to avoid both the joint surface and the physis. In type III or IV fractures, they should not be placed from the tip of the medial malleolus across the physis and into the metaphysis, as is done in adults, because this type of fixation in children is likely to further damage the physis.

After physeal injury, children should be followed until skeletal maturity.[7] Follow-up radiographs should be carefully checked for the presence of a growth disturbance line,[16] which normally appears and grows parallel to the physeal line. If the line appears angled toward the fracture site and is no longer parallel to the physis, bony bar formation should be suspected.[16] CT scan, MRI, or tomograms should be obtained for evaluation. Physeal bridging has been reported to occur as late as 2 years after injury, but usually is evident within 6 to 18 months of injury.[6]

Pitfalls

Soft-tissue interposition (usually the periosteum) may prevent anatomic reduction and may require removal, especially in Salter-Harris type II distal tibial fractures.

In Salter-Harris types III and IV injuries, failure to reduce the physeal and epiphyseal fracture to less than 2 mm may cause growth arrest and/or angular deformity.

Stripping of the periosteum around the physis may injure the perichondral ring and cause peripheral growth arrest.

Joint incongruity, especially after triplane fractures, frequently results in degenerative joint disease and arthrosis; if displacement and articular joint incongruity can be reduced to less than 2 mm with closed methods, a percutaneous pin or interfragmentary cannulated screw may be used for fixation of the articular surface only. If anatomic reduction cannot be obtained with closed methods, open reduction and fixation are indicated.

References

1. Mann DC, Rajmaira S: Distribution of physeal and nonphyseal fractures in 2,650 long-bone fractures in children aged 0-16 years. *J Pediatr Orthop* 1990;10:713-716.
2. Kärrholm J, Hansson LI, Laurin S: Supination-eversion injuries of the ankle in children: A retrospective study of radiographic classification and treatment. *J Pediatr Orthop* 1982;2:147-159.
3. Cooperman DR, Spiegel PG, Laros GS: Tibial fractures involving the ankle in children: The so-called triplane epiphyseal fracture. *J Bone Joint Surg* 1978;60A:1040-1046.
4. Peiró A, Aracil J, Martos F, et al: Triplane distal tibial epiphyseal fracture. *Clin Orthop* 1981;160:196-200.
5. Spiegel PG, Cooperman DR, Laros GS: Epiphyseal fractures of the distal ends of the tibia and fibula: A retrospective study of two hundred and thirty-seven cases in children. *J Bone Joint Surg* 1978;60A:1046-1050.
6. Kärrholm J, Hansson LI, Svensson K: Prediction of growth pattern after ankle fractures in children. *J Pediatr Orthop* 1983;3:319-325.
7. Kling TF Jr, Bright RW, Hensinger RN: Distal tibial physeal fractures in children that may require open reduction. *J Bone Joint Surg* 1984;66A:647-657.
8. Beaty JH, Linton RC: Medial malleolar fracture in a child: A case report. *J Bone Joint Surg* 1988;70A:1254-1255.
9. Cass JR, Peterson HA: Salter-Harris Type IV injuries of the distal tibial epiphyseal growth plate, with emphasis on those involving the medial malleolus. *J Bone Joint Surg* 1983;65A:1959-1070.
10. Kling TF Jr: Operative treatment of ankle fractures in children. *Orthop Clin North Am* 1990;21:381-392.
11. Dias LS, Giegerich CR: Fractures of the distal tibial epiphysis in adolescence. *J Bone Joint Surg* 1983;65A:438-444.
12. Letts RM: The hidden adolescent ankle fracture. *J Pediatr Orthop* 1982;2:161-164.
13. von Laer L: Classification, diagnosis, and treatment of transitional fractures of the distal part of the tibia. *J Bone Joint Surg* 1985;67A:687-698.
14 Manderson EL, Ollivierre CO: Closed anatomic reduction of a juvenile Tillaux fracture by dorsiflexion of the ankle: A case report. *Clin Orthop* 1992;276:262-266.
15. Schlesinger I, Wedge JH: Percutaneous reduction and fixation of displaced juvenile Tillaux fractures: A new surgical technique. *J Pediatr Orthop* 1993;13:389-391.
16. Hynes D, O'Brien T: Growth disturbance lines after injury of the distal tibial physis: Their significance in prognosis. *J Bone Joint Surg* 1988;70B:231-233.

CHAPTER 28

Arthroscopic Surgery of the Ankle

J. Whit Ewing, MD
James A. Tasto, MD
Joe W. Tippett, MD

Arthroscopic ankle surgery is an established technique for treatment of a variety of pathologic conditions.[1-4] Perhaps the clearest indication for ankle arthroscopy is the presence of an intra-articular loose body.[5,6] This relatively uncommon condition is most frequently the result of osteochondritis dissecans, often referred to as talar dome fracture. Anterior ankle impingement syndrome, either from soft tissue or osteophytic etiology, is probably the most common indication for ankle arthroscopy.[6,7] Arthroscopically assisted ankle arthrodesis is now recognized as an effective technique.[8] There have been sporadic reports of ankle arthroscopy as an adjunct to treatment of acute ankle fractures, stabilization procedures, rheumatoid synovectomy, and other pathologic conditions.[1,9-14] This chapter is limited to the discussion of a technique for ankle arthroscopy. The room setup, surgical instrumentation, noninvasive distraction method, and portal placements for diagnostic as well as surgical arthroscopy of the ankle are presented. Specific emphasis is placed on the indications for and the techniques of arthroscopic surgical management of talar dome fractures, anterior impingement lesions, and arthrodesis.

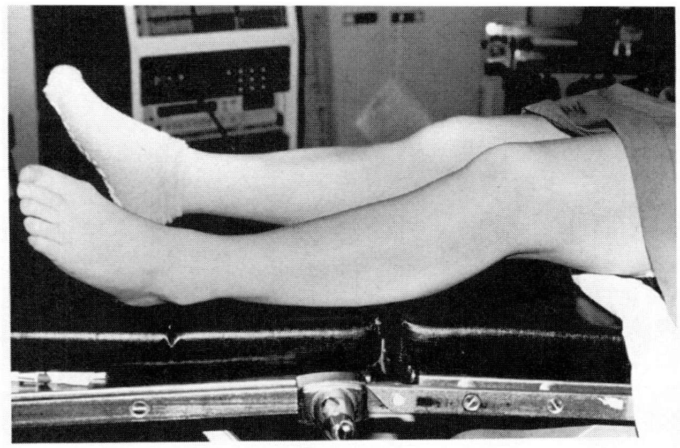

Fig. 1 The patient is positioned so that the midcalf is directly over the table break between the foot and body of the operating table.

Room Setup

A standard operating table with a head extension is used. The patient is placed in the supine position, and moved proximally on the table so that the mid-calf level rests at the break point for the foot of the table. The operating room should be large enough to accommodate the noninvasive distraction device, which protrudes approximately 60 inches beyond the foot of the table. A standard video arthroscopy cart is placed adjacent to the patient's left shoulder and angled to allow comfortable visualization by the operating room personnel. General or spinal anesthesia is preferred in order to overcome resistance to ankle joint distraction from muscular tension. A sterile draped surgical stand is positioned over the patient's midsection for placement of frequently used surgical instruments. The instrument table is situated distal to the operating table to allow easy passage of instruments. The arthroscopic fluid pump is placed at the head of the table, allowing the tubing to enter the surgical field in an unobtrusive manner.

Surgical Instrumentation

A 2.7-mm arthroscope is used for arthroscopic visualization. Both a 25° and a 70° fore-oblique lens should be available. The cannula used for the arthroscope should have a 3.5-mm diameter, which is 0.3 mm larger in diameter than the standard cannula offered with the smaller arthroscopes. Use of a cannula with a slightly larger diameter permits improved flow of the distending fluid. Sterile saline is used for joint distention, and an automated inflow device (pump) is employed. The inflow is directed through the arthroscope cannula by means of an adapter attached to the single side port of the sheath. A pressure of 50 mm Hg is used throughout the procedure. Standard video arthroscopic equipment is used, and electronic printing/recording devices can be used as desired. Instruments commonly used for knee and shoulder arthroscopy can also be used for ankle arthroscopy. The use of smaller instruments for ankle arthroscopy, however, promotes easier entry into the joint and less articular cartilage scuffing. Small joint instrument systems are available from a variety of manufacturers. The most frequently used instruments include a probe, grasping forceps, an intra-articular shaver, small arthroscopic knives, and curettes. A 3.5-mm diameter shaver blade works nicely within the ankle joint and does not require the use of a different hand piece from that used for knee arthroscopy. Some arthroscopists have reported that they can carry out

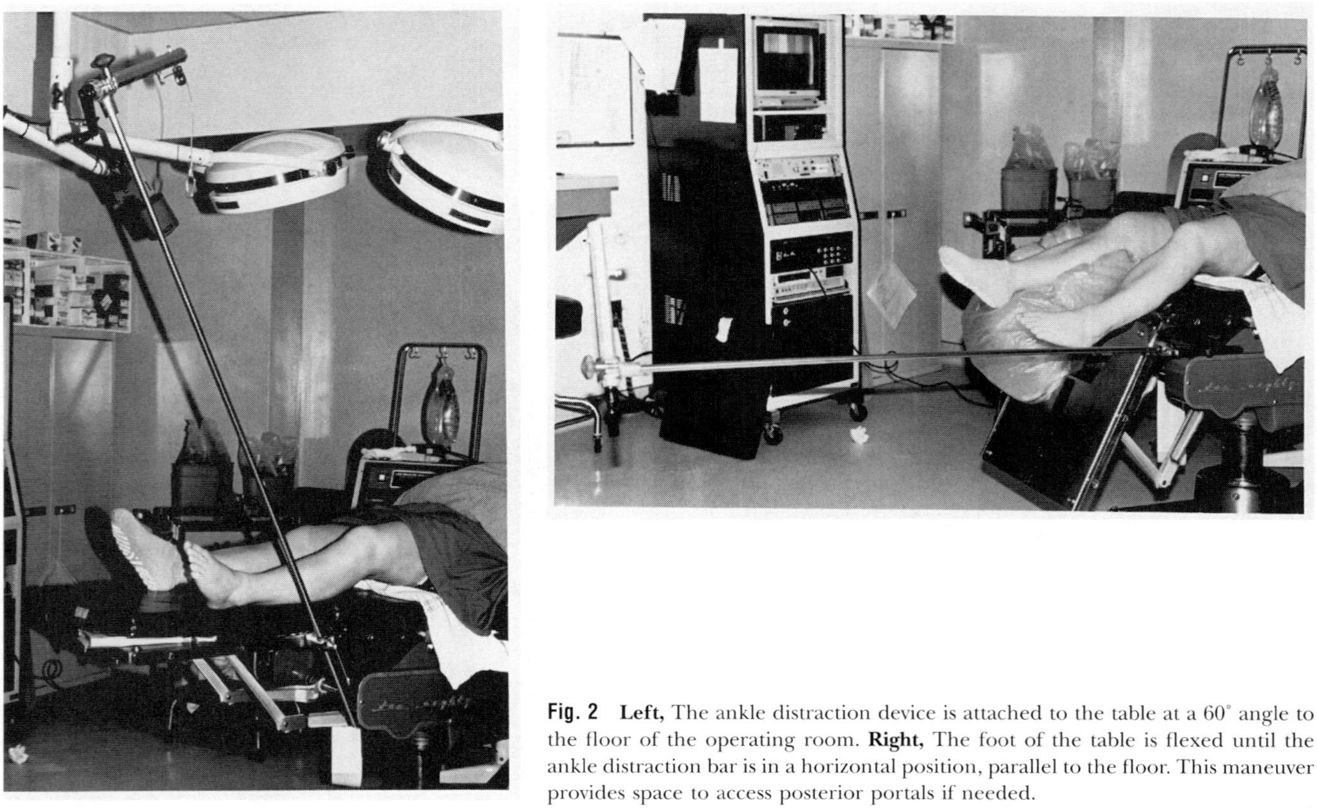

Fig. 2 **Left,** The ankle distraction device is attached to the table at a 60° angle to the floor of the operating room. **Right,** The foot of the table is flexed until the ankle distraction bar is in a horizontal position, parallel to the floor. This maneuver provides space to access posterior portals if needed.

arthroscopic ankle procedures without mechanical distraction of the joint.[15] For the most part, however, some form of mechanical ankle distraction device is preferred.[6,16] The distraction device may be either invasive or noninvasive. The invasive techniques require the drilling of pins into the tibia and the calcaneus. The noninvasive method depends on the use of a padded strap system that applies enough distraction to allow adequate entry into the ankle joint in all but a small percentage of cases.

Technique of Diagnostic Ankle Arthroscopy

The anesthetized patient is positioned with the midcalf level of the leg located over the break between the middle and the foot of the table (Fig. 1). A thigh tourniquet is inflated to 350 mm Hg after the leg has been elevated for 60 seconds. At this time, the noninvasive ankle distraction bar is affixed to the table on the side of the affected ankle. The bar is locked into position at a 60° angle to the floor (Fig. 2, *left*). The foot of the operating table is now flexed until the distraction bar is parallel to the floor of the operating room (Fig. 2, *right*). This allows free access to the ankle joint from both anterior and posterior approaches. The lower leg, including the foot and ankle, is now prepped and draped in a routine fashion. The anatomic landmarks for portal placement are outlined with a marking pencil prior to placement of the distraction straps. Finally, the prepackaged, presterilized ankle distraction straps are placed on the foot and, in turn, attached to the extension strap, the tensionometer, and to the distraction pulley cable (Fig. 3, *left*). The room circulating personnel can now apply traction to the ankle until 24 to 26 lbs traction is achieved as determined by reading the tensionometer. At this point, the entire nonsterilized portion of the apparatus is draped in a sterile fashion (Fig. 3, *right*).

Anteromedial and anterolateral portals are now created. The anteromedial portal is located immediately adjacent to the medial border of the anterior tibial tendon, at the level of the ankle joint line. This site is located with the use of an 18-gauge spinal needle. Several attempts may be necessary but, generally, the needle should be inserted easily into the ankle. Proper insertion is achieved when the needle rests within the joint, and the needle is not angulated in a cephalad or a caudad direction. Once proper needle placement is achieved, the ankle is distended with saline by means of syringe distention. The fluid should flow freely from the syringe with little resistance. When resistance is felt, the surgeon can appreciate a bulging soft spot in the location of the anterolateral aspect of the ankle. Pressure is maintained on the syringe to preserve the soft

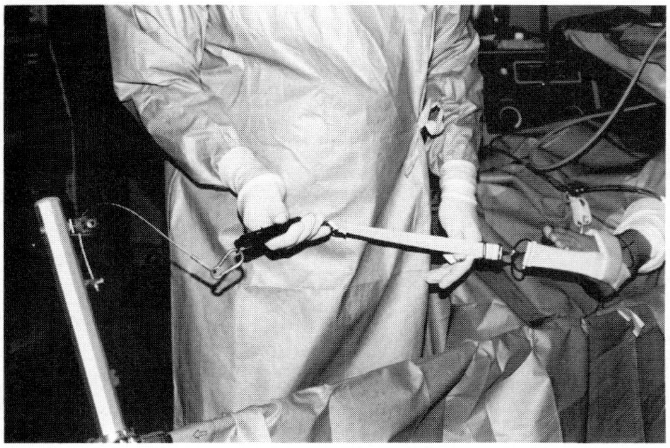

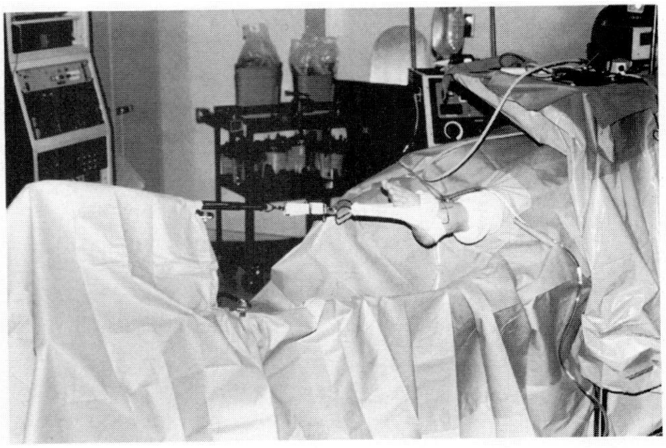

Fig. 3 **Left,** The traction assembly, including the foot straps, the extention strap, and the tensionometer are placed. The surgeon is seen to be holding the sterilized tensionometer. Traction has not yet been applied. **Right,** Final draping of the patient with traction applied to the ankle.

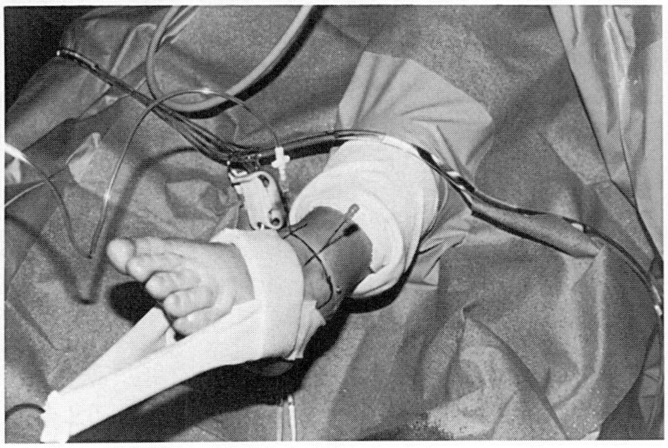

Fig. 4 Proper positioning of spinal needles into the anteromedial and anterolateral portals. The anteromedial portal needle is attached to a 50-cc syringe, which allows saline distention by manual means.

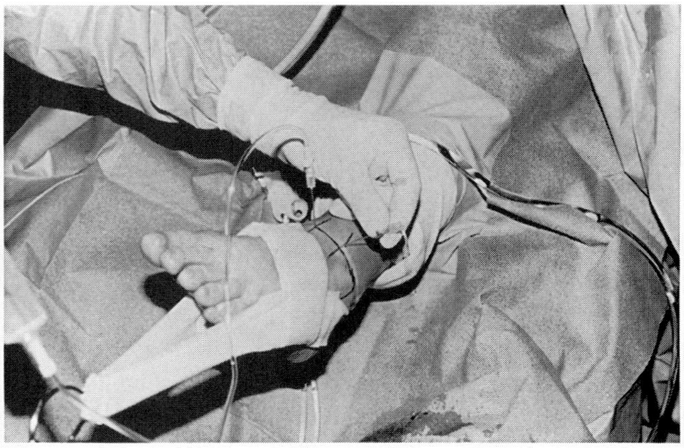

Fig. 5 Free flow of saline from the anterolaterally placed needle confirms accurate needle placement.

spot, and a second 18-gauge spinal needle is inserted into the joint anterolaterally (Fig. 4). This point of insertion is in the area of the soft spot, immediately adjacent to the medial border of the palpable peroneus tertius tendon, at the joint line level. An alternate placement position for this portal is immediately adjacent to the lateral border of the peroneus tertius tendon, again at the joint line level. More lateral portal placement increases the risk of damage to the intermediate dorsal cutaneous branch of the superficial peroneal nerve. By staying immediately adjacent to the medial border of the peroneus tertius tendon and using no sharp instruments to penetrate this area, avoidance of injury to both the intermediate dorsal cutaneous and the medial dorsal cutaneous branches of the superficial peroneal nerve is reasonably certain. Accurate placement of the spinal needle is confirmed by the free flow of saline from the laterally placed needle on removal of the needle stylus (Fig. 5).

Once accurate needle placement has been confirmed, the portals can be created. A number 11 knife blade is used for this purpose. A superficial skin incision is made at the point of entry of the spinal needle. Care is taken to incise the skin only, and effort is made to avoid subcutaneous penetration with the knife blade. The lateral portal is created initially. The spinal needle is maintained in the medial portal site in order to allow manual joint distention. After incising the skin at the portal site, a small hemostat is inserted into the incision. Spreading with the hemostat displaces neural elements from the field of action. The closed hemostat can then be used to penetrate the joint capsule; penetration is evidenced by the rapid return of saline from the distended joint (Fig. 6). The arthroscopic cannula fitted with a blunt trochar can then be introduced into

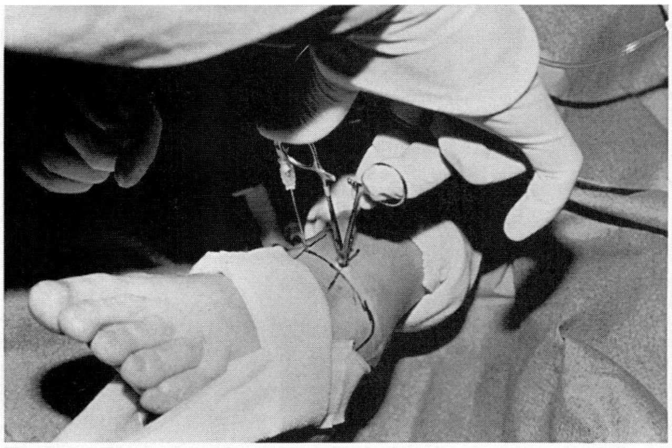

Fig. 6 The anterolateral portal is established with a hemostat. The hemostat is placed after simply nicking the skin with a surgical knife.

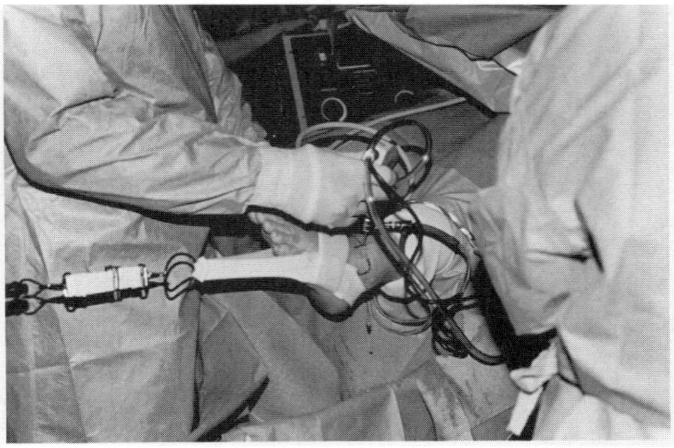

Fig. 7 Surgical arthroscopy is carried out. Note the placement of a spinal needle in the posterolateral portal. This maneuver permits outflow when the inflow is accomplished through the side arm of the arthroscope sheath.

the joint. The arthroscope is then inserted in a routine fashion, and the inflow tubing is attached to the side arm of the arthroscope cannula to provide automated inflow. At this point, the medial portal is created in the same fashion as the lateral, and instrumentation of the joint can be carried out. If outflow is desired, it can be accomplished by using a spinal needle in the posterolateral portal (Fig. 7). This portal is located immediately adjacent to the Achilles tendon at the ankle joint line level. The posteromedial portal should be avoided because of the risk of injuring the neurovascular bundle. Similarly, the anterocentral portal of the ankle should be avoided because of the increased risk of damage to the neurovascular bundle anteriorly.

Most surgical procedures in the ankle can be carried out with the use of the anterolateral and anteromedial portals. On occasion, the posterolateral portal may be used for visualization or instrumentation. Once the arthroscopic visualization is under way, the lateral and medial anterior portals can be used interchangeably. With the arthroscope introduced laterally and the probe placed through the medial portal, a systematic visual and tactile examination of the joint is carried out. The lateral sulcus, including visualization of the tip of the fibula, is best seen with the arthroscope placed into the anterolateral portal. Similarly, the medial sulcus and tip of the medial malleolus are best seen with the arthroscope placed anteromedially. Inspection of the anterior compartment of the ankle is enhanced on occasion by reducing the distraction tension. If difficulty is encountered in accessing the posterior compartment of the ankle, a gentle dorsiflexion of the ankle provided by the surgical assistant can be helpful. The use of a 70° fore-oblique lens aids in visualizing the posterior recesses of the joint. On occasion, the posterolateral portal is used to inspect the posterior compartment.

Arthroscopic Treatment of Transchondral Talar Dome Fracture (Osteochondritis Dissecans)

The terms talar dome fracture, osteochondritis dissecans of the talus, flake fracture, and transchondral talar dome fracture are synonymous. This uncommon condition was first described by Kappis[17] in 1922. He named the condition osteochondritis dissecans of the talus because of its pathologic similarity to osteochondritis dissecans of the knee. The etiology of this lesion remains unclear. Kappis believed that the lesions were the result of spontaneous avascular necrosis of subchondral bone. Rendu[18] and others have proposed a traumatic etiology for this peculiar abnormality. Berndt and Harty[19] were able to reproduce the lesion in cadaveric specimens and were the first to refer to these lesions as transchondral talar dome fractures. They went on to classify the condition into four stages: stage I, a small area of compression of subchondral bone; stage II, a partially detached osteochondral fragment; stage III, a completely detached osteochondral fragment that is not displaced from the crater; and stage IV, a displaced osteochondral fragment.

Stage I and II lesions are rarely seen by the orthopaedic surgeon, because they rarely cause symptoms. Stage III are the most frequently seen lesions, in part because they are quite symptomatic and because the fragments, although detached from their bed, infrequently dislodge as completely loose bodies into the ankle joint. Stage IV lesions are always best managed by surgical removal of the loose fragment. Lateral stage III lesions have almost no potential to heal with nonsurgical management.[20] Medial stage III lesions have only a slightly better chance of healing nonsurgically and are usually better managed by surgical means.[21]

Transchondral talar dome lesions occur either on the medial or the lateral surface of the dome of the talus.

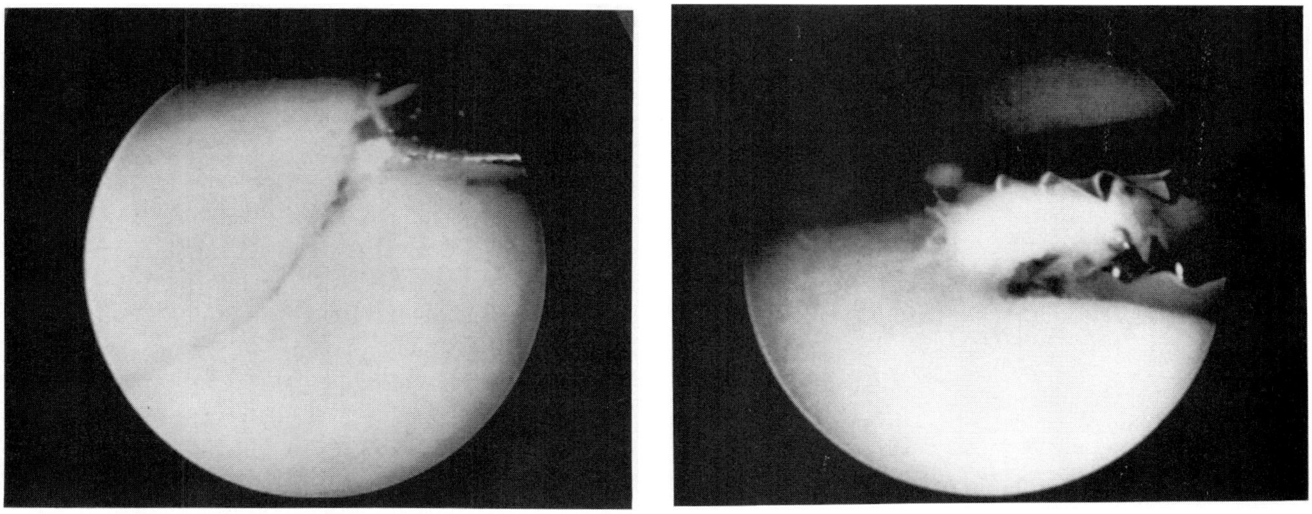

Fig. 8 **Left,** A large lateral talar dome lesion is seen. A blunt probe placed through the medial portal is seen about to be used to elevate the fragment. **Right,** A medial talar dome fragment is seen being grasped with a small grasping forceps. The arthroscope is placed anterolaterally, and the grasper is placed anteromedially. (Reproduced with permission from Ewing JW: Arthroscopic management of transchondral talar-dome fractures (osteochondritis dissecans) and anterior impingement lesions of the ankle joint. *Clin Sports Med* 1991;10:677-687.)

The medial lesions are located slightly posterior to the apex of the dome. The lateral lesions are located anterior to the apex and are, therefore, somewhat easier to remove arthroscopically. The lateral lesions are thin and wafer-like, whereas the medial lesions are much more cup shaped and have a deeper crater in the subchondral bone. Lateral talar dome fragments usually can be removed by means of an arthrotomy, but are relatively easy to remove arthroscopically. The medial talar dome fragments, however, usually require a medial malleolar osteotomy if they are to be approached nonarthroscopically. Arthroscopic removal of the medial fragments, therefore, reduces the morbidity of the surgical management of this particular lesion.

Technique

The arthroscopic approach to removal of the lateral fragment is as described earlier. Usually, the lesion can be seen to be elevated slightly. A probe is placed beneath the fragment, and the loosened fragment is elevated further (Fig. 8, *left*). A small grasping forceps is then used to remove the fragment (Fig. 8, *right*). Care is taken to enlarge the skin incision as necessary to avoid losing the fragment in the subcutaneous tissue or the back of the joint. A synovial reaction usually accompanies this pathology, necessitating a synovectomy of the anterior compartment of the ankle before removal of the fragment. Once the fragment is clear of the joint, the margins of the crater can be trimmed with a curette. The base of the lesion needs only to be debrided with an angled curette (Fig. 9). No drilling of the crater is required.

The medial lesion is more difficult to appreciate at first look. The use of a blunt probe is necessary to define the loosened fragment. With the arthroscope placed in the anterolateral portal, the blunt probe can be used through the anteromedial portal to feel for the softened area of articular cartilage. This area is usually easy to define by palpation, but can be difficult to identify visually. When the area has been located with the blunt probe, simply depressing the probe into the lesional area near its junction with normal tissue will cause the probe to drop into the crater without difficulty. When this occurs, simple rotation of the probe will produce a rather dramatic elevation of the entire medial loose fragment (Fig. 10). Once the fragment is

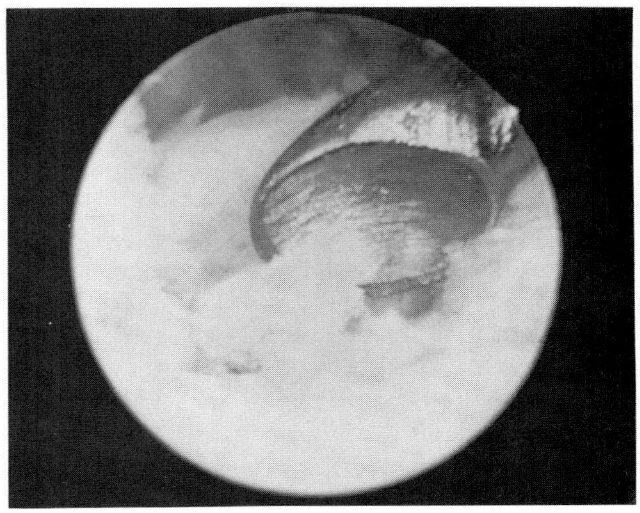

Fig. 9 The base of a medial talar dome lesion is being debrided with an angled curette to achieve a bleeding bone surface.

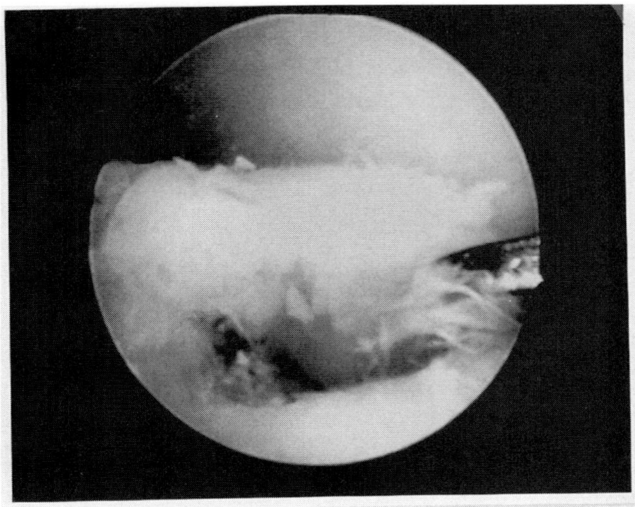

Fig. 10 A medial talar dome fragment is lifted from the crater with a blunt probe. (Reproduced with permission from Ewing JW: Arthroscopic management of transchondral talar-dome fractures (osteochondritis dissecans) and anterior impingement lesions of the ankle joint. *Clin Sports Med* 1991;10:677-687.)

elevated, it may be removed with the small grasping forceps. The surgeon must be alert to the fact that the necrotic fragment may be in more than one piece to avoid leaving an unrecognized fragment behind. It should also be recognized that there are occasions when the two standard anterior portals must be used interchangeably. Surgical situations dictate flexibility as far as the use of these portals is concerned. Again, once all loose fragments have been cleared from the joint, it only remains to curette the base of the lesion to stimulate a bleeding response. An angled curette is indispensable for this purpose. Drilling of the crater is not necessary, and no transosseous tunnels have been used in the arthroscopic management of these lesions.

Postsurgically, the ankle is dressed with a bulky soft-tissue dressing, and nonweightbearing crutch ambulation is advised for 1 week. At 1 week, partial weightbearing is allowed, and is progressed to full weightbearing at 2 to 3 weeks. The postsurgical dressing is left in place for the first week. The patient may return to full activities between 10 and 16 weeks.

Complications include those seen in any orthopaedic procedure, but they are quite rare. In particular, when dealing with the ankle, injury to the sensory nerves, especially the intermediate branch of the superficial peroneal, can be more than a nuisance. This hazard can be avoided by care in portal site selection and avoidance of the use of sharp instrumentation in the subcuticular tissue. The use of a bulky soft-tissue dressing, left in place for a week, will reduce the chance for development of a synovial fistula.

Clinical Material

In the course of 5 years, one of the authors (JWE) has performed 26 arthroscopic procedures for transchondral talar dome fracture in 24 skeletally mature patients. There were 12 males and 12 females. The average age of the patients was 32.2 years, with a range from 14 to 59 years. There were five teenagers, and five patients were in their fifties. Seventeen right ankles and nine left ankles were involved. Of the lesions, 22 were of the medial talar dome variety, and only four ankles presented with a lateral dome fracture. Fourteen of the 26 ankles had a longer than 2-year follow-up period. All but two of the remaining cases had a greater than 1-year follow-up. Twenty-four of the 26 ankles were regarded as satisfactory results. Two patients continued to have symptoms of pain with weightbearing activity. There were no significant complications in this group of patients.

Soft-Tissue and Osseous Impingement Lesions of the Ankle

Painful impingement lesions of the ankle can be broken down into osseous and soft-tissue lesions. These conditions are usually posttraumatic, but they can occur as manifestations of systemic disease.

Soft-tissue impingement lesions were first described by Wolin and associates[22] in a classic article in which they described a meniscoid type lesion that occurred in the lateral talofibular recess following repetitive ankle sprains. These lesions were recognized as early as 1937, when the first surgical procedure was done. The patients presented with a clicking painful ankle following multiple sprains, and many had complaints of instability. Exploration of this area revealed a large meniscoid type lesion that was excised and found quite prominently in the gutter of the lateral fibulotalar joint. In 1950, Wolin and associates[22] reported a series of nine patients with good to excellent results from open excision of this lesion.

Osseous lesions have not received as much attention, but have been noted by a number of authors[23,24] as a cause of painful conditions about the ankle joint. Posttraumatic osteophytes and loose bodies may cause osseous impingement and pain, leading to a syndrome similar to that of the classical soft-tissue lesion.

The osseous impingement types that fall into this category consist of osteophytes, loose bodies that may or may not be attached to the capsule, the Tillot fragment seen in anterior syndesmosis injuries, os trigonum syndrome, tibiotalar impingement, and a variety of others (Fig. 11, *left*). Probably the most prevalent of these lesions is the anterior tibiotalar osteophyte that is commonly noticed on the lateral radiograph of the ankle (Fig. 11, *right*). This syndrome may consist of an isolated tibial osteophyte, a talar

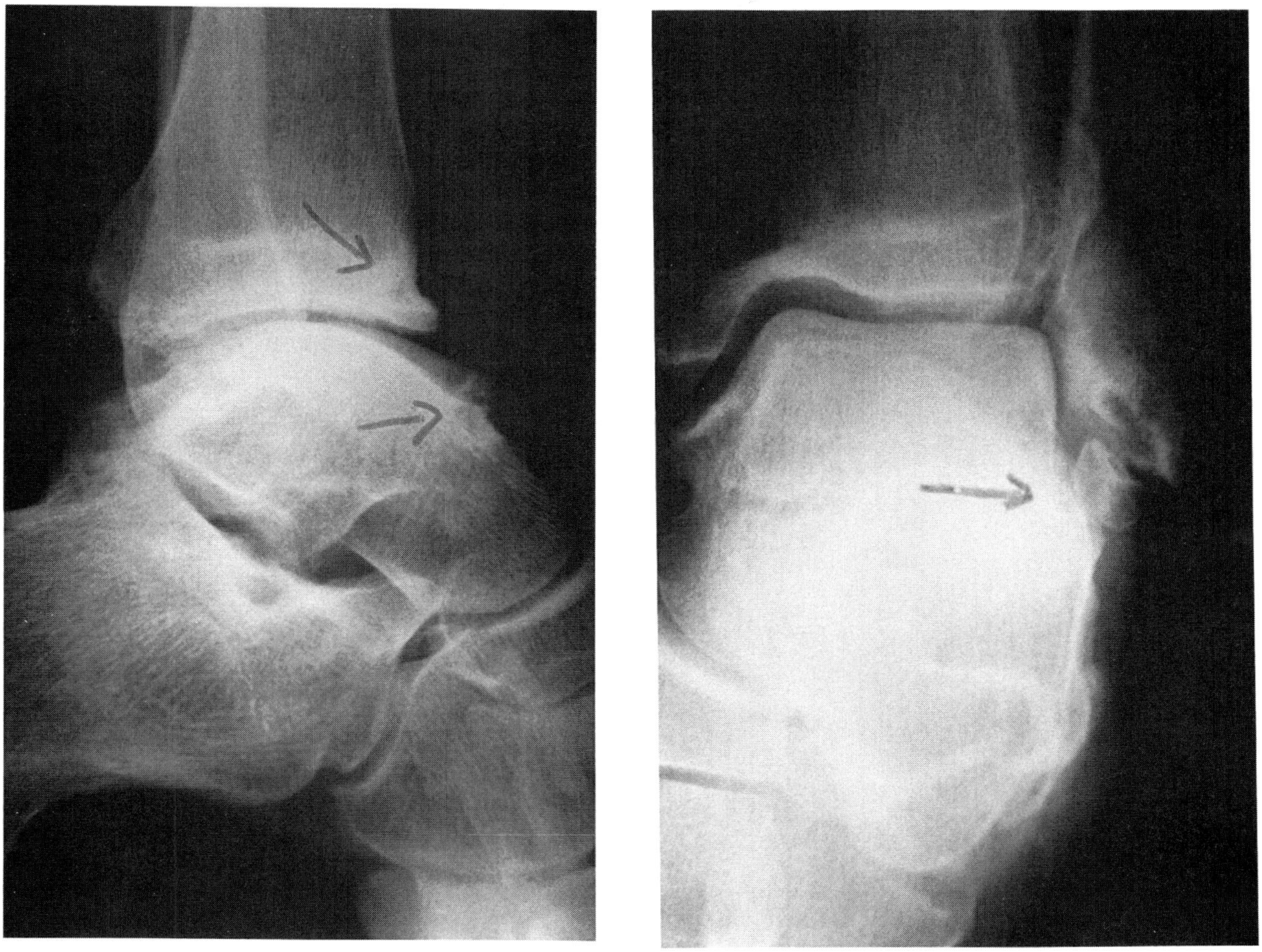

Fig. 11 **Left,** Radiograph of a loose body seen in the fibulotalar recess. **Right,** Lateral radiograph showing anterior impinging tibiotalar osteophytes.

osteophyte, or a combination of the two lesions. Athletes that have had repeated ankle sprains and anterior capsular injuries may be at greater risk for impingement. It develops slowly over the course of years and can produce significant symptoms. Occasionally, surgery will be required in those cases failing conservative management.

Osseous lesions can also present in both the medial and lateral gutters, as well as posteriorly. They can be found in combination with soft-tissue lesions. Posteriorly, the os trigonum can present as a posterior impingement lesion. This may be symptomatic in athletes, such as ballet dancers, who require significant plantarflexion. The surgeon may also find a chronic chip or avulsion fracture that has invaginated to cause bony impingement that may present both as an intra- and extra-articular problem.

Care must be taken to differentiate these intra-articular bony abnormalities from extra-articular pathology. Many authors have described their pathogenesis and treatment, both by arthroscopic and open surgical techniques.[6,7,9,25-27] The literature seems to place synovitic disorders and meniscoid lesions into the same category. Although these two lesions may be somewhat synonymous and may be part of the same pathologic process, we choose to differentiate the two for a clear understanding not only of pathogenesis, but also of treatment.

The soft-tissue impingement lesion occurs mainly after multiple repeated sprains, isolated fractures, syndesmotic injuries, and systemic illnesses. The pathogenesis of the classical anterolateral impingement lesion consists of a plantarflexion inversion injury with a tear of either the anterior talofibular ligament, calcaneofibular ligament, or posterior talofibular ligament. There is subsequent synovial hypertrophy and hyalinization with eventual production of a chronic synovitic or meniscoid type lesion that becomes fibrotic and firm. Therefore,

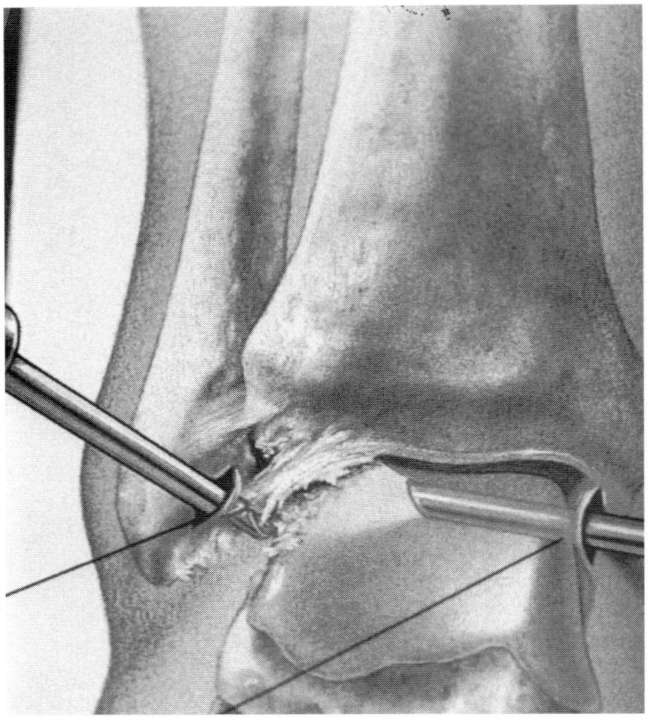

Fig. 12 Arthroscopic resection of a meniscoid lesion is depicted. (Reproduced with permission from Richard Ferkel, MD, Smith & Nephew Dyonics, Inc.)

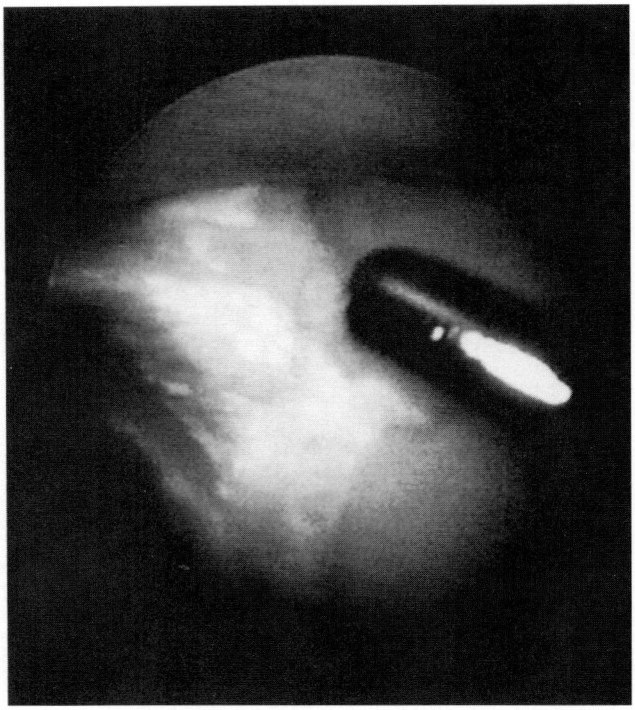

Fig. 13 Synovitis secondary to pseudogout is seen affixed to the posterior tibiofibular ligament.

these lesions may have a soft, chronic, classical synovitic appearance, or they may have the characteristics of hard, fibrotic meniscal tissue (Fig. 12).

Ferkel[1] has one of the largest series in the literature. He reviewed 100 patients who underwent ankle arthroscopy, 24 of whom presented with anterolateral pain, lateral gutter synovitis, and impingement. He later had a series of 31 patients who specifically underwent ankle arthroscopy for chronic intractable impingement syndrome.[7] The results of surgical excision were generally good to excellent. Patients whose corresponding chondromalacic changes were moderate or advanced did not do as well.

There are other mechanical and inflammatory soft-tissue conditions that should be included in this category. They consist of the classical impingement, as well as adhesions, synovitis, ligament disruption and hypertrophy, and a variety of extra-articular problems (Fig. 13).

Bassett and associates[28] and McCarroll and associates[29] have described a variety of other etiologies and lesions. Bassett and associates[28] found hypertrophy in the area of the accessory slip of the anterior tibiofibular ligament. This is sometimes associated with a chondromalacic lesion on the talus, and it can be responsible for impingement. McCarroll and associates[29] found impingement lesions in a series of soccer players who had sustained multiple ankle injuries.

The clinical presentation of the impingement syndrome is one of pain, tenderness, and swelling about the anterolateral aspect of the ankle. The patient presents with pseudo-instability or a history of the ankle giving way without supportive evidence of instability on stress radiographs. Typically, a patient will present with a clicking and catching sensation, as well as a history of multiple minor or major ankle injuries. This syndrome does not, however, limit itself to soft-tissue injuries of the ankle, for these lesions have been found following a variety of fractures.

The physical examination at this stage will demonstrate tenderness at the site of the impingement, which can be anterolateral, anteromedial, or posterior. In the case of the classical anterolateral impingement, the patient has tenderness and some localized swelling in this region. Pain is reproduced with the extremes of dorsiflexion and concomitant eversion of the ankle joint. The clinical examination for instability, which consists of passive inversion and an anterior drawer test, will be negative.

The differential diagnosis for the impingement syndrome can be lengthy, and the surgeon must consider all the osseous conditions that have been mentioned. Instability patterns have been confused with this lesion. Osteochondritis dissecans can be ruled out through routine radiographs or a magnetic resonance imaging (MRI) scan. Stress fractures of the fibula usually have a different location. Subtalar pathology, as well as the sinus tarsi syndrome, can present with symptoms that are similar to those of an impingement lesion. Tarsal coalition and peroneal tendon subluxation can be confused with this syndrome. Neurologic disorders, such as the superficial neurapraxias of the dorsal intermediate cutaneous branch of the peroneal nerve and other forms of reflex sympathetic dystrophy (RSD), can present with anterolateral pain. A careful history and physical examination will differentiate these conditions.

The workup for painful lesions of the ankle that are of a soft-tissue and bony origin can be performed in a cost-effective environment. The history and physical as well as a series of plain radiographs can bring the surgeon close to a correct diagnosis. When the question of instability arises, both anteroposterior and lateral stress films are necessary to rule this out. Tomography has been useful in isolating the exact location of bony impingement lesions prior to surgical resection. Differential subtalar and tibiotalar injections with or without cortisone can be helpful in isolating pathology, particularly around the complex anterolateral aspect of the ankle. Short-term response to this injection can help confirm the diagnosis. Bone scans have been helpful for both isolation and confirmation.[27] We have found MRI to be of limited value in the ankle, except for occasional occult osteochondritic lesions, subchondral fractures, and inflammatory tendinopathies that have not been evident on plain radiographs.[7,30,31] The confirmation of these conditions by MRI has been varied; therefore, it does not appear that it is a cost-effective diagnostic tool. Diagnostic arthroscopy is an excellent method of confirmation, but the physician should be confident of the presence of these lesions clinically before submitting a patient to surgery.

The conservative treatment of both of these conditions consists of the use of nonsteroidal anti-inflammatories, activity modification, heel wedges, and shoe modification. The use of cortisone injections should be limited and directed specifically at the pathologic lesion. Sometimes, patients that have not reached a chronic stage will respond to physical therapy modalities that include peroneal strengthening exercises and a flexibility and strengthening program, as well as ultrasound and phonophoresis. Immobilization has not proven to be effective and may aggravate the condition by leading to atrophy of the ankle musculature.

Surgical treatment of osseous and soft-tissue lesions is effective if the appropriate preoperative diagnosis is confirmed.[6,7] A conventional ankle arthroscopy is performed using a soft-tissue distraction system as described earlier in this chapter. A two-portal technique is used, and although an accessory posterolateral portal is seldom necessary, it may be used to improve fluid-flow characteristics. Following a complete diagnostic arthroscopy of the anterior and posterior compartments and the medial and lateral gutters, and upon confirmation of the impingement lesion, a resection of the lesion is carried out. Generally, small joint arthroscopic equipment is used. This allows adequate resection of pathologic tissue and reduces the chances of articular cartilage scuffing. A synovectomy is performed at the site of the lesion. Resection of the synovitic and meniscoid lesions can be done with a variety of small basket forceps and powered instrumentation. Synovectomy and full-radius blades, and a small burr or abrader are the most commonly used instruments. Only the lesional tissue needs to be resected; therefore, caution is exercised to avoid being overly aggressive. Excessive resection of capsule and soft tissue can lead to damage of normal structures, as well as development of fistulae and continued pain. It is alright to resect the separate fascicle of the anterior inferior tibiofibular ligament, but resection of the ligament proper should be avoided.

Other pathology may be addressed concomitantly. Occasionally, there is an area of chondromalacia in the region of the impingement that may be addressed with a chondroplasty. When patients have a chronic syndrome, they may also have some element of anteromedial or posterolateral impingement or synovitis, which must also be addressed. When separate or associated bony impingement is confirmed preoperatively as well as arthroscopically, the appropriate resection of the bony lesion can be done using small joint burrs or abraders. It is important to confirm the location of the osseous spur prior to surgery, because at the time of arthroscopy the amount of bone that needs to be resected can be unclear. The surgeon needs to address the tibial as well as the talar components, but a thorough resection of the anterior lesion on the tibia occasionally will be sufficient.

Complications of ankle arthroscopy and impingement surgery are the same as those with other arthroscopic procedures involving the ankle.[24,32,33] These complications include neurologic and vascular damage, fistula formation, broken instrumentation, reflex sympathetic dystrophy, fractures with invasive distraction devices, infection, arthrofibrosis, and chondral scuffing. Complications in ankle arthroscopy are relatively rare. With caution, most of them can be avoided. The most common of the complications is damage to the superficial cutaneous nerves about the ankle during portal placement.

It is the surgeon's choice whether to suture the portals, or simply to employ paper-tape closure. The advantage of the paper strip is the avoidance of catching a subcutaneous nerve with a suture. The postoperative care for most arthroscopic procedures of the ankle, other than arthrodesis, consists of the use of a bulky dry compressive bandage for the first 5 days, followed by early motion and weightbearing as tolerated. Return to full activity and sports is not encouraged until a minimum of 6 weeks has passed from the date of surgery. The patient should have a pain-free and normal examination before full sports activity is permitted. When bony resection has been necessary, full activity is frequently delayed until 8 to 10 weeks after surgery.

Arthroscopically Assisted Tibiotalar Arthrodesis With Autogenous Bone Graft

Albert[34] described the first arthrodesis of the ankle in 1879. Over the past 90 years, 30 different open fusion techniques have been described in the medical literature.[35] Tibiotalar arthrodesis by conventional open techniques has resulted in many complications, including pseudoarthrosis ranging from 0% to 37.5%,[36,37] infection that has led to amputation,[38] and injuries to neurovascular structures, such as posterior tibial nerve transection and laceration of the posterior tibial and dorsalis pedis arteries.[38]

Ankle arthrodesis fixation is divided into external[39] and internal with grafts, plates, and screws.[40-53] A comparative study of the two methods by Moeckel and associates[54] revealed that external fixation has a higher incidence of nonunion, delayed union, and infection than does internal fixation.

Myerson and Quill[8] compared arthroscopic and open methods for tibiotalar arthrodesis, reporting a postoperative period of 8.7 weeks for arthroscopic arthrodesis as compared to 14.5 weeks for open arthrodesis. It was their conclusion that arthroscopic arthrodesis was more appropriate than arthrotomy and malleolar resection, using similar methods of internal fixation. A recent article by Ogilvie-Harris[55] reports on 19 cases with a 2-year follow-up period. Satisfactory results were achieved in 16 of the 19 procedures, using the Mazur scoring system. There were two nonunions that required open arthrodesis. Tasto reported on 30 arthroscopically assisted ankle arthrodesis procedures at Specialty Day of the 1994 American Academy of Orthopaedic Surgeons meeting, in New Orleans, LA. His follow-up of 29 of these procedures revealed solid fusion in 27 and nonunion in 2 cases. In this group of osteoarthritic, rheumatoid arthritic, and posttraumatic arthritic patients, the fusion rate was 96%.

The indication for arthroscopically assisted tibiotalar arthrodesis is pain in the degenerative arthritic joint, from osteoarthritis, rheumatoid arthritis, or posttraumatic arthritis, that cannot be controlled by nonsurgical means (Fig. 14). The contraindications of arthroscopically assisted arthrodesis of the ankle are infection, excessive malalignment, severe bone loss, osteonecrosis of the talus, Charcot joint, and severe vascular insufficiency.

Advantages of arthroscopically assisted arthrodesis of the ankle include decreased postoperative morbidity, rapid fusion rate, and reduced patient hospitalization period.[8,55] Other benefits of the procedure are the need for smaller incisions with less tissue destruction, decreased infection potential, early weightbearing with faster rehabilitation, and decrease in time lost from the workplace.

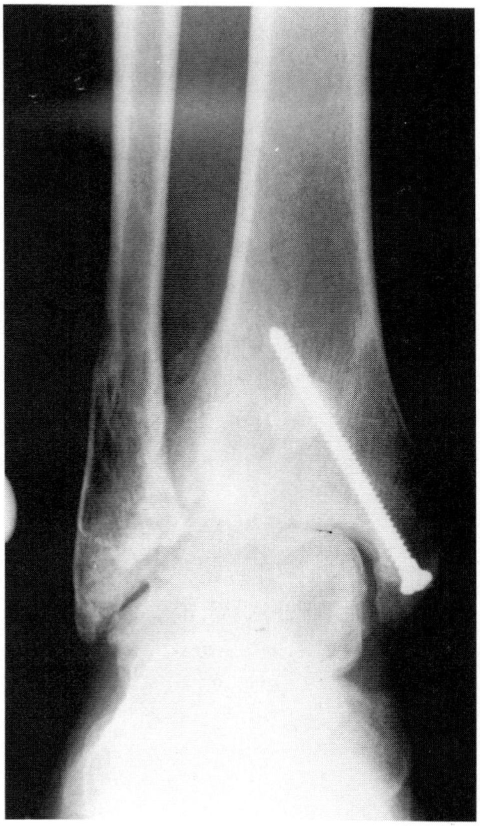

Fig. 14 A degenerative tibiotalar joint that is amenable to arthroscopic arthrodesis.

Technique

The patient is placed on the operating table with the unaffected leg flexed over two pillows for protection of the peroneal nerve. Following the sterile prep of the affected leg from toes to knee, the noninvasive ankle distractor is applied with 20 to 26 pounds of traction.[6] The anterolateral and anteromedial portals are used for arthroscopic surgical intervention. These portals are established as described by Ewing.[6] Once the arthroscope is placed into the joint by way of the anterolateral portal, joint distention is achieved with the aid of a pump through the arthroscopic cannula. The pump offers the advantages of being able to distend the soft tissues, provide a clear field of vision, diminish venous bleeding by exerting hydrostatic pressure when large bony surfaces are exposed, and permitting aggressive use of the power shaver with suction.

Once the diagnostic portion of the ankle surgery has been completed, an arthroscopically assisted arthrodesis is performed on the tibiotalar joint. Arthrodesis may be carried out in conjunction with the use of an

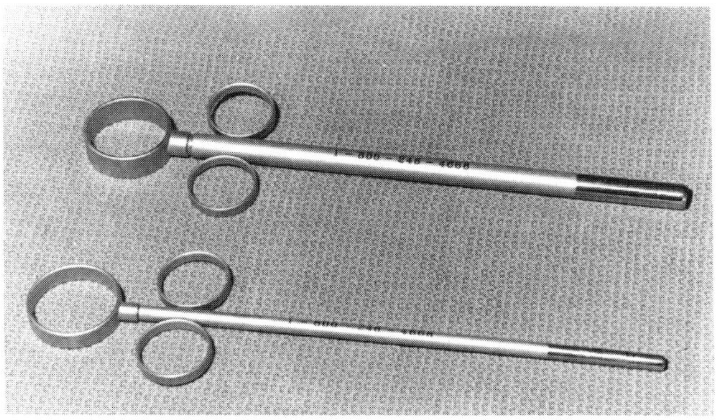

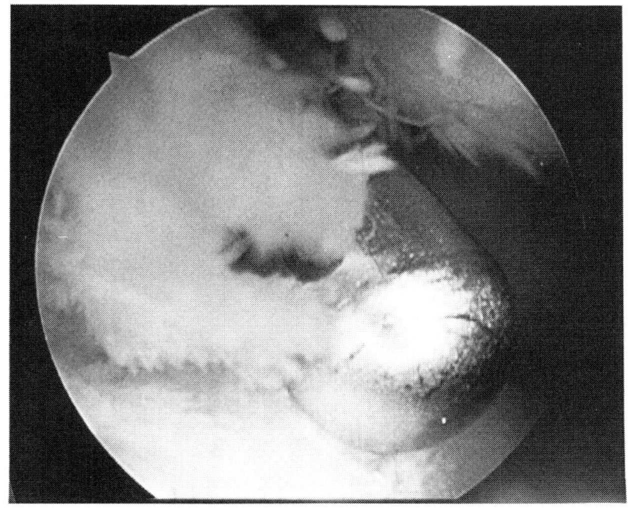

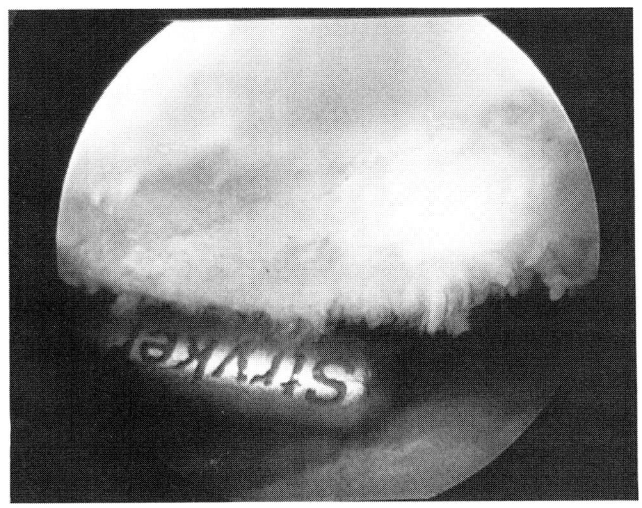

Fig. 15 **Left,** Bone syringe that facilitates insertion of cancellous bone into the tibiotalar joint. **Top right,** Synovium in the anterior aspect of the tibiotalar joint. **Bottom right,** Osteophyte seen on the anterior aspect of the tibia.

autogenous, cancellous bone graft, but the use of a bone graft is optional.

If the surgeon elects to use a bone graft, the patient's ipsilateral iliac crest is prepped and draped at the beginning of the procedure. An 8-cm incision is made over the anterior aspect of the iliac crest, exposing the bone. An 8-mm drill hole is placed in the superior portion of the crest between the inner and outer bony tables. The cancellous bone is removed with a curette and is placed in a bone syringe (Fig. 15, *left*) until time for insertion into the tibiotalar joint. A 4-mm full-radius resector is placed into the anteromedial portal to perform a partial synovectomy (Fig. 15, *top right*). Anterior tibial osteophytes will be found in the arthritic ankle (Fig. 15, *bottom right*). These must be removed to allow visualization and instrumentation of the tibiotalar space from anterior to posterior. The full radius resector is also used to remove the remaining articular cartilage from the medial dome of the talus, medial tibial plafond, and medial malleolus (Fig. 16, *left*). With the arthroscope in the anteromedial portal, a full-radius resector is placed in the anterolateral portal. The synovium and cartilage are removed from the anterolateral compartment, lateral talar dome, lateral tibial plafond, and fibula (Fig. 16, *right*).

Following removal of the soft tissue and cartilage, a 3.5- or 5-mm burr is inserted to perform a light decortication of sclerotic bone over the anterior to posterior aspects of the talar dome, articular surface of the tibia, medial malleolus, and fibula. A golf ball dimpling may be performed over the talar dome and the bony surface of the tibia. This provides increased surface area for osseous fusion (Fig. 17). Stabilization of the fusion is carried out by using cannulated 6.5-mm self-tapping cancellous screws. Before the arthroscopic surgery is begun, the landmarks for screw placement are marked on the medial aspect of the tibia at 5 to 7 cm proximal from the tip of the medial malleolus for distal screw placement, and 7 to 9 cm proximal from the medial malleolus for placement of the proximal

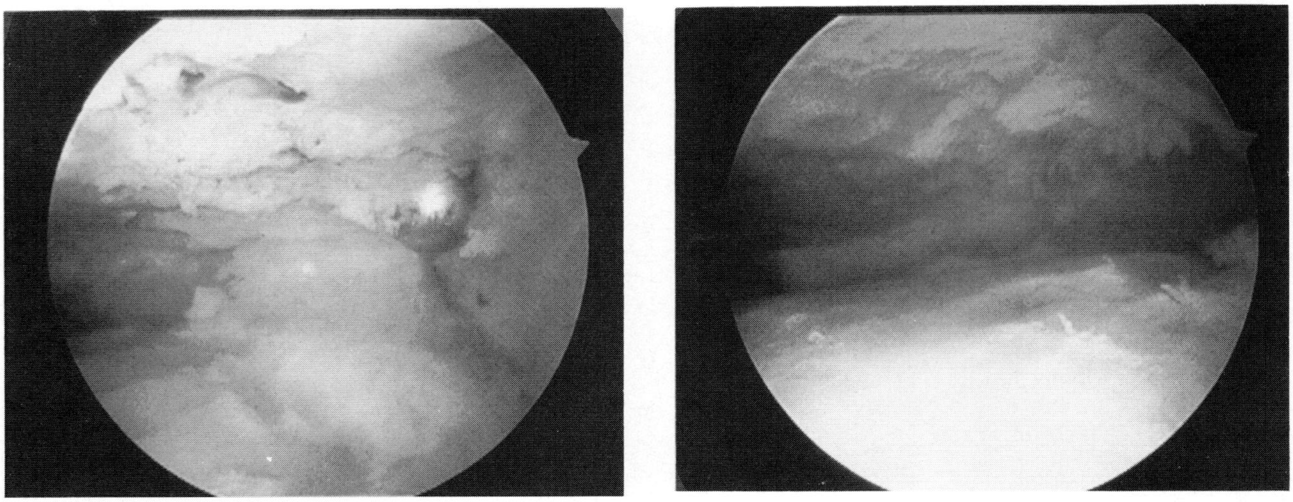

Fig. 16 **Left,** Articular cartilage removed from the medial talar dome, medial tibial plafond, and medial malleolus. **Right,** Articular cartilage removed from the lateral talar dome, lateral tibial plafond, and fibula.

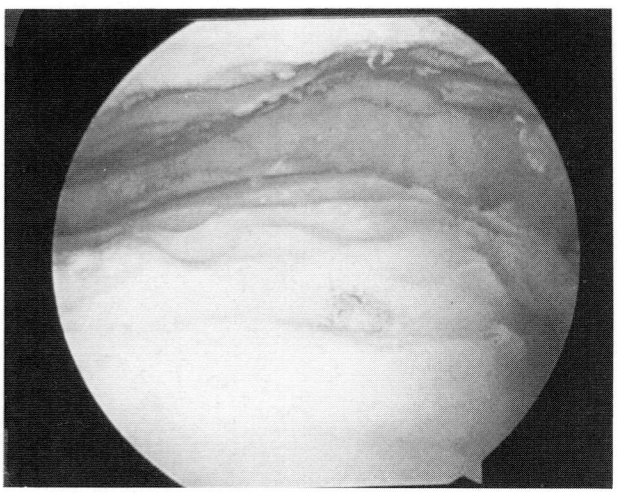

Fig. 17 Golf ball dimpling of the talar dome and the tibial plafond.

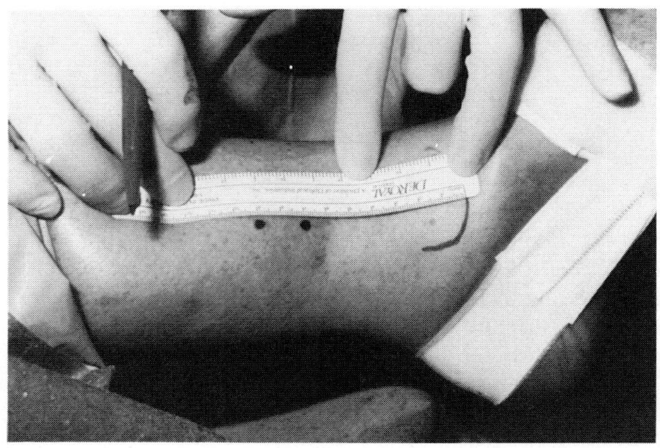

Fig. 18 External surface location for distal and proximal screw placement.

screw (Fig. 18). Small skin incisions are made over these previously marked sites on the anteromedial aspect of the tibia. The underlying soft tissue is spread bluntly with a hemostat in order to expose the periosteum of the tibia. This diminishes the risk of damage to neurovascular structures. The pin guide (Fig. 19, *top left*) is placed in the distal incision and secured to the periosteum at a 45° angle to the long axis of the tibia. The guide pin is inserted into the pin guide and drilled anteriorly just through the tibial surface. This aspect of pin placement is controlled by arthroscopic visualization (Fig. 19, *bottom left*). If the pin is not placed in the correct position; ie, the anterior aspect of the tibia near the center of the dome of the talus in the transverse plane, then correction of the placement is made by adjusting the angle of the pin guide and re-drilling the guide pin. The proximal pin is drilled into the tibia in a like fashion. This pin should be placed parallel to the distal pin, and should enter the tibia somewhat posterior to the initial pin.

After placement of the two parallel pins into the tibia (Fig. 19, *right*), traction is removed from the ankle. The tibiotalar joint is placed at 90° with neutral varus and valgus. Fluoroscopic control is used to aid in proper positioning of the ankle. At this point, the two guide pins are drilled into the talus. Again, fluoroscopic control is used to prevent unwanted penetration of the subtalar joint with the guide pins (Fig. 20, *top left*). A depth gauge is placed over the guide pins to determine

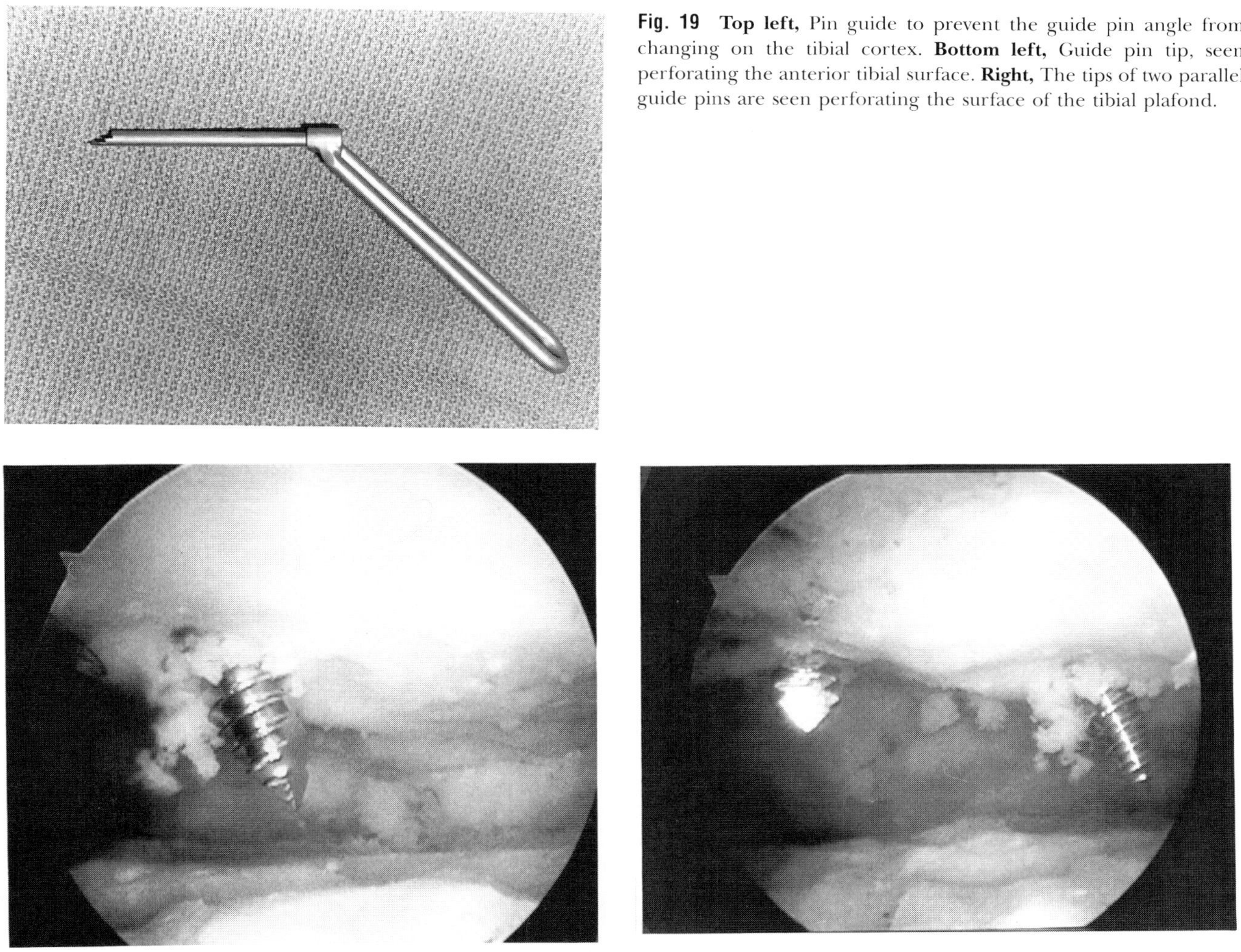

Fig. 19 **Top left,** Pin guide to prevent the guide pin angle from changing on the tibial cortex. **Bottom left,** Guide pin tip, seen perforating the anterior tibial surface. **Right,** The tips of two parallel guide pins are seen perforating the surface of the tibial plafond.

screw length. Five millimeters are subtracted from the original length determined by the depth gauge in order to prevent subtalar penetration and compensate for compression of the tibiotalar space. The bone graft is now placed into the tibiotalar space (Fig. 20, *top right*), followed by insertion of the screws over the guide pins. This portion of the procedure is controlled by fluoroscopy (Fig. 20, *bottom left*). It is important not to tighten the screws against the tibial cortex until the guide pins are removed and manual compression is applied to the calcaneus. Once the pins are removed, and compression against the calcaneus is applied, the cancellous compression screws are tightened to compress the tibiotalar joint (Fig. 20, *bottom right*).

The patient's wounds are closed in a routine fashion. A clinical inspection of the ankle at this point should reveal a 90° angle of the foot to the tibia and neutral varus and valgus positioning (Fig. 21). A bulky compression bandage is applied, and, the following day, a short-leg adjustable walking boot is fitted. The patient is permitted immediate partial weightbearing activity. Progressive weightbearing is permitted as the patient's level of discomfort diminishes.

Clinical Material (JWT)

Arthroscopically assisted tibiotalar arthrodesis procedures were performed by JWT on ten ankles using internal screw fixation and autogenous cancellous bone graft. The patients, eight men and two women, ranged in age from 33 to 72 years. The mean age was 54 years. Eight right and two left ankles were fused using this technique. All of the ankles were osteoarthritic with no osteonecrosis or neurologic disorders. One ankle had been infected, secondary to an open-fracture dislocation. This ankle fused, but one of the medial screw tracks drained, requiring screw removal and bony debridement. Primary arthrodesis occurred in nine ankles within a postoperative mean time of 10 weeks. There was one delayed union, which required the use of an external electrical bone stimulator. This ankle ultimately fused at 8 months. There were no surgical complications involving tendons, nerves, or vessels.

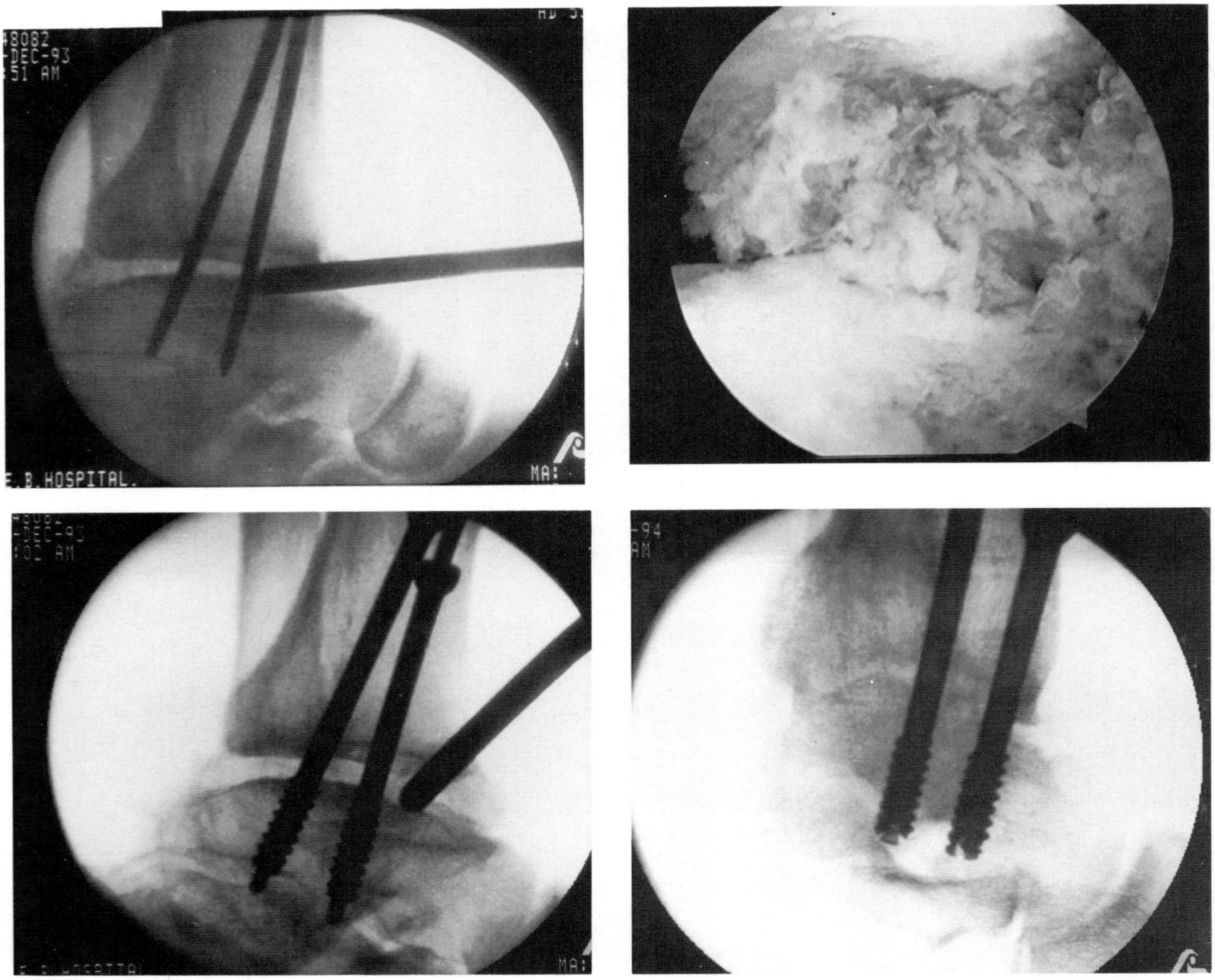

Fig. 20 **Top left,** Both guide pins are drilled into the talus with no penetration of the subtalar joint. **Top right,** Autogenous cancellous bone graft seen placed into the tibiotalar space. **Bottom left,** Self tapping cannulated cancellous screws are placed into the talus. **Bottom right,** Compression of the tibiotalar surfaces by use of the two parallel placed compression screws is seen on this radiograph.

Discussion

Arthroscopically assisted tibiotalar arthrodesis requires a high level of expertise in ankle arthroscopy with detailed understanding of the surface anatomy and portal placement. The surgeon should be aware of tourniquet time and fluid extravasation. If the procedure cannot be performed within a safe time frame, the surgeon should be prepared to perform an open conventional procedure.

The evolution from cross-screw fixation to two medial tibial parallel screws has decreased the risk of neurovascular damage and has offered better biomechanical compression with easier application. Use of autogenous bone graft is preferred by some authors, but others have had success without the use of bone grafting.

References

1. Ferkel RD, Fischer SP: Progress in ankle arthroscopy. *Clin Orthop* 1989;240:210-220.
2. Martin DF, Baker CL, Curl WW, et al: Operative ankle arthroscopy: Long-term followup. *Am J Sports Med* 1989;17:16-23.
3. Voto SJ, Ewing JW, Fleissner PR Jr, et al: Ankle arthroscopy: Neurovascular and arthroscopic anatomy of standard and trans-achilles tendon portal placement. *Arthroscopy* 1989; 5:41-46.
4. Barber FA, Britt BT, Ratliff HW, et al: Arthroscopic surgery of the ankle. *Orthop Rev* 1988;17:446-451.
5. Baker CL, Andrews JR, Ryan JB: Arthroscopic treatment of transchondral talar dome fractures. *Arthroscopy* 1986;2:82-87.
6. Ewing JW: Arthroscopic management of transchondral talar-dome fractures (osteochondritis dissecans) and anterior impingement lesions of the ankle joint. *Clin Sports Med* 1991;10:677-687.

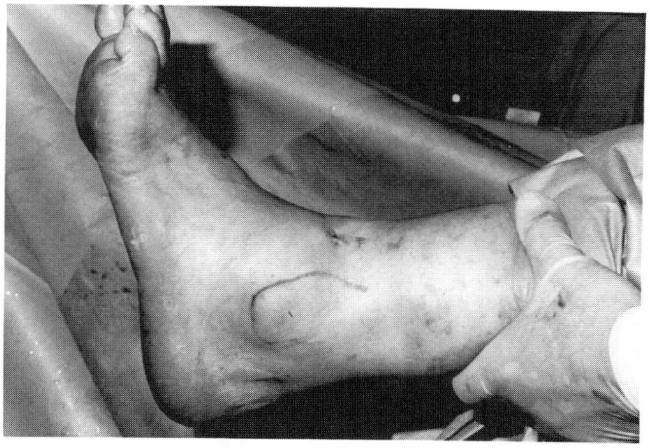

Fig. 21 The proper clinical position of a fused ankle.

7. Ferkel RD, Karzel RP, Del Pizzo W, et al: Arthroscopic treatment of anterolateral impingement of the ankle. *Am J Sports Med* 1991; 19:440-446.
8. Myerson MS, Quill G: Ankle arthrodesis: A comparison of an arthroscopic and an open method of treatment. *Clin Orthop* 1991; 268:84-95.
9. Martin DF, Curl WW, Baker CL: Arthroscopic treatment of chronic synovitis of the ankle. *Arthroscopy* 1989;5:110-114.
10. Parisien JS, Vangsness T: Operative arthroscopy of the ankle: Three years' experience. *Clin Orthop* 1985;199:46-53.
11. Parisien JS, Shaffer B: Arthroscopic management of pyarthrosis. *Clin Orthop* 1992;275:243-247.
12. Hanft JR, Kashuk KB, Schabler JA, et al: Pseudogout of the ankle: A case study and arthroscopic-assisted treatment. *J Foot Surg* 1991; 30:173-178.
13. Andrews JR, Tedder JL, Godbout BP: Simple bone cyst of the distal tibia: A case for ankle arthroscopy. *Arthroscopy* 1991;7:381-384.
14. Lundeen RO, Hawkins RB: Arthroscopic lateral ankle stabilization. *J Am Podiatr Med Assoc* 1985;75:372-376.
15. Baker CL: Video supplement: Ankle synovitis. *Arthroscopy* 1989, vol 1.
16. Guhl JF: New techniques for arthroscopic surgery of the ankle: Preliminary report. *Orthopedics* 1986;9:261-269.
17. Kappis M: Weitere Bieträge zur traumatisch-mechanischen entstehung der "spontenen" knorpelablösungen. *Deutsche Ztschrf Chir* 1922;171:13-29.
18. Rendu A: Fracture intra-articulaire parcellaire de la poulie astragalienne. *Lyon Méd* 1932;150:220-222.
19. Berndt AL, Harty M: Transchondral fractures (osteochondritis dissecans) of the talus. *J Bone Joint Surg* 1959;41A:988-1020.
20. Canale ST, Belding RH: Osteochondral lesions of the talus. *J Bone Joint Surg* 1980;62A:97-102.
21. Alexander AH, Lichtman DM: Surgical treatment of transchondral talar-dome fractures (osteochondritis dissecans): Long-term follow-up. *J Bone Joint Surg* 1980;62A:646-652.
22. Wolin I, Glassman F, Sideman S, et al: Internal derangement of talofibular component of the ankle. *Surg Gynecol Obstet* 1950; 91:193-200.
23. Scranton PE Jr, McDermott JE: Anterior tibiotalar spurs: A comparison of open versus arthroscopic debridement. *Foot Ankle* 1992;13:125-129.
24. Demaziére A, Ogilvie-Harris DJ: Operative arthroscopy of the ankle: 107 cases. *Rev Rheum Mal Osteoartic* 1991;58:93-97.
25. Stone JW, Guhl JF: Meniscoid lesions of the ankle. *Clin Sports Med* 1991;10:661-676.
26. Cerulli G, Caraffa A, Buompadre V, et al: Operative arthroscopy of the ankle. *Arthroscopy* 1992;8:537-540.
27. Thein R, Eichenblat M: Treatment of sports related synovitis of the ankle. *Am J Sports Med* 1992;20:496-498.
28. Bassett FH III, Gates HD, Billys JB, et al: Talar impingement by the anterior-inferior tibiofibular ligament: A cause of chronic pain in the ankle after inversion sprain. *J Bone Joint Surg* 1990; 72A:55-59.
29. McCarroll JR, Schrader JW, Shelbourne KD, et al: Meniscoid lesions of the ankle in soccer players. *Am J Sports Med* 1987;15:255-257.
30. Stone JW, Guhl JF: Ankle arthroscopy, in Pfeffer GB, Frey CC (eds): *Current Practice in Foot and Ankle Surgery*. New York, NY, McGraw Hill, 1993, pp 1-29.
31. De Smet AA, Fisher DR, Burnstein MI, et al: Value of MR imaging in staging osteochondral lesions of the talus (osteochondritis dissecans): Results in 14 patients. *Am J Radiol* 1990;154:555-558.
32. Barber FA, Click J, Britt BT: Complications of ankle arthroscopy (review). *Foot Ankle* 1990;10:263-266.
33. Small NC: Complications in arthroscopic surgery performed by experienced arthroscopists. *Arthroscopy* 1988;4:215-221.
34. Albert E: Zur resektion des kniegelenkes. *Wein Med Presse* 1879;20:705-708.
35. Scranton PE Jr: An overview of ankle arthrodesis. *Clin Orthop* 1991;268:96-101.
36. Chuinard EG, Peterson RE: Distraction-compression bone graft arthrodesis of the ankle: A method especially applicable in children. *J Bone Joint Surg* 1963;45A:481-490.
37. Mears DC, Gordon RG, Kann SE, et al: Ankle arthrodesis with an anterior tension plate. *Clin Orthop* 1991;268:70-77.
38. Johnson EW Jr, Boseker EH: Arthrodesis of the ankle. *Arch Surg* 1968;97:766-773.
39. Charnley J: Compression arthrodesis of the ankle and shoulder. *J Bone Joint Surg* 1951;33B:180-191.
40. Bingold AC: Ankle and subtalar fusion by a transarticular graft. *J Bone Joint Surg* 1956;36B:862-870.
41. Campbell CJ, Rinehart WT, Kalenak A: Arthrodesis of the ankle: Deep autogenous inlay grafts with maximum cancellous bone apposition. *J Bone Joint Surg* 1974;56A:63-70.
42. Gallie WE: Arthrodesis of the ankle joint. *J Bone Joint Surg* 1948;30B:619-621.
43. Graham CE: A new method for arthrodesis of an ankle joint. *Clin Orthop* 1970;68:75-77.
44. Hone MR: Dowel fusion of the ankle joint. *J Bone Joint Surg* 1968;50B:678.
45. Marcus RE, Balourdas GM, Heiple KG: Ankle arthrodesis by chevron fusion with internal fixation and bone-grafting. *J Bone Joint Surg* 1983;65A:833-838.
46. Kennedy JC: Arthrodesis of the ankle with particular reference to the Gallie procedure: A review of fifty cases. *J Bone Joint Surg* 1960;42A:1308-1316.
47. White AA III: A precision posterior ankle fusion. *Clin Orthop* 1974;98:239-250.
48. Scranton PE Jr: Use of internal compression in arthrodesis of the ankle. *J Bone Joint Surg* 1985;67A:550-555.
49. Yassine Z: Ankle arthrodeses with spoon plate. *Surg Rounds Orthop* 1987;1:15-22.
50. Weltmer JB, Choi SH, Shenoy A, et al: Wolf blade plate ankle arthrodesis. *Clin Orthop* 1991;268:107-111.
51. Müller ME, Allgöwer M, Schneider R, et al (eds): *Manual of Internal Fixation Techniques Recommended by the AO Group*, ed 2. Berlin, Springer-Verlag, 1979, p 10.
52. Morgan CD, Henke JA, Bailey RW, et al: Long-term results of tibiotalar arthrodesis. *J Bone Joint Surg* 1985;67A:546-550.

53. Maurer RC, Cimino WR, Cox CV, et al: Transarticular cross-screw fixation: A technique of ankle arthrodesis. *Clin Orthop* 1991; 268:56-64.
54. Moeckel BH, Patterson BM, Inglis AE, et al: Ankle arthrodesis (a comparison of internal and external fixation). *Clin Orthop* 1991;268:78-83.
55. Ogilvie-Harris DJ, Lieberman I, Fitsialos D: Arthroscopically assisted arthrodesis for osteoarthrotic ankles. *J Bone Joint Surg* 1993;75A:1167-1174.

CHAPTER 29

Reconstruction of the Lateral Ankle Ligaments

Mark R. Colville, MD

Injury of the ankle ligaments is one of the most common sports-related injuries and is among the most common of all injuries seen by physicians.[1,2] Although there is some debate as to the best initial treatment for an acute, complete tear of a lateral ligament, persistent functional instability of the ankle develops in approximately 20% of patients regardless of the type of initial treatment.[3-12] In these patients, late reconstruction of the lateral ankle ligaments may become necessary.

Indications

Most patients who have recurrent inversion instability of the ankle can be managed successfully with a rehabilitative exercise program and the use of a brace during hazardous endeavors, such as participation in sports activities and walking on rough or uneven terrain.[3,7] Bracing or taping may prevent recurrent injury during these activities, but many patients sustain injuries during day-to-day activities or in situations in which they are not able to wear an ankle brace. For these patients, reconstruction of the unstable lateral ligament complex with use of a variety of surgical techniques has had a high rate of success.

Candidates for reconstruction of the ankle ligaments should have increased laxity on anterior drawer and inversion stress-testing during the physical examination. In patients for whom nonsurgical management has failed and for whom reconstruction is contemplated, stress radiographs can demonstrate the degree of laxity in the ankle joint.[13-20] However, while increased laxity has been found to be associated with symptoms of functional instability, the absolute criteria for reconstruction of the ankle ligaments cannot be determined on stress-testing alone. In these patients, total inversion of the ankle and subtalar joints may be greater on the involved side than on the uninvolved side, indicating that the subtalar ligament complex is injured as well.[21-23] Carefully performed stress tests may influence the decision regarding the type of reconstructive procedure that is performed.

Stress-testing may be performed either manually or with the aid of a stress-testing device such as the Telos device (Austin and Associates, Fallston, MD), which may provide more consistent and reproducible results (Fig. 1).[20,24] Graded stress, to a maximum of 150 N of force, may be applied with this device. The ankle should be held in 10° of plantarflexion for both inversion and anterior drawer stress-testing. Care should be taken to allow the talus to rotate medially during the test, in order to relax the deltoid ligament so that it does not prevent anterior translation. Measurements of anterior drawer (anterior translation of the talus relative to the tibia) are made in the lateral plane. The distance to the articular surface of the talus is measured on the lateral radiograph (Fig. 2, *left*), on a line perpendicular to the posterior articular surface of the tibial plafond. Inversion stress radiographs are made

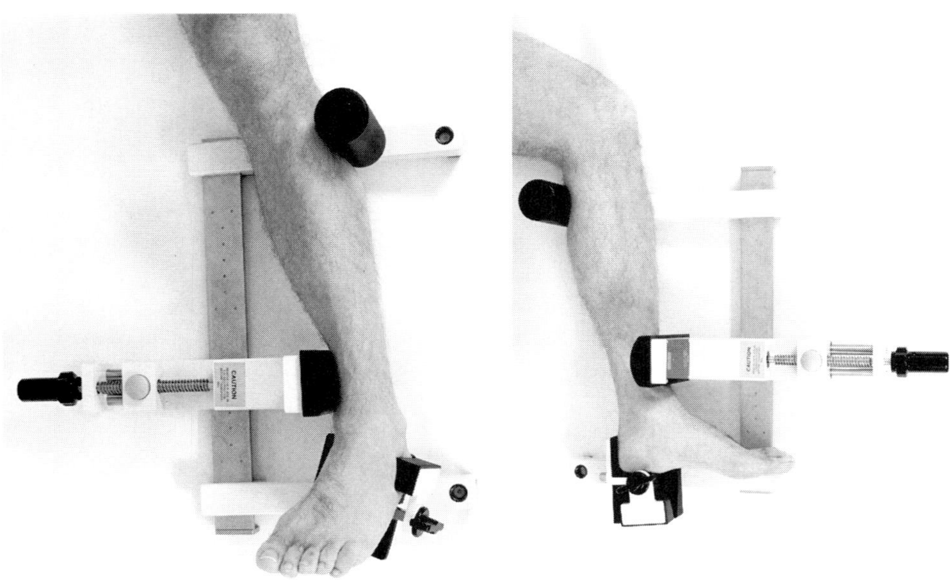

Fig. 1 The Telos device, which may be used to provide consistent measurements of talar tilt (**left**) or anterior talar translation (**right**) in patients who have chronic lateral instability of the ankle.

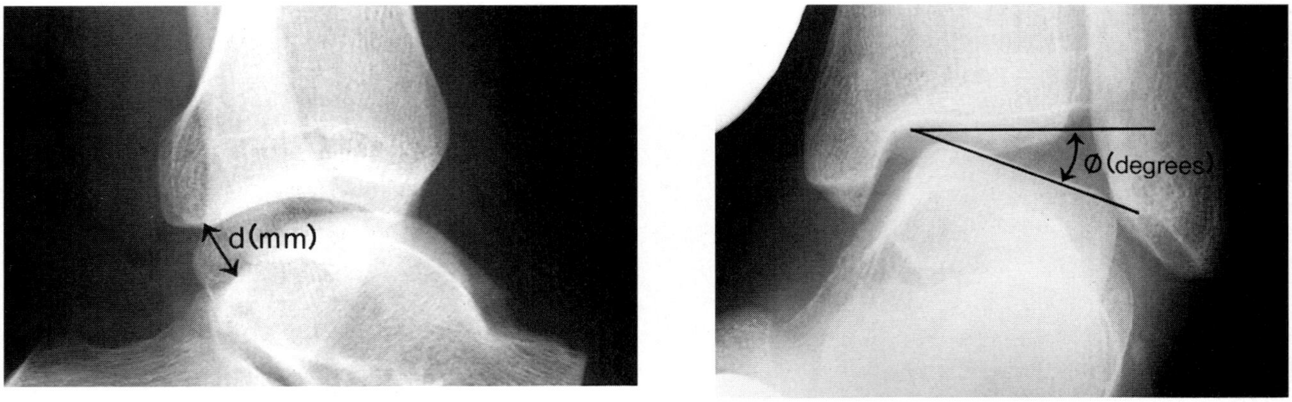

Fig 2 **Left,** The anterior translation of the talus is determined from lateral stress radiographs by measurement of the perpendicular distance (d) from the talus to the posterior articular margin of the tibial plafond. **Right,** A talar tilt radiograph, made with the ankle internally rotated 30°, gives a mortise view.

with the ankle in 30° of internal rotation to provide a mortise view so that talar tilt may be measured accurately (Fig. 2, *right*). Measurement of the angle created by lines drawn parallel to the tibial plafond and the superior surface of the talus demonstrates the degree of talar tilt. Stress radiographs of the uninvolved ankle are made routinely for comparison. While Rubin and Witten reported a wide range in laxity in patients who had normal ankles and called into question the validity of stress radiographs of the ankle,[19] others have found consistently reproducible results with stress-testing in patients who have a chronic ligamentous injury.[12,24,25] Anterior talar translation of 10 mm (or 5 mm more than that on the contralateral, uninjured side) has been generally accepted as indicating injury to the lateral ankle ligament complex. On inversion stress radiographs, 10° of talar tilt (or 5° more than that on the uninvolved side) is also indicative of pathological laxity of the ankle.[26]

Anatomy and Pathological Findings

The mechanism of injury of the lateral ankle ligaments in inversion ankle sprains is one of progressive inversion of the plantarflexed foot and ankle. As the injury progresses, the anterolateral aspect of the capsule is torn first, followed by sequential injury to the anterior talofibular ligament and the calcaneofibular ligament. The posterior talofibular ligament is rarely injured unless complete dislocation occurs. In cadaveric sectioning studies, Johnson and Markolf[27] found the anterior talofibular ligament to be the primary restraint to inversion and anterior talar translation at all angles of ankle flexion. Strain-gauge analysis by several authors has shown the anterior talofibular and the calcaneofibular ligaments to function in a synchronous fashion to resist inversion at all angles of flexion of the ankle.[28-30] Strain rates are highest in the calcaneofibular ligament in dorsiflexion, with strain increasing in the anterior tibiofibular ligament as the ankle is flexed plantarly.

At the time of the operation, Brostrom[31] found that all patients who had recurrent inversion instability had a tear of the anterior talofibular ligament. He also found that 27% of these 60 patients had evidence of an injury of the calcaneofibular ligament.

More recent studies have demonstrated a higher rate of combined injuries to the anterior talofibular ligament and the calcaneofibular ligament than that reported by Brostrom.[31] Moller-Larsen and associates[10] found combined injuries in 59% of their 175 patients. Meyer and associates[32] found serious injury to both the calcaneofibular ligament and the subtalar joint ligaments (the lateral talocalcaneal and the interosseous ligaments) in 32 of 40 patients. Kjaersgaard-Andersen and associates[33,34] found the calcaneofibular ligament to be an important structure in the rotatory stabilization of the hindfoot in a cadaveric study. Clinically, total inversion of the foot is increased in patients who have chronic, severe instability of the ankle, indicating injury of both the ankle and the subtalar joints. From these studies, it is apparent that while the anterior talofibular ligament must be reconstructed in all patients, most will also need reconstruction of the calcaneofibular ligament (or of its function) in order to regain stability of both the ankle and the subtalar joints and to avoid recurrence of the symptoms of instability. Instability of the subtalar joint may be isolated or it may be combined with lateral instability of the ankle. Patients who have subtalar instability may be indistinguishable, on the basis of history and physical examination alone, from those who have instability of the ankle, and stress radiographs of the subtalar joint as well as of the ankle may determine the site of the instability. In patients who have combined instability, reconstruction of the

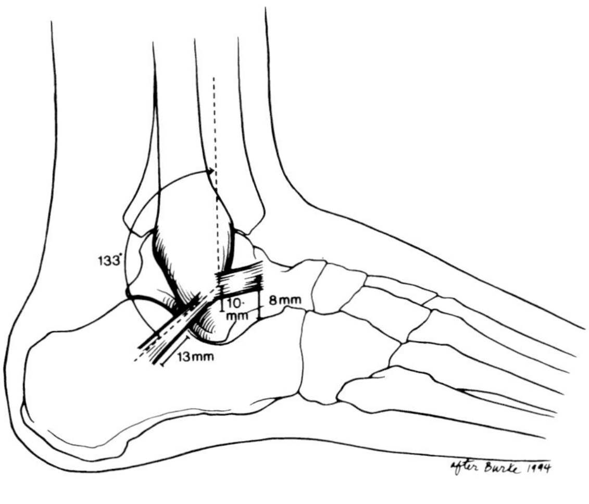

Fig. 3 The critical anatomy of the lateral ligament complex.

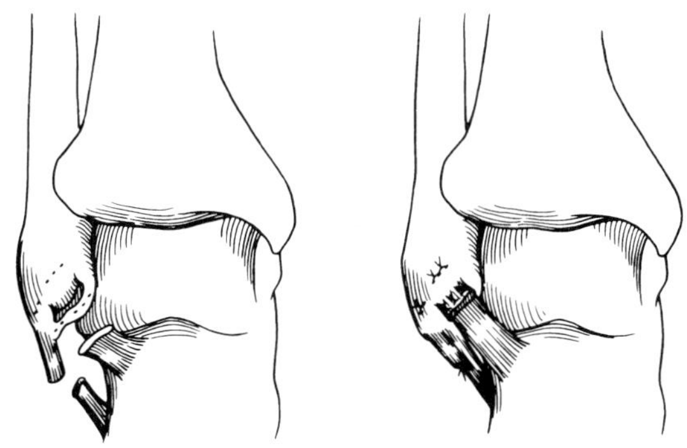

Fig. 4 The Karlsson modification of the Brostrom technique. **Left,** The anterior talofibular ligament and the calcaneofibular ligament are divided 3 to 5 mm distal to their fibular attachments. **Right,** The distal parts of the ligaments are shortened and attached to the roughened fibula through drill-holes. The proximal flaps are oversewn to reinforce the reconstruction.

lateral talocalcaneal ligament and, occasionally, of the cervical ligament may be necessary.[35-37]

A thorough understanding of the complex anatomy and function of the ankle and subtalar joints and their ligaments is important when reconstruction is considered. Articles on the technique of reconstruction of the ankle frequently lack precise descriptions of the sites of origin and insertion of the lateral ankle ligaments. Anatomic drawings in textbooks also frequently depict these ligaments inaccurately. In a recent anatomic study, Burks and Morgan[38] measured the orientation and areas of attachment of the lateral ligaments (Fig. 3). They found that the distance from the tip of the fibula to the center of the fibular attachment of the anterior talofibular ligament is 10 mm, that the calcaneofibular ligament attaches posteriorly on the calcaneus to form a 133° angle with the fibula when the ankle is in neutral dorsiflexion-plantarflexion, that the calcaneal attachment of the calcaneofibular ligament is 13 mm from the subtalar joint, and that the insertion of the anterior talofibular ligament onto the talus is 18 mm posterior to the subtalar joint. Burks and Morgan noted that, with the use of these specific reference points, the anatomic sites for ligament attachment can be located more precisely during reconstruction of the ankle.

Reconstruction Techniques

The goal of reconstruction of the lateral ligaments of the ankle is to restore functional stability. A wide variety of reconstructive techniques have had a high degree of success. After reconstruction, recurrent symptoms of instability are rare, with most authors reporting a good or excellent result in 80% to 85% of patients.[7,10,22,31,39-58] The methods of reconstruction fall into two general types: non-augmented and augmented.

Non-Augmented Reconstruction

Late direct repair of the lateral ankle ligaments was advocated by Brostrom for patients who had recurrent lateral instability of the ankle.[31] Brostrom recommended a mid-substance repair of the free ends of the ligaments with fine continuous sutures. Karlsson and associates[24] noted that, in patients who had a chronic injury, the lateral ligaments are usually elongated rather than disrupted. In a modification of the Brostrom technique, Karlsson and associates recommended shortening of the ligaments with reinsertion onto the fibula through drill-holes (Fig. 4). To reinforce the repair, Sjolin and associates[54] advocated the use of periosteal flaps taken off the distal aspect of the fibula and sutured over the repaired ligaments. Gould and associates[59] modified the Brostrom technique to include repair of the lateral talocalcaneal ligament and reinforcement of the repair with suturing of the lateral extensor retinaculum to the distal aspect of the fibula. This modification is important in patients who have excessive inversion and laxity of the subtalar joint (Fig. 5).

There are several advantages to the Brostrom or the modified Brostrom procedure. The normal anatomy is restored along with the normal joint mechanics. Motion of the subtalar joint is preserved. Unlike with augmented reconstructions, there is no associated donor-site morbidity or weakening of eversion strength due to sacrifice of a peroneal tendon. A single, smaller, more cosmetically acceptable incision may be used. The disadvantages are the inability to achieve stability with only the weak and attenuated local tissues, the

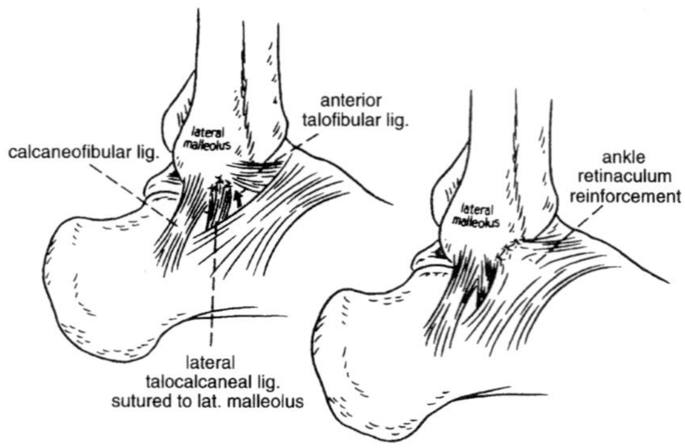

Fig. 5 The Gould modification of the Brostrom technique. The ligaments are repaired, and the repair is then reinforced by suturing of the lateral extensor retinaculum to the distal aspect of the fibula. (Reproduced with permission from Gould N, Seligson D, Gassman J: Early and late repair of lateral ligament of the ankle. *Foot Ankle* 1980;1:84-89.)

failure to reconstruct the calcaneofibular ligament adequately, and the failure to address the relatively frequent problem of subtalar instability.[24,60] Karlsson and associates[24] thought that the relative contraindications to late, direct, non- augmented repair were generalized hypermobility of the joints, a long-standing ligamentous tear that had been present for 10 years or more, and previous surgical repair of the ankle ligaments.

Some authors[24,54,55] have recommended a longitudinal incision for the performance of a Brostrom or modified Brostrom procedure, instead of the transverse oblique incision originally described. A longitudinal incision decreases the likelihood of injury to branches of the superficial peroneal nerve and it also allows extension of the incision to expose the peroneal tendons if the surgeon determines that an augmented reconstruction is necessary. As noted by Sobel and associates,[61] the longitudinal incision also permits routine opening of the peroneal tendon sheath for inspection of the peroneal tendons in patients who have posterolateral tenderness.

Augmented Reconstruction

Numerous techniques for augmented reconstruction of the lateral ankle ligaments have been described. They vary widely with regard to the choice of graft material and the exact site of placement of the graft. The widely used procedures described by Evans,[47] Watson-Jones,[42,62,63] and Chrisman and Snook[45,55] employ the peroneus brevis tendon to limit instability of the ankle. In the Evans procedure (Fig. 6, *top left*), the peroneus brevis tendon is anchored to the fibula, limiting inversion of the ankle and anterior talar translation indirectly, while also limiting motion of the subtalar joint.[47] With the Watson-Jones procedure (Fig. 6, *top right*), in addition to tenodesis of the peroneus brevis tendon to the fibula, the graft is routed anteriorly through the talar neck to reconstruct the anterior talofibular ligament.[42,62,63] Chrisman and Snook[45] demonstrated the importance of reconstruction of both the anterior talofibular ligament and the calcaneofibular ligament in an experimental study, and they devised a tenodesis procedure that used a split peroneus brevis tendon graft (Fig. 6, *center left*). In their reconstruction, the graft is brought through the fibula from anterior to posterior to reconstruct the anterior talofibular ligament and is then brought posteriorly and inferiorly to the calcaneus to reconstruct the calcaneofibular ligament. Although all three of these procedures have had a high rate of clinical success, they have been criticized because the sites of graft placement are anatomically incorrect and they restrict normal motion of the subtalar joint.[24,31,41,44,64]

My colleagues and I performed biomechanical testing of cadaveric ankle specimens treated with these three methods of reconstruction and found that the ability to control pathological motion at the ankle varies with each procedure and that each procedure, when performed as originally described by the authors, excessively limits subtalar motion.[64] We also found that alteration of the attachment sites of the tendon graft can improve stability of the ankle joint without excessive restriction of subtalar motion.

In 1985, Snook and associates[55] reported a modification of the Chrisman-Snook procedure that redirects the posterior limb of the graft more posteriorly, to achieve a more anatomic placement of the graft. The Chrisman-Snook procedure can be made even more anatomically correct by movement of the fibular tunnel distally and orientation of it more obliquely, so that it is similar to the fibular tunnel used by Anderson[41] (Fig. 6, *center right*) or by Elmslie.[46] Leach and associates[22] modified the procedure by suture of the anterior limb of the graft to the talar neck, in order to duplicate the anatomic orientation of the anterior talofibular ligament more closely. With this modification, the anterior limb of the graft still crosses the subtalar joint perpendicular to its axis of motion, so care must be taken not to overtighten the graft, except perhaps in a patient who has severe subtalar instability or a peroneal nerve palsy and in whom the tenodesis effect of the peroneus brevis across the subtalar joint may be necessary to ensure stability.

Several augmented reconstruction techniques have been described that do not restrict motion of the subtalar joint. On the basis of anatomic studies,[64] my colleagues and I developed a reconstruction that uses a split peroneus brevis tendon graft to reinforce the anterior talofibular and calcaneofibular ligaments anatomically (Fig. 6, *bottom left*). The graft is brought from the base of the fifth metatarsal to the calcaneus, emerging from an osseous tunnel at the insertion of the calcaneofibular ligament. The graft is then brought up through an oblique fibular tunnel, passing deep to the peroneal tendons. The graft emerges from the fibula anteriorly, at the origin of the anterior talofibular ligament, and inserts at the attachment of the anterior talofibular ligament on the talus. If there is sufficient length, the anterior limb is doubled back to reinforce the anterior talofibular ligament. Before the graft is passed, the anterior talofibular ligament and the anterolateral aspect of the joint capsule of the ankle are divided, the joint is inspected, and any intra-articular lesion is addressed. The anterior talofibular ligament and the anterolateral aspect of the capsule are reefed in a vest-over-pants fashion to tighten these usually lax and attenuated tissues. The graft is then used to augment this direct repair and is sutured to the calcaneofibular ligament, the anterior talofibular ligament, and the edges of the tunnel. We have used this procedure since 1986 and are encouraged by the clinical results in a small number of patients.[65]

Some authors have recommended the use of free tendon grafts to augment the anterior talofibular and the calcaneofibular ligaments. Anderson[41] used the plantaris tendon (Fig. 6, *center right*). The tendon is harvested with a tendon-stripper through small posterior incisions. It is left attached to the calcaneus and brought through a drill-hole to emerge at the attachment of the calcaneofibular ligament. Anderson emphasized the use of an oblique fibular tunnel so that the graft duplicates the orientation of the calcaneofibular ligament and the anterior talofibular ligament. In 1934, Elmslie[46] described a similar procedure with use of the fascia lata as a free graft. On the basis of their previously described anatomic study, Burks and Morgan[38] developed a method of reconstruction that also uses a free tissue graft (Fig. 6, *bottom right*).

The advantage of use of a tissue graft to augment the reconstruction of the lateral ligaments of the ankle is the increased strength of the repair, which enables the surgeon to stabilize an ankle that has had severe, long-standing ligamentous laxity. The disadvantages include the morbidity associated with the harvest of the graft, particularly the larger incisions needed and the associated risk of formation of a neuroma, and the weakness of eversion created by the sacrifice of part or all of the peroneus brevis tendon.

Results of Reconstruction of the Lateral Ankle Ligaments

Late reconstruction of the lateral ankle ligaments has a high rate of success. Brostrom[31] reported that 51 of 60 patients managed with his technique had minimum or no symptoms of functional instability at the follow-up examination. Similarly, Karlsson and associates[24] reported an 86% rate (128 of 148 patients) of good or excellent functional results after use of a modification of the Brostrom technique. On follow- up stress-testing, Karlsson and associates found that the functional result was roughly associated with the degree of stability achieved. They found that failures were more common in patients who had had long-standing instability, hypermobility of the joints, and failed previous reconstruction of the ankle. They also noted that most failures were in patients in whom only the anterior talofibular ligament had been reconstructed and they recommended routine reconstruction of both the anterior talofibular ligament and the calcaneofibular ligament. Brostrom[31] reported one failure in a patient who had Charcot-Marie- Tooth disease. Weakness or dysfunction of the peroneal muscles probably necessitates the use of a reconstruction, which restricts subtalar motion at least to some degree.

Augmented reconstructions appear to have a low rate of failure in terms of functional instability. Anderson[41] reported no failures in nine patients who had had an augmented reconstruction with the plantaris tendon. Snook and associates[55] reported recurrent instability in three of 48 patients at an average of 10 years postoperatively. Two of the three patients were asymptomatic until they sustained a severe reinjury, while the third patient had severe, generalized ligamentous laxity. Other surgeons who have used the Chrisman-Snook procedure have also achieved satisfactory stability in more than 90% of patients.[22,66,67] None of the 12 patients evaluated at a minimum of 2 years after an anatomic augmented reconstruction, in the series described by Grondel and me,[65] reported recurrent symptoms of instability.

While symptoms of instability may be well controlled with these techniques, pain frequently persists after reconstruction of the ankle ligaments. In the series reported by Grondel and me,[65] we found that, while pain was decreased postoperatively, only four of 12 patients reported no pain in the ankle at the follow-up examination. Barbari and associates[42] reported residual pain in 17 of 42 patients after a modified Watson-Jones procedure. Snook and associates[55] reported on three patients who were not included in their study but who had marked and painful limitation of inversion due to overtightening of the graft with use of the Chrisman-Snook procedure. Brunner and Gaechter[44] "repeatedly observed that excessive tension of the graft can lead to discomfort in the lateral ankle" after the Watson-Jones procedure.

It is unclear whether degenerative osteoarthrosis of the ankle will eventually develop in patients who have recurrent inversion instability. Thus, I do not know if ligamentous reconstruction will prevent the progression of osteoarthrosis. Harrington[68] noted degenerative

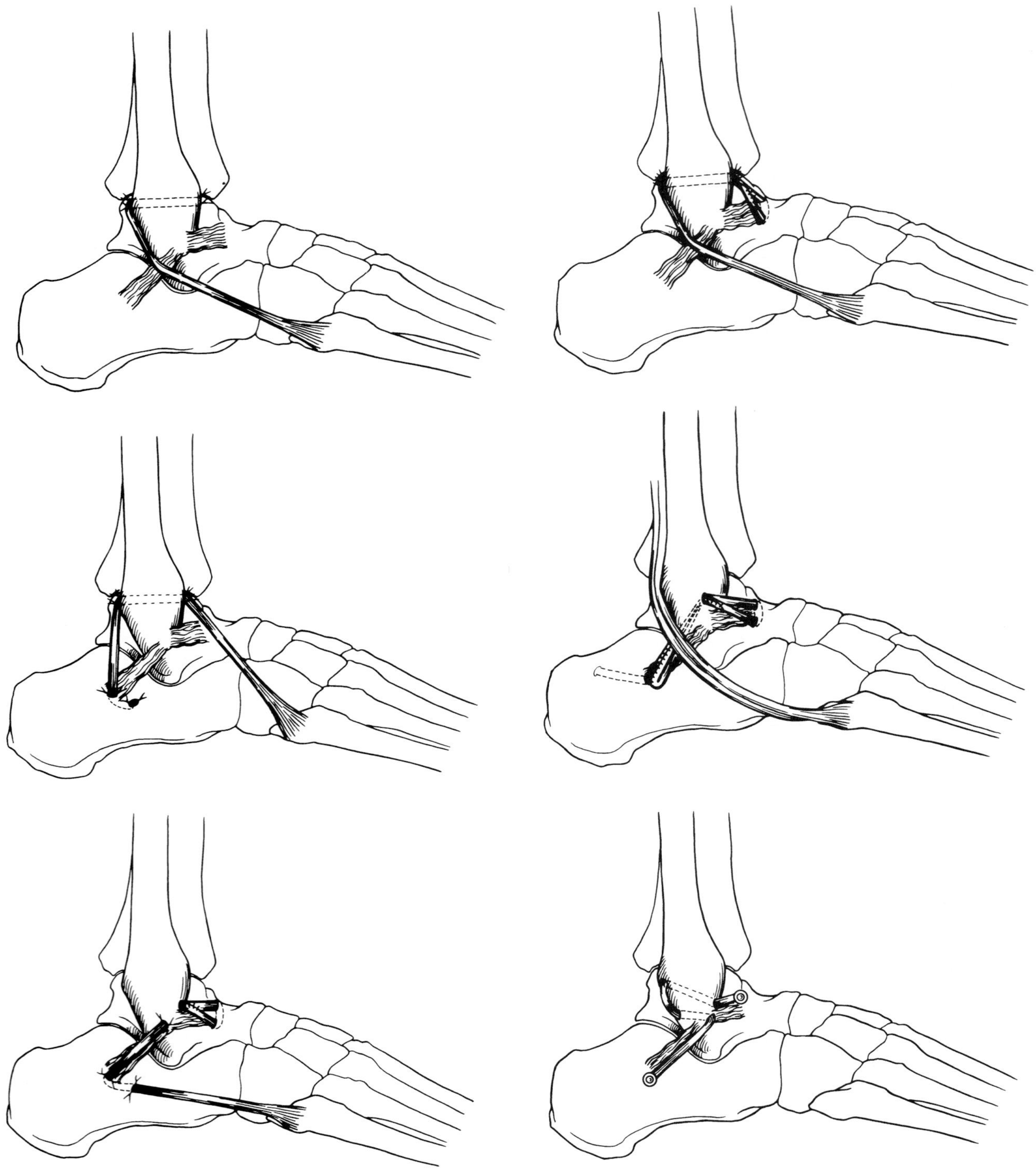

Fig. 6 Various augmented reconstructions. The orientation of the grafts and their effects on motion of the ankle and subtalar joint vary widely. **Top left,** The Evans reconstruction[47] involves tenodesis of the peroneus brevis tendon. **Top right,** The Watson-Jones reconstruction[63] involves tenodesis of the peroneus brevis tendon in addition to reconstruction of the anterior talofibular ligament. **Center left,** The Chrisman-Snook procedure[45] involves reconstruction of the anterior talofibular ligament and the calcaneofibular ligament with use of a split peroneus brevis tendon. The procedure may be modified to reconstruct the anterior talofibular ligament more closely by suturing of the graft to the talar attachment of the ligament, with use of an oblique fibular tunnel, and direction of the posterior limb of the graft posteriorly at 133° from the fibula. **Center right,** The Anderson procedure[41] uses the plantaris tendon to reconstruct the anterior talofibular and calcaneofibular ligaments anatomically. **Bottom left,** The technique that my colleagues and I use involves reconstruction of the anterior talofibular and calcaneofibular ligaments with a split peroneus brevis tendon graft without restriction of subtalar motion. **Bottom right,** The reconstruction proposed by Burks and Morgan[38] uses a free tissue graft and duplicates the anatomic attachments to the anterior talofibular and calcaneofibular ligaments.

changes at the time of arthroscopy in 36 patients who had long-standing instability of the ankle and reported improvement in symptoms following stabilization; however, most authors have not discussed the rate of degenerative osteoarthrosis of the ankle in their reports.

Recommendations for Treatment

As a result of a review of the literature and my laboratory and clinical studies, I do not believe that augmentation of the ligament repair with tendon grafts is necessary in most patients. For most patients, a late modified Brostrom reconstruction of the lateral ankle ligaments, similar to that described by Karlsson and associates[24] (Fig. 4), has a high rate of success, preserves motion of the ankle and subtalar joints, and avoids the potential morbidity associated with use of a tendon graft.

I use a longitudinal incision, running just posterior to the prominence of the lateral malleolus. This incision can be extended to allow harvest of the peroneus brevis tendon if augmentation of the reconstruction is found to be necessary. In most patients, the anterior talofibular ligament and the calcaneofibular ligament are both injured and both are usually reconstructed. The ligaments are divided just distal to their fibular attachments. The joint is inspected and debrided as necessary. Occasionally, one or both ligaments are avulsed from the fibula with a piece of bone. This so-called os subfibulare[69] should be excised. The bone at the anatomic attachment sites of the anterior talofibular and calcaneofibular ligaments is roughened, and the ligaments are reefed and reattached to the fibula with the use of drill-holes. The repair is oversewn with the proximal stump of the ligament to reinforce the repair. During the repair, the ankle is held in neutral and the foot is held in eversion. If the anterior talofibular ligament and the calcaneofibular ligament are so disrupted and frayed that they cannot be repaired, then an augmented reconstruction with the peroneus brevis tendon is performed (Fig. 6, *bottom left*). I also use an augmented reconstruction when there is a history of severe, long-standing instability or evidence of hypermobility of the subtalar joint or to treat a previous failed reconstruction of the ankle. Patients who have paralysis or severe weakness of the peroneal muscles may need a nonanatomic procedure, such as that described by Evans,[47] Watson-Jones,[63] or Chrisman and Snook.[45]

Regardless of the method of reconstruction, postoperatively the ankle should be immobilized for 2 weeks in a rigid compressive dressing with the ankle in neutral and the foot in eversion. At 2 weeks postoperatively, a below-the-knee cast is applied and the patient is allowed to bear weight as tolerated. At 6 weeks postoperatively, immobilization is discontinued and range-of-motion exercises, progressive resistance exercises, and proprioceptive exercises are begun. The patient should wear a lace-up ankle brace for outdoor activities for an additional 6 weeks. At 3 months, full sports activities can be resumed with the ankle taped or braced. Most athletes should continue to use tape or a brace indefinitely during sports activities, but bracing is not routine after 3 months for most work-related activities or activities of daily living.

With use of the principles outlined in this paper, it should be possible to restore stability in a high proportion of patients. However, care must be taken not to overlook the subtalar joint as a cause of instability. The reconstruction should not be done simply to prevent osteoarthrosis, and pain may persist despite relief of the symptoms of instability.

References

1. Brand RL, Black HM, Cox JS: The natural history of inadequately treated ankle sprain. *Am J Sports Med* 1977;5:248-249.
2. Glick JM, Gordon RB, Nishimoto D: The prevention and treatment of ankle injuries. *Am J Sports Med* 1976:4:136-141.
3. Balduini FC, Vegso JJ, Torg JS, et al: Management and rehabilitation of ligamentous injuries to the ankle. *Sports Med* 1987;4:364-380.
4. Boruta PM, Bishop JO, Braly WG, et al: Acute lateral ankle ligament injuries: A literature review. *Foot Ankle* 1990;11:107-113.
5. Freeman MAR: Treatment of ruptures of the lateral ligament of the ankle. *J Bone Joint Surg* 1965;47B:661-668.
6. Freeman MAR: Instability of the foot after injuries to the lateral ligament of the ankle. *J Bone Joint Surg* 1965;47B:669-677.
7. Freeman MAR, Dean MRE, Hanham IWF: The etiology and prevention of functional instability of foot. *J Bone Joint Surg* 1965; 47B:678-685.
8. Kannus P, Renström P: Current concepts review: Treatment for acute tears of the lateral ligaments of the ankle. Operation, cast, or early controlled mobilization. *J Bone Joint Surg* 1991;73A:305-312.
9. Lassiter TE Jr, Malone TR, Garrett WE Jr: Injury to the lateral ligaments of the ankle. *Orthop Clin North Am* 1989;20:629-640.
10. Moller-Larsen F, Wethelund JO, Jurik AG, et al: Comparison of three different treatments for ruptured lateral ankle ligaments. *Acta Orthop Scand* 1988;59:564-566.
11. Pennal GF: Subluxation of the ankle. *Can Med Assoc* 1943;49:92-95.
12. Rijke AM, Jones B, Vierhout PA: Injury to the lateral ankle ligaments of athletes: A posttraumatic followup. *Am J Sports Med* 1988;16:256-259.
13. Ahovuo J, Kaartinen E, Slatis P: Diagnostic value of stress radiography in lesions of the lateral ligaments of the ankle. *Acta Radiol* 1988;29:711-714.
14. Bulucu C, Thomas KA, Halvorson TL, et al: Biomechanical evaluation of the anterior drawer test: The contribution of the lateral ankle ligaments. *Foot Ankle* 1991;11:389-393.
15. Laurin C, Mathieu J: Sagittal mobility of the normal ankle. *Clin Orthop* 1975;108:99-104.
16. Laurin CA, Ouellet R, St-Jacques R: Talar and subtalar tilt: An experimental investigation. *Can J Surg* 1968;11:270-279.
17. Raatikainen T, Putkonen M, Puranen J: Arthrography, clinical examination, and stress radiograph in the diagnosis of acute injury to the lateral ligaments of the ankle. *Am J Sports Med* 1992;20:2-6.
18. Rijke AM, Vierhout PA: Graded stress radiography in acute injury to the lateral ligaments of the ankle. *Acta Radiol* 1990;31:151-155.

19. Rubin G, Witten M: The talar-tilt angle and the fibular collateral ligaments: A method for the determination of talar tilt. *J Bone Joint Surg* 1960;42-A:311-326.
20. Sauser DD, Nelson RC, Lavine MH, et al: Acute injuries of the lateral ligaments of the ankle: Comparison of stress radiography and arthrography. *Radiology* 1983;148:653-657.
21. Agnholt J, Nielsen S, Christensen H: Lesion of the ligamentum bifurcatum in ankle sprain. *Arch Orthop Trauma Surg* 1988; 107:326-328.
22. Leach RE, Namiki O, Paul GR, et al: Secondary reconstruction of the lateral ligaments of the ankle. *Clin Orthop* 1981;160:201-211.
23. Parlasca R, Shoji H, D'Ambrosia RD: Effects of ligamentous injury on ankle and subtalar joints: A kinematic study. *Clin Orthop* 1979;140:266-272.
24. Karlsson J, Bergsten T, Lansinger O, et al: Reconstruction of the lateral ligaments of the ankle for chronic lateral instability. *J Bone Joint Surg* 1988;70A:581-588.
25. Cox JS, Hewes TF: "Normal" talar tilt angle. *Clin Orthop* 1979; 140:37-41.
26. Cass JR, Morrey BF: Ankle instability: Current concepts, diagnosis, and treatment. *Mayo Clin Proc* 1984;59:165-170.
27. Johnson EE, Markolf KL: The contribution of the anterior talofibular ligament to ankle laxity. *J Bone Joint Surg* 1983;65A:81-88.
28. Colville MR, Marder RA, Boyle JJ, et al: Strain measurement in lateral ankle ligaments. *Am J Sports Med* 1990;18:196-200.
29. Shybut GT, Hayes WC, White AA III: Normal patterns of ligament loading among the lateral collateral ankle ligaments. *Trans Orthop Res Soc* 1983;8:15.
30. Shybut GT, Lelli JL, Rubin JD, et al: The effect of anterior talofibular insufficiency on ligament loading patterns. *Trans Orthop Res Soc* 1983;8:289.
31. Brostrom L: Sprained ankles: V. Surgical treatment of "chronic" ligament ruptures. *Acta Chir Scand* 1966;132:551-565.
32. Meyer JM, Garcia J, Hoffmeyer P, et al: The subtalar sprain: A roentgenographic study. *Clin Orthop* 1988;226:169-173.
33. Kjaersgaard-Andersen P, Wethelund JO, Helmig P, et al: Effect of the calcaneofibular ligament on hindfoot rotation in amputation specimens. *Acta Orthop Scand* 1987;58:135-138.
34. Kjaersgaard-Andersen P, Frich LH, Madsen F, et al: Instability of the hindfoot after lesion of the lateral ankle ligaments: Investigations of the anterior drawer and adduction maneuvers in autopsy specimens. *Clin Orthop* 1991;266:170-179.
35. Clanton TO: Instability of the subtalar joint. *Orthop Clin North Am* 1989;20:583-592.
36. Harper MC: The lateral ligamentous support of the subtalar joint. *Foot Ankle* 1991;11:354-358.
37. Schon LC, Clanton TO, Baxter DE: Reconstruction for subtalar instability: A review. *Foot Ankle* 1991;11:319-325.
38. Burks RT, Morgan J: Anatomy of the lateral ankle ligaments. *Am J Sports Med* 1994;22:72-77.
39. Ahlgren O, Larsson S: Reconstruction for lateral ligament injuries of the ankle. *J Bone Joint Surg* 1989;71B:300-303.
40. Anderson KJ, Lecocq JF: Operative treatment of injury to the fibular collateral ligament of the ankle. *J Bone Joint Surg* 1954; 36A:825-832.
41. Anderson ME: Reconstruction of the lateral ligaments of the ankle using the plantaris tendon. *J Bone Joint Surg* 1985;67A:930-934.
42. Barbari SG, Brevig K, Egge T: Reconstruction of the lateral ligamentous structures of the ankle with a modified Watson-Jones procedure. *Foot Ankle* 1987:362-368.
43. Brand RL, Collins MD, Templeton T: Surgical repair of ruptured lateral ankle ligaments. *Am J Sports Med* 1981;9:40-44.
44. Brunner R, Gaechter A: Repair of fibular ligaments: Comparison of reconstructive techniques using plantaris and peroneal tendons. *Foot Ankle* 1991;11:359-367.
45. Chrisman OD, Snook GA: Reconstruction of lateral ligament tears of the ankle: An experimental study and clinical evaluation of seven patients treated by a new modification of the Elmslie procedure. *J Bone Joint Surg* 1969;51A:904-912.
46. Elmslie RC: Recurrent subluxation of the ankle-joint. *Ann Surg* 1934;100:364-367.
47. Evans DL: Recurrent instability of the ankle: A method of surgical treatment. *Proc Roy Soc Med* 1953;46:343-344.
48. Eyring EJ, Guthrie WD: A surgical approach to the problem of severe lateral instability at the ankle. *Clin Orthop* 1986;206:185-191.
49. Horibe S, Shino K, Taga I, et al: Reconstruction of lateral ligaments of the ankle with allogeneic tendon grafts. *J Bone Joint Surg* 1991;73B:802-805.
50. Lee HG: Surgical repair in recurrent dislocation of the ankle joint. *J Bone Joint Surg* 1957;39A:828-834.
51. Milachowski KA, Wirth CJ: The results of reconstruction of the lateral ligaments of the ankle. *Int Orthop* 1988;12:51-55.
52. Palladino SJ, Smith SB, Jackson JL: Plantaris tendon reconstruction of the lateral ankle ligaments. *J Foot Surg* 1991;30:406-413.
53. Ruth CJ: The surgical treatment of injuries of the fibular collateral ligaments of the ankle. *J Bone Joint Surg* 1961;43A:229-239.
54. Sjolin SU, Dons-Jensen H, Simonsen O: Reinforced anatomical reconstruction of the anterior talofibular ligament in chronic anterolateral instability using a periosteal flap. *Foot Ankle* 1991; 12:15-18.
55. Snook GA, Chrisman OD, Wilson TC: Long-term results of the Chrisman-Snook operation for reconstruction of the lateral ligaments of the ankle. *J Bone Joint Surg* 1985;67A:1-7.
56. Stören H: A new method for operative treatment of insufficiency of the lateral ligaments of the ankle joint. *Acta Chir Scand* 1959; 117:501-509.
57. Windfeld P: Treatment of undue mobility of the ankle joint following severe sprain of the ankle with avulsion of the anterior and middle bands of the external ligament. *Acta Chir Scand* 1953;105:299-304.
58. Younes C, Fowles JV, Fallaha M, et al: Long-term results of surgical reconstruction for chronic lateral instability of the ankle: Comparison of Watson-Jones and Evans techniques. *J Trauma* 1988;28:1330-1334.
59. Gould N, Seligson D, Gassman J: Early and late repair of lateral ligament of the ankle. *Foot Ankle* 1980;1:84-89.
60. Jaskulka R, Fischer G, Schedl R: Injuries of the lateral ligaments of the ankle joint: Operative treatment and long-term results. *Arch Orthop Trauma Surg* 1988;107:217-221.
61. Sobel M, Warren RF, Brourman S: Lateral ankle instability associated with dislocation of the peroneal tendons treated by the Chrisman-Snook procedure: A case report and literature review. *Am J Sports Med* 1990;18:539-543.
62. Gillespie HS, Boucher P: Watson-Jones repair of lateral instability of the ankle. *J Bone Joint Surg* 1971;53A:920-924.
63. Watson-Jones R: *Fractures and Other Bone and Joint Injuries*, ed 4. Edinburgh, E & S Livingstone, 1955, vol 2, pp 821-823.
64. Colville MR, Marder RA, Zarins B: Reconstruction of the lateral ankle ligaments: A biomechanical analysis. *Am J Sports Med* 1992;20:594-600.
65. Colville MR, Grondel RJ: Anatomic reconstruction of the lateral ankle ligaments using a split peroneus brevis tendon. *Am J Sports Med*, in press.
66. Rechtine GR, McCarroll JR, Webster DA: Reconstruction for chronic lateral instability of the ankle: A review of twenty eight surgical patients. *Orthopedics* 1982;5:46-50.
67. Riegler HF: Reconstruction for lateral instability of the ankle. *J Bone Joint Surg* 1984;66A:336-339.
68. Harrington KD: Degenerative arthritis of the ankle secondary to long-standing lateral ligament instability. *J Bone Joint Surg* 1979;61A:354-361.
69. Berg EE: The symptomatic os subfibulare: Avulsion fracture of the fibula associated with recurrent instability of the ankle. *J Bone Joint Surg* 1991;73A:1251-1254.

CHAPTER 30

Current Methods for the Evaluation of Ankle Ligament Injuries

Richard A. Marder, MD

The lateral ankle ligaments are frequently injured during athletic activities requiring pivoting and jumping.[1-6] Less commonly involved are the tibiofibular syndesmosis and the deltoid (medial) ligament.[2] Although most of these injuries heal uneventfully, prompt diagnosis and treatment can shorten the recovery time and reduce the prevalence of residual symptoms that can impair future athletic performance. An accurate diagnosis of an injury of these ligaments requires an understanding of the pertinent functional anatomy and biomechanics as well as a thorough history, physical examination, and appropriate radiographic studies, including stress radiographs. In selected patients, arthrography, magnetic resonance imaging, or bone scintigraphy may be useful for further evaluation of the injury. When evaluating an injured ankle, the physician must perform a careful examination for injuries other than those of the ligaments, such as subluxation of the peroneal tendon, osteochondral lesions of the talus, and injuries of the midfoot and subtalar joint, which can occur concomitantly with inversion injuries of the ankle or which can mimic them.

Functional Anatomy and Biomechanics

Lateral Ankle Ligaments

The lateral aspect of the ankle capsule is augmented by the anterior and posterior talofibular ligaments and the calcaneofibular ligament. Of these three structures, the anterior talofibular and calcaneofibular ligaments are the most important clinically.

The anterior talofibular ligament is a thickening of the ankle capsule that extends a relatively short distance from the anterior edge of the distal part of the fibula to the talar neck, anterior to its lateral articular facet. The orientation of the anterior talofibular ligament depends on the position of the ankle joint.[1] In plantarflexion, it is parallel to the long axis of the foot, whereas in dorsiflexion, it is aligned with the tibial and fibular shafts. Strain in the anterior talofibular ligament is minimum in dorsiflexion and neutral, and it increases as the ankle is moved progressively through plantarflexion.[7,8] Inversion[7] and internal rotation[7,8] moments applied to the ankle increase the strain in this ligament.

The calcaneofibular ligament is a discrete, extra-articular, round ligament that spans the ankle and subtalar joints as it courses obliquely from the inferior tip of the distal part of the fibula to insert posteriorly on the mid-lateral part of the calcaneus. This ligament is extra-articular but it has an intimate connection to the overlying peroneal-tendon sheath. Brostrom[2] thought that the calcaneofibular ligament was lax until a supination force was applied. Strain studies of the intact calcaneofibular ligament have demonstrated increasing strain as the ankle is moved from plantarflexion to dorsiflexion, with the greatest strain occurring when an inversion moment is applied with the ankle in dorsiflexion.[7,8] Because of its unique anatomic orientation, the calcaneofibular ligament also has a major role in the stabilization of the subtalar joint.[9,10]

Deltoid Ligament

This ligament consists of deep and superficial components. The deep fibers connect the medial malleolus to the medial border of the talus, while the superficial portion has a broad, fan-shaped attachment to the navicular, the sustentaculum tali, and the posterior part of the talus. The deep portion resists external rotation of the talus, while the superficial component resists abduction of the talus.[11]

Distal Tibiofibular Syndesmosis

The ankle mortise is stabilized by the anterior and posterior tibiofibular ligaments, the inferior transverse ligament, and the interosseous ligament. Strain increases in the anterior and posterior tibiofibular ligaments with dorsiflexion, and it increases in the anterior tibiofibular ligament with external rotation of the talus.[7]

Pathomechanics of Injury

Analysis of ankle stability under physiologic loading of the joint demonstrated that articular contact provides 100% of inversion stability and 30% of rotational stability.[12] In reality, however, inversion ankle injuries usually occur during loading or unloading of the ankle.

Lateral Ankle Ligaments

Typically, injuries of the lateral ankle ligaments occur from an inversion or an internal rotation force, or both, applied to the foot when the ankle is plantarflexed. Because these injuries occur during loading or unloading of the ankle and foot, the stabilizing effects of the tibiotalar articular surfaces[12] are less important than those of the lateral ligamentocapsular structures of the ankle joint. Injury of the anterior talofibular ligament occurs first, followed by a varying degree of injury of the calcaneofibular ligament.[2,11,13-15] Rarely, a continuation of the applied force ruptures the posterior talofibular ligament and can even produce a dislocation of the talus.[16] Clinically, isolated rupture of the calcaneofibular ligament is unlikely. Although isolated rupture of the calcaneofibular ligament has been produced experimentally,[10,17] Rasmussen[11] was unable to do so and Brostrom[2] did not observe any isolated ruptures of this ligament in the clinical setting.

Injuries of individual ligaments are traditionally graded as first, second, or third-degree, depending on the severity. However, because the lateral ligament complex of the ankle consists of more than one ligament, Black and associates[18] chose to describe injuries to it as single if one ligament was ruptured and as double if more than one ligament were ruptured. Singer and Jones[19] classified injuries of the lateral ankle ligaments as stable or unstable and subdivided unstable injuries according to the degree of the talar tilt and anterior drawer that is present under stress, as will be described.

Deltoid Ligament

An isolated frank rupture of the deltoid ligament is uncommon, representing less than 5% (three) of the 105 ankle injuries in Brostrom's series.[2] An eversion or external rotation force that is sufficient to tear the deltoid ligament completely most often also ruptures the tibiofibular syndesmosis or causes a fibular fracture.

Distal Tibiofibular Syndesmosis

Both dorsiflexion and external rotation forces have been implicated in injuries of the distal tibiofibular syndesmosis. The true prevalence of these injuries is unknown because they are often not recognized or reported. Brostrom[2] noted a prevalence of less than 10% (six of 105) in his series, while Hopkinson and associates[20] reported a prevalence of approximately 1% (15) of 1,344 ankle injuries. Complete rupture of the syndesmosis can cause either frank or latent diastasis of the ankle mortise.[21]

History

The patient's history is especially useful when the physician is attempting to reconstruct the mechanism of injury, to identify any previous ankle injury, and to establish the performance level of the individual. A competitive performance level or a history of previous ankle injuries might be decisive factors leading to the recommendation of an operation for an acute, severe injury of the lateral ankle ligaments. The history is less often helpful in the assessment of the severity of the injury. Following recurrent injuries, the patient may report a history of pain, swelling, giving-way, or functional instability.[22]

Mechanism of Injury

Although the overwhelming majority of ankle ligament injuries occur from an inversion force applied to a plantarflexed ankle, it is very important to attempt to identify injuries that have occurred from either an eversion or an external rotation force or that have occurred with the ankle in dorsiflexion. Such mechanisms of injury should alert the examiner to a high probability of an injury of the syndesmosis or the deltoid ligament, or both. Additionally, a dorsiflexion injury associated with a snapping sensation followed by rapidly diminishing pain after the injury may indicate an acute rupture of the peroneal retinaculum with tendon subluxation.[23] A patient with this problem may continue to complain of a clicking sensation over the lateral malleolus.

Severity of Injury

The patient may describe a tearing sensation or feel a distinct popping with an injury of a lateral ankle ligament. The ability to resume playing in an athletic event and minimum swelling suggest a mild or moderate injury, whereas the inability to bear weight, severe pain, and rapid swelling suggest a frank rupture of a ligament or a fracture.

Physical Examination

Although the history may suggest a particular injury, it is important to perform a comprehensive examination of the entire ankle and foot to avoid missing a concomitant or adjacent injury. This is especially important when the patient is not evaluated until several hours or days after the injury, by which time diffuse swelling can mask the specific site of the injury.

Inspection

Swelling always develops following a frank rupture of a lateral ankle ligament, and ecchymosis can be expected after nearly one-half of such ruptures.[24] Localized swelling can be observed if the patient is seen within the first hours after the injury, and diffuse swelling involving the entire lateral aspect of the ankle and foot occurs thereafter. Swelling immediately inferior to the lateral malleolus is characteristic of a serious injury of the lateral ankle ligaments and can usually be differentiated from the more distal swelling—over the sinus tarsi and midfoot—that is seen after an injury of the subtalar joint or the midfoot and after a fracture of the anterior process of the calcaneus. Supramalleolar swelling suggests a rupture of the syndesmosis or a fibular fracture, while swelling posterior to the lateral malleolus is usually noted after rupture of the peroneal retinaculum. The amount of swelling usually does not correspond well with the degree of injury, although Funder and associates[25] reported that the amounts of swelling and direct ligament tenderness were a more accurate indication of the severity of the injury than was the amount of joint laxity.

Palpation

The foot, ankle, and calf up to the knee should be palpated for tenderness or deformity, or both. Specifically, the course of the deltoid ligament and the individual lateral ligaments of the ankle, the malleoli, the anterior and posterior tibiofibular ligaments, the entire length of the fibula, the anterior and posterior margins of the tibiotalar joint, the sinus tarsi, the peroneal tendons, and the Achilles tendon should all be palpated. Tenderness of an individual lateral ankle ligament is suggestive of, but not specific for, injury of that particular ligament.[24] Passive ankle motion invariably produces pain, especially if marked swelling has occurred, and therefore is not helpful in the diagnosis. Tenderness of the peroneal tendons posterior to the lateral malleolus is suggestive of a disruption of the peroneal retinaculum; anterior and lateral pressure should be applied to these tendons to demonstrate any potential for their displacement from the fibular groove.

Neuromuscular Tests

The active range of motion of the ankle should be recorded. Pedal pulses should be palpated, and sensory and motor function should be assessed. Traction injuries of the peroneal and posterior tibial nerves[26] as well as peroneal compartment syndromes[19] have been described following severe injuries of the ankle ligaments and should not be overlooked. The function of the peroneal muscles should be assessed carefully. Active dorsiflexion and eversion may demonstrate subluxation of the peroneal tendons. Integrity of the peroneal tendons is tested by having the patient attempt active eversion of the foot. Peroneal muscle weakness is often a notable finding in patients with recurrent instability.[27]

Special Tests

Specialized testing is done to exclude rupture of the Achilles tendon, which can be misdiagnosed as an ankle ligament injury when there is diffuse swelling and ecchymosis. When the Achilles tendon is intact, squeezing of the muscle belly of the gastrocnemius-soleus passively causes plantarflexion of the ankle.[28]

Hopkinson and associates[20] described another squeeze test to aid in the diagnosis of syndesmosis injury. Compression of the fibula against the tibia at the mid-calf level elicits pain near the ankle when the syndesmosis has been injured. The test is considered positive for a syndesmosis injury only when a fracture of the fibula or tibia, a contusion of the calf, and a compartment syndrome of the leg have been excluded.

Clinical Stress Tests

While many studies[7,8,29-41] have been done to define the specific functions of the lateral ankle ligaments, one practical consideration remains: it is difficult to be certain which ligament is being evaluated with each of the clinical tests. The commonly used tests for evaluation of lateral ligament laxity of the ankle are the anterior drawer and the talar tilt tests. Anterior displacement of the talus in relation to the tibia, first described by Dehne[30] and by Anderson and associates,[13] is known as the anterior drawer of the ankle. The anterior talofibular ligament is the primary restraint in the anterior drawer test. Testing of the ankle in 10° of plantarflexion[33] results in the greatest amount of translation, although one cadaveric study showed that maximum anterior excursion occurs in dorsiflexion.[34] Injury of the calcaneofibular ligament does not increase the amount of the anterior drawer.[36]

Talar instability is also assessed with the talar tilt test, in which the angle formed by the tibial plafond and the talar dome is measured as an inversion force is applied to the hindfoot.[39] The talar tilt test is useful for evaluation of a combined injury of both the anterior talofibular and the calcaneofibular ligaments. Isolated rupture of the calcaneofibular ligament probably does not cause demonstrable ankle laxity.[11] Rubin and Witten[39] reported talar tilt to range from 0° to 23° in normal ankles, while Cox and Hewes[29] demonstrated, in a large study of midshipmen, that normal ankles had 5° of talar tilt or less with manual stress. This variability in results may be due to differences in such testing variables as the method of application and the duration of load, the position of the ankle, or the use of anesthesia.[1,33] Testing with the ankle in plantarflexion assesses the anterior talofibular ligament primarily and the calcaneofibular ligament secondarily. When the anterior talofibular ligament alone is ruptured, small increases in talar tilt are noted. This fact, together with the greater variability in talar tilt measurements, has led some to favor the anterior drawer test as a measurement of lateral ligament instability.[32,40] However, as combined rupture of the anterior talofibular ligament and the calcaneofibular ligament results in increased talar tilt, the talar tilt test remains an important tool for the examiner.

The anterior drawer test can be performed with the patient either sitting or supine. When the patient is sitting, the knee should be flexed over the edge of a bench or table and the ankle should be allowed to fall into equinus. The examiner then stabilizes the distal part of the leg with one hand and applies an anterior force to the heel with the other hand, in an attempt to subluxate the talus anteriorly from beneath the tibia. This maneuver usually is not painful if the patient has an acute injury. The modified anterior drawer test[42] can be used when the patient is supine. With the knee hyperflexed, the ankle in equinus, and the foot fixed by

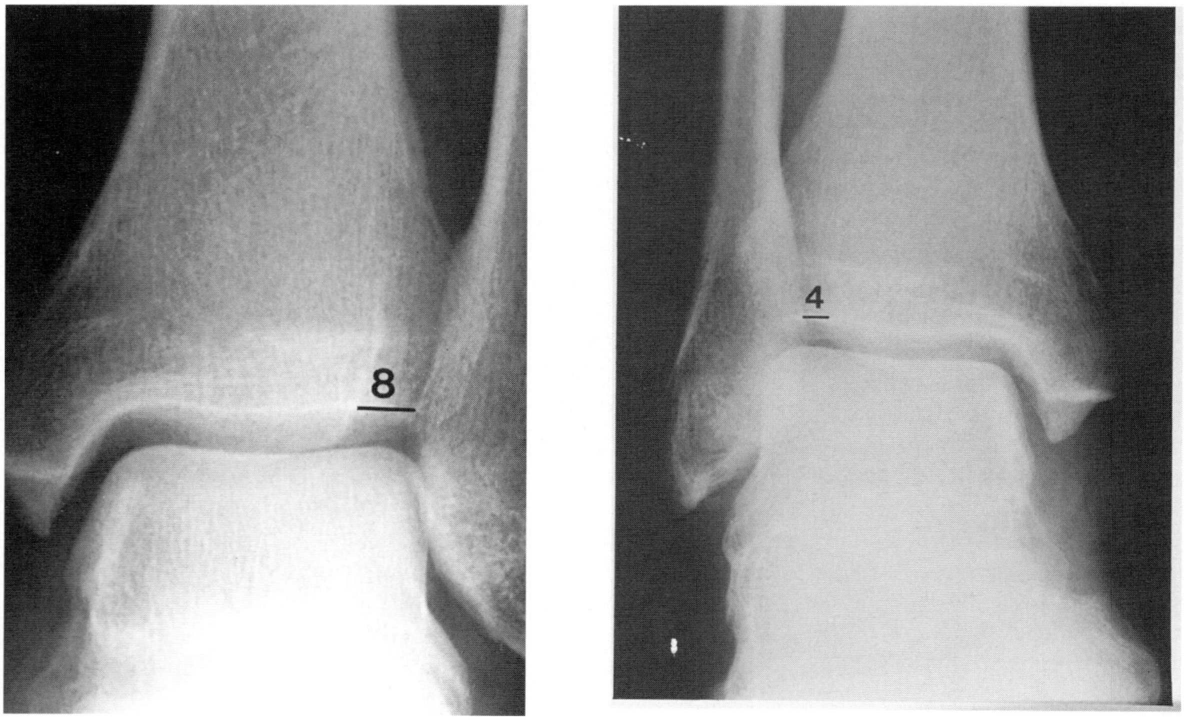

Fig. 1 Anteroposterior radiographs showing the clear space representing the tibiofibular syndesmosis to be 8 mm in the left, injured ankle compared with 4 mm in the right, uninjured ankle.

one of the examiner's hands to the ground or table, a force is applied with the other hand on the anterior aspect of the distal part of the leg, in an attempt to translate the tibia posteriorly.

The talar tilt test is performed with the patient seated and with the ankle and foot unsupported in 10° to 20° of plantarflexion. The examiner stabilizes the medial aspect of the distal part of the leg, just proximal to the medial malleolus, with one hand and applies an inversion force slowly to the hindfoot with the other hand. The lateral aspect of the talus should be palpated during inversion of the hindfoot to determine if tilting is occurring at the tibiotalar joint. Comparison with the normal ankle is helpful to detect any side-to-side difference. It has been noted that the talar tilt test may be positive only if gross instability is present.[43] If the anterior drawer or talar tilt test suggests abnormal laxity or if pain, swelling, and muscle spasm are present to a degree that prevents satisfactory clinical assessment, then stress radiographs are performed to measure laxity.

Radiographic Examination

Conventional Radiographs

As a rule, all joint injuries should be examined radiographically. For ankle injuries, anteroposterior, mortise, and lateral radiographs of the ankle are obtained routinely. Rarely, an inversion injury of the ankle produces an avulsion fracture of the tip of the fibula. Lateral talar shift, seen as an increase in the clear space between the medial malleolus and the talus, indicates disruption of the ankle mortise. This is a sign of disruption of the tibiofibular syndesmosis and should alert the examiner to the possibility of a proximal fibular fracture. Widening of the mortise in syndesmosis injuries can be subtle, and a comparison radiograph of the uninjured ankle can be helpful (Fig. 1). As a general guide, the clear space between the lateral aspect of the medial malleolus and the medial aspect of the talus should not be any greater than the distance between the talar dome and the tibial plafond (Fig. 2). The syndesmosis should be considered to be wider than normal if the medial clear space exceeds 6 mm on the anteroposterior and mortise radiographs.[44]

Additional radiographs are occasionally useful. An anteroposterior radiograph of the ankle in internal rotation may demonstrate an avulsion flake from the distal part of the fibula caused by acute peroneal subluxation.[45] When ankle injuries are associated with tenderness and swelling that involve the lateral part of the foot, a medial oblique radiograph of the foot can lead to a diagnosis of a fracture of the anterior process of the calcaneus, and routine radiographs of the foot may demonstrate a fracture of the base of the fifth metatarsal.

Ankle radiographs of patients with recurrent inversion injuries may demonstrate ossicles adjacent to the tip of the malleoli, heterotopic ossification of the distal

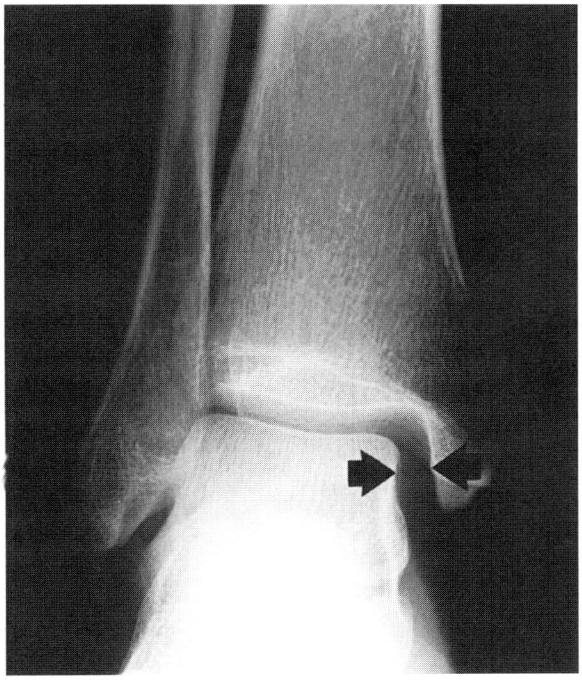

Fig. 2 Anteroposterior radiograph of the ankle, showing lateral talar shift as evidenced by an increase in the distance between the articular surfaces of the medial malleolus and the medial aspect of the talus (arrows) as compared with the distance between the articular surfaces of the tibial plafond and the talar dome.

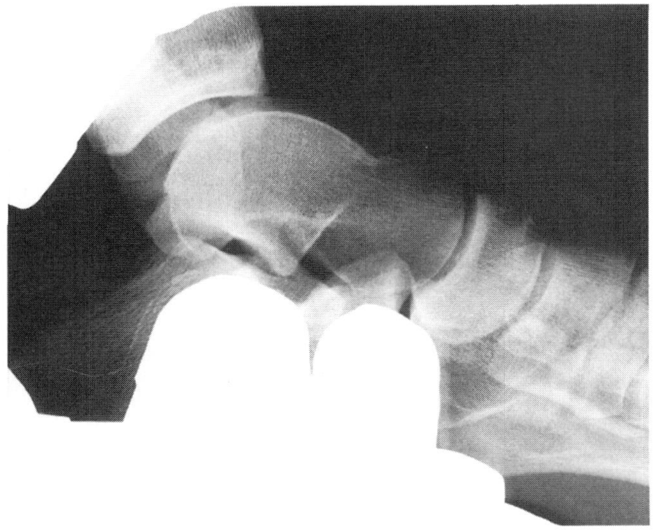

Fig. 3 Anterior drawer stress radiograph showing anterior talar subluxation of the injured ankle.

tibiofibular syndesmosis, and varying degrees of degenerative changes of the tibiotalar articulation.

Stress Radiographs

When 3 mm of anterior excursion or less is measured on the anterior drawer test and the clinical talar tilt test is clearly negative, only conventional radiographs are made. In all other cases, stress radiographs should be made to assess the various ankle and subtalar instabilities.

Lateral Ankle Instability

If a serious injury is suggested by either a positive anterior drawer test or a positive talar tilt test, then stress tests are performed with radiographic documentation to quantify the amount of anterior talar excursion and the degree of talar tilt. The anterior drawer stress test is performed with the ankle in approximately 10° of plantarflexion and the knee flexed. In order to assess the contributions of both the anterior talofibular and the calcaneofibular ligaments, the talar tilt test is performed with the ankle in neutral and the leg and foot internally rotated 15° to 20° (the ankle mortise radiograph). Having the patient seated with the hip and knee flexed may help the examiner to perform the talar tilt test.[29] Rarely, when necessary to relieve pain or achieve muscle relaxation, a local anesthetic can be injected into the ankle or a peroneal nerve block[46] can be performed. It is imperative to obtain similar stress radiographs of the normal ankle.

The amount of anterior displacement of the talus during the anterior drawer stress test is measured as the shortest distance from the posterior lip of the tibia to a constant point on the talar dome. A side-to-side difference of greater than 3 mm signifies a rupture of the anterior talofibular ligament (Fig. 3). A side-to-side difference of 10° or more on the talar tilt stress test (Fig. 4) probably indicates complete rupture of both the anterior talofibular and the calcaneofibular ligaments.[47-49]

Subtalar Instability

Differentiation of chronic subtalar instability from lateral ankle instability is rarely based on clinical evaluation alone. Not only do both conditions result in similar symptoms of giving way or recurrent inversion instability, but it is difficult to identify on physical examination whether increased motion of the hindfoot during the talar tilt test is occurring at the tibiotalar or the talocalcaneal joint alone or at both joints because of the coexistence of two instabilities.[16,50]

The use of stress radiography or stress tomography is indicated when subtalar instability is suspected. An anteroposterior stress radiograph, as described by Laurin and associates,[10] is made with the leg internally rotated 45°, the x-ray tube angled cephalad 45°, and the ankle and foot in neutral flexion-extension while manual inversion stress is applied. Loss of parallelism between the posterior facets of the talus and the calcaneus is indicative of subtalar instability. Initially described by Rubin and Witten,[39] stress tomography, which allows quantitative measurement of subtalar instability, has been advocated by Brantigan and associ-

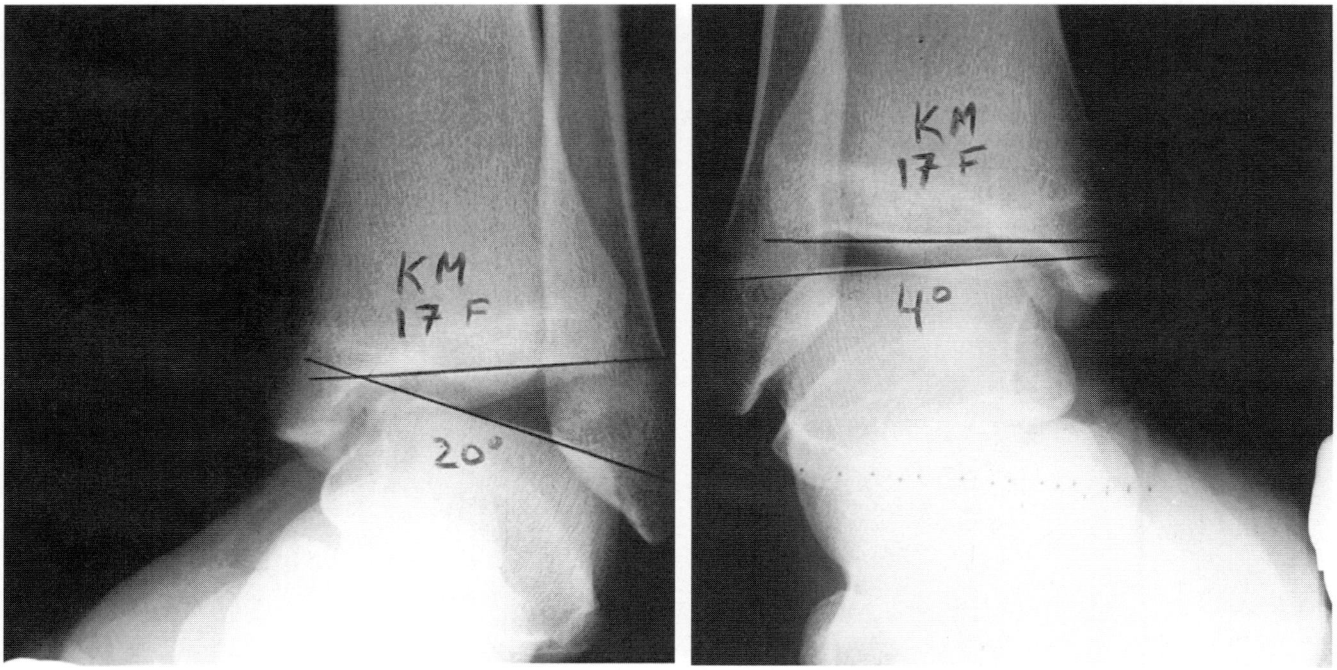

Fig. 4 Talar tilt stress radiographs showing 20° of talar tilt of the injured ankle compared with only 4° of tilt of the normal ankle.

ates[51] as being more practical than stress radiography of the subtalar joint.

Ankle Arthrography and Peroneal Tenography

Arthrography of the ankle, as popularized by Brostrom and associates,[52] is useful for detection of tears of the lateral, medial, and syndesmotic ligaments of the ankle.[53] Because of the intimate relationship of the anterior talofibular ligament with the lateral aspect of the ankle capsule, a tear of this ligament is readily demonstrated by leakage of contrast medium from the lateral aspect of the capsule at that site. Similarly, syndesmosis disruption can be demonstrated arthrographically (Fig. 5). Confirmation of a tear of the calcaneofibular ligament depends on the finding of contrast medium flowing into the peroneal tendon sheath (Fig. 6). However, with ankle arthrography, the contrast medium often fails to enter the peroneal sheath, despite surgically proven tears of the calcaneofibular ligament; therefore, the technique of peroneal tenography was developed.[18] It has proved to be more accurate in the diagnosis of disruption of the calcaneofibular ligament. Although their demonstration of the anatomic nature of the injury is an advantage, studies that employ contrast medium are rarely used because there are few indications for primary surgical repair of acute tears of the lateral ligaments.

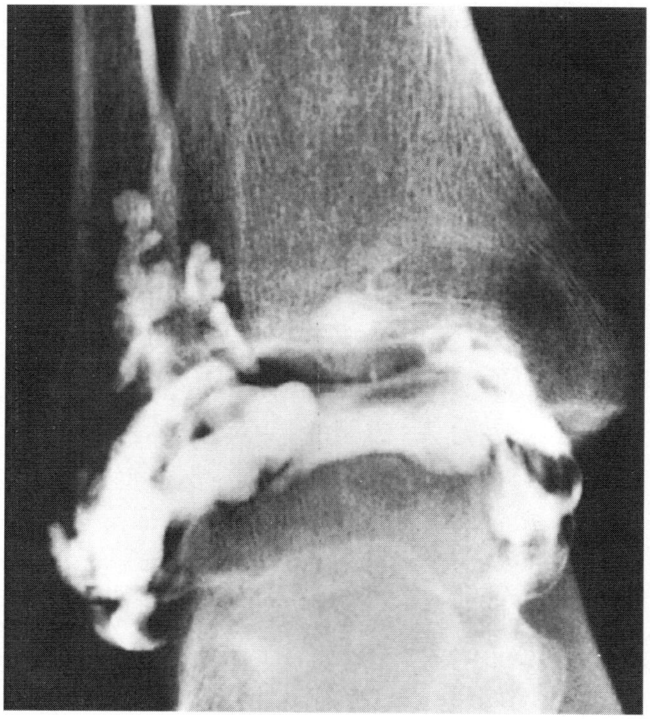

Fig. 5 Arthrogram of the ankle, showing leakage of contrast medium into the distal syndesmosis, confirming rupture of the tibiofibular ligaments. (Courtesy of Adam Greenspan, MD).

Magnetic Resonance Imaging

Magnetic resonance images can demonstrate accurately the normal and torn anterior talofibular and calcaneofibular ligaments (Fig. 7).[54] Despite its cost,

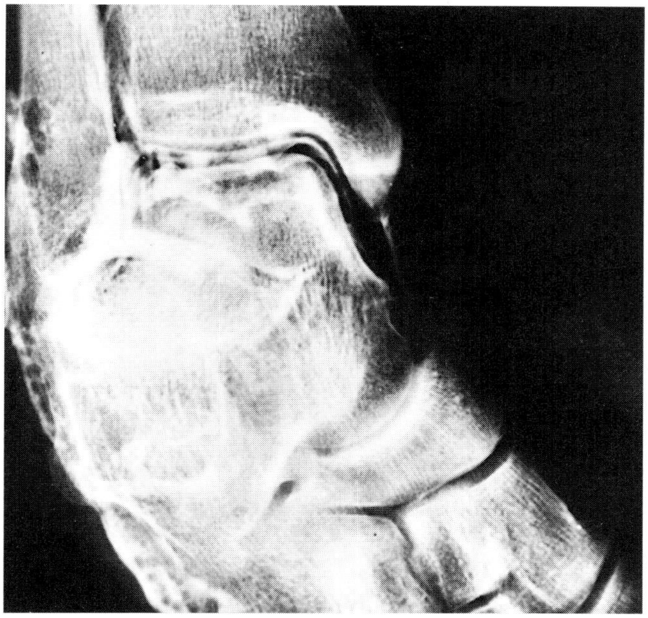

Fig. 6 Arthrogram of the ankle, showing extravasation of contrast medium into the peroneal tendon sheath, confirming rupture of the calcaneofibular ligament. (Courtesy of Adam Greenspan, MD).

magnetic resonance imaging can replace the invasive arthrogram and tenogram if demonstration of the extent of anatomic disruption is critical for the selection of treatment. If the treating physician always chooses a primary repair of acute, double (anterior talofibular and calcaneofibular) ligament ruptures in highly competitive athletes, then magnetic resonance imaging will help him or her to decide whether to perform surgery. However, as treatment is most often based on the demonstration of instability, magnetic resonance imaging has limited usefulness in the routine assessment of torn ankle ligaments.

Magnetic resonance imaging does have a major role in the evaluation of osteochondral lesions of the talus (Fig. 8), which can cause pain and a feeling of instability after an inversion injury of the ankle. Magnetic resonance imaging also can document partial and full-thickness tears of the peroneal tendons, which can occur in conjunction with inversion injuries or subluxation of the peroneal tendon.

Scintigraphy

There are few indications for the use of bone scans in the evaluation of acutely injured ankles. Notwithstanding the ability of radionuclide imaging to demonstrate occult injuries of the tibiofibular syndesmosis,[55] thorough clinical examination and conventional radiographs should be sufficient to establish the diagnosis in most patients. On the other hand, when symptoms persist, scintigraphy may aid in the diagnosis of conditions such as the os trigonum syndrome and occult fractures of the ankle, which can cause persistent symptoms of pain and functional instability.[56,57]

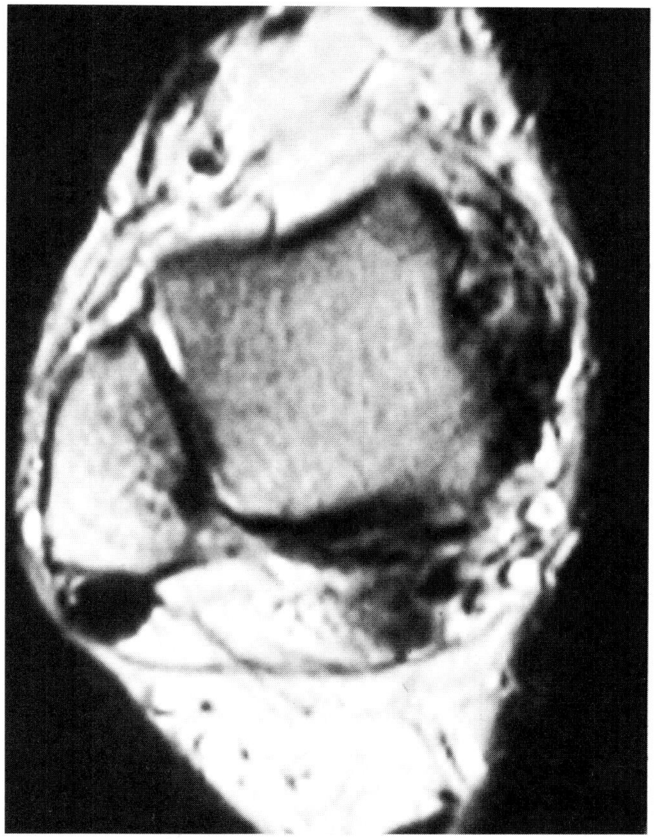

Fig. 7 Axial magnetic resonance image showing an intact anterior talofibular ligament (arrow).

Arthroscopy

Arthroscopy is useful in the treatment of certain conditions that may persist after an ankle injury, such as osteochondral defects of the talar dome, loose bodies, painful ossicles within the ankle ligaments, and the hypertrophied inferior border of the anteroinferior tibiofibular ligament.[58] However, arthroscopy does not play a role in the diagnostic workup of an acute ankle injury.

Overview

1. Most lateral injuries of the ankle involve the anterior talofibular ligament, alone or in combination with the calcaneofibular ligament.

2. The diagnosis of an injury of the lateral ligaments is suggested by the mechanism of injury and by the findings of localized tenderness and swelling.

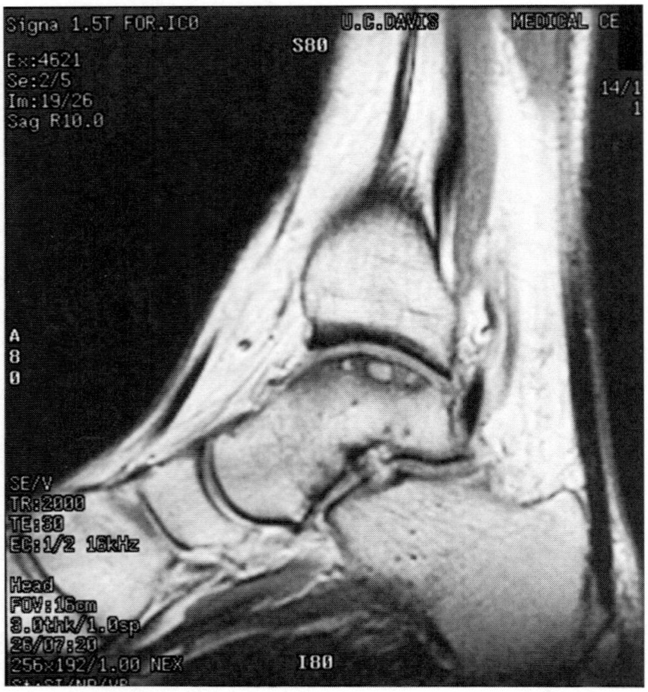

Fig. 8 Magnetic resonance image showing an extensive osteochondral lesion of the talar dome following an inversion injury.

3. The severity of the injury can be assessed with laxity testing and the use of radiographs for quantification. A positive anterior drawer test indicates a rupture of the anterior talofibular ligament, and a talar tilt test with a difference between the injured and uninjured ankles of 10° or more is consistent with a rupture of both the anterior talofibular and the calcaneofibular ligaments.

4. Anatomic confirmation of the injury can be achieved noninvasively by magnetic resonance imaging or invasively by arthrography, peroneal tenography, or direct observation at surgical exploration.

5. The differential diagnosis of an injury of the lateral ligament complex of the ankle should include injuries and fractures of the midfoot and subtalar joint, subluxation and tears of the peroneal tendon, malleolar fractures, syndesmosis injuries, and osteochondral fractures of the talus.

References

1. Boruta PM, Bishop JO, Braly WG, et al: Acute lateral ankle ligament injuries: A literature review. *Foot Ankle* 1990;11:107-113.
2. Brostrom L: Sprained ankles: I. Anatomic lesions in recent sprains. *Acta Chir Scand* 1964;128:483-495.
3. Ekstrand J, Tropp H: The incidence of ankle sprains in soccer. *Foot Ankle* 1990;11:41-44.
4. Garrick JG: The frequency of injury, mechanism of injury, and epidemiology of ankle sprains. *Am J Sports Med* 1977;5:241-242.
5. Hamilton WG: Sprained ankles in ballet dancers. *Foot Ankle* 1982;3:99-102.
6. Mack RP: Ankle injuries in athletics. *Clin Sports Med* 1982;1:71-84.
7. Colville MR, Marder RA, Boyle JJ, et al: Strain measurement in lateral ankle ligaments. *Am J Sports Med* 1990;18:196-200.
8. Renstrom P, Wertz M, Incavo S, et al: Strain in the lateral ligaments of the ankle. *Foot Ankle* 1988;9:59-63.
9. Heilman AE, Braly WG, Bishop JO, et al: An anatomic study of subtalar instability. *Foot Ankle* 1990;10:224-228.
10. Laurin CA, Ouellet R, St-Jacques R: Talar and subtalar tilt: An experimental investigation. *Can J Surg* 1968;11:270-279.
11. Rasmussen O: Stability of the ankle joint: Analysis of the function and traumatology of the ankle ligaments. *Acta Orthop Scand* 1985;211(suppl):1-75.
12. Stormont DM, Morrey BF, An KN, et al: Stability of the loaded ankle: Relation between articular restraint and primary and secondary static restraints. *Am J Sports Med* 1985;13:295-300.
13. Anderson KJ, Lecocq JF, Lecocq EA: Recurrent anterior subluxation of the ankle joint: A report of two cases and an experimental study. *J Bone Joint Surg* 1952;34A:853-860.
14. Dias LS: The lateral ankle sprain: An experimental study. *J Trauma* 1979;19:266-269.
15. Kannus P, Renström P: Treatment for acute tears of the lateral ligaments of the ankle: Operation, cast, or early controlled mobilization. *J Bone Joint Surg* 1991;73A:305-312.
16. Stephens MM, Sammarco GJ: The stabilizing role of the lateral ligament complex around the ankle and subtalar joints. *Foot Ankle* 1992;13:130-136.
17. Kleiger B: Injuries of the talus and its joints. *Clin Orthop* 1976;121:243-262.
18. Black HM, Brand RL, Eichelberger MR: An improved technique for the evaluation of ligamentous injury in severe ankle sprains. *Am J Sports Med* 1978;6:276-282.
19. Singer KM, Jones DC: Ligament injuries of the ankle and foot, in Nicholas JA, Hershman EB (eds): *The Lower Extremity and Spine in Sports Medicine.* St. Louis, MO, CV Mosby, 1986, vol 1, pp 475-497.
20. Hopkinson WJ, St Pierre P, Ryan JB, et al: Syndesmosis sprains of the ankle. *Foot Ankle* 1990;10:325-330.
21. Edwards GS Jr, DeLee JC: Ankle diastasis without fracture. *Foot Ankle* 1984;4:305-312.
22. Freeman MAR, Dean MRE, Hanham IWF: The etiology and prevention of functional instability of the foot. *J Bone Joint Surg* 1965;47B:678-685.
23. Eckert WR, Davis EA Jr: Acute rupture of the peroneal retinaculum. *J Bone Joint Surg* 1976;58A:670-672.
24. Broström L: Sprained ankles: III. Clinical observations in recent ligament ruptures. *Acta Chir Scand* 1965;130:560-569.
25. Funder V, Jorgensen JP, Andersen A, et al: Ruptures of the lateral ligaments of the ankle: Clinical diagnosis. *Acta Orthop Scand* 1982;53:997-1000.
26. Nitz AJ, Dobner JJ, Kersey D: Nerve injury and grades II and III ankle sprains. *Am J Sports Med* 1985;13:177-182.
27. Bosien WR, Staples OS, Russell SW: Residual disability following acute ankle sprains. *J Bone Joint Surg* 1955;37A:1237-1249.
28. Thompson TC, Doherty JH: Spontaneous rupture of tendon of Achilles: A new clinical diagnostic test. *J Trauma* 1962;2:126-129.
29. Cox JS, Hewes TF: "Normal" talar tilt angle. *Clin Orthop* 1979;140:37-41.
30. Dehne E: Die Klinik der frischen und habituellen Adduktionssupinationsdistorsion des Fusses. *Deutsche Ztschr f Chir* 1933;242:40-61.
31. Freeman MAR: Treatment of ruptures of the lateral ligament of the ankle. *J Bone Joint Surg* 1965;47B:661-668.
32. Glasgow M, Jackson A, Jamieson AM: Instability of the ankle after injury to the lateral ligament. *J Bone Joint Surg* 1980;62B:196-200.

33. Grace DL: Lateral ankle ligament injuries: Inversion and anterior stress radiography. *Clin Orthop* 1984;183:153-159.
34. Johnson EE, Markolf KL: The contribution of the anterior talofibular ligament to ankle laxity. *J Bone Joint Surg* 1983;65A:81-88.
35. Kjaersgaard-Andersen P, Frich LH, Madsen F, et al: Instability of the hindfoot after lesion of the lateral ankle ligaments: Investigations of the anterior drawer and adduction maneuvers in autopsy specimens. *Clin Orthop* 1991;266:170-179.
36. Larsen E: Experimental instability of the ankle: A radiographic investigation *Clin Orthop* 1986;204:193-200.
37. Leonard MH: Injuries of the lateral ligaments of the ankle: A clinical and experimental study. *J Bone Joint Surg* 1949;31A:373-377.
38. Pennal GF: Subluxation of the ankle. *Can Med Assoc J* 1943;49:92-95.
39. Rubin G, Witten M: The talar-tilt angle and the fibular collateral ligaments: A method for the determination of talar tilt. *J Bone Joint Surg* 1960;42A:311-326.
40. Seligson D, Gassman J, Pope M: Ankle instability: Evaluation of the lateral ligaments. *Am J Sports Med* 1980;8:39-42.
41. White RK, Kraynick BM: Surgical uses of the peroneus brevis tendon. *Surg Gynecol Obstet* 1959;108:117-121.
42. Nyska M, Amir H, Porath A, et al: Radiological assessment of a modified anterior drawer test of the ankle. *Foot Ankle* 1992;13:400-403.
43. Chapman MW: Sprains of the ankle: Part II, in Evans EB (ed): *American Academy of Orthopaedic Surgeons Instructional Course Lectures Volume XXIV.* St. Louis, MO, CV Mosby, 1975, pp 294-308.
44. Harper MC, Keller TS: A radiographic evaluation of the tibiofibular syndesmosis. *Foot Ankle* 1989;10:156-160.
45. Murr S: Dislocation of the peroneal tendons with marginal fracture of the lateral malleolus. *J Bone Joint Surg* 1961;43B:563-565.
46. Clayton ML, Trott AW, Ulin R: Recurrent subluxation of the ankle, with special reference to peroneal-nerve block as a diagnostic aid. *J Bone Joint Surg* 1951;33A:502-504.
47. Cass JR, Morrey BF: Ankle instability: Current concepts, diagnosis, and treatment. *Mayo Clin Proc* 1984;59:165-170.
48. Cox JS: Surgical and nonsurgical treatment of acute ankle sprains. *Clin Orthop* 1985;198:118-126.
49. Ryan JB, Hopkinson WJ, Wheeler JH, et al: Office management of the acute ankle sprain. *Clin Sports Med* 1989;8:477-495.
50. Chrisman OD, Snook GA: Reconstruction of lateral ligament tears of the ankle: An experimental study and clinical evaluation of seven patients treated by a new modification of the Elmslie procedure. *J Bone Joint Surg* 1969;51A:904-912.
51. Brantigan JW, Pedegana LR, Lippert FG: Instability of the subtalar joint: Diagnosis by stress tomography in three cases. *J Bone Joint Surg* 1977;59A:321-324.
52. Broström L, Liljedahl SO, Lindvall N: Sprained ankles: II. Arthrographic diagnosis of recent ligament ruptures. *Acta Chir Scand* 1965;129:485-499.
53. Raatikainen T, Putkonen M, Puranen J: Arthrography, clinical examination, and stress radiograph in the diagnosis of acute injury to the lateral ligaments of the ankle. *Am J Sports Med* 1992;20:2-6.
54. Verhaven EF, Shahabpour M, Handelberg FW, et al: The accuracy of three-dimensional magnetic resonance imaging in the diagnosis of ruptures of the lateral ligaments of the ankle. *Am J Sports Med* 1991;19:583-587.
55. Marymont JV, Lynch MA, Henning CE: Acute ligamentous diastasis of the ankle without fracture: Evaluation by radionuclide imaging. *Am J Sports Med* 1986;14:407-409.
56. Marotta JJ, Micheli LJ: Os trigonum impingement in dancers. *Am J Sports Med* 1992;20:533-536.
57. Paulos LE, Johnson CL, Noyes FR: Posterior compartment fractures of the ankle: A commonly missed athletic injury. *Am J Sports Med* 1983;11:439-443.
58. Bassett FH III, Gates HS III, Billys JB, et al: Talar impingement by the anteroinferior tibiofibular ligament: A cause of chronic pain in the ankle after inversion sprain. *J Bone Joint Surg* 1990;72A:55-59.

CHAPTER 31

Surgical Management of Fractures of the Os Calcis

Bruce J. Sangeorzan, MD
Stephen K. Benirschke, MD
James B. Carr, MD

Introduction

Fractures of the os calcis (calcaneus) account for about 60% of tarsal fractures and 1% to 2% of all fractures. Most of these injuries result from a fall, and working men in their prime years account for 80% to 90% of the injured. Because the bony architecture is complex and the soft-tissue envelope tenuous, open reduction is a relatively challenging and morbid undertaking. In the past, outcome from open treatment has failed to justify surgical intervention, yet results of closed treatment are poor in contrast to modern techniques of management of other intra-articular fractures. Open reduction with rigid internal fixation (ORIF) is standard for displaced intra-articular fractures in other weightbearing joints. Although it is hoped that ORIF will improve the outcome of calcaneus fractures, the ideal treatment is not clearly established.[1-17]

Anatomy

The calcaneus is a complex bone that acts as a major part of the platform for walking and standing and as a fulcrum that allows the calf musculature to propel the body forward. There are four clinically remarkable aspects of the bony anatomy. (1) Its lateral wall is relatively flat, covered primarily by skin and subcutaneous fat. This makes the lateral wall accessible and amenable to implantation of hardware but subject to soft-tissue vulnerability (Fig. 1). (2) The medial wall slopes more sharply and is closely approximated by the medial neurovascular structures and flexor group of tendons. It is therefore less accessible and is vulnerable to nerve or artery injury. (3) The superior surface has three articular facets; the large posterior facet and the smaller middle and anterior facets (Fig. 2). The three facets function as a single articulation with the talus. Changes in the relationships among the facets are analogous to an intra-articular fracture even when the fracture line does not traverse a cartilage surface. The relationship among the articular surfaces defies simple description. With this intricate relationship, restoration of a truly anatomic position is quite difficult. (4) The lesser facets, though smaller, bear more weight per unit area and are supported by the dense bone of the sustentaculum tali.[18] This dense bone provides a solid site for fixation of screws. In the intact joint, the three facets act together to allow an oblique rotation of the

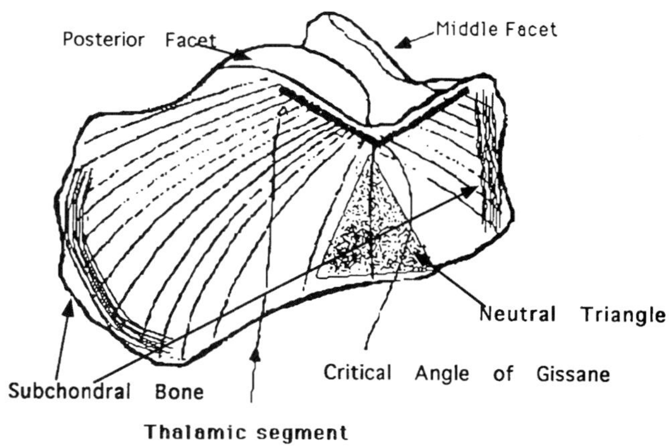

Fig. 1 A diagrammatic representation of a calcaneus viewed from the lateral side. The lateral wall is relatively flat. The bone is more dense in the darkened areas, and therefore better suited to internal fixation. The shaded area is the neutral triangle where there is little stress. The bone here is less dense and less suitable to internal fixation.

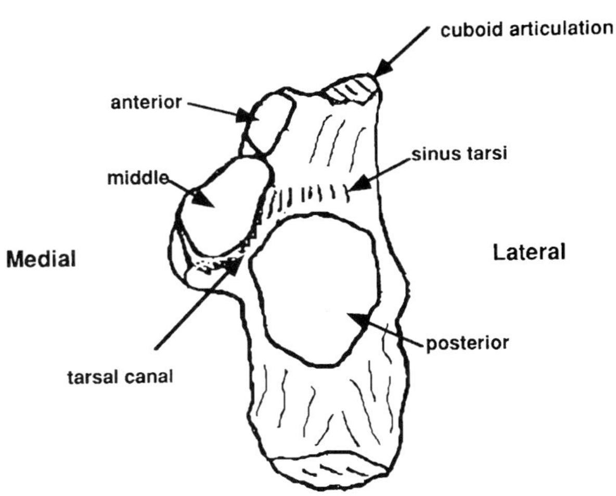

Fig. 2 A diagrammatic representation of a right calcaneus viewed from superiorly. In the majority of patients, the middle facet and anterior facet are contiguous.

hindfoot that accounts for most of the inversion and eversion of the foot.[18,19] The sinus tarsi is a recessed area anterior to the posterior facet that accommodates the lateral process of the talus. It funnels into the tarsal canal, which divides the posterior facet from the anterior and middle facets.[20]

Fracture Anatomy

To understand indications for and technique of surgical treatment, it is necessary to understand the fracture anatomy and the method of imaging it. Fracture of the calcaneus is most commonly caused by an axial load. The calcaneus is driven upward against the talus. The anterior part of the posterior facet of the talus, which includes the lateral process, acts as a fulcrum across which the calcaneus fractures. A fracture line is created that begins in the sinus tarsi near the lateral wall and propagates obliquely across the posterior facet to the medial wall. This fracture line, known as the primary fracture line or separation fracture, is common to most intra-articular fractures of the calcaneus.[12,21-24] The primary fracture line is less like a slice through the bone and more like the predominant part of a stellate fracture pattern centered on the sinus tarsi (Fig. 3). Although its position varies, the primary fracture line appears to be common to most calcaneus fractures. It proceeds from anterolateral to posteromedial across the posterior facet and out the medial wall posterior to the sustentaculum. It divides the tuberosity and lateral wall with a variable part of the posterior facet from the sustentacular fragment with the middle and anterior facet. In addition to this primary fracture line, many secondary fracture lines may occur. The location and number of these lines is presumably determined by the direction and force of impact, the quality of bone, and the position of the foot. Common secondary fracture lines include an anterior extension, which divides the anterior process, and a medial extension, which divides the middle facet from the posterior facet. The lateral edge of the posterior facet may be sheared off with the lateral wall.

The tuberosity is typically driven anteriorly and laterally along the oblique fracture line and assumes a lateral and anterior position beneath the fibula. The sustentacular fragment rotates downward away from the talus and locks into the posterior facet fragment.[23] Although this point is controversial, it is a common component of the high-energy fractures treated at our institution. Because it has strong soft-tissue attachments, it generally rotates back to its native position when the tuberosity fragment is disimpacted.

Classification

Several fracture classifications have been proposed, but none has been universally accepted, and none has demonstrated reproducible prognostic capability. Early classifications were based on (poor quality) lateral radiographs. The major classification systems are based on three features of the fracture pattern; whether it is displaced, whether it involves the posterior facet (intra-articular), and what degree of depression and comminution is present in the posterior facet. Computed tomography (CT) is suggested as a better method for assessing comminution. In general, the smaller the part of the posterior facet attached to the middle facet, the greater the comminution and the worse the prognosis. Although the ability of treating physicians to assess these parameters has never been validated, it is likely that the greater the comminution, the greater the energy and the worse the prognosis.[21,25-27]

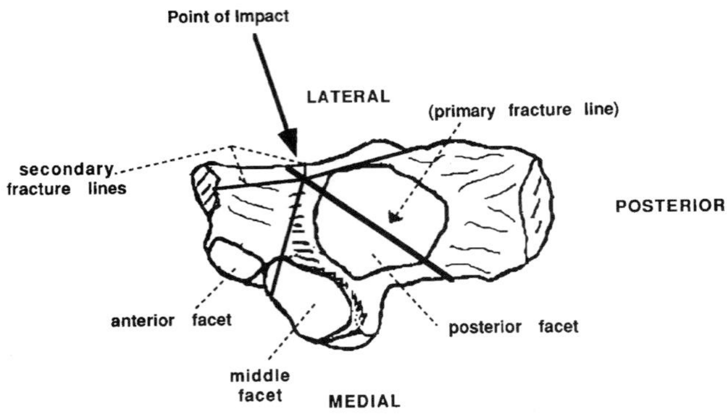

Fig. 3 A diagrammatic representation of idealized fracture lines on a right calcaneus viewed from above. The thick line represents the "primary fracture line" or separation fracture. The lesser lines represent typical positions of the secondary fracture lines. Taken together, the fractures make up a stellate pattern radiating outward from the point of impact on the talus located in the sinus tarsi. The two medialward fracture lines (the primary fracture line and the fracture distal and medial to it) isolate the sustentaculum tali from the rest of the calcaneus. Failure to recognize and reduce this component will result in an incongruous subtalar joint even if the posterior facet is reduced anatomically. (See Fig. 10, *bottom left*.)

Fractures are described as nondisplaced or displaced and intra- or extra-articular. Further classification is based on degree of depression of the posterior facet relative to the tuberosity (Bohler's angle),[24] and on the number of fracture lines separating the posterior facet articular surface. The last of these criteria can be assessed only by CT. Although the subtalar joint has three facets that function as a single complex articular surface, none of the current classifications give consideration to displacement that disturbs the relationships of the three facets. This independent variable may account for discrepancies in the reliability of the classification systems. In addition to these major groups, Essex-Lopresti[4] described two distinct fracture patterns. The first, joint depression type, involves actual depression of the posterior facet separately from the tuberosity. The second, the so-called tongue type fracture, involves a relative downward rotation of the posterior facet and tuberosity as one fragment (Fig. 4).

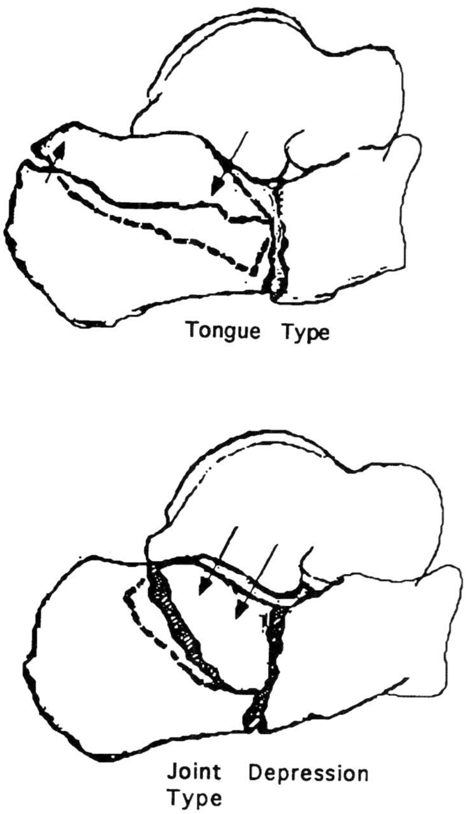

Fig. 4 A "tongue type" fracture is represented above. Note that the posterior facet is in continuity with the dorsal surface of the tuberosity. The amount of cartilage surface attached to the fragment can be estimated only by cross-sectional imaging. The bottom image represents a "joint depression" type injury. Again, the amount of cartilage surface of the posterior facet that is on the depressed fragment can only be estimated by cross-sectional imaging. This classification predates both standard tomography and computed tomography (CT).

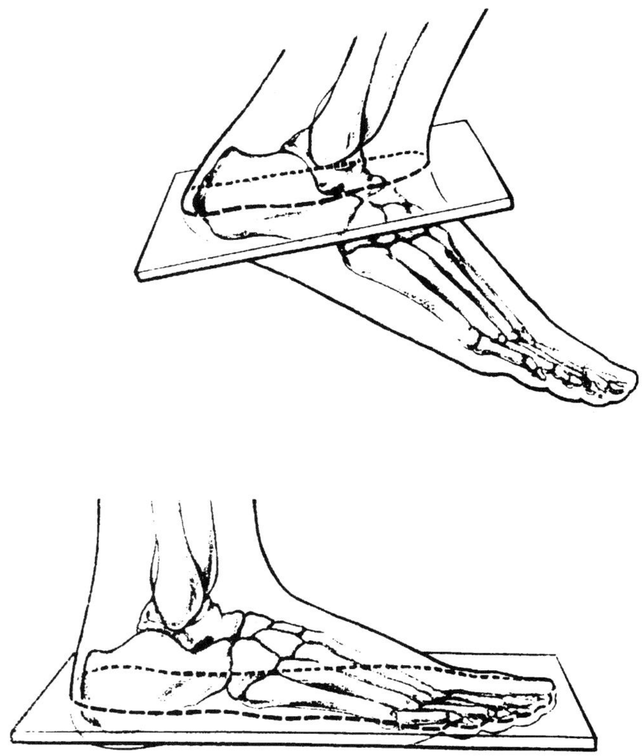

Fig. 5 Ideal planes of computed tomography (CT) scan are pictured here. The cuts should be 2 mm or less apart. The modified *coronal*, above, should be perpendicular to the posterior facet joint surface. The following parameters can be assessed; relationship of the posterior facet to the middle facet, position of the primary fracture line, the number of fragments of the facets, widening of the anterior process, widening of the heel (lateral translation of the tuberosity), and subfibular abutment. The *transverse* plane, below, approximately parallels the plantar surface of the foot. Widening of the anterior process, widening of the heel, heel varus, and the relationship between the posterior facet and the sustentacular fragment can be assessed.

Imaging

Acute radiographic evaluation of calcaneus fractures includes a dorsoplantar, lateral, axial (Harris), and oblique view of the foot. The lateral view is the most helpful in the assessment of the position of the posterior facet by way of the tuber joint angle of Bohler. The dorsoplantar view shows the calcaneocuboid joint, and the oblique view shows the calcaneocuboid joint as well as the lesser facets. The axial view demonstrates the direction and displacement of the tuberosity along the primary fracture line and gives information about the relationship between the posterior facet and the sustentacular fragment. The axial view also reveals lateral wall displacement and fibular abutment. Special oblique views may be helpful for displacing the surface of the posterior facet. Brodén,[28] Anthosen,[29] and Isherwood[30] each described an oblique view. The hindfoot oblique view is seen by placing the cassette behind the heel and distal tibia, rotating the foot inward and outward 45° and aiming the beam 20° to 40° cephalad. When contemplating surgical treatment, CT is also very helpful. If possible, CT should include two planes: a transverse plane, parallel to the plantar surface of the foot, and a semicoronal plane, perpendicular to the posterior facet (Fig. 5).[31,32] The transverse plane images provide a map of anterior process involvement, including the calcaneocuboid joint and secondary fracture lines that split the sustentacular segment. Sagittal plane reconstruction and 3-D images of the CT cuts may be useful as well, particularly for clinicians with limited experience in treating this injury.

Treatment

Indications and Rationale for Surgical Treatment

Principles of treatment of intra-articular fractures in weightbearing joints include anatomic reduction of the joint surface and restoration of the mechanical alignment of the involved bone. These principles have been slow to be applied to the calcaneus because of the complexity of the fracture anatomy, the poor soft-tissue envelope, the difficulty of achieving rigid fixation, and the historically high rate of morbidity.

Although it is probably safe to speculate that there are some instances in which open reduction is superior to closed treatment, exact indications remain elusive. Natural history studies demonstrate that most patients who have had displaced calcaneus fractures treated without surgery have long-term symptoms. Problems include a wide heel and short foot, an irregular subtalar joint with limited motion, and degenerative changes in the tibiotalar joint caused by the altered position of the talus during weightbearing activities. The majority continue to have a variable amount of pain and swelling at long-term follow up.[7,8,22,33-35]

The ideal method of determining treatment for any disease process is to first study the natural history and then to compare it to outcome in a group of patients randomly assigned to a specific treatment. Nothing approaching this standard has been done for the treatment of os calcis fractures. Further, the surgery is so technique-dependent that even a randomized study is unlikely to be definitive unless the surgical limb is performed by experienced fracture surgeons. The problem has been approached by other methods, however: retrospective studies; retrospective cohort matched studies;[36] computed tomography of the acute injury (for classification), followed by treatment;[25-27] CT assessment after open treatment;[37] and laboratory studies.[38] Retrospective clinical studies hint at several concepts. Higher energy injuries, as measured by the number of and displacement of fracture lines in the posterior facet and the degree of depression of the posterior facet, have worse outcome than lower energy injuries.[27,35,37] Also, pain in the subfibular area is an important and common clinical complaint following nonoperative treatment.[39] Although small numbers and multiple categories make the conclusions more empiric than scientific, these retrospective studies suggest that treatment that diminishes swelling, improves subtalar motion and decompresses the subfibular area (narrows the heel) is likely to lead to the best clinical outcome in a given group. In all studies, the percentage of patients who were free of pain was small, which suggests that an effort needs to be made on the part of clinicians to improve the outcome of this injury.[8,25,27,33,35,37]

When pain, activities, occupational function, gait, use of orthoses, and use of medications are correlated to findings on CT scans at the time of follow-up, incongruity and degeneration in the posterior facet of the subtalar joint have been associated with loss of subtalar motion, which in turn was associated with a poor clinical outcome. Interestingly, intra-articular hardware noted on CT scan was not significantly associated with a poor clinical score. The appearance of the middle or anterior facets was not examined to see if these correlated to that of the posterior facet.[37]

A laboratory model has also been used to study alteration in the congruity of the posterior facet. The empiric rule that displacement greater than 2 mm is an indication for open reduction is only loosely supported. In a simple calcaneus fracture, the joint area available for function diminishes significantly even with 2 mm of displacement. However, the area of the joint subjected to significant increases in high pressure does not increase until displacement exceeds 2 mm.[38]

The goal of surgical treatment is to improve on this natural history by addressing the anatomic causes. Restoring the height of the calcaneus improves the tibiotalar position, restores the relationships of the facets, and may diminish long-term degeneration in the ankle. Restoring the length of the heel may improve shoe fitting and the lever arm of the gastrocnemius-soleus complex. Because restoring the height and length requires placing the tuberosity beneath and posterior to the posterior facet, the widened heel will necessarily be narrowed. Narrowing relieves subfibular abutment.[39] Reduction of the joint surfaces and of the geometric relationships among the three facets of the talocalcaneal joint should diminish the stiffness and pain of the subtalar joint. These goals are meant to correct the things known to cause long-term morbidity. Significant controversy exists as to the indications for open treatment as well as the most effective means of achieving these goals.

Contraindications to surgical treatment include peripheral vascular disease, peripheral neuropathy, advanced age, sedentary lifestyle, inadequate soft-tissue envelope, and patient unwillingness to proceed with unproven treatment. None of these is an absolute contraindication. Bony prominence may force intervention in patients with peripheral neuropathy, vascular disease, or threatened soft tissue. Under these circumstances, reduction may be the safe and conservative thing to do. Likewise, advanced age and sedentary lifestyle are soft criteria that should be balanced against the degree of deformity and likelihood of poor outcome from closed treatment.

Surgical Approach

The patient is positioned in the true lateral position with the operative side up and the ipsilateral iliac crest accessible for bone graft if needed. The table beneath the operative limb is padded to provide a flat, stable platform for the limb and for intraoperative radiographs.

A lateral extensile approach, popularized by Benirschke,[40] is employed (Fig. 6). It differs from the classic lateral approach of Palmer in that it has an acute curve instead of following the peroneal tendons and is similar to that suggested by Gould.[40,41] It has an "L" shape when performed on the right foot and a reverse "L" or

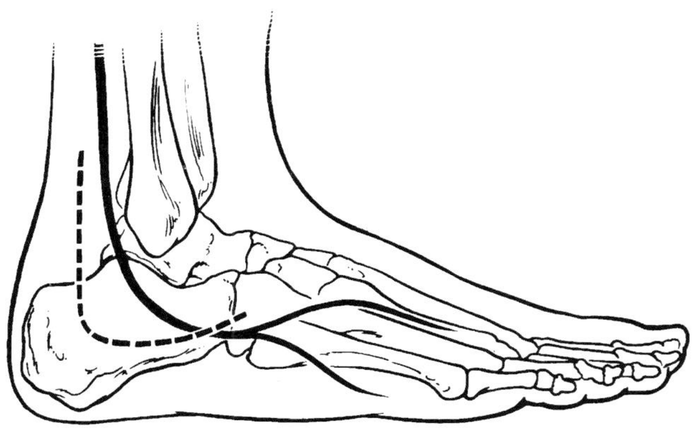

Fig. 6 Lateral view of the incision with the sural nerve drawn in. The dashed line indicates the direction of the incision. The dorsal limb of the incision parallels the Achilles tendon and is just posterior to the sural nerve (about equidistant between the peroneal and Achilles tendons). The plantar limb of the incision parallels the plantar surface of the foot. The incision is carried to bone directly, keeping the flap thick to protect the blood flow to the skin. The peroneal tendons and sural nerve cross the distal extension of the plantar incision. The posterior facet and calcaneocuboid joint can be seen through this extensile approach and a plate may be applied to the lateral wall.

flattened "J" shape on the left foot. The vertical limb parallels the Achilles tendon and is just posterior to the sural nerve. It curves sharply and parallels the plantar surface of the calcaneus and extends across the calcaneocuboid joint. In the apex of the flap, the incision is carried directly to bone, keeping a full thickness flap of skin, subcutaneous tissue, and periosteum. The peroneal tendons, sural nerve, and calcaneofibular ligament are left undisturbed in the flap. The flap is elevated upward until the subtalar joint can be seen and is elevated distally to the calcaneocuboid joint. Retraction of the flap may be maintained by inserting Kirschner wires (K-wires) into the talus to act as a barrier. This may protect against overly zealous retraction by an assistant.

Reduction

When the flap has been elevated, the lateral wall is reflected outward, exposing the comminuted posterior facet. The urge to reduce the suddenly visible posterior facet should be resisted. Typically, the central part of the calcaneus is compromised by the anterior and lateral position of the tuberosity (Figs. 7 and 8). The central part of the calcaneus should be decompressed before the posterior facet can be reduced. In a simple fracture pattern in which there is no fracture line separating the middle facet from the medial part of the posterior facet, pulling the tuberosity plantarward, medially, and out of varus accomplishes the decompression and makes room to allow reduction of the posterior facet (Fig. 9). A 4.0-mm Schanz pin is inserted into the tuberosity to provide direct control for the reduction maneuver. When the tuberosity is reduced to the medial wall of the sustentacular fragment, it is held with two 0.062-in K-wires placed from plantar posterior to dorsal anterior. This maneuver makes room to allow reduction of the posterior facet. In a more comminuted fracture, in which the medial part of the posterior facet is driven down beneath the middle facet and sustentaculum tali (which occurs in more than 50% of the fractures treated at our institution), this anterior fracture should be restored first and provisionally held with K-wires (Figs. 10 and 11). To accomplish this reduction, a head lamp is employed. The medial part of the posterior facet is elevated upward until it is aligned with the middle facet. It is difficult to see this relationship just posterior to the interosseous ligament, and almost impossible without a head lamp and adequate retraction. Intraoperative Harris axial and lateral views are done to assess reduction of the tuberosity and anterior process fractures. Broden's views may also be done intraoperatively.[27] The lateral part of the posterior facet may then be reduced to the medial part and the fragments held provisionally with K-wires. A second set of intraoperative radiographs is performed to determine if the bone is reduced before definitive fixation is done.

The most dense bone is in the sustentaculum tali, the thickened bone beneath the posterior facet, and in the bone deep to the heelcord insertion and calcaneocuboid joint (Fig. 2). These points of fixation should be employed. A pelvic reconstruction plate contoured into a "frown" is applied along the lateral wall. It is kept straight in the sagittal plane to reduce the varus of the tuberosity. The most distal screw should course just proximal to the calcaneocuboid joint and be directed cephalad to take advantage of the thickened bone beneath the anterior process. The most posterior screws should be inserted in the tuberosity to resist varus. The posterior facet itself is secured with two 3.5-mm cortical lag screws directed slightly anteriorly toward the middle facet. Supplemental fixation with screws, K-wires, or second plates may be required in highly comminuted fractures. In fractures that involve multiple small fragments of the posterior facet, the small fragments may be assembled extracorporally, held with 0.045-in K-wires, and then reduced to the intact surface of bone.

Even within our institution, the indications for bone graft are controversial. It is agreed that bone graft should be used when the area beneath the posterior facet is vacuolated, with no support for the joint. It is also agreed that graft should be used whenever enough bone is missing or impacted that a buttress situation is present, ie, cortical defects exist that need to be bridged by plates.[42] Under these circumstances, it seems unlikely that healing could occur before implant failure without graft. At our institution these high-energy fractures are common. The lower energy injuries have

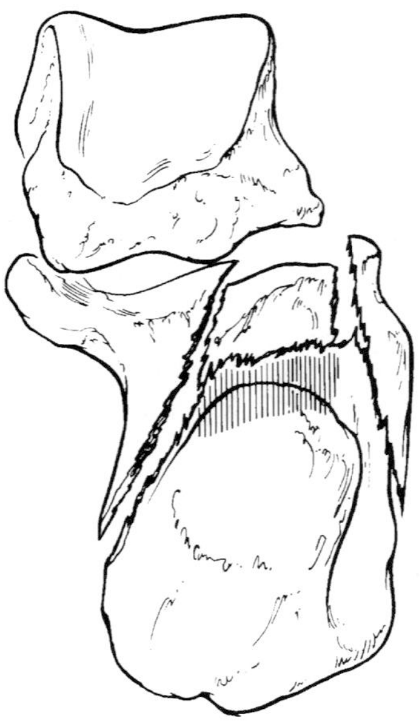

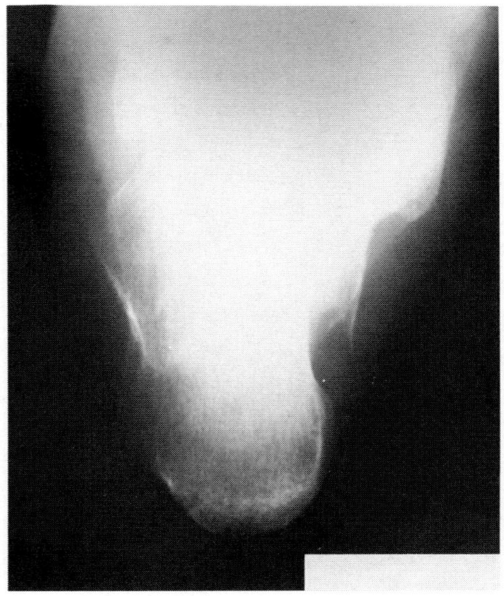

Fig. 7 **Top left,** Artist's conception of an axial view of a right calcaneus fracture. The shaded area represents depression of the posterior facets into the substance of the body. The lateral wall is sheared off at the outer border of the talus and the sustentacular fragment containing a small part of the posterior facet is minimally displaced. The line separating the two major fragments is called the "primary fracture line" or "separation fracture". **Top right,** An actual radiograph demonstrating the same view in a left calcaneus fracture. Note the comminution of both medial and lateral wall and the shortening of the tuberosity fragment. **Bottom left,** A diagrammatic lateral view of the same fracture pattern. The shaded area represents the posterior facet, which is now depressed below the outer lateral wall and into the substance of the calcaneus. The anterior process is tilted upward and the posterior process is tilted downward, as a result of the conflicting pull of the heel cord and depression of the talus. The primary fracture line exists right through the angle of Gissane. **Bottom right,** Lateral radiograph demonstrating similar features as shown in the illustration.

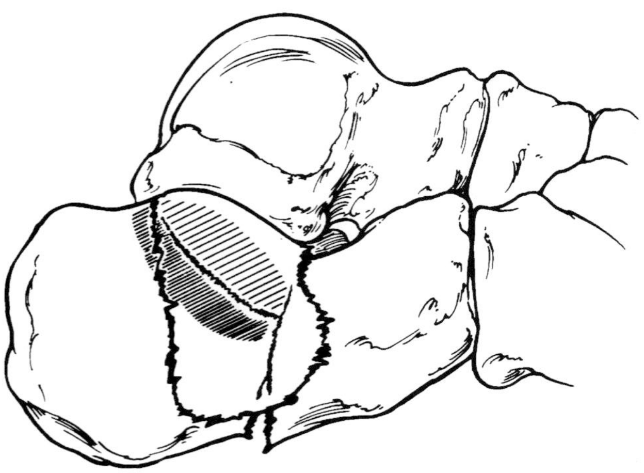

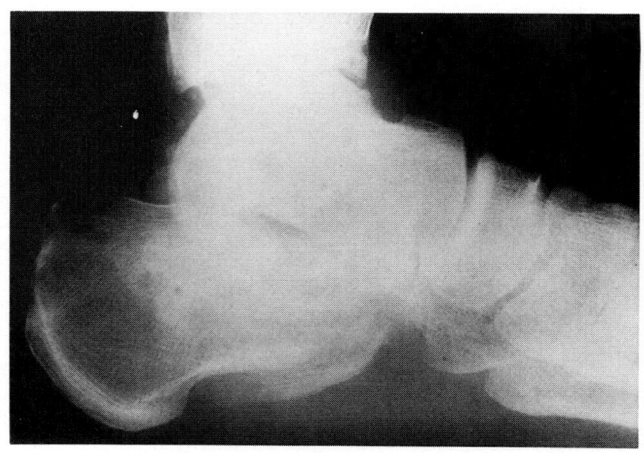

intact bone segments that can be compressed using lag screws and probably do not require graft. The so-called "neutral triangle" is an area with scant bone density. When it is impacted it does not need bone graft.

A one-eighth inch closed-suction drain is placed in the wound and brought out anteriorly. Closure of the wound is performed using layers of interrupted absorbable suture. When a significant amount of height is restored intraoperatively, the flap will have to be advanced, and there may be substantial tension at the beginning of the closure. Interrupted sutures are placed beginning at the ends of the wound, and the flap is advanced slightly with each stitch. The skin wound is closed with a nylon flap stitch.

Postoperative Management

The operated limb is splinted and elevated with the foot and ankle in the neutral position for 72 hours. Drains are removed 24 to 48 hours after the operation. During this time the patient may be up for limited periods of time such as bathroom privileges or trials of crutch walking. Smoking is prohibited. Oxygen is administered by nasal cannula to reinforce the principles of wound healing over nicotine drive.

Upon removal of the plaster splint, the limb is placed in a removable splint of aluminum lined with sheepskin. When the incision is dry (in 3 to 5 days), active range-of-motion exercises of the ankle and subtalar

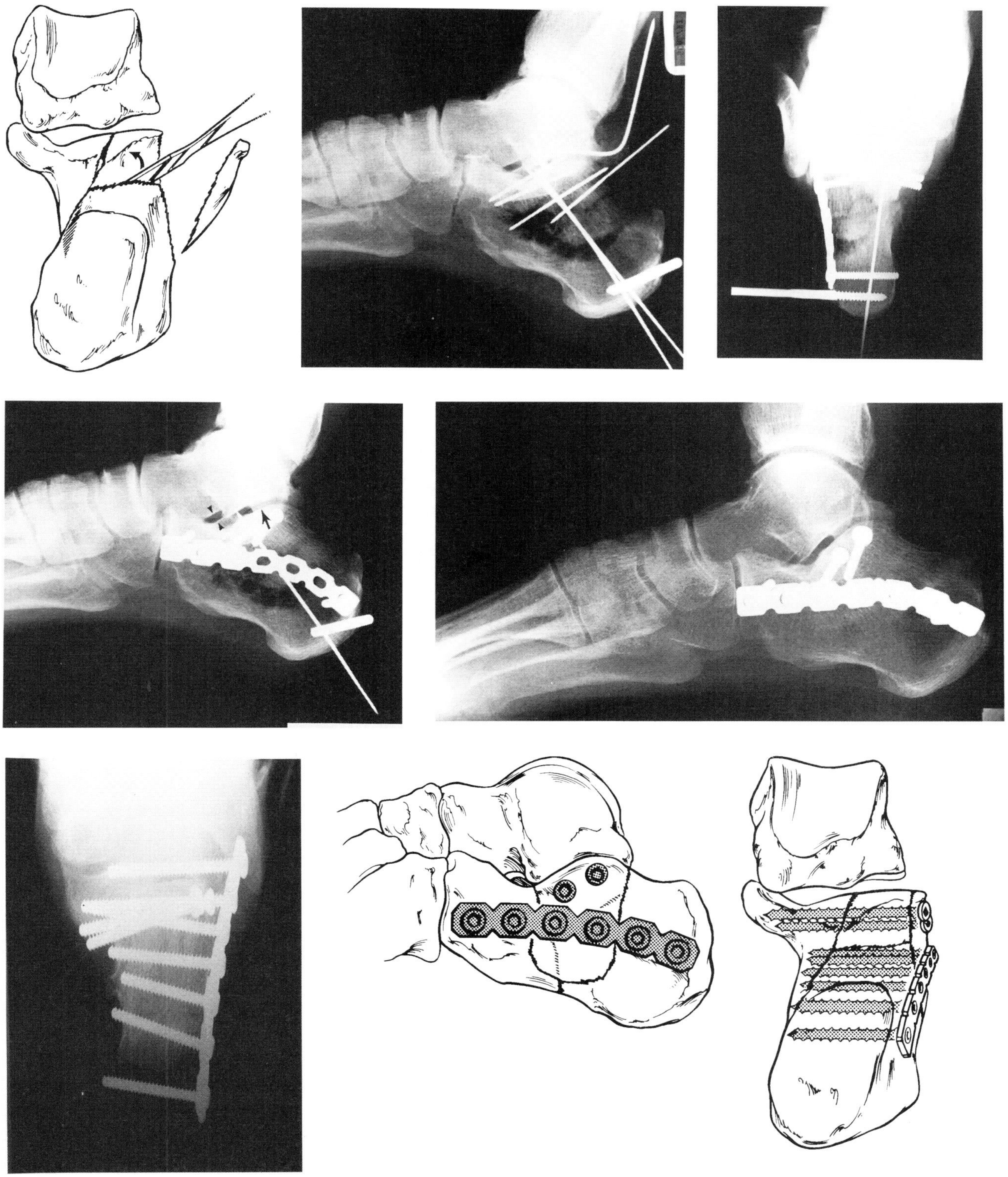

Fig. 8 Reduction technique for a simple fracture. **Top left,** With this tuberosity fragment reduced, the posterior facet can be elevated up into its native position. The lateral wall can then be reduced along the outer part of the posterior facet. **Top center,** An intraoperative lateral radiograph obtained after elevation of the posterior facet and provisional fixation with K-wires. The length of the heel has been restored and the joint surfaces reduced. **Top right,** In this axial radiograph, the Schantz pin has not been removed and a plate is held with two screws, demonstrating the indirect reduction of the medial wall. One K-wire continues to support the reduction of the medial wall until the remaining screws are inserted. Note that the plate is straight on this view, which prevents a drifting of the calcaneus into a varus position. **Center left,** Lateral view of the reduced calcaneus. The two screws that are outside of the plate are in the dense bone beneath the posterior facet and directed into the dense bone of the sustentaculum tali. The 3.5-mm reconstruction plate has been contoured into a "frown" type of position. It begins adjacent to the calcaneocuboid joint and extends to the thickening cortex of the tuberosity fragment. The middle facet (small arrowheads) and posterior facet (larger arrows) have been reduced. **Center right,** Lateral view of the same patient's heel 1 year later at final follow-up. **Bottom left,** Axial view of the same patient's heel at final follow up. **Bottom center** and **right,** Schematic representations of the lateral and axial views.

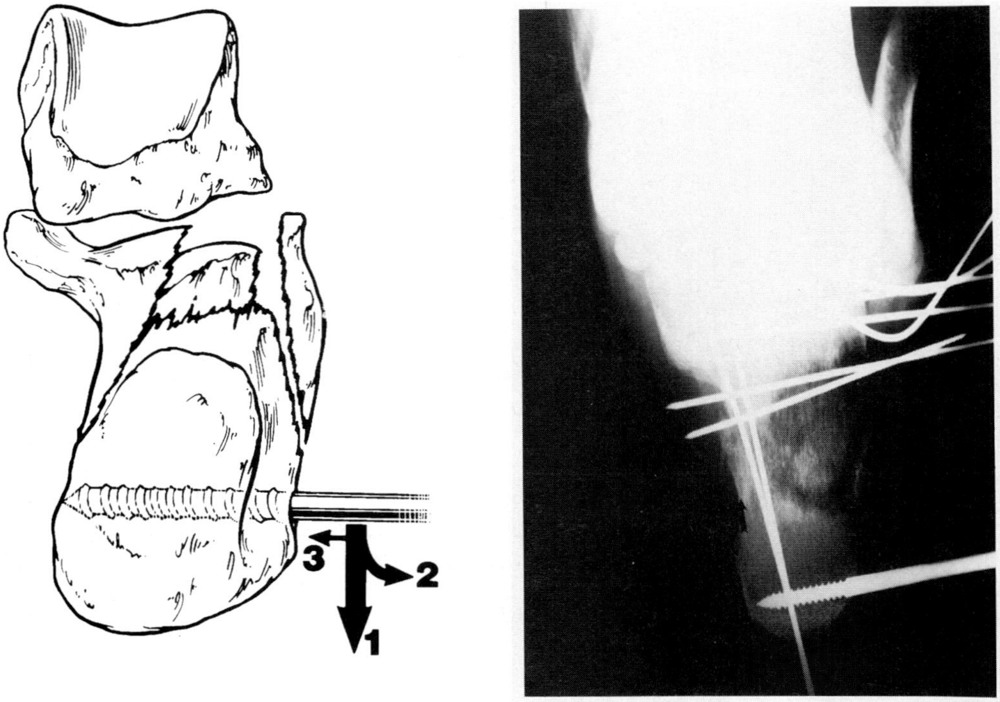

Fig. 9 **Left,** The reduction technique used in a simple fracture to reduce the tuberosity. This is the same representation as in Figure 7, *top left.* A Schanz pin has been placed into the tuberosity fragment. The three arrows indicate the relative motion of the Shantz pin, with the densest arrow indicating the greatest displacement. Traction is directed with three components on the Schanz pin to bring the tuberosity fragmented plantarly, medially, and into slight valgus position. **Right,** An intraoperative axial radiograph demonstrating the maneuver pictured in the schematic. The medial wall is reduced indirectly (arrow) and held provisionally with two K-wires directed from the heel upward into the sustentaculum.

joints are begun. Sutures are removed 2 to 3 weeks after surgery. Patients are fitted with support stockings as needed to control foot and ankle edema and are encouraged to wear them for at least 6 months. In general, analgesics are discontinued 3 to 4 weeks after surgery.

Weightbearing is not allowed for 10 to 12 weeks, depending on the fracture pattern. When the fracture is simple and the fragments can be compressed with lag screws, walking may be begun earlier than in fractures that depend on buttress plates to maintain the reduced position. Active range-of-motion exercises of the ankle and subtalar joints are continued during this nonweightbearing period. Patients with bilateral fractures are confined to bed-to-wheelchair transfers for 12 weeks. Weightbearing is then resumed according to patient tolerance. The use of ambulation aids is discontinued by 16 weeks. After healing, patients are encouraged to use shoes with a cushioned or shock-absorbing sole.

Results

A limited decrease in ankle range of motion is expected but not commonly noted by the patients. There is no way to accurately measure subtalar range of motion, but it is diminished in the majority of patients. Approximately 20% of patients have subtalar motion similar to the noninjured side (75% or more), 60% have significantly diminished motion (50% to 75%), and 20% have limited or no motion. The more than 85% of patients who worked at the time of injury return to work within 9 months. Patients with bilateral calcaneus fractures or other injuries and patients who do heavy labor may take longer and often alter employment. Patients who are self employed or who work in sedentary occupations return much sooner.[43]

Some patients may require shoe inserts or modification for ambulation, but shoe fitting (custom shoes or a different sized shoe for the injured foot) is rarely necessary. Most commonly patients complain that they need to wear a soft shoe because of swelling or heelpad pain. The majority either returned to previous shoe wear, or adopted use of a shoe with a shock-absorbing sole.

Thirty percent of patients significantly modify activity, changing to a more sedentary occupation. There is often a modification in recreational pursuits. Patients followed for more than 2 years noted continued improvement in subtalar symptoms. A subgroup of patients, presumed to be those with the severely injured subtalar joints, may not experience this improvement and will have ongoing pain.

Complications

Major and minor complications attributable to open reduction and internal fixation through a lateral approach are found in 10% to 20% of patients. These complications include infection, wound-healing prob-

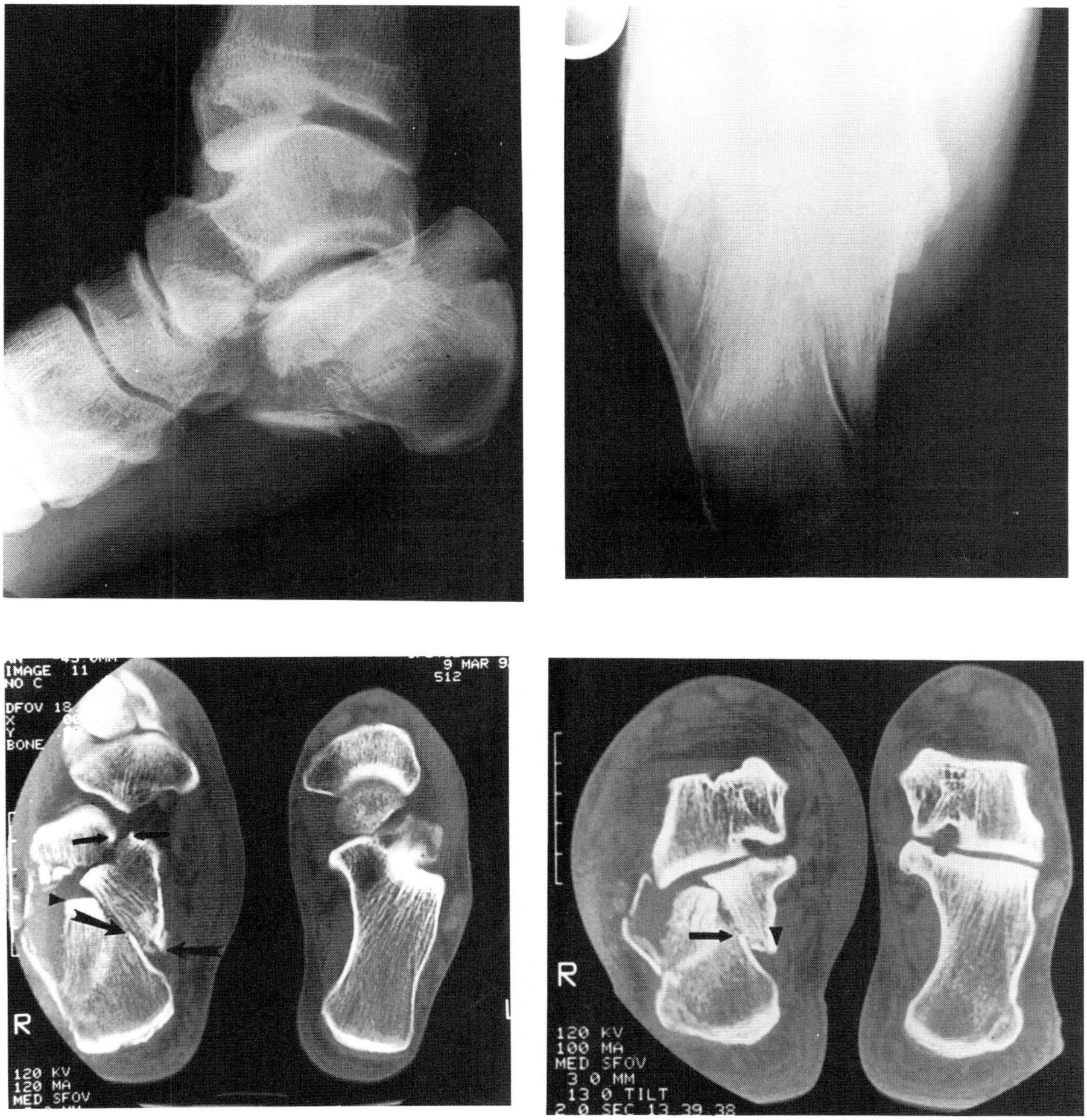

Fig. 10 A slightly more comminuted fracture with a "tongue" pattern that demonstrates the need to reduce the anterior process first. **Top left,** Lateral view of the acute injury. The top of the posterior facet of the subtalar joint is rotated plantarly and the posterior aspect of the tuberosity is rotated cephalad, resulting in a negative Böhler's angle. There is a fracture through the middle facet as well that is more apparent on CT. **Top right,** Axial view of the same fracture. Medial is on the right. As in a joint depression type the tuberosity is displaced laterally and the lateral wall is "buckled" outward. **Bottom left,** Transverse plane CT. The primary fracture line and a secondary fracture line have isolated the section of the calcaneus containing the sustentaculum tali. The primary fracture line (large arrows) divides the posterior facet. A secondary fracture line (small arrows) splits the middle facet and divides the sustentaculum tali from the anterior fragment containing the calcaneocuboid joint. This results in a widened heel and incongruity of the various facets of the subtalar joint. The tongue segment, which contains a large part of the posterior facet articular surface (arrowhead), is a separate segment. Until the entire medial wall is reduced (large and small arrows "matched up"), there is no space in which to properly reduce the posterior facet. Reducing the posterior facet without reducing the other fracture line will result in an incongruous subtalar joint. **Bottom right,** Semicoronal plane CT through the posterior facet, tibia, and fibula. The posterior facet has limited comminution. This cut is used in some classification schemes. In comminuted fractures it does not determine congruity of the subtalar joint. The medial wall of the tuberosity segment (arrow) must be reduced to the medial wall of the sustentacular segment (arrowhead) before there is room to reduce the posterior facet. This is the same fracture line shown in bottom left with large arrows.

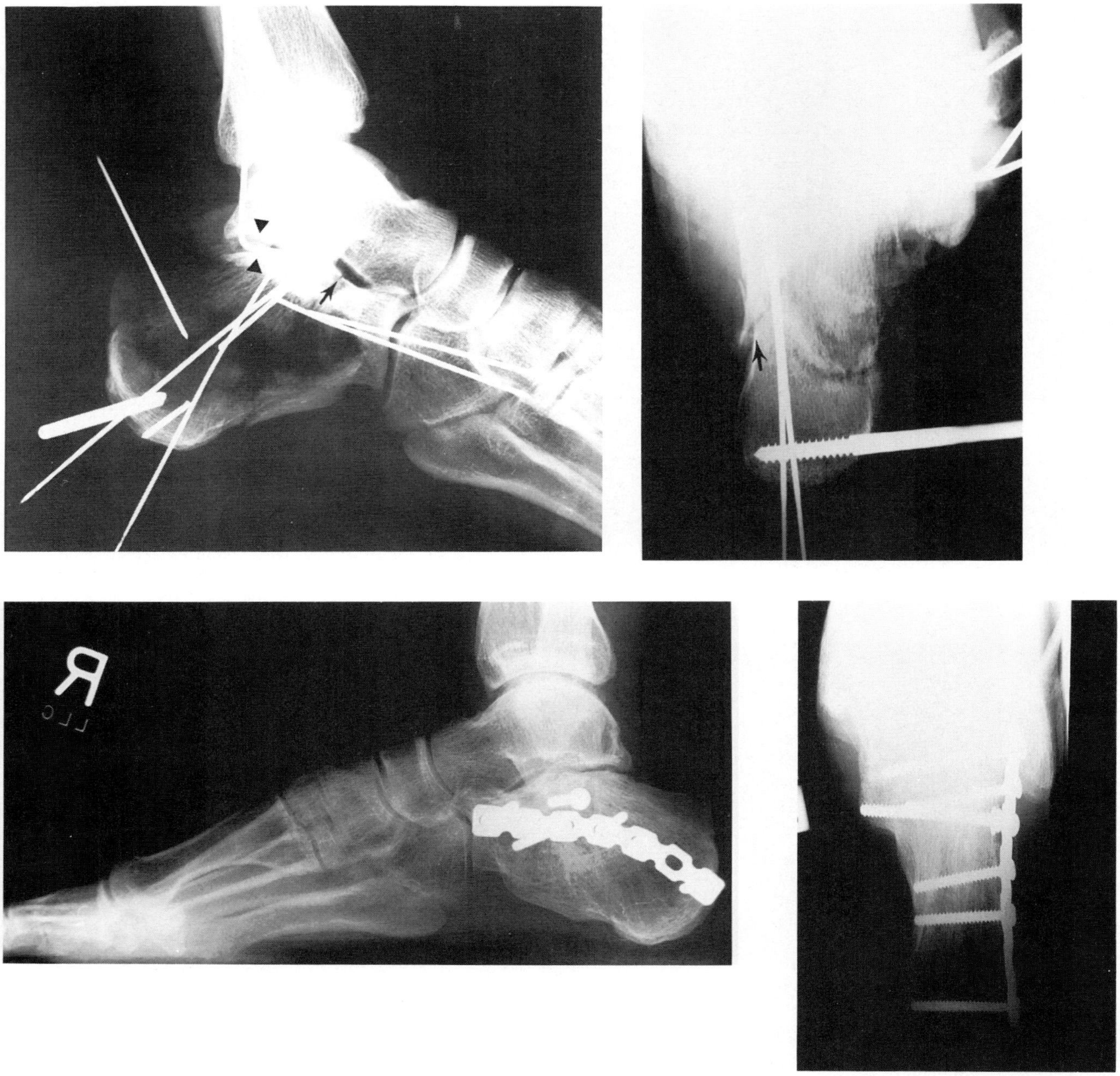

Fig. 11 The same fracture as Figure 10. **Top left**, Lateral view after preliminary reduction. Kirschner wires maintain a provisional reduction. Two K-wires are directed from the heel cephalad and ventrally maintaining the reduction of the medial wall. One is directed across the middle facet fracture line from anterior to posterior, holding the reduction of the middle facet (small arrow) that is slightly under-reduced. The posterior facet is reduced (arrowheads) and held with K-wires. **Top right,** Axial view after preliminary reduction. The arrow points to the reduced medial wall. **Bottom left,** Lateral view 1 year after healing. The subtalar joint is slightly narrow. **Bottom right,** Axial view 1 year after healing.

lems, sural nerve symptoms, and failure to achieve reduction.

The infection rate is 2% to 3%. In most cases, these infections resolve after healing of the fracture, when hardware is removed. Wound complications, including any wound that does not heal primarily, requires dressing changes or other local wound care, further surgery, or exhibits any signs of skin necrosis, occur in 8% to 9%. This is most often marginal necrosis at the corner of the skin flap. No free flaps have been needed in patients with closed injuries.[43] The number of wounds that develop marginal skin loss at the apex of the incision has diminished since the more gently curving approach described by Palmer and Letournel was modified to include a sharper curve. This is presumably because tension is avoided at the corner of the wound and undermining of the skin is not needed when applying the plate through the modified incision. When the calcaneal length and height are restored in surgery, the shape of the hindfoot may change as much as 2 cm. This adds to increased tension at the apex of the incision and may also be a contributing factor to the healing problems seen in these injuries.

Sural nerve symptoms occur in a small number of patients and resolve within a few months in most. Patients who present with neurapraxia of the tibial nerve usually have return of nerve function by 8 months. No patients have been made neurologically worse secondary to operative intervention. The majority of the mild nerve symptoms resolve soon after surgery, when the tension is removed.

Conclusions

The ideal treatment for calcaneus fractures is unknown. The natural history of calcaneus fractures is unfavorable compared with other fractures treated by contemporary techniques. For fractures with significant intra-articular displacement likely to lead to subtalar stiffness or arthrosis, subfibular abutment, anterior ankle impingement, pressure points, or difficulty in shoe fitting, open reduction may be appropriate. A careful lateral extensile approach allows reduction of all of the key elements of the fracture with sufficient rigidity to allow early motion. The morbidity of open treatment is comparable to similar injuries.

References

1. Brindley HH: Fractures of the os calcis: A review of 107 fractures in 95 patients. *South Med J* 1966;59:843-847.
2. Cave EF: Fracture of the os calcis: The problem in general. *Clin Orthop* 1963;30:64-66.
3. DeLee JC: Fractures and dislocations of the foot, in Mann RA (ed): *Surgery of the Foot*, ed 5. St. Louis, MO, CV Mosby, 1986, pp 592-808.
4. Essex-Lopresti P: The mechanism, reduction technique, and results in fractures of the os calcis. *Br J Surg* 1952;39:395-419.
5. Giachino AA, Uhthoff HK: Intra-articular fractures of the calcaneus. *J Bone Joint Surg* 1989;71A:784-787.
6. Harty M: Anatomic considerations in injuries of the calcaneus. *Orthop Clin North Am* 1973;4:179-183.
7. Lance EM, Carey EJ Jr, Wade PA: Fractures of the os calcis: Treatment by early mobilization. *Clin Orthop* 1963;30:76-90.
8. Lindsay WRN, Dewar FP: Fractures of the os calcis. *Am J Surg* 1958;95:555-576.
9. McFarland B: Industrial aspect of fractures of the os calcis. *Br Med J* 1937;1:607-610.
10. Nade S, Monahan PR: Fractures of the calcaneum: A study of the long-term prognosis. *Injury* 1973;4:200-207.
11. O'Connell F, Mital MA, Rowe CR: Evaluation of modern management of fractures of the os calcis. *Clin Orthop* 1972;83:214-223.
12. Heckman JD: Fractures and dislocations of the foot, in Rockwood CA Jr, Green DP (eds): *Fractures in Adults*, ed 2. Philadelphia, PA, JB Lippincott, 1984, pp 1703-1832.
13. Rowe CR, Sakellarides HT, Freeman PA, et al: Fractures of the os calcis: A long-term follow-up study of 146 patients. *JAMA* 1963;184:920-923.
14. Stephenson JR: Treatment of displaced intra-articular fractures of the calcaneus using medial and lateral approaches, internal fixation, and early motion. *J Bone Joint Surg* 1987;69A:115-130.
15. Tanke GM: Fractures of the calcaneus: A review of the literature together with some observations on methods of treatment. *Acta Chir Scand Suppl* 1982;505:1-103.
16. Widén A: Fractures of the calcaneus: A clinical study with special reference to the technique and results of open reduction. *Acta Chir Scand Suppl* 1954;188:5-119.
17. Zayer M: Fracture of the calcaneus: A review of 110 fractures. *Acta Orthop Scand* 1969;40:530-542.
18. Wagner UA, Sangeorzan BJ, Harrington RM, et al: Contact characteristics of the subtalar joint: Load distribution between the anterior and posterior facets. *J Orthop Res* 1992;10:535-543.
19. Mann RA: Biomechanics of the foot and ankle, in Mann RA (ed): *Surgery of the Foot*, ed 5. St. Louis, MO, CV Mosby, 1986, pp 1-30.
20. Sarrafian SK: *Anatomy of the Foot and Ankle*. Philadelphia, PA, JB Lippincott, 1983.
21. Letournel E: Open reduction and internal fixation of calcaneus fractures, in Spiegel PG (ed): *Topics in Orthopaedic Trauma*. Baltimore, MD, University Park Press, 1984, pp 173-192.
22. Carr JB, Hamilton JJ, Bear LS: Experimental intra-articular calcaneal fractures: Anatomic basis for a newa classification. *Foot Ankle* 1989;10:81-87.
23. McReynolds IS: The case for operative treatment of fractures of the os calcis, in Leach RE, Hoaglund FT, Riseborough EJ, et al (eds): *Controversies in Orthopaedic Surgery*. Philadelphia, PA, WB Saunders, 1982, pp 232-254.
24. Böhler L: Diagnosis, pathology, and treatment of fractures of the calcaneus. *J Bone Joint Surg* 1931;13:75-89.
25. Lowrie IG, Finlay DB, Brenkel IJ, et al: Computerised tomographic assessment of the subtalar joint in calcaneal fractures. *J Bone Joint Surg* 1988;70B:247-250.
26. Crosby LA, Fitzgibbons T: Computerized tomographic scanning of acute intra-articular fractures of the calcaneus: A new classification system. *J Bone Joint Surg* 1990;72A:852-859.
27. Sanders R, Fortin P, Thomas D, et al: Operative treatment of 120 displaced intraarticular calcaneal fractures. *Clin Orthop* 1993;290:87-95.
28. Brodén B: Roentgen examination of the subtaloid joint in fractures of the calcaneus. *Acta Radiol* 1949;31:85-91.
29. Anthonsen W: An oblique projection for roentgen examination of the talo-calcanean joint, particularly regarding intra-articular fracture of the calcaneus. *Acta Radiol* 1943;24:306-310.
30. Isherwood IA: Radiological approach to the subtalar joint. *J Bone Joint Surg* 1961;43B:566-574.
31. Segal D, Marsh JL, Leiter B: Clinical approach of computerized axial tomography (CAT) scanning of calcaneus fractures. *Clin Orthop* 1985;199:114-123.
32. Smith RW, Staple TW: Computerized tomography (CT) scanning technique for the hindfoot. *Clin Orthop* 1983;177:34-38.
33. Pozo JL, Kirwan EO, Jackson AM: The long-term results of conservative management of severely displaced fractures of the calcaneus. *J Bone Joint Surg* 1984;66B:386-390.
34. Leonard MH: Treatment of fractures of the os calcis. *Arch Surg* 1957;75:990-997.
35. Paley D, Hall H: Calcaneal fracture controversies: Can we put Humpty Dumpty together again? *Orthop Clin North Am* 1989;20:665-677.
36. Buckley RE, Meek RN: Comparison of open versus closed reduction in intra-articular fractures of the calcaneus: A matched cohort in workmen. *J Orthop Trauma* 1992;6:216-222.

37. Janzen DL, Connell DG, Munk PL, et al: Intra-articular fractures of the calcaneus: Value of CT findings in determining prognosis. *Am J Roentgenol* 1992;158:1271-1274.
38. Ananthakrishnan D, Tencer AF, Sangeorzan BJ: The effect of intra-articular displacement of calcaneus fractures on contact characteristics of the subtalar joint. *Orthop Trans* 1993;17:727.
39. Isbister JF: Calcaneo-fibular abutment following crush fracture of the calcaneus. *J Bone Joint Surg* 1974;56B:274-278.
40. Benirschke SK, Sangeorzan BJ: Intraarticular fractures of the foot: Surgical management of calcaneal fractures. *Clin Orthop* 1993;292:128-134.
41. Gould N: Lateral approach to the os calcis. *Foot Ankle* 1984;4:218-220.
42. Palmer I: The mechanism and treatment of fractures of the calcaneus: Open reduction with the use of cancellous grafts. *J Bone Joint Surg* 1948;30A:2-8.
43. Grujic L, Macey LR, Early JS, et al: Incidence of morbidity associated with open reduction and internal rigid fixation of displaced intra-articular calcaneus fractures using a lateral approach. Presented at the American Academy of Orthopaedic Surgeons 61st Annual Meeting, New Orleans, LA, Feb 24-Mar 1, 1994.

CHAPTER 32

The High Price of High-Fashion Footwear

Michael J. Coughlin, MD
Francesca M. Thompson, MD

Shoes have been an important part of attire since early civilization. Eons have passed since humans began to walk in an upright fashion, but the main purpose of footwear, protection of the foot, has remained virtually unchanged. The earliest footwear prototype was a primitive moccasin crafted from animal hide. Through the centuries, fashion has played an important role both in the manufacture of shoes and in the success of certain styles of shoes. Footwear has evolved a great deal—from the soft, flexible moccasins of early humans to the rigid, high-fashion footwear that is prevalent in Western society today.

It has been estimated that one in six persons (43.1 million people) in the United States has foot problems.[1] The prevalence of these foot problems dramatically increases in persons who are older than 30 years of age, while foot problems are relatively infrequent in persons who are younger than 15 years of age. Thirty-six per cent (15.5 million) of these persons have regarded their foot problems as serious enough to warrant medical attention.[1] In 1980, Gould and associates[2] estimated that 12% of the population of the United States had had an operation on the foot.

Proving a causal relationship between high-fashion footwear and foot problems has been difficult. Hundreds of published studies on the treatment of individual foot problems have reported a high proportion of female patients; however, most of these investigations covered a short period of time (1 to 2 years) and were biased because they reported on one specific surgical procedure only.

While the rate of foot problems in shoe-wearing societies is relatively high, investigations in societies where shoes are not worn have reported a paucity of foot problems.[3,4] In studies involving barefoot natives of the Belgian Congo,[5] of West Africa,[6] and of New Guinea,[7] there was no demonstrable tendency toward the formation of a hallux valgus deformity in either men or women. Bunions did not occur as the individuals aged.

In a study from mainland China,[8] two groups (those who wore shoes [118 subjects] and those who did not [107 subjects]) were compared regarding the effects of footwear. Chinese natives who had worn shoes were reported to have a 33% prevalence of bunions, while those who had never worn shoes had a 2% prevalence of bunions. Kato and Watanabe[9] reported on their experience with hallux valgus in Japanese women. Before 1972, very few operations for hallux valgus had been performed in Japan. After that date, such operations became much more frequent. Before 1948, Japanese women had worn a tabi, or thong, that did not constrict the foot. Following World War II, constricting leather footwear had been introduced in Japan and the tabi had fallen into disuse. The investigators concluded that the introduction of constricting footwear had made a marked difference in the prevalence of bunion formation and subsequent operations.

Some of the most incriminating evidence that foot deformities can be caused by compression of the foot comes from mainland China.[10-14] For over 1,000 years, the process of binding of the foot was performed on young (2- to 7-year-old) Chinese girls in order to compress the foot to a smaller size. This painful process of wrapping the foot over time could reduce the length of the foot to a mere 3 inches (7.6 cm). While the bound foot was the object of great sensuality in Chinese society, binding caused severe deformities of the feet of young girls and created serious difficulty with walking in their later years. The process eventually came to be reserved for the wealthy, who had servants to carry the women around and to wait on them.

We think that the same process occurs, to a much more limited degree and at a slower rate, in Western society. The binding of feet in China could alter the shape of the foot over the course of 3 to 4 years in childhood, while the use of high-fashion footwear in Western society can cause deformities of the foot over several decades. The desire to make the foot appear smaller, daintier, and narrower is as prevalent today in Western society as it was over 1,000 years ago in Eastern cultures. High-heeled shoes tend to make the foot appear smaller because they place the foot in a more vertical position. Likewise, most shoes constrict the width of the foot by ½ to 1 in (1.3 to 2.5 cm),[15] making it appear narrower. Along with these considerations, it is not known what effect a positive familial history has on the development of hallux valgus or other foot deformities.

The Difference between Men's and Women's Shoes

In general, the outline of a man's foot is comparable to the outline of a man's shoe; the shoe conforms to the outer dimensions of the foot. As a result, the typical man's shoe does not compress or constrict the foot. One would thus expect the prevalence of compressive foot problems in the American male population to be relatively low. Hewitt and associates,[16] in a study of 23,000 military recruits, noted that there was an extremely small prevalence (less than 4%) of bunions, hammertoes, and other deformities in this population.

In contrast, the typical woman's high-fashion shoe does not conform to the outer dimensions of a woman's foot. Frey and associates[15] found that 88% of 356 women (73% of whom were patients in an orthopaedic office and 80% of whom had foot pain) wore shoes that were an average of 1.2 cm narrower than the size of the foot. Women who wore shoes that had a discrepancy of only 0.5 cm had very few symptoms and less deformity. Frey and associates concluded that the deforming effects of improper shoes on a normal foot frequently can lead to hallux valgus, bunionette, hammertoes, and other problems.

Snow and associates[17] reported markedly increased pressure beneath the forefoot when a shoe with an elevated heel was worn compared with when no shoe was worn. A low heel (1.9 cm) increased the peak pressure by 22% in the forefoot, a 5-cm heel increased the peak pressure by 57%, and an 8.3-cm heel increased the peak pressure by 76%. Those authors also showed that a narrow toe box places a laterally directed force on the hallux and a medially directed force on the fifth toe.

To investigate the relative frequency of foot disorders occurring in the practice of a busy foot surgeon, the overall profile of patients who had had a forefoot operation between January 1979 and January 1994 was quantitated in the orthopaedic practice of one of us (M. J. C.). All of the cases of patients who had had surgical correction of forefoot problems were reviewed. Patients who had rheumatoid arthritis and other systemic arthritic disorders were excluded from the study. During this 15-year period, the prevalence of hallux valgus, hammertoe deformity, interdigital neuroma, and bunionette in women was extremely high in comparison with that in men. In contrast, during the same period of time, an approximately equal number of male and female patients had an ankle arthrodesis or surgical treatment of an ankle fracture, two procedures that are used to treat conditions that have little if any relation to footwear (Table 1).

The age of the patient at the time of the onset of the forefoot deformities was evaluated as well. There was no increase in the prevalence of hallux valgus, hammertoe deformity, or neuroma formation in men with increasing age (Fig. 1). In women, however, the prevalence of all of these conditions increased dramatically during the fourth, fifth, and sixth decades.

Table 1
Indications for Operations on the Foot in One Orthopaedic Practice, 1979 to 1994

	Women	Men	Total	Prevalence in Women (%)
Hallux valgus	785	53	838	94
Hammertoes	827	194	1,021	81
Neuromas	278	36	314	89
Bunionettes	96	11	107	90
Degenerative osteoarthrosis of the ankle	38	30	68	56
Ankle fractures	52	44	96	54

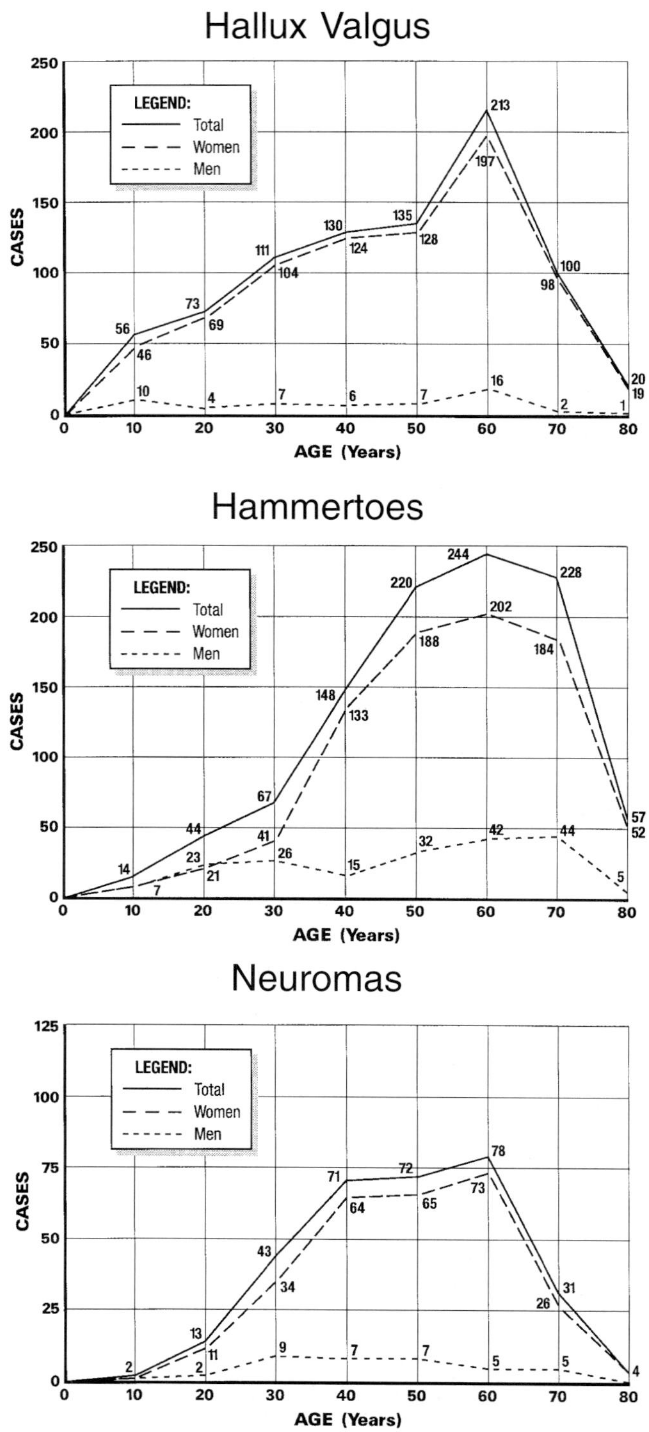

Fig. 1 These three graphs demonstrate the prevalence of hallux valgus, hammertoes, and neuromas. The peak prevalence occurs in the fourth, fifth, and sixth decades in women. There is no marked increase in men with increasing age.

Cost to Society

It is difficult to calculate the nationwide cost of the treatment of forefoot problems because of the extreme variations in hospital charges and physician fees across the country. No comparable figures are available on the frequency of bunionectomies, hammertoe repairs, neuroma excisions, and bunionette repairs in the United States; therefore, estimating the number of surgical procedures performed is extremely difficult. For patients who are older than 65 years of age, however, Medicare figures are readily available.[18] In 1991, 56,500 bunionectomies, 84,000 hammertoe procedures, 12,650 neuroma excisions, and 17,800 bunionette corrections were done for Medicare patients in the United States. In the present series, 27% of hallux valgus repairs, 40% of hammertoe repairs, 19% of neuroma excisions, and 15% of bunionette repairs were performed for Medicare patients. Applying these percentages to the total numbers of Medicare patients, it can be estimated that the following numbers of surgical corrections on the forefoot were performed in the United States in 1991: bunionectomy, 209,000; hammertoe repair, 210,000; neuroma excision, 66,500; and bunionette correction, 119,000.

It is our best estimate that 75% of these problems either result from or are greatly aggravated by the use of high-fashion footwear. The average cost per procedure (in hospital and physician charges) varies greatly, depending on the type of procedure, geographic location, and other factors. Use of $3,000 per procedure for simplicity's sake yields an estimated total direct cost of almost $1.5 billion for the treatment of the 75% of these four conditions that are caused by the use of high-fashion footwear. The indirect costs for these procedures (calculated as an average of 4 weeks off from work per person) approach an additional $1.5 billion. When one considers that several other problems (soft corns, hard corns, claw toes, intractable plantar keratoses, sesamoid abnormalities, hallux rigidus, and toenail problems) were excluded from this calculation, an estimated total cost resulting from the wearing of high-fashion footwear of $3 billion per year is undoubtedly a conservative one.

Clinical Approaches: How to Talk to Patients about Shoes

When one looks at the rectangular shape of the foot and the triangular shape of the toe box in high-fashion footwear, it is obvious that the forefoot becomes constricted in the toe box. The addition of a high heel to this shoe increases the downward pressure with which the forefoot is forced into the constricting, triangular toe box. Over time, this deforming force leads to bunion deformity of the great toe and bunionette formation on the lateral aspect of the foot. As the lesser toes become contracted, hammertoes develop. This constriction of the forefoot can cause injury to the interdigital nerves and neuroma formation.

While surgical intervention often is needed for the correction of these deformities, prevention is a reasonable objective. Preventive care can have a substantial effect on the reduction of the severity as well as the frequency of these problems.

The lower rate of foot problems in men demonstrates that forefoot problems can be reduced or even eliminated with the use of roomy, non-constricting footwear.

Achievement of this objective for many female patients means moving quickly into an area that many male orthopaedic surgeons often feel diffident about broaching in detail; experience has shown them that female patients often roll their eyes heavenward, shrug, and tell them they just don't understand the problems of shoe fit and the cultural or work requirements of shoe style. One of the authors (F. M. T.) has been consulted on many occasions about this problem and will review here the techniques that have helped her to engage patients in a substantive discussion of the contribution that shoes make to pain and deformity.

Step One: Observing a Discrepancy between the Size of the Foot and the Size of the Shoe

The starting point for a discussion of the patient's shoes is to observe the relationship between the size and shape of the foot and the size and shape of the shoe that the patient is wearing. Do this as you get the gist of the patient's chief complaint and examine her feet.

In the course of examining her feet, ask the patient to stand on a footstool. It is important for the patient to be in a weightbearing position when you measure the width of the foot, so that the width will be the same as when the patient is bearing weight in a shoe.

Next, take an old-fashioned ruler and hold it over each foot (Fig. 2) and then announce your observation, "Let's see now, this right foot measures 3¾ inches across, and this left foot measures 3⅞ inches across." Write down these measurements on the patient's chart.

Next, pick up the patient's shoe and turn it over so that both of you are looking at the sole, across the widest part of the toe box where the metatarsal heads lie (Fig. 3). Place the ruler across the shoe at that point and announce your observation, "This shoe measures 2⅞ inches across." Write this measurement on the chart. If she came in with both dress shoes and sneakers, measure both types.

Put your thumb on the ruler to mark the greatest width of the foot, hold it up and say, "See, this is how wide your foot is when you are standing on it." Then put the ruler, thumb in place, across the metatarsal area of the sole of the shoe (Fig. 4) and say, "Look, this is

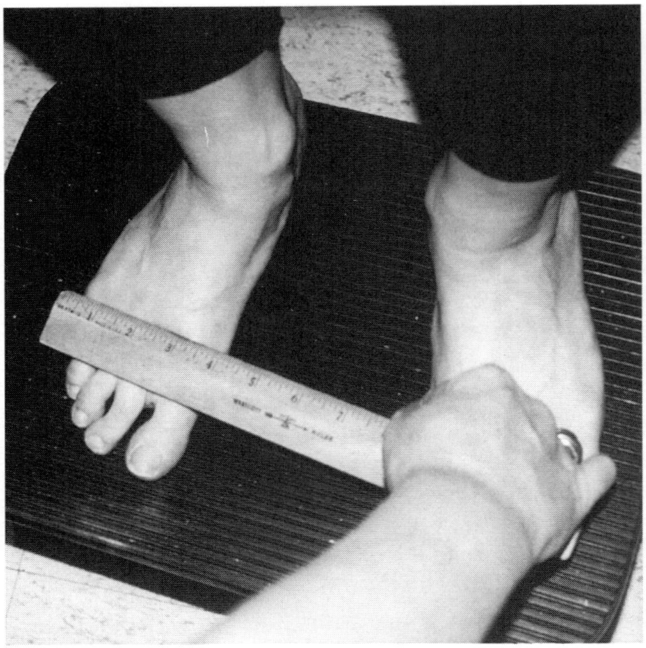

Fig. 2 How to measure each weightbearing foot with a ruler from the first to the fifth metatarsal. Announce the measurements to the patient and record the foot-width measurements in the chart.

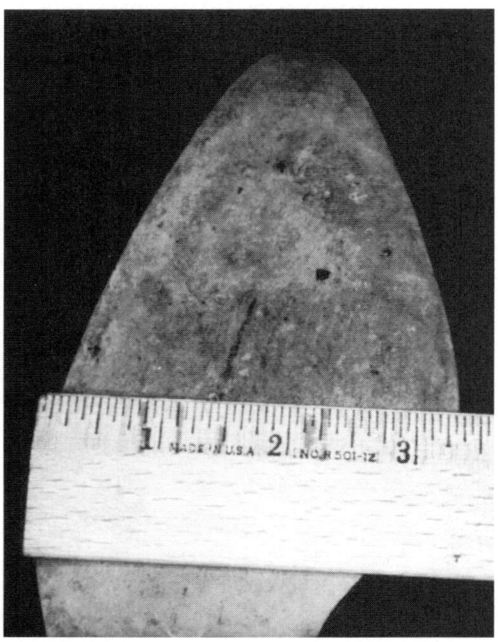

Fig. 3 How to measure the patient's shoe across the sole at the widest part. Announce the measurement to the patient and record the shoe-width measurement in the chart.

how wide your foot is, and this is how wide your shoe is. There is an inch of difference."

At this point, there can be no disagreement: her shoes are smaller than her feet.

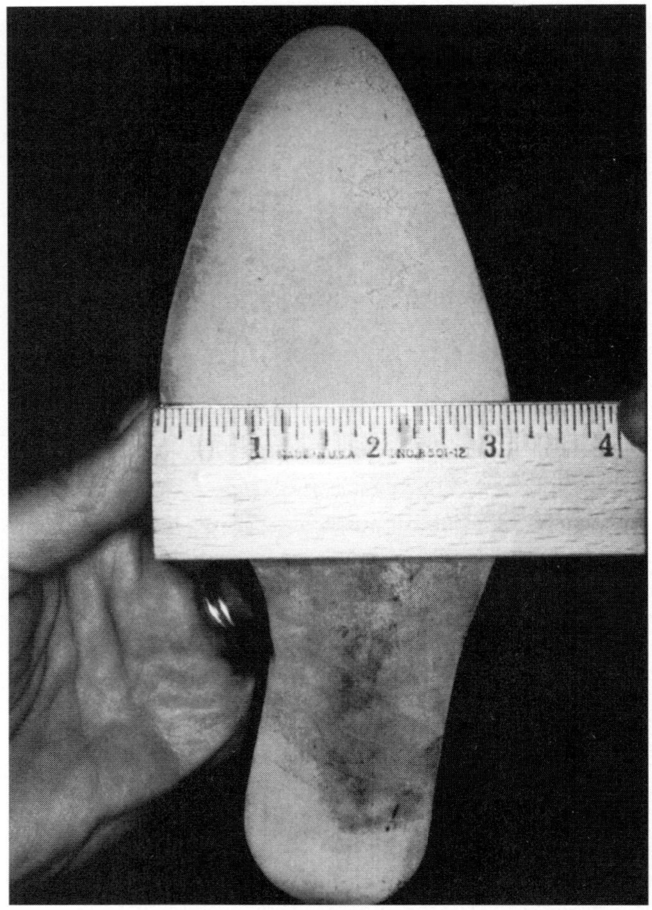

Fig. 4 How to place the ruler against the shoe, with your thumb on the ruler at the patient's foot width, to indicate the difference.

Step Two: Discussing What We Know about Shoe-Width Discrepancy, Foot Pain, and Deformity

Tell the patient about the findings of the Council on Women's Shoewear survey regarding women's feet, foot pain, foot deformity, and shoe width.[15] The average foot width was found to be 3⅔ inches (9.3 cm) (range, 3 to 4½ inches [7.6 to 11.4 cm]). Women who had no pain or deformity tended to wear shoes that were about ¼ inch (0.6 cm) narrower than the foot. Women who had pain and deformity tended to wear shoes that were more than ½ inch (1.3 cm) narrower than the foot. The study concluded that "an inch of pinch" is enough to cause foot pain and deformity. We recommend that a woman should wear sports shoes that are the same width as her foot and dress shoes that are no more than ¼ to ½ inch (0.6 to 1.3 cm) narrower than her foot.

Step Three: What You Can Do for Your Patient

Your patient needs a shoe sizer. Although the metal shoe sizer, called the Brannock device, that is found in stores looks official and has a lateral flare that is marked A, B, C, and so on, there is absolutely no relationship between the width of any shoe and the width of the foot as indicated by the Brannock device. The patient needs some way of determining whether the shoe proffered in the store or the shoes in her closet meet the basic requirement of being within ¼ to ½ inch (0.6 to 1.3 cm) of the foot width for a dress shoe and the same width as the foot for a sports shoe.

We recommend that the orthopaedist make a shoe sizer for the patient. A stamp may be made that says, just below the orthopaedist's name and address:

My foot is ___ inches wide.

My dress shoe should be ___ to ___ inches wide.

My sport shoe should be ___ inches wide.

This can be imprinted on a 3 x 5-inch index card, with the width of the patient's foot drawn on the card and the card marked to that width (Fig. 5, top). Two lines should be drawn to indicate the range from ¼ to ½ inch smaller than the foot width, and the card should be cut off at these lines (Fig. 5, center). The patient should be shown how to use the shoe sizer on the shoe that she is wearing (Fig. 5, bottom).

Give this customized card to the patient, saying, "This is your shoe sizer; put it in your wallet and keep it with you at all times in case you get a shoe-buying attack. But first take it home and check all the shoes in your closet. If they don't measure up, put them in the back of the closet until you are ready to throw them away."

Step Four: Stepping Out of the Heel

Many patients will be quick to point out that when they wear wider shoes, their heels lift out and they step out of the shoe (Fig. 6). They think that they are the only one with this problem and that it is a sign of abnormal feet. This is the most common problem that American women have with shoes, because the size and shape of their foot changes decade by decade: the heel does not widen, but the forefoot does. Shoes should fit the forefoot rather than feel snug in the heel. Manufacturers who split sizes (that is, those who make shoes that have a narrow heel and a wider toe box) should be sought out. These shoes are made on what is called a combination last. Tell your patients that shoes with laces, straps, or buckles on the vamp (the top part of the shoe) also will stay on better.

Step Five: Where to Buy Shoes

This is information that you and your staff can compile over time for your local area. Start by collecting brand names and shoe store names from patients themselves. Whenever you find a patient wearing a shoe that measures at least 3¼ inches (8.3 cm) across, and especially one that measures 3½ inches (8.9 cm) across, note the brand and ask the patient where she bought the shoes. In this way, you can develop a "Wide Shoe List" that you can give to every patient, along with the shoe sizer. Describe this as only a place to start, and warn her that she should anticipate shopping at a number of stores in order to find the appropriate shoes.

You should find out what facilities in your area are staffed by certified pedorthists; call the Pedorthic Footwear Association at 1-800-673-8447 for this information. In addition to being able to fit prescriptions for specialized orthoses, these stores tend to have a selection of off-the-shelf wide or extra depth shoes, or both, that might give your patient at least one pair of shoes that she can wear every day or when she must spend a long time on her feet. You can also give the patient a prescription for a bunion last shoe that will more easily accommodate a severe bunion deformity. You should point out to the patient that seams in the toe box that

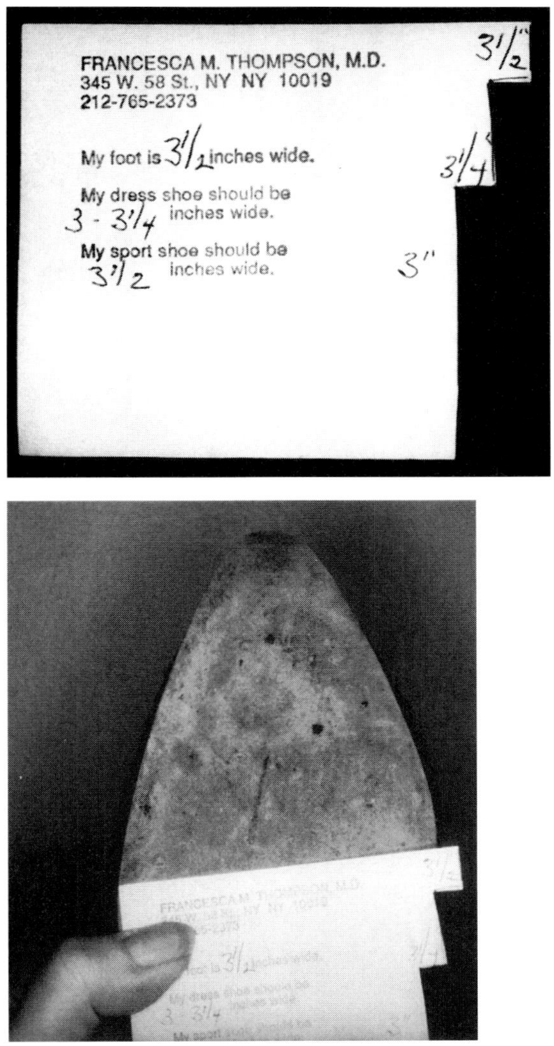

Fig. 5 The shoe-sizing card is a simple 3 x 5-in index card overprinted as shown. **Top**, Mark the card to the patient's foot width and draw a line down, stepping in two ¼-inch increments. Then cut the card along the line and give it to the patient. **Bottom**, Show the patient how to use the sizer against the sole of the shoe to see if it is within ½ inch of the width of her weightbearing foot, but preferably closer to the actual size of her foot.

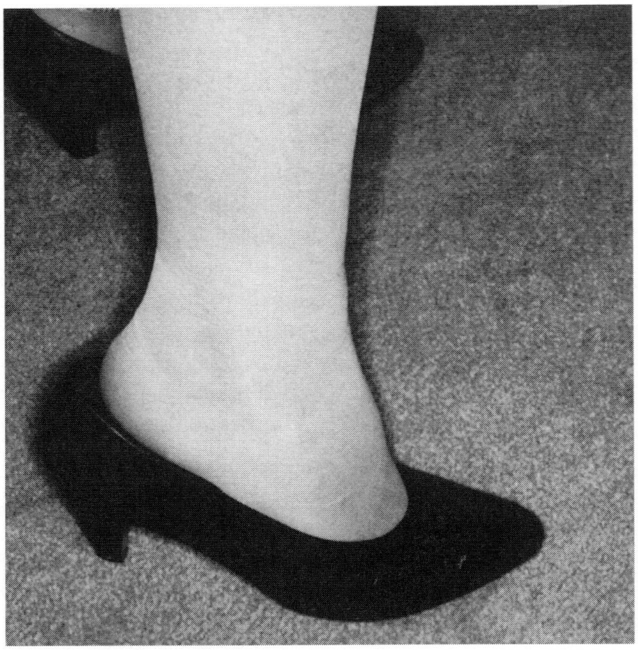

Fig. 6 Patients frequently observe that if the shoe fits the forefoot, it is too loose at the heel, as shown here.

Outline 1
Handout on the Subject of Wide Feet

Wide Feet and Your Shoes

Many common foot problems that orthopaedic surgeons see are caused or aggravated by improper size and fit of shoes.

Women's Shoe Survey

The Council on Women's Shoewear of the American Orthopaedic Foot and Ankle Society recently reported on a series of 356 women.[15] The width of the bare foot while the woman was standing was compared with the width of the shoe that she was wearing at the time that she was seen. The authors found that 88% of those studied had shoes that were more narrow than the foot by more than ½ in (1.3 cm). Eighty per cent of the women stated that they had some foot pain. Of those who had no pain, the shoe measured only ¼ in (0.6 cm) smaller than the width of the foot, on average. Seventy-six per cent of the women had some forefoot deformity such as a bunion, hammertoes, calluses under the metatarsals, or some other deformity. Of those who had no deformity, the average discrepancy between weightbearing foot width and shoe width again was only ¼ in (0.6 cm). The average foot width was 3⅔ in (9.3 cm), with a range of 3 to 4½ in (7.6 to 11.4 cm).

Do American women have a Cinderella Complex when it comes to high-fashion shoes? This is a tempting analogy, but most women state that the shoe has to be snug in the front to stay on the back! This makes sense anatomically, because the foot has only one bone in the heel, and this bone does not enlarge after the growth of the foot is complete (between the ages of 12 and 14 years). Therefore, the heel stays narrow throughout life. The front of the foot, in contrast, is made up of many bones connected by ligaments. Over the years, these ligaments stretch; as a result, the front part of the foot widens, the arch may sag, and the foot becomes longer as well. The women's shoe survey revealed that with every decade, more women noted that their foot size had increased. Remember that the average foot width was 3⅔ in (9.3 cm) and the range of widths was 3 to 4½ in (7.6 to 11.4 cm). As it is very hard to find shoes that measure more than 3 in (7.6 cm) in width, many women have a problem buying proper shoes.

A person's feet vary in width and length from foot to foot. The women's shoe survey found that 66% of the women felt that one foot was bigger than the other, divided equally between right and left feet.

Every trip to the shoe store is a compromise; some guidelines may help in shopping for shoes. Know the width of your weightbearing foot. Take a 6-in (15.2 cm) ruler to the store with you. Fit the larger foot. Shop at the end of the day when whatever swelling may occur will be present. Buy shoes that are within ¼ to ½ in (0.6 to 1.3 cm) of the width of your foot. Avoid shoes that have seams in painful areas. Exercise shoes should be as wide as your foot. Often boy's or men's shoes are cut more generously in the forefoot. There is no standardization of sizes, so you must measure the shoe you are offered in the store and try it on. Shoes don't "break in," but feet do.

High Heels

What happens when high heels are worn? Irish orthopaedic surgeons recently studied the effect of heel height on the forefoot.[19] They compared the metatarsal loading of 60 feet when the subjects were barefoot, wearing a shoe with a ¾-in (1.9-cm) heel, and wearing a shoe with a 1¾-in (4.4-cm) heel. They found that the higher heel increased the pressure under the ball of the foot by 50%, and, in addition, in many feet, the pressure was shifted from the middle of the foot to the bunion area.

press on the dorsomedial aspect of the first metatarsal will irritate a bursa in that area. Softer leather such as suede also conforms to the shape of the foot more readily than does patent leather or plastic, and cushioned inner soles decrease pressure in the metatarsal area. All of these elements will create a more comfortable shoe.

Many women whose feet are wider than average will be more comfortable in men's sports shoes, which usually are two sizes smaller; a woman's size 9 is a man's size 7.

Step Six: High Heels

As already noted, elevation of the heel increases forefoot pressure markedly. Advise your patients to limit the time that they spend wearing high heels, particularly those that elevate the heel more than two inches (5.1 cm). In New York City, it has been common for years for women to commute to work in running shoes, carrying their high heels with them.

Your patient must understand that you are talking about something real: the discrepancy between the width of her foot and the width of her shoe (Step 1). Next, you must convince her that there is clinical relevance to this finding (Step 2). Then, you must give her a shoe sizer to help rectify the problem (Step 3). Acknowledge the difficulty of keeping the shoes on her heels, and suggest ways of getting around this problem (Step 4). Give her a list of specific stores and brands of shoes that other patients have found that seem to meet the basic requirements, as well as a list of stores in your area where there are certified pedorthists to help with fitting (Step 5). Finally, recognizing that she may not be able to give up high heels entirely, suggest that she wear them sparingly (Step 6).

This information may be summarized in a handout on the subject of wide feet, like the one shown in Outline 1. You may use this as your handout or modify it as you see fit to help your patients.

The American Orthopaedic Foot and Ankle Society has developed ten points of proper footwear that can educate the public to the importance of a wellfitting shoe (Outline 2). These steps will add no great cost to the price of shoes but will make it clear that tight shoes have a long-term deleterious effect on foot comfort and on a person's ability to walk.

In conclusion, there is a much greater frequency of forefoot problems in women than in men. These problems peak in the fourth, fifth, and sixth decades. Studies of barefoot populations have demonstrated no tendency toward forefoot problems in women, and we conclude that the shoe-wearing patterns in the United States have a distinct and unequivocal influence on the development of forefoot problems in women. If we are to change societal footwear habits, we must make the public aware of the dangers of and damage done by ill-fitting, tight shoes. Proper shoe fit is critical for good foot health. Increased public awareness is the most important preventive step in reducing the prevalence of foot problems in women and in decreasing the huge expenditure of health care dollars for these forefoot problems. Finally, direct, informative discussions can provide female patients with insight into these problems and with practical guidance in the purchase of appropriate footwear.

Outline 2
Ten Points of Proper Footwear Provided by the American Orthopaedic Foot and Ankle Society*

1. Sizes vary among shoe brands and styles. Don't select shoes based on the size marked inside the shoe. Pick the shoe by how it fits your foot.
2. Select a shoe that conforms as nearly as possible to the shape of your forefoot.
3. Have your feet measured regularly. The size of your feet may change as you grow older.
4. Have both feet measured (often one foot is larger than the other). The shoe should be fitted to the larger foot.
5. Have your shoes fitted at the end of the day when your feet are the largest.
6. Stand during the fitting process because the foot lengthens as you are standing. There should be one fingerbreadth (½ in [1.3 cm]) between your longest toe and the end of the shoe.
7. The ball of your foot should fit snugly into the widest part of the shoe, but the shoe should not be too tight.
8. If the shoes don't fit, don't purchase them. Don't expect them to "stretch to fit."
9. Your heel should fit comfortably in the shoe with a minimum amount of pistoning.
10. While you are still in the shoe store, walk to make sure that the fit feels correct.

*Brochures are available from the American Orthopaedic Foot and Ankle Society, 701 16th Avenue, Seattle, Washington 98122.

References

1. Greenberg L, Davis H: Foot problems in the US: The 1990 national health interview survey. *J Am Podiatr Med Assoc* 1993; 83:475-483.
2. Gould N, Schneider W, Ashikaga T: Epidemiological survey of foot problems in the continental United States, 1978-1979. *Foot Ankle* 1980;1:8-10.
3. Hoffman P: Conclusions drawn from a comparative study of the feet of barefooted and shoe-wearing peoples. *Am J Orthop Surg* 1905;3:105-136.
4. James CS: Footprints and feet of natives of the Solomon Islands. *Lancet* 1939;2:1390-1393.
5. Engle ET, Morton DJ: Notes on foot disorders among natives of the Belgian Congo. *J Bone Joint Surg* 1931;13:311-318.
6. Barnicot NA, Hardy RH: The position of the hallux in West Africans. *J Anat* 1955;89:355-361.
7. MacLennan R: Prevalence of hallux valgus in a neolithic New Guinea population. *Lancet* 1966;1:1398-1400.
8. Sim-Fook L, Hodgson AR: A comparison of foot forms among the non-shoe and shoe-wearing Chinese population. *J Bone Joint Surg* 1958;40A:1058-1062.
9. Kato T, Watanabe S: The etiology of hallux valgus in Japan. *Clin Orthop* 1981;157:78-81.
10. Blakeslee TJ, Chan RJ: Chinese bound foot: A literature review and case report. *J Am Podiatr Med Assoc* 1986;76:502-505.
11. Chan LM: Foot binding in Chinese women and its psycho-social implications.*Can J Psychiatry* 1970;15:229-231.
12. Chew MB: Chinese bound foot. *Radiography* 1973;39:39-42.
13. Jackson R: The Chinese foot-binding syndrome: Observations on the history and sequelae of wearing ill-fitting shoes. *Int J Dermatol* 1990;29:322-328.
14. Levy H: *Chinese Foot Binding: History of a Curious Erotic Custom.* New York, NY, W Rawls, 1966.
15. Frey C, Thompson F, Smith J, et al: American Orthopaedic Foot and Ankle Society women's shoe survey. *Foot Ankle* 1993;14:78-81.
16. Hewitt D, Stewart AM, Webb JW: The prevalence of foot defects among wartime recruits. *Br Med J* 1953;2:745-749.
17. Snow RE, Williams KR, Holmes GB Jr: The effects of wearing high heeled shoes on pedal pressure in women. *Foot Ankle* 1992; 13:85-92.
18. United States Health and Welfare 1991 Medicare Figures, courtesy of The American Academy of Orthopaedic Surgeons [computer disk].
19. Corrigan JP, Moore DP, Stephens MM: Effect of heel height on forefoot loading. *Foot Ankle* 1993;14:148-152.

Women and Their Shoes: Unrealistic Expectations?

Karen S. Seale, MD

Introduction

Gender specific differences in shoewear have been implicated in the fact that a higher incidence of foot pain and foot deformity is seen in women than in men. A recent study indicated that almost half of the women surveyed were dissatisfied with their inability to buy shoes that are both fashionable and comfortable. Although this compromise between comfort and style is probably generally accepted, the reasons behind the discrepancy are poorly understood. Consumers need to learn why shoes that are fashionable may have inherent design characteristics that preclude comfort. This discussion will assist consumers and physicians in making educated decisions about the compromises involved in selecting shoes for comfort and fashion.

Comfort Versus Fashion

Many studies have shown that societies that wear constricting shoes have a higher incidence of foot deformities than do unshod societies.[1-6] Mounting evidence has confirmed the intuitively obvious and clinically apparent impression that the gender-specific higher incidence of foot pain and deformity in women may be directly related to their wearing of constricting shoes.[7-10] The decision by women to wear the fashionable shoes implicated in contributing to these statistics is clearly their choice. Why do women wear shoes that cause pain and deformity?

In a study performed by the American Orthopaedic Foot and Ankle Society's Council on Women's Shoewear to investigate the shoe-buying habits and attitudes of women, 620 questionnaires were distributed among women shoe buyers. The survey population was not limited by age, and no attempt was made to eliminate either those women who had or those who had not been under treatment by a physician for any orthopaedic problem. Some of the surveys were distributed and returned by members of the National Shoe Retailers Association, who were sent a copy of the survey in the Association's newsletter. Approximately 300 surveys were also completed by members of the Junior League of Little Rock.

The survey questions pertained to respondent age, occupation, length of time at current job, estimated number of hours per pay spent standing and/or walking, shoe size, and the number of pairs of shoes bought per year. The survey included 20 multiple-choice questions, which inquired about the factors that influence the decision to buy shoes to be worn at work, frequency of foot measurement when buying shoes and the technique used to have their feet measured, the types and frequency of various shoes worn, the frequency of foot pain, and satisfaction with their ability to find shoes that are both fashionable and comfortable. The respondents were also asked what changes they would like to see in the shoes that are available for purchase.

All data were analyzed using Statistical Analysis System Institute software. The χ^2 test of independence was used to compare all frequency data. Single measurement parametric data were compared using an unpaired t-test. The significance level used in all comparisons was 0.05. Two-tailed p values are reported. To facilitate broad comparisons by age, respondents were separated into two groups: women 40 years of age and older, and those 39 years of age and younger.

Findings from that study included the following. (1) The overall average number of shoes bought per year was 5.6 pairs (±4.5 pairs). Number of pairs purchased ranged from one pair to 40 pairs per year. (2) When queried about the amount of money generally paid for shoes, 366 (60%) said they paid between $50 to $200 for a pair of dress shoes, and 293 (49%) paid that same amount for a pair of recreation shoes. (3) When asked about their overall satisfaction with their ability to find shoes that are fashionable and comfortable, 263 (44%) responded that they were not satisfied. (4) Of those who wore heels higher than two inches, 78% did so because the shoes are fashionable. (5) Of the 620 surveyed, 173 (28%) responded when asked for their comments regarding what changes they would like to see in the shoes that are available to purchase. The three most frequent comments were summarized as more comfortable shoes that are at the same time fashionable; a greater variety of sizes; and a greater variety in styles. Their single most frequent desire could be summed up in the following statement: "We want the comfort of a tennis shoe with the style of a fashion shoe."

One very interesting conclusion derived from this study was that despite their willingness to spend a considerable amount of money on numerous pairs of shoes each year, almost half of the women surveyed were frustated because they had been unable to find shoes that were both comfortable and fashionable. Why can't women have what they say they want, which is the comfort of a tennis shoe with the fashion of a dress shoe? Can they not find shoes that are comfortable as well as fashionable? Are the two concepts mutually exclusive? If so, why?

This discussion must be prefaced with the clarification that the "comfort" of a particular shoe is a highly subjective concept. What may be comfortable for one person may be totally unacceptable for another. In addition, personal preference, work demands, social situation, and current fashions also influence the selection of shoewear. This discussion is intended to help consumers in general, and our patients in particular, make more educated decisions about their choices of shoewear.

Style and Fashion

It is helpful to clarify and understand the difference between style and fashion. Style is basic. It is the shoe's essential design character, its particular architecture and profile, its identity as a special category of footwear.[11] Style is the combination of characteristics that make a shoe unique.

There are really only seven basic shoe styles. These are the pump, moccasin, oxford, sandal, mule, boot, and clog (Fig. 1).[11] Of these seven basic footwear styles, which have emerged from all the fashions and designs introduced over the centuries, the newest is 300 years old. Ironically, not one of those seven basic designs was developed by or for a woman. To make women's shoes, adaptations of shoes originally designed by and for men were made. For example, the pump was a thin soled slip-on shoe worn by carriage footmen in pre-Elizabethan England. They were called pumps because the footmen pumped the carriage pedals with their feet.[11]

Fashion is a current or popular version or variation of a particular style.[11] The variations that can exist for any given shoe style are numerous and seem limited only by the imagination of the designer and the desires of the buyer.

Entire books, not to mention regularly published fashion magazines and magazines for the working woman, have been written about the choice of clothing and accessories for women in the work force. Although flats have become more widely accepted in the workplace in recent years, the consistently recommended shoe is "the heeled power pump."[12,13] Although women work and compete in the male-dominated power structure, they nonetheless feel obliged to wear shoes that not only are not as comfortable as a pair of men's dress shoes, but that have been implicated in producing foot pain and such deformities as bunions and hammertoes. One is compelled to wonder why, when all seven shoe styles were originally designed by and for men, the evolution of fashions has rendered men's shoes more comfortable while the trend in women's fashions have, to a great extent, failed to follow the trend toward increased comfort. Common sense dictates the recognition of this inherent discrimination.

Anatomy of the Shoe

Knowledge of the basic anatomy of the shoe is necessary to help understand whether women's shoes can be fashionable as well as comfortable. Figure 2 illustrates the five basic parts of the shoe: toe box, quarter, counter, vamp, and sole.[11,14]

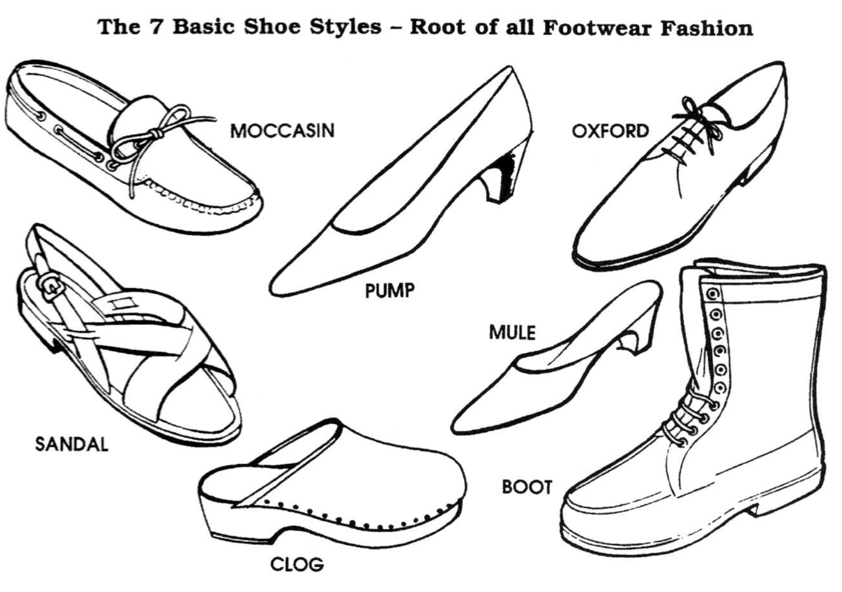

Fig. 1 The seven basic shoe styles — root of all footwear fashion. (Reproduced with permission from the National Shoe Retailers Association.)

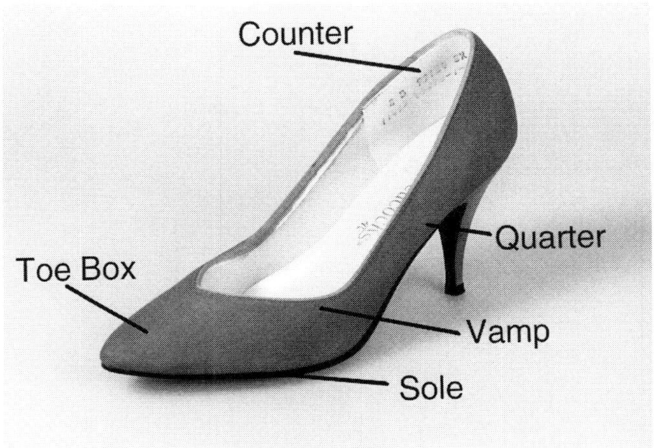

Fig. 2 Five basic shoe components: Toe box, vamp, quarter, counter, and sole. (Reproduced with permission from the National Shoe Retailers Association.)

Toe Box

The toe box is the forepart of the shoe's upper that covers the toe area.[14] Its prime function is to permanently retain the shape of the shoe's toe and to allow room for the toes. The volume of the toe box can be altered by changing both its height and shape.

Quarter and Counter

The quarter is the back half of the shoe's upper. The top edge of the quarter is the part of the shoe that wraps around either side of the ankle. The rear part of the quarter, which encases the heel, is called the counter. Inside the shoe, the security of the whole foot is largely influenced by the fit of the shoe's counter and quarter.

Vamp

The part of the shoe that covers the instep is the vamp. Many fashionable pumps and flats have relatively little vamp so that very little of the instep is covered by the shoe.

Sole

The sole is composed of two parts, the outsole and the insole, which make up the protective barrier between the foot and the ground. The outsole provides traction, insulation, and shock absorption and helps hold the shape of the shoe with wear. The degree to which the outsole performs these functions is dependent on its design, its workmanship, and the materials used in its construction.[11]

The insole is one of the "hidden" components of the shoe, the footbed upon which the foot rests.[11] The insole should provide a comfortable surface for the foot.

Shoe Fit, Design, and Comfort

Proper shoe fit is attained when shoe shape is properly matched to foot shape. As elementary as this may seem, it may be easier said than done. Although a complete discussion of shoe fit and design is beyond the scope of this chapter, it is important that the consumer be educated to some extent about achieving proper shoe fit.

Proper shoe size goes a long way in attaining comfort, regardless of shoe style. Obtaining assistance in getting the right size and fit is helpful, but not all shoe salesmen are professionally trained shoe fitters. In spite of the fact that 10% to 15% of the price of the shoe goes to cover the cost of shoe-fitting service, it is estimated that only 5% of retail shoe salespeople have received any formal, in-depth training in shoe fitting.[11] Clearly, the consumer must become aware of some of the pitfalls in fit and shoe design.

A valuable service that physicians can provide is to inform the public of the availability of trained shoe fitters. The Pedorthic Footwear Association (Columbia, MD) is a nonprofit organization of individuals and companies from a variety of disciplines who work closely with physicians. One of the main objectives of the Pedorthic Footwear Association is to advance the knowledge and skills of those responsible for the fitting of footwear. Many members of the Pedorthic Footwear Association are Certified Pedorthists—allied health professionals with demonstrated competence in shoe fitting and the fitting of prescription footwear.[15]

The National Shoe Retailers Association (Columbia, MD) is an organization that represents traditional footwear retailers. Some of the association's members specialize in an expanded variety of sizes and widths of shoes. Consumers should be encouraged to inquire about the qualifications and education levels of salespeople in the community and to seek skilled assistance in attaining proper shoe fit whenever necessary.

Shoe Shape

Although proper shoe size is one key element in attaining proper fit, shoe shape is equally important. The shape of a shoe, including the shape of the sole and the upper, depends primarily upon the shape of the last, the mold over which the shoe is made.[14] Lasts are made in a wide range of shapes and sizes, but the particular last used for any given shoe is determined solely (no pun intended) by the manufacturer. The two lasts shown in Figure 3 are exactly the same size, but it is obvious that the shape and, thus, the fit and comfort afforded by these different lasts differ radically. There are essentially three types of lasts. (1) The standard last, used for most popularly priced, mass-produced shoes, comes in limited sizes and often only in a single "medium" width. (2) The combination last has a heel

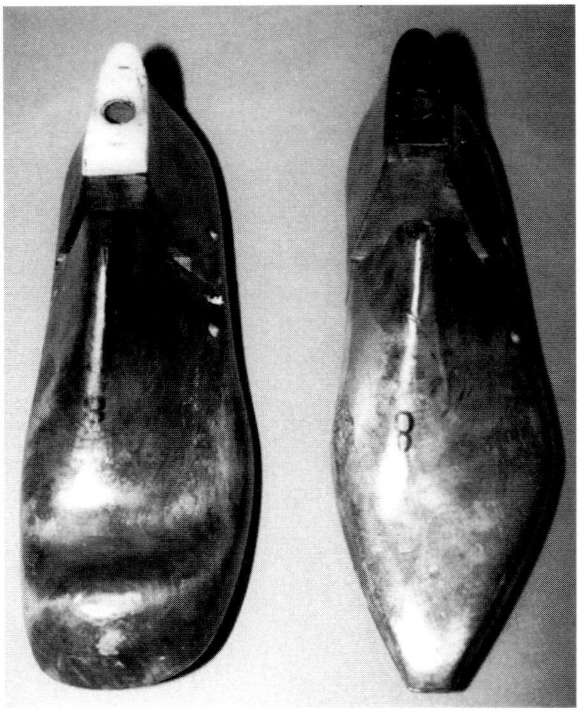

Fig. 3 Two lasts of exactly the same size, but significantly different shoe shape. (Courtesy of Dennis Janisse, C Ped, OST.)

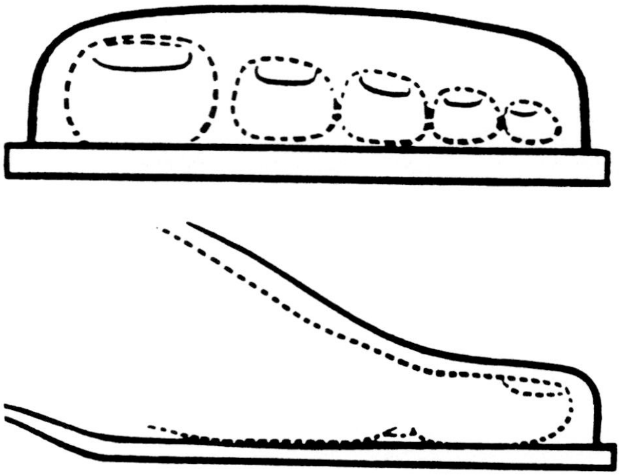

Fig. 4 The toe box walls should be shaped to allow adequate room for the toes. (Reproduced with permission from the National Shoe Retailers Association.)

that is narrower than the forefoot, which provides room for the metatarsals and toes and, at the same time, maintains a good heel fit. The heel width is often two widths narrower than the ball of the foot. For example, a shoe with an 8C/A designation means that the shoe size is 8 with a C-width ball combined with an A-width heel.[16] (3) The extra-depth last is designed to allow extra volume for the foot inside the shoe. Although there is no visible difference in appearance among the three lasts, the extra-depth shoe is the most versatile in achieving a good shoe fit.

Shoe retailers who specialize in orthopaedic shoes are more likely to carry shoes made from extra-depth and/or combination lasts. Many of these shoes are made not only in a wide range of sizes and widths, but in many shapes as well.

Traditionally, shoes made from extra-depth lasts have been made in styles, such as the oxford, that have limited contemporary appeal for adults. Now, however, manufacturers have expanded the designs to include pumps in a broad range of sizes and widths.

Toe Box

A shoe that has a high toe box provides more vertical room for the toes.[11] Figure 4 shows a toe box with a more vertical wall, which allows more accommodation for the toes. This contrasts with the shoe shown in Figure 5, which has a toe box that recedes to create a silhouette with a long, slender look.

In addition, the shape of the front of the toe box can vary. As is shown in Figure 6, a rounded toe box provides more room for the width of the toes, and a pointed toe box provides less room. Obviously, a narrow, pointed, receding toe box can apply pressure to the toes and force them into an unnatural shape. This pressure can cause calluses and discomfort and may eventually lead to deformity.[11,14] Therefore, both the height and the shape of the toe box affect the ability of the shoe to accommodate the toes comfortably.

Shoe Vamp

The more ample the vamp, that is, the more of the instep that is covered by the shoe's upper, the less snug the toe box needs to be to secure the shoe to the foot. Ideally, the vamp should be high enough to cover a substantial part of the instep, be snug enough to secure the shoe to the foot, but not be snug enough to cause undue pressure over the instep. Shoes with laces provide the greatest amount of adjustability, but elastic, buckle, velcro, or "T"-strap closures can also provide a comfortable, reasonably secure fit.

If the vamp is not ample enough to hold the shoe onto the foot, the shoe must depend on the toe box and the heel counter to keep from falling off. Therefore, the toe box and heel must fit snugly. This lack of an adequate vamp, in and of itself, may lead to discomfort.

Heel Height

The primary reason for adding heel height to the shoe is cosmetic. Heel height creates an optical illusion of "shortening" the foot, slenderizes the ankle, contributes to a long-legged look, creates a sensuous look to the stride, and increases height to generate the

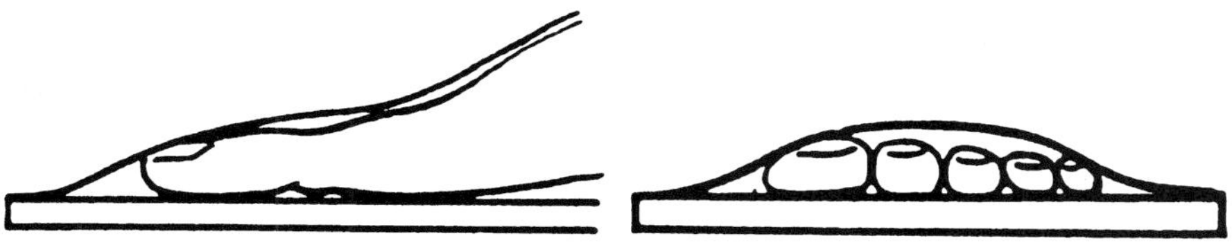

Fig. 5 Toe box with walls that are shallowly slanted or "recede" to create a silhouette that accentuates the long, slender look. (Reproduced with permission from the National Shoe Retailers Association.)

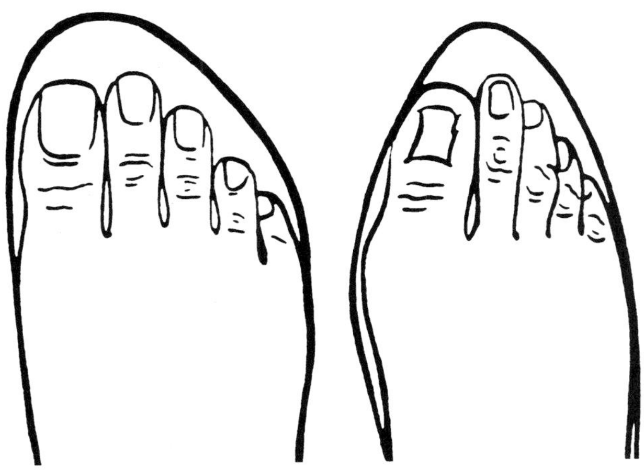

Fig. 6 The shape of the toe box affects the position of the toes within the shoe. The rounded toe box provides more room for the width of the toes as opposed to a pointed toe box. (Reproduced with permission from the National Shoe Retailers Association.)

sensation and appearance of power and status.[6,11,17-19] The down side is that when elevated heels are worn, the body weight is shifted forward in the shoe, which crowds the toe into the end of the shoe and creates even more cramped quarters for the toes.[11] In addition, more pressure is borne by the metatarsal heads and less is borne by the heel.[7,9,10] There is evidence to suggest that the great toe is disproportionately affected, which may be a primary cause of the bunion deformity and associated metatarsalgia.[7,9] A discussion of the many other documented deleterious effects on bipedal gait of high-heeled shoes is beyond the scope of this chapter.

As a general rule, lowering the height of the heel makes a shoe more wearer-friendly. The body's weight is more evenly distributed over the bottom of the foot in a low-heeled shoe, whereas in a high-heeled shoe the weight is concentrated over the ball of the foot.[7,9,10] If "heels" must be worn, the lower the heel, the better. Many women wisely wear comfortable sneakers to commute to their workplace and change to their work shoes upon arrival, thus limiting the length of time the higher-heeled shoes are worn and the distance walked in them. The same principle is applied when an extra pair of more comfortable, low-heeled shoes is kept at the workplace and is worn whenever possible.

Insole and Outsole

Most "fashionable" dress shoes have very thin insoles and outsoles, which help to accentuate the optical illusion of minimizing the size of the foot. This illusion works in concert with the elevated heel height, which shortens the appearance of the foot. Unfortunately, the lack of cushioning provided by minimal protective barrier between the shoe and the ground decreases the ability of the shoe to absorb shock and to provide comfort.

Placing an additional soft, cushioned insert in the shoe will help to provide foot support and increase comfort. Of the wide spectrum of inserts available for purchase over the counter, not all are created equal. The ideal insert would be a custom-molded orthotic device composed of durable, firm, moldable, breathable material. Unfortunately, most fashionable dress shoes lack the volume inside the shoe to accommodate such an insert. A few manufacturers do make an extra-depth pump especially designed to accommodate an insert of greater volume. Such a shoe greatly enhances comfort while maintaining some "acceptable" level of fashion.

An alternative compromise is to obtain a lower-profile, flat insole made from a material that provides cushioning and breathability. Although this type of insert will not distribute the forces at the bottom of the foot as well as does a custom-molded insert, it will help cushion the heel and forefoot. To place an insole into a shoe, there must be enough room in the shoe to accommodate the foot as well as the extra volume of the insole. For this reason, it is important to obtain the insert first and place the inserts into the shoes while trying them on before the shoes are purchased.

Summary

Is it unrealistic for a woman to consistently expect fashion and comfort in the same shoe? Probably so, unless, of course, the current fashion is shoes with a low heel, round toe, and cushioned sole. But, if the fashion trends of the last 300 years are any indication, it is doubtful that this will be the case any time soon.

However, a woman who is willing to compromise with a properly fitting, low-heeled, extra-depth or combination last pump augmented with a good quality cushioned insole has a better chance of finding comfort in a shoe. Although it is possible to have an orthopaedically sound shoe in a reasonably fashionable style, there is still room for the manufacturers and designers of shoes to improve the details of design.

It is important to recognize that as long as society defines "fashionable" as a thin-soled, stiletto-heeled, narrow-pointed shoe, comfort and fashion are, to some extent, mutually exclusive. Any woman who wants the comfort of a tennis shoe will probably have to wear a tennis shoe.

References

1. Barnicot NA, Hardy RH: The position of the hallux in West Africans. *J Anatomy* 1955;89:355-361.
2. Craigmile DA: Incidence, origin and prevention of certain foot defects. *Brit Med J* 1953;2:749-752.
3. Kato T, Watanabe S: The etiology of hallux valgus in Japan. *Clin Orthop* 1981;157:78-81.
4. Engle ET, Morton DJ: Notes on foot disorders among natives of the Belgian Congo. *J Bone Joint Surg* 1931;13;311-318.
5. Sim-Fook L, Hodgson AR: A comparison of foot forms among the non- shoe and shoe-wearing Chinese population, *J Bone Joint Surg* 1958;40A:1058-1062.
6. Stewart SF: Footgear—its history, uses and abuses. *Clin Orthop* 1972;88:119-130.
7. Corrigan JP, Moore DP, Stephens MM: Effect of heel height on forefoot loading. *Foot Ankle* 1993;14:148-152.
8. Frey CC, Thompson F, Smith J, et al: American Orthopaedic Foot and Ankle Society women's shoe survey. *Foot Ankle* 1993;14:78-81.
9. McBride ID, Wyss UP, Cooke TD, et al: First metatarsophalangeal joint reaction forces during high-heel gait. *Foot Ankle* 1991;11:282-288.
10. Snow RE, Williams KR, Holmes GB Jr: The effects of wearing high heeled shoes on pedal pressure in women. *Foot Ankle* 1992; 13:85-92.
11. Rossi WA, Tennant: *Professional Shoe Fitting.* New York, NY, National Shoe Retailers Association, 1984.
12. Pearce CA (ed): *Career Chic: What Every Woman Should Know About Getting Ahead in Style.* New York, NY, Putnam Publishing Group, 1990.
13. Molloy JT (ed): *The Woman's Dress for Success Book.* New York, NY, Warner Books Edition, 1987.
14. Janisse DJ: The art and science of fitting shoes. *Foot Ankle* 1992;13:257-262.
15. Directory of Pedorthics, 1992-1993; Pedorthic Footwear Association and Board for Certification in Pedorthics.
16. Wu KK: Principles and practice of pedorthics, in Wu KK (ed): *Foot Orthoses: Principles and Clinical Applications.* Baltimore, MD, Williams & Wilkins, 1990, pp 49-95.
17. Camper P: The classic: Dissertation on the best form of shoe. *Clin Orthop* 1975;110:2-5.
18. Opila-Correia KA: Kinematics of high-heeled gait with consideration for age and experience of wearers. *Arch Phys Med Rehabil* 1990;71:905-909.
19. Opila-Correia KA: Kinematics of high-heeled gait. *Arch Phys Med Rehabil* 1990;71:304-309.

CHAPTER 34

Trends in Women's Shoewear

Carol C. Frey, MD

For thousands of years, people have worn shoes. It has always been recognized that shoes can protect the feet from the environment. But, in more recent times, shoes have also been implicated as the principal cause of forefoot pathology seen in women. The harmful effects of footwear have been reported by several authors,[1-15] and the greatest single factor is a shoe that is improperly manufactured or fit.[6,7] Ill-fitting shoes can deform the normal foot, resulting in hammer toes, hallux valgus, bunionettes, corns, and other disabling problems (Fig. 1). The purpose of this chapter is to review trends in women's shoe wear and their effect on women's feet and health.

One recent study[6] evaluated 356 healthy females between 20 and 60 years of age. Information was collected on occupation, foot size, shoe preference, shoe comfort, shoe size, and the presence of foot pain and/or deformity. All women were evaluated by an orthopaedic foot and ankle surgeon, who noted any foot deformities and obtained shoe and weightbearing foot tracings (Fig. 2). Foot tracings were measured by bisecting the center of the heel with the center of the second toe. The widest perpendicular line that could be drawn in the forefoot was measured and recorded as the width of the foot. The shoe tracing was measured by drawing a line bisecting the center of the heel with the center of the most distal aspect of the toe box. The widest perpendicular line in the forefoot was measured and recorded as the width of the shoe. Any discrepancy between the measurements of the shoe and the foot was recorded.

The reported results revealed the subjects to have an average age of 42 years (range, 20 to 60 years). Twenty-three percent were 20 to 29 years old, 27% were 30 to 39 years old, 24% were 40 to 49 years old, and 26% were 50 to 60 years old. The participants had occupations that included professionals (23%), nurses and other health-care workers (19%), clerical and sales (19%), homemakers (19%), teachers (5%), students (5%), and entertainers, artists, and sports professionals (4%).

Of the participants, 60% noted that their shoe size had increased since they were 20 years old but 75% had neglected to have their foot measured in more than 5 years. If the increase in shoe size is reported by age group, 18% of the 20- to 29-year-old women, 43% of the 30- to 39-year-old women, 69% of the 40- to 49-year-old women, and 95% of the 50- to 60-year-old women had an increase in shoe size since the age of 20 years. Sixty-six percent had one foot that was larger than the other (36% right and 30% left).

Seventy-two percent of the women considered themselves a B width, and in this group the average width was 9.11 cm (8.0 to 11.0 cm range). Eighteen percent of the

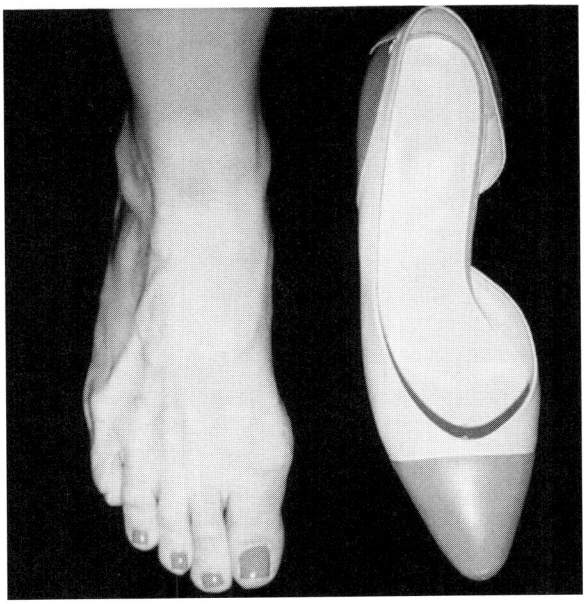

Fig. 1 Ill-fitting shoes have been implicated as the principal cause of the majority of forefoot problems seen in women. The majority of women in this study wore shoes that were smaller than their feet.

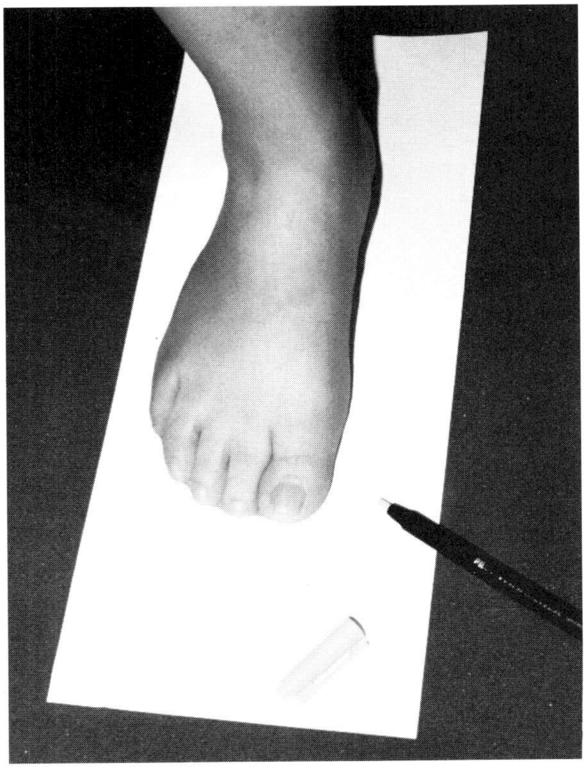

Fig. 2 Tracings and measurements were made of the weightbearing foot and the shoe. These values were compared.

women considered themselves a C width, and in this group the average width was 9.56 cm (8.0 to 11.5 cm range), and 10% considered themselves an A width or less with an average width in this group of 8.89 cm (7.8 to 10.0 cm range). The average width for all the women studied was 9.21 cm (7.8 to 11.5 cm range).

Seventy-two percent of the women stated that their work shoes were comfortable (19% wore sneakers, 27% wore high heels, and 54% wore flats). Twenty-eight percent stated that their work shoes were not comfortable (4% wore sneakers, 62% wore heels, and 34% wore flats). As a group, 14% of the women wore sneakers to work, 37% wore heels and 49% wore flats. Eighty-seven percent stated that their leisure shoes were comfortable (39% wore sneakers, 10% wore heels, and 51% wore flats).

Eighty percent of the women reported significant foot pain while wearing shoes. The pain was located in the toes in 58%, in the ball of the foot in 27%, in the arch in 10%, and in the heel in 5%. Seventy-six percent of the women had one or more forefoot deformities, with hallux valgus being the most common (71% of this group had hallux valgus, 50% had hammer toes, 18% had bunionettes, 13% had prominent metatarsal heads, and 4% had miscellaneous deformities). The incidence of hallux valgus overall was 54%.

Eighty-eight percent of the women in this study were wearing shoes that were smaller in width than their feet (average 1.2 cm smaller). In those women who had no foot pain (20%), the average foot-shoe discrepancy was only 0.56 cm. In those women without any deformity (23%) the average discrepancy was 0.60 cm (Table 1).

Table 1
Results of AOFAS Women's Shoe Survey[6]

Age Groups:	
20-29 years	23%
30-39 years	27%
40-49 years	24%
50-60 years	26%
Biggest Foot	
Right	36%
Left	30%
Equal	34%
Change in shoe size since age 20	
Shoe size increased	60%
Shoe size not changed	40%
Data by age group:	
20-29 years	18% increased in size
30-39 years	43% increased in size
40-49 years	69% increased in size
50-60 years	95% increased in size
Last time foot measured:	
< 5 years	25%
5-10 years	39%
10-20 years	36%
Type of work shoe used:	
Sneakers	14%
Heels	37%
Flats	49%
Type of leisure shoe used:	
Sneakers	39%
Heels	10%
Flats	51%
Are your work shoes comfortable?:	
Yes	72%
Sneakers	19%
Heels	27%
Flats	54%
No	28%
Sneakers	4%
Heels	62%
Flats	34%
Are your leisure shoes comfortable?:	
Yes	87%
No	13%
Foot pain:	
Yes	80%
No	20%
Where is pain?:	
Heel	5%
Arch	10%
Ball	27%
Toes	58%
Foot deformity:	
Yes	76%
No	24%
Type of foot deformity:	
Hallux valgus	71%
Hammer toes	50%
Bunionette	18%
Prominent MT	13%
Miscellaneous	4%
Foot-shoe size discrepancy:	
Foot bigger than shoe	88%
Foot same size as shoe	6%
Foot smaller than shoe	6%
Average discrepancy if foot bigger than shoe:	
1.2 cm (0.1 - 2.7 cm range)	
Of those with foot smaller than or equal to shoe:	
64% had pain	
57% had deformity	
Of those with foot larger than shoe:	
84% had pain	
79% had deformity	

In the above study,[6] measurements were only reported on the discrepancy of forefoot width and shoe width. Although forefoot widths vary widely among women, little is known about heel width. Women who have a large discrepancy between forefoot width and heel width require a combination last for good shoe fit. Because the combination last is not widely available, these may be the women who suffer most from poor shoe fit.

A recent study measured forefoot width and heel width and evaluated how these measurements vary with foot length and how this affects shoe fit and foot health.[7] The study evaluated 255 healthy females aged 20 to 60 years, with an average age of 41 years.[7] Foot and shoe tracings were measured by the method described above, and the widest line perpendicular to the bisecting line in the forefoot and the heel was recorded. No heel width measurements could be made from a tracing of the shoe, because the tracing only reflects the width of the outer sole of the heel, which is tapered in most shoes. An index was developed to compare forefoot and heel width (forefoot/heel width). The women with the higher indices were those with the largest variations between the forefoot width and the heel width.

The results of this study indicated that women with wider forefeet tend to have the wider heels. As foot length increased, forefoot width increased somewhat, but heel width did not increase significantly (especially above size 7). Yet as shoe length increases, manufacturers typically enlarge all the key internal dimensions in fixed proportions, a process called scaling. Unfortunately, a longer foot may not necessarily be wider and thicker in all areas.

Women with bigger feet (size 8 and above) had more pain and deformities than the study group as a whole. It may be that this group of women have a more difficult time with shoe fit than the smaller women. Notably, the heel counter of the shoe may not grip the heel unless a smaller shoe size is selected. The smaller shoe, chosen to provide the proper heel fit, may be too snug for the forefoot, which can result in deformity and pain. These women require a combination last for proper shoe fit.

Women need to be instructed in proper shoe fit and shoes of proper fit should be made available. The shoe designer and manufacturer need to keep in mind that feet that are long are not necessarily wider.

It is apparent that women need to be instructed in proper shoe fit. The shoe fitter usually takes two basic measurements, foot length and foot width at the ball of the foot. However, feet of identical linear measurements often differ in volume size. This is why a shoe of a given size and width in one last (the foot-like form over which a shoe is made) will fit and another last will not. The difference is in volume distribution.

To insure good fit, shoes should always be fit to the weightbearing foot and should be fit at the end of the day, when the feet are at their largest. The toe box should not wrinkle with flexion of the foot, and the foot should not bulge over the welt (the strip of leather or other material that joins the upper with the outer sole). The end of the longest toe of the biggest foot should be within one half inch (a finger's breadth) from the end of the toe box. The forefoot should not be crowded and the toes should be allowed to extend. There should be a relatively snug grip of the counter about the heel.

Studies indicate that the majority of women wear shoes that are too small for their feet and suffer from the resultant pain and deformities. Even women without foot pain or deformity wear shoes that are smaller than their feet, but to a lesser degree. Furthermore, even though women with wider forefeet tend to have wider heels and forefoot width increases somewhat with an increase in foot length, women with longer feet do not always have a wider heel. However, women select their shoe size not only to accommodate the length of the foot but also to make sure that there is adequate room in the toe box and a relatively snug grip of the counter about the heel so that the shoe stays on the foot. If correct sizing isn't available to women, compromises are made, proper shoe fit is not obtained, and painful foot deformities may be the result.

References

1. Bendix T, Sorensen SS, Klausen K: Lumbar curve, trunk muscles, and line of gravity with different heel heights. *Spine* 1984;9:223-227.
2. Brooke COSB: Foot health. *Med Officer* 1948;80:146-147.
3. Corrigan J, Moore D, Stephens M: The effect of heel height on forefoot loading. *Foot Ankle* 1991;11:418.
4. Didia BC, Omu ET, Obuoforibo AA: The use of footprint contact index II for classification of flat feet in a Nigerian population. *Foot Ankle* 1987;7:285-289.
5. Engle ET, Morton DJ: Notes on foot disorders among natives of the Belgian Congo. *J Bone Joint Surg* 1931;13:311-318.
6. Frey C, Thompson F, Smith J, et al: American Orthopaedic Foot and Ankle Society Women's Shoe Survey. *Foot Ankle* 1993;14:78-81.
7. Frey C, Smith J, Thompson F: American Orthopaedic Foot and Ankle Society Women's Shoe Survey Update. Presented at the AOFAS Specialty Day, Washington, DC, 1992.
8. Hoffmann P: Conclusions drawn from a comparative study of the feet of barefooted and shoe-wearing peoples. *Am J Orthop Surg* 1905;3:105-136.
9. Mann RA, Coughlin MJ: Hallux valgus and complications of hallux valgus, in Mann RA (ed): *Surgery of The Foot*, ed 5. St. Louis, MO, CV Mosby, 1986, pp 65-131.
10. Opila-Correia KA: Kinematics of high-heeled gait. *Arch Phys Med Rehab* 1990;71:304-309.
11. Opila KA, Wagner SS, Schiowitz S, et al: Postural alignment in barefoot and high-heeled stance. *Spine* 1988;13:542-547.
12. Sim-Fook L, Hodgson AR: A comparison of foot forms among the non-shoe and shoe-wearing Chinese population. *J Bone Joint Surg* 1958;40A:1058-1062.
13. Souther R: Shoes and feet. *Boston Med Surg J* 1906;154:40-42.
14. Staheli LT: Shoes for children: A review. *Pediatrics* 1991;88:371-375.
15. Stewart SF: Footgear: Its history, use and abuses. *Clin Orthop* 1972;88:119-130.

Knee

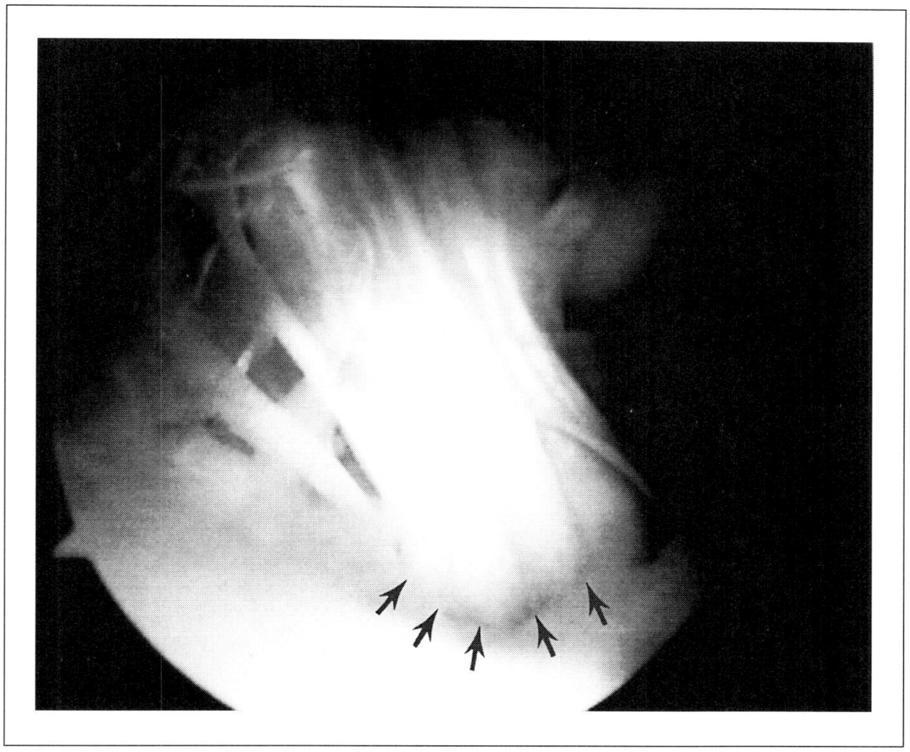

CHAPTER 35

Anterior Cruciate Ligament Reconstruction: Why Do Failures Occur?

Darren L. Johnson, MD
Freddie H. Fu, MD

Over the last 10 to 20 years, our understanding of the knee with a deficient anterior cruciate ligament (ACL) has improved dramatically as a result of numerous basic science and clinical studies performed during this period. Our improved ability to diagnose, to intervene through surgical or nonsurgical means, and to rehabilitate these patients has led to a better understanding of the natural history and the functional consequences of an ACL-deficient knee.[1,2] Most orthopaedic surgeons agree that intra-articular reconstruction of the ACL is the treatment of choice for the functionally unstable knee in the skeletally mature athletic individual.

It is difficult to accurately estimate the incidence of ACL injuries. In the general population, the incidence of acute ACL disruption has been estimated to be 1 in 3,000, which translates to roughly 75,000 ACL injuries and another 20,000 combined ACL/medial collateral ligament (MCL) injuries per year in the United States alone.[3] In the treatment of these injuries, it is estimated that over 50,000 ACL reconstructions are performed per year. Although our current methods of surgical treatment appear to achieve satisfactory results in a majority of patients, there remain a certain number of patients whose intra-articular ACL reconstruction fails in one mechanism or another.

A failed ACL reconstruction needs to be clearly defined. A knee that demonstrates recurrent anterior laxity, as was present prior to surgery, is obviously a failure. In addition, a stable knee that has a range of motion limited to only 10° to 120° of flexion, and that is stiff and painful even with activities of daily living, may also be classified as a failure. The absence of a universally accepted definition of ACL reconstruction failure makes it difficult to calculate the incidence of failures. Unsuccessful long-term results of ACL reconstruction have ranged from 5% to 52% depending on the criteria used to define failure.[4-8] Failures can generally be divided into one of four categories with potential overlap among them: (1) arthritis or recurrent pain;[4,6] (2) arthrofibrosis or loss of motion;[9-12] (3) extensor mechanism dysfunction;[11,13] and (4) recurrent patholaxity.[4-6,8] The purpose of this chapter is to discuss the potential mechanism of failures of primary intra-articular ACL reconstruction in the hope that this will decrease the number of patients requiring revision surgery.

Arthritis or Recurrent Pain

The onset and progression of degenerative articular changes after ACL reconstruction is often multifactorial in etiology. Whether or not this type of degenerative change should be classified as a "failed" ACL reconstruction is controversial. There are many rating systems that are used to evaluate the long-term outcome after ACL reconstruction. One of the most universally accepted systems is that of the International Knee Documentation Committee (IKDC) (International Knee Society Meeting, Toronto, Canada, 1991). Using these guidelines, the overall final rating for each patient includes subjective assessment, symptoms, range of motion, and laxity. The worst grade for any of the four categories determines the overall final rating. Final ratings are described as normal, nearly normal, abnormal, or severely abnormal. Using this rating system, a patient who has a stable knee 5 years after ACL reconstruction, but who has developed medial compartment arthritis secondary to a large irreparable medial meniscus tear that occurred at the time of injury can be graded as severely abnormal, despite having a stable knee (Fig. 1). Thus, the final rating is not indicative of the result of the ACL reconstruction, per se.

When an acute injury to the ACL occurs, other structures within the knee are often damaged. A recent prospective study was undertaken to define the initial osseous, articular, and meniscal lesions in acute ACL tears as determined by magnetic resonance imaging (MRI) and arthroscopy in an effort to elucidate prognostic risk factors for late degenerative changes.[14] In this study, as well as others,[15] MRI showed that up to 70% of patients had an acute osteochondral injury (a bone bruise). This lesion is most often found in the lateral compartment located at the middle portion of the lateral femoral condyle (sulcus terminalis) and the posterolateral portion of the tibial plateau. This bone bruise, or trabecular microfracture, may represent an acute blunt injury not only to the bone marrow but also to the subchondral bone and overlying articular cartilage. This injury may produce profound changes in the histologic, biomechanical, and ultrastructural characteristics of the articular cartilage. These changes may adversely affect the energy-absorbing capacity of the

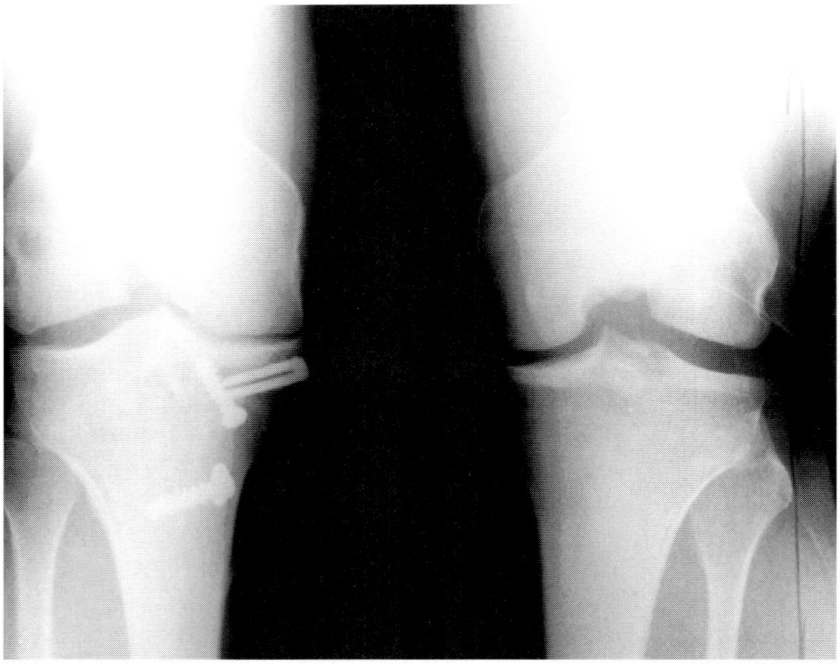

Fig. 1 This flexion-weightbearing radiograph (45° posteroanterior) illustrates decreased articular cartilage space after restoration of anterior stability following intra-articular ACL reconstruction and a sub-total medial meniscectomy.

cartilage and may be a predictor of future degeneration. In summary, the functional significance of a trabecular microfracture demonstrated on an MRI remains to be determined by the presence or absence of degenerative changes at a 5- and 10-year follow-up.

Although the natural history of the ACL-deficient knee has become better defined over the last 10 years, our selection criteria (age, sex, time from injury, associated injury, lifestyle, degree of instability, and patient cooperation) for patients requiring ACL reconstruction are still being defined. Patients who are treated nonsurgically and who then sustain repeated episodes of micro-subluxation with cumulative damage to the secondary and tertiary restraints, eventually requiring ACL reconstruction, may be predisposed to "arthritis" because of our surgical delay. This patient may be destined for the development of gonarthrosis irrespective of our surgical capability. Future studies, to determine which factors are important in determining final outcome, will improve our ability to select patients for surgical/nonsurgical treatment of the ACL-deficient knee.

After an acute ACL injury, the percentage of knees with a detectable meniscal tear ranges from 45% to 68%.[16-19] Furthermore, the incidence of meniscal pathology increases over time after ACL injury, with studies of chronic ACL-deficient knees reporting meniscal pathology in 88% to 91%. It is thought that lateral meniscal tears are more common in the acute situation, and that medial meniscus injuries predominate in the chronic ACL-deficient knee.[20] This variance is most likely caused by the increased concavity and lack of collateral attachment of the lateral meniscus (ie, increased mobility) and the increased stress on the posterior horn of the medial meniscus, which contributes to knee stability as a secondary restraint in the chronic ACL-deficient knee. Over the last decade, our treatment of meniscal pathology has changed dramatically. This change has come about through an increased understanding of the functions of the human meniscus, which are force transmission, contact area enlargement, contact stress reduction, shock absorption, joint lubrication, nutrition of chondrocytes, and stabilization. Loss of the meniscus, in part or entirely, significantly alters these functions and predisposes the joint to degenerative changes. It has been suggested that an unrepairable tear of the meniscus is the beginning of the end to an ACL-deficient knee.[21,22] This has led some surgeons to make the statement that the most important reason for reconstructing a torn ACL is to save the meniscus.

Of the knees that undergo early ACL reconstruction and in which there is a meniscal injury, approximately 40% to 50% of the meniscal tears are repairable.[16] Criteria used to determine the repairability of a meniscal tear include: size, location, chronicity, tissue quality, and type of meniscal tear. Tears located 3 mm or greater from the meniscal synovial junction can be repaired using adjunctive techniques that stimulate a biologic healing environment. Adjuncts used are parameniscal synovial abrasion, exogenous fibrin clot, and vascular access channels. Baratz and associates[23] showed that repair of simulated peripheral meniscal tears resulted in a near-normal return to contact area and peak local contact stress. Although further prospective studies will be needed to determine if healed meniscal repairs function as normal menisci and prevent the early degenerative changes seen in ACL reconstructed knees following meniscectomy, at present, every attempt should be made to save the meniscus at the time of ACL reconstruction. Partial meniscectomy is still indicated in many instances, but further research in the biology of meniscal repair (cytokines, growth factors, cyanoacrylate glue) may one day make this procedure obsolete.

Tears of the lateral meniscus are worthy of special consideration. It is well accepted that the lateral meniscus transmits more load than the medial meniscus (70% versus 50%) and that the long-term results of isolated lateral meniscectomy are worse than those of medial meniscectomy. Therefore, when performing an ACL reconstruction, every attempt should be made to preserve the lateral meniscus via repair (or by nontreatment in select tears that are posterior to the popliteal hiatus).[24] Even radial tears, which, by disrupting the circumferential tie fibers vital to the load-bearing function of the meniscus may render the meniscus biomechanically functionless, should have an attempt at repair.

Recent studies by Daniel[25] and McConville and associates[26] have shown the importance of the integrity of the menisci to the overall outcome in the ACL-reconstructed knee. Daniel[25] reported an increased incidence of degenerative joint disease in ACL-reconstructed patients, compared to patients treated without ACL surgery. He concluded this could be explained only in part by the higher incidence of meniscus injury in the ACL-reconstructed patients prior to their reconstruction. McConville and associates[26] have reported that individuals who have undergone meniscal excision at the time of ACL reconstruction reported subjective complaints and activity limitations more commonly than those whose menisci were intact. Significant positive correlations were found with pain, swelling, partial giving way, full giving way, and reduced postsurgical activity status (high level). The presence of Fairbank's changes was significantly more common in patients with partial or complete meniscectomy.[26] Although a large pool of evidence details the untoward effects of meniscectomy in the ACL-deficient knee, these studies provide valuable information on the relationship between meniscal status and outcome in the ACL-reconstructed knee. Rating scales must be developed that will separate the outcome of the return of static stability from the untoward effects of meniscal injury. Using IKDC guidelines, both of these parameters are used to develop a final rating for each patient.

Finally, our ability to restore functional stability to the ACL-deficient knee is high; however, whether or not this equates with physiologic stability with the restoration of normal articular cartilage contact stress is unknown. The relationship between clinical, functional, and physiologic stability has not been established, and there is often a low correlation between the physician's evaluation (objective) and the patient's perception (subjective) of knee function and stability.[4,27] These findings were also seen in the study reported by McConville and associates.[26] Many patients who underwent meniscectomy at the time of ACL reconstruction had a subjective sensation of giving way, despite the fact that clinical examination uncovered no discernible increase in laxity. This seems to suggest that although ACL reconstruction may restore functional stability, true physiologic stability may, in large part, be determined by meniscal status at the time of reconstruction. Even when primary stability has been restored, the overall kinematics of the reconstructed joint probably differ from those of the uninvolved knee, making the joint susceptible to degenerative joint disease, perhaps initiated and propagated by abnormal joint motions. Our current methods of objectively evaluating the function of a reconstructed ACL include only the restoration of the ACL function as a primary restraint. Surgical reconstruction techniques may be improved so as to address the additional roles (secondary restraints) the ACL plays in the kinematics of the normal knee as we increase our understanding of the multiple roles played by the ACL in the maintenance of joint stability. Improvements in the clinical evaluation of normal kinematics, which include multi-degree-of-freedom testing, will then be required to assess the eventual success of our reconstructive procedures.

In summary, the development of traumatic arthritis after ACL reconstruction depends on a multitude of variables. Etiologic factors include osteochondral injury at the time of the initial traumatic event, delayed stabilization from the time of injury with progressive damage to the secondary and tertiary restraints, previous meniscectomy, and restoration of functional stability without physiologic stability. The current standard of successful surgical reconstruction of an ACL-deficient knee is restoration of laxity equal to the contralateral uninjured knee. This may not represent the single, ideal objective assessment of the success or failure of surgical intervention, because the knees of some patients may manifest an active progression of degenerative changes even after static stability is restored. It is hoped that future studies will further define how these factors determine the overall outcome of ACL reconstruction, thus enabling the surgeon to intervene in a preventive fashion.

Loss of Motion

Loss of motion (LOM) has recently been recognized as the most common complication following ACL reconstruction.[9-13] While flexion and extension can both be lost, loss of extension is functionally more detrimental. Clinical experience indicates that tolerance to extension loss is extremely limited, and even minimal amounts of extension loss constitute an unacceptable result in the high-performance athlete. Often, loss of extension can be more disabling than the preoperative instability. Patients with loss of extension fail to progress with physical therapy, ambulate with a bent knee gait, have associated patellofemoral pain, demonstrate quadriceps weakness, and have poor functional results.[13] These patients often require additional surgery and prolonged rehabilitation to regain their motion. [28,29] Clinically, extension loss seems to occur more frequently in small hyperextensile females, such as gymnasts, than in other athletes. The etiologic factors known to contribute to loss of motion after ACL surgery include: primary and secondary capsulitis, including infrapatellar contracture syndrome (IPCS) and patella infera syndrome; "cyclops" lesion; intercondylar notch scarring (ICNS); concomitant ligament surgery; technical errors involved in the ACL reconstruction (graft placement, notchplasty, etc); reflex sympathetic dystrophy; prolonged postoperative immobilization; and infection. Current treatment is directed at prevention through the known pathways of pathogenesis.

The terms capsulitis or arthrofibrosis are used to imply periarticular inflammation and swelling. Affected patients often complain of pain and stiffness which result in quadriceps inhibition and weakness, and a quadriceps lag can develop. On physical examination, these patients are found to have lost more than 10° of knee extension and more than 25° of knee flexion, with significantly reduced patellar mobility. The knee is actively inflamed and diffuse swelling is present. If the diffuse inflammatory process is not recognized and treated, it may progress to patella baja associated with end-stage IPCS as described by Paulos and associates (Fig. 2).[10]

Primary capsulitis is a diagnosis of exclusion caused by an iatrogenic exaggerated healing response to injury or surgery. It is characterized by excessive pain, edema of tissues, warmth about the knee, and a limitation of knee motion. This diagnosis is made after secondary causes of capsulitis are ruled out (acute surgery, surgical technique errors, and delayed rehabilitation). Once it is recognized, the appropriate treatment depends on the stage of the disease process and the inflammatory state of the knee. Treatment goals include reduction of inflammation and pain, the use of therapeutic modalities to achieve a full painless range of motion (extension before flexion), patellar mobilization to increase patellar mobility, and muscle reeducation to gain active control of the passive motion that has been developed through stretching.[30]

Secondary causes of capsulitis can be prevented by appropriate surgical timing, surgical technique, and rehabilitation. Multiple studies have identified reconstruction soon after the injury (< 3 weeks) to be a significant risk factor for developing LOM. During the acute stage of the knee injury, the knee may still be actively inflamed. Performing surgery during this period can further inflame the knee and may accelerate the healing response of the surrounding tissue, resulting in excessive formation of fibrotic tissue. In knees that are immobilized by a large displaced bucket-handle meniscal tear, repair of the meniscus and restoration of motion may be staged from the ACL reconstruction to avoid the chance of LOM.[29] In most cases, surgery should be delayed until the acute symptoms of inflammation have resolved and the patient has recovered range of motion and muscle function.

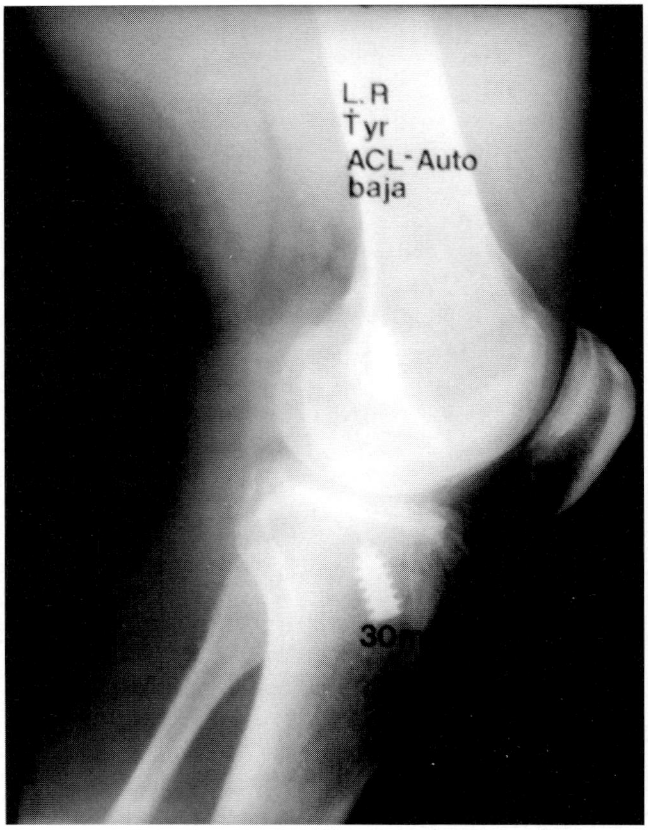

Fig. 2 Lateral radiograph showing patella baja (infera) after ACL reconstruction.

Technical errors that can lead to secondary causes of LOM include nonanatomic placement of the graft, excessive graft tension at the time of fixation, graft impingement within the intercondylar notch, and concomitant nonanatomic extra-articular ligament surgery. Nonanatomic placement of the graft will effectively "capture the knee" and result in LOM and/or failure of the graft with recurrent patholaxity. Graft placement anterior to the flexion axis (anterior placement of the femoral tunnel) will increase tension in flexion, with possible loss of motion. Conversely, grafts placed posterior to the flexion axis ("over-the-top") will tighten with extension and cause loss of extension. Graft impingement within the notch may be prevented through anatomic placement of the graft and performance of an appropriate notchplasty. The notchplasty should allow adequate clearance of the graft in the intercondylar notch as the knee is taken through a complete range of motion. Excessive tension placed on the graft at the time of fixation will overly constrain the knee and can lead to loss of flexion and/or extension. At the completion of the surgical procedure, the knee must be taken through a complete, unlimited range of motion to ensure that technical factors will not contribute to postoperative LOM.

Concomitant extra-articular reconstruction and collateral ligament repair should be minimized in order to reduce the incidence of LOM. The risk associated with concomitant ligament surgery is primarily related to procedures that involve the medial capsule (medial collateral ligament and posterior oblique ligament).[9] In some individuals, surgery that involves the medial capsule may accentuate the healing response of the knee joint, resulting in greater scar tissue formation. Additional surgical time and dissection can increase postoperative pain, possibly impeding motion. If concomitant ligament reconstruction is to be performed, it is imperative that motion be started immediately afterward with an emphasis on full extension.

Failure to remove excessive debris created during the drilling and preparation around the intra-articular opening of the tibial tunnel may result in formation of a cyclops lesion. This lesion often presents with a pathognomonic, painless, palpable and audible "clunk" that is heard upon terminal extension. Forman and Jackson[31] have described this lesion as an intra-articular intercondylar notch fibrous proliferation. It results in a fibrous nodule anterior to, and associated with, the tibial graft insertion site. Measures to avoid development of a cyclops lesion include posterior placement of the tibial tunnel within the native ACL footprint, adequate notchplasty, meticulous removal of overhanging cartilaginous margins and bony debris around the graft after insertion and fixation, and early restoration of full extension following surgery.

In intercondylar notch scarring (ICNS), scar tissue forms within the intercondylar notch and produces a mechanical block to full extension. Patients whose LOM is secondary to ICNS usually have a minimally swollen knee with normal patellar mobility, full flexion, and loss of terminal extension. These patients often complain of painless stiffness in the morning that gradually improves throughout the day with motion. Attempts to reduce the incidence of this problem have primarily involved an adjustment of rehabilitation protocols. Shelbourne and Nitz[32] compared an accelerated rehabilitation program that emphasized full extension with a rehabilitation program that immobilized the knee in flexion and restricted early extension of the knee. Emphasis on obtaining full extension immediately after surgery significantly decreased extension loss. An aggressive postoperative physical therapy protocol that emphasized early restoration of motion, early quadriceps activity, and immediate weightbearing enabled Fu and associates[33] to reduce the incidence of LOM from 11.1% to 1.7%. These two studies have shown conclusively that obtaining full extension immediately after surgery significantly decreased extension loss at follow-up. Placing the knee in full extension engages the graft in the intercondylar notch; this will minimize hemorrhage formation and the development of ICNS. Postoperative management protocols must be structured to emphasize reduction of inflammation, early restoration of extension symmetrical to the uninvolved knee, early range of motion, quadriceps exercises, and early resumption of normal gait.

Loss of motion after ligament reconstruction is increasingly recognized as a significant complication of knee surgery. The incidence has been reported to be as high as 35% in one group of patients undergoing acute ACL reconstruction or repair.[34] It has been shown that a significant residual loss of extension can be more disabling than the preoperative instability. Our treatment protocols must be tempered by the statement, "First, do no harm." Currently, the most effective method of treating arthrofibrosis is to prevent its occurrence by delaying ACL surgery until full preoperative range of motion has been achieved, by avoiding technical errors in the operating room, and by early postoperative extension exercises. If LOM occurs, early recognition and institution of aggressive physical therapy is imperative.

Extensor Mechanism Dysfunction

As discussed previously, extensor mechanism dysfunction after intra-articular ACL reconstruction is often associated with knee LOM. This section will focus on patellofemoral problems in the absence of loss of passive motion. A significant amount of literature has been written regarding the incidence of patellofemoral problems after ACL reconstruction using both autografts, either bone-patellar tendon-bone (BPTB) or hamstring tendons, and allografts.[9,10,13,35] The exact etiology of extensor mechanism dysfunction is often multifactorial and may include early morbidity associated with BPTB harvest (patellar fracture, patellar tendinitis, patellar tendon rupture, quadriceps tendon rupture, diminished structural properties of the remaining patellar tendon), abnormalities of patellar tracking, lateral patellar compression syndrome (LPCS), postmanipulation arthrosis, and patellar tendon contracture with associated patella baja.

The morbidity unique to BPTB harvest often manifests itself within the first year following surgery. However, there have been conflicting reports on whether or not quadriceps strength and functional capacity return to acceptable levels after disruption of the extensor mechanism with BPTB harvest. Lephart and associates[35] have recently shown there to be no statistical difference in thigh circumference, quadriceps strength and power, or functional performance testing between those patients who underwent ACL reconstruction using BPTB autograft or BPTB allograft. In contrast, other investigators have reported significant deficits in quadriceps strength after ACL reconstruction using patellar tendon autograft. It should be noted that the patients in the Lephart study were predominantly young, highly motivated, athletic individuals who underwent an intensive rehabilitation program with high compliance. The differences in patient characteristics and rehabilitation programs may explain this disparity in end results when comparing studies.

The exact etiology of patellar tendon contracture with associated patella baja is not completely understood, although strict immobilization of the knee after surgery has been implicated. While patella baja may often be seen as an end-stage phenomenon of developmental patella infera syndrome as described by Noyes and associates[36] and of infrapatellar contracture syndrome as described by Paulos and associates,[10] it may also occur in isolation with normal knee motion. It is possible that an exaggerated inflammatory process that develops within the patellar fat pad causes a proliferative healing response that leads secondarily to a shortening of the patellar tendon. A shortened patellar tendon, which increases patellofemoral contact forces and the anterior translation force on the tibia near full extension, requires a greater quadriceps muscle force to generate the same extensor moment toward terminal extension. Clinically, these patients often have decreased patellar mobility when measured in extension. This is manifested by the loss of positive passive patellar tilt, less than one quadrant of medial and lateral patellar glide, and less than 5 mm of superior and inferior patellar glide. If conservative measures fail, treatment may require a proximal transposition of the tibial tubercle.

The most effective method of prevention is the use of a rehabilitation program that does not limit motion and that stresses active quadriceps control. When there is quadriceps atonia and dyskinesia, the patellar tendon loses its inherent tension, which may predispose it to shortening and secondary contracture. Active quadriceps activity through straight leg raises maintains the physiologic stress across the patellar tendon. In addition, knee flexion is important in tensioning the patellar tendon along its length with associated retinacular attachments. Pain and inflammation must be controlled aggressively, through such rehabilitation modalities as cryotherapy, to allow for early recovery of the extensor mechanism.

Postoperative patellar malalignment (subluxation or instability) or LPCS, both acute and chronic, can be secondary to chronic patellar problems on which the ACL reconstruction is superimposed. There may also be a secondary phenomenon to some aspect of the reconstruction. Abnormalities of patellar tracking should be delineated through a careful history, patellofemoral examination, and appropriate radiographs. Failure to recognize and treat these associated maladies may compromise the overall function of the knee and lead to an apparent "failure" of the ACL reconstruction.

Recurrent Patholaxity

At the University of Pittsburgh, a classification system has been developed in an attempt to define the etiologic factors that lead to recurrent patholaxity after primary intra-articular ACL reconstruction (Outline 1).[37] Any of these mechanisms alone, or in combination, may result in graft attrition and recurrent patholaxity. Surgical errors may be subdivided into technical pitfalls, mechanical/biomechanical factors, or failure to address secondary/tertiary restraints. Failure of the graft to incorporate may be related to problems of graft biology (healing, vascularity), immunologic rejection (primarily allografts), or stress shielding from prosthetic ligaments or extra-articular procedures. Within the category of trauma, failures may result from premature return to ACL-dependent activities, an overly aggressive rehabilitation program, or significant reinjury.

Outline 1
University of Pittsburgh's proposed classification of mechanism/etiology of primary intra-articular ACL failures leading to recurrent patholaxity.

- I. Surgical Technique
  - 1. Technical errors
    - a. tunnel location
    - b. graft impingement
    - c. graft tension
    - d. graft fixation
  - 2. Mechanical/biomechanical
    - a. graft strength
    - b. synthetics
  - 3. Secondary stabilizers
    - a. combined ligament involvement
    - b. meniscal/articular cartilage loss
- II. Failure of graft incorporation
  - 1. Avascularity
  - 2. Immunology
  - 3. Stress shielding
- III. Trauma
  - 1. Traumatic re-injury
  - 2. Aggressive rehabilitation

(Reproduced with permission from Johnson DL, Harner CD, Maday M, et al: Revision ACL surgery, in Fu FH, Harner CD, Vince K, et al (eds): *Knee Surgery.* Baltimore, MD, Williams & Wilkins, 1994, pp 877-896.)

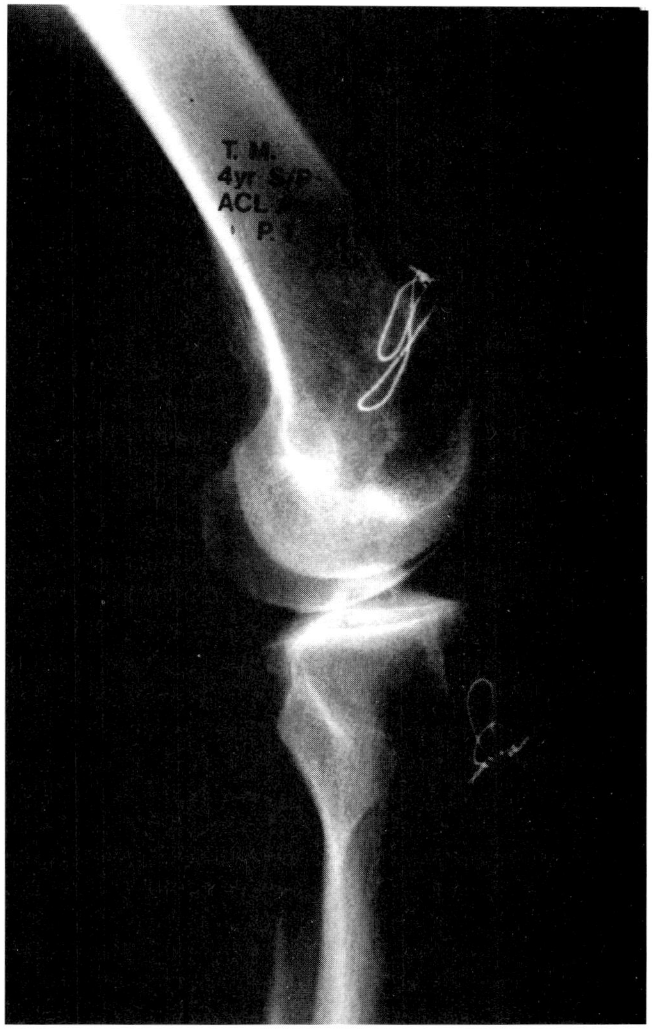

Fig. 3 Lateral radiograph showing anterior placement of the femoral and tibial tunnels.

Surgical Technique

Technical errors in the operating room which may lead to graft failure include: inappropriate graft tension, inadequate graft fixation, graft impingement, and what has been reported as the most common error, nonanatomic graft placement.[38-41] Any of these, alone or in combination, may lead to graft failure and recurrent laxity.

Numerous studies have documented the deleterious effects of nonanatomic tunnel placement.[11,42,43] A malpositioned femoral or tibial tunnel can cause excessive length changes of the ACL graft substitute as the knee is taken through a complete range of motion. Because a graft can accommodate only small changes in length prior to material property changes, a malpositioned graft will either capture the knee with resultant LOM, or the graft will lengthen, with the possibility of recurrent patholaxity.[44,45] Kinematic studies of the knee have shown that, secondary to the cam effect of the femoral condyles, the instant center of rotation of the knee is closer to the femoral insertion site than to the tibial insertion site. This explains why errors in femoral tunnel placement result in more deleterious effects on knee kinematics.

In order to achieve optimum placement of the femoral tunnel, one must avoid placing the tunnel too far anterior, yet not so posterior as to result in cortical breakout, ideally leaving a 2- to 3-mm cortical rim posteriorly. We have found the most common pitfall of tunnel placement using an endoscopic, one-incision technique has been anterior placement of the femoral tunnel (Fig. 3).[38,40] If the tunnel site is too anterior, there will be length changes with knee flexion (ie, increased tension), whereas posterior displacement or "over-the top" positioning causes ACL length increases with knee extension. Either situation is detrimental to graft function. If too tight, the graft will either stretch and ultimately fail or remain a check-rein, inhibiting motion. Poor placement of the tunnel in the coronal plane may lead to potential impingement on the medial femoral condyle, lateral femoral condyle, superior roof of the notch, or posterior cruciate ligament.

Variations in tibial tunnel placement have less of an effect than altered femoral tunnel placement on normal knee kinematics. When ACL reconstruction is performed via a one-incision endoscopic technique, placement of the tibial tunnel often dictates femoral tunnel location.[46] Although earlier studies stressed relative anterior placement within the footprint, current techniques emphasize posterior placement.[47,48] A tibial tunnel that is too anterior may affect graft tension in flexion and result in graft impingement.[41,45,47,49,50] Posterior placement will affect graft tension in extension and may cause impingement on the posterior cruciate ligament. Medial or lateral misorientation may lead to articular cartilage damage, graft impingement, or tunnel divergence with graft abrasion and wear. In order to prevent pitfalls in tunnel placement, it may be beneficial to obtain a lateral intraoperative radiograph of the knee, with the guide wires in place, to confirm the position of the drill holes prior to reaming.

The two tunnels should be as colinear as possible to mimic the orientation of the natural ACL fibers and to avoid graft impingement on the tunnel edges. The edges of both tunnels should be chamfered to avoid impingement and possible failure. Graf and associates[51] have recently shown that straight-line femoral tunnels are significantly less likely to result in graft failure than are unchamfered transverse tunnels. However, chamfering the edges of transverse tunnels significantly increases the likelihood of graft survival although the grafts still have more localized abrasion damage than those in straight-line tunnels. Wear avoidance is important today, because current rehabilitation protocols subject grafts to more flexion cycles in the early postoperative period than ever before, which increases the likelihood of wear-related failure.

Positioning the tunnels incorrectly and/or performing an inadequate notchplasty may cause graft impingement.[47,49,52] These technical pitfalls can lead to graft failure secondary to repetitive trauma, recurrent effusions, ligament attrition, and/or dislodgement of the femoral or tibial attachment (Fig. 4). Correct placement of the tibial tunnel and an adequate notchplasty prevent graft impingement. It is the responsibility of the primary surgeon to preoperatively assess individual notch architecture, anterior and posterior outlet stenosis, and intercondylar osteophytes for notchplasty requirements, using standard radiographs, computed tomography, or magnetic resonance imaging (MRI).[52-56] Intraoperatively, placement of the tibial tunnel within the posterior footprint of the native ACL, verified radiographically by showing the entire articular opening of the tunnel to be posterior to the slope of the intercondylar roof in full extension, helps eliminate the possibility of graft impingement.[44] A lateral radiograph in full extension will identify the location of the tibial and femoral tunnels and their relationship to the intercondylar roof, demarcated by Blumensaat's line. In addition, performance of the impingement test, as described by Johnson and associates,[57] will avoid excessive bone removal and ensure that once the graft is inserted and secured, there will be no need for further notchplasty, thereby avoiding iatrogenic graft injury. Removal of excessive bone can lead to articular incongruence between the patellofemoral/tibiofemoral articulation and can lateralize the normal anatomic attachment site of the ACL.

Graft tensioning during ACL reconstruction is another potential cause of failure. Factors that affect graft tension include physiologic joint laxity, anatomic placement of the graft, material/viscoelastic properties of the graft, length of the graft, type of fixation, and knee flexion angle at the time of fixation.[58] Unfortunately, the optimum tension for placing a graft intraoperatively is not currently known.[59,60] Animal studies have shown that graft tension and load can affect the mechanical properties of the transplanted graft, but the exact mechanisms by which this occurs are not well understood.[61,62] Over-tensioning of a graft has been associated with delayed vascularization with resultant myxoid degeneration (animal model), over constraining of the knee with possible LOM, decreased anterior tibial translation, high tibiofemoral contact forces, elongation of the graft, and fixation failure. Over-tensioning of the graft may allow the secondary restraints to relax, which adversely affects remodeling of the collagen fibers. Under-tensioning can lead to persistent pathological laxity and a non-functioning graft. Cadaveric model studies have shown that an initial graft tension of 20 to 40 N is required to maintain normal knee kinematics and physiologic laxity.[63,64] Clinically, controlling the amount of graft tension with resultant in vivo load on the graft substitute remains a challenge. Although some research has been reported, the further understanding of the molecular basis by which force (tension and load) affects the remodeling of soft tissue will allow for improved reconstruction techniques, which, in combination with rehabilitation programs,

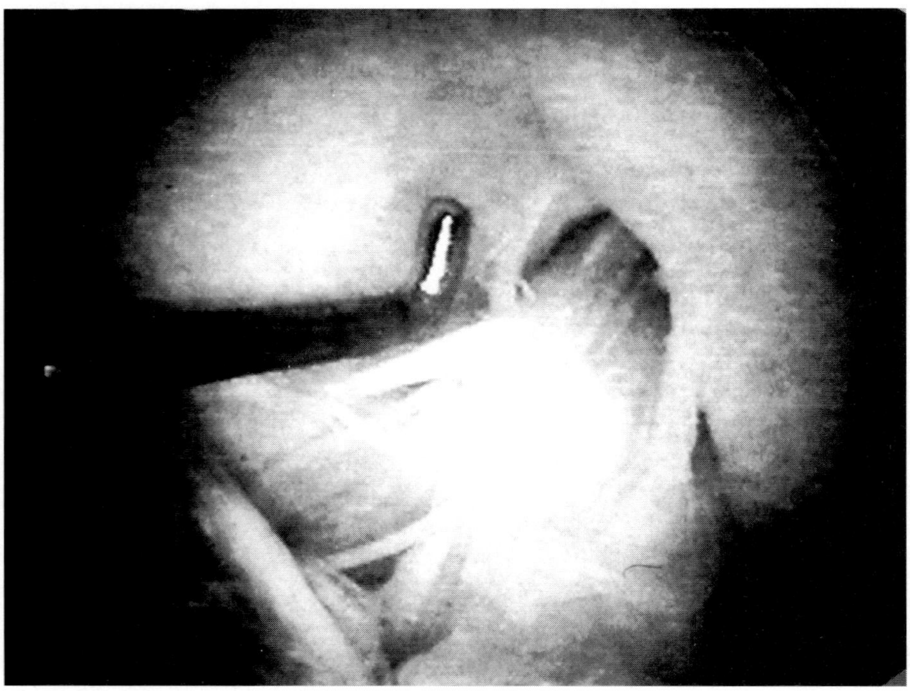

Fig. 4 Arthroscopic view of frayed ACL replacement secondary to graft impingement within a stenotic intercondylar notch.

could optimize the final biomechanical functioning of the graft.

Initial graft fixation is critical to the success of ACL reconstruction. Numerous studies have documented the advantages of early motion and aggressive postoperative rehabilitation in reducing morbidity and improving the results of ACL surgery. A major limiting factor in the early postoperative rehabilitation of patients after ACL reconstruction is the initial fixation strength of the ACL graft. In the first few weeks after ACL reconstruction, the fixation of the graft (either in bone tunnels or to the metaphysis of the femur/tibia) is the weakest link when the reconstruction is stressed. Graft fixation must be secure enough to prevent changes in graft position while graft incorporation occurs (Fig. 5).[65-67]

Fixation strength depends on the amount of surface area in contact with the graft, the fixation device used, the bone quality, and the type of material being fixed. Studies have shown that an interference screw provides the most secure fixation when using a BPTB graft via a one-incision "endoscopic" or two-incision technique.[68,69] Fixation strength depends on bone quality, compression of the bone plug in the tunnel, length of screw-thread bone contact, and the direction of the forces. Interference screw fixation is superior to a screw and washer, staple, suture fixation through a bone block, or the use of a 6.5-mm AO screw. However, potential pitfalls of interference screw fixation include: incorrect screw size, graft/screw tunnel mismatch, tunnel/screw divergence or convergence, graft advancement, graft translocation, graft fracture, and laceration of tensioning sutures.[25,70] Ideal placement of the interference screw within the femoral osseous tunnel is anterior to the bone block, which allows the collagen fibers to be positioned posteriorly in the most anatomic position. When an endoscopic technique is used, extreme caution must be exercised to avoid lacerating the graft during placement. On the tibial side, the screw should be positioned anterior to the bone block to avoid potential abrasion of the graft over the tip of the screw and to allow increased surface area of bone-to-

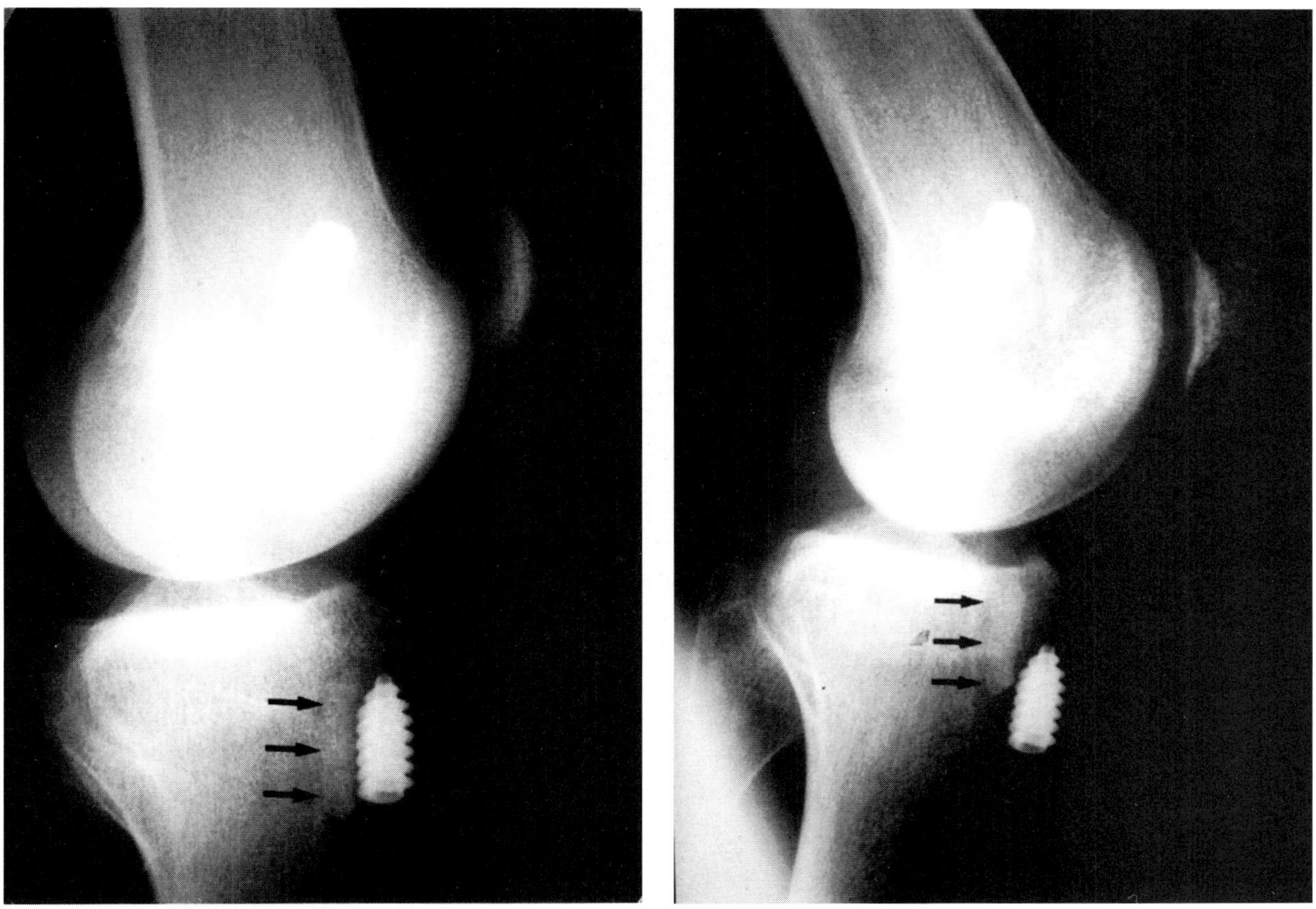

Fig. 5 **Left** and **right,** Lateral radiographs showing proximal migration of the tibial bone plug prior to bone and soft tissue incorporation. This resulted in recurrent anterior patholaxity. Also note relative anterior position of femoral tunnel. (Reproduced with permission from Johnson DL, Harner CD, Maday M, et al: Revision ACL surgery, in Fu FH, Harner CD, Vince K, et al (eds): *Knee Surgery.* Baltimore, MD, Williams & Wilkins, 1994, pp 877-896.)

bone contact for maximum strength and healing. The optimal orientation of the interference screw within the tunnel for maximum fixation strength is parallel to the graft. If the screws diverge or converge, fixation strength may be compromised.[71] Angling of the screw may be difficult to ascertain in the operating room, and it can cause fixation failure. A converging screw that angles into the bone block may result in fracture or graft transection. These pitfalls are avoided by carefully verifying the orientation of the tunnel and by obtaining an intraoperative radiograph after graft fixation if any doubt exists. In addition, to avoid insufficient fixation or a graft that is fixed too loose, an instrumented laxity exam (KT-1000) may be performed in the operating room after graft fixation prior to patient awakening.

The structural and material properties of the ligament substitute selected by the surgeon play a role in the possible failure of the reconstructed ACL. One of the primary biomechanical criteria used in the selection of an ACL replacement should be the reproduction of the structural and material properties of the normal ACL. This is a consideration not only at the time of implantation but also during the processes of inflammation, repair, and remodeling, all of which result in significant changes in the structural properties of the graft with time after surgery. The temporal remodeling behavior of the different autografts and allografts must be known in order to individualize our rehabilitation programs. Currently, autogenous BPTB remains the most common ligament substitute to which other replacements are compared. The roles played by allografts, other sources of autogenous tissue, and prosthetic ligaments in primary ACL reconstruction are still being defined.[72-74] Different soft-tissue replacements have different structural stiffness and ultimate failure load values. Consequently, once implanted, each soft-tissue replacement will have a different effect on knee joint kinematics.

While early results of ACL replacement using a variety of synthetic ligaments appeared promising, many recent series have shown an unacceptable high failure rate with increasing follow-up.[75-80] The mechanical properties have been shown to be too stiff, to have a low ultimate strain before rupture, and to have a poor resistance to abrasion. Ligament rupture through attrition has been the most common defect necessitating synthetic graft removal. Other reported causes of failure include recurrent or massive synovitis, infection, mechanical failure/loosening, and osteolysis.[78,81] Replacements that use the ligament augmentation device (LAD) have had a somewhat better success rate than pure replacements,[82-84] but the value of the LAD in improving final outcome has not been proven conclusively.[85] The role the LAD plays in stress shielding the biologic graft, which can potentially affect collagen remodeling, needs to be better defined.[86,87] The stress-shielded graft may be mechanically weaker and hence more susceptible to ligament failure. Even a surgeon who has not implanted any artificial ligaments may at sometime be required to take one out. In doing so, it is important to be aware of the potential problems often seen with artificial ligaments, which are complex joint laxity problems, the presence of synovitis, less than ideal positioning of the bone tunnels, residual ligament fixation hardware, and some degree of articular cartilage degeneration.[88]

The role of allografts in primary ACL reconstruction is currently being defined. The drive to use allograft tissue is fueled by its theoretical advantages over autogenous tissue, which are absence of donor site morbidity, increased tissue availability, decreased operative/tourniquet time, improved cosmesis, and a wide range of graft sizes.[38,40] In selected cases, allograft tissue is preferred over autogenous tissue. These include patients who have a narrow patellar ligament, malalignment of the extensor mechanism, or pre-existing degenerative changes in the patellofemoral or tibiofemoral articulations. The most commonly used allograft tissues are irradiated fresh frozen BPTB and Achilles tendon.[9,72,85] With careful screening and testing of donors, as well as treatment of allograft tissue with irradiation according to the standards set by the American Association of Tissue Banks, the risk of disease transmission remains acceptably low.[89] Clinical results comparing autograft and allograft tissue at 3- to 5-year follow-up have failed to show a significant difference using non-irradiated tissue.[74] However, irradiation has a dose-dependent effect on the material properties of the allograft tissue,[90] and the extent to which this will affect graft healing, incorporation, mechanical properties and clinical outcome remains to be determined.

Failure of the surgeon to appropriately diagnose and treat a combined instability pattern that involves damaged secondary and tertiary restraints may result in ligament attrition and stretch with eventual return of pathological laxity.[91-93] A missed ligament injury, resulting in a combined rotary instability pattern, or removal of an irreparable meniscus tear can cause increased loads on the ACL graft substitute. Although the meniscus is not a primary stabilizer to anterior translation of the tibia, the subtle alteration in knee joint kinematics may create unfavorable conditions for the ACL graft substitute. This increase in force may have a detrimental effect on graft incorporation and final material properties that can increase the likelihood of graft rupture. Is the biology of the incorporation process and final material properties the same after reconstruction in a knee with an isolated ACL versus a knee with a combined grade III ACL-MCL tear?[93-96] The answer to this question has yet to be determined, underlining the need for further research in the area of overlap between biomechanics and biology.

Failure of Graft Incorporation

Failure of incorporation of the biologic ACL graft substitute into the host tissue will lead to failure and recurrent patholaxity. The graft incorporation process has been studied extensively in primate, canine, goat, and rabbit models, using a variety of graft substitutes. These results must be interpreted cautiously because of the lack of similarity to the human knee joint. In addition, most animals have an uncontrolled rehabilitation regimen. Potential mechanisms of failure include avascularity (autograft and allograft), immunologic rejection (allograft), and stress shielding associated with use of an augmentation device (autograft and allograft).[97]

Second look arthroscopies of successful ACL autograft and allograft reconstructions have documented graft incorporation with gross revascularization of the graft.[9,98] Animal studies have conclusively shown that although allograft and autograft tissue are similar biomechanically, biochemically, and histologically, and although their vascular responses are also similar, allograft incorporation proceeds at a slower rate.[99] Both types appear to undergo the same biologic transformation of the collagen scaffold, which is revascularized and is then remodeled into a tissue that appears viable and has biomechanical characteristics similar to those of the anterior cruciate ligament. Applying this basic science data to the clinical situation has raised some interesting questions. Should we as surgeons use a similar rehabilitation protocol for allografts and autografts? The basic science information suggests that patients undergoing allograft ACL reconstruction need to be protected to a greater extent than those undergoing autograft reconstruction. Clinical data, however, demonstrates no deleterious effect associated with early motion and return to functional activities for patients receiving allografts.[74]

Some failed ACL reconstructions that have required revision surgery for patholaxity appear to be intact but nonincorporated. In these situations, the primary graft appears avascular and without a synovial envelope (Fig. 6). Although the graft appears intact, it is unable to maintain tension on probing and manual laxity testing. In several animal studies, a persistent central core of necrosis was seen in both autografts and allografts. Clinically, this type of necrosis is often seen in cases in which technical errors contributed to ligament failure. It may be that the poor intra-articular environment provided in the postoperative period secondary to inappropriate graft placement, tensioning, or weak fixation renders the graft nonfunctional and prevents graft incorporation into the host tissue. For whatever reason they occur, persistent large portions of unaltered donor graft may lead to failure and fragmentation due to mechanical wear.

The role of the immunologic response in the success or failure of allograft use in knee ligament surgery has yet to be determined.[100] Animal models have been used in an attempt to define the difference between allograft and autograft biologic incorporation; however, they only indirectly assess the role of the immune response

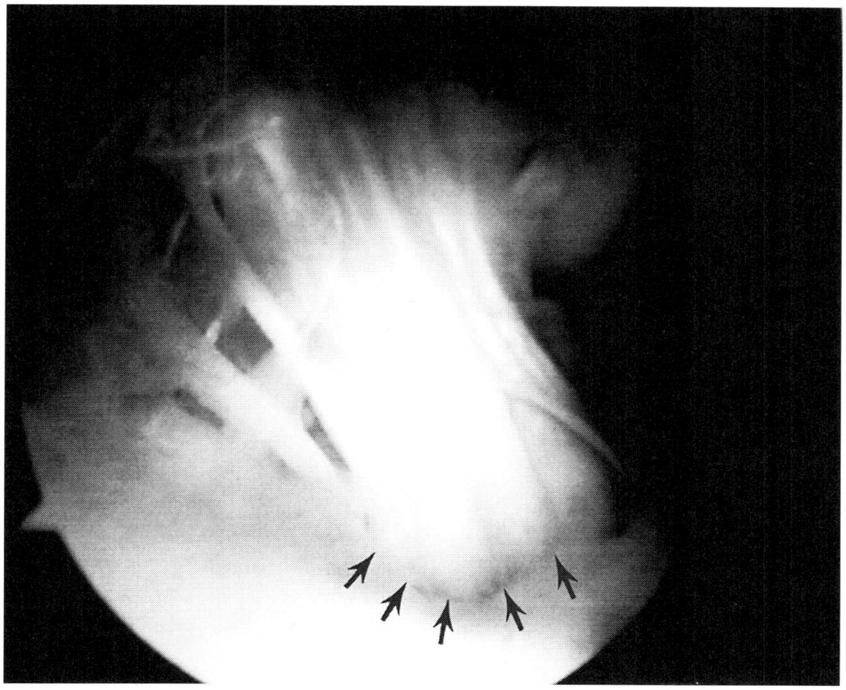

Fig. 6 Arthroscopic view of a failed patellar tendon allograft 6 months after surgery. The graft was incompletely synovialized, lax on palpation, and appeared to contain the original collagen fibers. Arrows demarcate the interface between the tibial tunnel and the failed graft.

in healing.[99,101] Clinically, two studies have attempted to assess directly the immune response in human allograft ACL reconstruction.[97,102] Thompson and associates[97] found evidence of a humoral immune response in 60% of cases that had undergone ACL reconstruction using non-irradiated fresh frozen allograft tissue.[97] Rodrigo and associates [102] found that three of 18 patients developed an anti-human lymphocyte antibody reaction 3 to 12 months after undergoing ACL reconstruction using freeze-dried, ethylene oxide-treated BPTB allografts. In two of the three patients the graft failed, requiring revision surgery, but it is not known if this was secondary to an adverse immunologic reaction or the known adverse side effects of ethylene oxide.[103,104] These studies seem to suggest that an immunologic reaction is present, but it is not known whether this mounted response is beneficial in terms of graft healing/incorporation or detrimental with potential bony tunnel resorption and ligament failure.[105-107] Most surgeons have seen grafts that did not undergo the remodeling process and that on second-look arthroscopy looked much as they did when originally implanted. Such allografts will stretch and fail, but most surgeons have also witnessed the same lack of remodeling response in autograft material. Until the existence and degree of the cellular and molecular mechanism of the immune response is better defined, the exact effect of the immunologic response in allograft ligament surgery remains undetermined.

Traumatic Failure

Etiologic factors that can lead to traumatic rupture and recurrent patholaxity include over-aggressive rehabilitation, premature return to athletic activities, and significant reinjury after initial functional stability was restored. The common etiologic factor in this category is the inability of the ACL graft substitute to withstand the physiologic tensile loads placed on it in that particular stage of healing.[11] The graft substitute may undergo plastic deformation and lengthening with possible rupture and return of patholaxity. Biomechanical studies have shown that, 1 year after reconstruction, strength and stiffness of the graft is 30% to 50% that of the native ACL.[108,109] Even though the graft looks like a normal ligament, it does not function like the native ACL. At present, tendon graft fibers are parallel and of uniform length, unlike the nonparallel, different length fibers of the native ACL. The collagen fibril pattern and diameter differ, replacement cells are not capable of re-establishing the inherent characteristics of the native ACL, and the neurovascular supply is variable.

Despite the research which has been done, little is known about the ability of the graft to withstand loads and strain during healing, maturation, and remodeling. While the use of early motion and aggressive rehabilitation has gained wide acceptance in improving functional results and minimizing complications,[12] the risk of injury to a partially revascularized graft remains a significant concern. Currently, it is difficult to base rehabilitation following ACL reconstruction strictly on the time required for maturation of the graft, and clinical experience has been used to justify accelerated rehabilitation programs. Additional research is necessary to document the long-term effects of accelerated rehabilitation following ACL reconstruction in terms of joint structure (ie, stability, strength, range of motion, and degenerative changes) as well as functional outcome from the patient's perspective in terms of functional abilities, symptoms, and return to activity. While we know that the healing and maturation time sequence for autografts and allografts differ,[99] current rehabilitation protocols used are very similar. Perhaps rehabilitation protocols for allograft and autograft tissue should be different. Patients receiving an allograft should be progressed at a slower pace than those receiving an autograft. The effects of an accelerated rehabilitation program on outcome following ACL reconstruction using allograft tissue requires further study.

An additional group of patients are those who have returned to their previous level of activity after completion of an appropriate rehabilitation program, who have exhibited complete restoration of functional stability, and who now experience a recurrent traumatic injury with an immediate hemarthrosis and increased anterior laxity. In the absence of an identifiable cause for graft failure, it is assumed that the previous graft had incorporated and was providing functional stability at the time of the reinjury. The question remains to be answered as to whether or not the restoration of functional stability equates with control of the anterior translation of the tibia relative to the femur (knee AP load-displacement behavior), and to a lesser degree internal-external and varus-valgus laxity of the knee joint. Future long-term, prospective studies need to be undertaken to determine the incidence of reinjury after apparently successful ACL reconstruction and the changes in survival rates with longer follow-up. In 1994, our ability to improve the function of an ACL-deficient knee is good; however, restoration of complete normal kinematics is questionable.

Conclusion

In summary, failure of an ACL reconstruction may be attributed to multiple etiologic factors including arthritis or recurrent pain, LOM or arthrofibrosis, extensor mechanism dysfunction, and recurrent patholaxity. Patients who have failed ACL surgery must be carefully analyzed by obtaining a careful history, including a detailed review of previous surgical records, intraoperative photographs and video, performance of a thorough physical examination, and analysis of all previous radiographs. In each patient, one or more mechanisms of failure can usually be identified.[110] The determination of the etiology of failure is the first step in a carefully constructed treatment plan.

In an effort to decrease the incidence of ACL failure, future research should attempt to prevent primary ACL reconstruction failures. First, investigations need to be performed in the area of ACL injury prevention. Within the sport of skiing alone, it is estimated that 10 ACL injuries per day occur on the four slopes in the Aspen, Colorado, area. When this figure is multiplied by the approximately 570 registered ski slopes in operation in the United States today, the seriousness of the problem becomes apparent. Work needs to be done on the modification of such sport-specific equipment as ski boots and bindings. Studies should also extend to other aspects of specific sport injury (surfaces, rules, coaching, training, etc). The questions surrounding the indications and effects of prophylactic bracing need to be answered. Each individual's unique genetic makeup, including hamstring/quadriceps ratio, notch size, joint shape, predisposing laxity, and collagen architecture, requires further study as it relates to ACL injury prevention.

Potential improvements in surgical equipment and surgical technique may further refine anatomic and appropriate biologic replacement of the ACL. These require input from the basic science arena in the following areas: a better definition of the ACL microstructure, a better definition of ACL mechanical functions (primary and secondary restraints),[111] the role of the ACL neurovascular supply as it pertains to proprioception in controlling the biomechanics of the knee,[112] a better understanding of revascularization and collagen remodeling, the potential role of growth factors and cytokines, further study of the interface between biology and biomechanics as they relate to graft incorporation, and a better understanding of the host inflammatory or immunologic (humoral and cellular) response. Improved surgical techniques for primary reconstruction include the development of absorbable graft fixation, the use of biosynthetic or biodegradable grafts made of exogenous or expanded endogenous (cultured host tissue) material, and a focus on weak secondary restraints at the time of initial surgery (role of meniscal replacement).

Finally, the use of allograft tissue in primary ligament surgery is still being defined as problems of purification, disease transmittal, and graft incorporation are being resolved. The effect of the immune response with allografts, the effect of irradiation on allograft mechanical properties, and the rate and extent of allograft incorporation need to be better understood. It is fairly well accepted that although allograft ACL reconstruction has met with reasonably good success, it is less predictable in both its time course of healing and its clinical outcome. Research efforts should be directed at an increased understanding of the cellular and molecular mechanism of the immune response in order to permit enhancement of the process of incorporation of the allograft in knee ligament surgery and to make it more predictable. Possibilities here include methods of processing the graft or impregnating or coating it with cellular-specific or bioactive factors to promote a more robust biologic response.

References

1. Caborn DN, Johnson BM: The natural history of the anterior cruciate ligament-deficient knee: A review. *Clin Sports Med* 1993; 12:625-636.
2. Johnson DL, Warner JJ: Diagnosis for anterior cruciate ligament surgery. *Clin Sports Med* 1993;12:671-684.
3. Miyasaka KC, Daniel DM, Stone ML, et al: The incidence of knee ligament injuries in the general population. *Am J Knee Surg* 1991; 4:3-8.
4. Harter RA, Osternig LR, Singer KM, et al: Long-term evaluation of knee stability and function following surgical reconstruction for anterior cruciate ligament insufficiency. *Am J Sports Med* 1988; 16:434-443.
5. Holmes PF, James SL, Larson RL, et al: Retrospective direct comparison of three intraarticular anterior cruciate ligament reconstructions. *Am J Sports Med* 1991;19:596-600.
6. Howe JG, Johnson RJ, Kaplan MJ, et al: Anterior cruciate ligament reconstruction using quadriceps patellar tendon graft. Part I. Long term follow-up. *Am J Sports Med* 1991;19:447-457.
7. Kaplan MJ, Howe JG, Fleming B, et al: Anterior cruciate ligament reconstruction using quadriceps patellar tendon graft: Part II. A specific sport review. *Am J Sports Med* 1991;19:458-462.
8. Kornblatt I, Warren RF, Wickiewicz TL: Long-term follow-up of anterior cruciate ligament reconstruction using the quadriceps tendon substitition for chronic anterior cruciate ligament insufficiency. *Am J Sports Med* 1988;16:444-448.
9. Harner CD, Irrgang JJ, Paul J, et al: Loss of motion after anterior cruciate ligament reconstruction. *Am J Sports Med* 1992;20:499-506.
10. Paulos LE, Rosenberg TD, Drawbert J, et al: Infrapatellar contracture syndrome: An unrecognized cause of knee stiffness with patella entrapment and patella infera. *Am J Sports Med* 1987; 15:331-341.
11. Graf B, Uhr F: Complications of intra-articular anterior cruciate reconstruction. *Clin Sports Med* 1988;17:835-848.
12. Shelbourne KD, Wilckens JH, Mollabashy A, et al: Arthrofibrosis in acute anterior cruciate ligament reconstruction. The effect of timing of reconstruction and rehabilitation. *Am J Sports Med* 1991; 19:332-336.
13. Sachs RA, Daniel DM, Stone ML, et al: Patellofemoral problems after anterior cruciate ligament reconstruction. *Am J Sports Med* 1989;17:760-765.
14. Spindler KP, Schils JP, Bergfeld JA, et al: Prospective study of osseous, articular, and meniscal lesions in recent anterior cruciate ligament tears by magnetic resonance imaging and arthroscopy. *Am J Sports Med* 1993;21:551-557.
15. Speer KP, Spritzer CE, Bassett FH III: Osseous injury associated with acute tears of the anterior cruciate ligament. *Am J Sports Med* 1992;20:382-389.
16. DeHaven KE: Diagnosis of acute knee injuries with hemarthrosis. *Am J Sports Med* 1980;8:9-14.
17. Gillquist J, Hagberg G, Oretorp N: Arthroscopy in acute injuries of the knee joint. *Acta Ortho Scand* 1977;48:190-196.
18. Noyes FR, Bassett RW, Grood ES, et al: Arthroscopy in acute traumatic hemarthrosis of the knee: Incidence of anterior cruciate tears and other injuries. *J Bone Joint Surg* 1980;62A:687-757.

19. Warren RF: Meniscectomy and repair in the anterior cruciate ligament deficient patient. *Clin Orthop* 1990;252:55-63.
20. Wickiewicz TL: Meniscal injuries in the cruciate deficient knee. *Clin Sports Med* 1990;9:681-694.
21. O'Brien WR: Degenerative arthritis of the knee following anterior cruciate ligament injury: Role of the meniscus. *Sports Med Arthro Rev* 1993;1:114-118.
22. Henning CE: Current status of meniscus salvage. *Clin Sports Med* 1990;9:567-576.
23. Baratz ME, Fu FH, Mengato R: Meniscal tears: The effect of meniscectomy and of repair on intraarticular contact areas and stress in the human knee: A preliminary report. *Am J Sports Med* 1986;14:270-275.
24. FitzGibbons RE, Shelbourne KD: Aggressive nontreatment of lateral meniscus tears in anterior cruciate ligament reconstruction. Presented at the 61st Annual Meeting of the American Academy of Orthopaedic Surgeons, New Orleans, LA, 1994.
25. Daniel DM: Selecting patients for ACL Surgery, in Jackson DW, Arnoczky SP, Woo SLY, et al (eds): *The Anterior Cruciate Ligament: Current and Future Concepts.* New York, NY, Raven Press, 1993, pp 251-258.
26. McConville OR, Kipnis JM, Richmond JC, et al: The effect of meniscal status on knee stability and function after anterior cruciate ligament reconstruction. *Arthroscopy* 1993;9:431-439.
27. Lephart SM, Perrin DH, Fu FH, et al: Relationship between selected physical characteristics and functional capacity in the anterior cruciate ligament-insufficient athlete. *J Orthop Phys Ther* 1992;16:174-181.
28. Cosgarea AJ, DeHaven KE, Lovelock JE: The surgical treatment of arthrofibrosis of the knee. *Am J Sports Med* 1994;22:184-191.
29. Shelbourne KD, Johnson GE: Outpatient surgical management of arthrofibrosis after anterior cruciate ligament surgery. *Am J Sports Med* 1994;22:192-197.
30. Paulos L, Meislin R: Patellar entrapment following anterior cruciate ligament injury, in Jackson DW, Arnoczky SP, Woo SLY, et al (eds): *The Anterior Cruciate Ligament: Current and Future Concepts.* New York, NY, Raven Press, 1993, pp 357-363.
31. Forman SK, Jackson DW: Cyclops lesions, in Jackson DW, Arnoczky SP, Woo SLY, et al (eds): *The Anterior Cruciate Ligament: Current and Future Concepts.* New York, NY, Raven Press, 1993, pp 365-372.
32. Shelbourne KD, Nitz P: Accelerated rehabilitation after anterior cruciate ligament reconstruction. *Am J Sports Med* 1990;18:292-299.
33. Fu FH, Irrgang JJ, Harner CD: Loss of motion following anterior cruciate ligament reconstruction, in Jackson DW, Arnoczky SP, Woo SLY, et al (eds): *The Anterior Cruciate Ligament: Current and Future Concepts.* New York, NY, Raven Press, 1993, pp 373-380.
34. Strum GM, Friedman MJ, Fox JM, et al: Acute anterior cruciate ligament reconstruction: Analysis of complications. *Clin Orthop* 1990;253:184-189.
35. Lephart SM, Kocher MS, Harner CD, et al: Quadriceps strength and functional capacity after anterior cruciate ligament reconstruction: Patellar tendon autograft versus allograft. *Am J Sports Med* 1993;21:738-743.
36. Noyes FR, Wojtys EM, Marshall MT: The early diagnosis and treatment of developmental patella infera syndrome. *Clin Orthop* 1991;265:241-252.
37. Johnson DL, Harner CD, Maday M, et al: Revision ACL surgery, in Fu FH, Harner CD, Vince KG (eds): *Knee Surgery.* Baltimore, MD, Williams & Wilkins, 1994, pp 877-896.
38. Maday MG, Fu FH, Harner CD, et al: Revision ACL reconstruction using fresh frozen allograft tissue. Presented at the 60th Annual Meeting of the American Academy of Orthopaedic Surgeons, San Francisco, CA, 1993.
39. Sherman OH, Minkoff J: Complications of arthroscopic anterior cruciate ligament technique, in Sherman OH, Minkoff J (eds): *Arthroscopic Surgery.* Baltimore, MD, Williams & Wilkins, 1990, pp 87-103.
40. Johnson DL, Harner CD, Swenson TM, et al: Revision anterior cruciate ligament reconstruction using fresh frozen allograft tissue: Classification, indications, techniques, results, and controversies. Presented at the 61st Annual Meeting of the American Academy of Orthopaedic Surgeons, New Orleans, LA, 1994.
41. Howell SM, Taylor MA: Failure of reconstruction of the anterior cruciate ligament due to impingement by the intercondylar roof. *J Bone Joint Surg* 1993;75A:1044-1055.
42. Graf B: Isometric placement of substitutes for the anterior cruciate ligament, in Jackson DW, Drez D Jr (eds): *The Anterior Cruciate Deficient Knee: New Concepts in Ligament Repair.* St. Louis, MO, CV Mosby, 1987, pp 102-113.
43. Hoogland T, Hillen B: Intra-articular reconstruction of the anterior cruciate ligament: An experimental study of length changes in different ligament reconstructions. *Clin Orthop* 1984;185:197-202.
44. Howell SM, Clark JA: Tibial tunnel placement in anterior cruciate ligament reconstructions and graft impingement. *Clin Orthop* 1992;283:187-195.
45. Romano VM, Graf BK, Keene JS, et al: Anterior cruciate ligament reconstruction: The effect of tibial tunnel placement on range of motion. *Am J Sports Med* 1993;21:415-418.
46. Olson EJ, Fu FH, Harner CD, et al: Optimal tibial tunnel starting point in endoscopic anterior cruciate ligament reconstruction. Presented at the 60th Annual Meeting of American Academy of Orthopaedic Surgeons, San Francisco, CA, 1993.
47. Howell SM, Clark, JA, Blasier RD: Serial magnetic resonance imaging of hamstring anterior cruciate ligament autografts during the first year of implantation: A preliminary study. *Am J Sports Med* 1991;19:42-47.
48. Jackson DW, Gasser SI: Tibial tunnel placement in ACL reconstruction. *Arthroscopy* 1994;10:124-131.
49. Tanzer M, Lenczner E: The relationship of intercondylar notch size and content to notchplasty requirement in anterior cruciate ligament surgery. *Arthroscopy* 1990; 6:89-93.
50. Fullerton LR Jr, Andrews JR: Mechanical block to extension following augmentation of the anterior cruciate ligament: A case report. *Am J Sports Med* 1984;12:166-168.
51. Graf BK, Henry J, Rothenberg M, et al: Anterior cruciate ligament reconstruction with patellar tendon: An ex-vivo study of wear-related damage and failure at the femoral tunnel. *Am J Sports Med* 1994; 22:131-135.
52. Howell SM, Clark JA, Farley TE: A rationale for predicting anterior cruciate graft impingement by the intercondylar roof: A magnetic resonance imaging study. *Am J Sports Med* 1991;19:276-282.
53. Anderson AF, Lipscomb AB, Liudahl KJ, et al: Analysis of the intercondylar notch by computed tomography. *Am J Sports Med* 1987;15:547-552.
54. Harner CD, Paulos LE, Greenwald AE, et al: Detailed analysis of patients with bilateral anterior cruciate ligament injuries. *Am J Sports Med* 1994;22:37-43.
55. Houseworth SW, Mauro VJ, Mellon BA, et al: The intercondylar notch in acute tears of the anterior cruciate ligament: A computer graphics study. *Am J Sports Med* 1987;15:221-224.
56. LaPrade RF, Burnett QM II: Femoral intercondylar notch stenosis and correlation to anterior cruciate ligament injuries: A prospective study. *Am J Sports Med 1*994;22:198-203.
57. Johnson DL, Miller MD, Fu FH: The arthroscopic "impingement test" during anterior cruciate ligament reconstruction. *Arthroscopy* 1993;9:714-717.
58. Gertel TH, Lew WD, Lewis JL, et al: Effect of anterior cruciate ligament graft tensioning direction, magnitude, and flexion angle on knee biomechanics. *Am J Sports Med* 1993;21:572-581.
59. Burks RT, Leland R: Determination of graft tension before fixation in anterior cruciate ligament reconstruction. *Arthroscopy* 1988;4:260-266.
60. Bylski-Austrow DI, Grood ES, Hefzy MS, et al: Anterior cruciate ligament replacements: A mechanical study of femoral attach-

ment location, flexion angle at tensioning, and initial tension. *J Orthop Res* 1990;8:522-531.
61. Yoshiya S, Andrish JT, Manley MT, et al: Graft tension in anterior cruciate ligament reconstruction: An in vivo study in dogs. *Am J Sports Med* 1987;15:464-470.
62. Muneta T, Lewis JL, Stewart NJ: Load affects remodeling of transplanted, autogenous bone-patellar tendon-bone segments in a rabbit model. *J Orthop Res* 1994;12:138-143.
63. Burks RT, Daniel D: Anterior cruciate graft preload and knee stability. *Orthop Trans* 1984;8:52.
64. Grood ES, Butler DL, Hefzy MS: Biomechanics of implantation of anterior cruciate substitutes, in Langrana NA (ed): *1985 Advances in Bioengineering*. New York, NY, American Society of Mechanical Engineers, 1985, pp 103-104.
65. Doerr AL Jr, Cohn BT, Ruoff MJ, et al: A complication of interference screw fixation in anterior cruciate ligament reconstruction. *Orthop Rev* 1990;19:997-1000.
66. Kurosaka M, Yoshiya S, Andrish JT: A biomechanical comparison of different surgical techniques of graft fixation in anterior cruciate ligament reconstruction. *Am J Sports Med* 1987;15:225-229.
67. Matthews LS, Soffer SR: Pitfalls in the use of interference screws for anterior cruciate ligament reconstruction: Brief report. *Arthroscopy* 1989;5:225-226.
68. Manaster BJ, Remley K, Newman AP, et al: Knee ligament reconstruction: Plain film analysis. *Am J Roentgenol* 1988;150:337-342.
69. Brown CH Jr, Hecker AT, Hipp JA, et al: The biomechanics of interference screw fixation of patellar tendon anterior cruciate ligament grafts. *Am J Sports Med* 1993;21:880-886.
70. Bach BR Jr: Potential pitfalls of Kurosaka screw interference fixation for ACL surgery. *Am J Knee Surg* 1989;2:76-82.
71. Jomha NM, Raso VJ, Leung P: Effect of varying angles on the pullout strength of interference screw fixation. *Arthroscopy* 1993; 9:580-583
72. Olson EJ, Harner CD, Fu FH, et al: Clinical use of fresh, frozen soft tissue allografts. *Orthopedics* 1992;15:1225-1232.
73. Shino K, Nakata K, Horibe S, et al: Quantitative evaluation after arthroscopic anterior cruciate ligament reconstruction: Allograft versus autograft. *Am J Sports Med* 1993;21:609-616.
74. Johnson DL, Harner CD, Irrgang JJ, et al: Matched pair analysis of three to five year results following allograft vs. autograft anterior cruciate ligament reconstruction. Presented at the 61st Annual Meeting of the American Academy of Orthopaedic Surgeons, New Orleans, LA, 1994.
75. Shelbourne KD, Whitaker HJ, McCarroll JR, et al: Anterior cruciate ligament injury: Evaluation of intra-articular reconstruction of acute tears without repair: Two to seven year followup of 155 athletes. *Am J Sports Med* 1990;18:484-489.
76. Barrett GR, Line LL Jr, Shelton WR, et al: The Dacron ligament prosthesis in anterior cruciate ligament reconstruction: A four-year review. *Am J Sports Med* 1993;21:367-373.
77. Paulos LE, Rosenberg TD, Grewe SR, et al: The Gore-Tex anterior cruciate ligament prosthesis: A long-term follow-up. *Am J Sport Med* 1992;20:246-252.
78. Seemann MD, Steadman JR: Tibial osteolysis associated with Gore-Tex grafts. *Am J Knee Surg* 1993;6:31-38.
79. Wilk RM, Richmond JC: Dacron ligament reconstruction for chronic anterior cruciate ligament insufficiency. *Am J Sports Med* 1993;21:374-380.
80. Woods GA, Indelicato PA, Prevot TJ: The Gore-Tex anterior cruciate ligament prosthesis: Two versus three year results. *Am J Sports Med* 1991;19:48-55.
81. DiGiovine NM, Shields CL: Synthetic ligaments in ACL reconstruction: A review. *Am J Knee Surg* 1991;4:42-48.
82. Amendola A, Fowler P: Allograft anterior cruciate ligament reconstruction in a sheep model: The effect of synthetic augmentation. *Am J Sports Med* 1992;20:336-346.
83. Fowler PJ: Semitendinosus tendon and the Kennedy ligament augmentation device in anterior cruciate ligament reconstruction. *Operative Tech in Orthop* 1992;2:117-124.
84. Jackson DW, Grood ES, Arnoczky SP, et al: Cruciate reconstruction using freeze-dried anterior cruciate ligament allograft and a ligament augmentation device (LAD): An experimental study in a goat model. *Am J Sports Med* 1987;15:528-538.
85. Noyes FR, Barber SD: The effect of a ligament-augmentation device on allograft reconstructions for chronic ruptures of the anterior cruciate ligament. *J Bone Joint Surg* 1992;74A:960-973.
86. Chen EH, Balduini FC, Smith GK, et al: Absorbable augmentation of a bone-patellar tendon-bone graft for reconstruction of the anterior cruciate ligament in canines. Presented at the ACL Study Group, January 1992, Vail, Colorado.
87. Majima T, Yasuda K, Yamamoto N, et al: Deterioration of mechanical properties of autograft in controlled stress-shielded augmentation procedures: An experimental study. Presented at American Orthopaedic Society for Sports Medicine 19th Annual Meeting, July 14, 1993, Sun Valley, Idaho.
88. Greis PE, Johnson DL, Fu FH: Revision anterior cruciate ligament surgery: Causes of graft failure and technical considerations of revision surgery. *Clin Sports Med* 1993;12:839-852.
89. Buck BE, Malinin TI, Brown MD: Bone transplantation and human immunodeficiency virus: An estimate of risk of acquired immunodeficiency syndrome (AIDS). *Clin Orthop* 1989;240:129-136.
90. Rasmussen TJ, Feder SM, Butler DL, et al: The effects of 4 Mrad of gamma irradiation on the initial mechanical properties of bone-patellar tendon-bone grafts. *Arthroscopy* 1994;10:188-197.
91. Muller W (ed): *The Knee: Form, Function, and Ligament Reconstruction*. Berlin, Springer-Verlag, 1983, pp 63-66, 179.
92. Paulos LE, Rosenberg TD, Parker RD: The medial knee ligaments: Pathomechanisms and surgical repair with emphasis on the external-rotation pivot-shift test. *Techniques Orthop* 1987;2:37-46.
93. O'Brien SJ, Warren RF, Pavlov H, et al: Reconstruction of the chronically insufficient anterior cruciate ligament with the central third of the patellar ligament. *J Bone Joint Surg* 1991;73A:278-286.
94. Andersson C, Gillguist J: Treatment of acute isolated and combined ruptures of the anterior cruciate ligament: A long-term follow-up study. *Am J Sports Med* 1992;20:7-12.
95. Shapiro MS, Markolf KL, Finerman GAM: The effect of medial instability on measured force in the ACL. *Trans Orthop Res Soc* 1990;15:517.
96. Shelbourne KD, Porter DA: Anterior cruciate ligament-medial collateral ligament injury: Nonoperative management of medial collateal ligament tears with anterior cruciate ligament reconstruction. A preliminary report. *Am J Sports Med* 1992;20:283-286.
97. Thompson WO, Harner CD, Jamison JP: Immunologic response to fresh frozen patellar tendon allograft anterior cruciate ligament reconstruction. Presented at the 61st Annual Meeting of the American Academy of Orthopaedic Surgeons, New Orleans, LA, 1994.
98. Johnson LL: The outcome of a free autogenous semitendinosus tendon graft in human anterior cruciate reconstructive surgery: A histological study. *Arthroscopy* 1993;9:131-142.
99. Jackson DW, Grood ES, Goldstein JD, et al: A comparison of patellar tendon autograft and allograft used for anterior cruciate ligament reconstruction in the goat model. *Am J Sports Med* 1993;21:176-185.
100. Harner CD, Fu FH: Editorial: The immune response to allograft ACL reconstruction. *Am J Knee Surg* 1993;6:45-46.
101. Vasseur PB, Stevenson S, Gregory CR, et al: Anterior cruciate ligament allograft transplantation in dogs. *Clin Orthop* 1991; 269:295-304.

102. Rodrigo JJ, Jackson DW, Simon TM, et al: The immune response to freeze dried bone-tendon-bone ACL allografts in humans. *Am J Knee Surg* 1993;6:47-53.
103. Jackson DW, Windler GE, Simon TM: Intra-articular reaction associated with the use of freeze-dried, ethylene oxide-sterilized bone-patella tendon-bone allografts in the reconstruction of the anterior cruciate ligament. *Am J Sports Med* 1990;18:1-11.
104. Silvaggio VJ, Fu FH, Georgescu HI, et al: The induction of IL-1 by freeze-dried ethylene oxide-treated bone-patellar-tendon-bone allograft wear particles: An in vitro study. *Arthroscopy* 1993; 9:82-86.
105. Berg EE: Tibial bone plug nonunion: A cause of anterior cruciate ligament reconstructive failure. *Arthroscopy* 1992;8:380-384.
106. Fahey M, Indelicato PA: Bone tunnel enlargement after anterior cruciate ligament replacement. *Am J Sports Med* 1994;22:410-414.
107. Linn RM, Fischer DA, Smith JP, et al: Achilles tendon allograft reconstruction of the anterior cruciate ligament deficient knee. *Am J Sports Med* 1993;21;825-831.
108. Clancy WG Jr, Narechania RG, Rosenberg TD, et al: Anterior and posterior cruciate ligament reconstruction in rhesus monkeys. *J Bone Joint Surg* 1981;63A:1270-1284.
109. Drez DJ Jr, DeLee J, Holden JP, et al: Anterior cruciate ligament reconstruction using bone-patellar tendon-bone allografts: A biological and biomechanical evaluation in goats. *Am J Sports Med* 1991;19:256-263.
110. Johnson DL: Revision ACL surgery. *Adv Op Ortho* 1994;2:21-48.
111. Fu FH, Harner CD, Johnson DL, et al: Biomechanics of knee ligaments: Basic concepts and clinical application. *J Bone Joint Surg* 1993;75A:1716-1727.
112. Nyland J, Brosky T, Currier D, et al: Review of the afferent neural system of the knee and its contribution to motor learning. *J Orthop Sports Physical Therapy* 1994;19:2-11.

CHAPTER 36

Revision ACL Surgery: Technique and Results Utilizing Allografts

Marc R. Safran, MD
Christopher D. Harner, MD

Introduction

The chapter by Johnson and Fu discussed the evaluation and classification of anterior cruciate ligament (ACL) reconstruction failure. This chapter covers three different approaches to treatment of failed ACL reconstructions and includes technique pearls that we have learned from our collective experiences. The first section outlines our approach to the evaluation of the patient with a failed ACL reconstruction and to preoperative planning. The second section outlines the technique for revision ACL surgery using allografts, and the third section describes the technique and results for autograft reconstruction. The last section includes the pearls and procedures for revision of failed synthetic ligament reconstruction.

The purpose of this chapter is to help the orthopaedic surgeon plan revision surgery in such a way that the repetition of errors can be avoided. Techniques of revision ligament surgery that we have found to be most beneficial will be outlined in detail. Finally, our clinical experience with the use of fresh frozen allograft tissue in the treatment of these difficult cases will be presented. Before any revision surgery is attempted, a good preoperative evaluation and thorough planning are necessary to avoid complications and to ensure success.

Preoperative Evaluation

As with primary ACL reconstruction, an appropriate history, a physical examination, and a radiographic evaluation are required. The examiner must determine if the previous surgery has truly failed, and if the patient is a candidate for revision surgery. We consider a failed ACL reconstruction one in which the patient complains of functional instability with activities of daily living or sports and demonstrates increased laxity on physical examination and instrumented knee testing. Our current indications for revision surgery are a failed reconstruction in an active, well-motivated individual. The single most important factor to be considered is what activities the patient wishes to return to, not the patient's previous athletic history. Time must be spent in evaluating the patient as an individual and identifying the "knee abuser" who will undoubtedly fail revision surgery as well. In counseling the patient, it is imperative that the surgeon's treatment recommendations and description of potential results be realistic. These cases are technically complex and difficult, so care must be taken not to promise the patient too much. Because it is difficult to achieve results equal to those of primary ACL reconstruction, results should not be compared between the two groups (primary versus revision). False expectations will certainly lead to subjective failure even if the procedure is technically successful. Preoperative counseling should also inform the patient of the possibility that a staged procedure may be required to deal with bony deficiency or loss of motion.

A careful history should be obtained regarding the cause of the primary injury, subsequent symptoms prior to reconstruction, surgical technique used (endoscopic versus two-incision, intra-articular versus extra-articular), postoperative treatment, rehabilitation program (including timing of progression of specific modalities), ability to return to preinjury activity, history of significant re-injury, and exact time at which the patient felt that he or she was no longer improving. Review of all previous records including the operative note is helpful to define exactly what was done at the time of the primary surgery. Information about the type of graft used, the status of the menisci, and the condition of the articular surfaces is very helpful in planning revision surgery and in predicting prognosis. Also, the exact hardware used in graft fixation can be determined from the operative note, which can make planning and removal easier. The sequence of events leading up to the patient presentation should be examined with emphasis on defining whether the chief complaint is pain or instability. The patient whose chief complaint is increasing pain with activities of daily living (ADLs) and sports is very different from the patient who experiences recurrent instability while participating in vigorous sports. Potential causes of increasing pain include delayed stabilization, meniscectomy, osteochondral injury, and restoration of functional, but not physiologic, stability to a sports-active patient. Although both types of patient may demonstrate increased laxity on physical examination or instrumented knee testing, their primary problem, required treatment, and prognosis are very different.

Physical examination should include an evaluation of gait, overall lower extremity alignment, previous skin incisions, and a comprehensive knee examination with particular attention paid to the status of secondary restraints. Failure to recognize and treat a combined instability pattern will result in recurrent failure. All patients, especially athletes with ACL injuries, should be told of the importance of the other stabilizers in the knee (ligaments, menisci, articular cartilage) before they undergo revision surgery. Any change in range of motion is important—both acute changes due to recurrent trauma and residual loss of range of motion from the original injury and operation. Simultaneous revision ligament surgery with restoration of motion should not be performed. Loss of motion should be addressed prior to revision surgery. A staged procedure should be performed with surgical intervention as needed to gain motion, followed by revision surgery if goals are obtained. If restoration of complete knee extension within 5° of the contralateral knee is unobtainable, revision surgery is contraindicated.

Radiographic evaluation should include anterior-posterior, lateral, 45° posteroanterior flexion weightbearing and merchant views.[1,2] If clinically indicated, standing long cassette views are taken to evaluate varus or valgus alignment. The position and size of the femoral and tibial tunnels on the anteroposterior and lateral radiographs should be noted. Review of the lateral radiograph will often show the most common nonisometric placement of the graft (ie, anterior placement of the femoral tunnel). Anterior placement of the tibial tunnel (Fig. 1) will lead to impingement of the graft in full extension with resultant ligament attrition and failure.[3,4] Previous radiographs should be compared to check for potential enlargement of the bony tunnels. The location and type of retained hardware should also be noted. Merchant and flexion weightbearing views should be examined for joint space narrowing or evidence of early arthritic changes. Patella alta or baja should also be assessed, because either of these can affect the preoperative plan with respect to graft selection.[5] Significant varus or valgus alignment may require correction by osteotomy prior to or in conjunction with ACL revision.[6,7] Notch architecture should be closely examined, because some problem in this area may have predisposed the patient to ACL failure.[8,9]

Other imaging modalities that may be of use in selective cases include magnetic resonance imaging (MRI), bone scintigraphy, and computerized tomography (CT). Recent technological advances have made MRI increasingly accurate and more valuable in its role of providing the information on which diagnosis, treatment, and prognosis can be based. MRI will show the post "bone bruise" sequelae of the original cartilage injury, which, because it affects long-term prognosis, is an important consideration in revision surgery.[10] CT is helpful in defining the extent of bone tunnel widening or osteolysis previously described with the use of autografts, allograft, and synthetic ligaments.[2] Bony scintigraphy, which can detect radiographically silent early arthritic changes, has been used extensively to assess chronic knee pathology.[11]

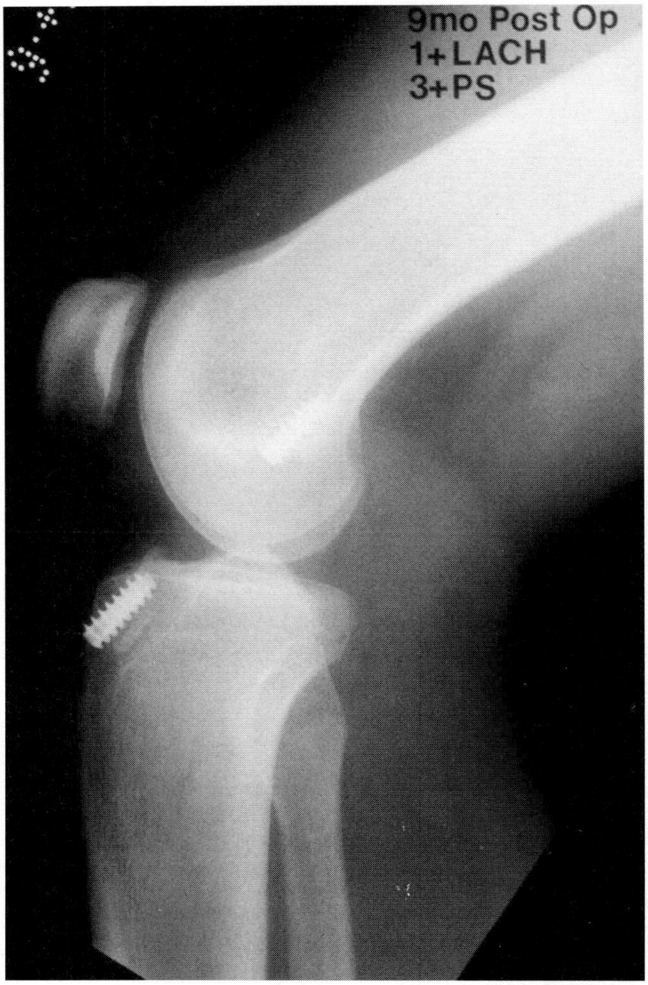

Fig. 1 Lateral radiograph of a functionally unstable patient 9 months after an autograft patellar tendon ACL reconstruction. Notice the anterior tibial tunnel and screw.

Graft Selection

As with primary ACL reconstruction, graft selection involves one of three options: synthetics, autograft, or allograft. While each type of graft has advantages and disadvantages that are patient specific, the major advantage of autograft over allograft is the elimination of the potential for disease transmission, immunologic reaction, and delayed graft incorporation.[12] Potential disadvantages of autograft include: prolonged operative time and donor site morbidity. Disadvantages specific to the patellar tendon are quadriceps weakness, donor site pain, patellar tendon weakness/rupture, and patellar fracture. Autograft tissues available include ipsilateral patellar tendon, contralateral patellar tendon, and semitendinosus/gracilis tendons. Disadvantages of hamstring tendon include decreased fixation strength and the necessity for tendon-to-bone healing.[13] Contraindications to the use of ipsilateral patellar tendon include patella-femoral arthritis, questionable viability of the anterior skin, and recent (less than 2 years) harvest of the tendon.[14] Some authors have recommended repeat use of the patellar tendon if more than 2 years have elapsed since the original surgery; however, the mechanical qualities of this tissue have not been studied. MRI may be helpful in evaluating the previously harvested patellar tendon.[15]

We believe the use of synthetic ligaments is contraindicated because of the high complication rates recently reported with primary and revision ACL surgery.[16-19] These complications include effusion, synovitis, mechanical loosening with potential rupture, infection, accelerated arthritis, and tunnel osteolysis. Because of these reported complications, we no longer consider the use of synthetic ligaments for primary or revision surgery.

The use of allograft tissue in revision surgery has many advantages: tissue availability, no donor site morbidity, decreased operative time, smaller incisions, larger graft sizes available (increased strength), and ability to fashion bone plugs corresponding to large tunnel sizes in cases of tunnel osteolysis.[20] With careful screening and testing of donors as well as treatment of allograft tissue with irradiation, the risk of disease transmission remains acceptably low.[21] The most commonly used allograft tissues at present are bone-patellar tendon-bone and Achilles tendon.[22-24] In reviewing our 3- to 5-year results comparing autograft versus allograft in primary ACL reconstruction using non-irradiated tissue, we could find no objective or subjective differences between the two groups.[25] Currently, all our allograft tissue is being irradiated on the recommendation of the American Association of Tissue Banks and the effects of radiation on the mechanical properties of the ligament are being investigated.

The ultimate choice of graft selection is patient and surgeon dependent. Patients must be educated in the choices available to them with potential advantages and disadvantages explained in detail. Often, the graft material selected will be dictated by the type of original surgery performed.

Staging of Revision Surgery

If loss of motion of the affected knee is present or a bony deficiency of either tunnel is significant enough to require bone grafting, serious consideration should be given to staging of the revision procedure. Often, the use of arthroscopic debridement, manipulation, and use of an extension drop out cast can be successful in restoring full motion.[26] If osteolysis or cystic change that will compromise graft placement or fixation has occurred at the tunnel sites (Fig. 2, *left*), the first stage should include graft removal and bone grafting of the lesion (Fig. 2, *right*). Following the 10 to 16 weeks necessary for incorporation of the bone graft, revision ACL surgery can be performed.

After performing a careful history, a detailed physical examination, a review of the previous operative and postoperative notes and radiographs, and patient counseling with respect to the possibility of a staged procedure and prognosis/expectations, a preoperative plan can be formulated that will allow for successful revision surgery without any unexpected complications.

Technical Considerations of Revision ACL Surgery

General

Technical considerations specific to revision surgery include: placement of skin incisions, removal of graft fixation devices, removal of prosthetic ligaments, revision of notchplasty, placement and size of bony tunnels, graft fixation, and postoperative rehabilitation. With careful preoperative planning, these technical difficulties of revision surgery can be anticipated and contingency plans made that will avoid potential complications in the operative suite.

Revision ACL surgery requires all the instruments used for primary surgery plus additional equipment for hardware removal and several possible options for graft fixation. Examination under anesthesia and arthroscopy should be confirmatory to the preoperative evaluation. Associated meniscal and articular injury, as well as other ligament insufficiencies, should be noted and addressed.

Skin Incisions

Incisions around the knee must be carefully planned in order to avoid skin slough and potential infection. Previous skin incisions should be used only if they allow for hardware removal and placement of the new graft and fixation. Small incisions, usually through previous ACL incisions, can be used for hardware removal and allograft placement. Allograft reconstruction can be done through a smaller incision. In the knee with previous intra-articular and extra-articular reconstruction undertaken through multiple incisions where skin viability is in doubt, the use of allograft tissue is preferred, to minimize subcutaneous dissection and unnecessary flap production. Care should be taken when elevating the periosteum covering the tibial tunnel to allow for anatomic closure.

Hardware Removal

Arrangements should be made with the operating room staff to have the specific equipment available for removal of hardware during the surgical procedure. Complete removal of bone and soft tissue around staples and interference screws is imperative for proper seating of instruments. Care must be taken because the density of bone differs in each revision case. A large

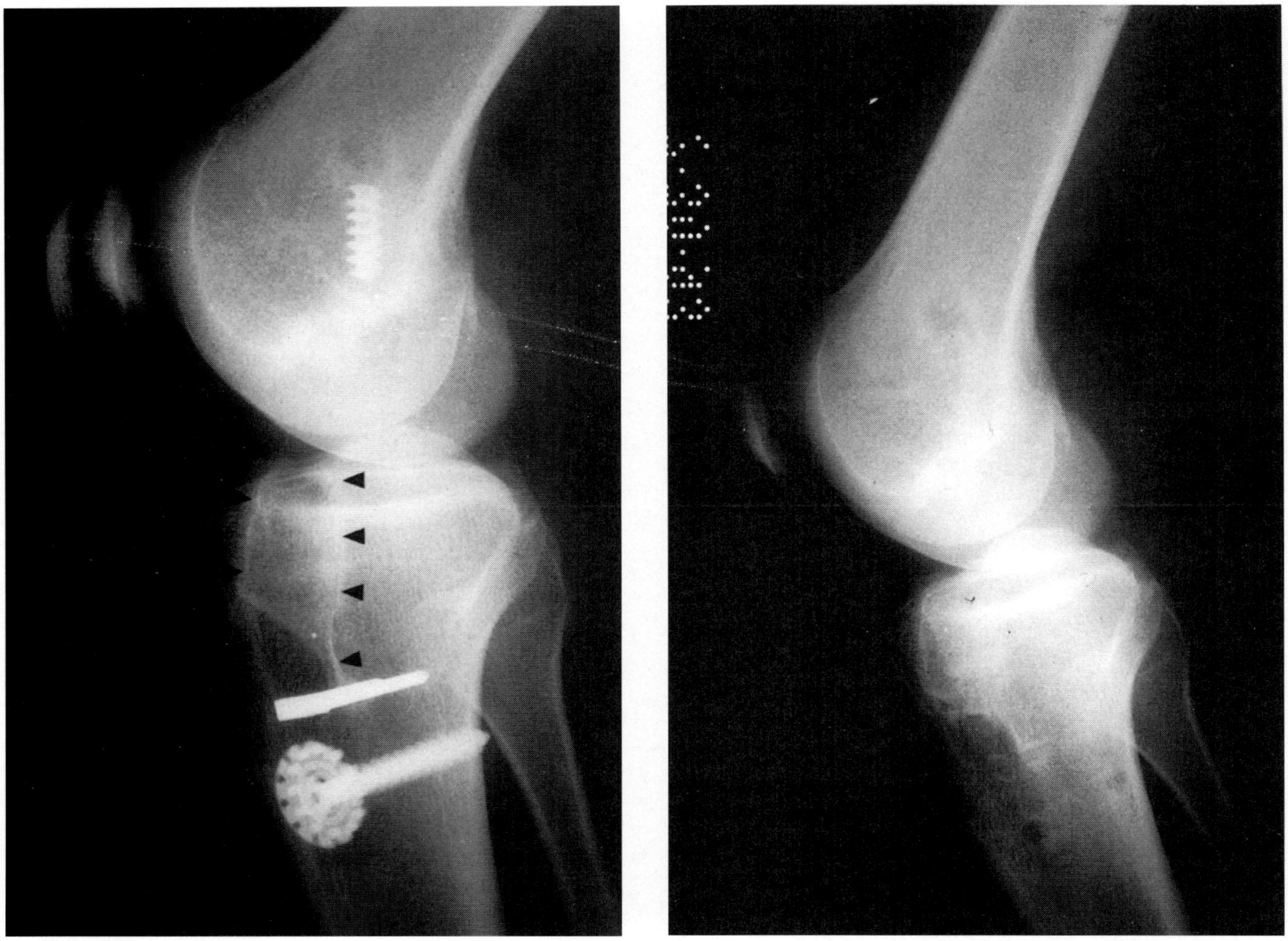

Fig. 2 **Left,** Lateral radiograph of a patient with a failed Achilles tendon allograft ACL reconstruction with large cystic changes of the tibial tunnel. These changes have also been seen following autograft ACL reconstruction. **Right,** Lateral radiograph following bone grafting of enlarged cystic tibial tunnel at the first stage of revision ACL reconstruction.

bony defect that compromises graft fixation requires bone grafting. Staples can be removed with appropriate staple extractors or osteotomes.

Interference screws that had been placed endoscopically must be removed with the appropriately sized screwdriver to avoid potential stripping. Clear identification of the screwhead by removal of bone and soft tissue and clearing of bone from around the outer threads prior to removal are necessary to allow complete seating of the screwdriver. If the screw threads were damaged during original placement or are damaged during removal, it will be necessary to remove excessive bone to retrieve the screw, often necessitating a staged reconstruction or placement of the graft in the over-the-top position. When revision surgery is performed endoscopically, hardware previously placed in the femur through a two-incision technique can often be left in place, thereby avoiding an additional incision with associated morbidity. Tibial hardware is usually removed without difficulty unless the screwhead has been stripped.

Prosthetic Ligament Removal

Prior to performing revision surgery for a prosthetic ligament, complete knowledge of the technique used for implantation must be known. Otherwise, a failed prosthetic graft will be replaced with a failed autograft or allograft. Unfortunately, these grafts were placed in the early 1980s, and many of the techniques used then have become obsolete. Over time, most of these artificial ligaments eventually fail, necessitating revision.[18,27] In suspected cases of tunnel osteolysis, seen with the use of Gore-Tex grafts, consideration should be given to preoperative MRI or CT scan to evaluate the extent of bone loss and determine the potential need for bone grafting.[18]

Removing synthetic ligament augmentation devices (LADs) has been found to be technically the most difficult. LADs, if appropriately placed, are anchored at only one end. If anchored at both ends, the LAD serves as a permanent prosthesis that causes stress shielding to the graft, eventually leading to failure (Fig. 3). An

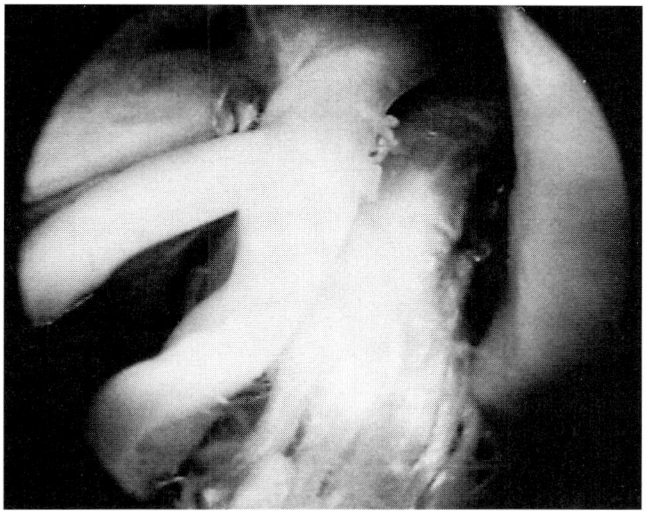

Fig. 3 Arthroscopic view of a failed primary ACL reconstruction using an LAD. Stress shielding led to the failure of this autograft.

attempt should be made to remove the prosthesis in total (Fig. 4), as the use of synovial and meniscal resectors is not aggressive enough to resect LAD remnants in a piecemeal fashion. The previous operative record will indicate at which tunnel the graft was secured and will allow attempted removal from that site. Gore-Tex ligaments present special problems of potential creation of synthetic fiber particles during removal. These particles have been shown to stimulate the inflammatory process, which can lead to the destruction of bone and cartilage.[28] Removal begins with preoperative planning, including a review of the operative technique used in placement. Finding and removing the proximal and distal attachments is the initial operative step. The ligament often fails via mechanical rupture, which can be verified arthroscopically (Fig. 5). The ligament must be removed en bloc, without the use of drills, which, by creating tiny particles, could lead to further tunnel widening. A bone gouge that matches the size of the original bony tunnel is selected and is passed down over the graft to loosen the intraosseous attachments. A large Kocher clamp can then be wrapped around one end of the ligament and it can be removed in total.

Revision Notchplasty

We have found that most cases of revision surgery require a repeat notchplasty for a variety of reasons. Preoperative review of flexion weightbearing radiographs will reveal notch architecture and serve as a guide to the amount of bone that should be removed. A revision of the notchplasty is necessary in cases in which failure may have been caused by graft impingement from an inadequate notchplasty or in which the lateral femoral condylar bone has regrown, narrowing the notch. Potential areas where impingement can lead to graft failure include the lateral femoral condyle, the superior roof, the anterior aspect of the femoral tunnel, the posterior aspect of the tibial tunnel, and the tibial spines. When performing ACL reconstruction endoscopically, placement of the tibial tunnel determines the need and extent of notchplasty required.[4] An incorrectly positioned tunnel often requires a large notchplasty to avoid intraoperative impingement; however, up to 1 cm of notch regrowth can occur, which will lead to postoperative impingement and graft failure.

In addition to eliminating potential graft impingement, a revision of the notchplasty allows the adequate visualization of the posterior arch of the notch that is required for correct placement of the femoral tunnel. Complete visualization of the over-the-top position, confirmed by palpation with an arthroscopic probe, is required prior to tunnel placement. When performing the notchplasty, it is important to remove only the amount of bone necessary to prevent impingement. Removal of an excessive amount of bone is relatively easy to do in revision cases because of the absence of normal arthroscopic anatomic landmarks. Excessive bone removal may interfere with the patellofemoral and femoral tibial articular surfaces. Finally, to ensure adequate notchplasty prior to final graft placement and fixation, the use of an appropriately sized commercially available tunnel expander (Instrument Makar, Inc, Okemos, MI), placed within the notch after tunnel placement while moving the knee through a complete range of motion will allow assessment of graft impingement (Fig. 6).

Tunnel Placement

The most important technical consideration in revision surgery is placement of the new tunnels. An evaluation of the old tunnels is done after complete removal of the old ligament substitute and adequate notch debridement to allow complete visualization of the borders of both previous tunnels. If, based on preoperative radiographs, the old tibial and femoral tunnels are in a suboptimal position, then new tunnels must be drilled, taking the position of the old tunnels into consideration. We have found that placement of the new femoral tunnel, which is the most technically demanding, requires innovative solutions to complex problems.

In general, when revision surgery is performed endoscopically, femoral tunnel hardware that has been placed on the outer femoral cortex can usually be left alone, while hardware placed endoscopically must be removed. The most common technical error we have seen following endoscopic placement of the femoral tunnel is anterior placement (Fig. 7). In these cases, new femoral tunnels can often be drilled so that they do not interfere with the old tunnels.

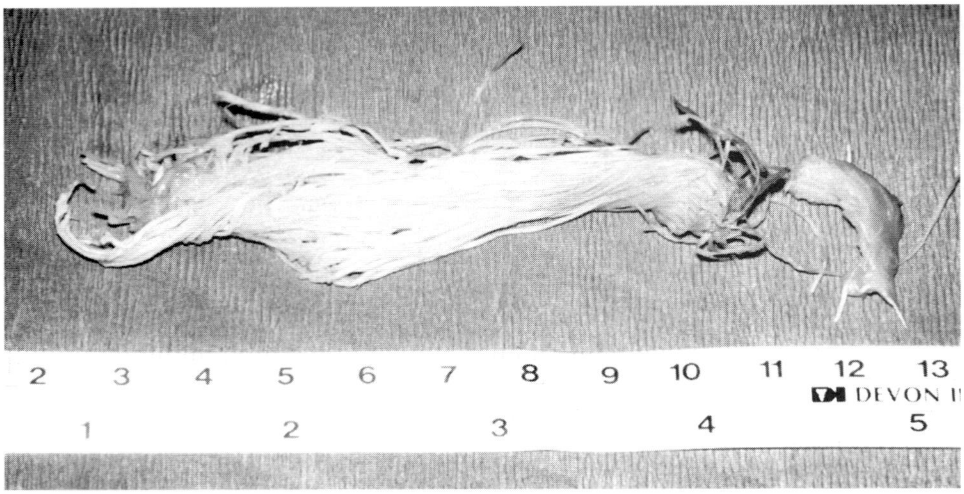

Fig. 4 Photograph of a synthetic ACL graft removed in toto. Removal in toto is important, because synovial and meniscal resectors are not aggressive enough to resect the graft in a piecemeal fashion.

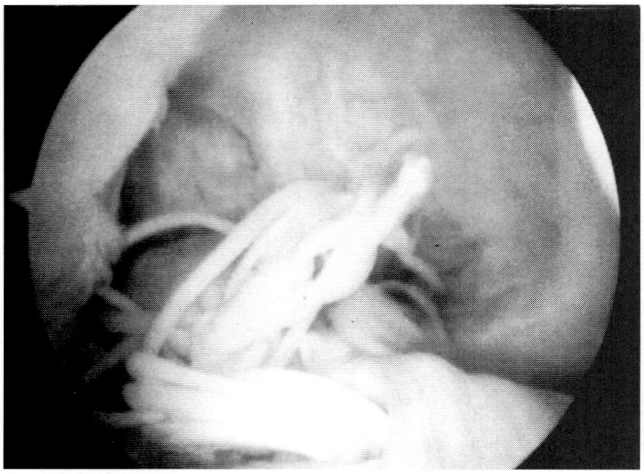

Fig. 5 Arthroscopic view of a failed primary synthetic ACL graft.

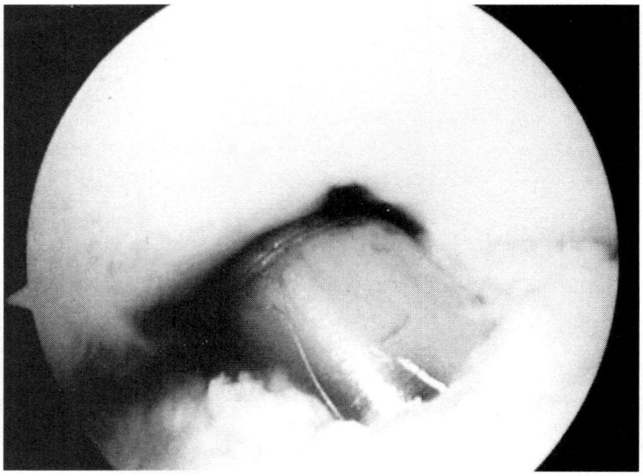

Fig. 6 Arthroscopic view of the tunnel expander placed through the tibial tunnel into the joint to assess for an adequate notchplasty. The knee is brought through a range of motion, here in extension, to check for impingement.

If previous tunnel location does not allow for a completely new tunnel to be drilled, many options are available. If enlargement of the old tunnel will adequately position the graft 1 to 2 mm anterior to the posterior cortex, an allograft with a large bone block can be used to fill the femoral defect. Positioning of the tendinous collagen fibers posteriorly will allow anterior fixation of the interference screw. Another option that can be used in cases of cystic widening of the femoral tunnel is the "over-the-top" revision procedure. When this technique is used with an Achilles tendon allograft, the soft-tissue end is fixed to the femur with a screw and washer.

Similar techniques can be applied to the tibial tunnel. In cases in which previous tunnel placement was too anterior and if it does not affect new tunnel placement, the old hardware may be left in place with no detrimental effect. If bony deficiency requires that a staged procedure be performed, tricortical iliac crest bone graft is used to fill tunnel defects. The graft is meticulously fashioned to press-fit into the tibial tunnel defect, using arthroscopic visualization to ensure placement to the articular surface level. Once radiographs reveal graft incorporation (at 10 to 16 weeks), ACL revision can be performed.

We have found the use of variable size tunnel expanders to be invaluable in revision surgery cases (Fig. 8). These expanders allow the surgeon to drill tunnels of a smaller diameter into existing tunnels and expand in a progressive fashion, decreasing the chance of posterior breakout of the femoral cortex or anterior breakout of the tibial cortex, while impacting the often osteopenic

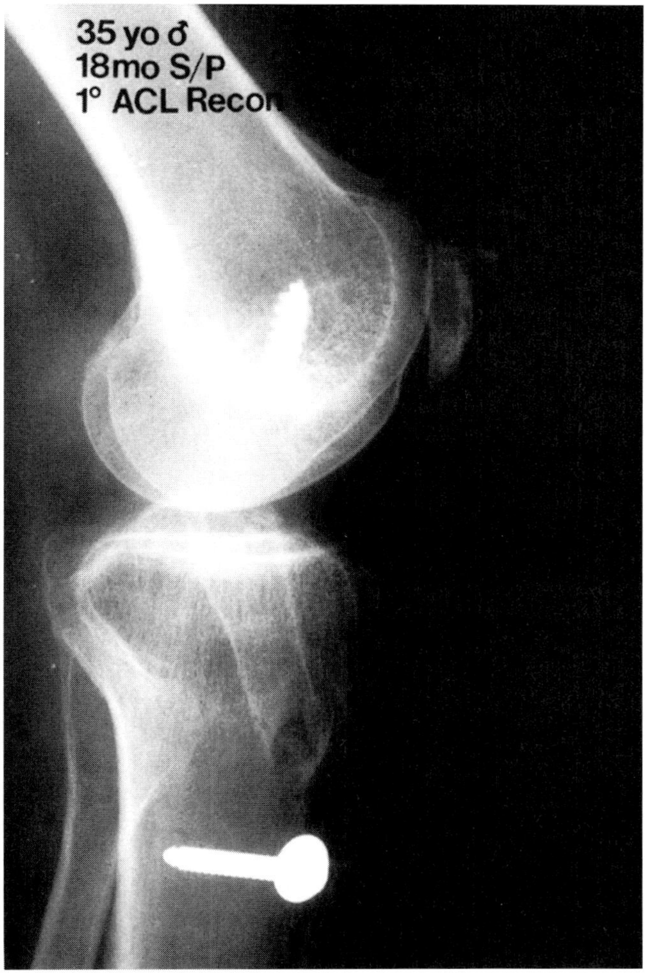

Fig. 7 Lateral radiograph of a patient 18 months following an endoscopically assisted Achilles tendon allograft ACL reconstruction. Note the anterior placement of the femoral screw indicating anterior femoral tunnel placement.

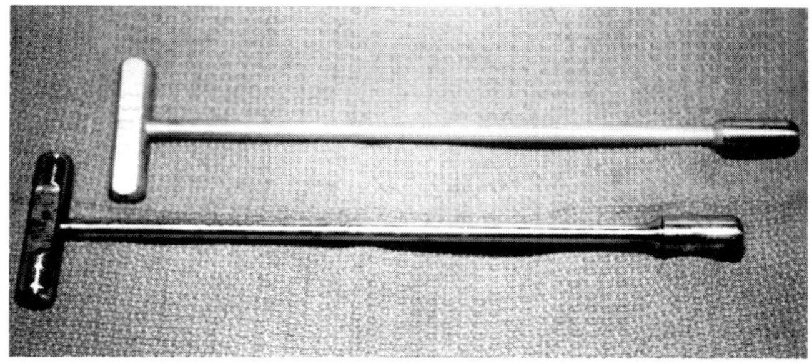

Fig. 8 Variable size tunnel expanders (two shown here) are used to dilate the tunnels, to compress intratunnel bone to assist in interference screw graft fixation, and to allow radiographic evaluation of tunnel position.

bone to enhance graft fixation. In this manner, it is possible to take advantage of bone that has already been compromised by the previous tunnels. If the tunnel location must be verified or if blow-out of the posterior cortex may have occurred, an intraoperative lateral radiograph with the bone tunnel expander in place can be extremely valuable (Fig. 9).

Graft Fixation

In the first few weeks after ACL reconstruction, the fixation of the graft (either in bone tunnels or to the lateral metaphysis of the femur) is the weakest link when the reconstruction is stressed. It is important to remember that fixation strength is proportional to the surface area in contact with the graft and is affected by the fixation device and the type of material being fixed. Although it has been shown that bone-to-bone fixation is much stronger than tendon and suture to bone and that interference screw use is much stronger than fixation acquired by tying sutures to hardware,[13,29] prior tunnel placement may compromise the quality of the bone and make the use of interference screws inadequate. If there is a question as to the fixation provided by the interference screw technique, alternative modes of fixation can be employed, including screw and spiked washer fixation, suturing over a post, or staple fixation into a bony trough. It is the responsibility of the surgeon to be familiar with all fixation techniques and to make sure that the appropriate instrumentation is available in the operating room.

Before Closing

Following placement and fixation of the graft, the knee is taken through a full range of motion to rule out impingement and to document the adequacy of the notchplasty. Additional bone is removed if necessary to ensure full, unrestricted range of motion. In order to ensure adequate fixation and return of acceptable laxity, some surgeons have recommended using a KT-1000 measuring device in the operating room prior to closure. Forty pounds of force is applied to the fixation to see if it will pull out. It is estimated that in 5% of primary cases, the reconstruction must be redone because the side-to-side differences, measured on the operating table, are greater than acceptable.

Rehabilitation

We consider postoperative rehabilitation in revision ACL surgery separately from the rehabilitation program designed for patients with a primary reconstruction. The goals of the patient and the nature and extent of the revision surgery will determine the rehabilitation progression and protocol. Protocols must be designed to protect the graft/patient from acute bending angles, weak fixation, inconsistent tension through healing, weak secondary restraints, and excessive recovery forces. Important surgical variables to be considered include type of graft used, adequacy of fixation, graft position,

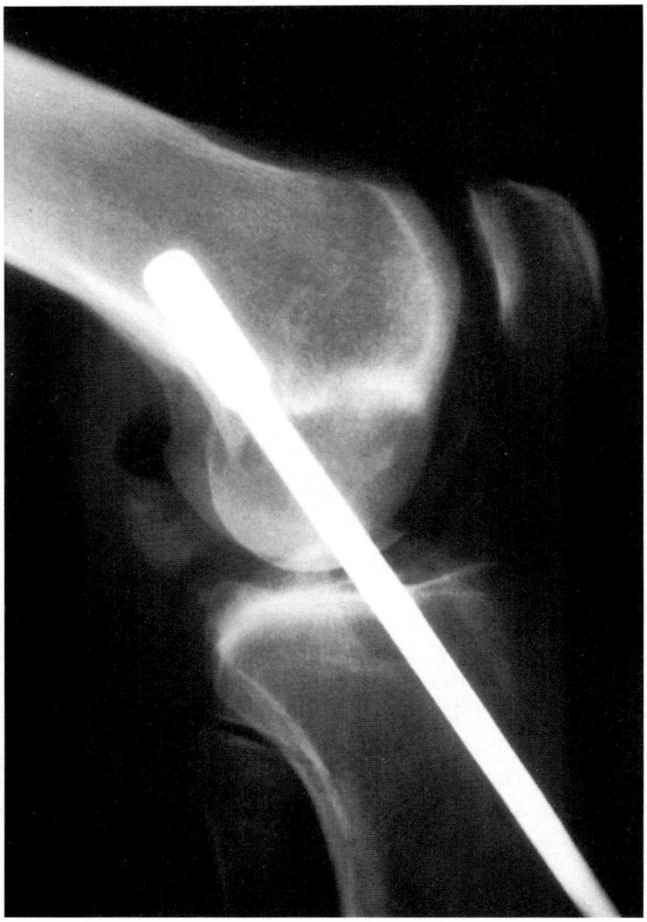

Fig. 9 Intraoperative lateral radiograph of a case of revision ACL reconstruction using the tunnel expander to assess tunnel placement.

and any other concomitant surgery that may have been performed (secondary restraints). Patient variables include demand, activity level, size, limb alignment, and hyperelasticity. These variables will help the surgeon to determine the need to restrict the range of motion, to delay weightbearing, or to delay active motion. Our current philosophy is to consider a revision ACL reconstruction as a "salvage" operation and, therefore, to use a less aggressive rehabilitation protocol. If the secondary restraints were also reconstructed, postoperative brace use is continued and weightbearing is delayed for 6 weeks. After motion has been established, a rehabilitation protocol is customized to the specific pathology addressed at the time of surgery.

Results of University of Pittsburgh Revision Experience

Over the last 5 years we have seen an increasing number of patients with failed ACL reconstruction.[20] A failed ACL reconstruction is defined as one in which the patient complains of functional instability with activities of daily living or sports and has evidence of increased knee laxity on physical examination. We recently reviewed our short-term follow-up results for 35 patients who met specific criteria for revision surgery using fresh frozen allograft tissue (bone-patellar tendon-bone and Achilles tendon) after failed intra-articular ACL reconstruction.

Primary reconstruction involved 24 autografts, nine allografts, and two synthetic ligaments. The mechanism of failure most commonly identified was surgical technique (21 patients), with erroneous tunnel placement being the most frequent. At an early follow-up average of 2 years, all patients indicated that they would have repeat revision surgery, if necessary. Each patient showed improvement in results of Lachman, Pivot-Shift, and KT-1000 testing. Subjectively, all patients were improved in terms of functional stability with ADLs and pain. However, only 70% could return to their pre-primary ACL reconstruction activity level. This is why preoperative counseling of the patient with respect to postoperative goals is of paramount importance. If the goals of the patient are unrealistic, revision surgery should not be offered to that patient. Serial radiographs have failed to reveal any cystic enlargement of the bony tunnels. Allograft tissue offers many advantages in technically demanding cases: shorter tourniquet time, smaller incisions, no donor site morbidity, availability of larger graft sizes, and it can be used even when autogenous tissue was used previously. Over the last seven years, we have used allograft tissue in over 500 cases, with no complications secondary to disease transmission or graft rejection.[23]

Conclusion

Revision ACL surgery will become more common as the number of primary ACL reconstructions performed by a greater number of surgeons with different training and using various techniques increases. We are also seeing increasing numbers of patients who had ACL reconstruction using synthetic ligaments and other non-anatomic techniques that are no longer used.

In our experience, preoperative planning is imperative for a successful outcome. This planning begins with a determination of the mechanism of failure for each patient. It is often possible to determine a primary, as well as a secondary, cause for failure. The determination of the etiology of failure is the first step in a carefully constructed preoperative plan, including the type of revision, skin incision, graft removal, hardware removal, tunnel placement, graft selection, graft fixation, and rehabilitation. Our precise preoperative plan should have enough flexibility to accommodate unanticipated findings in the operating room. Rehabilitation protocols must be designed specifically for each revision surgery patient, and they must be flexible enough to accommodate changes based on surgical findings and techniques.

Finally, it is of vital importance that each patient be counseled preoperatively regarding the potential results. This is perhaps one of the most difficult areas for the surgeon, whose expectations must be adjusted to match realistically the potential for success. Failure to do so will result in subjective failure and patient dissatisfaction even with a technically correct operative procedure. With proper planning and attention to detail, revision ACL surgery can provide a satisfying solution to difficult knee instability cases.

References

1. Burnstein MI, Ellis BI, Teitge RA, et al: Radiographic features of anterior cruciate ligament reconstruction. *Henry Ford Hospital Med J* 1986;34:270-274.
2. Rosenberg TD, Paulos LE, Parker RD, et al: The forty-five degree posteroanterior flexion weight-bearing radiograph of the knee. *J Bone Joint Surg* 1988;70A:1479-1483.
3. Howell SM, Clark JA: Tibial tunnel placement in anterior cruciate ligament reconstructions and graft impingement. *Clin Orthop* 1992;283:187-195.
4. Olson EJ, Fu FH, Harner CD, et al: Optimal tibial tunnel starting point in endoscopic anterior cruciate ligament reconstruction. Presented at the 60th Annual Meeting of the American Academy of Orthopaedic Surgeons. San Francisco, CA, 1993.
5. Paulos LE, Rosenberg TD, Drawbert J, et al: Infrapatellar contracture syndrome: An unrecognized cause of knee stiffness with patella entrapment and patella infera. *Am J Sports Med* 1987;15:331-341.
6. Noyes FR, Barber SD, Simon R: High tibial osteotomy and ligament reconstruction in varus angulated anterior cruciate ligament-deficient knees: A two- to seven-year follow-up study. *Am J Sports Med* 1993;21:2-12.
7. O'Neill DF, James SL: Valgus osteotomy with anterior cruciate ligament laxity. *Clin Orthop* 1992;278:153-159.
8. Harner CD, Paulos LE, Rosenberg TD, et al: Bilateral anterior cruciate ligament injuries: A detailed analysis of 30 patients. *Am J Sports Med* 1989;17:711-712.
9. Houseworth SW, Mauro VJ, Mellon BA, et al: The intercondylar notch in acute tears of the anterior cruciate ligament: A computer graphics study. *Am J Sports Med* 1987;15:221-224.
10. Vellet AD, Marks PH, Fowler PJ, et al: Occult posttraumatic osteochondral lesions of the knee: Prevalence, classification, and short-term sequelae evaluated with MR imaging. *Radiology* 1991;178:271-276.
11. Mooar P, Gregg J, Jacobstein J: Radionuclide imaging in internal derangements of the knee. *Am J Sports Med* 1987;15:132-137.
12. Jackson DW, Grood ES, Goldstein JD, et al: A comparison of patellar tendon autograft and allograft used for anterior cruciate ligament reconstruction in the goat model. *Am J Sports Med* 1993;21:176-185.
13. Robertson DB, Daniel DM, Biden E: Soft tissue fixation to bone. *Am J Sports Med* 1986;14:398-403.
14. Berg EE: Intrinsic healing of a patellar tendon donor site defect after anterior cruciate ligament reconstruction. *Clin Orthop* 1992;278:160-163.
15. Coupens SD, Yates CK, Sheldon C, et al: Magnetic resonance imaging evaluation of the patellar tendon after use of its central one-third for anterior cruciate ligament reconstruction. *Am J Sports Med* 1992;20:332-335.
16. Barrett GR, Line LL Jr, Shelton WR, et al: The Dacron ligament prosthesis in anterior cruciate ligament reconstruction: A four-year review. *Am J Sports Med* 1993;21:367-373.
17. Karzel RP, Diefendorf DR, Fox JM, et al: Four year experience with the Gore-Tex prosthetic ligament in anterior cruciate deficient knees. *Orthop Trans* 1990;14:618.
18. Seemann MD, Steadman JR: Tibial osteolysis associated with Gore-tex grafts. *Am J Knee Surg* 1993;6:31-38.
19. Wilk RM, Richmond JC: Dacron ligament reconstruction for chronic anterior cruciate ligament insufficiency. *Am J Sports Med* 1993;21:374-380.
20. Maday MG, Fu FH, Harner CD, et al: Revision ACL reconstruction using fresh frozen allograft tissue. Presented at the 60th Annual Meeting of the American Academy of Orthopaedic Surgeons. San Francisco, CA, February 1993.
21. Buck BE, Malinin TI, Brown MD: Bone transplantation and human immunodeficiency virus: An estimate of risk of acquired immunodeficiency syndrome (AIDS). *Clin Orthop* 1989;240:129-136.
22. Noyes FR, Barber SD: The effect of a ligament-augmentation device on allograft reconstructions for chronic ruptures of the anterior cruciate ligament. *J Bone Joint Surg* 1992;74A:960-973.
23. Olson EJ, Harner CD, Fu FH, et al: Clinical use of fresh, frozen soft tissue allografts. *Orthopedics* 1992;15:1225-1232.
24. Shino K, Inoue M, Horibe S, et al: Reconstruction of the anterior cruciate ligament using allogeneic tendon: Long term follow-up. *Am J Sports Med* 1990;18:457-465.
25. Lephart SM, Kocher MS, Harner CD, et al: Quadriceps strength and functional capacity after anterior cruciate ligament reconstruction: Patellar tendon autograft versus allograft. *Am J Sports Med* 1993;21:738-743.
26. Harner CD, Irrgang JJ, Paul J, et al: Loss of motion after anterior cruciate ligament reconstruction. *Am J Sports Med* 1992;20:499-506.
27. DiGiovine NM, Shields CL: Synthetic ligaments in ACL reconstruction: A review. *Am J Knee Surg* 1991;4:42-48.
28. Olson EJ, Kang JD, Fu FH, et al: The biochemical and histological effects of artificial ligament wear particles: In vitro and in vivo studies. *Am J Sports Med* 1988;16:558-570.
29. Kurosaka M, Yoshiya S, Andrish JT: A biomechanical comparison of different surgical techniques of graft fixation in anterior cruciate ligament reconstruction. *Am J Sports Med* 1987;15:225-229.

CHAPTER 37

Revision Ligament Reconstruction of Failed Prosthetic Anterior Cruciate Ligaments

J. Richard Steadman, MD
Mitchell D. Seemann, MD
Kirk S. Hutton, MD

The natural history of the anterior cruciate ligament (ACL) deficient knee is generally incompatible with an active, athletic lifestyle.[1-3] Recurrent instability with pivoting activities as well as the inevitable associated degenerative changes make reconstruction of the ACL the most viable option in this group of patients.[1-3] Several methods to attain a stable knee have evolved over the last 30 years. Most recently, autogenous tissue, such as patellar tendon and medial hamstrings, allografts, and prosthetics have been employed to reconstruct the ACL. Each of these grafts has specific advantages and disadvantages, and although the patellar tendon is the most popular at this time, it may not be the "gold standard" it was once thought to be.

The development of prosthetic ligaments was driven by the desire to minimize the adverse effects of harvesting autogenous tissue to act as the ACL graft. Indeed, despite its popularity, the patellar tendon graft has been associated with several potential complications. Arthrofibrosis,[4-6] patellar entrapment,[7,8] anterior knee pain,[9] patellar fractures,[10] patellar tendon ruptures,[11] and quadriceps weakness[12-14] are risks associated with disruption of the extensor mechanism. Use of the medial hamstrings, another popular ACL graft, also carries a defined morbidity linked to procuring autogenous tissue from around the knee joint.[15,16] The use of synthetic ligaments avoids sacrificing the patient's own tissue and the associated subsequent morbidity.

Another advantage of prosthetic ligaments is their biomechanical superiority over autogenous tissue, which allows immediate weightbearing, range-of-motion, and subsequent earlier return to sport. The ultimate strengths of the synthetic ligaments discussed here range from 1,730 N to 4,448 N, as compared to the normal ACL strength of 1,730 N as reported by Noyes,[17] or 2,160 N reported by Woo.[18] Noyes' study showed that a 14-mm patellar tendon graft was the only autogenous graft with an ultimate strength greater than that of the ACL (168%). Other studies have suggested that the ultimate strength of the patellar tendon may be as high as 2,900 N.[19] These ultimate strengths, however, are at time of harvest. During revascularization and remodeling, the strengths in vivo are much less, and by 1 year the graft may have regained only 80% of its strength.[20] Because of this delay in maturation of the graft, return to vigorous sporting activities is not encouraged for several months. Our current protocol allows return to easy skiing at 5 months and competitive skiing at 6 months. The use of prosthetic ligaments, however, allows an almost immediate return to full activities.

Despite these advantages, prosthetic ligaments have come under close scrutiny recently because of increasing failure rates and complications.[21-25] In the early 1980s, there were great expectations that prosthetic ligaments would become a viable option for ACL reconstructions. Indeed, Kennedy[26] stated that "eventually, an ideal synthetic intra-articular material will . . . totally replace the ACL . . ." And the early results from synthetics such as Gore-Tex were encouraging. However, as has happened with hip and knee arthroplasties, we are seeing an increase in failure rates and complications with time. Friedman[22] states, "It is inconceivable to think that a permanent prosthesis will last a lifetime of athletic use." The rising numbers of prosthetic ligament failures have led several authors to advise against further placement of these grafts.[27-29]

It is estimated that in the 1980s over 56,000 prosthetic ligaments were used in ACL reconstructions worldwide.[22] Considering this substantial number, and the significant rate of failures reported, it is inevitable that numerous revision reconstructions of prosthetic ligaments will be undertaken in the future. The purpose of this chapter is to aid in the understanding of prosthetic ligament failures and to convey technical tips for use in revising these ligaments.

Overview of Prosthetic Ligaments

History

Although there was an explosion of interest in prosthetic ligaments in the 1980s, artificial ligaments have been around for some time. In one of the first reported cases, silver wire was used to replace the ACL in a soccer player in 1914.[23,30] Four years later, Alwyn-Smith used silk strands for reconstruction of the ACL, but he had to remove them at 11 weeks due to a severe inflammatory reaction.[23,30] Von Mironova, in the 1940s, reported on a 15-year experience with Lavasan and claimed a 91% satisfactory rate in 262 athletic patients.[23,30]

More recently, Proplast was approved by the FDA in 1973. This synthetic ligament was intended to act as a temporary stent while an extra-articular reconstruction was healing. Two separate studies[23,30] revealed only a 50% satisfactory rate, and a significant number of failures occurred during the first 13 months of implantation. In 1974, Richards Marketing Company introduced the Polyflex, an ultra-high-molecular-weight polyethylene and steel tube construct, meant to act as an ACL substitute. A two-year clinical trial was established, but biomechanical data that revealed a 50% failure rate within the first year forced cancellation of further clinical trials.[23,30] Several other synthetic ligaments have been developed, the most common of which will be discussed.

Classification of Prosthetic Ligaments

Friedman and associates[22] categorized prosthetic ligaments into three separate classes: permanent prostheses, scaffolds, and augmentation devices. Permanent prostheses, such as the Gore-Tex (Gore & Company, Flagstaff, AZ) and Stryker Dacron (Stryker Endoscopy Company, Sunnyvale, CA), generally exhibit high ultimate tensile strengths and are meant to act as permanent replacements for the ACL. Scaffolds, such as the Leeds-Keio and carbon fiber ligament, allow the ingrowth of autogenous tissue over a period of time, tissue that ultimately increases in strength. Augmentation devices, such as the LAD, act as stents to protect autogenous tissue during the crucial revascularization and remodeling phase, when it is relatively weak.

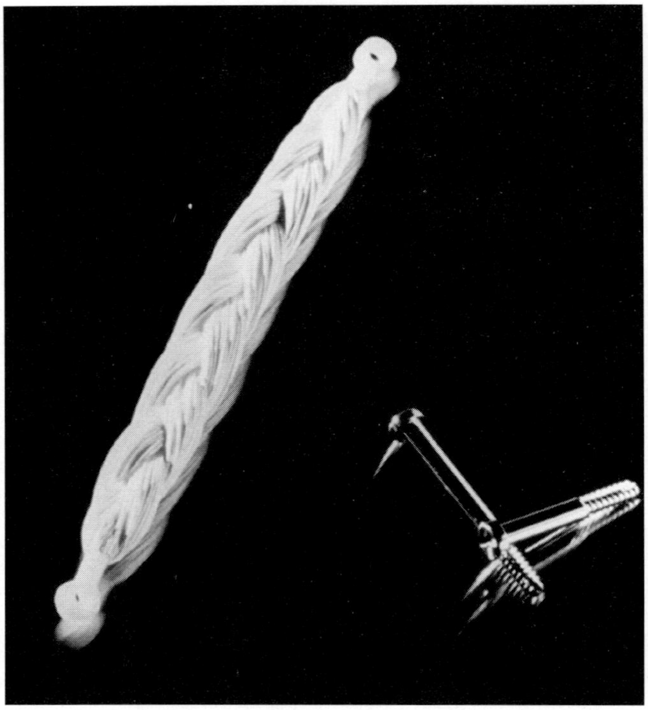

Fig. 1 The Gore-Tex ligament prosthesis and fixation screws.

Permanent Grafts

Gore-Tex (Polytetrafluoroethylene) The Gore-Tex ligament prosthesis is one of the most popular in the United States with more than 6,000[22] having been implanted since its approval by the FDA in 1986 for failed intra-articular reconstruction. Several clinical trials, dating back to 1983, preceded the FDA approval. Since then, various centers have published regular reports of objective and subjective results and complications. Over time, the rates of complications and failures have steadily increased.

The Gore-Tex ligament is a triple helical multifilament strand composed of polytetrafluoroethylene (PTFE). The strands terminate in loops on each end of the graft, which allow initial fixation to bone with the help of a screw (Fig. 1). The ultimate strength of the prosthesis, 5,300 N, is significantly higher than that of the normal ACL. It is very stiff, with 2% to 5% strain at yield as compared to 25% for the normal ACL. The amount of elongation prior to failure is 8% to 9%.[23]

In an 18-month follow-up evaluation of 82 patients from the Kerlan-Jobe Clinic,[31] improvement in objective scores in pain, swelling, giving way, and stairclimbing was observed. Return to activities of daily living occurred at 3 months and return to athletics at 8 months. Despite an early nonprogressive shift toward loosening, final follow-up showed improvements in Lachman, pivot shift, and KT-1000 measurements. Complications included four ruptures, four chronic sterile effusions, one infection, and one loose body.

Indelicato and associates[32] reported satisfactory results in 34 of 39 patients (87%) after 2 years follow-up. The average KT-1000 measurements improved from 5 mm preoperatively to 2 mm maximum difference postoperatively. Nine patients had one or more episodes of sterile effusion. Of six with recurrent effusions, five were noted to have partial tears of the prosthesis at arthroscopy. In a minimum 36-month follow-up of the same patients, Woods and associates[33] identified seven additional failures, bringing to 11 the total failures in a series of 33 grafts available for follow-up.

Karzel and associates[27] reported on 61 patients with at least 4 years of follow-up. Subjective categories established by Lysholm scores, as well as objective findings of Lachman and pivot shift, all showed improvement. Five grafts had complete ruptures, three were removed for infection, and 16 had nontraumatic sterile effusions that became chronic in five.

Grewe and Paulos[34] reported on 188 cases with a minimum of 4 years follow-up. Eighty-nine (47%) reported subjective improvement, but only 43% showed objective improvement. Twenty-two patients (12%) had three or more effusions. Graft rupture occurred in 23 patients (12%). Twenty-three had intermediate loosening (5 mm to 8 mm), and ten had severe (> 8 mm) loosening. Of note, the patients with a previous intra-articular reconstruction had a 76% complication rate (33% loosening, 24% effusions, and 14% ruptures).

Finally, Sledge and associates[29] reported on 66 patients with a minimum of 5 years follow-up. There were 19 (29%) documented failures. Complications included one superficial infection, three sterile effusions, and painful, symptomatic hardware in 12 patients. In addition to the failure patients, there was a subgroup of 10 patients with asymptomatic looseness (grade II-III Lachman and grade II pivot shift) who did not meet the strict criteria for failure, but who did display abnormal laxity over time and may represent impending failures. Inclusion of these patients would raise the failure rate to 44%.

In an attempt to address the rising complication and failure rate, Gore-Tex developed a Compact Diameter Cruciate Ligament (CDCL) (Fig. 2). This second generation Gore-Tex ligament, whose cross-sectional diameter was reduced by over 40% and wrapped with a PTFE covering, was intended to decrease abrasion in the bony tunnels. In a prospective multicenter clinical investigation in Canada and Europe, in which 110 patients were presented at the International Knee Society meeting in Copenhagen (1993), the CDCL demonstrated significantly better postoperative stability than the first-generation ligament and fewer overall adverse events at 31 months. Despite these improvements, Gore-Tex elected to remove both ligaments from the market in June, 1993.

Dacron (Stryker) Dacron has been used successfully in the past for arterial reconstructions and for extra-articular repair of such structures as the Achilles and patellar tendons. It was originally meant to be used as an augmentation device or a scaffold, but because of its high strength characteristics, it is more commonly used today as a permanent prosthesis. The prosthesis is composed of four strands of Dacron tape, which act as a core, surrounded by a knitted Dacron velour tube. The ends are covered with plastic tips to facilitate insertion. The woven pattern of the Dacron is designed to contribute tensile strength and to resist fraying under cyclic loading. Another goal of this distinctive pattern is to allow fibrous ingrowth, which adds to the overall strength.

The ultimate strength of the ligament has been tested at 3,613 N.[23] It is considerably less stiff than the normal ACL at 42kN/m.[23] The ultimate strain before rupture is 18%.[23,35] Canine model studies showed adequate ingrowth of type I and III collagen, although the fibers were not functionally aligned.[36] Intra-articular abrasion has been diminished by beveling the tunnel edges and by wrapping the ligament in fascia lata.[36]

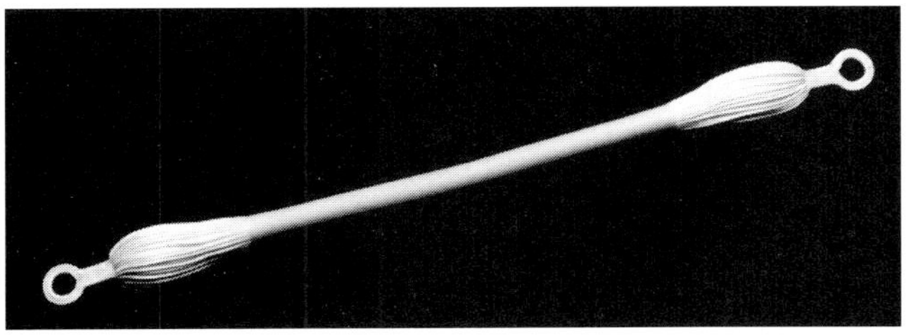

Fig. 2 The Gore-Tex CD ligament. Note the small cross-sectional diameter in the intra-articular portion of the graft.

Lukianov and associates[37] reported on a large series of Dacron ligament reconstructions in acute, chronic, and salvage cases. In the first part of the study, 137 patients were available for greater than 2 years follow-up. Complication rates in this predominantly nonsalvage series was relatively low: synovitis 2%, septic arthritis 2%, extra-articular infection 1%, and graft failure 4%. The second part of the study involved mainly salvage cases, and 80 patients were available for at least 21 months follow-up. This study reported good stability in more than 70% of failed autologous reconstructions and 80% of failed primary repairs. Despite this, 59% of the patients still had pain, 47% still had swelling, and 10% of the grafts failed.

Lopez-Vazquez and associates[38] reported on 54 Dacron ligament reconstructions with 2- to 5-year follow-up. At their follow-up only 23 (43%) were symptom free. Early subjective scores were acceptable, but ligament failures began occurring during the second year and peaked at the third year. A total of 26 (48%) prostheses failed or elongated. Most of the failures occurred at the femoral insertion of the ligament and were felt to be secondary to abrasion of the ligament on the leading edge of the tunnel. The authors recommended against the use of this graft for ACL reconstruction.

Richmond and associates[39] conducted a single-center prospective study on 35 patients with ACL insufficiency who underwent a Dacron reconstruction. Twenty-six had isolated ACL deficiency, and nine had multiple instabilities or failed reconstruction. The mean follow-up was 50 months. The overall failure rate was 37%. The failure rate for isolated ACL insufficiency was 23%, but for the salvage group it was 78%. All failures occurred at least 2 years after implantation. Anderson and associates[40] reviewed 57 patients with a 34-month follow-up. These patients had primary chronic, functional ACL instability and were treated with a Dacron reconstruction. Although subjective scores improved, only 22% had a negative Lachman postoperatively and the graft failure rate was 17.5%.

Gillquist and Odensten[41] reported on 69 Dacron ligament reconstructions with 5-year follow-up. Patients in this group were treated for chronic anterior unstable knees and included 34 with combined medial instability and 22 with failed previous ACL surgery. Although subjective scores improved, the stability that was gained at surgery was gradually lost at a rate of 11% per year. The rupture rate was 23%, and most ruptures occurred proximal to the tibial insertion. Factors influencing the rupture rate included an anterior tibial tunnel and a nontreated MCL tear.

Barrett and associates[42] used the Dacron ligament prosthesis augmented with iliotibial band in a modified Macintosh over-the-top technique. The average follow-up was 47.5 months on 40 patients, 30 of whom had undergone prior procedures. Subjective and objective scores improved markedly, but in 47% the prostheses were considered failures based mainly on such subjective symptoms as residual pain, inability to squat, and failure to return to athletic activities. Complications (27%) included graft failure (12%), infection, and synovitis. The authors recommended against the Dacron prosthesis in the salvage cases because of a higher failure rate.

Finally, Wilk and Richmond[43] reported on a prospective multicenter trial with an average 78-month follow-up in 84 patients with both isolated laxity and failed prior ligament surgery or combined laxities. The subjective scores had improved at 2 years but had plateaued or declined slightly at the 5-year mark. The overall failure rate at 5 years was 35.7%, which was a significant deterioration compared to the two-year rate of 20%.

In summary, as was true with the Gore-Tex reconstructions, there has been a definite trend towards early acceptable results with the Dacron ligament followed by increasing, unacceptable failure rates as time progresses. Despite improvement in Lysholm and Tegner scores, objective measures failed to produce such acceptable results. Revision of a failed prior procedure or multiple ligament laxity contributes to a higher failure rate than isolated ligament laxity. Despite these facts, the Stryker Dacron ligament prosthesis may still have potential for future ACL revision surgery.

Scaffolds

Despite their mechanical superiority, the permanent prostheses are invariably short lived and prone to failure. Scaffolds, which were developed in response to this fact, have an open weave structure that promotes the ingrowth of fibrous tissue. Initially, they are biomechanically inferior to permanent prostheses, but their strength increases as host collagenous ingress ensues. Although technically a permanent prosthesis, scaffolds have biomechanical characteristics that change over time to more closely resemble those of an autogenous graft. Despite these theoretic advantages, these synthetic ligaments are not popular in the United States at this time, but a scaffold prosthesis might conceivably be encountered in a revision situation.

Leeds-Keio The Leeds-Keio prosthesis is popular outside the United States, and over 14,000 have been implanted.[22] It is composed of polyester, with an open-weave tube to promote fibrous ingrowth (Fig. 3). A unique feature of this ligament is the mode of fixation. A tubular bone graft, harvested from the tunnel, is inserted in a loop on one end of the prosthesis and is press fit back into the tunnel. Another bone plug secures the other, flat end of the ligament in a similar fashion in the opposite tunnel. The initial protocol called for 4 to 6 weeks of immobilization until fibrous ingrowth occurred. Prior to implantation, the ultimate strength of the Leeds-Keio is 840 to 870 N.[44-46] As fibrous tissue invades the open weave and aligns itself along the lines of stress, the strength increases to 2,000 N.

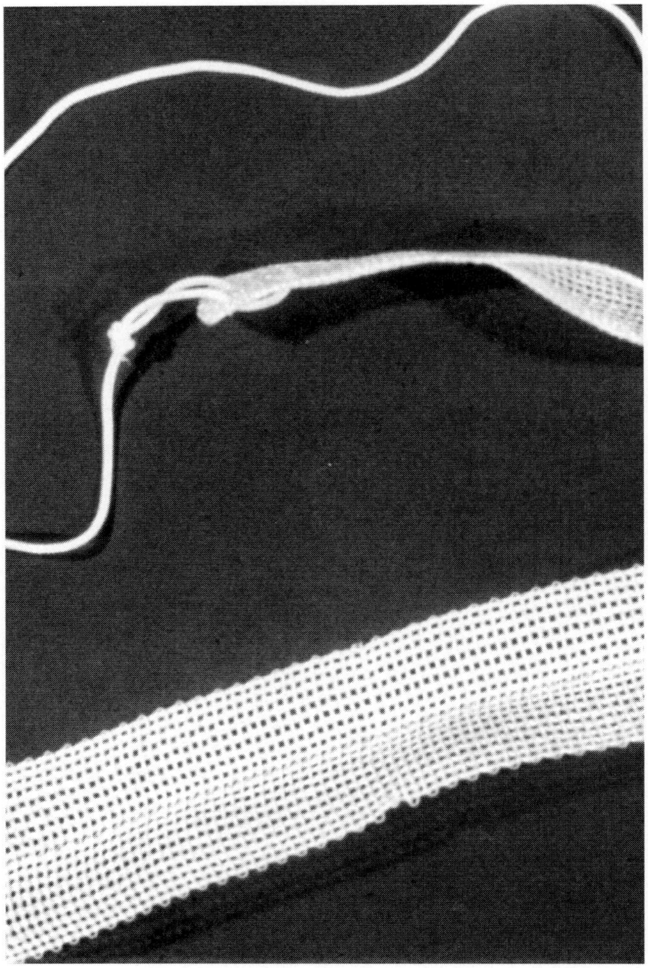

Fig. 3 The Leeds-Keio ligament prosthesis is designed to have bone plugs inserted in both ends, which cause eventual fibrous tissue ingrowth into the open weave polyester.

Denti and associates[44] reported on 26 patients with a mean follow-up of 33 months. Postoperatively, the patients showed significant improvement in pivot shift, KT-1000 displacement, and Lysholm scores. Two ruptures occurred, one at 12 months and the other at 20 months. One of these was caused by a technical error; the other was secondary to subsequent trauma. Follow-up has been too short to allow definitive conclusions.

Fujikawa and associates[45] reviewed 152 cases that had more than 4 years follow-up. Postoperative Lachman, anterior drawer, and jerk tests were negative in 80% to 90% of these patients. Arthroscopy was performed at various intervals in 42 cases. At 3 months, new random tissue with a rich vascular network was observed around the ligament. By 12 months, a nearly mature ligament resembling a normal ACL was observed. Complications were rare; no synovitis, infection, or effusions were noted. Only five reconstructions (3.3%) resulted in a rupture.

Carbon Fiber Carbon fiber implants are strong and bioinert, and they have been shown to induce fibrous ingrowth.[35,47,48] Subsequently, they have been popular in augmenting or replacing structures such as the Achilles tendon or the medial collateral ligament. They were first used in knee ligament surgery in South Africa in 1979.[49] Their function was to act as an inert intra-articular stent until they were transformed by fibrous ingrowth into a biologic, functioning ligament. Initial histologic studies[47,50] reported the formation of a new vascularized, innervated ligament. Subsequent studies, however, have shown the ingrowth of fibroblasts and collagen to be slow and incomplete.[50-52]

Other problems plague the carbon fiber ligament and limit its usefulness today. In reconstructions where the ligament was not surrounded by autogenous tissue, little neotendon was formed and a significant amount of synovitis was seen in reaction to carbon fiber particles.[35,50,53] Because of its high modulus, carbon fibers cannot tolerate significant shear stresses. They also have low elasticity[35] and little tolerance for repeated dynamic loading, especially the kind seen in athletic endeavors.[53] Encasing the ligament in fascia lata has eased some of these difficulties.[35,50,53]

Rushton and associates[54] reported on 39 patients who underwent a carbon fiber reconstruction without a sheath of autogenous tissue. Ten of those patients underwent a second operation 16 months later for persistent pain, effusion, and synovial thickening. Arthroscopy revealed carbon fibers scattered through the knee, and the repaired ligament was surrounded only by a thin fibrous sheath. Weiss and associates[55] reported on an FDA-approved study of 82 patients with a 24-month follow-up, using a copolymer-carbon fiber ligament prosthesis in predominantly chronically unstable knees. Results showed increased function and stability and decreased pain in this short follow-up study. Only five ruptures were reported.

In his series, J. Norgrove Penny[56] used carbon fiber ligaments for augmentation, rather than as lone prosthesis. His group included 93 patients (45 carbon fiber and 48 controls) followed for a minimum of 2 years. The carbon fiber ligament was sandwiched between either an ITB graft or split-thickness patellar tendon graft, taking care to completely enclose the carbon fiber ligament with a water tight closure. He found chronic effusions twice as often in the carbon fiber group as compared to the control group. Knee scores and KT-1000 showed no difference between carbon fiber and controls. Follow-up arthroscopies, done in 22 patients, showed satisfactory fibrogenesis in 75%, while 25% showed a flimsy fibrous membrane covering the carbon fiber with little ingrowth. Overall, 33% of his cases exhibited carbon fiber debris at this early follow-up.

Augmentation Devices

The Ligament Augmentation Device (LAD) was introduced by JC Kennedy[26] in 1979.[57] Kennedy hoped the LAD would overcome some of the difficulties inherent in the use of autogenous tissue, such as initial loss of strength due to revascularization and the eventual failure of prosthetic ligaments. By acting as a load-sharing device, the LAD deflects a portion of the force on the ligament during the early healing phase. As the graft matures, it takes on more of the force than the LAD, thus decreasing the chances of failure we have seen with other prosthetic ligaments.[57] Because the graft is protected early, there is less chance that it will stretch and eventually rupture. The LAD has been used with patellar tendon, semitendinosus, quadriceps tendon, and allograft.

The LAD, a permanent, woven type of prosthesis, is composed of nine strands of braided polypropylene, the ends of which are heat treated to prevent unraveling (Fig. 4). The ultimate strength has been tested at 1,500 to 1,730 N.[57] It has an elongation of 22% at failure and a stiffness of 200 N/m.[57] The LAD is secured to the autogenous graft with nonabsorbable suture, and an effort is made to tube the latter around the former. This composite is then attached at only one end. If both ends are secured, significant stress shielding and subsequent interim stretching could occur.[57]

Initial animal studies were encouraging. In several, augmented ACL reconstructions were found to be stronger than nonaugmented ACL reconstructions. In one, the LAD was found to take up 45% of the force in a gracilis-semitendinosus reconstruction.[57] In a much stiffer construct, which used the patellar tendon, the

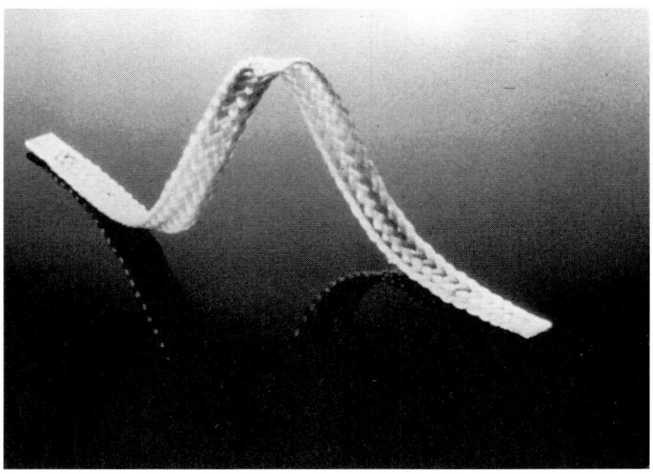

Fig. 4 The Kennedy ligament augmentation device.

LAD only diverted 28% of the force.[57] Another study showed significant rupture rates (100%) if stress shielding from dual fixation occurred.[57]

Kennedy compared 43 augmented and 45 nonaugmented reconstructions, using the modified Marshall Macintosh technique.[57] At 4 years, objective laxity and functional testing showed a trend toward better results in the LAD group and significantly better results in subjective evaluation, clinical examination, and radiographic analysis. Fowler and Capra[57] gave further follow-up on the patients (mean, 7.5 years). Overall evaluation revealed 91% good to excellent results. Ninety-six percent stated that they would undergo the procedure again.

Roth and associates[58] compared 45 augmented modified Marshall Macintosh reconstructions with 38 nonaugmented reconstructions, with a mean follow-up of 50 months. The augmented group fared better in objective laxity, physical examination, functional testing, and subjective symptoms. Of the augmented group, 11% complained of recurrent giving way, compared with 32% of the nonaugmented group. Del Pizzo[59] reported on patients with a 3-year minimum follow-up of augmented ACL reconstructions. In this group, 95% had a 0 to 1+ pivot shift, 72% had ≤ 3 mm of anterior laxity with KT-1000 testing, and 93% had < 5° of extension restriction. There was a 0.7% rate of infection, 1% of sterile effusion, and 1.4% of ruptures.

Modes of Failure

Surgical revision of a failed prosthetic ligament can be a very demanding task. Because several types of prosthetic ligaments have been used, many different types of revisions may be encountered. Basic mechanisms of failure common to all include effusions/synovitis, ruptures, infections, and osteolysis. Because the incidence of failure increases with time after prosthetic replacement, standard methods of addressing these complications will be discussed.

Synovitis

Synovitis and chronic effusion are two of the more common complications associated with prosthetic ligaments, with an incidence that ranges from 5% to 47%.[27,29,31,34] Clinically, these entities are characterized by swelling, warmth, pain, and increased white blood cells in the absence of infection. Transient synovitis can be readily treated, but chronic synovitis can be debilitating and may eventually require removal of the prosthetic ligament. Most synovial irritation occurs as a reaction to particulate debris released by the prosthetic ligaments by abrasion or rupture.[60] Pathologic biomechanics emanating from a failed ligament and degenerated cartilage debris may also contribute to synovial inflammation. Although further research is needed regarding the pathophysiology of particulate matter-induced synovitis, recent basic science studies have given us insight into possible etiologies.

Working with animal models, Olson and associates[60] studied the effect on synovial cells in vitro and in vivo of particulate matter from seven prosthetic ligaments. The ligaments tested were: Gore-Tex (PTFE), Stryker Dacron, Versigraft, LAD, carbon fiber, Leeds-Keio, and xenograft, as well as human patellar tendon. Morcellized particulate matter placed in an in vitro lapine cell culture was observed to activate synovial cells, with subsequent release of enzymes such as gelatinase, collagenase, and interleukin-1, that are catabolic to cartilage and bone. This foreign body response was dependent on material type, particle dose, and particle size. Xenografts and carbon fiber grafts showed statistically greater enzyme production.

In vivo histologic analysis of rabbit knee synovium 14 weeks after intra-articular injection of the same particulate matter revealed "synovial hypertrophy and a vigorous foreign body response with dense macrophage and foreign body giant cell accumulations around the wear particles." Although the authors felt there was not enough experimental evidence to indict particulate matter from prosthetic ligaments in failed human reconstructions, they urged caution in using these materials and suggested technical considerations, such as adequate notchplasty and tunnel chamfering, to decrease the liberation of wear particles.

Rupture

Rupture of a prosthetic graft is another common factor leading to revision surgery. Despite their inherently high ultimate tensile strengths, these ligaments are subjected to cyclic loading at the relatively large loads seen in athletic activity. Abrasion of the prosthesis under such conditions can eventually lead to failure. Factors that can predispose the graft to abrasion in the notch include inadequate notchplasty, nonphysiometric tunnel placement, sharp tunnel entrances, and notch regrowth.

The amount of notchplasty to be performed depends in part on tibial tunnel placement and chronicity of the ACL insufficiency. Our tibial tunnel placement aligns with the articular surface-notch junction in the coronal plane, and is just lateral to the apex of the medial tibial spine in the sagittal plane. Through experience, we have determined that 18 mm is the optimal size for the majority of notches when using a 10-mm patellar tendon graft. A pituitary rongeur is a useful guide to determine notch size (Fig. 5). An inadequate notch abrading a prosthetic ligament over thousands of cycles can lead to eventual rupture.

Improper tunnel placement can result in abnormal forces and impingement on the graft (Fig. 6). Nonphysiometric placement of the femoral tunnel can lead to graft failure by placing excessive stress on the graft at the extreme of motion. If the tunnel is placed too far

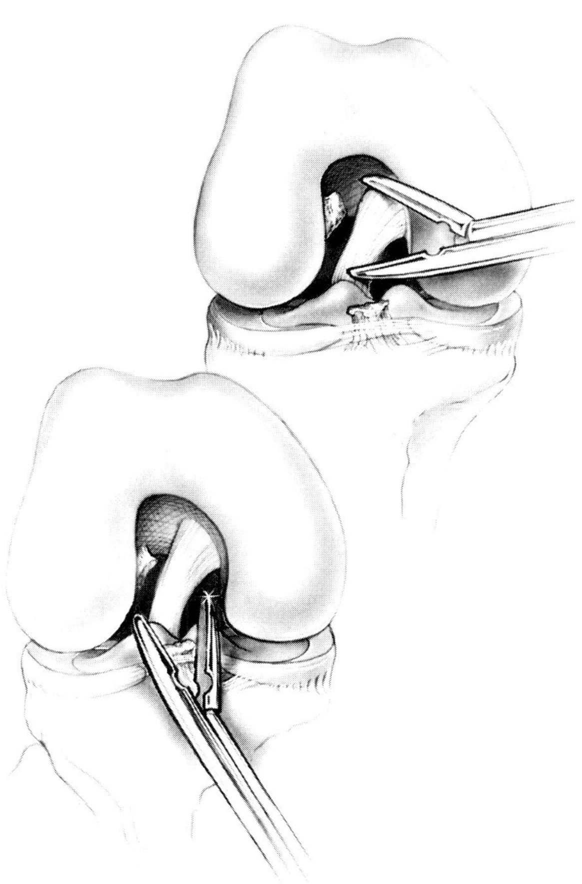

Fig. 5 A pituitary rongeur that measures 18 mm when fully opened can be used to measure the notch height and width. (Reproduced with permission from Steadman JR, Seemann MD: ACL injuries in the elite skier, in Feagin JA Jr (ed): *The Crucial Ligaments: Diagnosis and Treatment of Ligamentous Injuries About the Knee,* ed 2. New York, NY, Churchill Livingstone, 1994, pp 759-772.)

anteriorly, the graft will tighten in flexion. Similarly, if the tunnel is placed too far posteriorly, it will tighten in extension. Athletic activities that repetitively place the knee in extreme flexion or terminal extension predispose an improperly placed graft to fatigue failure.

Howell[61-63] has done considerable research on the roof impingement that can occur on an ACL substitute from an anteriorly placed tibial tunnel. During terminal extension (Fig. 7), the intercondylar roof impinges prematurely on the anteriorly placed graft, leading to compression of its distal two thirds. Repetitive terminal extension can lead to graft failure. Extension deficit, activity-induced effusions, and graft failure with instability are clinical signs of impingement that can be diagnosed on a true lateral radiograph of the knee in full passive extension. If the anterosuperior aspect of the tibial tunnel passes anterior to the intercondylar roof, impingement is likely. Howell feels that magnetic resonance imaging (MRI) is able to diagnose impingement more clearly because it can show increased signal in the region of the ACL under impingement.

Notch regrowth is a poorly understood phenomenon that can lead to impingement. Generally occurring months after the initial reconstruction, it is thought to be caused by overzealous notchplasty, which results in excessive bleeding, leading to subsequent new bone and fibrocartilage formation. Clinically, the patients experience a click in terminal extension. This click, which appears late in rehabilitation, may be associated with effusions and pain. It sometimes appears in patients who have difficulty obtaining full extension, such as those who have undergone meniscus repair in association with an ACL reconstruction. Theoretically, a graft that fills up the notch will inhibit the growth of neocartilage and bone and avoid resultant impingement. Notch regrowth is an unpredictable and, fortunately, rare event.

Finally, an acute angle on the intra-articular portion of the femoral and tibial tunnels can abrade the graft, increasing the likelihood of rupture. The sharp edge of bone on the posterior aspect of the tibial tunnel and the inferoanterior aspect of the femoral tunnel should be adequately chamfered to decrease the abrasion on the graft. The causes of an initial graft failure are invariably present at revision and must be adequately addressed to prevent another failure with the revision graft.

Infection

Infection, another complication necessitating revision, has been reported in approximately 2% to 3% of prosthetic ligament reconstructions.[27,29,31,34,48] A postoperative infection in any situation can be a disaster, but it is even more so when the operation is intra-articular and foreign material has been implanted. Much of our knowledge about musculoskeletal infections comes from patients with infected total joint or fracture fixation devices, but the symptoms can be similar in all patients. The pathogens most commonly involved in biomaterial infections include *Staphylococcus aureus, Pseudomonas aeruginosa,* and *Escherichia coli.*[64] It has been shown that when these bacteria adhere to surfaces, phenotypic changes occur that affect the bacteria's virulence. These changes may explain a unique property of biomaterial-centered infections, which is the transformation of a normal, nonpathologic bacteria, such as *Staphylococcus epidermidis,* into a serious infection-causing pathogen.[64] Patients with infected prosthetic ligaments commonly present with a painful, swollen knee. Because this can mimic a sterile effusion, joint aspiration with Gram stain and culture and sensitivity testing of the aspirate is necessary to confirm a septic arthritis.

Osteolysis

Tibial osteolysis in association with a Gore-Tex graft has recently been reported as another complication of prosthetic ligaments that may necessitate revision.[28] In

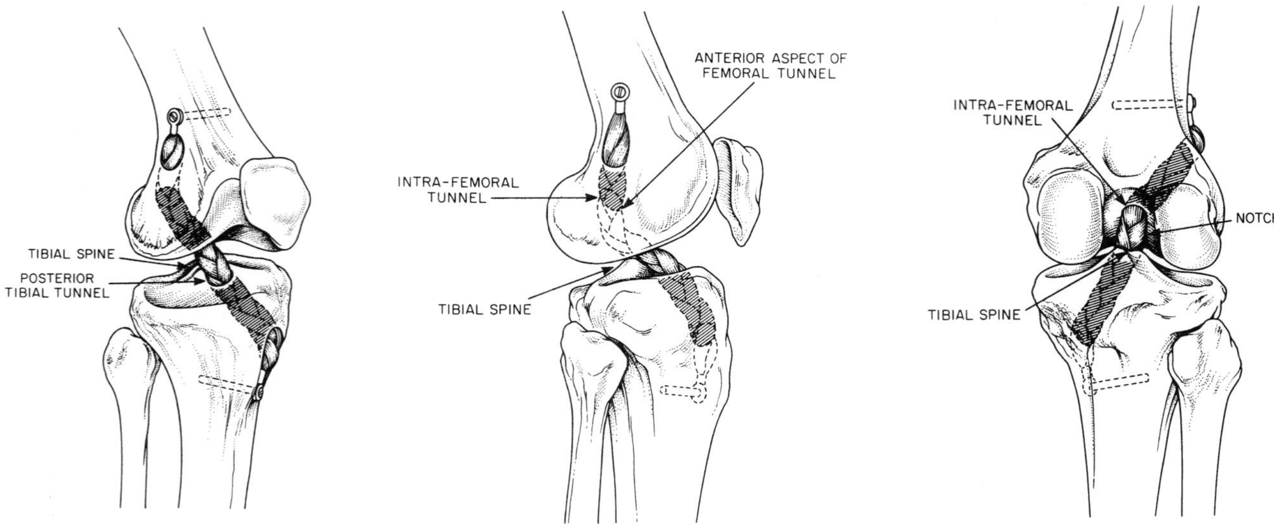

Fig. 6 Pictures of a Gore-Tex ligament prosthesis showing potential areas of graft abrasion.

a small number of patients who underwent Gore-Tex graft ACL reconstruction, progressive widening of the tibial tunnel has been observed. Failure of these grafts is seen late (> 6 years), as the tunnel widening causes functional incompetency of the graft. The precise etiology of the osteolysis is unclear, but it is hypothesized that wear debris particles stimulate release of interleukin-1 from the synovial cells. The interleukin-1 gravitates to the intra-articular tibial tunnel, where it stimulates bony resorption.[28] In a standard Gore-Tex ACL reconstruction, the femoral tunnel is not located within the notch, and it therefore seems to be more resistant to wear-debris osteolysis. Prosthetic materials that use a femoral tunnel located within the notch may be predisposed to femoral tunnel osteolysis.

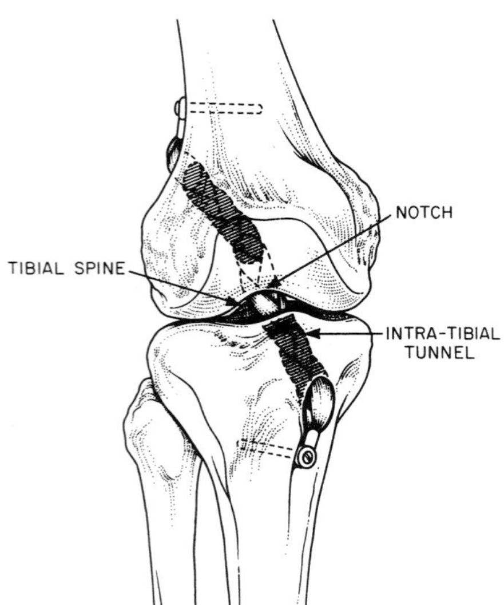

Fig. 7 Knee in full extension shows Gore-Tex graft impinging on the intercondylar roof, as well as on the tibial spine and tibial tunnel.

Osteolysis induced by wear particles should be suspected in anyone about to undergo a prosthetic ACL revision. Tibial osteolysis can be recognized as widening of the bone tunnel on plain radiographs. Often, the widening is subtle and difficult to see. CT scan or MRI can be helpful in these instances and can more accurately predict the true size of the defect. Adequate preoperative workup is essential, because, if a large cystic space is noted on preoperative diagnostics, it may be necessary to bone graft the defect, making it a two-stage procedure. If the osteolysis is overlooked and is not adequately addressed intraoperatively, the fixation of the revised graft can be severely compromised.

Preoperative Planning

When contemplating revision of a prosthetic ligament, preoperative planning is crucial. As with the approach to any surgical patient, the initial step in preoperative planning is taking a thorough history. This history will help formulate a good differential diagnosis as to the cause of the failure of the prosthetic ligament, as well as delineate other symptoms that may mimic graft failure. It is important to know what symptoms the patient has, how long they have been present, what makes them worse or better, and the degree of disability these symptoms cause. When questioning the patient, it is also important to document if there have been any signs or symptoms of infection such as purulent drainage, cellulitis, or fevers and chills. The patient who comes in with problems after a traumatic event may likely have a pathology different from that of a patient who presents with a chronic effusion and progressive laxity.

Another key piece of information is what type of prosthetic material was used, the location of the bone tunnels through which it was passed, and the type of fixation used to fix the prosthetic material. Because many patients are unable to give accurate answers to these questions, operative reports and arthroscopy videos of the previous surgery can be very valuable.

When presented with a patient who has a complex problem, the surgeon should discuss with the patient his/her lifestyle, activity level, degree of disability, and future expectations. Answers to these questions will help you and the patient decide whether revision surgery even needs to be undertaken and, if so, which type of surgery will offer the greatest benefit for the patient.

A physical examination will determine the amount of instability and the possibility of infection. If a small amount of instability is present, such as less than 5 mm displacement on the KT-1000 arthrometer, revision may not be able to give a more stable knee.[65] Septic knees react with extreme pain to any type of motion, are swollen, and generally are warm. However, a subclinical infection may be less dramatic and, thus, an aspiration is indicated. The aspirate should be sent to the laboratory for cell count, Gram's stain, culture/sensitivity, glucose, protein, and crystals. The laboratory results can be used to determine which is present, infection or sterile effusion. Effusions can elevate the white count in the absence of infection. Blood chemistry, white blood cell count, sedimentation rate, and C-reactive protein determination can further delineate the possibility of infection.

Routine radiographs are useful in the preoperative workup. The presence or absence of degenerative arthritis can be determined and may affect operative planning. Femoral and tibial tunnel positioning can be ascertained on the lateral radiographs (Fig. 8). Osteolysis often can be seen on both the AP and lateral radiographs. The type of hardware used for graft fixation needs to be addressed and the proper equipment for removal ordered preoperatively. CT scans or MRI can be used to further delineate the extent of the osteolysis (Fig. 9).

An extremely important part of the preoperative planning is determination of the type of graft to be employed. Present options include: ipsilateral medial hamstrings, contralateral or ipsilateral patellar tendon, allograft, or another prosthetic graft. The patient's expectations and activity level, as well as the surgeon's experience, are important in choosing the appropriate revision graft. All have advantages and disadvantages, and these must be discussed with the patient preoperatively. If allograft tissues are used, the surgeon must give careful consideration to the supplying tissue bank. It should be emphasized that current screening techniques, while very good, are not perfect. A small risk of disease transmission exists.

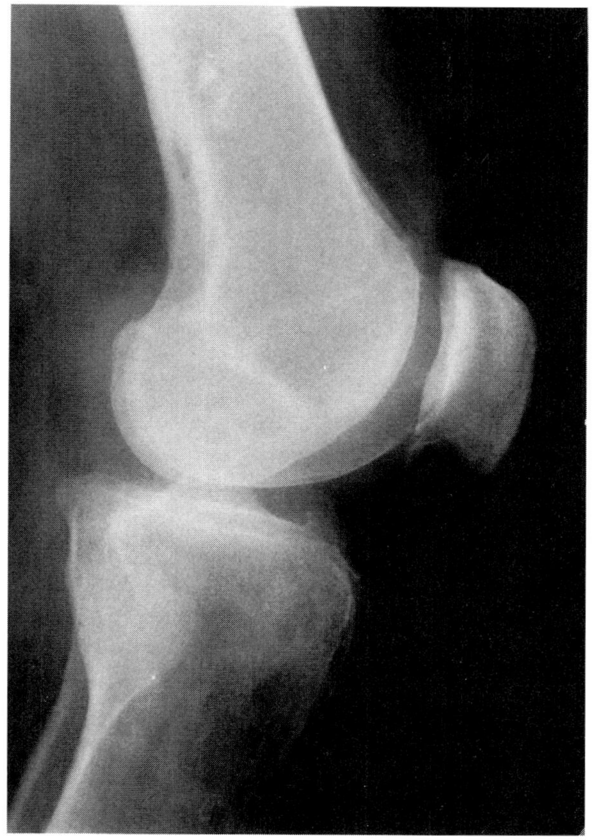

Fig. 8 Lateral radiograph showing position of tibial and femoral tunnels, as well as tibial tunnel widening. (Reproduced with permission from Seemann MD, Steadman JR: Tibial osteolysis associated with Gore-Tex grafts. *Am J Knee Surg* 1993;6:31-38.)

If significant osteolysis exists, bone grafting of the defect may be necessary to provide an optimal environment for revision. A period of 3 to 6 months is needed for the bone graft to mature, and this time delay makes the revision a two-stage procedure. Therefore, patients should be counseled thoroughly preoperatively.

Surgical Technique

Revision of a prosthetic ACL reconstruction can be technically demanding and fraught with opportunities for error. Adequate preoperative workup, precise surgical technique, and individually tailored rehabilitation are required for a successful outcome. The decision to proceed with a revision reconstruction should not be taken lightly and, at this time, the procedure should be attempted only by surgeons with extensive experience in routine ACL reconstructions.

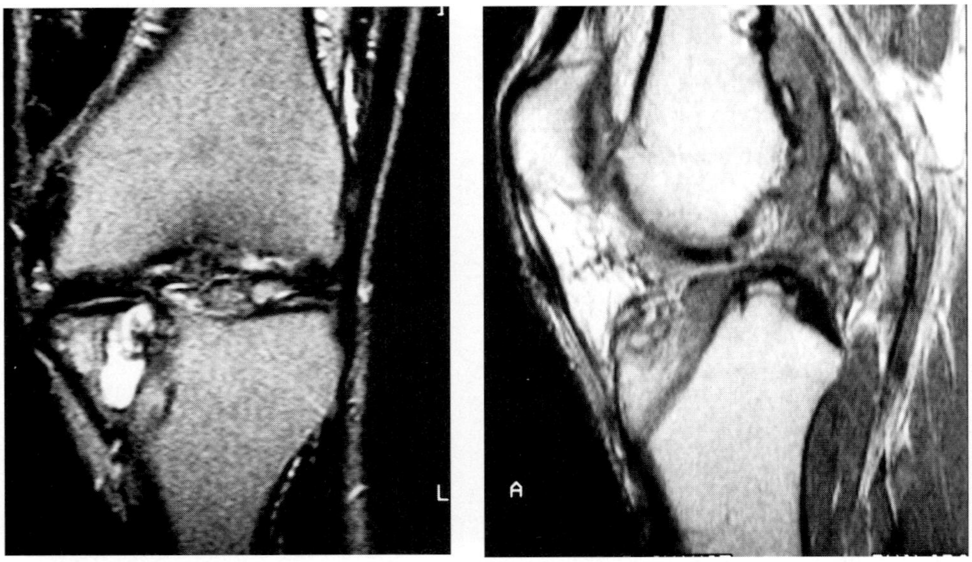

Fig. 9 MRI scan showing extent of tibial tunnel osteolysis. (Reproduced with permission from Seemann MD, Steadman JR: Tibial osteolysis associated with Gore-Tex grafts. *Am J Knee Surg* 1993;6:31-38.)

If a patient presents with true septic arthritis, a protocol similar to one used for an infected total knee replacement is instituted. This involves isolation of the causative bacteria, early surgical debridement, and administration of appropriate intravenous antibiotics. If the infection is diagnosed early, the debridement may be done arthroscopically. Otherwise, an arthrotomy may be necessary to ensure that all the loculated areas are adequately drained, and all the prosthetic material has been removed from the bony tunnels. If the knee joint is grossly infected, the use of antibiotic beads may be considered. As with any musculoskeletal infection, the white blood cell count, erythrocyte sedimentation rate, and C-reactive protein should be followed to determine the patient's response to treatment. If after 6 weeks of antibiotics the patient's laboratory values are normal and the clinical examination reveals no signs of infection, revision may be contemplated.

When infection has been ruled out, the initial step in a revision entails removal of all of the failed prosthetic ligament. It is imperative that all residual ligament be removed from the bony tunnels, as well as the joint, to decrease the risk of recurrent effusions or infection in subsequent reconstruction. First, fixation hardware must be removed. Generally, interference screws, a screw used as a post, staples, or buttons will be encountered. Use of the appropriate instruments for each will ease hardware removal.

Once the hardware is extracted, the ligament device is removed from the tunnels. We have found an 8-mm gouge to be extremely useful in loosening the fibers from the walls of the tunnel. The extra-articular portion of the prosthesis is grasped with a Kocher clamp and the gouge is inserted in the tunnel wall/ligament interface. Circumferential release with the gouge helps free the fibers for eventual removal. After this procedure has been performed on both the femoral and tibial side, the ligament is wound in a circular fashion around the clamp, creating a sufficient uniform force to withdraw most fibers from the tunnel. A curette can then dislodge residual fibers from the tunnel wall surface. The arthroscope inserted into the tunnels, both intra-articular and extra-articular, can verify complete excision of all ligament debris and may also be used to check for tunnel expansion due to osteolysis.

If osteolysis is present, the surgeon must determine if the tunnel can accept a revision ligament. Excessive widening can compromise fixation of the new graft. In such cases, bone grafting is required, and the surgery should be staged in two parts. After 6 to 8 weeks, the bone graft should be mature enough to accept a revision graft in the standard fashion. In cases with less widening, a large bone plug on the graft and/or a 10-mm screw may provide adequate fixation. If the graft fixation in the revision reconstruction is compromised, subsequent failure is likely.

In the absence of osteolysis, the surgeon must determine whether the intra-articular tunnel positions are adequate for replacement of the revision graft. In failed ligaments in which the tibial site is placed too far anterior, the tunnel can be reamed to a larger size or the posterior aspect of the tunnel chamfered to displace the ligament more posteriorly. In rare instances, the tunnel site can be completely changed, if the original tunnel was so misplaced that a new tunnel can be created that will still allow an adequate bony bridge between the new and old tunnels.

The femoral tunnel is handled in a similar fashion. In failed ligaments, the femoral site is often too far anterior. If a new tunnel cannot be made that is posterior to the existing one, an over-the-top position may be used. With a Gore-Tex graft, the femoral tunnel is outside the notch, and a new femoral tunnel can be drilled in the standard fashion. Finally, because the femoral bony tunnels from a "two-incision" ACL reconstruction traverse a more acute angle than is used for an endoscopic approach, a different femoral tunnel angle may be used if necessary in a revision situation.

Fixation of the revision graft is another technical consideration. In routine reconstructions, various methods are employed. Interference screws, buttons, staples, and screws used as a post are all still in use. Several studies[66,67] have shown superior pullout strengths with interference screws. Some concern has been voiced that use of interference screws on both sides of the graft could potentially "capture" the knee and lead to stiffness or eventual arthritis. We feel that if the tunnels are placed in a "physiometric" fashion, this should not happen and need not be a concern. For these reasons, our fixation of choice is a 9-mm cannulated interference screw. We use a 6.5-mm AO cancellous screw post as a backup if fixation with the interference screw is not adequate.

The type of graft used in revision surgery depends on individual preference. Because of its superior biomechanical characteristics over medial hamstrings, we prefer ipsilateral patella tendon. If the contralateral patellar tendon is harvested, it is recommended that an initial arthroscopy be performed to assess the patella and rule out chondromalacia. If a significant amount of chondromalacia is present, we recommend against using that patellar tendon as a graft. If neither patellar tendon is viable, our next choice is a patellar tendon allograft. We do not use allogeneic tissues as first-line grafts because of the small but definite risk of disease transmission. Also we have noticed variability in the quality of grafts, and biomechanical studies have confirmed this with regard to their ultimate strength (personal communication, Jack McCarthy, 1987.) Finally, we feel that some patients may have an immunologic reaction to allografts, which can affect the final outcome. Because of their record of eventual long-term complications, we have not employed prosthetic ligaments in revisions.

Postoperatively, rehabilitation should be individualized depending on graft type, security of fixation and patient reliability. Our baseline protocol calls for aggressive ACL rehabilitation, including immediate full range-of-motion, with emphasis on extension, weight-bearing as tolerated, and closed chain quadriceps strengthening. The majority of our revision patients follow this protocol.[68]

Conclusion

Several thousand ACL reconstructions with prosthetic ligaments have been performed since the early 1980s. With time, we are seeing increasing numbers of failures of these grafts due to varying causes. Experience with total joint arthroplasties has taught us that nonbiologic implants do not hold up to a lifetime of use in a biologic environment. Synthetic ligaments are often placed in athletic individuals, and the physical demand in competitive athletes may accelerate their deterioration. Revision of a failed prosthetic ligament may be a difficult undertaking. Careful preoperative planning, sound intraoperative judgment, and appropriate rehabilitation enhance the likelihood of acceptable results. Further studies need to be performed regarding outcomes of prosthetic anterior cruciate ligament revision reconstructions.

References

1. Daniel DM: Selecting patients for ACL surgery, in Jackson DW, Arnoczky SP, Woo SLY, et al (eds): *The Anterior Cruciate Ligament: Current and Future Concepts.* New York, NY, Raven Press, 1993, pp 251-258.
2. Jackson RW: The torn ACL: Natural history of untreated lesions and rationale for selective treatment, in Feagin JA Jr (ed): *The Crucial Ligaments: Diagnosis and Treatment of Ligamentous Injuries About the Knee,* ed 2. New York, NY, Churchill Livingstone, 1994, pp 485-493.
3. Jackson RW, Peters RI, Marczyk RL: Late results of untreated anterior cruciate ligament rupture. *J Bone Joint Surg* 1980;62B:127.
4. Harner CD, Irrgang JJ, Paul J, et al: Loss of motion after anterior cruciate ligament reconstruction. *Am J Sports Med* 1992;20:499-506.
5. Mohtadi NG, Webstor-Bugaerts S, Fowler PJ: Limitation of motion following anterior cruciate ligament reconstruction: A case-control study. *Am J Sports Med* 1991;19:620-625.
6. Shelbourne KD, Wilckens JH, Mollabashy A, et al: Arthrofibrosis in acute anterior cruciate ligament reconstruction: The effect of timing of reconstruction and rehabilitation. *Am J Sports Med* 1991;19:332-336.
7. Paulos LE, Meislin R: Patellar entrapment following anterior cruciate ligament injury, in Jackson DW, Arnoczky SP, Woo SLY, et al (eds): *The Anterior Cruciate Ligament: Current and Future Concepts.* New York, NY, Raven Press, 1993, pp 357-363.
8. Paulos LE, Rosenberg TD, Drawbert J, et al: Infrapatellar contracture syndrome: An unrecognized cause of knee stiffness with patella entrapment and patella infera. *Am J Sports Med* 1987; 15:331-341.
9. Friedman MJ, Re LP, Rintz KG, et al: Incidence of anterior knee pain after treatment for ACL rupture. *Orthop Trans* 1993;17:1005.
10. McCarroll JR: Fracture of the patella during a golf swing following reconstruction of the anterior cruciate ligament: A case report. *Am J Sports Med* 1983;11:26-27.
11. Bonamo JJ, Krinick RM, Sporn AA: Rupture of the patellar ligament after use of its central third for anterior cruciate reconstruction: A report of two cases. *J Bone Joint Surg* 1984; 66A:1294-1297.
12. Shino K, Nakagawa S, Inoue M, et al: Deterioration of patellofemoral articular surfaces after anterior cruciate ligament reconstruction. *Am J Sports Med* 1993;21:206-211.

13. Eilerman M, Thomas J, Marsalka D: The effect of harvesting the central one-third of the patellar tendon on patellofemoral contact pressure. *Am J Sports Med* 1992;20:738-741.
14. Sachs RA, Daniel DM, Stone ML, et al: Patellofemoral problems after anterior cruciate ligament reconstruction. *Am J Sports Med* 1989;17:760-765.
15. Kramer J, Nusca D, Fowler P, et al: Knee flexor and extensor strength during concentric and eccentric muscle actions after anterior cruciate ligament reconstruction using the semitendinosus tendon and ligament augmentation device. *Am J Sports Med* 1993;2:285-291.
16. Marder RA, Raskind JR, Carroll M: Prospective evaluation of arthroscopically assisted anterior cruciate ligament reconstruction: Patellar tendon versus semitendinosus and gracilis tendons. *Am J Sports Med* 1991;19:478-484.
17. Noyes FR, Grood ES, Zernicke RF, et al: Biomechanical analysis of human ligament grafts in knee ligament repairs and reconstruction. *J Bone Joint Surg* 1984;66A:344-352.
18. Woo SL, Hollis JM, Adams DJ, et al: Tensile properties of the human femur-anterior cruciate ligament-tibia complex: The effects of specimen age and orientation. *Am J Sports Med* 1991;19:217-225.
19. Cooper DE, Deng XH, Warren RF, et al: Strength of the central third patellar tendon graft: A biomechanical study. Presented at the 59th Annual Meeting of the American Academy of Orthopaedic Surgeons, Washington, DC, 1992.
20. Clancy WG Jr, Narechania RG, Rosenberg TD, et al: Anterior and posterior cruciate ligament reconstruction in Rhesus monkeys: A histological, microangiographic and biomechanical analysis. *J Bone Joint Surg* 1981;63A:1270-1284.
21. Arnoczky SP, Warren RF, Minei JP: Replacement of the anterior cruciate ligament using a synthetic prosthesis: An evaluation of graft biology in the dog. *Am J Sports Med* 1986;14:1-6.
22. Friedman MJ: Prosthetic anterior cruciate ligament. *Clin Sports Med* 1991;10:499-513.
23. McCarthy DM, Tolin BS, Schwendeman L: Prosthetic replacement for the anterior cruciate ligament, in Jackson DW, Arnoczky SP, Woo SLY, et al (eds): *The Anterior Cruciate Ligament: Current and Future Concepts.* New York, NY, Raven Press, 1993, pp 343-356.
24. Schepsis AA, Greenleaf J: Prosthetic materials for anterior cruciate ligament reconstruction. *Orthop Rev* 1990;19:984-991.
25. Woods GW: Synthetics in anterior cruciate ligament reconstruction: A review. *Orthop Clin North Am* 1985;16:227-235.
26. Kennedy JC: Application of prosthetics to anterior cruciate ligament reconstruction and repair. *Clin Orthop* 1983;172:125-128.
27. Karzel RP, Diefendorf DR, Fox JM, et al: Four-year experience with the Gore-Tex prosthetic ligament in anterior cruciate deficient knees. *Orthop Trans* 1990;14:618.
28. Seemann MD, Steadman JR: Tibial osteolysis associated with Gore-tex grafts. *Am J Knee Surg* 1993;6:31-38.
29. Sledge SL, Steadman JR, Silliman JF, et al: Five-year results with the Gore-Tex anterior cruciate ligament prosthesis. *Am J Knee Surg* 1992;5:65-70.
30. Larson RL: Gore-tex anterior cruciate ligament reconstruction, in Scott WN (ed): *Ligament and Extensor Mechanism Injuries of the Knee: Diagnosis and Treatment.* St. Louis, MO, Mosby Year Book, 1991, pp 319-329.
31. Glousman R, Shields C Jr, Kerlan R, et al: Gore-Tex prosthetic ligament in anterior cruciate ligament deficient knees. *Am J Sports Med* 1988;16;321-326.
32. Indelicato PA, Pascale MS, Huegel MO: Early experience with the Gore-Tex polytetrafluoroethylene anterior cruciate ligament prosthesis. *Am J Sports Med* 1989;17:55-62.
33. Woods GA, Indelicato PA, Prevot TJ: The Gore-Tex anterior cruciate ligament prosthesis: Two versus three year results. *Am J Sports Med* 1991;19:48-55.
34. Grewe SR, Paulos LE: Prosthetic replacement of the anterior cruciate ligament with expanded polytetrafluoroethylene, in Tullos HS (ed): *Instructional Course Lectures Volume XL.* Park Ridge, IL, American Academy of Orthopaedic Surgeons, 1991, pp 213-217.
35. Claes L, Neugebauer R: In vivo and in vitro investigation of the long-term behavior and fatigue strength of carbon fiber ligament replacement. *Clin Orthop* 1985;196:99-111.
36. Park JP, Grana WA, Chitwood JS: A high strength Dacron augmentation for cruciate ligament reconstruction: A two-year canine study. *Clin Orthop* 1985;196:175-185.
37. Lukianov AV, Richmond JC, Barrett GR, et al: A multicenter study on the results of anterior cruciate ligament reconstruction using a Dacron ligament prosthesis in "salvage" cases. *Am J Sports Med* 1989;17:380-386.
38. Lopez-Vazquez E, Juan JA, Vila E, et al: Reconstruction of the anterior cruciate ligament with a Dacron prosthesis. *J Bone Joint Surg* 1991;73A:1294-1300.
39. Richmond JC, Manseau CJ, Patz R, et al: Anterior cruciate reconstruction using a Dacron ligament prosthesis: A long-term study. *Am J Sports Med* 1992;20:24-28.
40. Anderson HN, Bruun C, Sondergard-Petersen PE: Reconstruction of chronic insufficient anterior cruciate ligament in the knee using a synthetic Dacron prosthesis: A prospective study of 57 cases. *Am J Sports Med* 1992;20:20-23.
41. Gillquist J, Odensten M: Reconstruction of old anterior cruciate ligament tears with a Dacron prosthesis: A prospective study. *Am J Sports Med* 1993;21:358-366.
42. Barrett GR, Line LL Jr, Sheldon WR, et al: The Dacron ligament prosthesis in anterior cruciate ligament reconstruction: A four-year review. *Am J Sports Med* 1993;21:367-373.
43. Wilk RM, Richmond JC: Dacron ligament reconstruction for chronic anterior cruciate ligament insufficiency. *Am J Sports Med* 1993;21:374-380.
44. Denti M, Arosio A, Monteleone M, et al: Preliminary assessment of anterior cruciate ligament reconstruction with the Leeds-Keio artificial ligament. *Am J Knee Surg* 1990;3:181-186.
45. Fujikawa K, Iseki F, Seedhom BB: Anterior cruciate reconstruction with the Leeds-Keio artificial ligament, in Scott WN (ed): *Ligament and Extensor Mechanism Injuries of the Knee: Diagnosis and Treatment.* St. Louis, MO, Mosby Year Book, 1991, pp 311-318.
46. Schindhelm K, Rogers GJ, Milthorpe BK, et al: Autograft and Leeds-Keio reconstructions of the ovine anterior cruciate ligament. *Clin Orthop* 1991;267:278-293.
47. Goodship AE, Wilcock SA, Shah JS: The development of tissue around various prosthetic implants used as replacements for ligaments and tendons. *Clin Orthop* 1985;196:61-68.
48. Tayton K, Phillips G, Ralis Z: Long-term effects of carbon-fibre on soft tissues. *J Bone Joint Surg* 1982;64B:112-114.
49. Jenkins DHR: The repair of cruciate ligaments with flexible carbon fibre: A longer term study of the induction of new ligaments and of the fate of the implanted carbon. *J Bone Joint Surg* 1978;60B:520-522.
50. Mendes DG, Iusim M, Angel D, et al: Histologic pattern of biomechanic properties of the carbon fiber-augmented ligament tendon: A laboratory and clinical study. *Clin Orthop* 1985;196:51-60.
51. Mäkisalo S, Paavolainen P, Holmstrom T: Carbon fiber as a prosthetic anterior cruciate ligament: A biochemical and histological analysis in pigs. *Am J Sports Med* 1989;17:459-462.
52. Mäkisalo S, Skutnabb K, Holmstrom T, et al: Reconstruction of anterior cruciate ligament with carbon fiber: An experimental study on pigs. *Am J Sports Med* 1988;16:589-593.
53. Strover AE, Firer P: The use of carbon-fiber implants in anterior cruciate ligament surgery. *Clin Orthop* 1985;196:88-98.

54. Rushton N, Dandy DJ, Naylor CPE: The clinical, arthroscopic and histological findings after replacement of the anterior cruciate ligament with carbon-fibre. *J Bone Joint Surg* 1983;65B:308-309.
55. Weiss AB, Blazina ME, Goldstein AR: Ligament replacement with an absorbable copolymer carbon-fiber scaffold: Early clinical experience. *Clin Orthop* 1985;196:77-85.
56. Penny JN: The role of synthetics in ACL surgery. Presented at the University of British Columbia, October 17, 1992.
57. Fowler PJ, Capra SW Jr: Anterior cruciate ligament reconstruction with the Kennedy ligament augmentation device, in Scott WN (ed): *Ligament and Extensor Mechanism Injuries of the Knee: Diagnosis and Treatment.* St. Louis, MO, Mosby Year Book, 1991, pp 301-310.
58. Roth JH, Kennedy JC, Lockstadt H, et al: Polypropylene braid augmented and nonaugmented intraarticular anterior cruciate ligament reconstruction. *Am J Sports Med* 1985;13:321-336.
59. Del Pizzo W: U.S. Kennedy LAD Clinical Experience. Presented at the Sixth International Symposium on Advances in Cruciate Ligament Reconstruction of the Knee. Los Angeles, CA, March 3-5, 1989.
60. Olson EJ, Kang JD, Fu FH, et al: The biochemical and histological effects of artificial ligament wear particles: In vivo and in vitro studies. *Am J Sports Med* 1988;16:558-570.
61. Berns GS, Howell SM: Roofplasty requirements in vitro for different tibial hole placement in anterior cruciate ligament reconstruction. *Am J Sports Med* 1993;21:292-298.
62. Howell SM: Arthroscopic roofplasty: A method for correcting an extension deficit caused by roof impingement of an anterior cruciate ligament graft. *Arthroscopy* 1992;8:375-379.
63. Howell SM: Roof impingement of ACL grafts: Diagnosis, cause, prevention, and late surgical correction, in Feagin J Jr (ed): *The Cruciate Ligaments: Diagnosis and Treatment of Ligamentous Injuries About the Knee,* ed 2. New York, NY, Churchill Livingstone, 1994, pp 637-648.
64. Gristina AG, Naylor PT, Myrvik QN: Molecular mechanisms of musculoskeletal sepsis, in Esterhai JL Jr, Gristina AG, Poss R (eds): *Musculoskeletal Infection.* Park Ridge, IL, American Academy of Orthopaedic Surgeons, 1992, pp 13-28.
65. Maday MG, Harner CD, Fu FH: Revision ACL surgery: Evaluation and treatment, in Feagin JA Jr (ed): *The Crucial Ligaments: Diagnosis and Treatment of Ligamentous Injuries About the Knee,* ed 2. New York, NY, Churchill Livingstone, 1994, pp 711-728.
66. Kurosaka M, Yoshiya S, Andrish JT: A biomechanical comparison of different surgical techniques of graft fixation in anterior cruciate ligament reconstruction. *Am J Sports Med* 1987;15:225-229.
67. Paschal SO, Seemann MD, Ashman RB, et al: Interference fixation versus postfixation of bone-patellar tendon-bone grafts for anterior cruciate ligament reconstruction: A biomechanical comparative study in porcine knees. *Clin Orthop* 1994;300:281-287.
68. Steadman JR, Seemann MD: ACL injuries in the elite skier, in Feagin JA Jr (ed): *The Crucial Ligaments: Diagnosis and Treatment of Ligamentous Injuries About the Knee,* ed 2. New York, NY, Churchill Livingstone, 1994, pp 759-772.

CHAPTER 38

The Anatomic and Surgical Considerations for Posterior Cruciate Ligament Reconstruction

Mark D. Miller, MD
Christopher D. Harner, MD

Introduction

The posterior cruciate ligament (PCL) has been a topic of keen interest in orthopaedic surgery recently. Perhaps this is because injuries to this ligament are being recognized with increasing frequency, and recent long-term follow-up studies have suggested that nonoperative treatment is not as "benign" as once believed.[1,2] A myriad of surgical procedures for reconstruction of the PCL have been proposed over the years, many with a nonanatomic basis.[3-5] Because we feel that most successful orthopaedic procedures are based on reproducing normal anatomy, comprehensive anatomic and biomechanical studies were completed at the University of Pittsburgh over the past several years to first define the normal characteristics of the PCL, and then to develop surgical procedures in an attempt to reproduce these characteristics. In this article, we will first review the functional anatomy of the PCL, discuss the gross and microscopic anatomy, review the relevant biomechanics, and then attempt to apply these principles to surgical reconstruction of the PCL.

Anatomy

Functional Anatomy

The PCL serves two major functions: (1) It is a primary restraint against posterior tibial displacement,[6] and (2) it works in conjunction with the anterior cruciate ligament to regulate the "screw home" mechanism of the knee.[7,8]

The PCL is located near the center axis of the knee and is composed of two components—a thick anterolateral portion and a smaller posteromedial portion (Fig. 1). These components are named based on their relative positions at their respective insertions (ie, the anterolateral portion of the PCL is more anterior at its origin on the medial femoral condyle, and more lateral in its insertion in the fovea of the tibia).[9] The anterolateral component is tight in flexion and relatively lax in extension. The posteromedial component (more posterior at the medial femoral condyle and medial at the tibia) is tight in extension and relatively lax in flexion (Fig. 2).[10,11]

In addition to the two components, there are two variable meniscofemoral ligaments: (1) anterior (ligament of Humphry) and (2) posterior (ligament of Wrisberg) (Fig. 3). Although the size of these ligaments is highly variable, they average approximately 20% the size of the PCL.[12] The reported presence of these two ligaments is also quite variable in the literature; most knees will have one or the other but rarely both.[13,14] The meniscofemoral ligaments serve as a secondary restraint to posterior tibial translation. In fact, with less severe injuries to the PCL, the presence of these ligaments may obscure the examination and make the diagnosis more difficult.

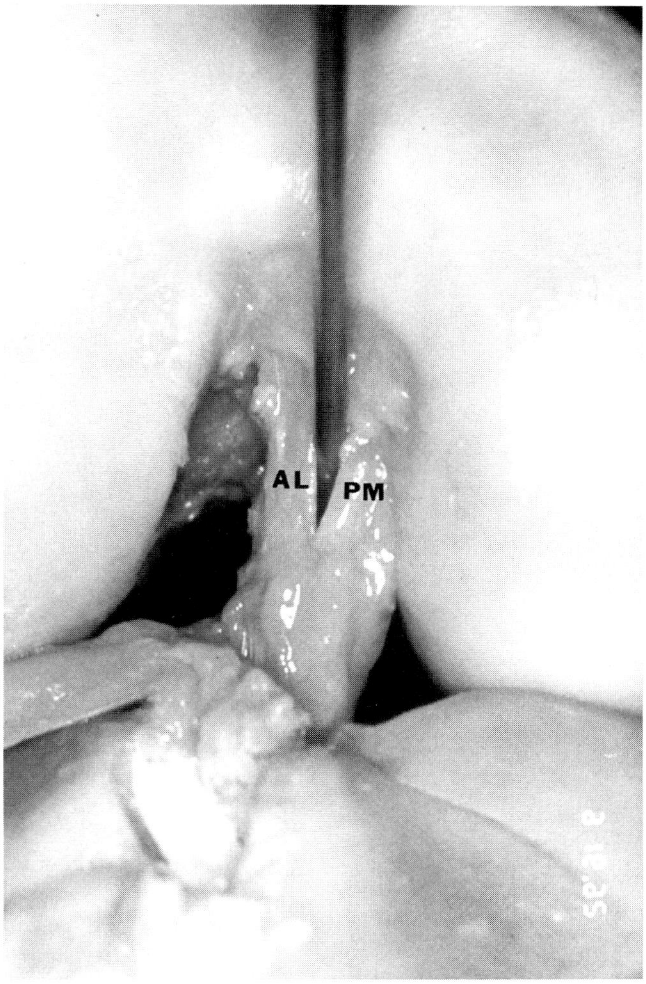

Fig. 1 Dissection specimen showing the anterolateral (AL) and posteromedial (PM) components of the PCL. (Reproduced with permission from Miller MD, Johnson DL, Harner CD, et al: Posterior cruciate ligament injuries. *Orthop Rev* 1993;22:1201-1210.)

Neurovascular Anatomy

The primary blood supply to both cruciate ligaments is via branches of the middle geniculate artery.[15] The

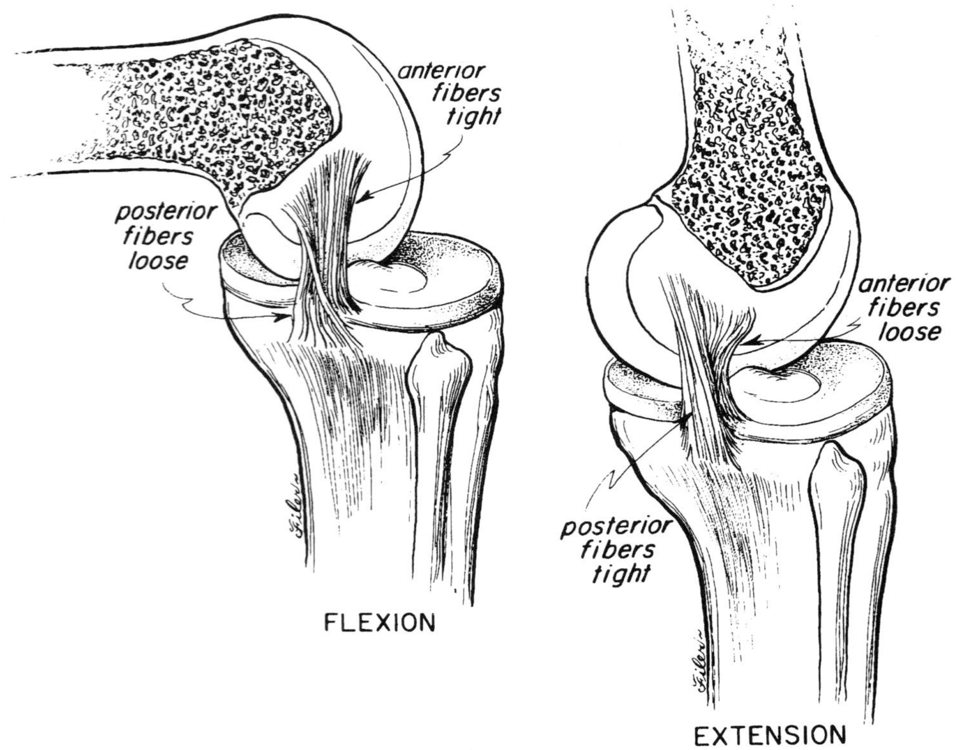

Fig. 2 Illustration demonstrating tensioning of different components of the PCL during range of motion. **Left**, Note tension in the anterolateral portion of the PCL in flexion, and **Right**, tensioning of the posteromedial portion in extension. (Reproduced with permission from Girgis FG, Marshall JL, Monajem A: The cruciate ligaments of the knee joint: Anatomical, functional, and experimental analysis. *Clin Orthop* 1975;106:216-231.)

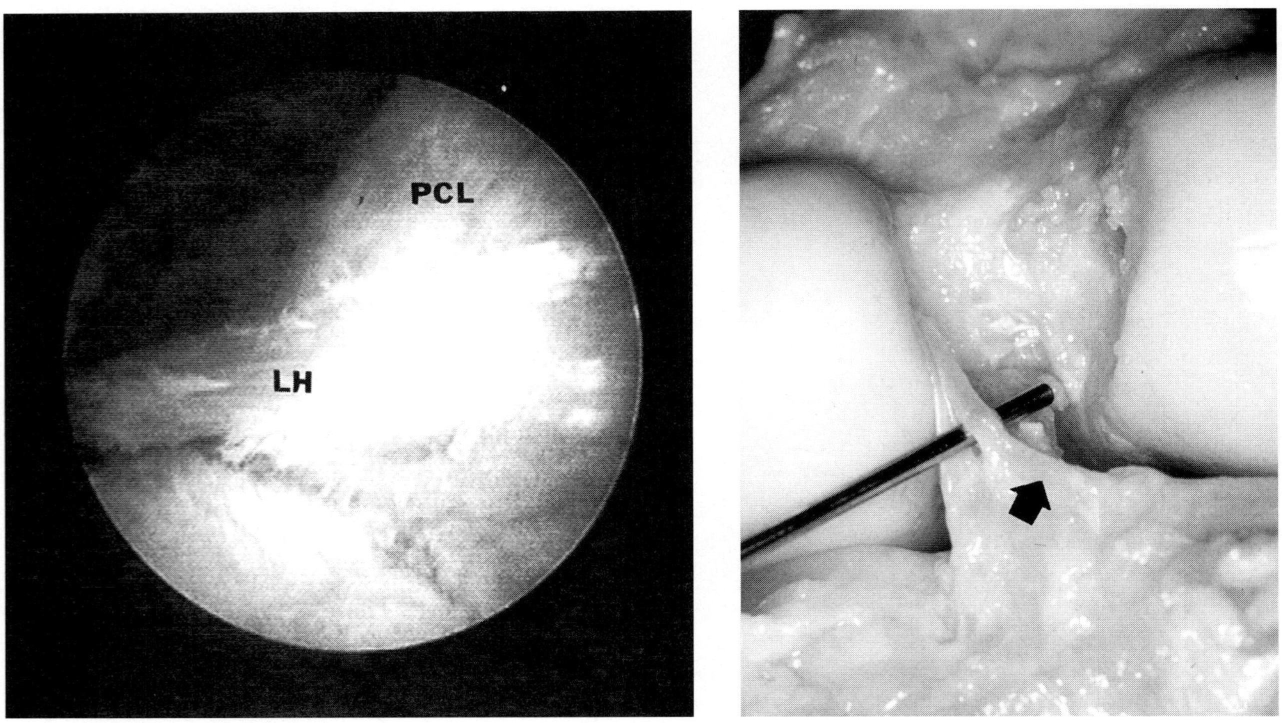

Fig. 3 Meniscofemoral ligaments. **Left,** Arthroscopic view of the anterior meniscofemoral ligament, or ligament of Humphry (LH). **Right,** Dissection specimen showing the posterior meniscofemoral ligament or ligament of Wrisberg (arrow).

nerve supply to the PCL is via the posterior articular branch of the posterior tibial nerve.[16] Although little is known regarding the function of nerves in the cruciates, receptor organs that have been identified (primarily at the femoral origin of the ligaments) are thought to have a proprioceptive function.[17]

Cross-Sectional Anatomy

In order to define the in-vivo size and shape of the cruciate ligaments, a laser micrometer was used to measure their cross-sectional dimensions at various locations.[12] The results of this study of fresh frozen cadavers revealed that the PCL is approximately 1.5 times as large as the ACL at the femoral and midsubstance levels. There was no statistically significant difference between the ACL and PCL at the tibial level. Further, these studies demonstrated that the cross-sectional area did not change with knee motion. Finally, the PCL increased in size from the tibial to the femoral insertion, and the ACL demonstrated the exact opposite trend (Fig. 4).

Insertion Site Anatomy

According to Girgis, the PCL has a broad femoral origin that forms a semicircle on the medial femoral condyle with an average width of 32 mm.[11] Its tibial insertion lies in a depression (fovea) 1 cm below the medial tibial articular surface (Fig. 5). The ligament is oriented vertically in the frontal plane and angles forward 30° to 45° in the sagittal plane (depending on the amount of knee flexion).[14]

In order to better characterize the insertion site anatomy of the cruciate ligaments, a three-dimensional digitizing system, nicknamed "the bird" was used to perform insertion site mapping.[18] The results of this study demonstrated that the insertion sites were approximately three to four times the cross-sectional area of the ACL and PCL in their midsubstance.[18] These findings led to further investigation of the ligaments' ultrastructural make-up.

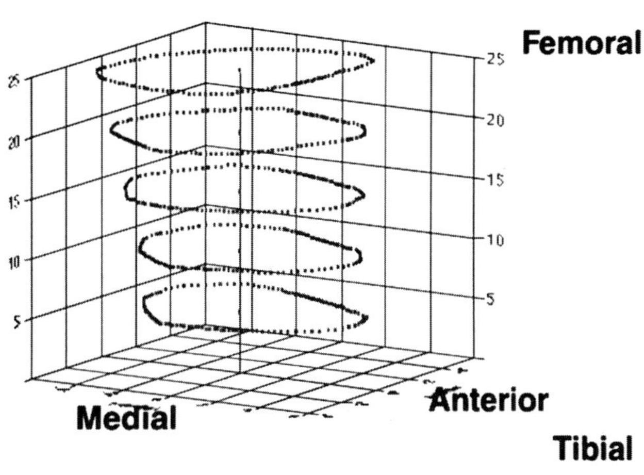

Fig. 4 Cross-sectional area of the PCL.

Ultrastructural Morphology

Like all ligaments, the PCL is composed primarily of type I collagen with variable amounts of elastin and reticulin. The sinusoidal collagen pattern, called "crimp," has less amplitude in the cruciate ligaments than in the medial collateral ligament.[19] Light microscopy fails to reveal any other significant differences between the cruciate ligaments.

Quantitative electron microscopy of the cruciate and meniscofemoral ligaments was carried out in order to help explain the relative differences in cross-sectional and insertion site anatomy (Fig. 6).[20] In this study of young (20- to 22-year-old) fresh cadaver ligaments, the mean collagen fibril cross-sectional area was found to vary from the femoral to the tibial insertion sites.

The PCL fibrils increased from the tibial to the femoral insertion; the ACL showed the opposite trend. These findings correlated with our laser cross-sectional study. The meniscofemoral ligaments demonstrated the largest collagen fibrils, and these did not vary in size from the tibia to femur. It appears then that each cruciate ligament demonstrates a unique gross and ultrastructural morphology. These differences may help explain their biomechanical differences. In addition, commonly used graft substitutes (patellar tendon, semitendinosis, Achilles tendon allograft) may not demonstrate these patterns, making them less than ideal for ligament reconstruction. Future research should be directed to address more accurate reproductions of the gross and ultrastructural morphology of the cruciate ligaments.

Ligament Biomechanics

The PCL is the primary restraint to posterior tibial translation, sustaining from 85% to almost 100% of the load at 90° of flexion.[6,21,22] Posterior laxity of 4 to 5 mm is seen with the application of a 100 N posterior force.[8,21] Isolated loss of the PCL results in an increase in posterior laxity, with the maximum being 15 to 20 mm at 90° of flexion.[6,8,21]

Tensile studies of the PCL have yielded imprecise results and have led to such general statements as "The PCL is twice as strong as the ACL."[23] Because there are actually three components to the PCL (ie, the anterolateral, posteromedial, and meniscofemoral ligaments), we feel that it is important to understand the relative structural and mechanical properties of each. In order to investigate this, nine fresh frozen human cadaver knees were studied.[24] The results of these studies demonstrated that each component had unique biomechanical properties. The anterolateral portion of the PCL was significantly stronger than the posteromedial portion (1,600 vs 450 N). The meniscofemoral ligaments had an ultimate yield strength of approximately 350 N. Additionally, the linear stiffness of the antero-

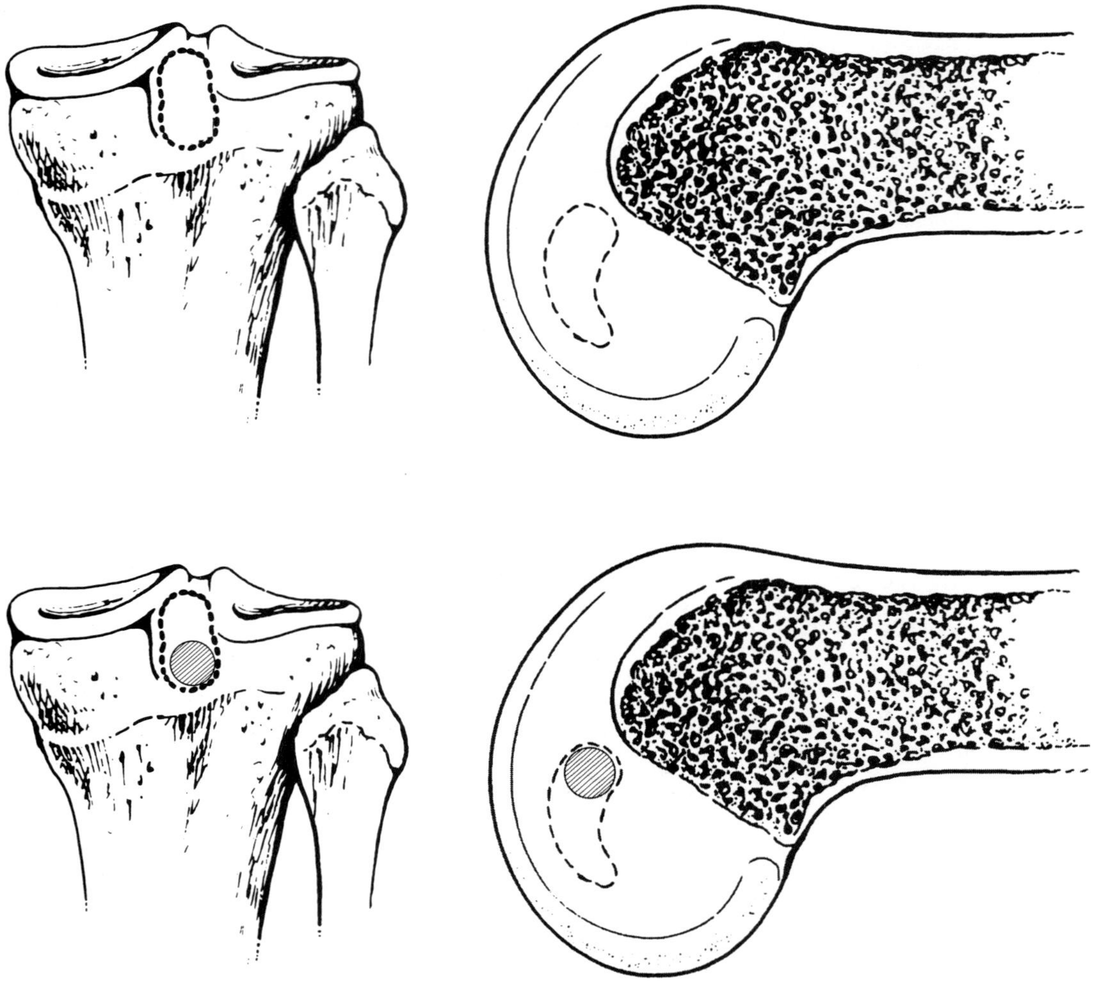

Fig. 5 Origin and insertion site anatomy for the PCL. (Reproduced with permission from Miller MD, Johnson DL, Harner CD, et al: Posterior cruciate ligament injuries. *Orthop Rev* 1993;22:1201-1210.)

lateral component was significantly higher than those of the posteromedial component and the meniscofemoral ligament. The modulus of elasticity (stiffness) of both the anterolateral component and meniscofemoral ligament were significantly greater than that of the posteromedial component.[24] Because the anterolateral component has superior biomechanical properties, we feel it has a more important role in controlling knee kinematics. This becomes important with respect to the surgical technique used to reconstruct the PCL.

Other Considerations

Significant bending around the tibial tunnel will undoubtedly affect graft pressure and tension (Fig. 7, Table 1).[25] However, the full implications of this work with regard to vascular ingrowth and cellular repopulation is still unknown. The proper amount of tension to apply to the graft prior to fixation is another unknown. Most authors indicate that the graft should be pulled taut or tensioned prior to fixation.[26,27]

Pretesting or "preloading" of PCL grafts has been advocated by many surgeons. This is frequently done by placing the prepared graft in a tensioning device on the back table before it is inserted into the knee. This has the theoretical advantage of avoiding late "stretching out" of the graft in situ. However, optimum prefixation tension has not been characterized.[26] The tension in the graft decreases within minutes by stress relaxation.[28] Additionally, there have been reports of decreased vascularization of autografts with higher levels of graft tensioning.[29] Despite the lack of proven efficacy and risks associated with autograft pretensioning, allograft pretensioning with cyclic stretching (practically done by repeated in situ range of motion prior to graft fixation) may help eliminate the histological crimping that occurs in the freezing process.[30]

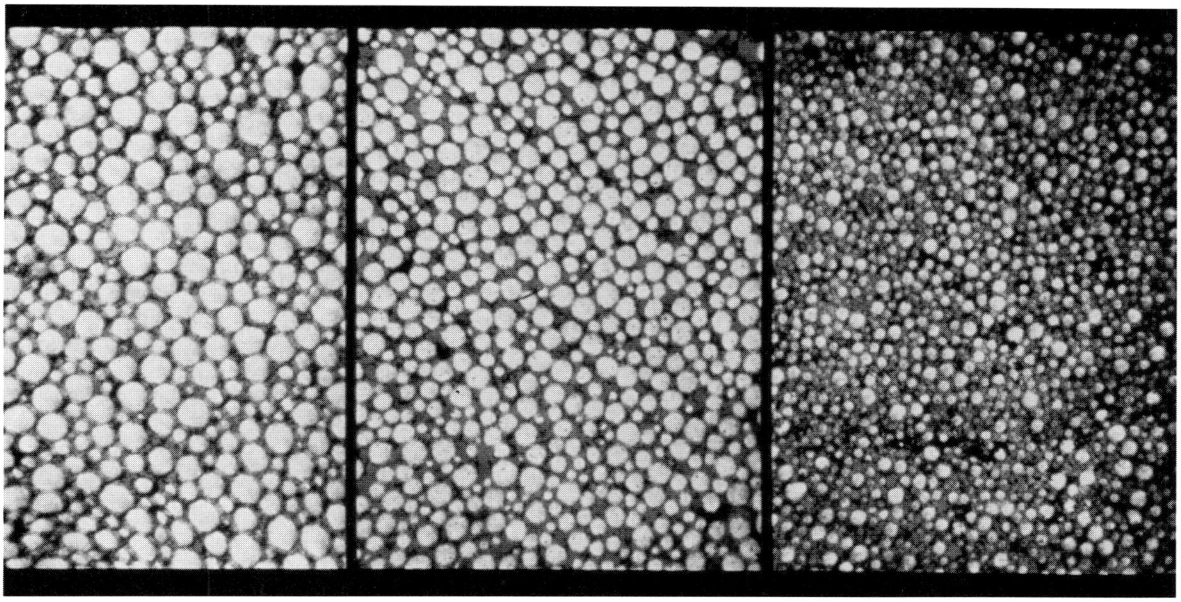

Fig. 6 Electron microscopy of **(left)** ACL, **(center)** PCL, **(right)** Meniscofemoral ligaments.

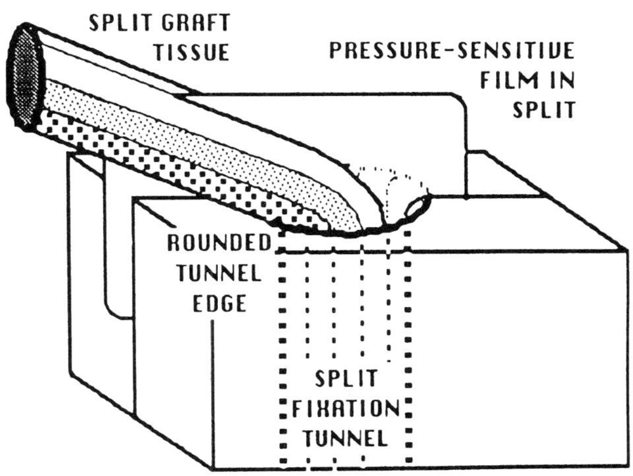

Fig. 7 Experimental set-up for measurement of internal graft pressures. (Reproduced with permission from Sidles JA, Clark JM, Garbini JL: A geometric theory of the equilibrium mechanics of fibers in ligaments and tendons. *J Biomech* 1991;24:943-949.)

Current Techniques

Rationale

We feel that restoration of the normal anatomy yields the most consistent results. It is because of this belief that current research has been directed to defining the normal anatomy and developing surgical techniques to recreate this anatomy. With current grafts and techniques, it is possible to accurately reconstruct only one of the two bundles of the PCL. We choose to attempt to reproduce the anterolateral bundle because it is anatomically and biomechanically a more substantial structure.[24] In doing so, it is critical that the surgeon visualize the entire insertion site of the ligament on the tibia and femur and position the tunnels in the anterior half of the PCL femoral insertion and the distal and lateral portion of the tibial insertion. We also have attempted to reduce graft bending by locating the junction of the graft and bone plug flush with the posterior cortex of the tibia (Fig. 8, *top*). This results in graft orientation similar to the normal PCL without excess bending at the tunnel interface (Fig. 8, *center* and *bottom*). Other techniques, developed in conjunction with intensive laboratory research, will be described in detail below. Because of its high tensile strength, ease of passage, and lack of donor site morbidity, we currently favor Achilles tendon allograft for use in PCL reconstruction. However,

Table 1
Experimental measurements and theoretical predictions of internal pressures

		Maximal Internal Pressure	
Load (N)	Bending angle (°)	Experiment	Theory
50	45	0.6 Mpa	0.6 Mpa
50	90	0.9	1.0
100	45	1.3	1.3
100	90	1.7	2.0

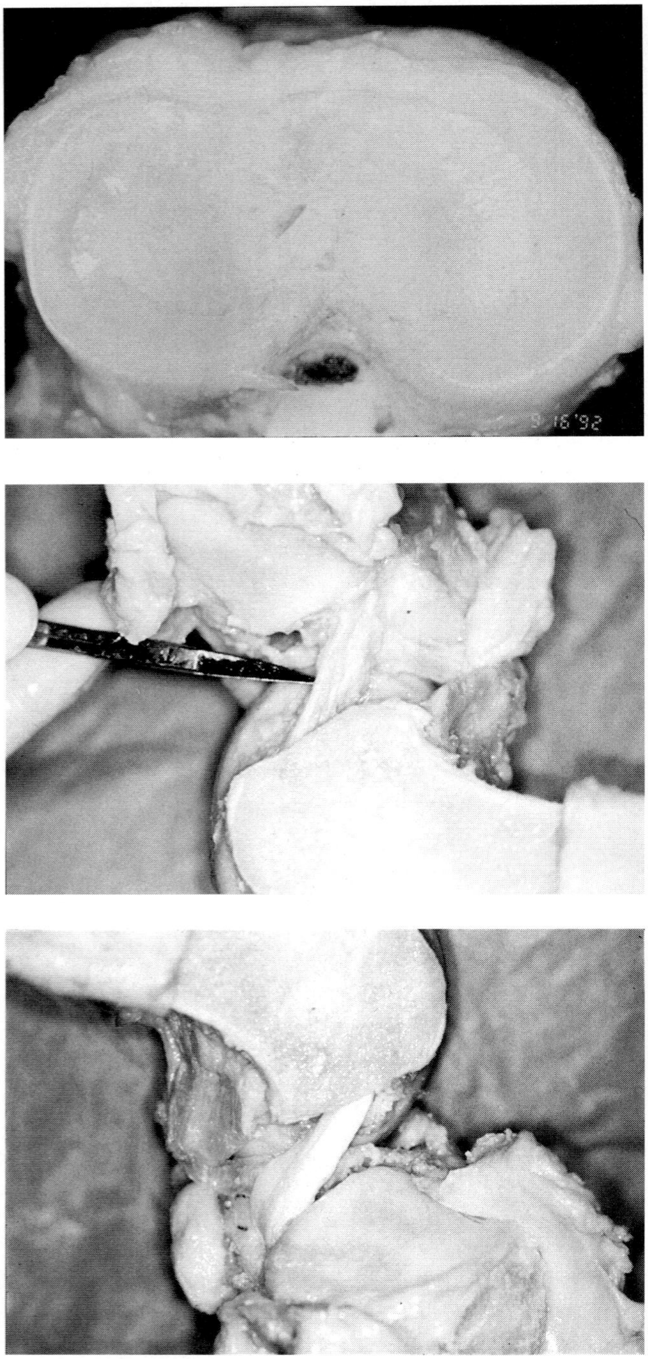

Fig. 8 **Top,** Axial view of bone plug (painted dark) flush with posterior tibial cortex. **Center,** Normal orientation of PCL. **Bottom,** Orientation of PCL graft.

patellar tendon allograft or autograft may also be used. Although there is a theoretical risk of disease transmission associated with allograft use, the risk of receiving an HIV-infected soft-tissue allograft has been estimated to be 1:1,667,700.[31] Current screening techniques, combined with irradiation, theoretically reduces this risk even further. Allografts are procured in accordance with standards outlined by the American Association of Tissue Banks (AATB).[32]

Following successful induction of anesthesia, we perform a thorough examination, focusing particularly on the posterior drawer test. The degree of displacement and the quality of the endpoint is noted. Of critical importance is palpation of the anteromedial tibial plateau "step-off." If no step-off is present and the anterior tibial crest is flush with the medial and lateral femoral condyles, then there is at least a 2+ posterior drawer present. If the tibia is subluxed posterior to the medial femoral condyle, it is considered to be a 3+ posterior drawer. When even a 3+ posterior drawer is present, it is critical to rule out concomitant pathological posterolateral rotatory laxity. If present, then a posterolateral procedure is also indicated.

Surgical Technique

Examination under anesthesia, followed by arthroscopic preparation of the intercondylar notch, is performed first. It is important to note that the normal anterior cruciate ligament (ACL) will appear to be lax in PCL-injured knees. This "pseudolaxity" is caused by tibial subluxation posteriorly when the knee is flexed 90°. This phenomenon, along with the impression of PCL being intact arthroscopically (due to "healing" behind the ACL) may lead the inexperienced surgeon to proceed with unnecessary ACL reconstruction in PCL-injured knees.

The allograft or autograft is prepared to fit a 10 to 12 mm tunnel. It is important to fashion the soft-tissue end of the Achilles tendon allograft as tight as possible so that it will not bind during passage (Fig. 9). Debridement of the tibial attachment site of the torn PCL is carried out with the arthroscope in the anterolateral portal. Although a 30° arthroscope can be used in certain situations (larger knees and knees with altered anatomy), we routinely use a 70° scope to visualize the PCL insertion on the tibia. A posteromedial portal is utilized for debridement of the tibial insertion site with a full radius resector. In addition, a 30° arthroscope can be placed in this portal to further define the insertion site anatomy.

The tibial drill guide is inserted through the anteromedial portal and is placed in the posterolateral aspect of the tibial insertion. Careful attention is paid to the slope of the tibial guide pin. We have found that this slope is approximated by a line that is parallel to the slope of the proximal tibia-fibula joint. Ideally, the pin should exit at the junction of the middle and distal one third of the posterior slope of the posterior tibial eminence. The starting point of the anterior tibia is usually 1 to 2 cm below and 2 to 3 cm medial to the tibial tubercle. The pin should also be parallel to the posterior tibial cortex. A 3-cm skin incision is made for the tibial drill. The periosteum is incised and carefully elevated with an osteotome. The pin is inserted using

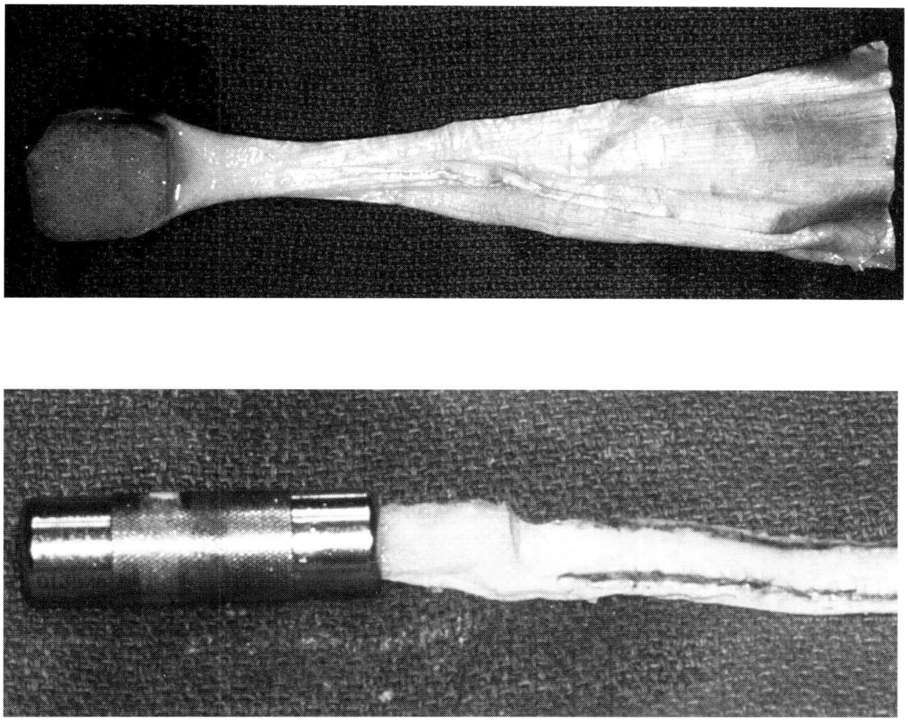

Fig. 9 Achilles tendon allograft (**top**) prior to and (**bottom**) following preparation.

drill guides designed for placement of PCL tunnels (Linvatec, Accufex). The guide wire is placed under direct arthroscopic visualization. After drilling the guide pin (3⁄32 inch) an intraoperative lateral radiograph is taken to evaluate placement of the pin (Fig. 10, *left*). After insuring that the pin is placed correctly, a 10 to 12 mm cannulated drill is used to create the tibial tunnel (Fig. 10, *right*). In order to protect the posterior neurovascular structures, the surgeon must exercise extreme care in completing the tibial tunnel. We routinely finish the tunnel by hand, and often will place an elevator or curette through the posteromedial portal behind the guide pin.

Placement of the femoral tunnel is technically easier, because the insertion site is readily identifiable with a 30° arthroscope. After identifying the insertion, a 3⁄32 inch guide wire is passed through the anterior half of the femoral insertion. This wire exits approximately 5 to 10 mm from the intra-articular cartilage of the medial femoral condyle. It is helpful to aim the guide wire toward the tibial insertion when drilling outside the knee (Fig. 11, *left*). A 3-cm skin incision centered over the medial femoral condyle is made after marking the ideal location with a commercially available ACL drill guide. On the extra-articular side of the femoral condyle, the K-wire should exit approximately 1.0 to 1.5 cm from the articular cartilage margin to avoid disrupting the subchondral bone. After the K-wire is passed (radiography is not necessary), a 10- to 11-mm cannulated drill is used to create the tunnel (Fig. 11, *right*). To avoid potential damage to the subchondral bone, we do not routinely use a 12-mm drill bit in this area.

A looped 18-gauge wire is inserted from the femoral tunnel and brought out the tibial tunnel to facilitate graft placement. We then carefully pass the graft from the tibia to the femur with the bone plug remaining in the tibia. Ideally, the bone plug should be advanced until its proximal edge is flush with the cortex of the posterior tibia prior to graft fixation. We have found in the lab that this results in the least amount of graft bending.

The tibial side of the graft is fixed with an interference screw that secures the bone block within the tibial tunnel. The knee is then checked for stability or pretensioning of the graft. The arthroscope can be used to check the position of the bone block within the tunnel.

The soft-tissue end of the graft can be fixed with a variety of techniques. Several studies have shown that fixation with a screw and spiked washer is the most secure fixation attainable when interference fixation is not possible.[33,34] We have recently developed a technique that allows interference fixation of soft tissue within bony tunnels, and we use this technique to fix the femoral tunnel in PCL reconstructions. On the back table we fashion a cortical-cancellous plug, which is inserted into the interval between the soft tissue and the tunnel periphery. The plug is placed snugly into the tunnel (sometimes a tamp is helpful to secure it), and an interference screw is inserted in the standard fash-

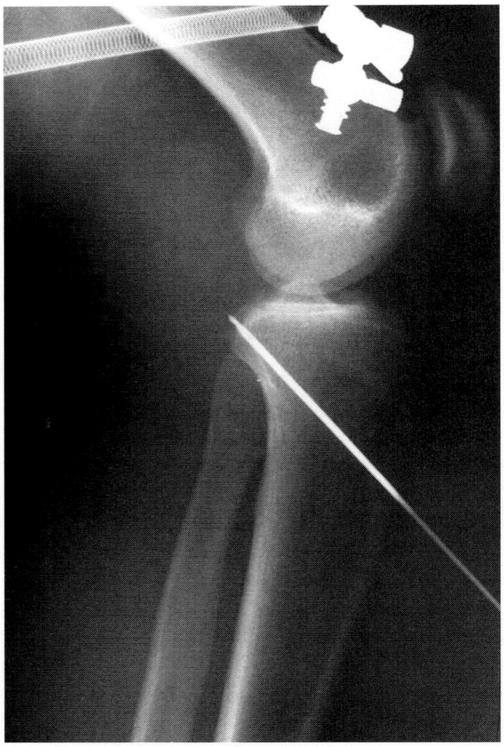

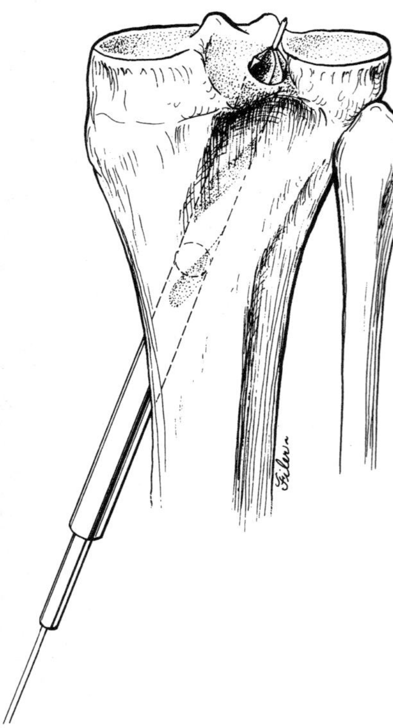

Fig. 10 **Left,** Lateral radiograph taken intraoperative to verify position of tibial tunnel prior to drilling. **Right,** Artist depiction of tibial tunnel preparation. Note location in lateral aspect of PCL "footprint."

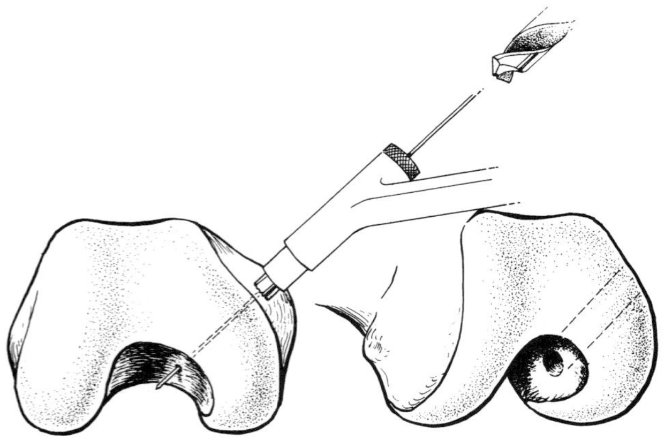

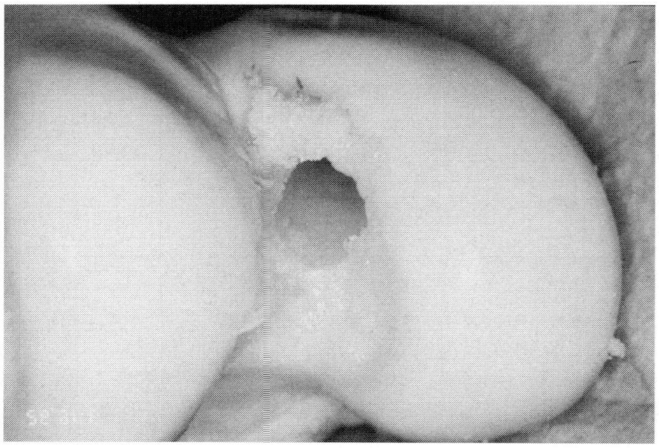

Fig. 11 **Left,** Femoral tunnel preparation. **Right,** Cadaver model demonstrating completed femoral tunnel.

ion (Fig. 12). Because we are unsure about the long-term stability of this method of fixation, we often supplement this with a screw and soft-tissue washer or a staple.

Although the ideal amount of tension that should be applied to the graft prior to fixation is unknown, we feel that it is important to reestablish the normal "step off" of the tibial plateau prior to final graft fixation. We routinely position the knee in 70° to 80° of flexion and apply 5 to 10 lbs of tension before we fix the femoral attachment of the graft as described above. The knee is flexed during fixation because the anterolateral bundle (which we attempt to reproduce) is under maximum tension in this position and, therefore, the risk of overtensioning the graft is reduced. After securing the graft, excess graft is removed and the knee is placed through a range of motion and tested for stability. The graft is also viewed arthroscopically prior to closure. The periosteum and subcutaneous tissues are closed in layers, with absorbable sutures, and a drain is placed

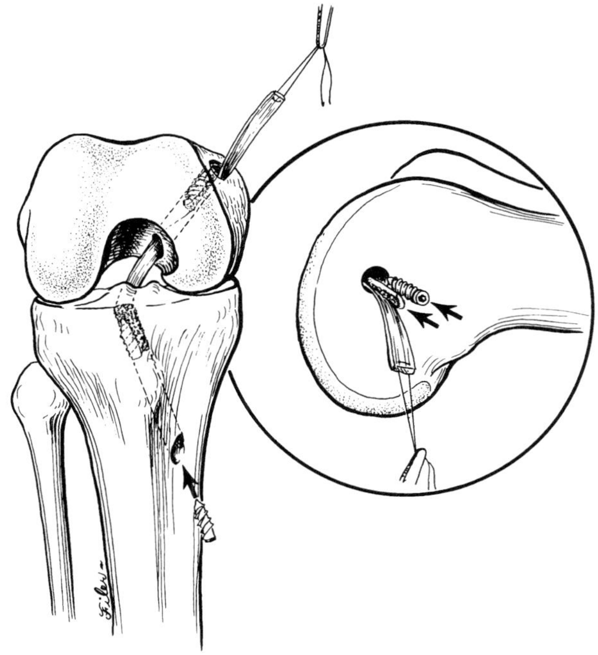

Fig. 12 Composite drawing demonstrating current technique and method of fixation in the femoral tunnel. (Reproduced with permission from Miller MD, Johnson DL, Harner CD, et al: Posterior cruciate ligament injuries. *Orthop Rev* 1993;22:1201-1210.)

between the layers. Dry sterile dressings, a brace, and a cold compression device are applied. Radiographs can be taken intraoperatively or postoperatively (Fig. 13).

Postoperatively, the knee is placed in a hinged knee brace, which is initially locked in extension. The tibia is supported posteriorly to prevent posterior sag. Range of motion exercises and continuous passive motion are started soon after surgery. The patient ambulates with crutch assistance. In the early rehabilitation period, emphasis is placed on avoiding posterior tibial translation, and therapists play an active role in controlling the leg during the early rehabilitation period.

Future Directions

It is difficult to determine if our technique for PCL reconstruction is any real improvement over the numerous other surgical techniques described in the literature. Our belief that reconstruction of the normal anatomy is an important consideration in knee ligament reconstruction led to the development of our current techniques, techniques that have been, and will continue to be, modified as our appreciation of the anatomy of the human PCL evolves. Several initiatives are now underway to better define the ultrastructure of the PCL and to identify the ideal graft for reconstruction of this ligament. Additionally, in our laboratory, we are actively investigating the role of the PCL in knee kinematics. We hope that continued research will yield improvements in grafts, techniques, and materials.

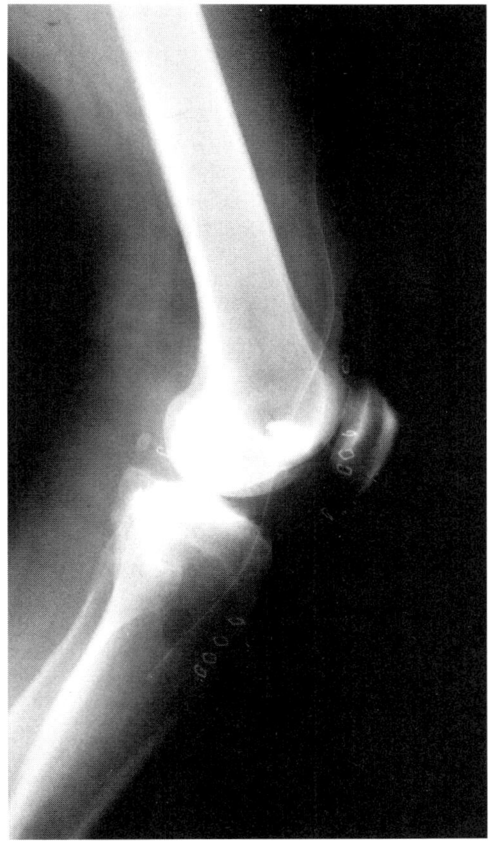

Fig. 13 Postoperative radiograph of PCL reconstruction case.

References

1. Dejour H, Walch G, Peyrot J, et al: The natural history of rupture of the PCL. *French J Orthop Surg* 1988;2:112-120.
2. Keller PM, Shelbourne KD, McCarroll JR, et al: Nonoperatively treated isolated posterior cruciate ligament injuries. *Am J Sports Med* 1993;21:132-136.
3. Hughston JC, Degenhardt TC: Reconstruction of the posterior cruciate ligament. *Clin Orthop* 1982;164:59-77.
4. McCormick WC, Bagg RJ, Kennedy CW Jr, et al: Reconstruction of the posterior cruciate ligament: Preliminary report of a new procedure. *Clin Orthop* 1976;118:30-31.
5. Wirth CJ, Jager M: Dynamic double tendon replacement of the posterior cruciate ligament. *Am J Sports Med* 1984;12:39-43.
6. Butler DL, Noyes FR, Grood ES: Ligamentous restraints to anterior-posterior drawer in the human knee: A biomechanical study. *J Bone Joint Surg* 1980;62A:259-270.
7. Detenbeck LC: Function of the cruciate ligaments in knee stability. *J Sports Med* 1974;2:217-221.
8. Fukubayashi T, Torzilli PA, Sherman MF, et al: An in vitro biomechanical evaluation of anterior-posterior motion of the knee: Tibial displacement, rotation, and torque. *J Bone Joint Surg* 1982;64A:258-264.

9. Hughston JC, Bowden JA, Andrews JR, et al: Acute tears of the posterior cruciate ligament: Results of operative treatment. *J Bone Joint Surg* 1980;62A:438-450.
10. Brantigan OC, Voshell AF: The mechanics of the ligaments and menisci of the knee joint. *J Bone Joint Surg* 1941;23:44-66.
11. Girgis FG, Marshall JL, Monajem A: The cruciate ligaments of the knee joint: Anatomical, functional and experimental analysis. *Clin Orthop* 1975;106:216-231.
12. Harner CD, Livesay GA, Choi NY, et al: Evaluation of the sizes and shapes of the human anterior and posterior cruciate ligaments: A comparative study. *Trans Orthop Res Soc* 1992;17:123.
13. Heller L, Langman J: The menisco-femoral ligaments of the human knee. *J Bone Joint Surg* 1964;46B:307-313.
14. Van Dommelen BA, Fowler PJ: Anatomy of the posterior cruciate ligament: A review. *Am J Sports Med* 1989;17:24-29.
15. Scapinelli R: Studies on the vasculature of the human knee joint. *Acta Anat (Basel)* 1968;70:305-331.
16. Kennedy JC, Alexander IJ, Hayes KC: Nerve supply of the human knee and its functional importance. *Am J Sports Med* 1982;10:329-335.
17. Johansson H, Sjolander P, Sojka P: A sensory role for the cruciate ligaments. *Clin Orthop* 1991;268:161-178.
18. Harner CD, Kashiwaguchi S, Livesay GA, et al: Insertion site anatomy of the human anterior and posterior cruciate ligaments. *Trans Orthop Res Soc* 1993;18:341.
19. Amiel D, Billings E Jr, Akeson WH: Ligament structure, chemistry, and physiology, in Daniel DM, Akeson WH, O'Connor JJ (eds): *Knee Ligaments: Structure, Function, Injury, and Repair.* New York, NY, Raven Press, 1990, pp 77-91.
20. Marks PH, Harner CD, Livesay GA, et al: Quantitative electron microscopy of the human cruciate and meniscofemoral ligaments. *Trans Orthop Res Soc* 1994;19:604.
21. Gollehon DL, Torzilli PA, Warren RF: The role of the posterolateral and cruciate ligaments in the stability of the human knee: A biomechanical study. *J Bone Joint Surg* 1987;69A:233-242.
22. Piziali RL, Seering WP, Nagel DA, et al: The function of the primary ligaments of the knee in anterior-posterior and medial-lateral motions. *J Biomech* 1980;13:777-784.
23. Kennedy JC, Hawkins RJ, Willis RB, et al: Tension studies of human knee ligaments: Yield point, ultimate failure, and disruption of the cruciate and tibial collateral ligaments. *J Bone Joint Surg* 1976;58A:350-355.
24. Harner CD, Kusayama T, Carlin GJ, et al: Structural and mechanical properties of the human posterior cruciate and meniscofemoral ligament. *Trans Orthop Res Soc* 1994;19:629.
25. Sidles JA, Clark JM, Garbini JL: A geometric theory of the equilibrium mechanics of fibers in ligaments and tendons. *J Biomech* 1991;24:943-949.
26. Clancy WG Jr: Repair and reconstruction of the posterior cruciate ligament, in Chapman MW, Madison M (eds): *Operative Orthopaedics.* Philadelphia, PA, 1988, vol 3, pp 1651-1665.
27. Whipple TL, Ellis FD: Posterior cruciate ligament injuries. *Clin Sports Med* 1991;10:515-527.
28. Woo SLY, Adams DJ: The tensile properties of human anterior cruciate ligament (ACL) and ACL graft tissues, in Daniel DM, Akeson WH, O'Connor JJ (eds): *Knee Ligaments: Structure, Function, Injury and Repair.* New York, NY, Raven Press, 1990, pp 279-289.
29. Yoshiya S, Andrish JT, Manley MT, et al: Graft tension in anterior cruciate ligament reconstruction: An in vivo study in dogs. *Am J Sports Med* 1987;15:464-470.
30. Haut RC, Powlison AC: The effects of test environment and cyclic stretching on the failure properties of human patellar tendons. *J Orthop Res* 1990;8:532-540.
31. Buck BE, Malinin TI, Brown MD: Bone transplantation and human immunodeficiency virus: An estimate of risk of acquired immunodeficiency syndromes (AIDS). *Clin Orthop* 1989;240:129-136.
32. American Association of Tissue Banks (ed): *Standards for Tissue Banking,* revised. Arlington, VA, American Association of Tissue Banks, 1987.
33. Daniel DM, Robertson DB, Flood DL, et al: Fixation of soft tissue, in Jackson DW, Drez D Jr (eds): *The Anterior Cruciate Deficient Knee: New Concepts in Ligament Repair.* St. Louis, MO, CV Mosby, 1987, pp 114-126.
34. Robertson DB, Daniel DM, Biden E: Soft tissue fixation to bone. *Am J Sports Med* 1986;14:398-403.

CHAPTER 39

Posterolateral Instability of the Knee

Major Daniel M. Veltri, MD
Russell F. Warren, MD

Acute or chronic isolated posterolateral instability of the knee is uncommon. Posterolateral instability of the knee occurs more commonly in association with an injury to the anterior or posterior cruciate ligament. Recognition of posterolateral instability of the knee is important clinically, as it may affect the treatment of associated ligamentous instabilities. O'Brien and associates[1] noted that failures of reconstructions of the anterior cruciate ligament (ACL) may be a result of unrecognized and untreated posterolateral instability of the knee.

Confusion concerning the diagnosis and treatment of posterolateral instability is caused by the great variety of ligamentous injuries that may be associated with posterolateral injury. It is difficult to isolate the effect of a posterolateral injury on instability of the knee when these combined instability patterns are present. In most reports of posterolateral instability, the majority of patients have had combined ligamentous instabilities. Baker and associates[2] noted 11 tears of the ACL among 17 consecutive patients who had acute posterolateral rotatory instability. Baker and associates[3] also reported a series of 13 consecutive patients who had acute combined posterior cruciate ligament (PCL) and posterolateral instabilities. Hughston and Jacobson[4] noted that 77 of 96 patients who were managed with reconstruction for chronic posterolateral instability had associated instability patterns. In a review of 39 patients who underwent surgical procedures for posterior problems in the knee, Fleming and associates[5] noted that several had combined PCL and posterolateral injuries of the knee. As stated, these associated ligamentous injuries often make it difficult to identify the contribution of a posterolateral injury to overall knee instability.

In this chapter, the anatomy of the posterolateral corner will be described. The resultant instability of the knee from injury to the posterolateral corner will be detailed with a review of selective ligament-cutting studies. This information will be used to correlate the mechanism of injury, symptoms, and physical findings in posterolateral instability of the knee. Thorough knowledge of the anatomy and function of the posterolateral corner will allow accurate diagnosis and treatment of isolated as well as of combined injuries of the posterolateral corner.

Anatomy of the Posterolateral Corner

The principal anatomic structures of the posterolateral corner of the knee include the lateral collateral ligament (LCL), the arcuate ligament, the popliteus tendon, the popliteofibular ligament, the short lateral ligament, the fabellofibular ligament, and the posterolateral part of the capsule. Confusion exists regarding the anatomy of the posterolateral corner because inconsistent terminology has been used to describe the posterolateral structures. When reviewing clinical reports, one must differentiate the arcuate ligament from the arcuate ligament complex. The arcuate ligament is a Y-shaped structure, the lateral limb of which arises from the fibular head and courses over the popliteus muscle. Baker and associates[2] described the arcuate ligament complex as the arcuate ligament, the LCL plus the tendinous and aponeurotic portions of the popliteus, and the lateral head of the gastrocnemius. The variation in terminology used to describe the posterolateral corner is compounded by the fact that there is wide variability in the anatomy of the structures of the posterolateral corner.[6-13]

In an effort to simplify our understanding of the anatomy of the posterolateral corner, Seebacher and associates[9] organized it into three layers. The most superficial layer, layer I, consists of the iliotibial tract and its expansion anteriorly and the superficial portion of the biceps and its expansion posteriorly (Fig. 1). At the level of the distal part of the femur, the peroneal nerve is deep to layer I and lies posterior to the biceps tendon. Layer II is formed anteriorly by the quadriceps retinaculum coursing anterolaterally adjacent to the patella. Posteriorly, layer II is incomplete and is represented by the two patellofemoral ligaments. The proximal patellofemoral ligament joins the terminal fibers of the lateral intermuscular septum. The distal patellofemoral ligament ends posteriorly at the fabella, when the fabella is present, or at the femoral insertion of the posterolateral part of the capsule and the lateral head of the gastrocnemius.

Layer III is the deepest layer of the posterolateral corner and forms the lateral part of the capsule (Fig. 2). The capsular attachment to the periphery of the lateral meniscus is called the coronary ligament. The popliteus tendon passes through a hiatus in the coronary ligament to attach to the femur anterior to the femoral attachment of the LCL. The area of the lateral meniscus with no coronary ligament attachment is called the bare area of the lateral meniscus. Posterior to the overlying iliotibial tract, the capsule divides into two laminae: superficial and deep. The superficial lamina encompasses the LCL. This superficial lamina ends posteriorly at the fabellofibular ligament or the short lateral ligament. When a fabella is present, the fabellofibular ligament will be found coursing parallel to the LCL from the fabella to the fibula, inserting posterior to the insertion of the biceps tendon. Kaplan[6] noted

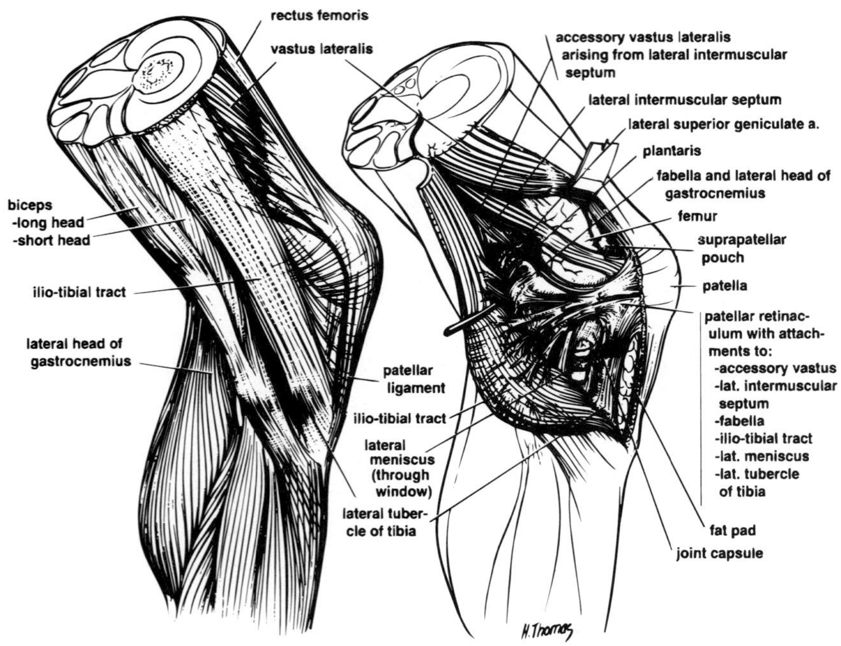

Fig. 1 The anatomy of the posterolateral corner of the knee (layers I and II). (Reproduced with permission from Seebacher JR, Inglis AE, Marshall JL, et al: The structure of the posterolateral aspect of the knee. *J Bone Joint Surg* 1982;64A:536-541.)

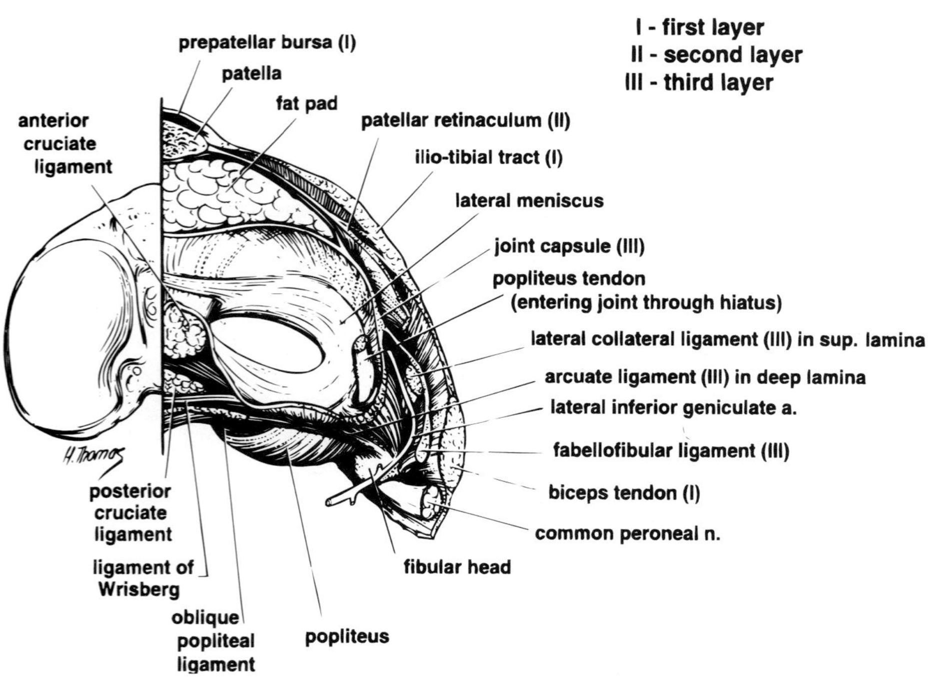

Fig. 2 A coronal section of the anatomy of the posterolateral corner of the knee, including layer III. (Reproduced with permission from Seebacher JR, Inglis AE, Marshall JL, et al: The structure of the posterolateral aspect of the knee. *J Bone Joint Surg* 1982;64A:536-541.)

that, when the fabella is absent, the short lateral ligament may be absent or attenuated. If the short lateral ligament is present, it will be found adjacent to the lateral limb of the arcuate ligament, running from the femoral condylar origin of the lateral head of the gastrocnemius to the fibula.

The lateral inferior geniculate vessels lie between the superficial and the deep laminae of the posterolateral part of the capsule. The deep lamina of the posterolateral part of the capsule passes along the edge of the lateral meniscus to form both the coronary ligament and the hiatus for the popliteus tendon. This inner lamina terminates posteriorly at the Y-shaped arcuate ligament. When present, the arcuate ligament consists of a medial limb that arises from the posterior part of the capsule at the distal part of the femur and courses medially over the popliteus muscle to the oblique popliteal ligament. The lateral limb arises from the posterior part of the capsule and courses laterally over the popliteus muscle and tendon, deep to the lateral inferior geniculate vessels to insert on the posterior part of the fibula.

The final component of layer III is the popliteofibular ligament. It has also been called the popliteofibular fascicle and the fibular origin of the popliteus muscle.[10,12-14] This ligament is found deep to the lateral limb of the arcuate ligament. It arises from the posterior part of the fibula, posterior to the biceps insertion, and courses toward the junction of the popliteus muscle and its tendon. The popliteofibular ligament joins the popliteus tendon just proximal to its musculotendinous junction. We call this structure the popliteofibular ligament because it connects the fibula to the femur through the popliteus tendon. Thus, the popliteus muscle-tendon unit is a Y-shaped structure with a muscle origin from the posterior part of the tibia, a ligamentous origin from the fibula, and a united insertion on the femur (Fig. 3).

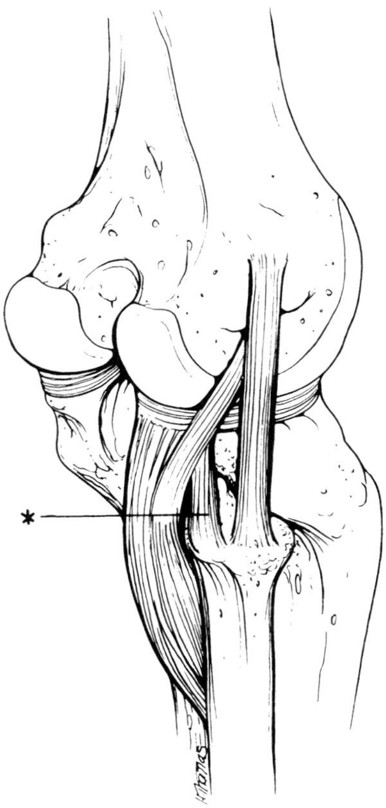

Fig. 3 Arising from the posterior part of the fibula, the popliteofibular ligament joins the popliteus tendon just above the musculotendinous junction.

Variability of the anatomy of the posterolateral corner has been found in cadaveric dissections. In 35 dissections, Seebacher and associates[9] noted that the arcuate ligament alone reinforced the capsule in 13% of knees, the fabellofibular ligament alone reinforced the capsule in 20%, and both of these ligaments reinforced the capsule in the remaining 67%. When a large fabella was present, the fabellofibular ligament was prominent and the arcuate ligament was absent. Conversely, when no fabella was present, the fabellofibular ligament was absent and the arcuate ligament was prominent. Seebacher and associates[9] did not comment on the presence of the popliteofibular ligament.

The anatomy of the posterolateral corner of the knee was also found to be variable in cadaveric dissections by Sudasna and Harnsiriwattanagit[12] as well as by Watanabe and associates.[13] Sudasna and Harnsiriwattanagit dissected 50 cadaveric knees to study the posterolateral anatomy of the knee or the posterolateral corner. The fabellofibular ligament was found in 34 knees (68%) and the short lateral ligament, in two (4%). In 12 knees (24%), the arcuate ligament was found to be a thin membranous structure. The fibular origin of the popliteus, the popliteofibular ligament, was found in 49 knees (98%). Watanabe and associates dissected 115 knees to determine the supporting structures of the posterolateral corner. The LCL and popliteus tendon were found in all knees. They called the popliteofibular ligament the popliteus muscle with origin from the fibular head. This structure was found in 108 of the 115 knees. The posterolateral part of the capsule was reinforced by the popliteofibular ligament and the fabellofibular ligament in 44 knees; by the popliteofibular ligament and the arcuate ligament in 41 knees; by the popliteofibular ligament alone in 14 knees; by a combination of the fabellofibular ligament, the arcuate ligament, and the popliteofibular ligament in nine knees; by the fabellofibular and arcuate ligaments in four knees; by the fabellofibular ligament alone in two knees; and by the arcuate ligament alone in one knee. These cadaveric dissections showed that the fibular attachment of the popliteus, the popliteofibular ligament, is a common supporting structure of the posterolateral corner of the knee. The oblique anatomic orientation of the popliteofibular ligament suggests that it may act as a static restraint to varus and external rotation moments.

Biomechanics

In addition to anatomic dissections, biomechanical analysis of knee ligaments can be done with the use of a selective ligament-cutting technique in fresh cadaveric specimens. This technique involves measurement of laxity in response to applied forces in the intact knee. A specific ligament is then transected, and the resulting increase in laxity, compared with the intact knee, is measured. This increase reflects the loss of the sectioned ligament and also the change in interaction among the remaining knee ligaments. When multiple ligaments are tested, the resulting change in knee laxity depends on the sequence in which ligaments are sectioned; the order of ligament sectioning must be varied to determine the relative importance of each ligament. The major advantage of the selective-cutting technique is that it allows direct measurement of the change in knee motion after one or a combination of ligaments has been sectioned. These changes are measured throughout 90° of knee flexion, to allow comparison with clinical knee testing. The angle of knee flexion at which clinical laxity testing for a certain ligament is most specific can then be determined.

Some biomechanical studies of the selective-cutting technique involving the posterolateral corner have been reported.[15-19] Gollehon and associates[15] used selective-cutting techniques to examine the static contributions to knee stability of the PCL, the LCL, the popliteus tendon, and the arcuate ligament. The arcuate ligament, the popliteus tendon, the fabellofibular ligament, and the posterolateral part of the capsule were sectioned together as the "deep ligament complex." The LCL and the PCL were sectioned separately. The order of ligament-sectioning was varied to determine the role of each structure.

Anterior-posterior translation, internal-external rotation, and varus-valgus rotation are measured in response to applied forces and moments. Translations and rotations that occur along the axis of the applied force or moment are called primary translations and rotations. Thus, posterior translation in response to a posterior force is a primary posterior translation. Translations and rotations that do not occur along the axis of the applied force or moment are called coupled translations and rotations. Thus, external tibial rotation that occurs in response to a posterior force is called a coupled external rotation. The primary translations and rotations and coupled rotations after sectioning of specific ligaments are summarized in the following sections.

Primary Anterior-Posterior Translation With Anterior-Posterior Force

In the study of Gollehon and associates,[15] isolated section of either the LCL or the deep ligament complex did not increase posterior translation at any angle of knee flexion. Combined section of both the LCL and the deep ligament complex (that is, complete posterolateral section) resulted in small (3-mm) increases in posterior translation at all angles of knee flexion. Isolated section of the PCL increased posterior translation at all angles of knee flexion; the amount of posterior translation increased progressively as the knee was flexed from 0° to 90°. At 0° and 30° of knee flexion, the posterior translation from complete posterolateral section equaled that from isolated section of the PCL. Finally, combined section of the PCL, the LCL, and the deep ligament complex resulted in large (20- to 25-mm) increases in posterior translation at all angles of knee flexion when compared with intact knees or with knees with isolated section of the PCL.

Coupled Internal-External Rotation With Anterior-Posterior Force

When an anterior force was applied to the tibia of an intact knee, the tibia rotated internally.[15] Conversely, when a posterior force was applied to the tibia of an intact knee, the tibia rotated externally. These predictable rotations are called coupled rotations. Coupled internal rotation with anterior force did not change with isolated or combined section of the PCL, the LCL, or the deep ligament complex. However, isolated section of the PCL eliminated the coupled external rotation that was seen with application of a posterior force to the intact knee. Combined section of the LCL and deep ligament complex substantially increased coupled external rotation seen with posterior force at all angles of knee flexion, but the increase was maximum (20°) at 30° of knee flexion. Additional section of the PCL did not result in a further increase in coupled external rotation.

Primary Varus-Valgus Rotation With a Varus-Valgus Moment

In the intact knee, varus and valgus rotation is least in full extension and it progressively increases as the knee flexes to 90°. In the study of Gollehon and associates,[15] isolated or combined section of the PCL, the LCL, and the deep ligament complex did not change the amount of primary valgus rotation at any angle of knee flexion. Isolated section of the PCL did not increase primary varus rotation at any angle of knee flexion. Isolated section of the LCL produced a small increase (1° to 4°) in varus rotation at all angles of knee flexion. Combined section of the LCL and the deep ligament complex resulted in a larger increase (5° to 9°) in varus rotation at all angles of knee flexion, but the maximum increase was at 30° of knee flexion. Combined section of the PCL, the LCL, and the deep ligament complex resulted in an even larger increase in varus rotation (15° to 19°) at all angles of knee flexion, and the maximum increase was at 60° of knee flexion.

Primary Internal-External Rotation With an Internal-External Tibial Moment

The amount of primary internal rotation of the tibia on the femur did not change after isolated or combined section of the PCL, the LCL, or the deep ligament complex. Isolated section of the PCL did not change the amount of primary external rotation at any angle of knee flexion. Section of the deep ligament complex resulted in an increase in primary external rotation at 90° of knee flexion. Combined section of the LCL and the deep ligament complex resulted in primary external rotation that was increased at all angles of knee flexion and maximum at 30° of knee flexion. Additional section of the PCL allowed a further increase in primary external rotation at 60° and 90° of knee flexion.

Grood and associates,[16] Nielsen and Helmig,[18] Markolf and associates,[17] and Wascher and associates[19] also performed selective-cutting studies on the posterolateral structures. Different experimental methods of force application were used, and different magnitudes of force and moments were applied in each of the studies. Although the magnitudes of change in rotation and translation were different, the direction of the change in rotation and translation after section of the posterolateral structures was consistent among the various studies. In all of the studies, section of the posterolateral structures resulted in increased primary posterior translation, primary varus rotation, primary external rotation, and coupled external rotation.

Clinical Application

Biomechanical studies allow one to determine the angle of knee flexion at which the function of specific knee ligaments can best be tested. This information can facilitate the clinical examination of the injured knee. The results of multiple selective-cutting studies suggest that increases in primary posterior translation, primary varus rotation, primary external rotation, and coupled external rotation are most useful for the detection of an injury of the posterolateral structures.[15-19] An isolated PCL injury results in posterior translation that is increased at all angles of flexion but is maximum at 70° to 90°. Therefore, the posterior drawer test should be most sensitive for the detection of a PCL injury when performed at 90° of knee flexion. An isolated PCL injury would not result in a change in primary varus rotation or primary external rotation.

Isolated injury of the LCL results in an increase in varus rotation (1° to 4°) that is maximum at 30° of knee flexion. However, this amount may be too subtle to be detected on clinical examination. Complete posterolateral injury associated with an intact PCL should result in a maximum increase in posterior translation, varus rotation, and external rotation at 30° of knee flexion. When one suspects posterolateral injury, varus and external rotation stress tests should be performed at 30° and 90° of knee flexion and compared with the results in the contralateral knee. An increase in primary varus rotation and external rotation at 30° of knee flexion that decreases at 90° of knee flexion when external rotation and varus moments are applied indicates an isolated injury of the posterolateral corner. When combined injuries of the PCL and the posterolateral corner are present, varus rotation, posterior translation, and external rotation are increased at all angles of knee flexion. Thus, an increase in varus rotation and external rotation at both 30° and 90° of knee flexion when external rotation and varus moments are applied indicates combined injuries of the PCL and the posterolateral corner.

Mechanism of Injury

The mechanism that commonly leads to posterolateral injury can also cause injury of the cruciate ligaments. In a review of 17 patients who had acute posterolateral instability, Baker and associates[2] reported that six patients had sustained a posterolaterally directed blow to the medial part of the tibia that caused knee hyperextension, an additional six patients had sustained a noncontact hyperextension and external rotation force to the knee, two patients had sustained a pure hyperextension injury, and three patients had been involved in a motor-vehicle accident. These authors also reviewed the cases of 13 patients who had acute combined PCL and posterolateral instability of the knee.[3] The mechanism of injury was an anteromedial blow to the flexed knee in six patients, a fall on the knee in two patients, and an unknown mechanism in five. In a large review of 140 patients who had chronic posterolateral instability of the knee, Hughston and Jacobson[4] attributed the mechanism of injury to a direct blow to the tibia with the knee flexed or extended or to a twisting injury of the knee. Flynn and associates[20] found that, in their experience with acute combined ACL and posterolateral injuries, most patients had sustained a hyperextension injury.

Clinical Presentation

In patients who have acute isolated posterolateral instability of the knee, the major symptom is pain in the posterolateral aspect of the knee. In addition, dysesthesias and weakness of the leg and foot may be present because of associated injury of the peroneal nerve. When the initial swelling and pain from an acute injury have resolved and walking has been resumed, a patient may note instability of the knee in extension. The knee may buckle into hyperextension with weightbearing.[4] The patient may also complain of instability when ascending and descending stairs and may walk with the knee in flexion to avoid this instability. The gait may demonstrate a varus thrust of the affected knee and instability with cutting activities. Chronic posterolateral instability may produce pain localized along either the lateral or the medial joint line.[4] Finally, there may be associated injury of the ACL or PCL, and symptoms related to the absence of the cruciates may predominate. Careful physical examination is needed to document both isolated posterolateral injury and posterolateral injury combined with additional ligamentous injuries.

Physical Findings

Posterolateral injury is often associated with cruciate injury. Injuries of the PCL and posterolateral corner are commonly missed at the initial evaluation. Initially, the posterolateral aspect of an acutely injured knee should be examined for swelling, tenderness, ecchymosis, or induration. Inspection of the anteromedial part of the tibia may reveal an abrasion or ecchymosis, providing supporting evidence for an injury of the posterolateral structures. When multiple acute ligamentous instabilities are present with a posterolateral injury, one must be suspicious that the knee has dislocated and spontaneously reduced. If a knee dislocation is suspected, an arteriogram should be done to rule out an arterial injury such as an intimal tear. Finally, peroneal nerve injury occurs often with lateral and posterolateral knee injury. Baker and associates[2] noted two patients who had complete peroneal-nerve palsy among 17 patients who had acute posterolateral instability of the knee. In a recent review of 14 patients who had acute reconstruction for combined ACL and posterolateral injuries, four patients had an injury of the peroneal nerve and surgical exploration revealed intact nerves with variable amounts of hemorrhage in all four.[20] Thorough evaluation of peroneal nerve function is mandatory in all patients who have acute posterolateral injury or chronic posterolateral instability.

After initial documentation of the neurovascular function, it is important to observe the gait and limb alignment of patients in whom a posterolateral injury is suspected. Examination of gait is more useful for patients who have chronic posterolateral injury, as patients who have an acute injury may walk with an antalgic gait. Patients who have a chronic posterolateral injury may demonstrate a varus thrust or a hyperextension varus thrust of the injured knee during the stance phase of gait. Hughston and Jacobson[4] attributed this finding to an apparent tibia vara that occurs because of external rotation of the tibia in full extension in the stance phase. Similarly, the injured knee may demonstrate a varus alignment in stance. During the stance phase of gait, an adduction moment is normally present at the knee. Varus limb alignment may contribute to an increased adduction moment, exacerbating the symptoms of posterolateral instability. Anteroposterior radiographs of the hips to the ankles, made with the patient standing, can document limb alignment. Also, radiographs of the knee in full extension, made with the patient supine and with the application of varus and valgus stress, may be needed to determine the role of posterolateral laxity in the creation of varus limb alignment. Formal gait analysis may assist in the evaluation of patients who have varus limb alignment and chronic posterolateral instability of the knee.

Anterior-Posterior Translation

After gait and limb alignment have been assessed, direct examination of the knee is performed. Anterior-posterior translation is documented at 30° and 90° of knee flexion. Slightly increased posterior translation at 30° but not at 90° indicates posterolateral injury. Increased posterior translation at both 30° and 90° indicates injury of the PCL. A Lachman test is performed to document the integrity of the ACL. With isolated posterolateral injury, a Lachman test will demonstrate increased anterior-posterior translation with a firm end-point. Finally, a quadriceps active test should be performed to assess the integrity of the PCL.[21]

Varus-Valgus Rotation

Varus and valgus stress testing is performed with the knee in full extension and in 30° of flexion. An isolated cruciate-ligament injury does not affect varus or valgus stability. Combined injuries of the LCL and the posterolateral corner increase varus opening with varus stress at both 0° and 30° of flexion, but the increase is maximum at 30°. A large degree of varus instability in full extension may indicate combined injuries of the posterolateral corner, the PCL, and possibly the ACL.

Tibial External-Rotation Test

When a knee is examined for posterolateral injury, external rotation of the tibia on the femur is assessed at both 30° and 90° of knee flexion. This test can be performed with the patient supine or prone, but we prefer the prone position. The medial border of the foot in its neutral position is used as a reference point for external rotation. At the desired degree of knee flexion, the foot is externally rotated forcefully by the examiner. The degree of external rotation of the foot relative to the axis of the femur is assessed and compared with that on the contralateral side (Fig. 4). External rotation is measured with use of the foot-thigh angle, as is commonly done to assess tibial torsion in children. In addition to measuring the degree of external rotation, the tibial plateaus are palpated to determine their relative positions compared with the femoral condyles. This is done to determine if the external rotation is caused by the lateral tibial plateau moving posteriorly (posterolateral instability) or by the medial plateau moving anteriorly (anteromedial instability). There is a wide variability in the degree of

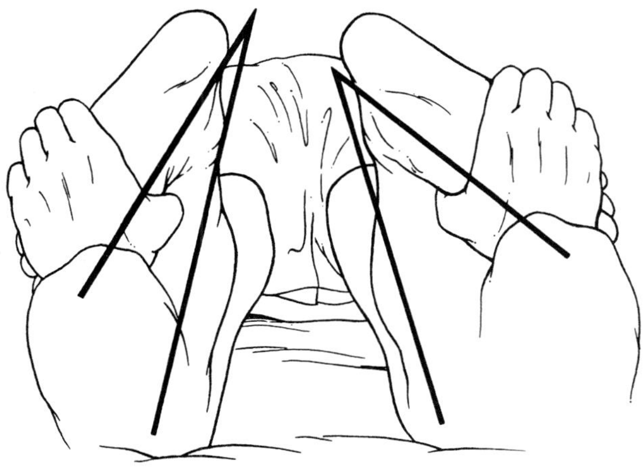

Fig. 4 The prone external-rotation test is performed at both 30° and 90° of knee flexion. Forceful external rotation is exerted by the examiner, and the amount of external rotation is measured by comparing the axis of the medial border of the foot with the femur. (Reproduced with permission from Veltri DM, Warren RF: Isolated and combined posterior cruciate ligament injuries. *J Am Acad Orthop Surg* 1993;1:67-75.)

external rotation at 30° and 90° among people who have normal knees, so one must always compare the degree of external rotation to that on the contralateral side.[22] We consider a 10° difference in the amount of external rotation to be evidence of a pathological condition. An isolated injury of the posterolateral corner increases external rotation at all angles of knee flexion, but the maximum increase is at 30°. Thus, more than a 10° increase in external rotation compared with that on the contralateral side at 30° of knee flexion, but not at 90° of knee flexion, indicates an isolated injury of the posterolateral corner. An increase in external rotation of more than 10° compared with that on the contralateral side at both 30° and 90° of knee flexion indicates injury of both the PCL and the posterolateral corner.

External-Rotation Recurvatum Test

This test can be performed by two methods, as originally described by Hughston and Norwood.[23] In the first method, with the patient lying supine, the examiner grasps the great toes of both feet at the same time and lifts the lower limbs off of the table. If the knee has posterolateral instability, there will be relative hyperextension on its lateral side, external rotation of the tibia, and apparent tibia vara of the medial aspect of the knee (Fig. 5). In the second method, the examiner holds the heel of the foot in his or her hand while extending the knee from 30° of flexion to full extension. The examiner's other hand grasps the posterolateral aspect of the knee, and any relative hyperextension and external rotation that occurs in comparison with the uninjured knee is noted. In our experience, this test may give a mildly positive result for a varus knee with isolated posterolateral injury. When there is substantial hyperextension and varus rotation, the ACL is probably also injured and the PCL is possibly also injured.

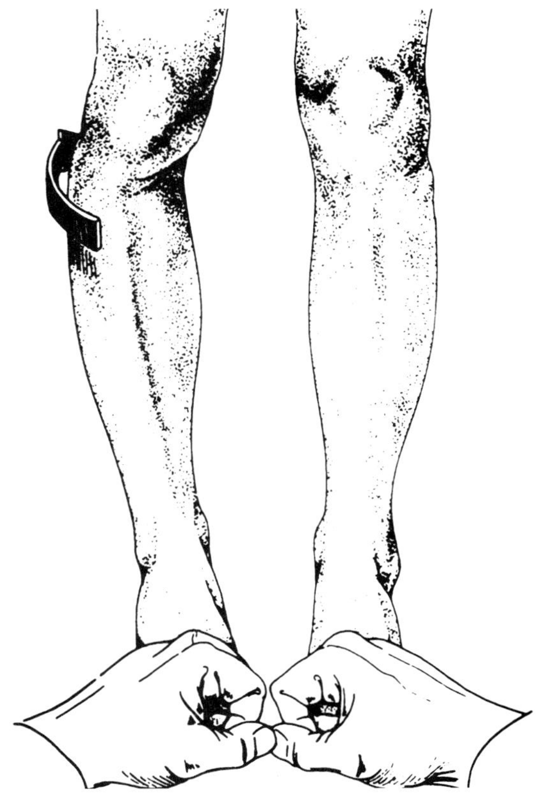

Fig. 5 The external rotation recurvatum test. (Reproduced with permission from Hughston JC, Norwood LA Jr: The posterolateral drawer test and external rotational recurvatum test for posterolateral rotatory instability of the knee. *Clin Orthop* 1980;147:82-87.)

Posterolateral Drawer Test

The posterolateral drawer test is performed with the patient supine and the hip flexed 45°, the knee flexed 80°, and the tibia in 15° of external rotation.[23] As the foot is fixed, a posterior drawer is performed. Hughston and Norwood[23] consider the test positive for posterolateral instability when the lateral tibial condyle externally rotates relative to the lateral femoral condyle (Fig. 6). In our experience, this test is difficult to quantitate. In the normal knee, the end-point to posterior translation is firm, but the end-point to external rotation is variable. Biomechanical studies of knee stability have documented that external rotation is normally coupled with posterior translation, and substantially increased external rotation at 90° of knee flexion is correlated with injury of both the PCL and the posterolateral corner.[15] If the posterolateral drawer is grossly positive, we think that injury of both the PCL

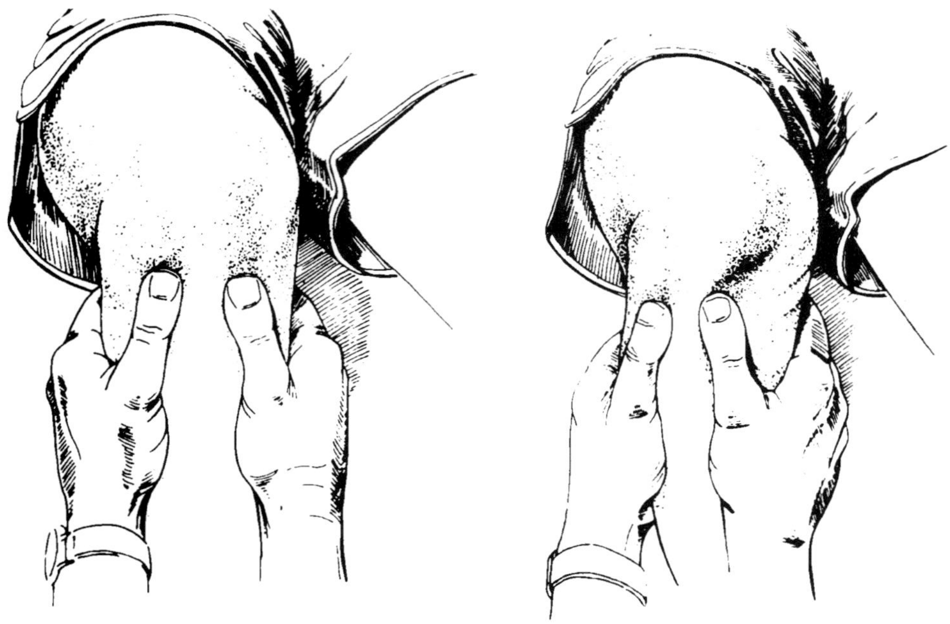

Fig. 6 The posterolateral drawer test. (Reproduced with permission from Hughston JC, Norwood LA Jr: The posterolateral drawer test and external rotational recurvatum test for posterolateral rotatory instability of the knee. *Clin Orthop* 1980;147:82-87.)

and the posterolateral corner should be suspected. The posterolateral drawer test is not specific for injury of the posterolateral corner, and comparison with the contralateral knee is necessary to assess qualitatively any degree of increased external rotation.

Reversed Pivot-Shift Test

The reversed pivot shift is performed by the examiner applying a valgus force to the tibia while bringing the knee from 90° of flexion to full extension with the foot in external rotation. In knees with posterolateral instability, the lateral tibial plateau is subluxated posteriorly relative to the lateral femoral condyle when the knee is in flexion. As the knee is brought into extension, the lateral tibial plateau reduces and a shift or jerk can be palpated. Jakob and associates[24] examined 100 military recruits who had asymptomatic, normal knees and found that three had a bilateral, grossly positive reverse pivot shift and eight had a bilateral, weakly positive reverse pivot shift. Cooper[22] examined 100 asymptomatic knees with the patients under anesthesia and found that 35% had a positive reverse pivot shift. A positive reverse pivot shift correlated strongly with increased generalized ligamentous laxity and mild varus alignment of the knee. As with other tests for posterolateral instability, the reverse pivot shift is not a specific test. In the original description of the reverse pivot-shift test, Jakob and associates[24] clarified the importance of a positive test. They considered a positive test to be clinically important when it was found in one knee only, when the maneuver was painful and reproduced the patient's symptoms, when there were other signs of posterolateral instability, and when there was an appropriate history of trauma.

As outlined, many tests for the diagnosis of posterolateral instability of the knee have been described. In our experience, the most useful are the prone external rotation test at 30° and 90° of knee flexion and varus stress testing at 0° and 30° of flexion. The other tests, such as the reverse pivot-shift test, are used to supplement the diagnosis of posterolateral instability. The Lachman and the pivot-shift tests are used to determine the integrity of the ACL, and the posterior drawer and the quadriceps active tests are used to determine the integrity of the PCL. Complete documentation of ligamentous integrity is necessary before treatment can be recommended.

Treatment

When the ACL or PCL is torn after a posterolateral injury, we recommend reconstruction of all injured ligaments. We believe that all components of the instability should be addressed surgically to achieve the best opportunity for success. O'Brien and associates[1] documented that failures of ACL reconstruction can be caused by unrecognized and untreated posterolateral instability. Several clinical reports of surgical reconstruction of acute and chronic posterolateral instability have suggested that reconstruction of acute instability is more successful than that of chronic instability. The clinical experience of Flynn and associates[20] in the treatment of posterolateral instability supports this conclusion. Acute reconstruction is recommended for both isolated posterolateral instability and acute posterolateral instability combined with a cruciate injury.

Several operations have been designed for the treatment of posterolateral instability. These include popliteus tendon recession, arcuate advancement, biceps tenodesis, and popliteus tendon reconstruction with use of a patellar ligament autogenous graft. Baker and associates[2] performed acute posterolateral reconstruction by primary repair of the injured structures. For acute injuries with insufficient tissue for primary repair, or in reconstructions of chronic posterolateral injuries, anterior and superior advancement of the arcuate complex was performed. When the injury of the popliteus tendon and posterolateral structures was distal to the level of the joint line and it was thought that femoral advancement alone would not restore adequate tension to the posterolateral corner, Hughston and Jacobson[4] recommended distal primary repair and proximal advancement of the arcuate complex. The advancement of the arcuate complex may shift the insertion sites of the popliteus and the LCL anterior to the center of knee rotation. This may lead to stretching and ultimate failure of the reconstruction.

Jakob and associates[24] also recommended a recession of the popliteus tendon at its femoral insertion to restore posterolateral stability. This may suffice for mild instability but, as with advancement of the arcuate complex, proximal recession will not restore adequate tension to the popliteus if there is distal injury at the musculotendinous junction or if there is injury of the popliteofibular ligament.

Clancy[25] used a biceps tenodesis to reconstruct the posterolateral corner. The biceps tendon is transferred to the lateral femoral epicondyle while its distal attachment to the fibula is left intact. In this procedure, the biceps tendon is freed from the lateral head of the gastrocnemius and from the peroneal nerve. It is then passed under the split in the iliotibial band and attached with a ligament screw and washer to the lateral femoral epicondyle. This transfer recreates an LCL and may also tighten the arcuate complex. The reconstruction does not anatomically recreate the popliteus tendon or the popliteofibular ligament and, thus, represents only a partial reconstruction of the injured structures. Wascher and associates[19] demonstrated, in a cadaveric model, that biceps tenodesis to a point 1 cm anterior to the insertion of the LCL on the femoral epicondyle can restore varus and external rotation stability equal to that of the intact knee. While this reconstruction has proved to be successful clinically, we prefer to reconstruct the posterolateral injury anatomically.

Biomechanical selective-cutting studies have demonstrated that the LCL and the popliteus tendon are the major structures that prevent posterolateral instability of the knee.[15,18] Recently, renewed attention to the anatomy of the posterolateral corner has revealed a consistently strong attachment of the popliteus tendon to the fibula, the popliteofibular ligament. We think that the popliteofibular ligament is an important component of the popliteal muscle-tendon unit and that its anatomic orientation performs a static stabilizing function to resist varus and external rotation moments. We completed a selective-cutting study of the LCL, the popliteus attachment to the tibia, and the popliteofibular ligament. Section of the LCL and popliteus attachment to the tibia resulted in limited increases in primary varus rotation and primary external rotation because of the remaining, intact popliteofibular ligament. Therefore, for both acute and chronic posterolateral injuries, we attempt to repair, or reconstruct, the LCL, the popliteus tendon and its attachment to the tibia, and the popliteofibular ligament.

Acute Reconstruction

In acute posterolateral instability, associated ACL or PCL tears are reconstructed first, with the use of arthroscopic techniques. At the time of the arthroscopy, injury of the popliteus tendon can be assessed. Through a curvilinear skin incision, the posterolateral corner is then exposed. The popliteus tendon is followed proximally to its femoral insertion. It is then followed distally to the musculotendinous junction and its tibial and fibular insertions (the popliteofibular ligament). With complete exposure of the popliteus, the injury is evaluated with respect to its location and the quality of the remaining popliteus tissue. Surgical options include primary repair, advancement or recession, augmentation, or reconstruction. If the popliteus tendon is intact but the tibial or fibular attachments have been injured, we attempt to restore tension with suture fixation to bone. If the popliteus tendon is stretched but in continuity, one can remove the femoral insertion along with a bone plug and advance the tendon insertion by recessing the bone plug into a femoral drill-hole.

If the popliteus tissue is insufficient for direct repair, augmentation is warranted. The tibial component of the popliteus unit is augmented with a strip of iliotibial band (Fig. 7), while a strip of biceps tendon can be used to augment the popliteofibular ligament (Fig. 8). When the iliotibial band and biceps are injured, one can reconstruct the tibial and fibular attachments of the popliteus with patellar ligament autogenous graft or allograft or with Achilles tendon allograft.

An injury of the LCL is also addressed directly. Avulsions of the LCL are repaired with sutures. If needed, the LCL is augmented with a strip of biceps tendon (Fig. 9). When a direct repair or biceps augmentation cannot be accomplished, the LCL can be reconstructed with patellar ligament autogenous graft or allograft.

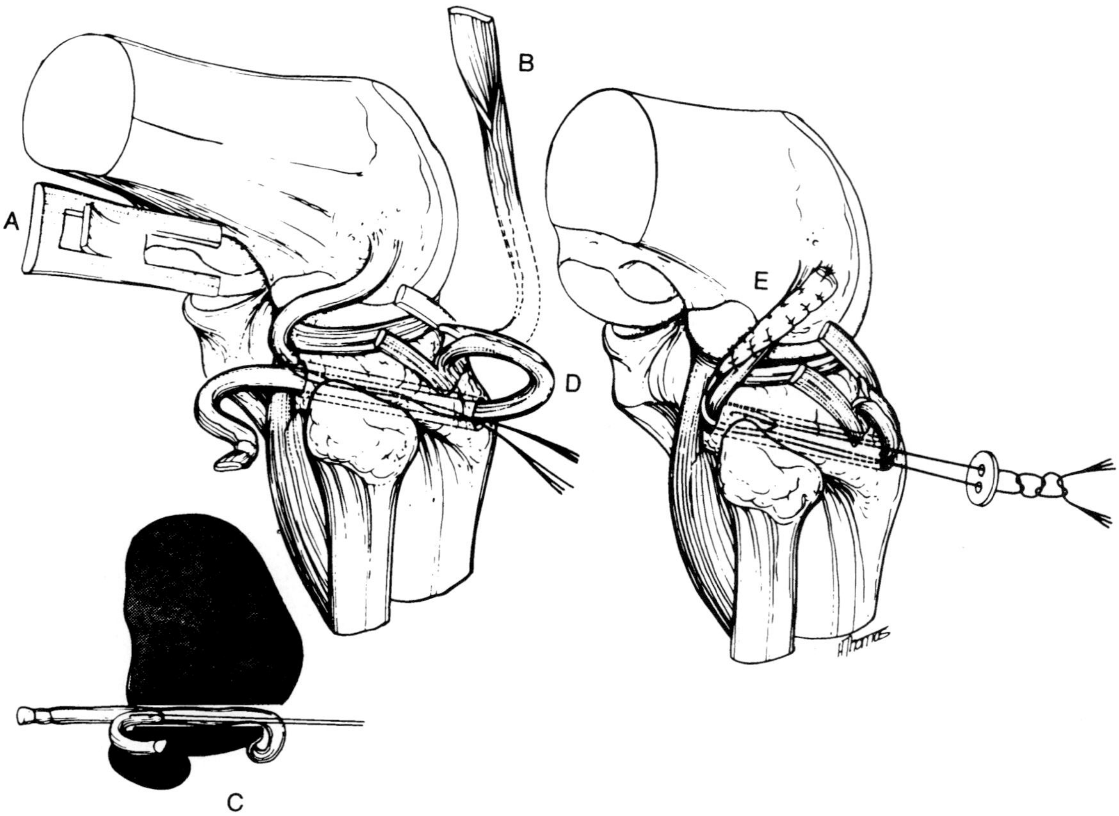

Fig. 7 Iliotibial-band augmentation of the popliteus. A strip of iliotibial band is harvested (A) and tubed with sutures (B). The strip is then passed through a tibial drill-hole from anterior to posterior (C and D) and secured to the remaining popliteus tendon with sutures (E). (Reproduced with permission from Bowen MK, Warren RF, Cooper DE: Posterior cruciate ligament and related injuries, in Insall J (ed): *Surgery of the Knee*, ed 2. New York, NY, Churchill Livingstone, 1993, pp 505-554.)

Chronic Posterolateral Injury

Initially, it is critical to evaluate limb alignment in a patient who has chronic posterolateral instability. If the patient has a varus knee alignment and a lateral thrust in the stance phase of gait, a valgus proximal tibial osteotomy is necessary to correct the alignment. Otherwise, with substantial varus alignment, surgical reconstruction of the posterolateral corner will fail because of chronic repetitive stretching of the reconstruction. The valgus osteotomy may be performed before, or combined with, posterolateral reconstruction. When it is done as a staged procedure, an osteotomy alone may alleviate the symptoms of posterolateral instability in some patients. If such symptoms persist after the osteotomy, a delayed posterolateral reconstruction can be performed.

If a chronic tear of the ACL or PCL is present in addition to posterolateral instability, the cruciate should be reconstructed first with a patellar ligament autogenous graft or allograft with use of an arthroscopic technique. After cruciate reconstruction, the posterolateral corner is exposed through a lateral incision. Treatment of a chronic popliteus injury can involve recession and advancement, augmentation, or reconstruction. For these chronic tears, an ipsilateral patellar-ligament autogenous graft is often used to reconstruct the associated cruciate deficiency, and the popliteus reconstruction necessitates the use of a contralateral patellar-ligament autogenous graft or allograft. When the popliteus tendon is reconstructed, both the tibial and the fibular attachments should be addressed. A single, split patellar-ligament or Achilles-tendon allograft can be used to reconstruct both components of the popliteus. The popliteofibular ligament should always be re-established because it plays such a critical role in the prevention of rotational instability (Fig. 10). In addition to reconstruction of the popliteus attachment to the fibula and tibia, the LCL may need to be reconstructed in these patients. Reconstruction can involve proximal or distal advancement and recession, augmentation, or reconstruction. In most patients who have chronic posterolateral instability, the LCL can be reconstructed with a strip of the biceps tendon. In rare cases, reconstruction with a patellar ligament autogenous graft or allograft may be necessary.

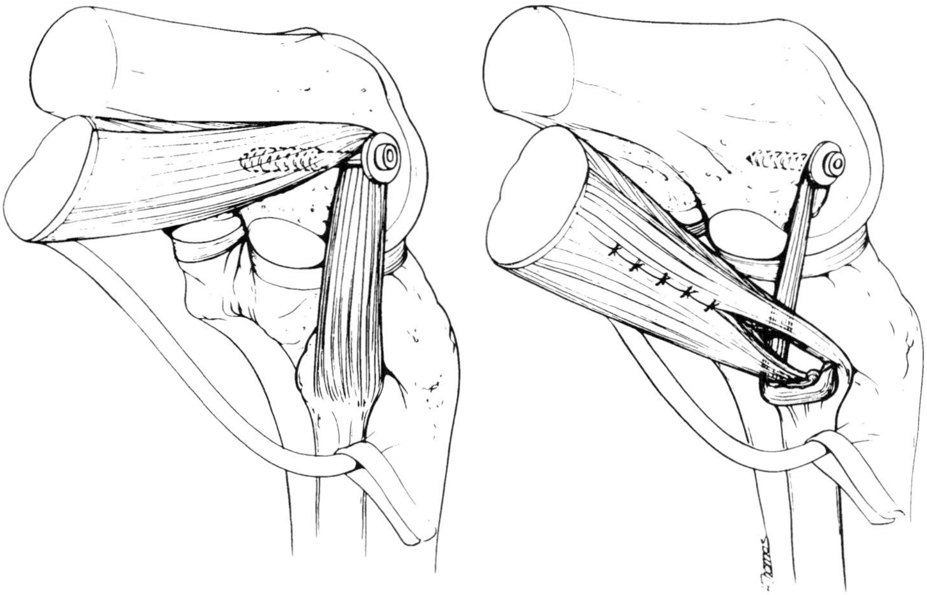

Fig. 8 For the biceps tenodesis of the posterolateral corner, usually the entire distal part of the tendon is moved to the femur and secured with a screw and ligament washer (**left**). We prefer to reconstruct the popliteofibular ligament anatomically with the central slip of the biceps tendon (**right**). This is tubed and sutured to the posterior part of the fibula. The strip is then passed under the remaining biceps tendon and secured to the lateral part of the femur with a screw and ligament washer. (Reproduced with permission from Veltri DM, Warren RF: Operative treatment of posterolateral instability of the knee. *Clin Sports Med*, in press.)

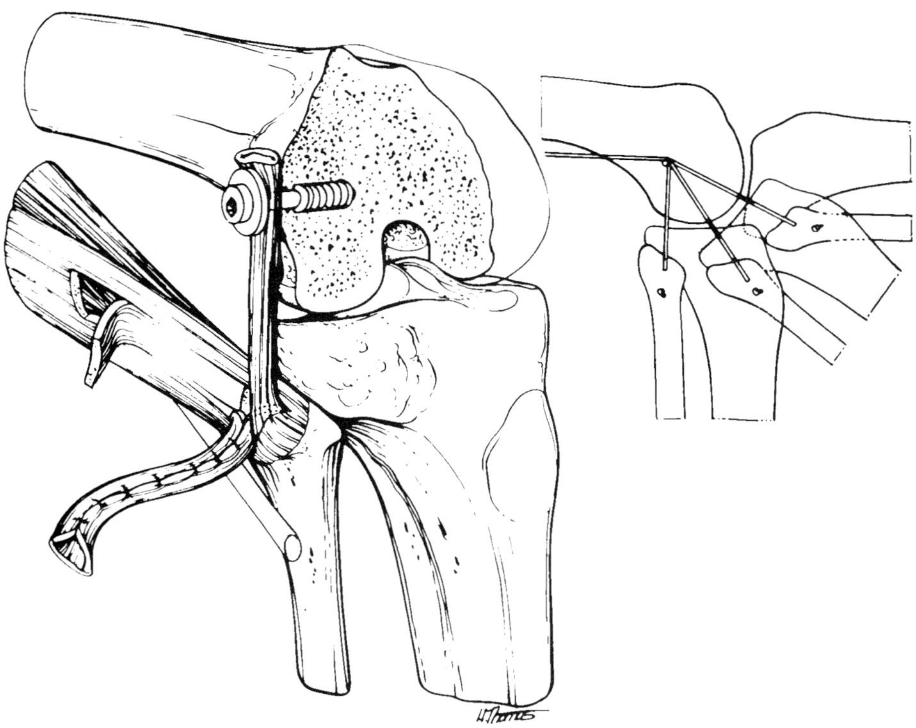

Fig. 9 Reconstruction of the LCL with a central strip of biceps tendon (**left**). Isometric femoral placement is achieved by examination of the position of the graft relative to a Kirschner wire placed at the proposed ligament-fixation site (**right**). (Reproduced with permission from Bowen MK, Warren RF, Cooper DE: Posterior cruciate ligament and related injuries, in Insall J (ed): *Surgery of the Knee*, ed 2. New York, NY, Churchill Livingstone, 1993, pp 505-554.)

Conclusion

Treatment of posterolateral instability of the knee requires a thorough knowledge of the variable anatomy of the posterolateral corner. Posterolateral instability is rarely an isolated finding, and one must be proficient in the diagnosis of all knee-ligament injuries. While many surgical procedures have been devised to treat posterolateral instability, we prefer to repair all ligamentous injuries as anatomically as possible. Repair and

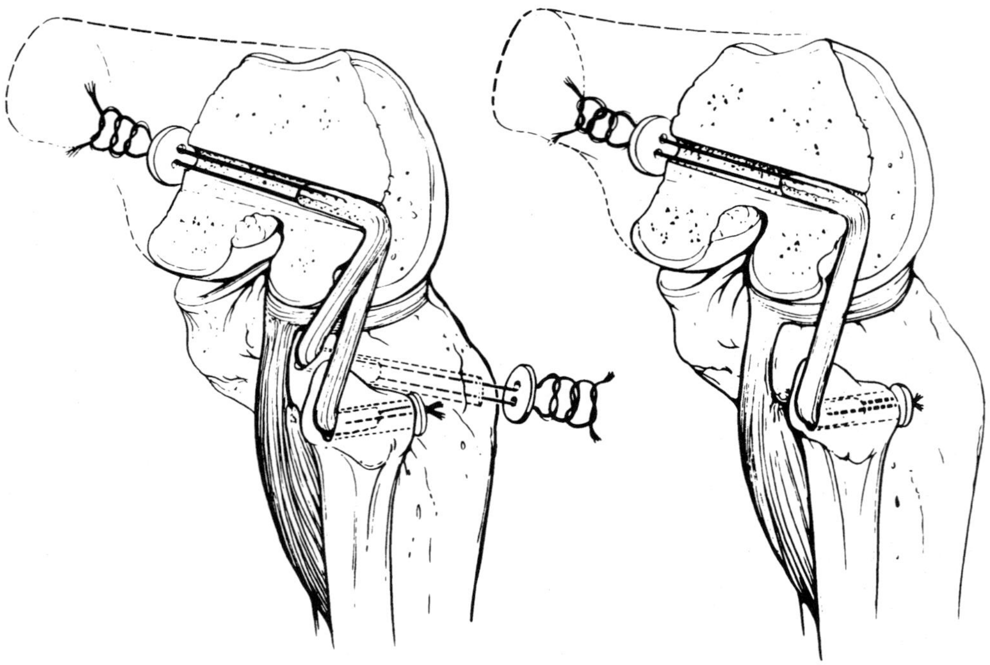

Fig. 10 Reconstruction of the popliteofibular ligament. **Left,** Reconstruction of the popliteofibular ligament and the tibial attachment of the popliteus with a split patellar-ligament graft. The graft is placed into the femoral tunnel proximally. The graft is then split and one end is placed in a tibial tunnel and the other, in a fibular tunnel. **Right,** Reconstruction of the popliteofibular ligament with a patellar ligament graft. (Reproduced with permission from Veltri DM, Warren RF: Operative treatment of posterolateral instability of the knee. *Clin Sports Med*, in press.)

reconstruction for the treatment of acute posterolateral instability results in greater success than do reconstructions for chronic posterolateral instability and, accordingly, we recommend acute repair or reconstruction when possible. When a major posterolateral injury is present, the popliteus muscle-tendon unit and the LCL can be repaired, augmented, or reconstructed primarily. Reconstruction of all ligamentous lesions leads to the greatest chance of success in the treatment of this problem.

References

1. O'Brien SJ, Warren RF, Pavlov H, et al: Reconstruction of the chronically insufficient anterior cruciate ligament with the central third of the patellar ligament. *J Bone Joint Surg* 1991;73A:278-286.
2. Baker CL Jr, Norwood LA, Hughston JC: Acute posterolateral rotatory instability of the knee. *J Bone Joint Surg* 1983;65A:614-618.
3. Baker CL Jr, Norwood LA, Hughston JC: Acute combined posterior cruciate and posterolateral instability of the knee. *Am J Sports Med* 1984;12:204-208.
4. Hughston JC, Jacobson KE: Chronic posterolateral rotatory instability of the knee. *J Bone Joint Surg* 1985;67A:351-359.
5. Fleming RE Jr, Blatz DJ, McCarroll JR: Posterior problems in the knee: Posterior cruciate insufficiency and posterolateral rotatory insufficiency. *Am J Sports Med* 1981;9:107-113.
6. Kaplan EB: The fabellofibular and short lateral ligaments of the knee joint. *J Bone Joint Surg* 1961;43A:169-179.
7. Last RJ: The popliteus muscle and the lateral meniscus with a note on the attachment of the medial meniscus. *J Bone Joint Surg* 1950;32B:93-99.
8. Lovejoy JF Jr, Harden TP: Popliteus muscle in man. *Anat Rec* 1971;169:727-730.
9. Seebacher JR, Inglis AE, Marshall JL, et al: The structure of the posterolateral aspect of the knee. *J Bone Joint Surg* 1982;64A:536-541.
10. Staubli HU, Birrer S: The popliteus tendon and its fascicles at the popliteal hiatus: Gross anatomy and functional arthroscopic evaluation with and without anterior cruciate ligament deficiency. *Arthroscopy* 1990;6:209-220.
11. Staubli H, Rauschning W: Popliteus tendon and lateral meniscus. *Am J Knee Surg* 1991;4:110-121.
12. Sudasna S, Harnsiriwattanagit K: The ligamentous structures of the posterolateral aspect of the knee. *Bull Hosp Joint Dis Orthop Inst* 1990;50:35-40.
13. Watanabe Y, Moriya H, Takahashi K, et al: Functional anatomy of the posterolateral structures of the knee. *Arthroscopy* 1993;9:57-62.
14. DeLee JC, Riley MB, Rockwood CA Jr: Acute posterolateral rotatory instability of the knee. *Am J Sports Med* 1983;11:199-207.
15. Gollehon DL, Torzilli PA, Warren RF: The role of the posterolateral and cruciate ligaments in the stability of the human knee: A biomechanical study. *J Bone Joint Surg* 1987;69A:233-242.
16. Grood ES, Stowers SF, Noyes FR: Limits of movement in the human knee: Effect of sectioning the posterior cruciate ligament and posterolateral structures. *J Bone Joint Surg* 1988;70A:88-97.
17. Markolf KL, Wascher DC, Finerman GA: Direct in vitro measurement of forces in the cruciate ligaments: Part II. The effect of section of the posterolateral structures. *J Bone Joint Surg* 1993;75A:387-394.
18. Nielsen S, Helmig P: The static stabilizing function of the popliteal tendon in the knee: An experimental study. *Arch Orthop Trauma Surg* 1986;104:357-362.
19. Wascher DC, Grauer JD, Markoff KL: Biceps tendon tenodesis for posterolateral instability of the knee: An in vitro study. *Am J Sports Med* 1993;21:400-406.
20. Flynn W, Warren RF, Marchand R, et al: Results of early reconstruction of combined injuries to the anterior cruciate ligament and the posterolateral corner of the knee. Presented at the Annual Meeting of The American Orthopaedic Society for Sports Medicine, San Diego, CA, July 9, 1992.

21. Daniel DM, Stone ML, Barnett P, et al: Use of the quadriceps active test to diagnose posterior cruciate-ligament disruption and measure posterior laxity of the knee. *J Bone Joint Surg* 1988; 70A:386-391.
22. Cooper DE: Tests for posterolateral instability of the knee in normal subjects: Results of examination under anesthesia. *J Bone Joint Surg* 1991;73A:30-36.
23. Hughston JC, Norwood LA Jr: The posterolateral drawer test and external rotational recurvatum test for posterolateral rotatory instability of the knee. *Clin Orthop* 1980;147:82-87.
24. Jakob RP, Hassler H, Staeubli HU: Observations on rotatory instability of the lateral compartment of the knee: Experimental studies on the functional anatomy and the pathomechanism of the true and the reversed pivot shift sign. *Acta Orthop Scand* 1981;191(suppl):1-32.
25. Clancy WG Jr: Repair and reconstruction of the posterior cruciate ligament, in Chapman MW (ed): *Operative Orthopaedics.* Philadelphia, PA, JB Lippincott, 1988, vol 3, pp 1651-1665.

CHAPTER 40

Alignment In Total Knee Replacement

David S. Hungerford, MD

Introduction

Although it is generally recognized that alignment is an important factor in the long-term survival of total knee replacement (TKR), a review of the literature contains little substantial validation for its importance. In fact, even a recent report suggests that varus-valgus alignment within a fairly wide range is not a very important contributor to aseptic loosening in TKR.[1] I believe that part of this problem is an oversimplification of the issues involved in alignment. Most reports that have analyzed the influence of malalignment on clinical and functional problems associated with TKR have been limited to a single degree of freedom, varus-valgus.

The purpose of this chapter is to define alignment in terms of both the normal anatomy and total knee arthroplasty; to define the methods for achieving alignment in TKR that are in common use with different instrumentation systems, giving both their advantages and their pitfalls; and to identify the problems with measuring alignment postoperatively. Although it is beyond the scope of this chapter to discuss the diverse instrumentation systems used today to carry out TKR, a comprehensive understanding of alignment should help each surgeon better understand and more intelligently use his or her instrumentation system. After all, the most important instruments for TKR are the human eye and brain.

Different methods are used to achieve alignment and ligament balance in TKR. It is important for the surgeon to have a clear understanding of the differences between these methods, the assumptions on which each is based, and their implications for TKR. Failure to understand these differences could lead the surgeon to combine different methodologies, thereby inadvertently introducing a variable that could contribute to prosthetic or clinical failure for the TKR. Proper component alignment is necessary to ensure symmetric bone loading, which contributes both to functional prosthetic stability and to the long-term survival of the bone-prosthesis or bone-cement-prosthesis interfaces (Fig. 1). Symmetric loading is also important for long-term polyethylene survival. When the contact area passes to only one condyle, catastrophic polyethylene wear will result (Fig. 2). Malalignment can impose strain in the retained ligaments, causing pain or functional instability (Fig. 3). Finally, in prostheses that depend on proper ligament balance throughout flexion, malalignment can contribute to gross instability (Fig. 4).

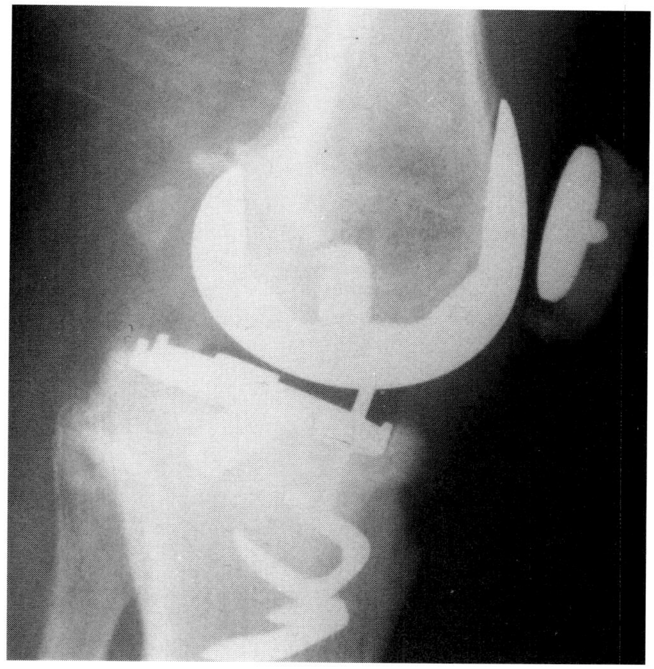

Fig. 1 Anterior subsidence of this cementless tibial component was a direct result of malalignment, in this case anterior sloping of the tibial cut.

What Is Alignment?

Alignment in reference to TKR is generally conceived as encompassing varus-valgus alignment and perhaps even flexion-extension alignment of the individual components. In fact, however, there are six degrees of freedom for each of the prosthetic components. There is a pair of rotational alignments around each of the three reference axes, X, Y, and Z, and a pair of translational alignments along each of these axes for proper positioning of the individual components (Fig. 5).

For both the femoral and tibial components, varus-valgus alignment is rotation around the Z axis, flexion-extension around the X axis, and internal and external rotation around the Y axis. The same six degrees of freedom apply to the patella, but, because the patella is oriented in the coronal plane, the common alignment nomenclature is different. Rotation around the vertical axis (Y) defines the medial-lateral resection orientation, the proximal and distal resection orientation takes place around the transverse axis (X), and the internal and external rotation of the prosthetic component takes place around the Z axis. The latter is not applicable for symmetrical dome-shaped prostheses that lack specific rotational orientation within the component.

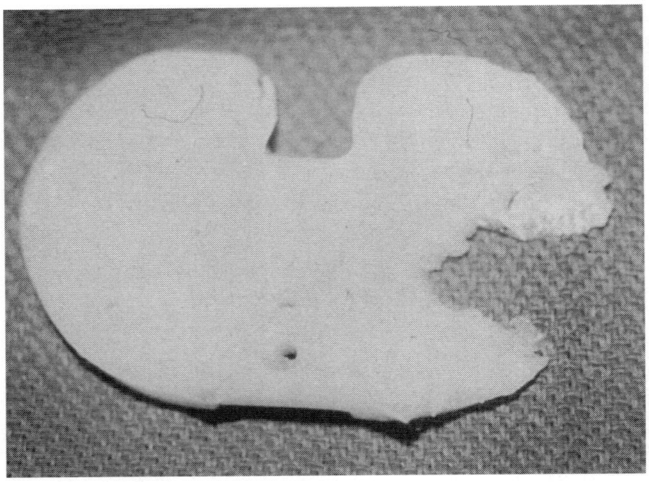

Fig. 2 Catastrophic wear, the result of varus malalignment, has caused this polyethylene insert to completely disappear on the medial side.

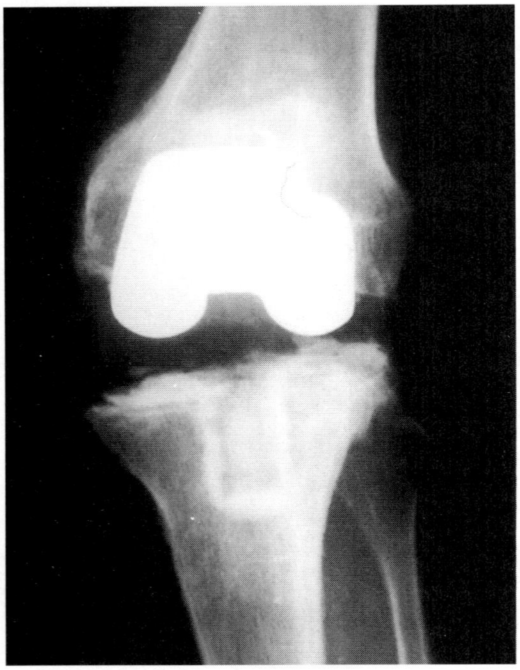

Fig. 3 Valgus malalignment has contributed to stretching of the medial ligaments, with resulting pain and instability.

However, many prostheses are eccentric or oval in shape, and, for these, some rotational orientation is required.

The remaining three degrees of freedom result from translation along the reference axes. For the transverse or X axis, this results in the proper medial-lateral positioning of each of the components. For the vertical axis, this refers to the proximal-distal position of the components or the quantity of distal resection of the femur and proximal resection of the tibia. For the patellar component, it involves the proximal or distal positioning of that component. Translation along the Z axis refers to the

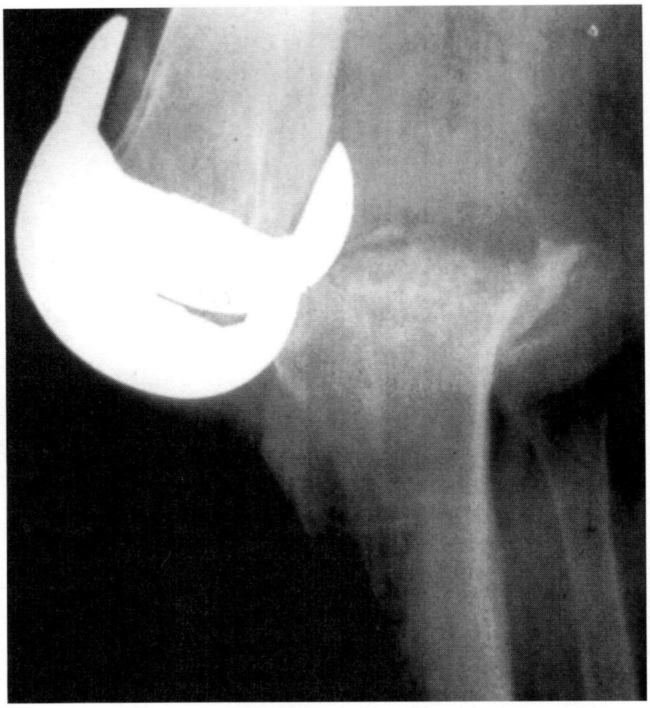

Fig. 4 Anterior translation of the femoral component caused instability in flexion and resulted in anterior femoral dislocation.

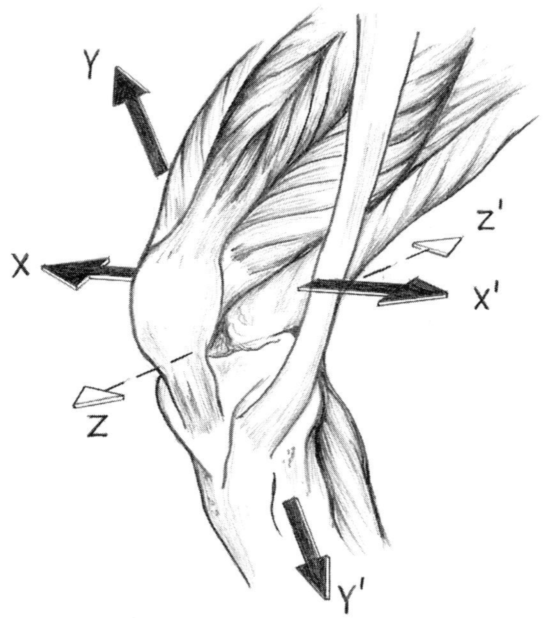

Fig. 5 The three axes of the knee.

anterior-posterior position of the femoral component and the tibial component and the depth of the patellar resection for the patellar component.

Part of the problem in assessing the true importance of alignment in total knee replacement is that not all of these alignments can be assessed equally well by traditional radiographs. On radiographs, the most common reference is the mechanical axis, which is defined as a line drawn from the center of the femoral head to the center of the ankle. This line should pass through the center of the normally aligned knee (Fig. 6). In the absence of significant tibial diaphyseal deformity, the mechanical axis coincides with the anatomic axis of the tibial shaft. Kapandji[2] first defined the relationship between the mechanical axis, the anatomic axis of the femur, and the joint line. The anatomic axis of the femur is a line drawn from the center of the knee through the center of the diaphysis of the femur with the leg in neutral rotation. This line normally makes an angle of 6° to the mechanical axis. The normal joint line, as measured through the bony radiographic projections of the distal femur, is at an angle to the mechanical axis of 87° on the lateral side and of 93° on the medial side. With the leg in the position of single leg stance, with the foot brought to the midline, the mechanical axis is inclined 3° in valgus to a vertical reference point and the joint line is horizontal.

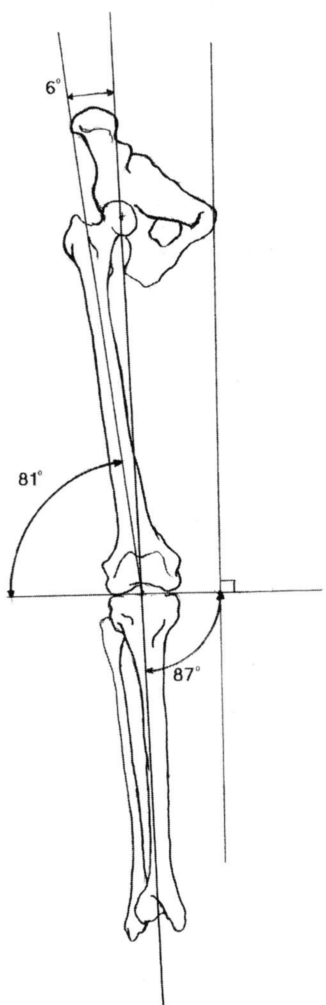

Fig. 6 In the normal knee, a line from the center of the femoral head to the ankle passes through the center of the knee. The axis of the femoral shaft intersects the center of the knee at an average angle of 6° to the mechanical axis and 9° to the vertical axis. The joint line intersects the mechanical axis at 87°.

For the normal knee, the joint line subtends a 9° valgus angle (99°) to the femoral shaft and a 3° varus angle (87°) to the tibial shaft. Common terminology for referring to varus or valgus deformity uses a normal femoral shaft/tibial shaft reference axis of 6° of valgus. This means that a knee with 4° of tibial shaft/femoral shaft valgus would actually be in 2° of varus deformity. In a more recent technique for measuring alignment, one line is drawn from the femoral head to the center of the knee and another line is drawn from the center of the ankle to the center of the knee. The angle formed by the two lines is measured on the medial side and subtracted from 180°. A straight line from the center of the hip to the center of the knee and the center of the knee to the center of the ankle is referred to as neutral alignment. A positive number indicates a varus deformity and a negative number a valgus deformity of the indicated degrees.

From the work done by Kapandji and confirmed by others, it is seen that the normal joint line makes an 87° angle to the mechanical axis, as measured on the medial side.[2-7] Although this is often referred to as 3° of varus, it should be noted that this is not a 3° deformity, it is neutral alignment. Therefore, angles greater than 3°are a varus deformity and those less than 3° are a valgus deformity. These will become important points in discussing the two current methods of alignment, namely, the classic method introduced by Insall and associates[5] and the anatomic method introduced by Hungerford, Krackow, and Kenna.[4]

The Classic Alignment Method

In the classic alignment method, introduced by Insall and associates,[5] the femoral and tibial components are cut perpendicular to the mechanical axis. A femoral cut perpendicular to the mechanical axis is actually a cut in 3° of varus deformity, whereas a tibial cut perpendicular to the mechanical axis is in 3° of valgus (Fig. 7). These are perfectly offsetting malalignments and leave the leg in neutral alignment, with the mechanical axis passing from the center of the femoral head to the center of the ankle through the center of the knee. Now, the joint line, however, is perpendicular to the mechanical axis and not perpendicular to the vertical axis.

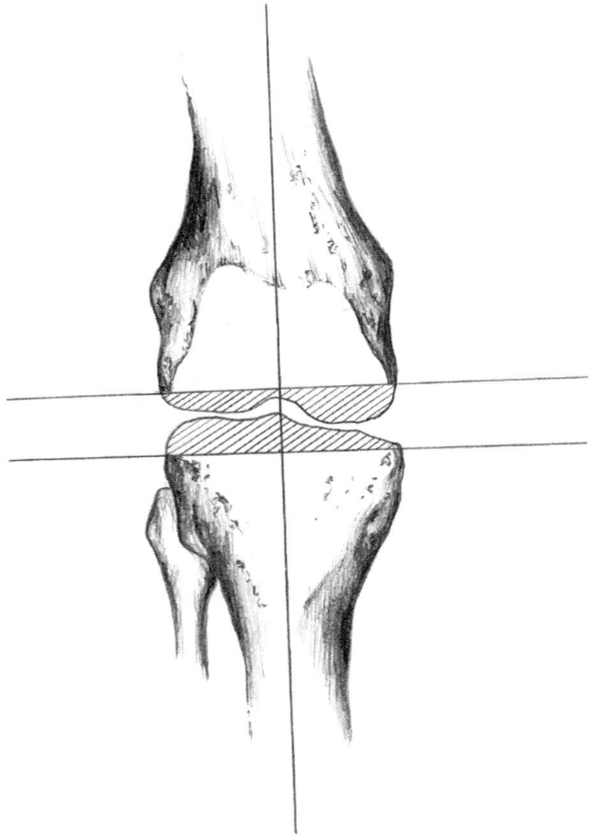

Fig. 7 This drawing depicts femoral and tibial cuts perpendicular to the mechanical axis. Note underresection of the lateral femoral condyle and compensatory overresection of the lateral tibial plateau.

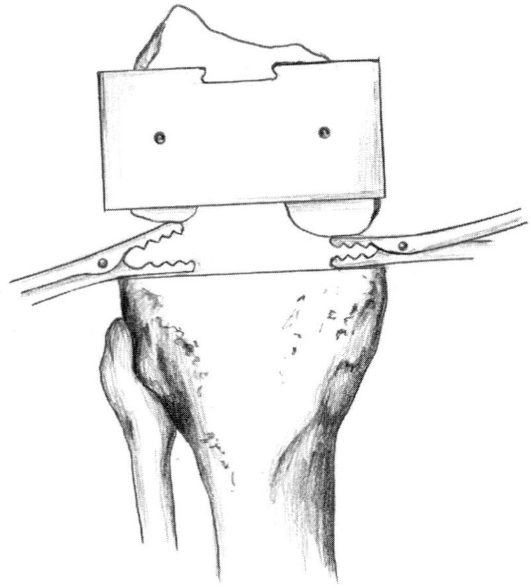

Fig. 8 Under the influence of the tensor, the femur is internally rotated, which leads to compensatory lateral rotation of the femoral component.

These references predate the introduction of comprehensive instrumentation systems, and they generally were used with the flexion-extension gap method for achieving ligamentous balance at the time of TKR. This method of ligamentous balance usually made a minimal cut on the tibia referenced to the tibial shaft (mechanical axis). Proportional cuts were then made on the posterior and distal femur, using a tensor device to place the medial and lateral collateral ligaments under tension (the former in flexion and the latter in extension) while adjusting for varus-valgus orientation but not for a fixed rotational orientation, or proximal-distal orientation.

As noted above, the classic alignment method leads to a valgus overresection of the lateral tibial plateau, which is compensated for by a relative underresection of the lateral femoral condyle. However, as the knee passes into flexion, this overresection of the lateral tibial plateau is not compensated for if the femoral component is placed in anatomic neutral rotation by any of the anatomic references. However, by combining the classic alignment method with the common flexion and extension gap method, when the tensor is applied to the joint space with the knee in flexion, the femur is characteristically internally rotated, which leads to a relative external rotation of the femoral component or relative underresection of the posterior lateral femoral condyle (Fig. 8). This offsets the relative valgus overresection of the tibial component by underresection of the lateral-posterior femoral condyle.

To my knowledge, the kinematic implications of this combination of offsetting malalignments have not been documented in an instrumented prosthesis or instrumented cadaveric preparation. However, the fact is that many series that have demonstrated long-term survival and good clinical results have used this method. The common flexion-extension gap method, however, combined with a minimal tibial resection, often led to both a proximal and an anterior displacement of the femoral component vis-a-vis the anatomic position of the joint space. This produces a relative patella baja and has been reported by Aglietti and associates[8] to be at least partially responsible for an increased incidence of extensor mechanism complication when compared to a group of patients in whom this displacement did not occur.

Currently, many instrumentation systems use a combination of the measured resection method (see below) and the common flexion-extension gap method. Those that combine the classic alignment method with the measured resection method characteristically externally rotate the femoral component from its anatomic reference by approximately 3°.

Anatomic Alignment Method

The anatomic alignment method, using Universal™ instruments, was introduced by Hungerford, Krackow, and Kenna[9] in 1978. This method drew on the work of Kapandji and sought to use the femoral shaft as a reference axis, the intact femoral condyle for the proximal-distal position of the femoral component, and the posterior femoral condyles for the anterior-posterior position of the femoral component. The anatomic reference method has always been associated with the measured resection method for ligament balance. In this method, the distal femoral resection and the posterior femoral resections equal the thickness of the components to be implanted, thus preserving the orientation of the prosthetic joint line as near as possible to the original (Fig. 9). This orientation preserves the relationship of the joint line to the femoral attachments of the collateral ligaments. This method has been demonstrated in a fresh cadaver instrumented model to reproduce nearly perfectly the kinematics of the intact knee using a minimally constrained prosthesis that preserves the posterior cruciate ligament.[4] Any ligament imbalance is caused by osteophytes, scar, contractures, or stretching out and is dealt with separately.

Either the medial or the lateral distal femoral condyle can be used for the proximal-distal position of the femoral component. The femoral shaft is used for the varus-valgus orientation, with a joint line-femoral shaft axis angle that approximates 9°. The space between the deficient condyle and the reference instrument represents the amount of bone lost through the disease process. In most instances, the posterior femoral condyles are preserved even in the face of advanced disease, particularly varus disease.

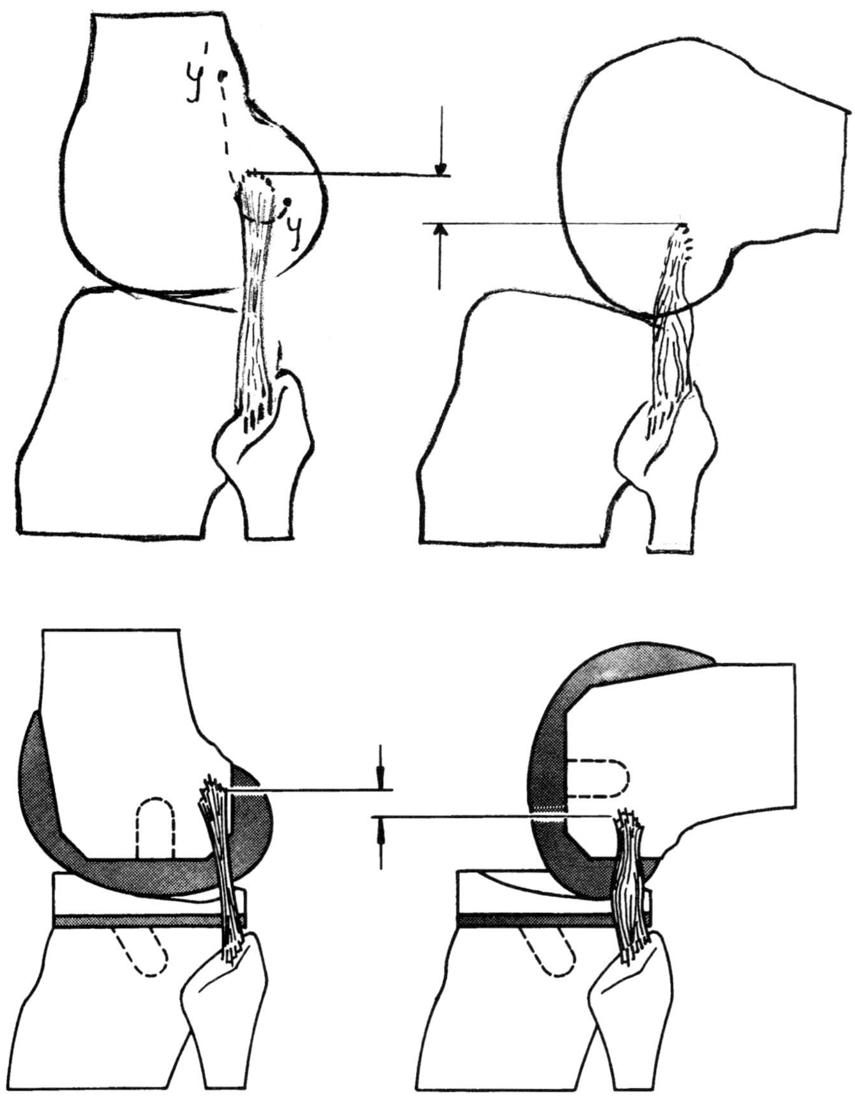

Fig. 9 **Top,** The attachment of the collateral ligaments within the concavity of a line connecting the intact radii of the contact areas of the femoral contour means that the collateral ligaments relax during flexion, allowing rotational movement. **Bottom,** Positioning the femoral component at the same level as the original joint line preserves normal collateral ligament function.

In some cases, however, the lateral posterior condyle is deficient. The medial femoral condyle is then used as the reference condyle for the anterior-posterior position of the femoral component, and secondary rotational references are used for the rotational orientation as opposed to using the lateral-medial posterior condylar plane as the sole rotational reference.

Ligament Balance

In the deformed knee, ligaments are often displaced by osteophytes that build on the concave side of the deformity (Fig. 10). All osteophytes, loose bodies, and scarred synovium must be removed before the ligaments can be balanced. The philosophy of the anatomic and measured resection method of alignment is as follows. If the prosthetic components are placed in anatomic relationship to the bony attachments of the retained ligaments, they will be balanced through a functional range of motion. That hypothesis is tested by the trial reduction. If the trial reduction shows that the ligaments are not stable, it may reveal a malalignment that must be identified and corrected. Of course, it is preferable to avoid the malalignment in the first place, and this requires a complete and detailed understanding of alignment. If the ligaments are not balanced, the tight side can be released, allowing the introduction of a thicker tibial spacer to tighten up the loose side; the loose side can be reconstructed; or a constrained prosthesis can be used to compensate for the instability. This subject is addressed comprehensively in several sources.[4-6] The measured resection method carries out all bony resections first and then balances ligaments. It can be used with either the classic or anatomic alignment methods.

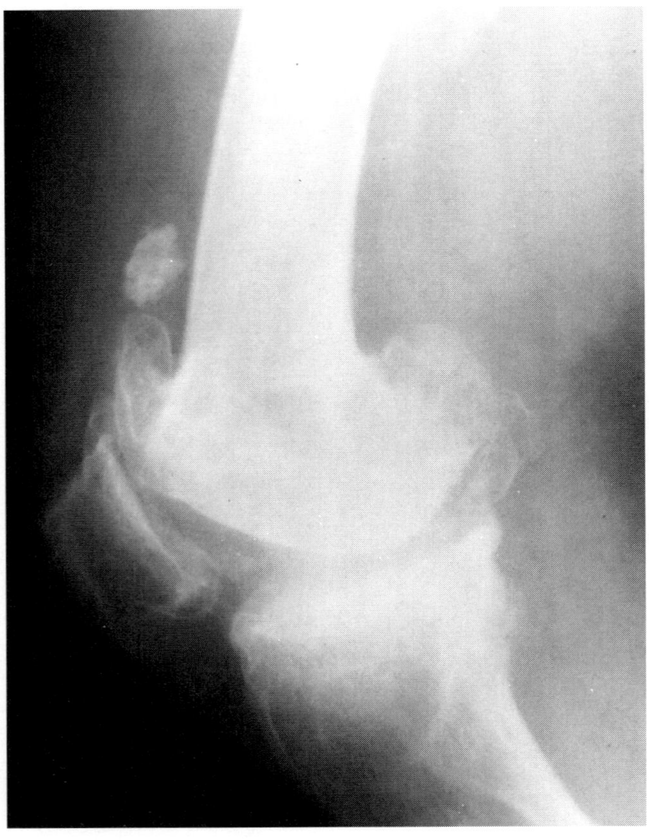

Fig. 10 Because the medial osteophytes in this varus osteoarthritic knee prevent passive correction, they must be removed before ligament balance can be evaluated intraoperatively.

The common flexion-extension gap method of ligament balance requires that all blocks to free and normal ligament movement be removed before bony resection is done. The rotational orientation of the femoral component and, to a lesser extent, the proximal-distal level of the femoral component are determined by the ligaments under the tension of the tensor. Therefore, the tension on the soft tissue must not be changed by the bony resection. For example, if the posterior capsule is contracted, it becomes the principal determinant of the space between the femur and the tibia when the knee is extended. This can lead to overresection of the distal femur. The knee would now be stable in full extension by virtue of posterior capsular tightness. However, when the knee is flexed and the posterior capsule is no longer under tension, the collateral ligament laxity, which was present in extension, is now evident, and the knee is unstable. With the common flexion-extension gap method of ligament balance, bone resection levels and ligament balance are determined at the same time. Therefore, the surgeon has to be careful that such problems as soft-tissue abnormalities, contracture blockages, and stretching out do not lead to the wrong resection levels. Some instrumentation systems now combine elements of the measured resection method and the common flexion-extension gap method to assure that the femoral component is near the original joint line.

Alignment References

Femoral Component

Varus-Valgus, Flexion-Extension In the past, a variety of alignment references have been used, including the estimated line from the center of the femoral head, as determined by its anatomic probability or as determined by radiographic confirmation intraoperatively, to the center of the knee. More commonly, the femoral shaft has been used, initially extraosseously and more recently using the intramedullary canal, from the center of the knee to the isthmus. For extramedullary alignment and flexion-extension of the component, a line between the greater trochanter and the lateral epicondyle has been used (Fig. 11). The intramedullary route determines both flexion-extension and varus-valgus. Most systems today use the intramedullary femoral route. When that is not possible because of defor-

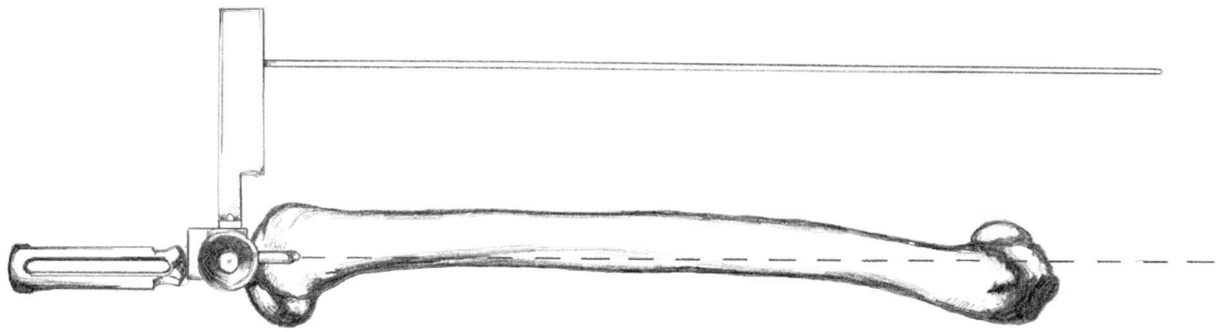

Fig. 11 Proper positioning of the extramedullary guide to assess flexion-extension alignment for the distal femoral cut.

mity, fracture with internal fixation device, or a long cemented femoral stem, the reference point between the femoral epicondyle and the trochanter is still valid for flexion-extension. The mechanical axis, using the femoral head as a reference, has to be used for varus-valgus if the femoral shaft is deformed, although an extramedullary guide can be used if the medullary canal is simply blocked and the shaft is not deformed.

It should be recognized, however, that significant deformity of the femoral shaft malaligns the soft-tissue attachments of the distal femur relative to the mechanical axis. This malalignment leads to a compensatory resection of the distal femur to compensate for the deformity of the shaft and can result in the introduction of a complex ligamentous instability. This problem is outside the context of this chapter but has been addressed elsewhere by Wolff, Hungerford, and Pepe.[10]

Proximal-Distal Position Because the flexion-extension gap method of ligament balancing uses ligament tension to determine the proximal-distal position for the femoral component, this position is relative, not fixed. As long as the femoral component is not significantly displaced proximally from the original level of the condyles, this method produces acceptable ligamentous stability and alignment throughout a functional range of motion. However, Martin and Whiteside[11] have shown in a cadaver model and Sidles and associates[12] in a computer model that, although significant proximal and compensatory anterior displacement of the femoral component produces ligament stability in full extension and in 90° of flexion, it produces relative instability in the mid-range of flexion.

If the level of the distal femoral cut, as determined by the tensor, is proximally displaced to a significant extent by excessive soft-tissue tightness of the posterior structures as opposed to tightness in the collateral ligaments, stability will be present only in full extension with the posterior capsular structures under tension. At only a few degrees of flexion, the posterior capsular structures relax, and ligament balance is lost. For this reason, many current instrumentation systems, although they use some aspect of the combined flexion-extension gap method, use the intact condyle of the distal femur to determine the distal femoral resection level in order to prevent excessive proximal displacement of the femoral component.

The measured resection method seeks to reestablish the anatomic level of the distal femoral cut. Therefore, the prominent condyle is used for the reference. The depth of the cut is determined by the instrument to equal the thickness of the distal femoral component. Because prostheses differ in thickness, this resection level is system specific.

Anterior-Posterior Position Several methods are currently used to determine the final anterior-posterior position of the femoral component. Some systems reference the anterior cortex, and, in these, the size of the component chosen determines how much posterior femoral condyle must be resected. If the component is too small, the posterior condyles will be overresected, creating too much space in flexion, hence instability. If too large a component is chosen, too little posterior condyle will be resected and the knee will be tight in flexion. Therefore, flexion stability depends on the choice of just the right size femoral component. For this reason, I prefer to use the posterior femoral condyles as a reference, and I resect the amount of condyle that will be replaced by the prosthesis. This procedure assures that flexion stability will not be compromised. If a prosthesis of the wrong size is chosen, the result will be overresection or underresection of the anterior femur, which is of less importance than flexion stability. Both of the above are variations of the measured resection method.

With the combined flexion-extension gap method, the level of the posterior resection is determined by the tensor, with all the caveats expressed regarding distal femoral resection. As long as the component does not end up too far from the original level, it should function satisfactorily.

Rotation There are three anatomic aspects of the distal femur that assist in determining correct rotation (Fig. 12). (1) In the normal femur, the posterior condyles define the coronal plane and, if these are not worn or destroyed by disease, they probably represent the most reliable reference for rotation. (2) In the normal anatomy, the lateral trochlear facet is projected more anterior than the medial trochlear facet, and all surgeons are familiar with the typical appearance of the patellofemoral joint in the "sky-line" radiograph. The plane of the lateral and medial trochlear facet is approximately 5° to 6° to the coronal plane or the plane of neutral rotation. (3) The epicondyles are available as a rotational reference, but they are less easily defined, because they are covered with the soft tissue of the collateral ligament attachments. The lateral epicondyle is posterior to the medial epicondyle and the medial epicondyle-lateral epicondyle axis is externally rotated about 10° referable to the neutral rotation or coronal plane.

The posterior condyles, in addition to being used as a reference for the anterior-posterior position of the femoral components, are also used as a rotational reference for the femoral component. Because the orientation of the anterior and posterior planes of resection also determines the rotational reference, these two references—level and rotation—are usually determined together.

The way the common flexion-extension gap method used the tensor to determine the anterior-posterior position of the femoral component was described earlier. In this method, the tensor also determines the rotational position of the femoral component. Because the lateral soft-tissue stabilizers are normally more lax than the medial soft-tissue stabilizers, the femur automatically rotates internally when the tensor is applied, leading to external rotation of the femoral component and femoral resection orientation. Thus, when the classic alignment scheme is used, the valgus overresection of the lateral tibial plateau tends to be compensated for automatically.

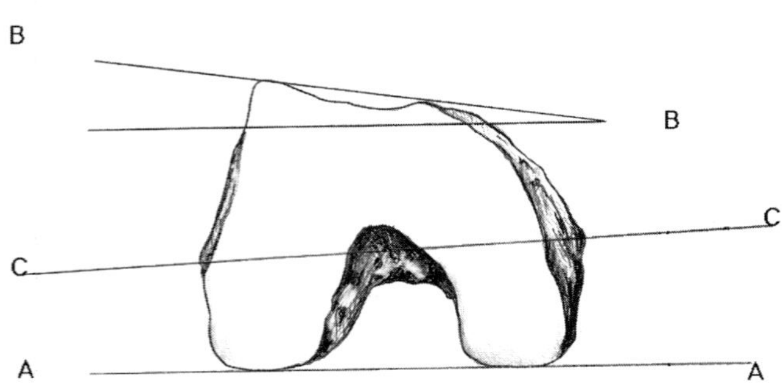

Fig. 12 This end-on drawing of the distal femur shows the three anatomic features used to assess rotation. **A** The posterior condylar axis is parallel to the neutral rotation plane. **B** The trochlea facet axis is inclined 20° to the neutral plane. **C** The transepicondylar axis is inclined 10° to the neutral rotation.

The measured resection method can be applied to either the anatomic or the classic alignment scenarios. If the classic alignment method is used and the posterior femoral condyle is used for rotation, the reference drill holes made in the distal femur can be externally rotated (Fig. 13). If the anatomic method of alignment is used, the reference drill holes will be equidistant from the posterior femoral condyles. It is important to recognize this difference between the classic and anatomic alignment philosophies, because combining the two can leave lateral instability in flexion if the femoral component is not relatively externally rotated. There does not appear to be any downside risk to external rotation of the femoral component.

In general, even in the diseased knee, the posterior femoral condyles are intact as a reliable reference for rotation. However, in severe valgus deformity, the lateral posterior condyle may be significantly eroded and, therefore, is not a reliable reference. In such cases, the secondary references of the orientation of the trochlea and the orientation of the epicondyles are used to determine rotation.

Medial-Lateral Position Five of the six degrees of freedom for the femoral component—varus-valgus, flexion-extension, rotation, proximal-distal, and anterior-posterior position—have now been covered. Medial-lateral position, the final degree of freedom, is simply determined by covering the cut surface of the distal femur. Usually, if the right size is chosen, this will cover completely. Medial displacement should be avoided, because medial displacement of the trochlea can compromise tracking of the patella. If the bone surface is wider than the prosthesis, the component should be coapted to the lateral margin of the distal femur. If the component is wider than the bone, any overhang should be on the lateral and not the medial side. If overhang is substantial, the anterior-posterior residual of the femur should be carefully assessed to see if the next smaller component could be used.

Tibial Component

Varus-Valgus, Flexion-Extension As in the distal femur, the plane of the proximal tibial cut defines the varus-valgus and flexion-extension alignment of the tibial component. The normal tibial shaft is coincident with the mechanical axis. Even in the deformed shaft, the center of the knee and the center of the ankle are both accessible at surgery and can be referenced with an extramedullary device, which determines the flexion-extension and varus-valgus orientation of the proximal tibial cut. If the classic alignment method is chosen, the varus-valgus orientation is perpendicular to the mechanical axis, which inherently leads to relative overresection of the lateral tibial plateau (Fig. 7). With the

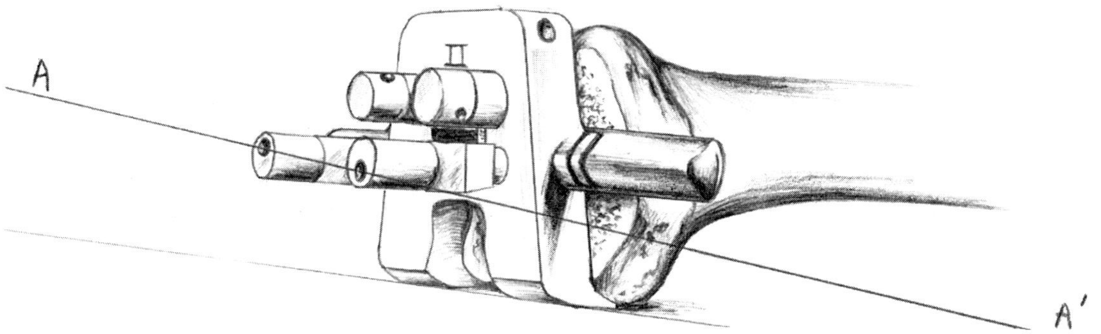

Fig. 13 Drill guide for the distal femoral reference holes, positioned using the posterior condyles as reference. The drill guide insert is available for neutral reference, equidistant from the posterior condyles, or for 3° external rotation, as in this instance (line A-A').

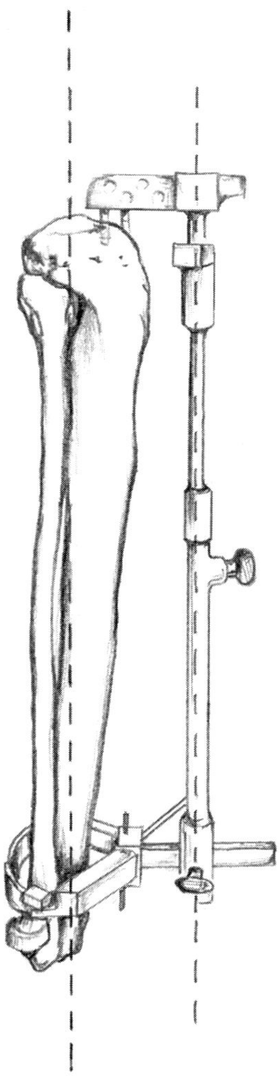

Fig. 14 Extramedullary tibial resection guide, aligned with the fibula for flexion-extension (posterior slope) orientation.

anatomic alignment method, the orientation will be an 87.5° angle on the medial side to the mechanical axis. Although this is referred to as a 2.5° varus cut, it should be noted that it is actually a neutral resection orientation, not a cut in varus malalignment. It should also be noted that when a tibial stem of significant length is being used in the tibial component, the classic alignment scenario must be chosen, because the only such components available have the tibial stem oriented perpendicular to the plateau.

The central axis of the tibial shaft, not the anterior crest of the tibia, constitutes the flexion-extension reference. With the extramedullary alignment instrument, the fibula serves as a reliable guide (Fig. 14). The flexion-extension orientation of the proximal tibia resection is usually referred to as the tibial slope. For some prostheses, this is built into the prosthetic design so that less posterior slope of the resection orientation is necessary than the 7° to 10° characteristic of the posterior slope of the normal knee. In some instrumentation systems, the correct posterior slope is built into the instruments. In others, the alignment rod must be drawn distally, away from the ankle, to increase posterior slope. This important alignment reference is related to prosthetic and instrument design and careful attention must be paid to it.

The disadvantage of excessive posterior slope is that, for prostheses that retain a posterior cruciate ligament, it resects the tibial attachment of the ligament. Also, the lower the resection level, the weaker the bone and the smaller the surface area. Excessive posterior slope represents a relative posterior overresection, and the replaced knee will be unstable in flexion.

Rotation The alignment references for tibial rotation, which are perhaps the least precise of any of the alignment references in TKR, are nonetheless important. For some systems, it is recommended that the tibial spacer be allowed to seek its own rotational level when the knee is placed in full extension. Some total knee designs in the past were completely unconstrained rotationally. With these implants, the tibia was allowed to seek its own rotational orientation, because the design of the component lacked rotational constraint. These prostheses were associated with a significant incidence of patellar instability.

The soft-tissue envelope around the knee should be properly balanced. If these soft tissues are allowed to dictate the rotational relationship between the tibial component and the femoral component, any soft-tissue imbalance can lead to rotational malalignment of the tibial component. This is particularly true in valgus deformity of the knee, because tight lateral structures tend to externally rotate the tibia in extension, resulting in an internal rotation malalignment of the tibial component.

It is, therefore, my opinion that, within the very narrow limits dictated by the anatomy and the position of the tibial tubercle, the rotational alignment of the tibial component should be chosen and tentatively fixed. The implications of that alignment are then determined by trial reduction, and the soft tissues are balanced with the tibial component in the selected rotational alignment. Currently, most TKRs create some rotational constraint, albeit incomplete, in full extension. With the final selection of rotational orientation and soft-tissue balance, the surgeon must assure that there is no conflict between the way the design of the tibial and femoral components lines up the respective components in extension and the way the soft tissues line up the components in extension. Any such conflict will produce excessive polyethylene wear, a phenomenon that has been noted at the time of reoperation in polyethylene components retrieved from failed knees (Fig. 15).

The most reliable rotational reference for the tibia is the transverse axis of the tibial plateau. When the entire tibial plateau is seen during good exposure of the tibia prior to resection, the articular surface of the tibia can be seen to be oval with a fairly obvious transverse axis (Fig. 16). When the appropriately sized tibial components are in the proper medial-lateral position, and correctly rotated, the center of the tibial component should be lined up between the middle and central thirds of the tibial tubercle. This is an important secondary reference.

However, the position of the tibial tubercle cannot, in and of itself, be the sole reference for rotation, because a combination of medial or lateral malposition and rotational malposition can still align the center of the tibial component with the tibial tubercle. Therefore, the rotation of the tibial component should first be selected in reference to the transverse axis of the tibial plateau and then adjusted to align with the tibial tubercle. There may be instances in which the tibial tubercle is abnormally laterally displaced. Some deformities, such as congenital dislocation of the patella, which can lead to the need for TKR, have as part of the deformity a severe lateral displacement of the tibial tubercle. If the distal fragment of a high tibial osteotomy has been externally rotated, the tibial tubercle may be laterally displaced. Rarely, in such instances, the tibial tubercle must be osteotomized and medialized in

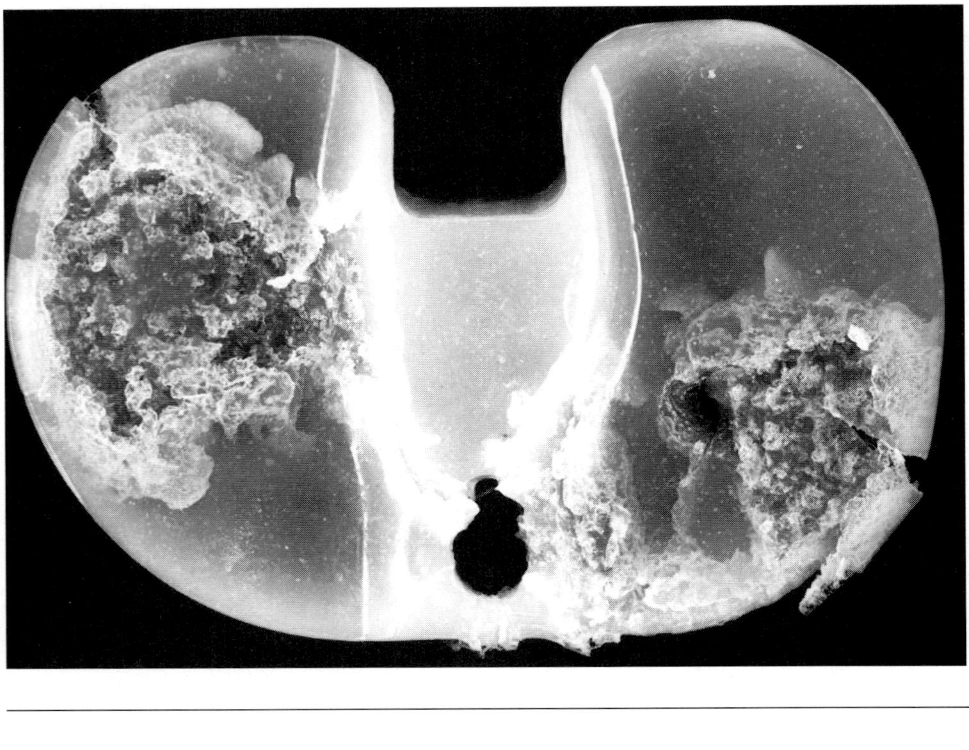

Fig. 15 Retrieved polyethylene insert showing anterolateral and posteromedial wear, a pattern which must indicate rotational malalignment.

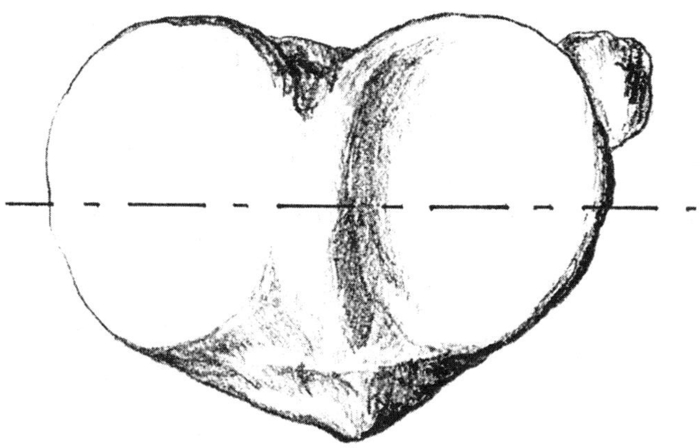

Fig. 16 Drawing of the top view of the fully exposed tibial plateau. The transverse axis is apparent.

order to achieve correct patellar tracking. In such instances, it is probably not acceptable to excessively externally rotate the tibial component to line it up with the tibial tubercle, because to do so would produce abnormal position of the collateral ligaments in regards to the tibial articulation and would result in faulty tibial-femoral mechanics.

Most current TKRs slope the tibial cut posteriorly, some by as much as 10°. For this reason, it is important to estimate accurately the proper rotational alignment of the tibial component before cutting the proximal tibia. If the tibial cut is made in an improper degree of rotation, then the posterior slope is not in the anterior-posterior plane, but is oblique. For example, if the tibia is inadvertently externally rotated when the tibial cutting jig is fixed in place, the posterior slope will be from anteromedial to posterolateral, rather than from anterior to posterior. Then, at the time of trial reduction, if the surgeon recognizes the internal rotation of the tibial component and seeks to correct it, external rotation of the component will rotate the posterior slope toward the lateral side of the knee, creating a valgus deformity. Thus, it is important to approximate the correct rotational alignment closely before the tibial cut is made. In an earlier surgical technique, which used the Universal instruments introduced in 1978, use of the transmalleolar axis was recommended for approximating tibial rotational alignment. However, the relationship between the transmalleolar axis and the true transverse axis of the tibia varies considerably. Although it averages 25°, it varies from 0° to 48°. Therefore, unless the surgeon knows the norm for the patient being treated, this reference is not reliable.

Medial-Lateral, Anterior-Posterior Position Most systems today have many tibial sizes so that the cut surface of the tibia can be completely capped, which defines both of these degrees of freedom. If the component is slightly undersized, it should be coapted to the lateral and posterior margins of the cut surface. If it is slightly oversized, it should overhang laterally and anteriorly. Medial overhang must be avoided so as not to cause painful conflict with the medial collateral ligament. Because the lateral collateral attaches to the fibula and not the tibia, slight lateral overhang is not a problem.

Proximal-Distal Position Because the tibial component, as opposed to the femoral component, is available in many thicknesses, the depth of the tibial cut is not a problem. Typically, the tibia is resected to the level of the bone defect and the proper thickness is chosen at the time of trial reduction. Minimal thickness is usually 8 or 9 mm. If bone erosion is less than that, the intact plateau can serve as a reference to assure that the cutting guide is positioned at the minimal depth.

Patellar Component

It may seem hard to think of six degrees of freedom for the patellar component, but they do exist. However, because the patella articular surface lies in a different plane, some of these degrees of freedom are commonly named differently than for the femoral or tibial component. The six degrees of freedom are proximal-distal slope, medial-lateral slope, rotation, proximal-distal position, medial-lateral position, and depth of cut or anterior-posterior position.

Proximal-Distal and Medial-Lateral Slope These slopes are defined by the plane of resection and should parallel the front of the patella so that the resected remnant is approximately the same thickness as the original bone. The resected articular surface should look like the skyline view of the patella (Fig. 17). The proximal-distal slope parallels the central ridge (Fig. 18).

Rotation Most systems have a symmetrical dome-shaped patellar button, and for these the rotational references are irrelevant. However, because the medial-lateral dimension of the patella is characteristically greater than the proximal-distal dimension, the cut surface of the

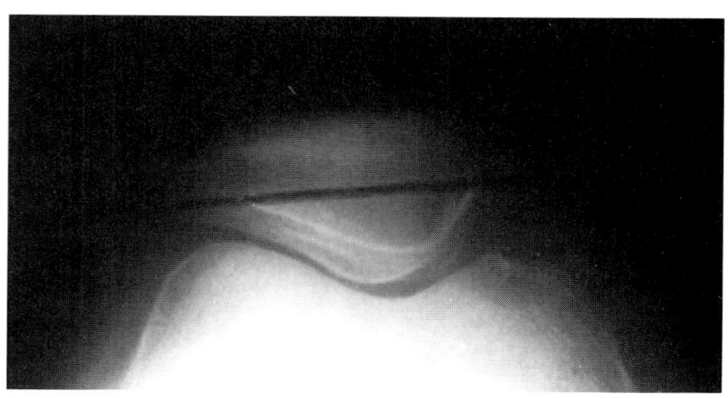

Fig. 17 Skyline view of the patella with resection orientation indicated.

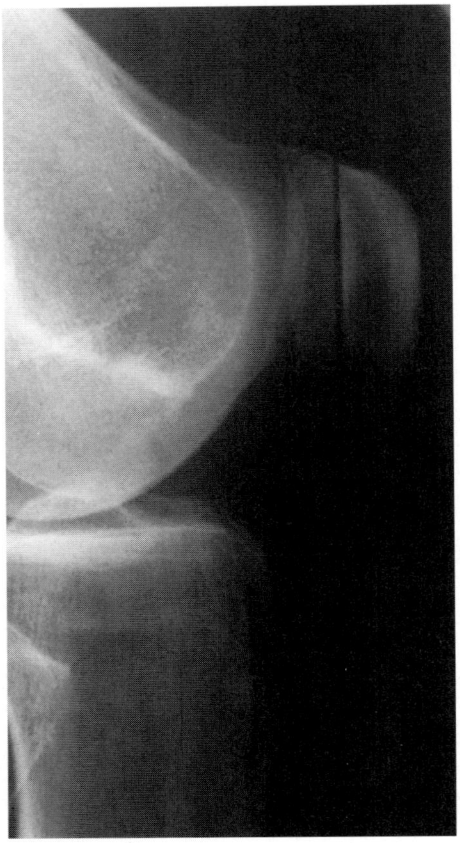

Fig. 18 Lateral radiograph of the patella indicating proximal-distal resection orientation paralleling the central ridge.

patella is oval. The symmetrical dome patella, therefore, sized to cover medially-laterally will overlap proximally-distally, and one sized for the proximal-distal dimension will not cover medially-laterally. For this reason, some systems provide an asymmetric dome-shaped patella, with medial-lateral and proximal-distal dimensions similar to those of the anatomic patella. For these prostheses, approximate rotational alignment is important even though these are not usually constrained in the rotational sense. The central ridge of the patella defines the rotational axis of the patella and, therefore, the longer medial lateral axis of the patellar component ideally should be implanted perpendicular to this longitudinal central ridge. However, because even the asymmetric patellar components are not rotationally constrained, the asymmetric dimension of the component can be aligned with the asymmetric contour of the resected surface of the patella.

Proximal-Distal and Medial-Lateral Position Normally the patellar component is sized to the proximal-distal dimension of the cut surface, so that proximal-distal malposition can occur only if the prosthesis overhangs the bony margin. However, a properly sized dome patella will never fully cover the medial-lateral cut surface of the patella. Because the central ridge of the patella is not centered on the patella, but is more medial than lateral, the prosthetic component should always be coapted to the medial margin of the cut surface. Any portion of the lateral patella that remains uncovered does not appear to be a problem.

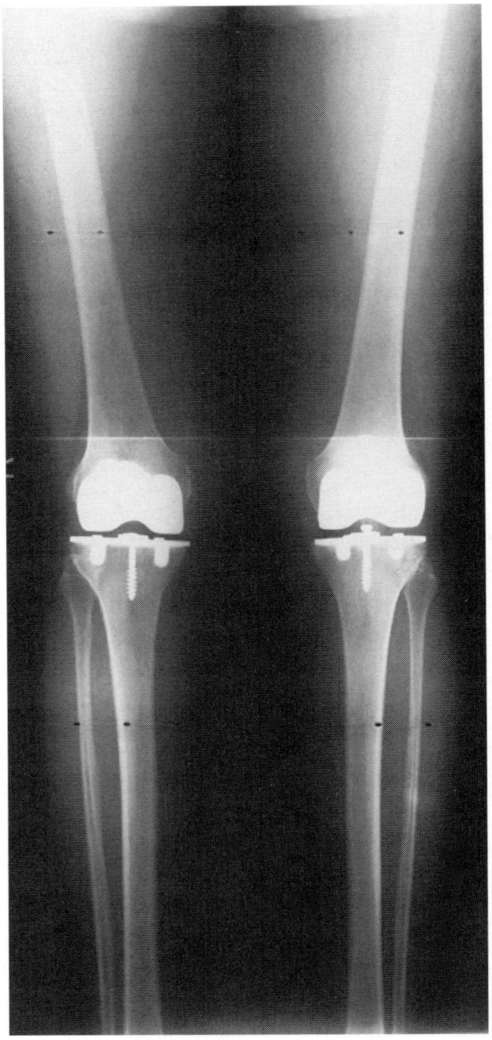

Fig. 19 AP radiograph of a perfectly aligned knee in neutral rotation.

Anterior-Posterior Position Level of resection or depth is the sixth degree of freedom. Most patellar components are 9 to 11 mm thick. A caliper should be used to measure patellar thickness prior to resection, measuring from the central ridge to the anterior surface. The thickness of the component is resected making sure that at least 12 mm of residual bone is left to support the prosthesis.

Assessing Alignment

It should be the responsibility of all orthopaedic surgeons to assess carefully the quality of their work. Only in this way can improvement take place. There

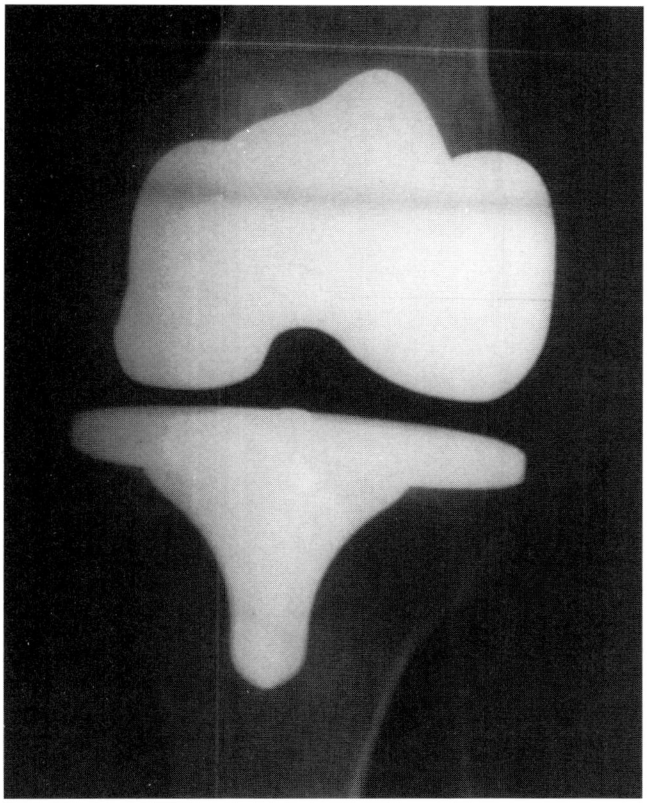

Fig. 20 Same knee as in Figure 19, positioned in 10° external rotation and 15° of flexion. Accurate varus-valgus alignment measurement is not possible.

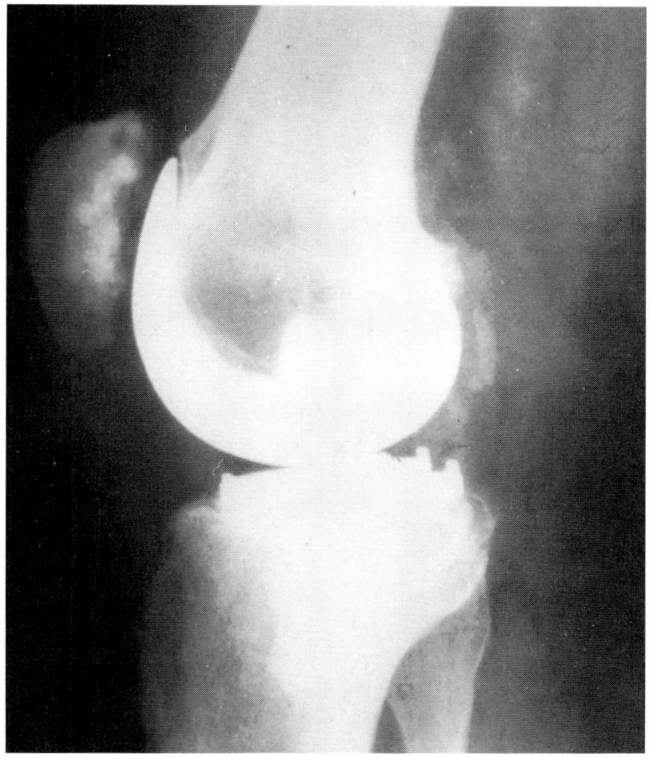

Fig. 21 Flexion-extension attitude of both components can be accurately measured on a standard lateral radiograph.

are, however, some caveats. Not all of the degrees of freedom can be equally effectively measured on radiographs. Rotational alignment, depth, anterior-posterior and proximal-distal alignment are hard to measure. Varus-valgus is most accurately measured on a long (36- or 40-inch) film, which includes the femoral head and ankle. The most common difficulty, however, is that even these parameters can be measured accurately only if the knee is in neutral rotation (Fig. 19). If the leg is externally rotated when the radiograph is taken, and particularly if it is externally rotated and flexed, it is not possible to measure accurately varus-valgus alignment (Fig. 20). Flexion-extension alignment can usually be measured easily on a standard lateral radiograph (Fig. 21).

Conclusion

Alignment in TKR is important to function. Any malalignment can lead to a clinical problem. Severe malalignments produce early clinical failure. More subtle malalignments may take years to manifest an adverse effect. However, the average patient undergoing TKR in my institution is 64 years old with a 19-year life expectancy. All aspects of alignment must be understood and addressed if we are to achieve a high degree of survival at the 20-plus year mark.

References

1. Ritter MA, Faris PM, Keating EM, et al: Postoperative alignment of total knee: Its effect on survival. *Clin Orthop* 1994;299:153-156.
2. Kapandji A: *The Physiology of the Joints.* New York, NY, Churchill Livingstone, 1970, vol 2.
3. Greenberg RL, Kenna RV, Hungerford DS, et al: Instrumentation for total knee arthroplasty, in Hungerford DS, Krackow KA, Kenna KA, et al (eds): *Total Knee Arthroplasty: A Comprehensive Approach.* Baltimore, MD, Williams & Wilkins, 1984, pp 35-70.
4. Hungerford DS, Krackow KA, Kenna RV (eds): *Total Knee Arthroplasty: A Comprehensive Approach.* Baltimore, MD, Williams & Wilkins, 1984.
5. Insall JN, Windsor RE, Scott WN, et al (eds): *Surgery of the Knee,* ed 2. New York, NY, Churchill Livingstone, 1993.
6. Krackow KA (ed): *The Technique of Total Knee Arthroplasty.* St. Louis, MO, CV Mosby, 1990.
7. Moreland JR, Bassett LW, Hankes GJ: Radiographic analysis of the axial alignment of the lower extremity. *J Bone Joint Surg* 1987; 62A:745-749.
8. Aglietti P, Buzzi R, Gaudenzi A: Patellofemoral functional results and complications with the posterior stabilized total condylar knee prosthesis. *J Arthroplasty* 1988;3:17-25.
9. Hungerford DS, Krackow KA, Kenna RV: Alignment in total knee arthroplasty, in Dorr LD (ed): *The Knee: Papers of the First Scientific Meeting of the Knee Society.* Baltimore, MD, University Park Press, 1985, pp 9-21.

10. Wolff AM, Hungerford DS, Pepe CL: The effect of extraarticular varus and valgus deformity on total knee arthroplasty. *Clin Orthop* 1991;271:35-51.
11. Martin JW, Whiteside LA: The influence of joint line position on knee stability after condylar knee arthroplasty. *Clin Orthop* 1990; 259:146-156.
12. Sidles JA, Matsen FA, Garbini JL, et al: Total knee arthroplasty: Functional effects of tibial resection level. *Trans Orthop Res Soc* 1986;11:263.

CHAPTER 41

Circular External Fixation in High Tibial Osteotomy

Vladimir Schwartsman, MD

Introduction

The biomechanical basis for a high tibial osteotomy in the management of unicompartmental osteoarthritis of the knee is to unload the diseased joint compartment by correcting malalignment and redistributing the loading forces on the knee. Proper surgical technique should alter the mechanical axis of the extremity, achieve normal knee and ankle joint orientation, and also correct any coexisting rotational deformity.

The two most critical factors that influence the long-term success of a high tibial osteotomy are proper patient selection and precise correction of the extremity's mechanical axis.[1] The majority of unsatisfactory results with high tibial osteotomy are caused by over- or undercorrection of the extremity's mechanical axis.[2] Conventional methods of high tibial osteotomy, which use bone wedge resection and various types of internal fixation, do not always offer the optimal solution for this problem. Measurements of the bone wedge to be removed for high tibial osteotomy are, at best, approximate preoperatively and are even less precise intraoperatively. About 1 or 2 mm of bone is usually lost because of bone compression if an osteotome is used, or, if a power saw is used, some bone is turned into dust.[1]

Preoperative and postoperative measurements depend on the position of the extremity at the time radiographs were taken. Internal or external rotation of the limb will affect the measured femorotibial angle. Furthermore, medial tibial torsion may cause a varus knee, and lateral tibial torsion may cause the appearance of a valgus knee.[3] The position of the weightbearing line of the extremity is also sensitive to the lengths of the femur and tibia and to abnormal lateral joint opening.[4] It may be possible, through elaborate trigonometric formulas, to calculate precisely the amount of correction needed, taking all important data into account. However, during surgery it may prove impossible to implement those calculations with any degree of precision.

Deformity correction is much more accurate if alignment can be altered after the operation, when standing full limb-length anteroposterior radiographs are available and appropriate measurements are obtained. The Ilizarov apparatus and Ilizarov's principles of deformity correction seem to offer several advantages over other methods of high tibial osteotomy.

Advantages of Circular External Fixation

The fact that the frame is infinitely adjustable allows precision and predictable accuracy of correction of the extremity's mechanical axis. The planned correction can be done acutely in the operating room or gradually during the postoperative period. In either case, it is important that fine adjustments of the degree of correction be possible later, after the operation is completed. The degree of achieved correction is measured postoperatively on a 5-foot standing anteroposterior radiograph and, if necessary, the correction can be easily changed for up to several weeks after surgery.

With the Ilizarov method, a distractional open-wedge technique is used to correct the knee deformity below the patellar tendon insertion, at the level of the lower border of the tibial tubercle. With conventional techniques, a closing-wedge osteotomy (often performed above the tibial tubercle) is used for most internal fixation methods, because this strategy has resulted in more predictable healing of the cancellous metaphyseal bone. On the other hand, a high closing-wedge osteotomy causes loss of bone stock, interferes with patellofemoral biomechanics by producing patella infera, and has an adverse effect on the results of a total joint arthroplasty if one has to be performed in the future.[5] Conversely, a distractional open-wedge osteotomy below the tibial tubercle (and the technically demanding dome-shaped osteotomy) do not interfere with patellar biomechanics. Use of the Ilizarov method assures uncomplicated and fast healing of the corrective corticotomy site.

Correction of the knee deformity with the Ilizarov apparatus is biomechanically sound. When the medial or lateral knee joint compartments are affected by degenerative arthritis, the limb angulates into either varus or valgus. The true apex of this deformity lies at the level of the joint line, and a corrective osteotomy at the true apex of the deformity is impossible because the apex is within the joint. Nonapical correction of such a deformity may result in an incorrect mechanical axis of the extremity, in which the axis of the distal tibial fragment is parallel to, but is not colinear with, the extremity's axis (Fig. 1). Special translational hinges of the Ilizarov apparatus, positioned at the true apex of the deformity at the level of the knee joint, restore the extremity's mechanical axis correctly by providing the appropriate amount of translation of the distal fragment. Furthermore, use of this eccentric hinge offers

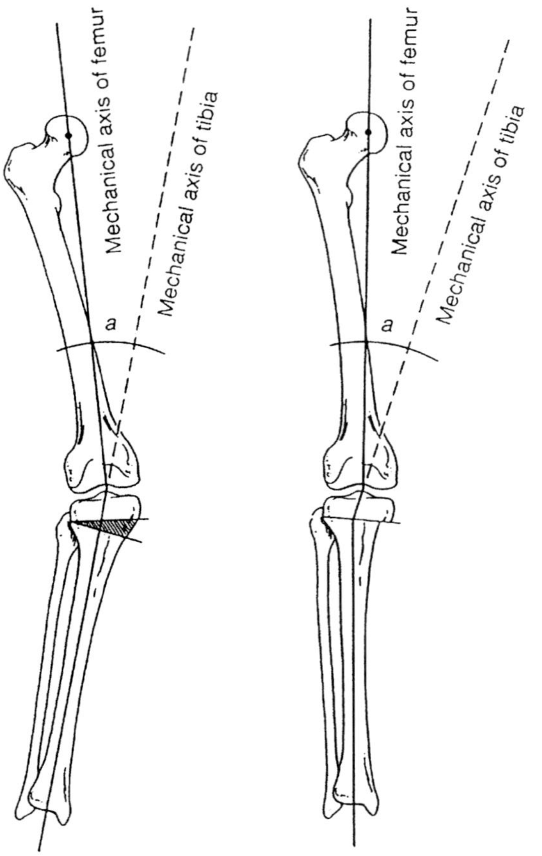

Fig. 1 **Left,** Preoperative tracing to calculate the size of the wedge for varus tibial osteotomy. (Reproduced with permission from Murray PB, Rand JA: Symptomatic valgus knee. *J Am Acad Orthop Surg* 1993;1:1-9.) **Right,** After deformity has been corrected, the jagged instead of straight appearance of the extremity mechanical axis is evident. (Adapted with permission from Murray PB, Rand JA: Symptomatic valgus knee. *J Am Acad Orthop Surg* 1993;1:1-9.)

some latitude in selecting the level of the corticotomy. This important point—translating the distal fragment to restore the extremity's proper mechanical axis—was not taken into consideration with conventional techniques of high tibial osteotomy. With the unilateral frame distraction technique, the apex of deformity correction is significantly below the joint line (the true apex of deformity), and there is no provision for translation of the distal fragment to correctly restore mechanical axis of the extremity.[6]

With conventional methods of high tibial osteotomy, the correction must be done at once, which causes more traumatic injury to the bone and soft tissues and, on occasion, can lead to nonunion. This problem is particularly serious when the deformity to be corrected is severe. Also, when correcting a valgus knee deformity, gradual correction has an advantage over acute correction, because it minimizes the risk of injury to the peroneal nerve.

In place of an open osteotomy, correction of the deformity with Ilizarov's method is performed with a corticotomy that is accomplished through a 1.0- to 1.5-cm incision, which minimizes the injury to soft tissues and to the bone's osteogenic elements. Conventional methods of deformity correction require more traumatic extensive soft-tissue dissection to achieve bone wedge resection and osteotomy stabilization.

Internal fixation methods of high tibial osteotomy may not provide adequate stability of the osteotomy site, and if instability is noted after surgery, it is impossible to correct. The Ilizarov apparatus, which uses thin tensioned wires placed in different directions and levels, offers multiplanar stable fixation of the relatively small proximal fragment. Tensioned transfixion wires are a more appropriate mode of fixation for this fragment than any type of cantilevered fixation, because stability of fixation can be enhanced easily by simply adding more wires or by using olive wires. Wires applied at several levels widen the area of fixation, thereby improving stability of fixation.

The ability to increase compression at the corrective corticotomy site speeds healing and also increases the stability of fixation. Compression at the site of the osteotomy, achieved by judicious shortening of the connecting rods, can be done either by the surgeon at an office visit or by the patient.

Conventional methods of high tibial osteotomy can lead to postoperative joint stiffness if prolonged cast immobilization is used to supplement internal fixation. This problem is avoided with the Ilizarov technique, because the range of motion of the knee joint in the apparatus is 0° to 90° and full weightbearing on the extremity is commenced on the first day after surgery.

Another, rather unusual advantage of the Ilizarov method for high tibial osteotomy is that the technique can be used just as successfully in large patients or when the deformity is so great that acute correction with conventional methods might be too traumatic for the soft tissues.

On rare occasions, limb length discrepancy and rotational deformity of the proximal tibia can be corrected with frame modifications done on an outpatient basis. This type of correction is not possible with internal fixation techniques of high tibial osteotomy.

Disadvantages of Circular External Fixation

As with any other method of treatment, the Ilizarov technique for high tibial osteotomy has its disadvantages as well. The main concern is the proximity of the wires to the joint and a fear that superficial pin tract infection will spread either into the joint or in the metaphyseal area, perhaps jeopardizing future total joint surgery. This has not happened in any of our cases. Furthermore, the Ilizarov wires are only 1.8 mm in diameter and, with good surgical technique, leave only a small hole in the bone that heals promptly after frame removal. It is easy to remove an infected Ilizarov wire and apply another one in a different location on the same ring. An infected half pin in close proximity to the knee joint may prove to be much more hazardous and technically challenging to change without interfering with stability of fixation and alignment.

The long learning curve associated with circular fixation method and the seemingly labor intense procedure are other considerations but, in our experience, this operation requires less time than internal fixation procedures.

Surgical Technique

Preoperative Measurements

Standing double stance 5-foot alignment radiographs are obtained preoperatively and the deviation of the mechanical axis of the extremity is measured. Calculations are made for correction and overcorrection of the extremity mechanical axis. It is important to position the patient correctly for those radiographs. Both patellae (not feet) must point directly forward. The most common mistake is to position the patient with the feet parallel and pointing forward, a maneuver that does not take into account the rotational deformity of the limb. Preoperative radiographic studies also include four views of the knee joint: anteroposterior, lateral, intercondylar notch, and tangential patellar views.

Frame Preassembly

Three rings are normally used for frame construction. One ring (usually a radiolucent carbon-fiber ring) is above the proximal tibial corticotomy, and a block of two rings is distal to the corticotomy site.

Construction and application of the translational hinges is the most important part of the frame assembly. In general, a hinge may be below a ring, on a ring, or above a ring (Fig. 2). As a rule, for high tibial osteotomy due to degenerative knee joint disease, hinges either at the level of the ring or above the ring are recommended. If varus knee deformity is to be corrected, the location of these hinges should be above and somewhat lateral to the planned corticotomy site. For valgus knee deformity correction, the hinge is placed proximally and medially to the corticotomy site. The more proximal the hinge from the corticotomy site, the more translation will be achieved. The more lateral (or medial in case of valgus knee deformity correction) the hinge is with respect to the corticotomy site, the more lengthening will be achieved with deformity correction. When correcting a varus knee deformity, a lateral placement of the hinges is better tolerated by the patient than if the hinges are positioned medially or at the apex of the deformity. This placement avoids crushing of the lateral tibial cortices during angular deformity correction. The location of the hinge determines the apex for deformity correction. Two hinges, one applied anteriorly and the other posteriorly, connect the proximal ring to the block of two distal rings. The limbs of the hinges are angled precisely to the calculated degree of desired correction and are then locked. This step tilts the proximal ring in relation to the middle ring at the angle chosen for deformity correction. A distraction rod is then applied medially (or laterally for valgus knee) to connect the proximal ring to the set of distal rings. The distraction rod should be located on the side of the rings opposite the hinges and halfway between them.

Fibular Osteotomy

Fibular osteotomy is not needed for a deformity of 10° or less. For greater deformities it is an important part of the procedure. The fibular osteotomy should avoid muscle damage and injury to the superficial peroneal nerve. Our complications with peroneal nerve palsy at the beginning of the learning curve were attributed to improper surgical technique of fibular osteotomy. The knee is flexed and the skin incision is made laterally in the upper third of the leg. The interval between the gastrocnemius-soleus muscles and the peroneal muscles is found and split, to reflect the peroneal muscles with the superficial peroneal nerve anteriorly and the gastrocnemius-soleus muscle group posteriorly. Using the intermuscular septum as a guide, the fibula is exposed in the upper third. A small oblique segment of the fibula, less than 1 cm, is excised. The wound is irrigated and closed in layers.

Frame Application

Usually five olive (beaded) wires and two smooth 1.8-mm Kirschner wires (K-wires) are used for frame application. The first wire (an olive wire) is inserted from the lateral side, parallel to the knee joint line. The preassembled frame is then connected to this wire. The position of the frame and hinges is checked in relationship to the leg and the wire is tensioned. By pivoting the frame on this single proximal wire, the anterior connecting rods of the frame are made parallel to the anterior tibial crest. The second olive wire is then applied to the distal ring in mediolateral direction and tensioned. Three more olive wires are applied, one medially on the proximal ring and two (laterally and medially) on the middle ring. One smooth wire is passed through both the tibia and the fibular head from the lateral side and is tensioned on the proximal ring. The second smooth wire is applied to the distal ring.

Corticotomy

Before the corticotomy is performed, the hinges and the distraction rod are removed temporarily. The tibial

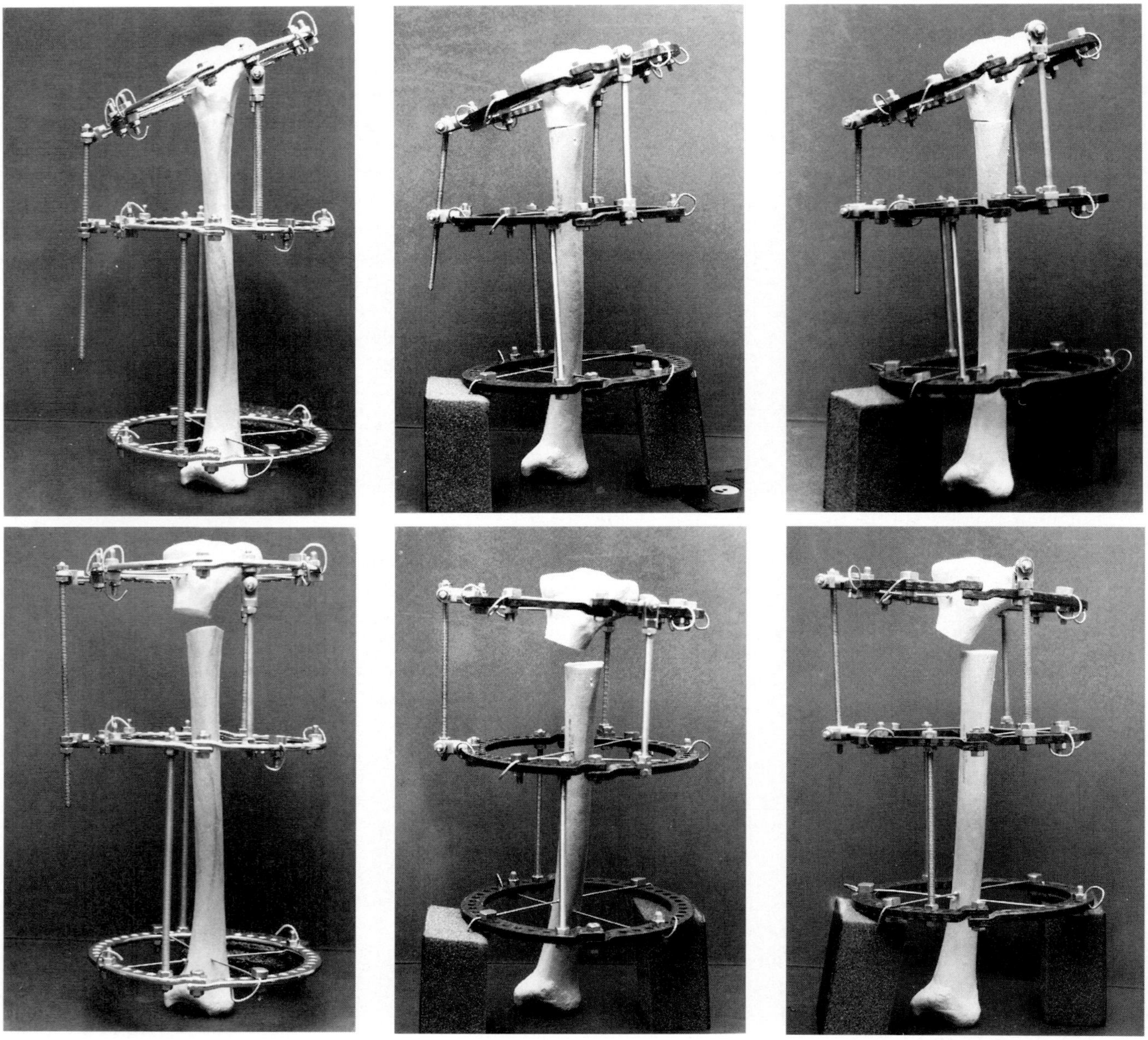

Fig. 2 Hinges for valgus high tibial osteotomy. **Top left** and **bottom left,** Correction with the hinge below the ring. **Top center** and **bottom center,** Correction with the hinge on the ring. **Top right** and **bottom right,** Correction with the hinge above the ring. Note that amount of translation of the distal fragment is increasing with more proximal location of the hinge.

corticotomy is performed proximally, at the level of the lower border of the tibial tubercle. The Ilizarov corticotomy technique is standard and has been described.[7] To assure that the corticotomy will be transverse and does not extend into wire holes that are in close proximity to the planned corticotomy, two or three holes are routinely made with a smooth K-wire in the posterior tibial cortex through corticotomy incision. Completeness of the corticotomy is verified under image intensifier control. The hinges and the distraction rod are then reapplied. The wire insertion sites and the operative wounds are dressed, and the foot is supported in neutral position with a stockinette attached to the frame.

Postoperative Management

The patient is discharged from the hospital on the first or second postoperative day. Before discharge, the patient is encouraged to ambulate on crutches with weightbearing as tolerated. Distraction of the corticotomy site and deformity correction is started on the seventh postoperative day. At that time, the hinges are

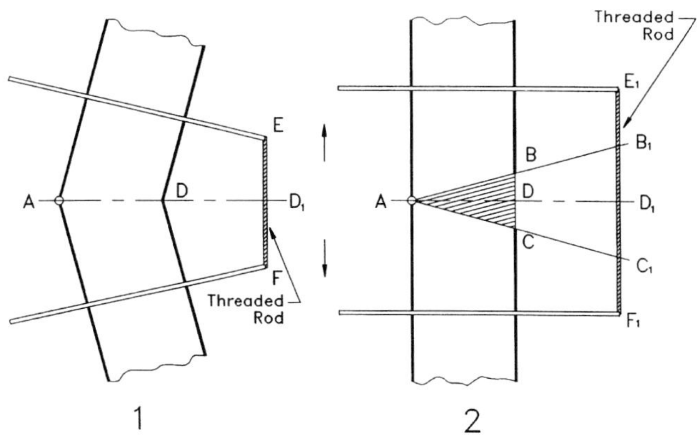

Fig. 3 The rule of triangles. **Left,** Before and **right,** after deformity correction. ABC = triangular bone regenerate. A = hinge at the apex of the deformity. EF = length of the distraction rod before correction. E_1F_1 = length of the distraction rod after correction. AD = width of the bone. AD_1 = distance from the hinge to the distraction rod. $\frac{AD}{AD_1} = \frac{BC}{B_1C_1}$ is the ratio used to calculate the rate of distraction.

loosened and the amount of deformity correction required is calculated according to the rule of triangles to determine how much and how often the nuts on the distraction rod should be turned.[8] The rule of triangles is used to calculate the amount of bone distraction required on the concave side of the deformity (Fig. 3). As the deformity is corrected, a triangular area of bone regenerate forms, with its apex at the hinge. The geometric relationship between the amount of distraction on the distraction rod and the amount of distraction on the concave site of the deformity is the same as relationship between the distance from the hinge to the distraction rod and distance from the hinge to the concave site of the deformity. To calculate the rate of daily correction, the distance from the hinge to the distraction rod and the distance from the hinge to the concave side of the bone are measured on an anteroposterior radiograph. For example, if the ratio between those two distances is 1 to 2, then in order to produce 1 mm of daily distraction on the concave site of the deformity the distraction rod has to be lengthened 2 mm.

Two to three weeks later, after the deformity has been corrected, standing 5-foot radiographs are obtained to verify and document the precision of deformity correction. The cosmetic appearance of the extremity is also considered. When deformity correction is complete, the proximal ring is usually parallel to the set of two distal rings. The hinges and distraction rod are now replaced by four threaded connecting rods to increase the stability of fixation. The corticotomy site can be slightly compressed at this time as well as later, when the patient visits the office for follow-up.

At the appropriate time, the frame is neutralized and then dynamized. The frame is removed 8 or 10 weeks after surgery, when bone healing is evident radiologically. A knee immobilizer may be applied for 2 to 3 days, mainly for patient confidence. There is usually no need for vigorous physical therapy after frame removal, because the patient has maintained a good range of knee motion (from 0° to 90°) and was able to ambulate with full weightbearing while in the frame.

Results

Between March 1989 and April 1993, 27 patients (18 men and nine women) underwent 30 high tibial osteotomies for varus deformity of the knee using the Ilizarov method. Three of the 27 had bilateral surgery, and another four patients also had high tibial osteotomy for valgus deformity of the knee. The age distribution for group was from 16 to 60 (mean 45.40 years). The main indication for surgery was medial joint pain and mechanical axis deviation of the extremity. Occasionally the indications for surgery were extended to include a young patient who had radiologic evidence of tricompartmental knee joint disease and who did not want either knee fusion or a total joint replacement.

The great majority of patients had a history of open or arthroscopic meniscectomy, multiple arthroscopic procedures, or an intra-articular fracture of the knee. One patient had 4 cm of tibial shortening and 25° of juxta-articular varus knee deformity as a result of polio in childhood. Total joint replacement with a custom-made prosthesis was offered to this patient in another institution as an alternative to treat degenerative arthritis and deformity of the knee joint. Another patient had 2 cm of tibial shortening as a result of two tibial fractures and 15° of varus knee deformity as a result of degenerative arthritis of the knee joint. In both instances, deformity was corrected with simultaneous limb lengthening.

The goal of treatment was achieved in all cases. Immediate and short-term results were excellent and good. There were no cases with recurrence of deformity. In one case, a high tibial osteotomy was done to a patient in his early 40s with advanced degenerative changes in the knee joint. The immediate result was good, with decreased pain and increased function. Three years later, due to progression of arthritis and knee injury, he underwent an uncomplicated total joint arthroplasty.

The functional level increased in all patients. Range of knee joint motion did not decrease after surgery. Some patients reported an increase in range of knee motion of up to 10°. In some patients, a mild flexion contracture (up to 10°) was present preoperatively but disappeared at the end of treatment.

Mild postoperative ankle swelling and pain was noticed in some cases. Two or three weeks of physical therapy treatments were usually enough to eliminate this problem.

Complications

There were no serious complications. The main problem was an occasional superficial wire tract infection that responded well to proper wire care and antibiotics. In no instances did a wire have to be removed or changed. There were no cases of knee joint or osteotomy site infection. There were no nonunions or fractures of the tibial plateau. With this technique, iatrogenic fracture of the tibial plateau is unlikely, because the fragment is already stabilized by three wires in different planes and levels before corticotomy is performed. Even more, the Ilizarov technique might be the optimal strategy to treat a tibial plateau fracture that happened as a complication of any other method of high tibial osteotomy. There were no cases of loss of fixation or loss of deformity correction. There were no cases of vascular injury or osteonecrosis of the tibial plateau. Likewise, there were no cases of lost or decreased joint motion. Two cases of transient peroneal nerve palsy, which occurred at the beginning of the learning curve, were attributed to the suboptimal technique of fibular osteotomy.

Conclusions

High tibial osteotomy is a procedure designed to prolong useful life span of the knee joint by redistribution of loading forces on the knee. The procedure is particularly good for a young, active patient who has medial or lateral knee joint arthritis and who is not yet a candidate for either knee arthroplasty or knee arthrodesis. Many of those patients had already undergone several arthroscopic surgeries that had given only short-lived pain relief. This report has focused on the principles of surgical technique of high tibial osteotomy using the Ilizarov apparatus and Ilizarov's methods of deformity correction. Our short-time follow up does not permit us to make any conclusions about the longevity of our results or recurrence of deformity. It is still to be proven that results of the high tibial osteotomy using this particular technique will outlast results of the operation performed by any other method. Furthermore, the long-lasting result of a high tibial osteotomy depends on many factors in addition to the particular surgical technique used. The most important factor is probably the rate of progression of the degenerative arthritis. Nevertheless, when compared with other techniques, a high tibial osteotomy using Ilizarov's principles offers a biomechanically sound, predictably accurate, and reproducible method of correcting an extremity's mechanical axis deviation. This technique does not interfere with patellofemoral biomechanics, does not deplete proximal tibial bone stock, does not leave any metal in the proximal tibia at the end of treatment, does not interfere with any future total joint replacement, and appears to be a low-risk operation with minimal possible complications.

References

1. Berman AT, Bosacco SJ, Kirshner S, et al: Factors influencing long-term results in high tibial osteotomy. *Clin Orthop* 1991;272:192-198.
2. Kettelkamp DB, Leach RE, Nasca R: Pitfalls of proximal tibial osteotomy. *Clin Orthop* 1975;106:232-241.
3. Coventry MB: Osteotomy about the knee for degenerative and rheumatoid arthritis. *J Bone Joint Surg* 1973;55A:23-48.
4. Dugdale TW, Noyes FR, Styer D: Preoperative planning for high tibial osteotomy: The effect of lateral tibiofemoral separation and tibiofemoral length. *Clin Orthop* 1992;274:248-264.
5. Windsor RE, Insall JN, Vince KG: Technical considerations of total knee arthroplasty after proximal tibial osteotomy. *J Bone Joint Surg* 1988;70A:547-555.
6. Elting JJ, Hubbell JC: Unilateral frame distraction: Proximal tibial valgus osteotomy for medial gonarthritis. *Contemp Orthop* 1993;27:435-440.
7. Schwartsman V, Schwartsman R: Corticotomy. *Clin Orthop* 1992;280:37-47.
8. Paley D: The principles of deformity correction by the Ilizarov technique: Technical aspects. *Tech Orthop* 1989;4:15-29.

Fracture Treatment

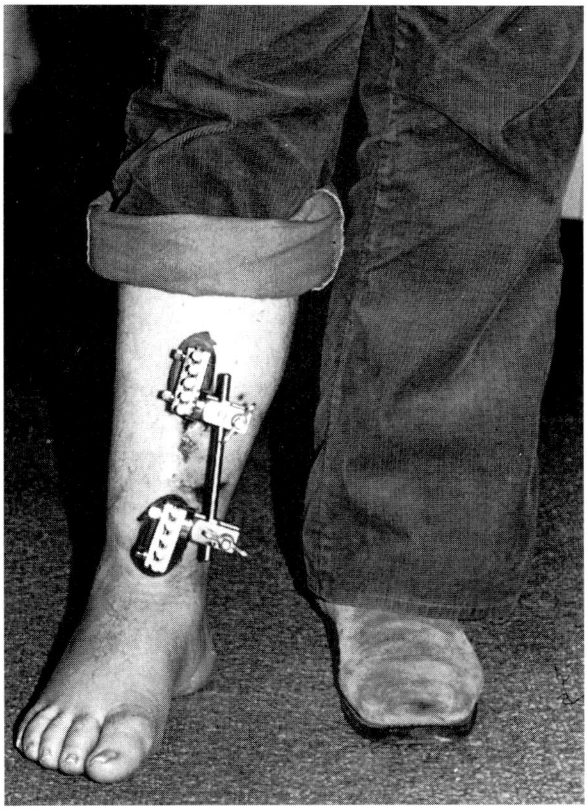

CHAPTER 42

Management of the Multiply Injured Patient with Fractures

Lawrence B. Bone, MD
Philip Stegemann, MD
George Babikian, MD

Because multiply injured patients require the expertise and skill of multiple surgeons and paramedical personnel, a team approach is necessary to coordinate resuscitation, diagnosis, and management of their multiple injuries. Initial resuscitation at the site of the accident is handled by the trained paramedical team, who do a preliminary evaluation, note the mechanism of injury, and start fluid resuscitation. Some patients may also need endotracheal intubation. The most critically injured patients are then triaged to a trauma center.[1-3]

In the trauma center, the general surgical team initiates cardiovascular and pulmonary resuscitation, following the Advanced Trauma Life-Support Guidelines of the Committee on Trauma, American College of Surgeons.[4,5] The orthopaedic surgeon is a vital member of the trauma team. Fractures are present in more than half of the multiply injured patients and their management may be life, as well as limb, saving. Protocols must be made for splinting fractures, reducing dislocations, managing open wounds, and obtaining appropriate diagnostic studies. A better understanding of the orthopaedic musculoskeletal injury gives the general surgeon a better appreciation of their importance. Communication between members of the trauma team is needed for optimal care of these patients.

Pelvic Injuries

Priorities for treating musculoskeletal injuries vary depending on the associated injuries. A pelvic injury with exsanguination into the pelvis can be life-threatening.[6] In a hemodynamically unstable patient, examination of the pelvis with pressure on the anterior iliac crests should be done as part of the initial examination. Movement of the wings of the pelvis is an indication of a pelvic disruption. An anterior to posterior radiograph of the pelvis, along with chest and cross table lateral cervical spine films, should be performed in the emergency room on all trauma patients. The pelvic radiograph will help diagnose pelvis fractures or ligamentous disruptions of the pelvis. A patient with a diastasis of the symphysis pubis (open book injury) (Fig. 1), who remains hemodynamically unstable after initial fluid resuscitation, should have an anterior ex-

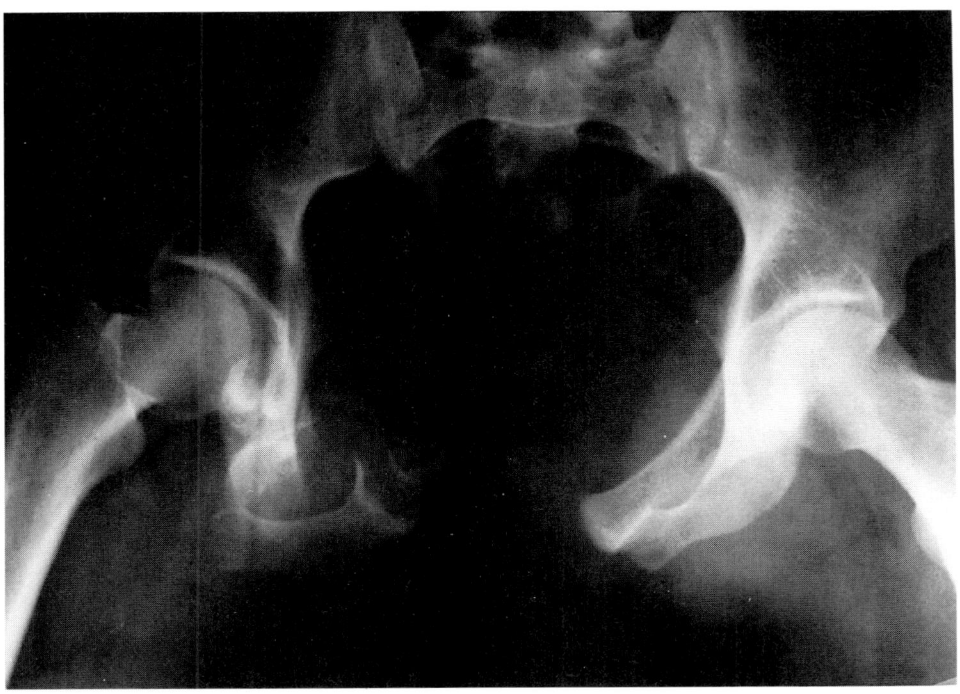

Fig. 1 AP radiograph of a pelvis with severe widening of the symphysis pubis, fracture of the right pubic rami and right sacroiliac disruption.

ternal fixator placed as an emergency procedure (Fig. 2).[7,8] A Schanz screw is placed in each anterior crest and, after manual closing of the widened pelvis, the screws are connected to an anterior frame (Fig. 3). Because this maneuver controls bleeding by reducing both the volume of the pelvis and the space that the patient can hemorrhage into, the tamponade effect can be lifesaving and dramatic. The external frame should be placed prior to exploratory laparotomy, perhaps while the surgical team is preparing the abdomen for exploratory laparotomy.

The anterior frame will not control posterior instability of the pelvis, but emergency posterior fixation (for sacroiliac disruption or sacral fractures) is rarely required to control bleeding. Only occasionally does bleeding from the fractured bone of the posterior ilium or sacrum need to be controlled urgently, and then open surgical stabilization may have to be performed. Stabilization, performed with threaded screws, bars, or plate fixation, should be done posteriorly without entering the retroperitoneal space. To enter this space could release the tamponade and cause further life-threatening, uncontrollable bleeding.

Management of an open pelvic injury[6] requires even greater team coordination, and the general surgeon, orthopaedic surgeon, urologist and, at times, the gynecologist must work together for diagnosis and treatment. Proper radiographs for diagnosis of the bony injury may not be possible in the patient who is hemodynamically unstable. Perineal wounds must be packed to control bleeding, and anterior pelvic fixation placed at once. Sigmoidoscopy and visual vaginal examination will reveal lacerations of the colon or vagina. Urologic diagnostic studies, including a voiding cystogram and urethrogram, should be obtained if the patient is stable hemodynamically. An exploratory laparotomy with colostomy should be performed. The placement of the colostomy should be in the left upper quadrant, rather than the left lower quadrant, in order to keep the stoma away from potential incisions in the lower abdomen required for pelvic reconstruction. A rectal washout is then performed, and the open pelvic wound is debrided, thoroughly irrigated, and packed open. Additional fracture stabilization is then coordinated with the general and urologic surgeons.

The majority of pelvic fractures and dislocations are not life threatening and can be stabilized electively. This is also true of acetabular fractures. In general, it is best to allow the patient to be restabilized and resuscitated following urgent surgeries on the head, chest, and abdomen when associated pelvic and acetabular fractures are present. Warming the patient and replacing platelets and clotting factors will control the bleeding around pelvic and acetabular fractures. The patient can be taken for reconstruction and stabilization of these injuries approximately 48 hours after the injury. Once stabilization is sufficient the patient is allowed to sit up in bed,[9,10] getting his or her chest into an upright position. This reduces the postinjury and postoperative atelectasis that occurs with the forced supine position and improves oxygenation. During this 36- to 48-hour time period, the patient can undergo special radio-

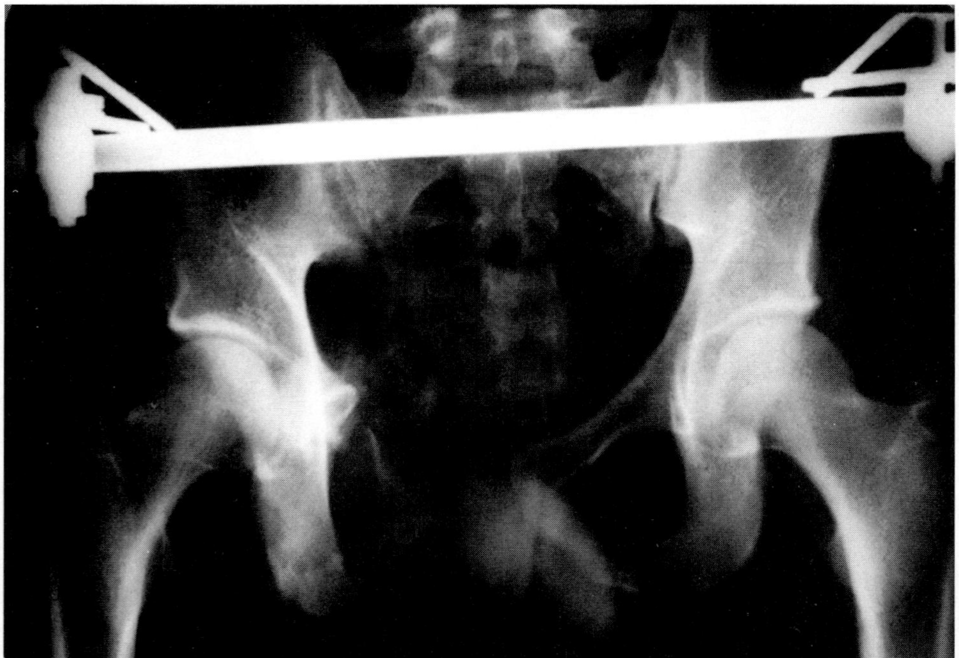

Fig. 2 AP radiograph after an anterior external fixator frame has been placed and the anatomy of the pelvis restored.

graphic procedures to obtain full views of the pelvis and acetabulum as well as computed tomographic (CT) scanning of the pelvis.

On rare occasions, surgical stabilization of the pelvic injury in a hemodynamically stable patient must be performed acutely or within 24 hours following the injury. These patients usually have an associated injury that is likely to cause major pulmonary failure and their oxygenation worsens progressively with time. Patients with pulmonary contusions or major chest trauma or who have had prolonged periods of hemorrhagic shock often develop severe pulmonary failure. This pulmonary failure may not allow the patient to be moved from the intensive care unit to the operating room for further stabilization of the pelvis and acetabulum. These patients, if hemodynamically stable, are usually best able to undergo stabilization in the early postinjury period.

Additional considerations for acetabular and pelvic stabilization must be made in patients who have spinal fractures or dislocations and femur and hip fractures on the ipsilateral side of the pelvic injury. The femur fracture must be stabilized early,[1,11,14] usually with proximal thigh incisions, by placement of an intramedullary rod.[15] This incision may interfere with subsequent posterior incisions for acetabular fixation. If acetabular stabilization is delayed, the hip incision may need to be reopened at two or three days, which can increase the risk of wound infection. Therefore, in patients with ipsilateral acetabular and femoral fractures, open reduction and internal fixation of the acetabulum may have to be done at the same time as femoral fracture stabilization or within the first 24 hours. The need for the early acetabular fixation, however, can be eliminated if the acetabular fracture can be reduced and stabilized via an ilioinguinal approach.

Spinal Injuries

Unstable spine injuries in the multiply injured patient with additional fractures present special problems. For posterior stabilization of the spine, the patient must be placed prone on the fracture table, and the presence of anterior pelvic external fixators complicates this process. For these patients, consideration should be given to plate stabilization of the anterior pelvis, either acutely or after initial external fixation of the pelvis. The anterior external fixator can be removed, the symphysis plated, and the patient rolled to the prone position for posterior spinal stabilization.

Patients with spinal injuries and femoral fractures require special cooperation between the orthopaedic traumatologist and the spinal surgeon. As a rule, these patients can be placed supine on a radiolucent operating table or a fracture table in skeletal traction. Cervical spine injuries can be stabilized with halo traction. In the supine position, the femoral fracture can be rodded or plated without risk to the cervical or thoracolumbar spinal injury. Once the femur fracture is stable, the patient may be placed prone for spinal fixation either acutely or at 48 hours postinjury. Most spinal fractures

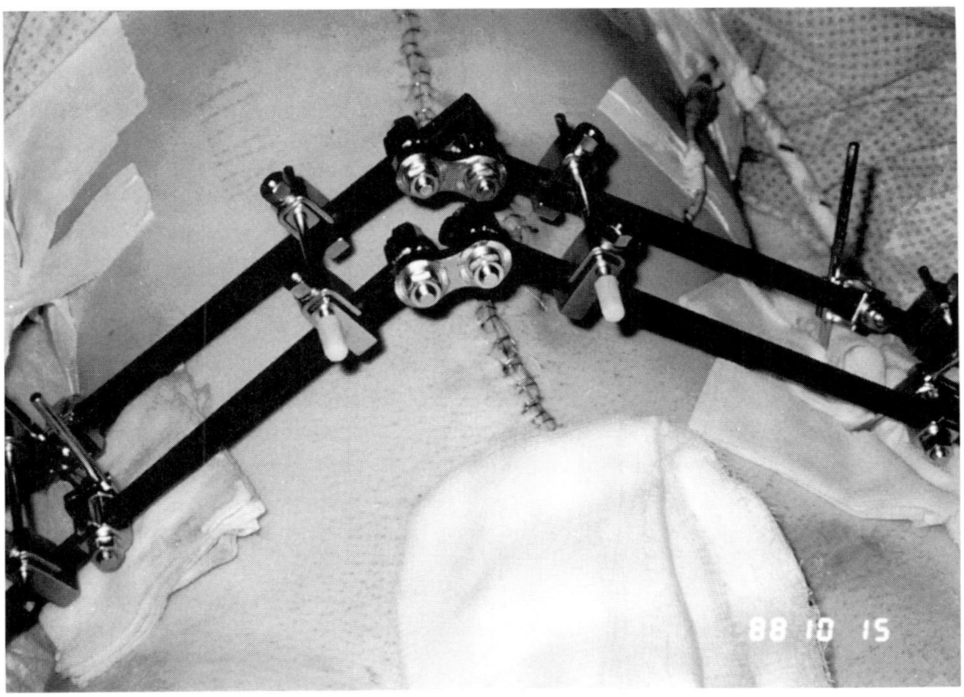

Fig. 3 Photograph of an anterior pelvis external fixator.

can be stabilized within 48 hours. The exception is the patient whose neurological condition is deteriorating.[16] A worsening neurologic injury requires urgent diagnosis, decompression, and spinal stabilization. A CT scan of the spine and, if possible, a myelogram with magnetic resonance imaging should be performed. Retropulsed vertebral body fragments, spinal dislocations, or hematomas causing cord compression can then be diagnosed. If the neurologic examination indicates additional neurologic loss, urgent decompression of the cords should be performed.[16]

Other Musculoskeletal Injuries

The remaining musculoskeletal injuries are not immediately life threatening, but their proper care can save limbs and can improve postinjury limb function. Dislocations, especially of the hip, should be reduced as early as possible, because the longer the hip remains dislocated, the greater the risk of osteonecrosis of the femoral head.[17] Knee dislocations should be reduced and splinted and an arteriogram performed to rule out popliteal artery intimal injuries, even if normal pulses are present. Shoulder and elbow dislocations should be reduced promptly, even in the multiply injured patient, to prevent potential nerve damage, to relieve pain, and to prevent damage of articular cartilage. Fracture-dislocations of the foot and ankle should be reduced and splinted to avoid further compromise to soft tissue.

As part of the trauma team, the orthopaedic surgeon must be alert to potential compartment syndromes associated with limb fractures. In any situation that suggests this complication, affected compartments should be monitored with compartment pressure readings. Compartment syndromes are more common in the lower leg and forearm, but they can occur in thigh and gluteal regions as well as in the foot and hand.

Vascular injuries are general surgical problems commonly associated with fractures of the distal femur and proximal tibia, with open fractures, and with supracondylar humerus fractures. These injuries must be looked for by the orthopaedic surgeon who examines the limb. Any diminution of pulse, compared to the uninjured extremity, must be investigated. If blood pressure in the injured extremity is less than 90% of that in the uninjured, investigation for vascular injury should proceed.[18,19]

Open fractures are an urgent surgical problem. Sterile dressings are placed over the open wound in the emergency room, and systemic antibiotics and tetanus toxoid are administered. The limb should be splinted and appropriate radiographs obtained. In the operating room, the wound is thoroughly debrided of necrotic and grossly contaminated tissue and is pulse lavaged, after which the fracture is stabilized.

In multiply injured patients, stabilization of the skeleton, especially femur fractures, has been shown to reduce pulmonary complications,[1,10-14] including adult respiratory distress syndrome (ARDS),[20] pulmonary dysfunction, fat emboli syndrome, and pneumonia. In addition, skeletal stabilization reduces systemic infections.[13] The patient with early femur fracture stabilization has a shorter period of endotracheal intubation,[11] which lessens the risk of pneumonia and possible multiple system organ failure.[9] In a multicenter study, mortality rates were also reduced when early total care of the multiply injured patient, including the musculoskeletal system, was undertaken within the first 48 hours postinjury.[12] The patient with a major head injury, ie, Glasgow Coma Scale of less than 8, also had a lower mortality rate with early total care.[3,21,22]

The two-team approach to the multiply injured patient allows the patient with a femoral fracture to be placed in skeletal traction on the fracture table and have the exploratory laparotomy performed on the fracture table. Following exploratory laparotomy, the femur fracture can be rodded without transferring the patient from an operating table to a fracture table. Likewise, a patient with a femoral fracture and a femoral artery injury that requires vascular repair can be placed in skeletal traction on a fracture table, stabilizing the fractured limb out to length and allowing easy access to the medial distal thigh and popliteal artery for vascular repair. With the fractured limb out to length and stabilized by traction, the vascular surgeon knows the length of the vessel and the vascular repair that must be performed. Following vascular repair, which should be done first, the femur fracture can be rodded or plated without further manipulation of the limb.

The floating knee, a femur fracture and ipsilateral tibia fracture, is best managed by surgically stabilizing both fractures.[11,23] While the femur is rodded, the tibia is stabilized temporarily with a short leg cast. Following femoral rodding, the tibia can be stabilized in any fashion. If an intramedullary rod is chosen, an unreamed rod should be used to avoid reaming the acutely swollen fracture. This reduces the risk of developing a compartment syndrome. After the femur fracture is stabilized, the patient can be placed in skeletal traction on a fracture table for intramedullary rodding of the tibia. An open tibia fracture should be debrided and irrigated before the femur is rodded. If an external fixator is to be used, the tibia can be stabilized following irrigation and debridement. However, if an unreamed rod is to be used, temporary casting of the debrided tibia fracture will allow the femur fracture to be rodded, followed by redebridement and unreamed rodding of the tibia fracture.[24]

Both the tibia and femur can be rodded without the use of a fracture table. If a femoral distraction device is used to reduce the fracture, all surgery can be performed on a standard radiolucent operating table.

In the multiply injured patient, a closed tibia fracture can be splinted initially and stabilized surgically after the swelling has subsided, at 48 to 72 hours postinjury. In the severely injured patient whose injuries, ie, a chest injury or a head injury, may prevent a return to the operating room, it is probably best to stabilize the tibia fracture acutely. Unreamed intramedullary rods can be safely placed in this situation.[24]

The intra-articular fracture is a special problem in the multiply injured patient. These injuries are usually associated with significant soft-tissue swelling. The risk of skin sloughing and wound infection is greatly increased if large open reduction and internal fixation procedures are performed acutely.[20] An external fixator that spans the joint can be used to reduce and temporarily stabilize the articular fragments.[25] It may then be possible to perform percutaneous cannulated screw fixation of the articular surface, or it may be necessary to wait until the soft-tissue swelling has gone down, to allow surgical incisions with less risk of skin devitalization. Initial indirect reduction brings the fractures out to length and greatly facilitates later reduction and internal fixation. If small wire, hybrid circular external fixators are used in certain articular fractures, it is possible to avoid crossing the joint with the external fixator. Open articular fractures, like any open fracture, require proper debridement.[13] Use of the external fixator allows the fractures to be managed through smaller incisions, often through the open wound. Additional incisions need to be carefully placed to avoid additional skin compromise and potential skin sloughs. If necessary, the combination of external fixation with limited internal fixation can then be converted to a more rigid construct once the soft tissues have healed.

Most upper extremity fractures, including humerus fractures, can be temporarily splinted and managed surgically at 48 to 72 hours postinjury. Isolated humerus fractures rarely need surgical stabilization, but in polytrauma patients they are best stabilized surgically.[26] Plating or rodding the humerus allows the patient greater use of that extremity. The arm can then be used to help transfer the patient when lower extremity injuries are present or to allow the patient to use crutches. In the patient with a floating elbow, ie, humerus and forearm fractures, best results have been achieved with surgical stabilization of the humerus fracture.[27]

In the patient with multiple extremity trauma, time can be saved by performing simultaneous surgery on upper and lower extremity fractures. This team approach can significantly reduce the operative time and allow more injuries to be managed acutely. Tourniquets should be used whenever possible to reduce blood loss, and, in order to maintain proper fluid balance, the anesthesiologist must be acutely aware of the blood loss from multiple surgical incisions.

Fractures and dislocations of the foot may seem to be minor injuries in the multiply injured patient with multiple fractures. However, if they are not properly managed, these injuries can often give the patient the most morbidity. Skeletal stabilization should be performed early to reduce and maintain normal bony and soft-tissue relationships. Late severe swelling makes reduction more difficult. The foot should also be monitored for compartment syndromes.

Table 1 outlines the general rule for timing of treatment of musculoskeletal injuries in the multiply injured patient. The goal is for all patients to have early total care of their injuries. Once the musculoskeletal system has been stabilized, the patient can be mobilized in an upright chest position. Nursing care is eased. Also, because the patient has less pain, the need for narcotic analgesics, which further depress the respiratory system, is reduced. Additionally, skeletal stabilization reduces the inflammatory mediators created by the trauma (interleukins, tumor necrosis factor), which have detrimental effects on the pulmonary system.[9,28-30] This lessens the risk for pulmonary failure, ARDS, and subsequent multiple system organ failure.[9]

Head Injuries

Multiply injured patients who have head injuries present special problems. Additional blood loss during surgical procedures can cause hypotension and further damage to brain tissue. A well-coordinated team approach between the neurosurgeons, anesthesiologists, general surgeons, and orthopaedic surgeons is needed. Intracranial ventricular monitoring should be performed. Proper hydration, with special attention to surgical blood loss and urinary output, is required, and good oxygen transport must be maintained. With proper oxygenation, proper hydration, and ventilation, patients with head injuries can safely have early total care of their injuries. Data have shown a decrease in mortality of severely injured patients with Glasgow Coma Scales of less than 8 when early total care is performed.[21,22]

Chest Trauma

Multiply injured patients with a major chest trauma (Abbreviated Injury Scale of 3 or greater) also need special consideration. These patients are at potentially greater risks for additional pulmonary insult during reaming of their femoral fractures for intramedullary rodding. While clinical data substantiating this problem are lacking, animal studies have documented increased pulmonary capillary leak and worsening of pulmonary failure with reaming of a femur in a patient with pulmonary contusion.[31] Therefore, in patients with chest injuries, special care must be given to maintaining high oxygenation and hydration during femoral rodding. The unreamed femoral rod may be the implant of choice in these patients.

Table 1
Optimal care of the injured patient with musculoskeletal trauma

	Prehospital Care			Acute Hospital Care			Post-Acute Care
		Acute Resuscitation Phase	Primary Phase		Secondary Phase	Tertiary Phase	Rehabilitation Phase
Optimal Care	0-60 minutes	1-2 hours	2-12 hours	12-48 hours	48-72 hours	72 hours-discharge	Varies
Clinical Goals	Focus on primary and secondary surveys and initial resuscitation—goals include (1) reduce external bleeding, (2) triage and transport to appropriate facilities, and (3) alert facility of impending arrival	Focus on life-threatening injuries—goals include (1) stop major blood loss (internal/external), (2) identify principal injuries, and (3) identify direction of impact	Focus on limb-threatening injuries—goals include (1) make limb salvage decisions (reconstruction versus primary amputation), (2) identify occult injuries, and (3) plan course of orthopaedic treatment	Focus on facilitating nursing care through sufficient fracture stabilization—principal goal is for the patient to sit up within a day to assist GI, pulmonary, and hemodynamic functioning	Focus on management of all fractures and injuries that have not been treated definitively by this time—goal is to initiate bedside therapy and injured extremity range-of-motion exercises	Focus on acute inpatient rehabilitation, quality improvement, and patient education—goals are to (1) increase mobility; (2) assess progress to date; and (3) advise patient and family of follow-up care, procedures, necessary therapies, and prognosis	Goals are to minimize chronic pain and to maximize functional independence; that is, return patient to preinjury functional state (for example, ability to attend work/school)
Essential Orthopaedic Diagnostic Procedures	Assess spine and extremities for open wounds, deformity, pain, alignment, and symmetry	Obtain spinal, pelvic, and femoral portable and/or CT films, if indicated; validate prehospital assessment		Assess neurovascular status		Reassess reductions and alignments	
Essential Orthopaedic Procedures	Stabilize/immobilize spine and injured extremities; cover open wounds with sterile dressing; apply traction splint for femoral fractures	Apply pelvic external fixation to help control unstable pelvic ring injuries and resultant retroperitoneal bleeding; reduce dislocations with neurovascular compromise	Obtain stable fixation of pelvic and long-bone fractures; reduce major joint dislocations; use casts, splints, and external fixators to support other areas until definitive fixation is obtained	Obtain operative fixation of all other fractures and joint injuries that may interfere with mobilization of patient	Reassess open wounds in OR and debride as necessary; address all remaining fractures (hand, foot, arm, acetabular, posterior pelvic, and complex articular)	Consider bone grafts for high-energy tibial fractures, other comminuted fractures, and fractures with bone loss; implement soft tissue repair/free muscle flaps	Consider bone grafts and need for bone-lengthening techniques (for example, Ilizarov)
Extra-Orthopaedic Clinical Concerns		Ensure correction of hypothermia and coagulopathy; assess respiratory function	Strive for concurrent OR procedures (OMF, ortho, neuro, plastics, and general) to minimize patient's OR and anesthesia time	Be aware of ARDS risk; schedule sufficient and convenient OR time	Assess metabolic and nutritional needs of patient; control pain without excessive sedation	Monitor patient mobility during recuperation	

Conclusion

During the initial management of the multiply injured patient, the patient's temperature and coagulation profiles, prothrombin time, partial thromboplastin time, platelets, and fibrin split products must be monitored. As long as the patient remains hemodynamically stable with good urine outputs and good oxygenation, and does not become hypothermic or coagulopathic, early total care can continue. If, following life-threatening surgeries, the patient is hypothermic or coagulopathic, musculoskeletal stabilization must be delayed.[3] These patients should be left intubated on a volume cycle ventilator and taken to the intensive care unit, where they are warmed and have appropriate factor replacement to correct the coagulopathy. Urgent skeletal procedures, open fractures care, femoral stabilization, and external fixation can be performed once the patient is reresuscitated. If the patient continues to be stable, tibial fractures and upper extremity fractures may be managed at that time. Spinal, pelvic, and acetabular fractures can be reevaluated and stabilized at 48 to 72 hours postinjury.

Postoperatively, these patients should have prophylactic treatment to prevent deep vein thromboses. Pneumatic compression devices are used initially, and low-dose Coumarin[32] can be started if there is no head injury or risk of ongoing hemorrhage. Indomethacin should be started to prevent heterotopic ossification.[33,34] Parenteral nutrition is started as early as possible to feed the gut and nourish these patients, who require large amounts of protein and calories.[9,12]

Treatment of multiply injured patients requires close coordination among the various physicians and paramedical staff who care for them. It is important to outline general principles and to understand the importance of early total care. Attention to these points will help these patients survive and, with the help of the rehabilitation service, become productive members of society again.

Clinical Case

A 24-year-old man was involved in a high-speed, head-on collision. He was hemodynamically unstable in the emergency department and was taken to the operating room for urgent exploratory laparotomy. He was found to have suffered major blood loss from a lacerated liver. He also had a closed head injury, a Glasgow Coma Scale score of 10, multiple rib fractures, a right femur

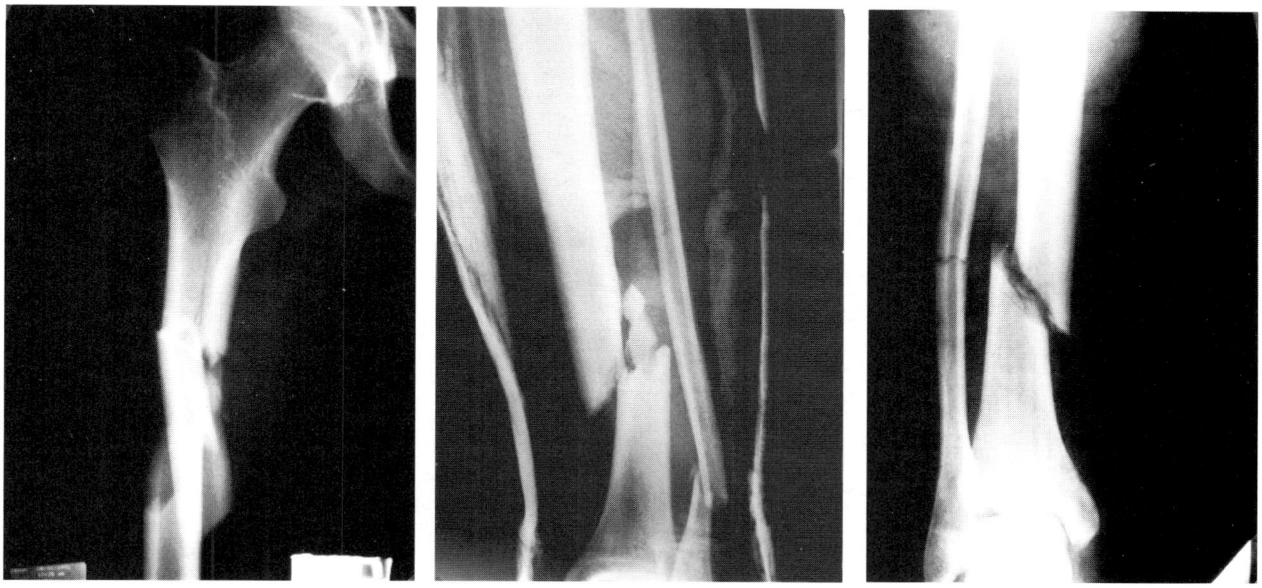

Fig. 4 **Left,** Right femur fracture, **Center,** Open left tibia fracture (grade II), **Right,** Closed right tibia fracture.

fracture (Fig. 4, *left*), an open left tibia fracture (Fig. 4, *center*), a right tibia fracture (Fig. 4, *right*), and a sacroiliac dislocation with pelvic fractures (Fig. 5). After exploratory laparotomy, during which 12 units of packed erythrocytes and a large volume of crystalloid was administered, the patient was hypothermic and had a coagulopathy. He was not a candidate for continued surgical intervention at that time. The patient remained intubated on a volume cycle ventilator and was taken to the intensive care unit, where he was warmed and hemodynamically stabilized, and his coagulopathy was corrected. Eighteen hours after the initial injury, he was taken back to the operating room for debridement of the open tibia fracture and placement of unreamed intramedullary rods in both the tibia and the right femur (Fig. 6). The right tibia was placed in a splint. The

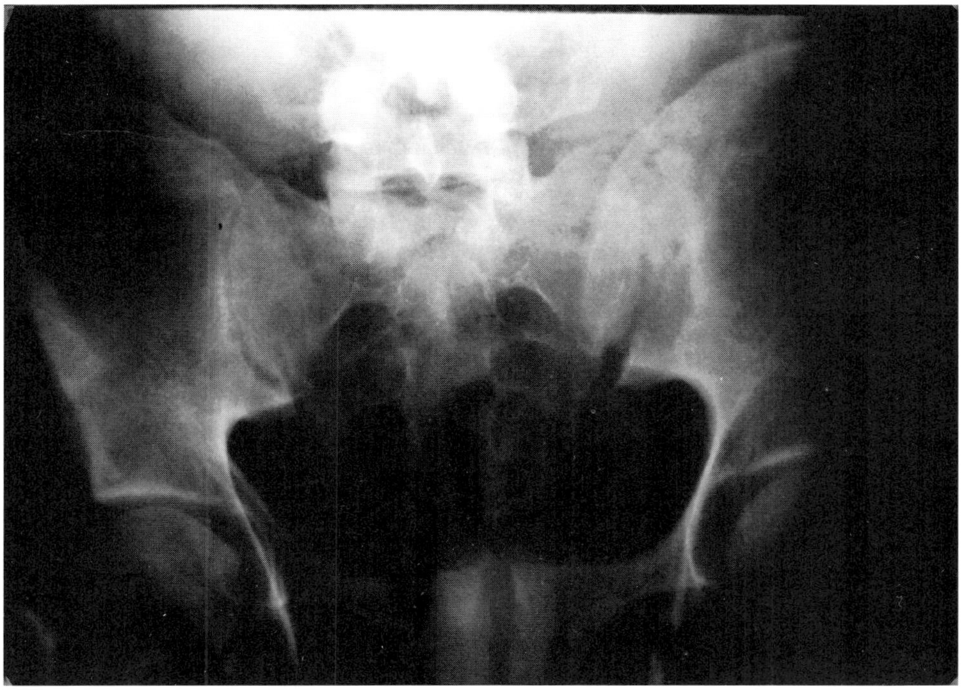

Fig. 5 AP radiograph of pelvis with left SI separation.

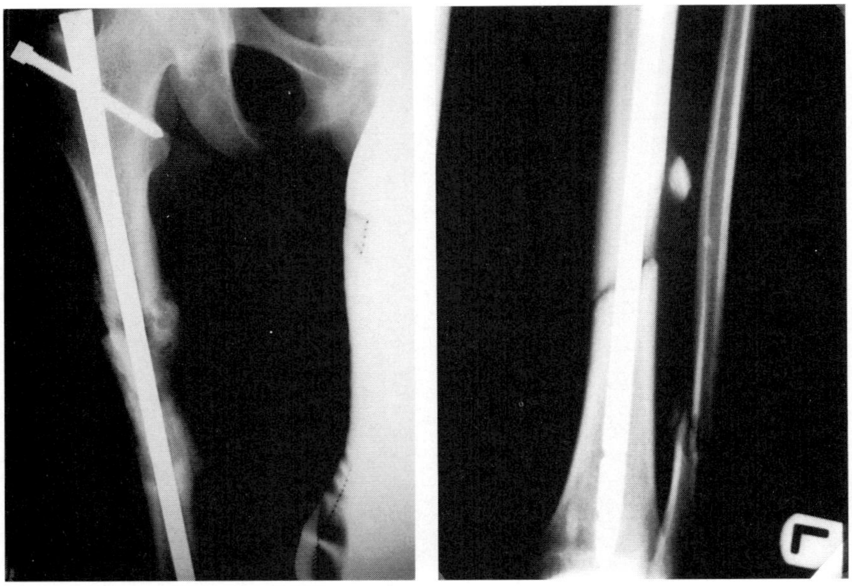

Fig. 6 **Left**, Right femur after unreamed intramedullary rodding. **Right,** Left tibia after unreamed tibial rodding.

patient's pelvic injuries were unstable, but they did not prevent him from being mobilized into an upright chest position. Therefore, he was taken back to the intensive care unit, where he was reevaluated over the next 36 hours. His oxygenation improved and he regained hemodynamic stability. The trauma team (the general surgeon, orthopaedic surgeon, and anesthesiologist) believed him to be stable enough to undergo further stabilization of his musculoskeletal system. He was taken back to the operating room 48 hours after his initial orthopaedic surgery and underwent plate fixation of the distal fracture of the right tibia and screw stabilization of the sacroiliac joint. Had the patient been stable following his exploratory laparotomy, the femur and open tibia would have been rodded acutely. However, the patient had a coagulopathy that required treatment. He was, however, stabilized as soon as possible.

References

1. Seibel R, LaDuca J, Hassett JM, et al: Blunt multiple trauma (ISS 36), femur traction, and the pulmonary failure-septic state. *Ann Surg* 1985;202:283-295.
2. Veith RG, Winquist RA, Hansen ST Jr: Ipsilateral fractures of the femur and tibia: A report of fifty-seven consecutive cases. *J Bone Joint Surg* 1984;66A:991-1002.
3. Bone LB, Chapman MW: Initial management of the patient with multiple injuries, in Greene WB (ed): *Instructional Course Lectures, Volume XXXIX.* Park Ridge, IL, American Academy of Orthopaedic Surgeons, 1990, pp 557-563.
4. Bone L, Bucholz R: The management of fractures in the patient with multiple trauma. *J Bone Joint Surg* 1986;68A:945-949.
5. *Advanced Life Support Course.* Chicago, IL, Committee on Trauma, American College of Surgeons, 1985.
6. Richardson JD, Harty J, Amin M, et al: Open pelvic fractures. *J Trauma* 1982;22:533-538.
7. Properties of musculoskeletal management, in *Resources for Optimal Care of the Injured Patient.* Committee on Trauma, American College of Surgeons, 1990, pp 45-49.
8. McMurtry R, Walton D, Dickinson D, et al: Pelvic disruption in the polytraumatized patient: A management protocol. *Clin Orthop* 1980;151:22-30.
9. Border JR, Rodriguez J, Bone L, et al: Role of immediate surgery in prevention of multiple organ failure, in Deitch EA (ed): *Multiple Organ Failure: Pathophysiology and Basic Concepts of Therapy.* New York, NY, Thieme Medical Publishers, 1990, pp 261-274.
10. Border JR, Allgöwer M, Hansen ST Jr, et al: Fracture management and pulmonary failure, in Border JR, Allgöwer M, Hansen ST Jr, et al (eds): *Blunt Multiple Trauma: Comprehensive Pathophysiology and Care.* New York, NY, Marcel Dekker Inc, 1990, pp 77-91.
11. Bone LB, Johnson KD, Weigelt J, et al: Early versus delayed stabilization of femoral fractures: A prospective randomized study. *J Bone Joint Surg* 1989;71A:336-340.
12. Border JR, Hassett J, LaDuca J, et al: The gut origin septic states in blunt multiple trauma (ISS=40) in the ICU. *Ann Surg* 1987; 206:427-448.
13. Johnson KD, Cadambi A, Seibert GB: Incidence of adult respiratory distress syndrome in patients with multiple musculoskeletal injuries: Effect of early operative stabilization of fractures. *J Trauma* 1985;25:375-384.
14. Riska EB, Myllynen P: Fat embolism in patients with multiple injuries. *J Trauma* 1982;22:891-894.
15. Johnson KD: Management of fractures of the femur, tibia, and upper extremity in the multiply injured patient, in Greene WB (ed): *Instructional Course Lectures, Volume XXXIX.* Park Ridge, IL American Academy of Orthopaedic Surgeons, 1990, pp 565-576.
16. Benson DR, Keenen TL: Evaluation and treatment of trauma to the vertebral column, in Greene WB (ed): *Instructional Course Lectures, Volume XXXIX.* Park Ridge, IL, American Academy of Orthopaedic Surgeons, 1990, pp 577-589.
17. Jacob JR, Rao JP, Ciccarelli C: Traumatic dislocation and fracture dislocation of the hip: A long-term follow-up study. *Clin Orthop* 1987;214:249-263.
18. Bliss B, Mansfield AO, Shepherd R, et al: Editorial: Vascular injuries. *J Bone Joint Surg* 1989;71B:738.

19. Drost TF, Rosemurgy AS, Proctor D, et al: Outcome of treatment of combined orthopedic and arterial trauma to the lower extremity. *J Trauma* 1989;29:1331-1334.
20. Pierce RO Jr, Heinrich JH: Comminuted intra-articular fractures of the distal tibia. *J Trauma* 1979;19:828-832.
21. Bone L, McNamara K, Border J: Mortality in the multiply trauma patient with fractures. *J Trauma* 1994;37:262-265.
22. Hofman PA, Goris RJ: Timing of osteosynthesis of major fractures in patients with severe brain injury. *J Trauma* 1991;31:261-263.
23. Shackford SR, Hollingworth-Fridlund P, Cooper GF, et al: The effect of regionalization upon the quality of trauma care as assessed by concurrent audit before and after institution of a trauma system: A preliminary report. *J Trauma* 1986;26:812-820.
24. Whittle AP, Russell TA, Taylor JC, et al: Treatment of open fractures of the tibial shaft with the use of interlocking nailing without reaming. *J Bone Joint Surg* 1992;74A:1162-1171.
25. Bone L, Stegemann P, McNamara K, et al: External fixation of severely comminuted and open tibial pilon fractures. *Clin Orthop* 1993;292:101-107.
26. Bone LB: Fractures of the shaft of the humerus, in Chapman MW, Madison M (eds): *Operative Orthopaedics*, ed 2. Philadelphia, PA, JB Lippincott, 1993, pp 425-438.
27. Lange RH, Foster RJ: Skeletal management of humeral shaft fractures associated with forearm fractures. *Clin Orthop* 1985: 195:173-177.
28. Carey PD, Leeper-Woodford SK, Walsh CJ, et al: Delayed cyclooxygenase blockade reduces the neutrophil respiratory burst and plasma tumor necrosis factor levels in sepsis-induced acute lung injury. *J Trauma* 1991;31:733-741.
29. Heideman M, Kaijser B, Gelin LE: Complement activation and hematologic, hemodynamic, and respiratory reactions early after soft-tissue injury. *J Trauma* 1978;18:696-700.
30. Weigelt JA, Chenoweth DE, Borman KR, et al: Complement and the severity of pulmonary failure. *J Trauma* 1988;28:1013-1019.
31. Pape HC, Dwenger A, Regel G, et al: Pulmonary damage after intramedullary femoral nailing in traumatized sheep—is there an effect from different nailing methods? *J Trauma* 1992;33:574-581.
32. Collins DN, Barnes CL, McCowan TC, et al: Vena caval filter use in orthopaedic trauma patients with recognized preoperative venous thromboembolic disease. *J Orthop Trauma* 1992;6:135-138.
33. Kaempffe FA, Bone LB, Border JR: Open reduction and internal fixation of acetabular fractures: Heterotopic ossification and other complications of treatment. *J Orthop Trauma* 1991;5:439-445.
34. Moed BR, Maxey JW: The effect of indomethacin on heterotopic ossification following acetabular fracture surgery. *J Orthop Trauma* 1993;7:33-38.

CHAPTER 43

Pin and Wire Technique for External Fixation

Stuart A. Green, MD

Introduction

During the past decade the potential indications for external skeletal fixation have decreased for some clinical problems and have substantially increased for others. Consider, for example, low-grade, long-bone open fractures. For a while it appeared that external skeletal fixation was the treatment of choice for virtually all such injuries. More recently, however, a number of reports have documented the safety, efficacy, and patient acceptance of locked intramedullary nails for primary stabilization of grade I, grade II, and even some grade III diaphyseal fractures.

Acute traumatology has long been the most frequent use of external fixators, and one would think that widespread nailing of open fractures would cause sales of fixator frames to decline. In fact, quite the contrary is true. The indications for external skeletal fixation have expanded during the past 5 years, especially since the introduction of Ilizarov's method of distraction osteogenesis. Patients who required limb lengthening, gradual deformity correction, stump elongation, and the filling of long bone defects have all benefited from Ilizarov's discoveries. Hinged external fixators are now routinely used to overcome joint contractures, to treat club foot, and to aid in the management of complex hip pathologies.

Even in the area of traumatology, external fixators have found new uses, this time as an adjunct in the treatment of fractures of the articular ends of long bones, and for the definitive management of severely comminuted diaphyseal fractures not amenable to internal stabilization. For these indications, attachment of the frame to the limb is accomplished with pins or tensioned wires in any combination. (When tensioned wires are used, a circular frame must surround the limb.) In many cases, external fixation techniques combine these two fixation methods. In general, surgeons using modern external fixation strategies employ tension wires in cancellous bone and threaded half-pins in the denser cortical regions. In some locations, pins and wires are used in geometric combinations designed to obtain the maximum stability with the least number of pin-skin interfaces.

Pin and Wire Technique

The advances in mounting strategies have paralleled improvements in pin and wire technique. Indeed, were it not for the steady improvements in the methods of pin and wire insertion, fixators would have retained their reputation for low patient tolerance.

One reason for this reduction in pin and wire site sepsis has been the recognition by a number of experts that implant site infections are often (but not always) related to the creation of necrotic tissue at the implant-tissue interface during pin or wire insertion. Such sepsis can be caused when tissues are wound up around a spinning drill-bit, wire, or pin (Fig. 1). Soft tissues are torn away (microscopically) as strands of cellular material adherent to the whirling implant. This disrupted tissue provides nutrition for the skin microflora that rapidly contaminate any transcutaneous implant site. Likewise, heat from drilling and soft-tissue tension after the implant is in place contribute to implant site sepsis. Implant site management is the final step in reducing the likelihood of an infected pin or wire site.

Pin Technique

Our clinical experience at Rancho Los Amigos Medical Center has convinced us that titanium alloy pins are better tolerated by soft tissues than are stainless steel implants. At first, we could not understand this phenomenon, which was characterized by a lower incidence of pin site sepsis when titanium pins were used. Moreover, when a titanium pin site did become infected, we almost never observed the extensive type of cellulitis that often surrounded infected steel pins.

A recently published article explains this observation. Researchers working with Dr. Raymond Gustillo were curious about the apparently lower incidence of infections following total hip arthroplasties when titanium implants were used, in comparison with the numbers that occurred with stainless steel prostheses.[1] Gustillo and associates ground up various metals (stain-

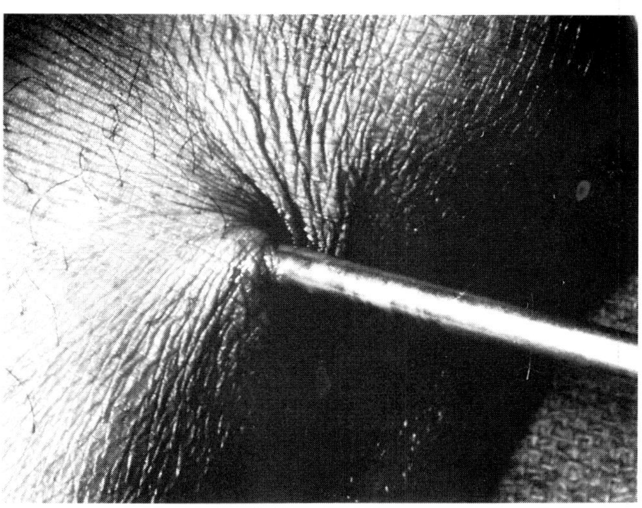

Fig. 1 A twirling implant can damage deep tissues, leading to implant site sepsis.

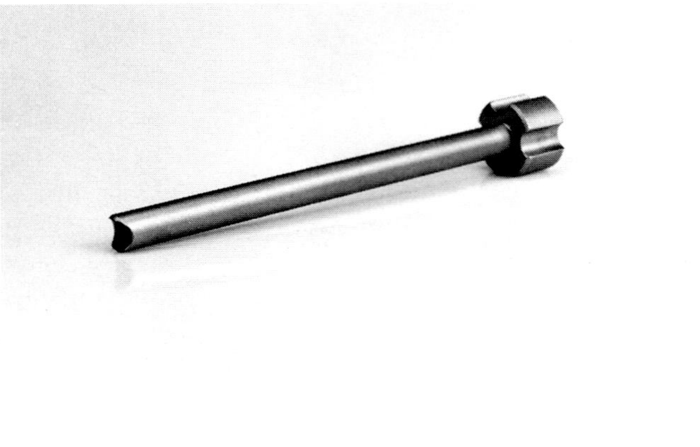

Fig. 2 A modern drill sleeve, shown without the trochar.

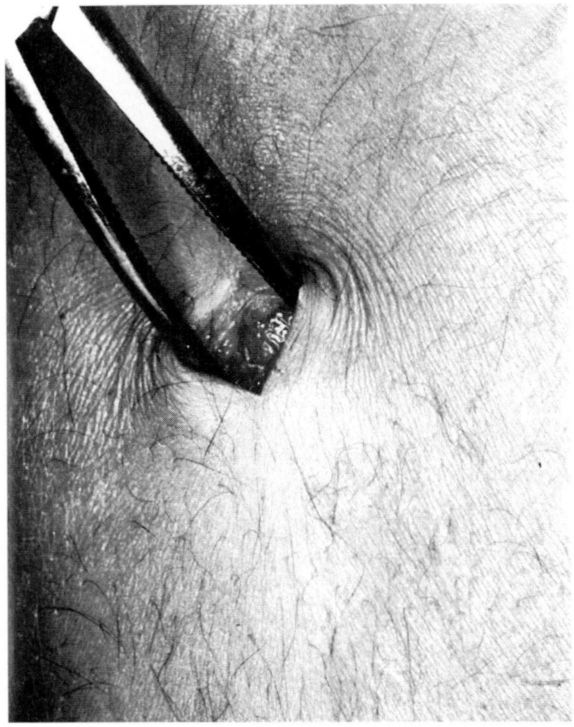

Fig. 3 Spreading the soft tissues prior to drill sleeve insertion.

less steel, cobalt-chromium-molybdenum, titanium, and titanium alloy) and added these powders to incubating white blood cells mixed with inocula of staphylococci. They found that stainless steel inhibits white blood cell bactericidal activity to a far greater extent than any of the other metals. This inhibition of normal cellular defenses explains the clinical differences observed between titanium and steel at the pin site interface. Unfortunately, titanium is about 10% more flexible than stainless steel, a factor that reduces the stability of the bone-fixator construct. Luckily though, pin stiffness is proportionate to the fourth power of pin diameter; thus a 1-mm increase in pin diameter enhances pin stiffness by about 250%. For this reason, substituting a 6-mm titanium pin for a 5-mm steel pin will result in a stiffer overall configuration.

Predrilling A trochar or hollow drill-sleeve (Fig. 2) must be used for pin insertion to prevent tissues from being wrapped up around a turning implant. Make an adequate skin incision before inserting the trochar and sleeve device. Spread the tissues apart (with a mosquito clamp) all the way down to the bone (Fig. 3). Likewise, use a joker or periosteal elevator (Fig. 4) to scrape the periosteum off the bone's surface at the site of pin insertion to reduce the possibility that the drill-bit tip will grind up the periosteal tissues.

Do not use a power drill to insert a threaded pin directly into bone, because heat build-up at the pin's point could cause a thermal injury to bone. Instead, predrill the bone hole with a sharp fluted drill-bit and a drill sleeve and then insert the pin by hand.

While drilling, stop the drill every few seconds to allow the cutting tip to cool down. The heat generated by drilling not only damages the bone, but also "work hardens" osseous tissue, which then resists further advancement. A worthwhile practice is to irrigate the exposed portion of the drill-bit to cool it and conduct heat away from the tip. Likewise, be sure to release the tourniquet before drilling into bone to allow circulating blood to help conduct heat away from the drill point.

If much resistance is encountered during drilling, remove and check the drill-bit tip between your fingers for excessive temperature build-up. If the tip cannot be comfortably held for a few seconds, do not insert a pin into that bone-hole, because there would be necrotic (thermally injured) bone in communication with the pin's bacteriologic environment; a set-up for chronic osteomyelitis. Instead, insert the pin elsewhere. Likewise, the bone in the drill-bit's flutes should be white, never black or brown, the signs of burnt bone. We routinely remove a drill-bit half way through dense cortical bone, specifically for the purpose of clearing bone chaff from the drill-bit flutes.

In 1984, Ripley and I observed that most cases of ring sequestra-associated chronic pin-tract osteomyelitis were related to intracortical (rather than transmedullary) pin insertion (Fig. 5).[2]

We advised that pins be inserted through a wide portion of a bone, advice that seems appropriate for smooth transfixion wires as well. (Two distinct cortices will be felt when a drill-bit crosses the medullary canal.) Moreover, whenever osseous resistance to drilling progress is encountered, a slow stop-and-start insertion technique is essential to avoid burning the bone.

Pin Insertion To insert the pin, press the drill sleeve firmly against the bone and carefully remove the drill bit. Place the pin through the sleeve with a hand-held

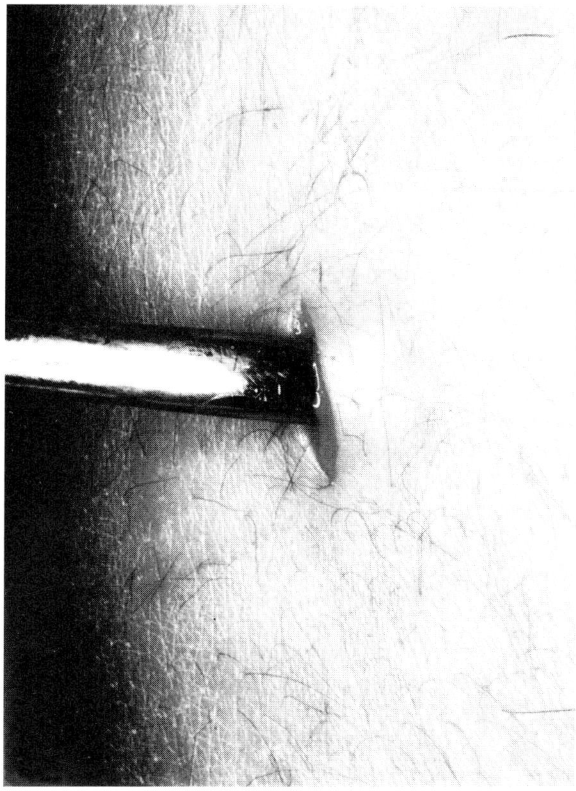

Fig. 4 A joker is used to elevate the periosteum prior to drilling.

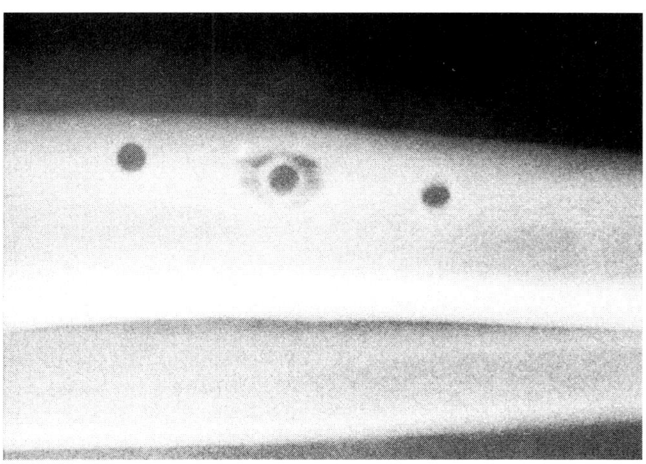

Fig. 5 A ring sequestrum. Note the intracortical location.

inserter. Once the pin is in place, test its stability by firmly wiggling the pin back and forth. It should hold securely. On rare occasions, a pin may slide off the surface of a long bone during insertion and be anchored in firm juxta-osseous soft tissues instead.

Transfixion Wire Technique

Whenever external fixators employ only smooth Kirschner wires for attachment to bone, fixation is not secure unless two or more wires are used at each level of fixation. For maximum stability, the two wires should cross each other at a right angle at each plane of fixation.[3] Unfortunately, anatomic considerations limit the surgeon's ability to insert wires crossing at 90° within the bone. For this reason, transfixion wires usually end up crossing each other at a more acute angle, thereby diminishing fixator stability. To overcome this problem, the surgeon must either use more than two wires at each plane of fixation or insert additional wires away from—or oblique to—the ring's plane of fixation. Alternatively, half-pins can be used in combination with wires. For added stability, tensioned wire fixation systems also use beaded wires, which prevent the bone from sliding along the wire.

Wire Placement Certain technical considerations are necessary for the successful application of any tensioned-wire circular external fixator. If they are inserted without regard to cross-sectional anatomy, transfixion wires can endanger neurovascular structures. In 1981, I described a "Zone System" atlas for pin placement to ensure safe application of transfixion and half-pins.[4] This same system can also be employed to aid placement of transfixion wires. Other atlases are also available.

A pin or wire that is directed at a neurovascular structure may push the nerve or vessel to the side, or it may impale it. When a nerve is first touched or irritated by a wire or drill-bit point, the muscle it supplies will twitch if the patient has not been subjected to the neuromuscular blockade. For this reason, any paralyzing agent should be reversed before the surgeon starts to insert a pin or wire. If a wire penetrates a vessel, excessive bleeding will be noted at either the entry or exit point of a wire. When this happens, the wire must be removed.

Wire Insertion As transfixion wires are being inserted, a spinning bayonet point can wind-up soft tissues in a manner similar to the flutes of a drill-bit, causing necrosis. To avoid this, push the transfixion wires straight through the tissues to bone before turning on the drill. If the wire misses the bone, withdraw it completely and reinsert it, do not try to redirect the wire within the limb's tissues.

When inserting a transfixion wire with a motorized chuck, the wire's flexibility can, at times, cause it to bend, reducing accuracy of placement. For this reason, whenever inserting a wire, manually grasp the wire close to its tip to stabilize it. To avoid having the spinning wire wrap up the surgical gloves, hold the wire with a small (2 × 2) gauze pad soaked in an antibiotic solution. This technique of stabilizing the spinning wire with a gauze pad has a second advantage: it allows the surgeon to hold the wire in the chuck close to its blunt end, thereby avoiding the possibility of nicking the wire in a region where the wire will be tensioned. (Such nicks can lead to wire breakage if they are located anywhere between the fixation bolts when the final frame assembly is completed.)

When transfixion wires are being inserted, dense cortical bone, which offers substantial resistance to the wire-point's progress, can cause heat build-up. The heat hardens the bone, which then resists additional progress of the wire-point. I suspect that the potential for heat build-up is even greater for pointed wires than for drill-bits because the wire has no flutes to conduct bone cuttings away from the worksite. For this reason, when drilling a transfixion wire through hard cortical bone, a safe practice is to stop the drill every few seconds, using a stop-start action to advance the wire slowly through hard osseous tissue. Furthermore, complete intracortical insertion of a wire—not accompanied by the "feel" of crossing the marrow to encountering a second cortex—is especially prone to excessive heat build-up, thermal damage and the possibility of wire-hole osteomyelitis.

As soon as a transfixion wire's point penetrates a bone's far cortex, it is important to stop drilling, because a slightly bent spinning wire-tip can act like an egg-beater and damage tissues on the limb's opposite side. Instead, grasp the wire with pliers and hit the pliers with a mallet to drive the wire through or, if the wire is thick enough, strike the end of the wire with a mallet while holding the wire in your hand.

A most important principle to follow with any transfixion implant is: if the tip of a wire (or transfixion pin) emerges from the opposite side of a limb either smoking, or too hot to be comfortably held between the surgeon's fingertips, the wire should be withdrawn, cooled, and reinserted elsewhere. (In the Soviet Union, whenever a wire is inserted into cortical bone, the assistant surgeons irrigate the wire with a cold antiseptic solution to conduct heat away from the wire.)[5]

With any transfixion wire or pin, it is necessary to check the range of nearby joint motion to make sure that no undue tension occurs while the fixator is on the limb. If necessary, an implant should be reinserted if movement of an adjacent joint causes excessive skin tension.

Certain important techniques of transfixion-wire insertion ensure maximum functional limb use and joint mobility. The surgeon should avoid impaling tendons, should avoid (whenever possible) transfixing synovium, and should take care to penetrate muscles at their maximum functional length. The last rule, critically important for a successful long-term application, means that the surgeon must change the position of a nearby joint as a wire is passed through the flexor and extensor muscle groups. When inserting a wire into the lower leg, for example, the surgeon must plantarflex the foot when transfixing the anterior compartment, invert the foot when inserting wires into the peroneal muscles, and dorsiflex the foot during triceps surae impalement.

The above considerations apply to the optimum position for muscle transfixion. The skin's position is another matter. Flexing the knee during femoral wire or pin insertion pulls the lower anterior thigh skin distalward, while, at the same time, the posterior thigh skin slides a bit proximally. Transfixion of anterior thigh skin during 90° of knee flexion (the best position for quadriceps impalement) might cause the skin to limit knee extension, restrict knee motion and decrease ambulation, leading, perhaps, to a knee flexion contracture. For this reason, before inserting a wire or even a half-pin, the surgeon should shift the skin in a direction appropriate to adjacent joint motion. In determining which way to move the skin before inserting a wire, consider the following:

First, when lengthening a limb, some redundant skin and subcutaneous tissue should, if possible, overlay the cortical osteotomy site, where stretching will be greatest. Thus, when inserting supracondylar wires or pins prior to lengthening a femur through a distal corticotomy, pull the skin and subcutaneous tissues proximally during wire or pin penetration and, at the same time, flex and extend the knee as described above. Likewise, shift the skin and subcutaneous tissues distally when mounting the fixator to the proximal thigh.

Second, when correcting a deformity by an opening-wedge corticotomy, the skin and subcutaneous tissues should be loose on the deformity's concave side. In a case of correction of a tibia with apex-lateral angulation, for instance, shift the medial cutaneous tissues first down and then up during proximal and distal wire insertion. (When shifting skin for the two reasons just described, the shifting movement should be slight—never enough to cause undue tension at any wire or pin insertion site.)

Third, try, whenever possible, to select wire or pin placement locations that normally have limited skin movement during flexion or extension of an adjacent joint. In the distal humerus, for example, when an elbow is flexed, the anterior lower arm skin moves up while the posterior skin moves down; with elbow extension, these same tissues move in the opposite directions. Between the flexor and the extensor surfaces, however, a fairly stationary tissue plane exists around which the upward-downward movement of anterior and posterior tissues revolve. This plane of limited skin motion lies along the medial and lateral supracondylar ridges of the humerus—an ideal location for transfixion wire or even half-pin placement. Unfortunately, the distal humerus flattens and widens above the elbow; two supracondylar transfixion wires (in the same transverse plane) will not have enough of an angle between them for stable fixation. A far better strategy is to cross the two wires in the frontal plane (Fig. 6). Insert wires into both epicondyles, in such a way that they exit the humerus proximally out the medial and lateral supracondylar ridges, with care taken not to transfix either the ulnar or radial nerves. A third wire straight across from one supracondylar ridge to the other completes this distal humerus mounting. Attach the cross wires to a half- or 3/5-ring with posts extending above and below the ring's plane. When the mounting is complete, the elbow should flex and extend fully without skin tension. (A mechanical block to full extension means that one or more wires has entered the olecranon fossa of the distal humerus.)

When a wire (or a pin) must be inserted near a tendon, a simple technique will help avoid tendon transfixion. First, palpate the tendon at risk to determine its exact course and location. Next, while holding the wire (or drill sleeve) in one hand, palpate the position of the tendon with the other hand. Then insert the wire (or drill-bit) through the skin down to, but not quite touching, the bone. Then, wiggle the structure ordinarily moved by tendon in question. For example, dorsiflex and plantarflex the ankle when a wire is inserted near the tibialis anterior tendon. If the wire tip or trochar point has impaled the tendon, the wire will move as the joint is put through a range of motion. If this occurs, withdraw the wire and reinsert it in a slightly different position.

Frame Attachment Bending a transfixion wire to reach the ring for attachment can cause excessive soft tissue damage, because the wire, being so narrow, concentrates pressure over a small area. Transfixion-wire fixator systems use special strategies to ensure that none of the wires are bent during frame attachment. Most circular fixators employ washers, posts, and other hardware to achieve this goal (Fig. 7). Indeed, the principle of not bending a wire when attaching it to a frame is a critical element to successful smooth-wire external fixation.

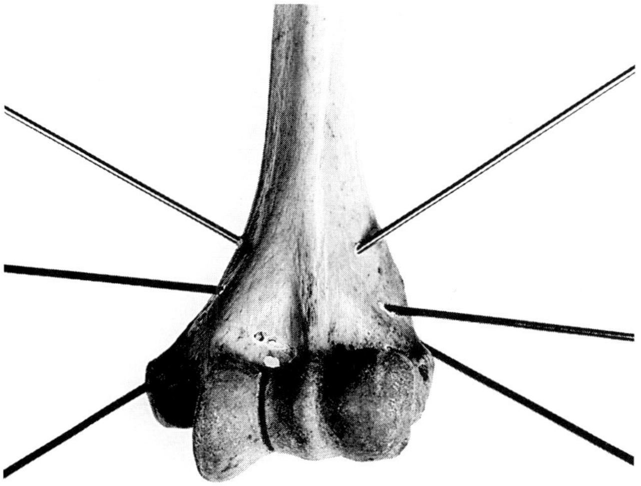

Fig. 6 Transfixion wires crossing in the coronal plane in the distal humerus.

The Implant Interface

Interface Skin Tension

After inserting a wire or pin, but before attaching it to the frame, check the implant-skin interface for evidence of tissue tension while the limb is in its most functional position—that is, with the knee extended, the ankle at neutral, etc. Interface tension will create a ridge of skin on one side of an implant (Fig. 8, *left*). When half pins are used, incise the ridge to enlarge the skin hole (Fig. 8, *right*). When the skin tension is caused by a wire (Fig. 9, *left*), however, slowly withdraw the wire (with pliers and a mallet) until its tip drops below the skin surface (Fig. 9, *center*). Allow the skin to shift to a more neutral location and advance the wire again until it passes through the skin in an improved position (Fig. 9, *right*).

If an olive wire causes skin tension on the side of the limb opposite the olive, simply back the wire out until the tip drops below the skin surface and make the correction described above. If the tension is on the olive side of the wire, enlarge slightly the skin incision originally made for olive insertion. I recommend closing the enlarged hole with a nylon suture on the side of the wire opposite the released ridge, because the skin hole will be enlarged on this side.

Limb Function

Once wires and pins are in place, after the final frame configuration is established, it is important to put the adjacent joints through a range of motion to be sure that the implants do not cause excessive soft tissue tension that interferes with joint motion. If such tension does exist, it may be necessary to either change the position of a wire or a pin or release skin tension with a scalpel.

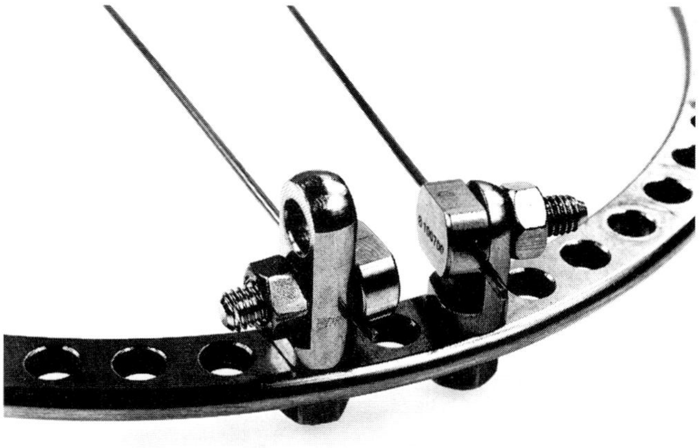

Fig. 7 Hardware used to capture wires that are not in the plane of a ring.

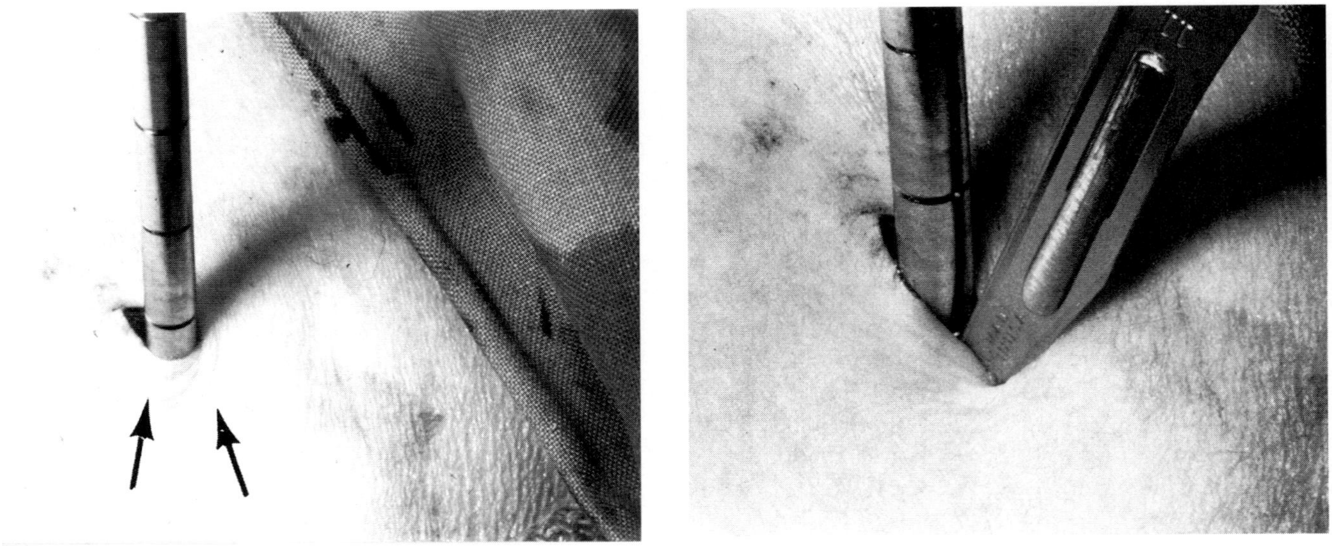

Fig. 8 **Left,** Skin tension (arrows) on the near side of a half-pin. **Right,** Release tension by inserting a knife into the ridge of skin.

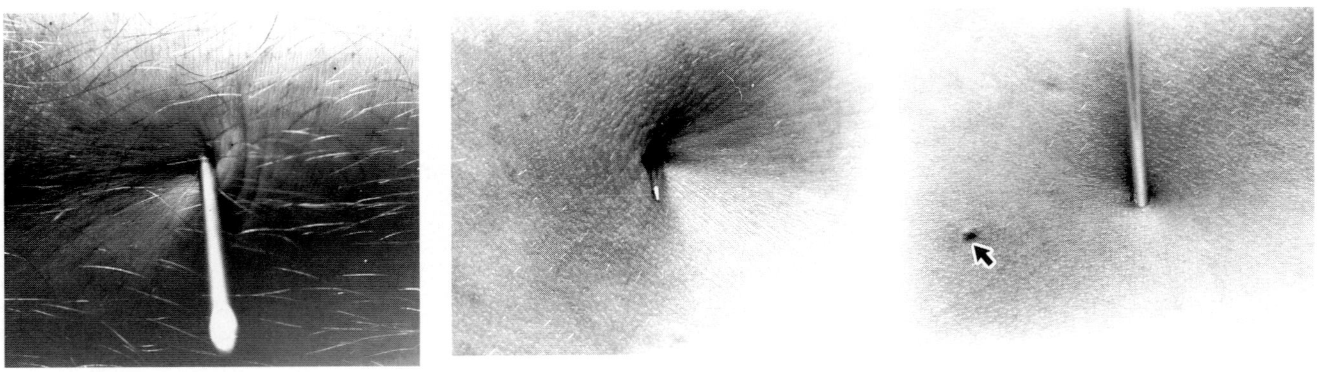

Fig. 9 **Left,** Skin tension at a wire site. **Center,** Backing the wire below the skin surface. **Right,** The skin has shifted into a more neutral position. (Arrow points to original wire hole.)

Pin-Site Care

A basic principle of pin-site care is to help the host tissues resist infection caused by the skin micro-organisms that ordinarily contaminate all transcutaneous implant sites. In an attempt to achieve this objective, patients have been taught to apply antiseptics to the pin site. Many such substances have been employed in this manner: hydrogen peroxide, alcohol, iodine preparations (including Betadine) and so forth. Although these antiseptics are lethal to many micro-organisms, they are also toxic to all mammalian cells—including phagocytic white blood cells. Thus, antiseptics lower both the inoculum size and the host resistive capacity at the same time. It is far better, I believe, to reduce the number of contaminating micro-organisms without impairing the antimicrobial activity of tissues lining the pin-hole. Because pin-site contamination most commonly includes staphylococcal skin organisms, I instruct my patients to use an antibiotic (rather than an antiseptic) ointment that is especially effective for the treatment of impetigo—a staphylococcal skin eruption. This ointment, called Bactroban®, is rather expensive, but it does the job better than any other preparation that I have tried. Because it is an antibiotic rather than antiseptic, it will not harm host tissues. Polysporin ointment, another antibiotic, is also affective.

My recommended pin-site care routine: at surgery, wrap the pin site with gauze pads and Kerlex® wrap soaked in an antibiotic irrigating solution. Fill the space between the skin and fixator completely with the bulky wrap (Fig. 10). Leave this dressing in place until the first postoperative visit, at which time the bulky wraps are removed and any sutures taken out. The patient is instructed to shower (preferably with Dial® soap), dry the limb and fixator and apply a small dab of Bactroban ointment at each interface site. In locations where little or no soft-tissue motion around the implant site is expected (eg, anterior tibia), no dressing is required. In places where the skin is expected to slide along the implant (eg, lateral thigh), a bulky wrap dressing is needed to stabilize the implant-skin interface. I also give my patients a prescription for oral anti-staphylococcal antibiotic, such as Keflex®, with instructions to start taking the medication whenever the pin site becomes inflamed, painful, reddened, or otherwise infected.

The pin and wire techniques described in this chapter will, I believe, do much to improve the longevity of a fixator's application, decrease patient discomfort, and reduce the likelihood of complications.

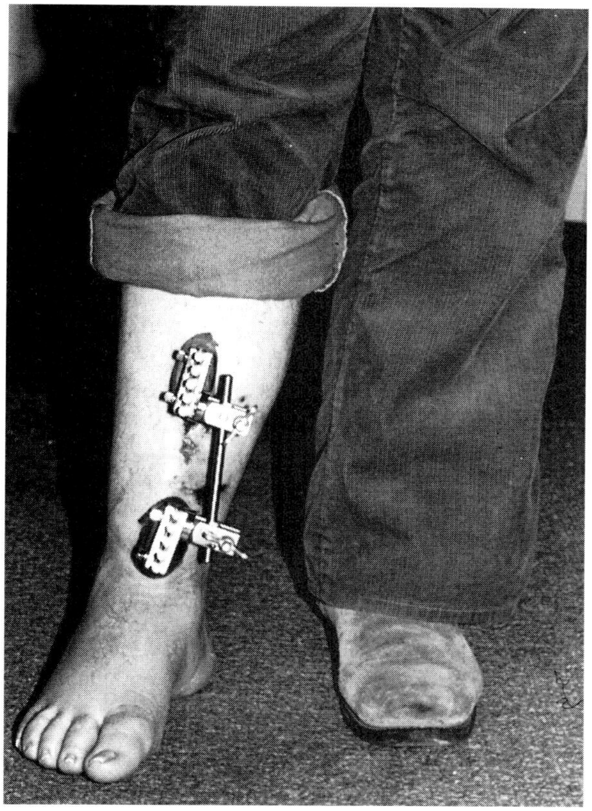

Fig. 10 Bulky wraps placed around the implants stabilize the implant-skin interface.

References

1. Pascual A, Tsukayama DT, Wicklund BH, et al: The effect of stainless steel, cobalt-chromium, titanium alloy, and titanium on the respiratory burst activity of human polymorphonuclear leukocytes. *Clin Orthop* 1992;280:281-288.
2. Green SA, Ripley MJ: Chronic osteomyelitis in pin tracts. *J Bone Joint Surg* 1984;66A:1092-1098.
3. Green SA, Wall DM: Ilizarov external fixation: Transfixion wire technique. *Mediguide to Orthopedics* 1989;4:1-4.
4. Green SA: *Complications of External Skeletal Fixation: Causes, Prevention and Treatment.* Springfield, IL, Charles C. Thomas, 1981.
5. Green SA: The Ilizarov method: Rancho technique. *Orthop Clin North Am* 1991;22:677-688.

Kinetics

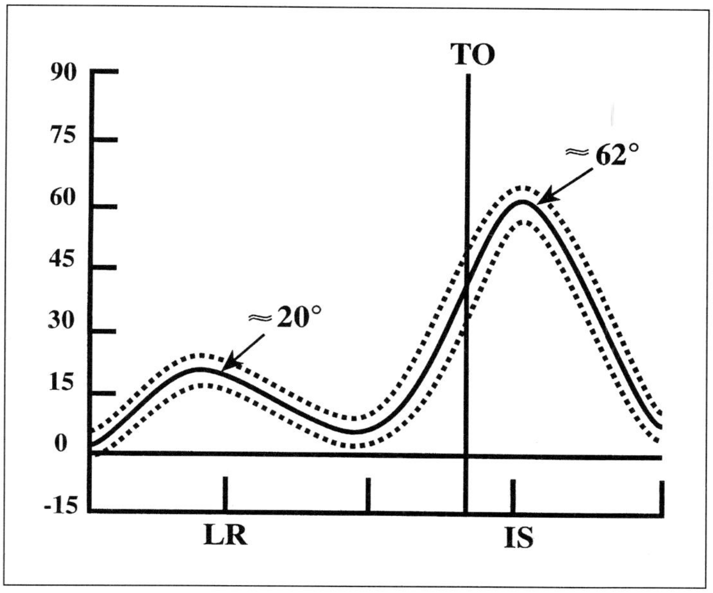

Walking, Running, and Sprinting: A Three-Dimensional Analysis of Kinematics and Kinetics

Tom F. Novacheck, MD

Introduction

The study of human locomotion is a fascinating one. In the past, videotapes were reviewed to evaluate joint positions and attempt to determine the muscles responsible for various movements. Later, dynamic electromyographic (EMG) analysis became available to substantiate or refute these speculative data. Then it became possible to time these findings in accordance with stance or swing phase through use of simple electronic timing switches affixed to the foot. Hand digitization of video data provided more accurate joint motion information, and the advent of computerized motion analysis techniques and force plate technology has revolutionized the study of human movement.

Normal walking and running have been well documented using these techniques. The body segment positions, joint motions, and the locations of energy generation and absorption are well known for these two activities. Sprinting, however, has not been fully evaluated. The evaluation of sprinting and the comparison of sprinting with walking and running are the purposes of this chapter.

Forward human locomotion can be divided into walking, running, and sprinting. Although these three conditions represent a continuum that ranges from extremely slow walking (velocity barely greater than zero) to sprinting at top speed, there are unique characteristics that distinguish each of these three states. Some basic definitions will be provided here, but the reader is referred to previous publications for a more formal introduction to the terminology and conventions of motion analysis.[1] To avoid confusion at the outset, several terms should be defined. One gait cycle, a stride, begins when one foot strikes the ground and ends when it strikes the ground the next time. The stride time is the time elapsed during one gait cycle. The gait cycle is commonly divided into two phases. Stance phase occurs when the foot is in contact with the ground. Conversely, swing phase occurs when the foot is not contacting the ground. Kinematics is the study of motion without regard to the forces which created it. Kinetics is the study of the forces responsible for that motion. The distinction between walking and running is made according to the percentage of stance, or ground contact, in the gait cycle. In walking there are two periods of double support in each gait cycle during which both feet are in contact with the ground simultaneously (Fig. 1). During running and sprinting, there are two periods of double float during which neither foot is in contact with the ground (Fig. 1). The necessary implication is that stance cannot equal or exceed 50% of the gait cycle in running; whereas in walking, it does. The differentiation between running and sprinting is based on which part of the foot strikes the ground first at initial contact. In running, heel contact occurs first. In sprinting, initial contact is with the forefoot.

Walking, running, and sprinting cycles can be divided into distinct phases, distinguished by the motion and muscle activity at that point in the cycle. All three have distinct stance phases, during which there is foot contact with the ground, and swing phases, during which the foot is not in contact with the ground. Figure 2 shows how these phases are divided into distinct periods.

In walking, stance phase is divided into initial contact, loading response, midstance, terminal stance, and preswing. Swing phase is simply divided into initial, mid-, and terminal swing. In running and sprinting the divisions of the stance and swing phases are different (Fig. 2). Stance phase is divided into two periods—absorption and propulsion. The instantaneous event that separates them has been referred to as midstance. This point represents the reversal between flexion and extension, ie, absorption and propulsion. I find this terminology confusing, because in walking the term midstance refers to a period of time, while in running and sprinting, it refers to an instantaneous event. For this reason, I prefer the term stance phase reversal.

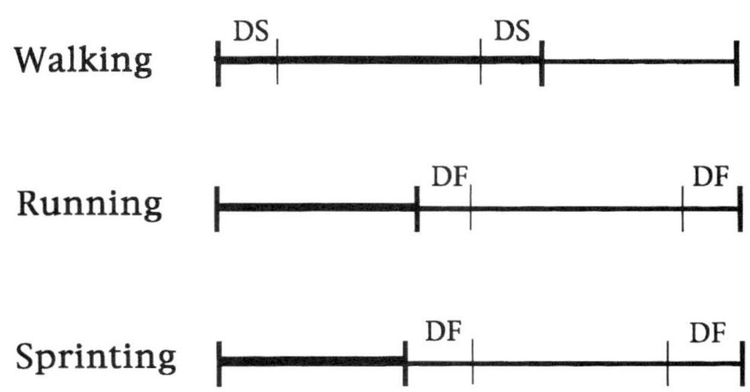

Fig. 1 Double stance (DS) and double float (DF). Stance phase for each condition is depicted by the thicker line and swing phase by the thinner line. Stance phase progressively shortens with increasing velocity. Length of double float time increases as speed increases from running to sprinting.

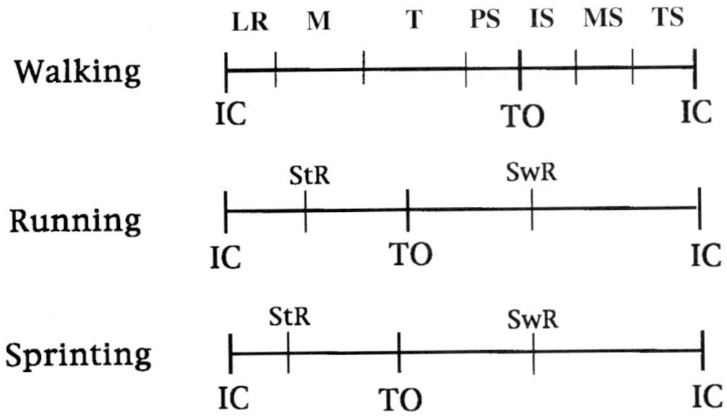

Fig. 2 Specific periods in walking, running, and sprinting gait cycles. (IC = initial contact, LR = loading response, M = midstance, T = terminal stance, PS = preswing, TO = toe off, IS = initial swing, MS = midswing, TS = terminal swing, StR = stance phase reversal.

Swing phase is likewise divided into two periods separated by an instantaneous event. Initial swing represents continued and progressive joint flexion. Terminal swing represents progressive hip and knee extension. The point in time that separates these two has similarly been referred to as midswing. Again, to avoid confusion with this well-accepted period in the walking cycle, I prefer the term swing phase reversal. The running and sprinting gait cycles can therefore be divided into four phases divided by four instantaneous events—initial contact, stance phase reversal, toe-off, and swing phase reversal.

It should be noted that walking gait has two periods of double support during which both feet are in contact with the walking surface. These occur at the beginning and end of the stance phase and coincide with loading response and preswing. It is during these periods that the two limbs are alternatively loaded and unloaded as body weight is transferred from one leg to the other. Running and sprinting, unlike walking, have no periods of double support. Instead, they have two periods of double float, one at the beginning and one at the end of swing phase (Fig. 3, point A). This is the distinction between walking and running in the continuum from stationary standing without any forward motion to an individual's fastest sprint. As mentioned previously, the separation between running and sprinting is based on whether initial contact is with the hindfoot or forefoot (Fig. 3, point B). As velocity increases from zero to maximum (as one moves from a standstill through walking, to running, and finally to sprinting), double support time progressively decreases until it gives way to double float which steadily increases in duration to maximum attainable velocity.

Running and sprinting have been studied in the past,[2-4] but, to the author's knowledge, a three-dimensional kinematic and kinetic evaluation of sprinting in untrained athletes has not been reported. Mann[2,3] studied adult trained athletes and used a two-dimensional system requiring hand digitization of video data. Joint moments were calculated using a Kistler force plate as in this report, but joint powers were not discussed. Ounpuu[4] studied running and specifically excluded sprinting in her study. For these reasons, this study was undertaken at the Motion Analysis Lab of Gillette Children's Hospital in an effort to evaluate sprinting and to compare it to walking and running.

Materials and Methods

Twenty-seven healthy children (eight boys and 19 girls) ranging in age from 5 to 18 years were tested. They were tested in normal walking. They were then asked to run as fast as they could during the running/sprinting collection. The data were then evaluated to determine whether the collection represented running or sprinting as described previously. Data determined to be representative of running rather than sprinting were included in the running file. A preliminary assessment was made after each collection to see if a sprinting collection had been obtained on the subject before their testing was completed. If one had not, the subject was simply asked to run faster. To avoid artifact, no reference was made to running on your toes. The data presented here are based on 17 sides in 10 children for the running file and 40 sides in 15 children for sprinting.

The Vicon system (Oxford Metrics), which has a standard retroreflective marker set and a series of four in-line AMTI force plates, was used to obtain and process the data. The remainder of the study was completed in accordance with the usual routine for the motion lab, including physical exam with anthropometric measurements. EMG data, which have been documented well in the past for running[4] and sprinting, were not collected during this study. Three-dimensional

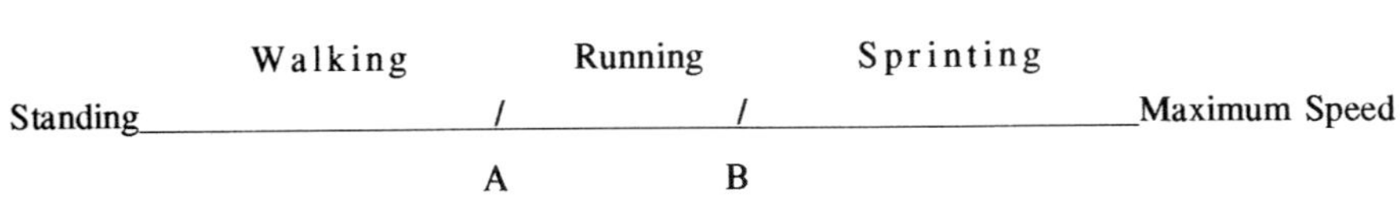

Fig. 3 Continuum from zero to maximum velocity. Point A, Start of double float distinguishes running from walking. Point B, initial contact with the forefoot distinguishes sprinting from running.

joint kinematics and kinetics were averaged across all subjects for walking, running, and sprinting. This study used three methods to determine whether initial contact was with the forefoot (sprinting) or the heel (running). First, the videotape of the data collection was reviewed visually. Second, the screen image of the applied retroreflective marker set was evaluated. Third, and most importantly, the kinetic plot of ankle moments was used. If the moment at initial contact was plantarflexor, then the collection was determined to represent sprinting. Conversely, a dorsiflexor moment represented running, because the dorsiflexors act to lower the forefoot to the ground following initial heel contact.

Results

Temporal and Stride Parameters

Table 1 and Figure 4, *top left* show that velocity increases from walking through running to sprinting. Running velocity was 2.72 times that of walking while sprinting velocity was 3.24 fold faster than walking speed. The change in speed from running to sprinting was only 19% in this study. As velocity increases, relative length of stance decreases from 62% to 37% while swing phase increases from 38% to 62% (Fig. 4, *center* and *bottom left*). This is the case because the stance phase periods of double support in walking give way to the running and sprinting swing phase periods of double float. Ounpuu reported a 43% stance phase.[4] The difference between that collection and this one is most likely related to the instructions given to the subjects. Our children were instructed to run as fast as they could. Ounpuu's group ran at a slower velocity (223 cm/sec) as they were instructed simply to run. Mann's highly trained athletes certainly ran at a much higher velocity. His subjects were instructed to attain a maximum sprint. In that study stance phase decreased to 30% of the gait cycle.

Stride length steadily increases and cycle time decreases with increasing speed. Figure 4, *top right* shows that an increase in cadence accounts for the main difference between walking and any of the runs or sprints. Increased running speed is apparently accomplished by increasing one's stride length (Fig. 4, *center right*). Most of the increase in velocity from running to sprinting was due to increases in cadence (Fig. 4, *top right*) and not to increases in stride length (Fig. 4, *center right*).

It should be noted that kinematic and kinetic results for all three conditions (walking, running, and sprinting) are depicted as a percentage of the gait cycle. Because the cycle time steadily decreases with increasing velocity (Fig. 4, *bottom right*), the events in sprinting occur much more rapidly than in walking.

Table 1
Comparison of walking, running and sprinting

Parameters	Walking	Running	Sprinting
Stance (% of stride)	62	39	37
Swing (% of stride)	38	61	63
Step length (cm)	57.5	97.5	99.5
Stride length (cm)	115	195	199
Cycle time (sec)	0.91	0.6	0.51
Cadence (step/min)	117	199	230
Velocity (cm/sec)	118	321	382

Kinematics

This study differed from some past studies in that joint rotations were calculated in all three planes for the hip, knee, and ankle joints of the lower extremities. The kinematic results are shown in Figure 5. A description of these findings follows.

Sagittal Plane Hip motion follows a nearly sinusoidal pattern with maximum hip extension occurring at toe-off and maximum flexion in terminal swing. Maximum hip extension is similar in timing and magnitude to both walking and running; however, maximum hip flexion is significantly increased in sprinting compared to both walking and running (p = 0.001 and 0.005, respectively). Therefore, as velocity increases, swing phase hip flexion increases. As stated earlier, much of the increase in velocity from walking to either running or sprinting resulted from increased stride length. Greater hip flexion would account for this increase in distance traveled with each step.

Although the knee motion pattern is very similar to that seen in running, the extremes of motion again differ. During the absorption period of stance phase in sprinting, the knee progressively flexes from 34° to 39°. There is much greater knee flexion in running (31° to 44°, p = 0.005). The progressive knee extension in the generation period leads to greater knee extension (20° as opposed to 25° in running, p = 0.01), which contributes to increased step length of the opposite side. These results show that in running the knee is much more important in shock absorption (decreasing vertical velocity). In sprinting, it is much more important in generating energy for forward propulsion. This difference will be discussed more extensively in the kinetics section. Maximum sprinting knee flexion at swing reversal is much greater than that which occurs with running (105° vs 89°, p = 0.001). Both are much greater than maximum knee flexion in walking (58°). The greater angular accelerations in sprinting account for the increased knee flexion (also to be discussed in the kinetics section).

Statistically significant sagittal plane changes in sprinting occur at the ankle. At initial contact, the foot is in a neutral position (0° dorsi/plantarflexion) compared to the tibia. During absorption, the ankle progressively dorsiflexes as the body weight is transferred to that leg.

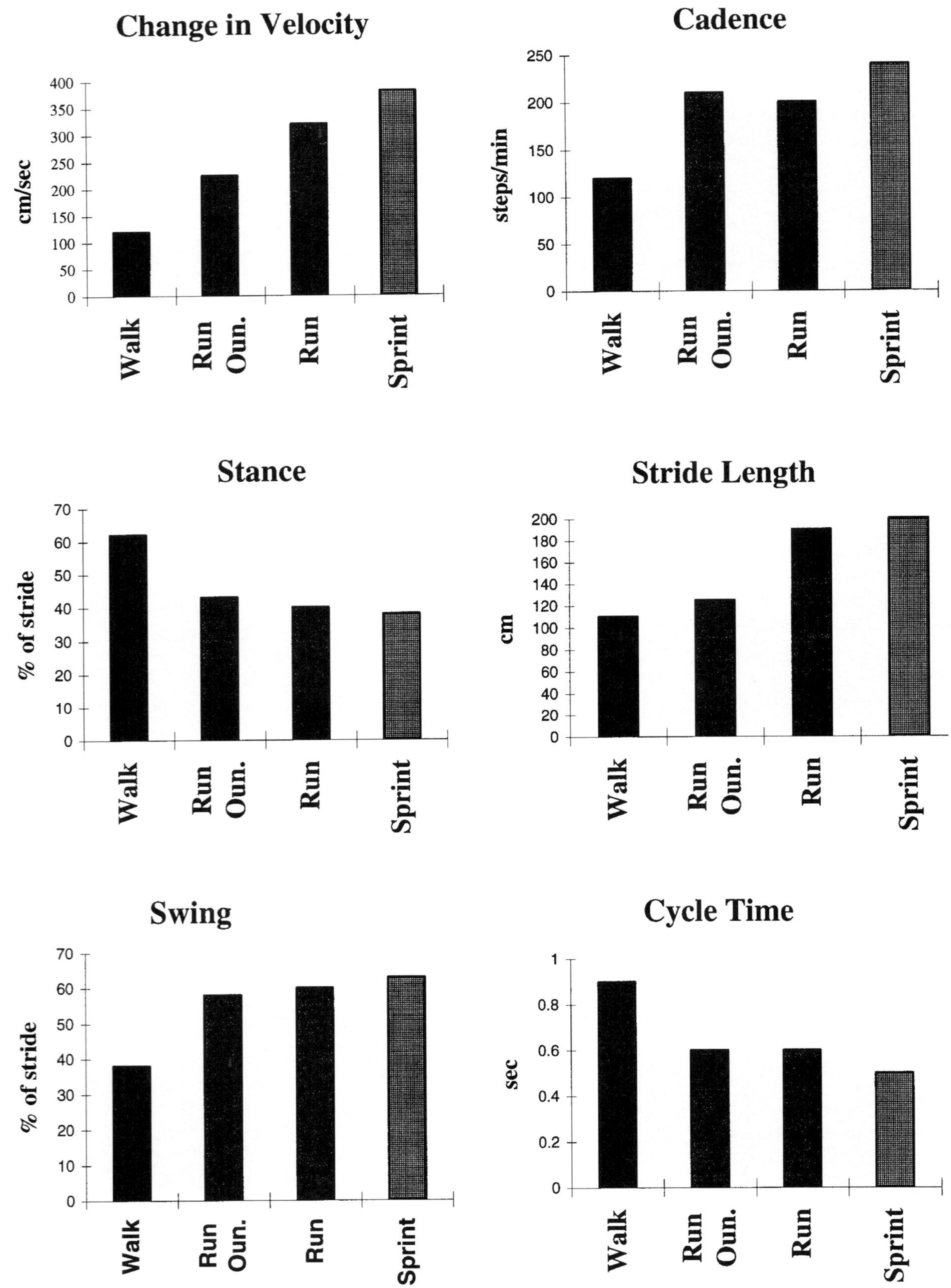

Fig. 4 Linear parameters for walking, running, and sprinting.

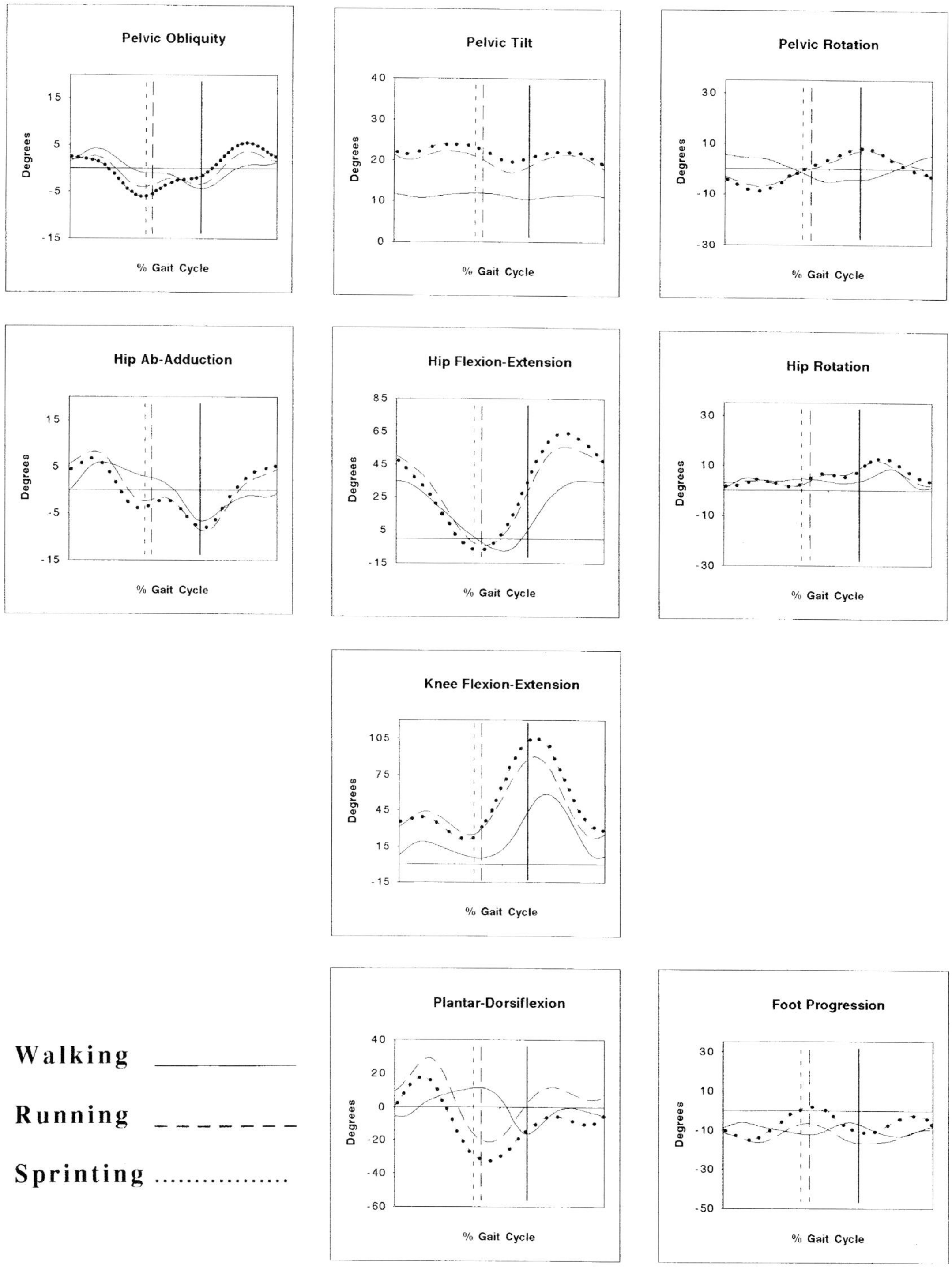

Fig. 5 Kinematic results for walking, running, and sprinting. Note that the data are presented according to plane of motion in each column and by joint in each row. In each plot, the vertical lines represent the toe-off point for each of the three conditions and correspond to the curve of similar line type.

Maximum dorsiflexion, however, is much more limited than in running, due in part to the shorter duration of the absorption period and to the relative plantarflexion at initial contact (IC). During generation, the ankle plantarflexes to a much greater degree than in running (33° vs 21°, p = 0.001). During swing phase, ankle dorsiflexion is less complete than in both walking and running. Dorsiflexion to neutral position is not necessary for toe clearance given the increased knee flexion. The results for ankle position at IC at first may seem both disturbing and perplexing. Initially, it seems incorrect to find that the ankle is in greater dorsiflexion at IC in sprinting than it is in walking. One must remember, however, that the ankle rotation is reported relative to the position of the tibia (or shank) segment. If one recalls that in sprinting the knee and hip are in greater flexion at this point and that the body is pitched forward, then it becomes apparent that IC can occur on the toe in sprinting and on the heel in walking (Fig. 6).

The pelvis is more anteriorly flexed with increasing velocity indicating a greater forward lean of the trunk. One might expect a greater amount of pelvic motion with faster velocities, but there is in fact little increased motion. Pelvic motion is minimized to conserve energy and maintain efficiency in running and sprinting.

Coronal Plane Joint rotation in this plane is overall very small. Given that the only lower extremity joint with significant motion in the coronal plane is the hip, it is the one of most importance. Generally, the hip is adducted in stance phase and abducted during swing. Hip motion in this plane mirrors pelvic motion to a great extent in such a way as to minimize the relative motion between the lower extremities and the body segments above. In other words, when the hip is adducted, the pelvis is elevated on that side. When the hip is abducted, the pelvis is lower. This nearly reciprocal motion combined with slight lumbopelvic motion minimizes shoulder motion in the coronal plane.

The pelvis is most oblique in terminal swing during double float. The forward limb preparing for initial contact is elevated. This maintains foot clearance at this point in the gait cycle, because both the hip and knee are more extended than they were at the reversal point. As the limb is loaded (during the absorption period in stance phase), the pelvis continues to drop and the hip progressively adducts relative to the pelvis. This shock-absorbing mechanism is similar to that seen at the knee in the sagittal plane during the absorption period of stance phase.

Transverse plane Joint rotations in this plane may be the most difficult to comprehend because the motions are relatively small and are difficult to perceive with the naked eye. The conventions used to report these motions must be appreciated in order to understand the motion plots in this plane. The pelvic and foot rotations are depicted relative to the line of progression. Thus, if the pelvis is externally rotated during stance phase on the right, the right hemipelvis is rotated away from or posterior to the direction of progression. The hip motion is reported relative to the pelvis. Further description will be provided in the following discussion to aid in the understanding of these concepts.

In general, in stance phase, the hemipelvis is externally rotated. In swing, the pelvis is internally rotated. It should be noted that, because the pelvis moves as a unit, its position at two points 50% of the gait cycle apart must be equal and opposite. In sprinting, for example, at 16% the pelvis is maximally externally rotated 9°. The simultaneous occurrence on the opposite side is at 66% of the cycle, at which point it can be seen that the pelvis is internally rotated to the same degree.

Pelvic motion during running and sprinting is interestingly opposite that of walking. In Ounpuu's chapter, the motion in running was intermediate between that seen in walking and sprinting. This difference is related again to the slower walking velocity in her group than in ours. In walking, the pelvis is internally rotated in stance phase to increase step length. The pelvis is no longer used as a stride lengthener in running and sprinting. The reason for the progressive changes in pelvic position with increasing velocity are undoubtedly related to an effort to minimize relative motion between the shoulders and the lower extremities. With the contribution of power from the moving arms and shoulders, it would be essential to transfer power from the upper body to the legs without wasteful motion between them. In a sense, the pelvis is used as a

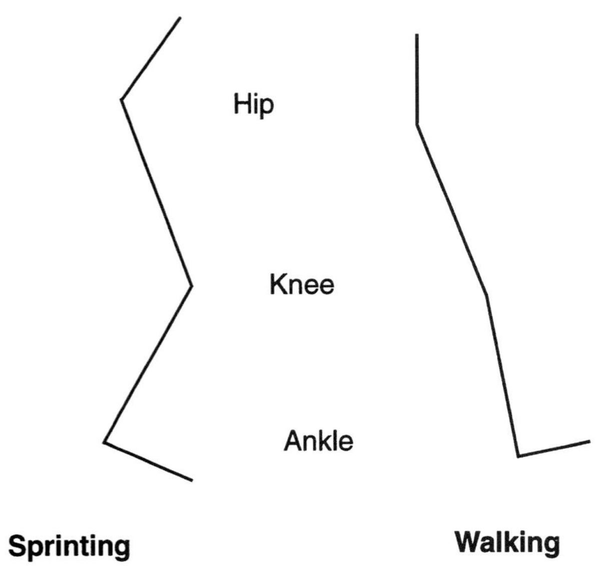

Fig. 6 Stick figure schematic for walking versus running. Initial contact occurs on the toe in sprinting and on the heel in walking despite ankle dorsiflexion in the former and plantarflexion in the latter.

transition point between the counter-rotating trunk and the forward-swinging leg. The motions in the transverse plane (as in the coronal plane) are small in magnitude compared to those in the sagittal plane. Maximum pelvic rotation occurs during single support. The pelvis is, however, nearly neutral during double float. The foot can be seen to progressively externally rotate in absorption and internally rotate later in stance phase.

Kinetics

Several important points should be made about the reporting of joint kinetic data.

The reported moment is a resultant net moment occurring at that joint at that particular point in the gait cycle. For example, if a pair of antagonistic muscles were contracting simultaneously, the result would represent only the net resultant moment. The predominant muscle group at that point would be shown. Certainly at zero crossover points, there is coexistent antagonistic muscle activity to smooth joint motion. When both the hamstrings and quadriceps contract simultaneously, only the more dominant one is reported. It should be noted that during the majority of the gait cycle, antagonistic muscles are not contracting.

The moment is named for the muscle group controlling the action. Some researchers name the moment by the external force creating it. It seems more straightforward clinically to name the moment for the muscle creating it. Because muscle moment and power generation are directly related to body weight, all data are normalized for reporting purposes by dividing by body weight.

Perhaps of greatest interest in sprinting is the area of kinetics. The combination of joint motion data (kinematics) with force plate information provides insight into joint moments as well as the sources and magnitudes of power generation or absorption. Information about joint loading (moments) can be derived. Armed with this information, the researcher can evaluate joint injuries caused either by acute stress or by chronic overload. Understanding the sources and timing of power generation and absorption may aid in developing training strategies to improve performance and to avoid injuries.

Sagittal Plane It is intuitive that the most important and significant kinetic findings are in the sagittal plane. The sagittal plane kinetic results are depicted in Figure 7.

At the ankle, there is a constant plantarflexor moment in the stance phase of sprinting. There is no initial dorsiflexor moment as seen in running and walking indicating initial contact on the forefoot. The magnitude of the plantarflexor moment in sprinting is 107% that in running and 194% that in walking (Fig. 8). The plantarflexor power in sprinting is one of immediate absorption (eccentric contraction) followed by generation (concentric contraction). This pattern is similar to that seen in running, except that in running there is an initial period of lowering of the forefoot to the ground controlled by eccentric contraction of the anterior tibial muscles. This accounts for the delay in the onset of the power absorption by the ankle plantarflexors until about 10% of the cycle. In swing phase, because the mass of the foot segment is minute and because the foot is not in contact with the ground, no moment or power is recorded at the ankle.

The knee moment in sprinting and running is very similar in pattern. Knee extension in swing phase (following the reversal point) is a passive phenomenon and is due to the inertia of the shank (tibial segment). It is resisted and controlled by eccentric hamstring contraction. This is seen as a knee flexor moment and a power absorption in terminal swing. The peak occurs during double float just prior to initial contact. The hamstring activity fades shortly after initial contact and is supplanted by a stance phase knee extensor moment (quadriceps). The magnitude of the stance phase quadriceps moment is greatest in running (Fig. 9). The quadriceps have significantly different functions in running and sprinting. In sprinting, they are almost exclusively a source of power generation. In running, the quadriceps contract both eccentrically and concentrically (therefore both absorbing and generating power). In the stance phase of running the quadriceps predominantly generate power, because the knee is progressively extending at this time. For sprinting the period of absorption (progressive knee flexion in early stance) is seen to be primarily a passive phenomenon at the knee. It is controlled by adjacent joint muscle activity in walking and sprinting and eccentric quadriceps contraction in running. In running, the absorption period is more prolonged. With greater knee extension at initial contact, the knee flexes more and is resisted by eccentric quadriceps contraction. Therefore, the stance phase quadriceps contraction in running is both eccentric and concentric; in sprinting it is almost exclusively concentric. The knee extensor moment is continuous into swing phase to the reversal point (eccentrically controlling knee flexion). The eccentric activity is seen as a power absorption during initial swing phase. The remainder of swing phase has been described above.

Kinetic evaluation at the hip reveals that the hip flexors and extensors are both responsible for increased power generation in sprinting. The moment pattern is similar in all conditions of forward locomotion—walking, running, and sprinting. The magnitude of the hip flexor moment in sprinting is significantly greater ($p = 0.001$) than that in running (Fig. 10). The hip extensor moment in both stance and swing phase is identical in pattern in running and sprinting. Comparing the hip power plots reveals large differences in magnitude between running and sprint-

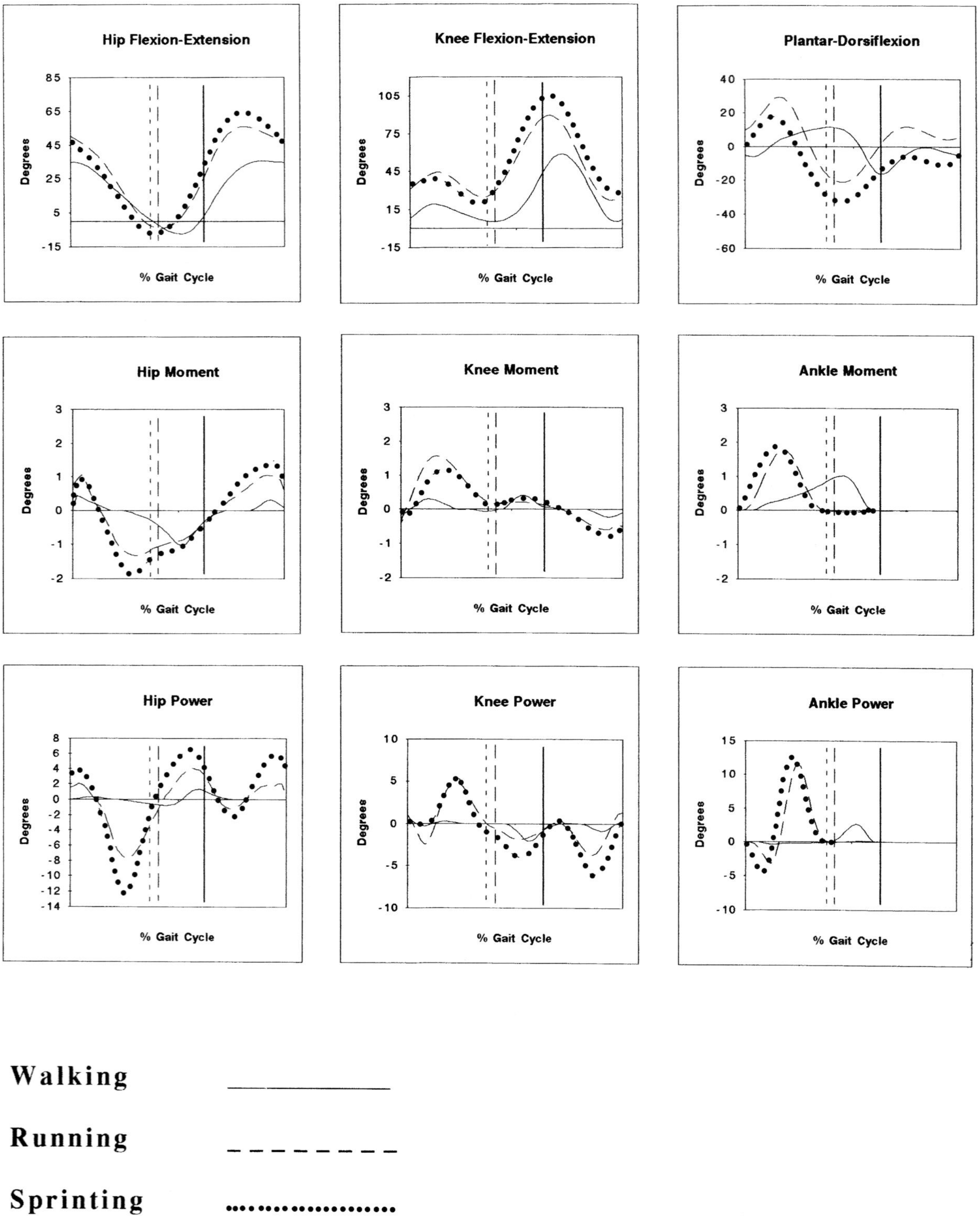

Fig. 7 Sagittal plane kinetics for walking, running, and sprinting. The sagittal plane motion is depicted in the top row. The joint moment data are in the middle row and the joint power in the bottom row. In evaluating and reporting the joint moments and powers, it is helpful to see the corresponding joint motion in the sagittal plane. It is therefore plotted directly above that joint's moment and power plots. Note that the scaling on the y-axis is identical in the reporting of the joint moments for the hip, knee, and ankle. Because of the large magnitude of power generation at the ankle, the scaling is expanded at that joint compared to the corresponding plots for the hip and the knee.

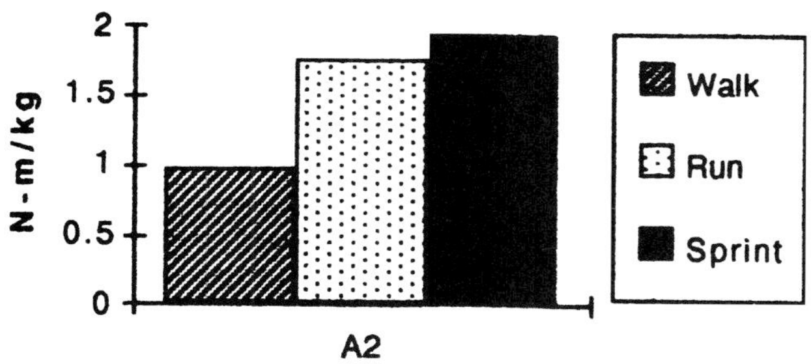

Fig. 8 Peak sagittal plane ankle moments.

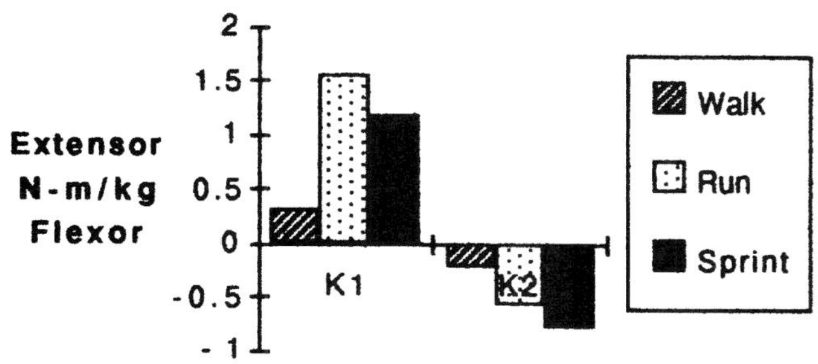

Fig. 9 Peak sagittal plane knee moments.

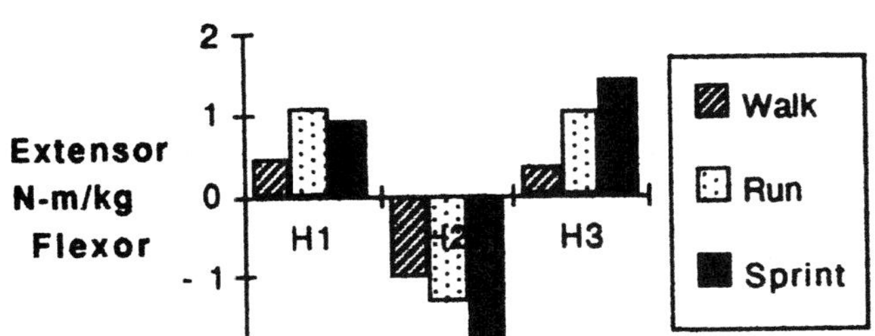

Fig. 10 Peak sagittal plane hip moments.

ing. The pattern, however, is the same. The hip flexor power generation propelling the swing limb forward in sprinting is 1.5 times that in running. The hip power generation in terminal swing preparing the swing limb for initial contact is 2.5 times that in running. (Fig. 11).

Coronal Plane The coronal plane moments and powers are very similar in running and sprinting. For a detailed description of these results, the reader is referred to Ounpuu's chapter in *Instructional Course Lectures, Volume XXXIX.*[4] Because the results of the two studies are similar, they are not repeated here.

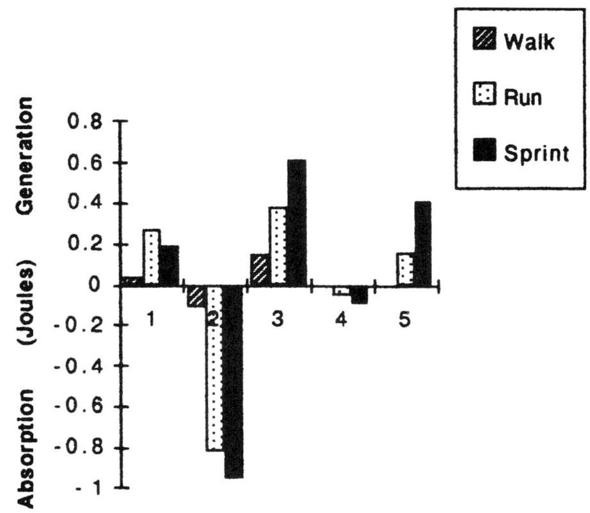

Fig. 11 Total work generated and absorbed at the hip.

Summary

Just as in running, the two-joint muscles acting at the hip and at the knee work to transfer energy efficiently between body segments. This can be seen in Figure 12. The powers at the hip and knee are overlaid to show that when power is generated at the hip, it is absorbed at the knee and vice versa. For example, a concentric contraction of the hamstrings proximally at the hip is coupled with an eccentric contraction at the knee just prior to initial contact in terminal swing. The rectus femoris functions in a similar way but in an opposite direction in initial swing.

For the three conditions discussed, the relative contribution of work occurring at each joint is different. Figure 13 shows that the muscles about the ankle are

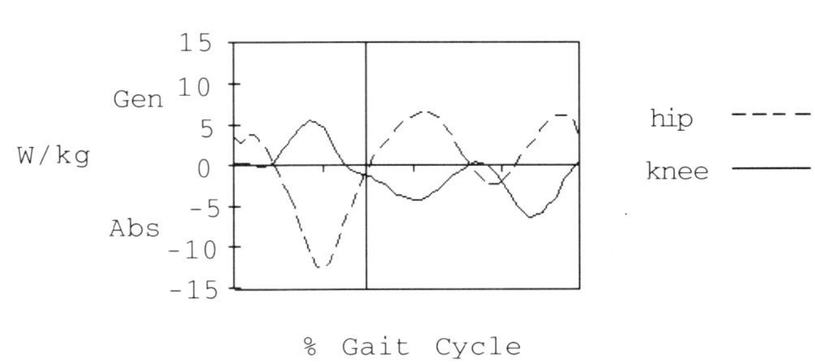

Fig. 12 Power overlays for sprinting. The knee (solid line) and hip (dashed line) power curves are overlaid to show how the two joint muscles (hamstrings and rectus femoris) efficiently transfer energy by simultaneously contracting eccentrically (absorption) at one joint and concentrically (generation) at the other.

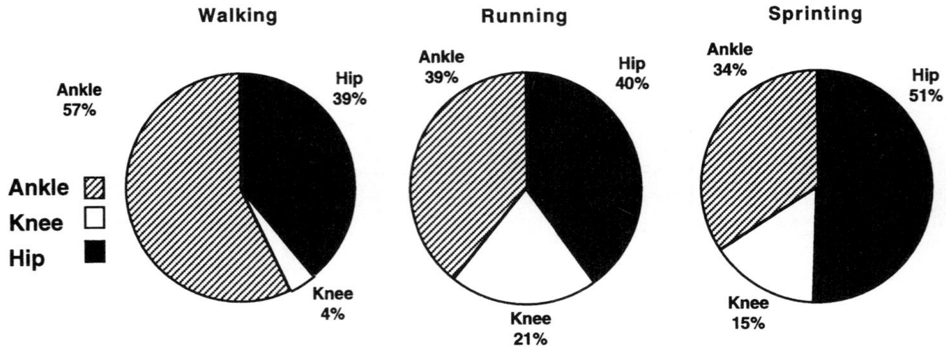

Fig. 13 Relative power generation by joint. The integrated areas under each peak of power generation were summed and are depicted for each joint for walking, running, and sprinting.

the most important source of work in walking and that the knee musculature does not significantly contribute to the work done for walking. In walking, the knee is felt to be important for the smoothing of gait. The quadriceps are a much more important source of energy at the knee in both running and sprinting, as can be seen in Figure 13. Finally, the hip musculature becomes the dominant source of work in sprinting in our group of untrained subjects with significant contributions from both the hip flexors and extensors. One would expect that the relative importance of each of the muscle groups about each of these joints in terms of sources of energy might change with training.

The intent of this work was to evaluate the three conditions of walking, running, and sprinting. I hope that it will stimulate further interest and research in this area in order to come to a greater understanding of human locomotion. As more knowledge and experience are gained, the motion analysis lab will be able to offer insight into training strategies, injury prevention, and the treatment of pathologic running and sprinting conditions.

References

1. Gage JR: An overview of normal walking, in Greene WB (ed): *Instructional Course Lectures, Volume XXXIX*. Park Ridge, IL, American Academy of Orthopaedic Surgeons, 1990, pp 291-303.
2. Mann RA, Hagy J: Biomechanics of walking, running, and sprinting. *Am J Sports Med* 1980;8:345-350.
3. Mann RV: A kinetic analysis of sprinting. *Med Sci Sports Exerc* 1981;13:325-328.
4. Ounpuu S: The biomechanics of running: A kinematic and kinetic analysis, in Greene WB (ed): *Instructional Course Lectures, Volume XXXIX*. Park Ridge, IL, American Academy of Orthopaedic Surgeons, 1990, pp 305-318.

CHAPTER 45

The Clinical Use of Kinetics for Evaluation of Pathologic Gait in Cerebral Palsy

James R. Gage, MD

Until very recently, gait problems in children who had cerebral palsy were treated empirically, and this empiricism was based only on observation of the child's gait and the clinical evaluation. However, in the more recent past, there have been efforts to approach gait disorders in cerebral palsy on a more scientific level, by assessing the child preoperatively and postoperatively with computerized gait analysis.

Kinesiology, which is the study of gait, can be divided into two areas: kinematics and kinetics. Kinematics is the study of motion without regard to the forces that produce it. An example of this is the sagittal plane graph of knee motion (Fig. 1). Kinematics, therefore, gives a precise description of the motions that are occurring in a particular joint in all three planes during the gait cycle, but the measurements are essentially descriptive and do not provide any insight into the cause of the motion. Kinetics, on the other hand, deals with the forces that produce the motion. These measurements include joint moments and joint powers. In 1987, Winter[1] described the way in which kinetics are calculated (a procedure known as inverse dynamics) and discussed some of the possible clinical uses for kinetics. Subsequently, Davis and associates[2] and Ounpuu and associates[3] developed clinical software that describes the moments and powers of each of the three major joints of the lower extremity in all three planes. Employment of these parameters for the assessment of normal and pathologic gait led to the discovery that these measurements can provide a great deal of insight into the specific gait abnormalities associated with cerebral palsy.

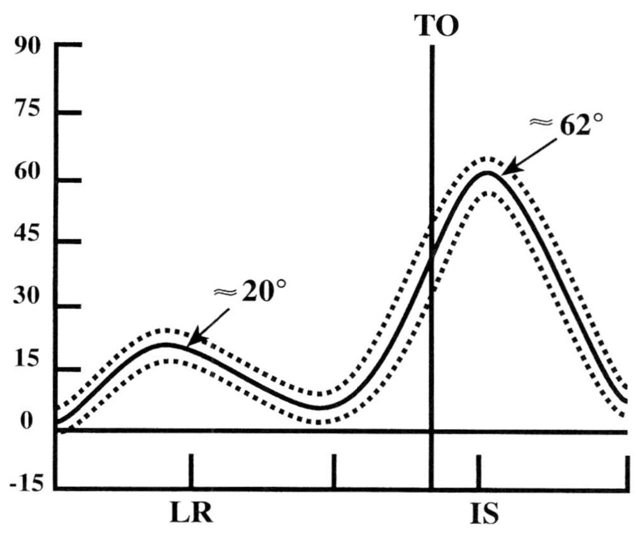

Fig. 1 Graph representing knee kinematics. The gait cycle is on the axis of the graph and the degrees of motion are on the abscissa. The vertical line represents toe-off (TO). The solid curve represents the mean and the dotted curves show one standard deviation. Stance phase represents approximately 60% of the gait cycle and swing phase, 40%. The two peaks of knee flexion are labeled. The first peak facilitates shock absorption during a period of gait called loading response (LR). The second wave of knee flexion occurs during initial swing (IS) and it provides clearance for the foot. (Reproduced with permission from Gage JR (ed): *Gait Analysis in Cerebral Palsy*. London, UK, Mac Keith Press, 1991, p 86.)

Before proceeding with the discussion of the clinical use of kinetics, it is necessary to have insight into how kinetic information is calculated. The process is known as inverse dynamics. In addition, to understand inverse dynamics, some concepts from basic physics must first be understood: specifically, the relationship between force and motion as expressed by Newton's second law. Newton's second law states that, at every instant in time, the sum of the forces acting on a body is equal to the mass of the body multiplied by the acceleration of the body: Σforce = mass × acceleration, or $\Sigma F = ma$. The scientific unit of force is the newton. One newton is the force that is needed to accelerate a mass of 1 kg at a rate of 1 m per square second ($1\ N = 1\ kg \times 1\ m/s^2$). Scientists make a distinction between mass and weight. Mass, which is generally measured in kilograms, tells about the inertia of an object (that is, how difficult the object is to accelerate). Weight, on the other hand, is measured in newtons and refers to the force that gravity exerts on the object. On the surface of the earth, an object falling freely in a vacuum has an acceleration of $9.8\ m/s^2$. Therefore, a mass of 1 kg has a weight of approximately 9.8 newtons.

If a force acts at a distance from a rotational axis, the moment of the force about the axis is given by the product of the force and the moment arm (also called the lever arm), where the moment arm is the shortest distance between the line of action of the force and the axis of rotation (Fig. 2). The force exerted by a muscle produces a moment about the axis of rotation of a joint that it crosses. Newton's second law can also be applied to express the relationship between moments and angular accelerations. Specifically, the sum of all moments of force acting on a body is equal to the mass moment of inertia of the body multiplied by the angular acceleration of the body: moments = mass moment of inertia × angular acceleration, or $\Sigma M = I\alpha$.

An additional concept that is used in inverse dynamics is described by Newton's third law, which states that for every action there is an equal and an opposite reaction. Thus, if I push down on the floor with my

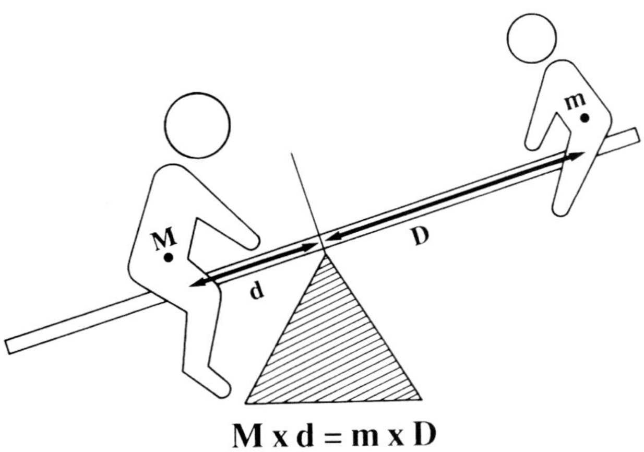

Fig. 2 The relationship between a child and an adult on a seesaw is exactly the same as that of the muscle and the ground-reaction force at each of the joints in the lower extremity. The pivot point (fulcrum) is always the center of the joint. M = weight of large subject, d = his distance from fulcrum, m = weight of small subject, and D = his distance from fulcrum. (Reproduced with permission from Gage JR (ed): *Gait Analysis in Cerebral Palsy*. London, UK, Mac Keith Press, 1991, p 80.)

foot, the floor pushes back with an equal force, known as the ground-reaction force. Ground-reaction forces and moments can be easily measured with use of a force-plate.

To illustrate how these concepts can be applied to the analysis of human movement, consider the sagittal view of the foot (Fig. 3). The ground-reaction force produces a moment around the ankle joint. The moment is referred to as the external joint moment. It is resisted by an internal joint moment produced by the muscles crossing the ankle: in this case, primarily the triceps surae. Both the internal muscle force and the external ground-reaction force act on the skeletal levers to produce rotation around the ankle joint. The internal muscle force is acting through the lever arm of the hindfoot, whereas the external ground-reaction force is acting through the lever arm provided by the forefoot. If these two moments are identical, there will be no motion around the ankle—that is, $\Sigma M = 0$, so the angular acceleration must also equal zero. However, if the internal muscle moment is slightly greater than the ground-reaction moment, the ankle will move into plantar flexion—that is, the angular acceleration will not be zero.

Inverse dynamics, as described by Winter,[1,4] involves solving for the forces and moments that will produce observed motions. It requires information from three sources: ground-reaction forces and moments measured with use of a force-plate; positions, velocities, and accelerations of all segments of the lower limb; and anthropometric data. The three types of information are used in an iterative application of Newton's second law in order to solve for the unknown forces and moments acting at the ankle, the knee, and the hip.

I will begin with the foot. The forces and moments acting on the foot are the known ground-reaction forces and moments (as measured with the force-platforms) and the unknown forces and moments acting at the ankle (for example, internal muscle forces). The accelerations of the foot are also known, and the mass and moment of inertia can be estimated from anthropometric data. If the equations are rearranged (Fig. 4), the unknown ankle forces and moments can be solved for. Once the forces and moments acting on the foot at the ankle joint have been solved for, the forces and moments acting on the shank at the ankle are also known (according to Newton's third law, these forces and moments are equal in magnitude but opposite in direction to the calculated forces acting on the foot).

Newton's second law can again be applied to determine the forces and moments acting on the shank at the knee. Similarly, the calculated knee forces and moments can be used to calculate the forces and moments acting on the thigh at the hip. In this manner, the internal joint moment can be determined for each joint in the lower limb.

With this insight into inverse dynamics, muscle function should be discussed next. Muscles provide all of the power needed for erect stance and propulsion, but they can function in only three ways: eccentric contraction, concentric contraction, and isometric contrac-

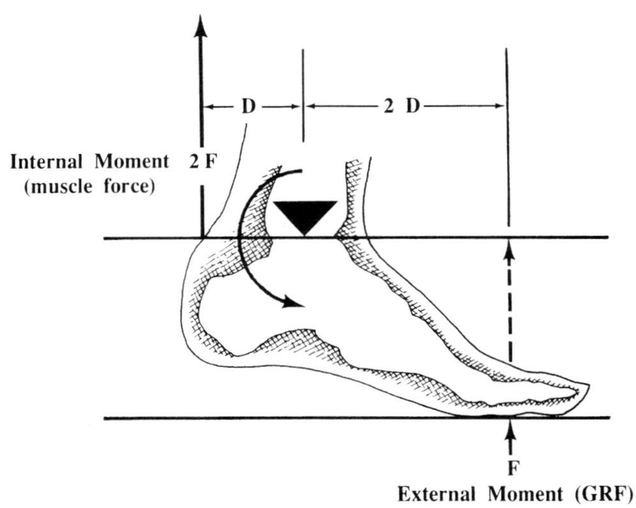

Fig. 3 Illustration of the relationship between the external moment produced by the ground-reaction force and the internal moment produced by the muscles. In each case, they act on a skeletal lever, and their fulcrum is the center of the joint. Because the length of the lever arm (D) of the ground-reaction force (GRF) is twice as long as that of the muscle force (mf), its magnitude is only half as much: D(mf) = 2D(GRF). Dividing by D gives the resultant equation: mf = 2(GRF). (Adapted with permission from Gage JR (ed): *Gait Analysis in Cerebral Palsy*. London, UK, Mac Keith Press, 1991, p 76.)

tion. Eccentric contraction, which is lengthening under tension, always implies shock absorption. Concentric contraction is shortening under tension; all accelerators work concentrically. Isometric contraction is muscle tension without a change in length; postural stabilizers work in this mode.

In gait analysis, it is very useful to have some estimate of muscle power. The kinetic concept that can be used to derive this estimate is joint power.[1,4] Joint power, measured in watts per kilogram, is the product obtained by multiplication of the joint moment of force by the angular velocity of the joint: joint power = joint moment × angular velocity, or $P = M\alpha$.

A positive value for joint power indicates that the muscle is shortening and producing an acceleration. A negative value indicates that the muscle is lengthening and producing a deceleration. If there is a moment but no power, the joint is being held motionless either by ligamentous forces or by isometric contraction of muscle (Fig. 5). Joint power is the single variable that best describes the concentric and eccentric phases of mechanical energy that muscles generate in order to accomplish movement. Because the power estimation is based on the concept of inverse dynamics, the estimates of power obtained by these methods are net power and, hence, do not provide any information about the power of specific muscles or muscle groups. Commercial computer software that generates graphs of joint moments and joint powers in all three planes can now be purchased with most gait-analysis systems.

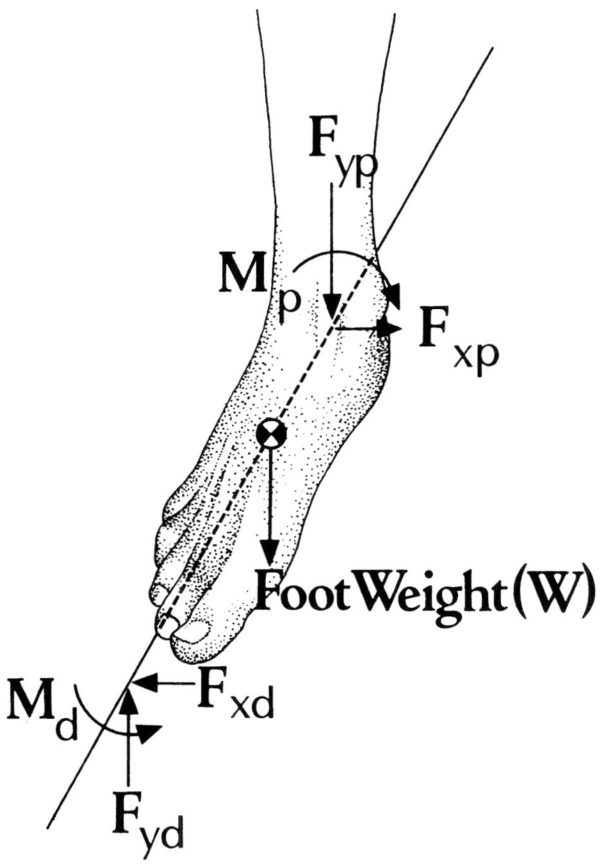

Fig. 4 An illustration of how Newton's second law is used in the calculation of inverse dynamics. The weight (W) of the foot, the location of its center of mass, and its moment of inertia are estimated from anthropometric data. For simplicity, in this illustration, the center of mass is assumed to be located along the axis of the foot, as shown. M_d, F_{xd}, and F_{yd} represent ground-reaction forces and moments measured with a force-plate. Newton's second law (represented schematically by $\Sigma F = ma$ and $\Sigma M = I\alpha$) allows the forces and moments to be related to the accelerations. The acceleration of the center of mass in the x and y directions (a_x and a_y), and the angular acceleration of the foot (α), are also known quantities, derived from position measurements ($F_{xd} - F_{xp} = ma_x$, $F_{yd} - F_{yp} - W = ma_y$, and $M_d - M_p = I\alpha$). The unknown forces and moments acting proximally at the ankle (M_p, F_{xp}, and F_{yp}) can be found by rearranging the expressions for Newton's second law and solving for M_p, F_{xp}, and F_{yp} ($M_p = M_d - I\alpha$, $F_{xp} = F_{xd} - ma_x$, and $F_{yp} = F_{yd} - W - ma_y$). Once these values are known, they can be used, along with anthropometric data and kinematic information for the shank, to calculate the forces and moments at the knee. Similarly, the calculated forces and moments at the knee can be used to calculate the forces and moments at the hip.

Clinical Applications of Kinematics and Kinetics

After an introduction to joint kinetics, kinematics and kinetics can be used to look at the function of the ankle joint in the sagittal plane. During normal walking, ankle function can best be described in terms of three rockers (Fig. 6). First rocker begins at initial contact of the heel with the ground and continues until the entire sole of the foot is in contact with the floor. First rocker is controlled by eccentric lengthening of the anterior tibial musculature. Its purpose is shock

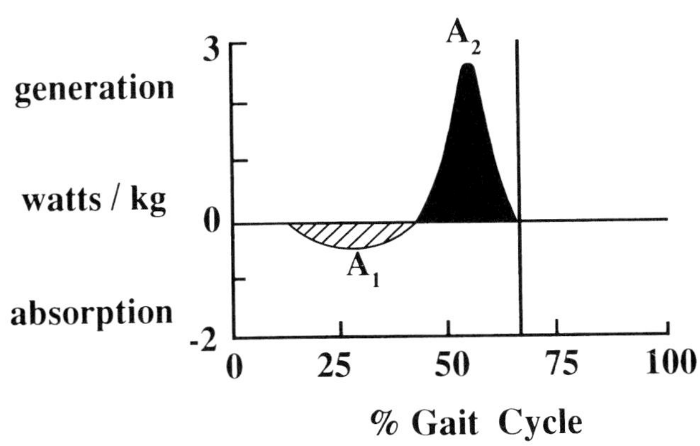

Fig. 5 Graph representing joint power at the ankle during normal gait. The numerical value for power is calculated by multiplication of the moment by the joint angular velocity. The sign convention is such that negative power indicates negative work—that is, the muscle is contracting eccentrically (A_1) (hatched area) and absorbing energy. Positive power indicates that the muscle is contracting concentrically (A_2) (solid area) and performing positive work—that is, producing an acceleration.

absorption—that is, deceleration of the inertia of the body at initial contact. Consequently, the terminology used at Rancho Los Amigos Medical Center refers to this portion of the gait cycle as loading response.[5] Loading response constitutes about 10% of the gait cycle.

Second rocker begins when the entire sole of the foot is in contact with the floor and ends when the heel rises off the floor. In the Rancho Los Amigos terminology, this portion of the gait cycle is known as mid-stance and constitutes about 35% of the gait cycle. Second rocker, like first rocker, is eccentric. Second rocker is largely under the control of the soleus. Its purpose is to conserve energy by controlling the rate of forward progression of the shank and, by so doing, controlling the position of the ground-reaction force referable to the knee. If the ground-reaction force is maintained slightly in front of the knee, an extension moment can be generated against the posterior aspect of the capsule that, in turn, relieves the quadriceps of the responsibility of stabilizing the knee. Therefore, energy conservation is realized by contraction of the quadriceps ceasing at the end of loading response and maintenance of the stability of the knee throughout the remainder of stance phase via the ground-reaction force. Because the ground-reaction force is actually generated by the action of the ankle plantar flexors, this phenomenon is referred to as a plantarflexion-knee extension couple.

Third rocker begins when the heel leaves the ground. During the latter part of mid-stance, the gastrocnemius joins the soleus as an active plantar flexor. The combined force of these two muscles is enough to arrest the forward progression of the tibia (ankle dorsiflexion) and begin ankle plantar flexion. Thus, third rocker is concentric, and concentric muscle action, by definition, produces an acceleration. If it is assumed that the individual is walking at a constant speed, the purpose of third rocker is to maintain a steady state by producing an acceleration sufficient to recover the inertial energy lost by the two previous rockers. The period during which this rocker acts is known as terminal stance and constitutes approximately 15% of the gait cycle.

In a graph of the kinematics and kinetics of the sagittal plane (Fig. 7), in which gait cycle is on the x axis

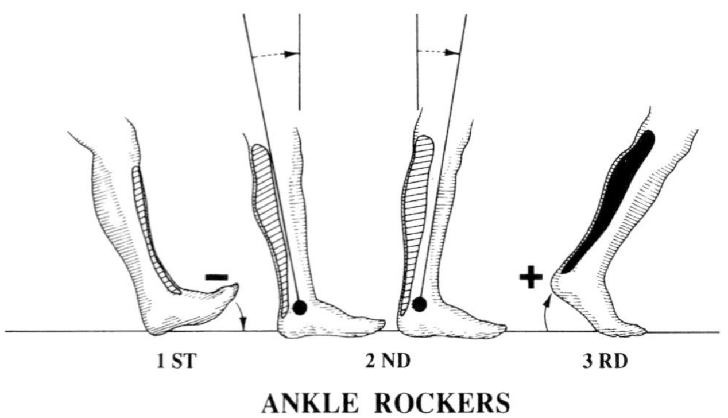

Fig. 6 Illustration of the three rockers of the ankle in stance. The first two are deceleration rockers, so the respective muscles are acting eccentrically—that is, doing negative work—by undergoing a lengthening contraction with energy absorption. Third rocker is an acceleration rocker, so the plantar flexors must act concentrically—that is, produce positive work (+). The point of application of the ground-reaction force is forced to move forward with each successive rocker, thus allowing the center of mass to move forward with it. The hatched areas represent eccentric muscle power and the solid areas, concentric muscle power. (Adapted with permission from Gage JR (ed): *Gait Analysis in Cerebral Palsy*. London, UK, Mac Keith Press, 1991, p 82.)

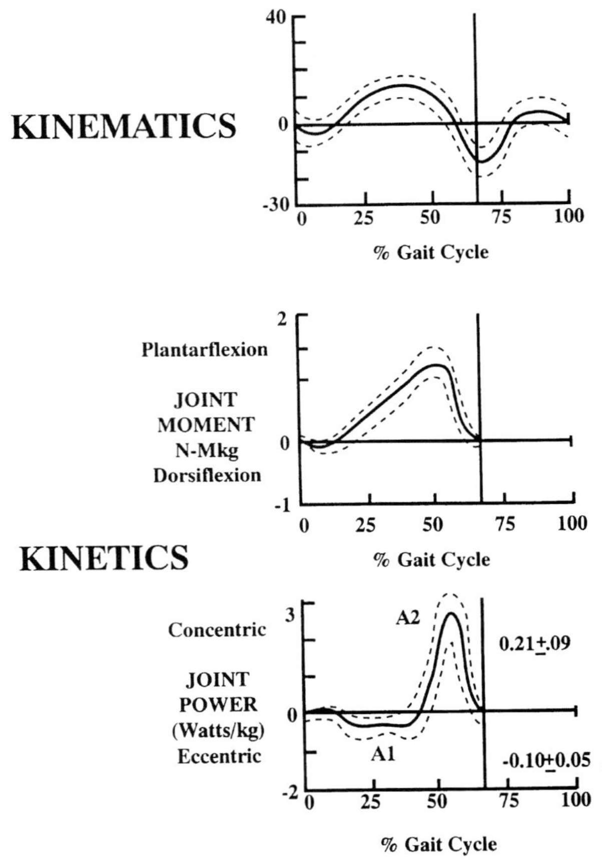

Fig. 7 Graphs of normal ankle kinematics and kinetics. The solid curves represent the mean and the dotted curves, one standard deviation. During first rocker, there is a small dorsiflexor moment. At the end of loading response, a plantar flexor moment begins that reaches its peak at terminal stance and then rapidly falls to zero at the end of stance during a period called pre-swing. The power graph indicates that power is eccentric (deceleration or negative work) during first and second rocker and concentric (acceleration or positive work) during third rocker. With use of the convention of Winters and associates,[7] the identification for each burst of ankle power on the graph begins with A, and the bursts are numbered successively from left to right. The numbers at the right of the bottom graph are an integration of all positive and negative powers and one standard deviation and represent the total work done in joules. Joint moment is shown in N·m/kg and joint power, in watts/kg.

and degrees of motion are on the y axis (the abscissa), the line at about 60% of the gait cycle represents toe-off and hence separates stance from swing. First rocker ends at about 10% of the gait cycle, second rocker ends at about 45% of the gait cycle, and third rocker ends at toe-off. The foot then is pulled back into dorsiflexion during swing. On a graph of joint moment measured in N·m/kg, the dorsiflexion moment is so small that it barely shows on the graph. The plantarflexion moment peaks early in third rocker and then rapidly falls to zero in the period of double support, so that by the time of toe-off, no substantial plantarflexion moment remains. On a graph of joint power, eccentric muscle action (power absorption) is always negative and hence is below the zero line. Concentric power (acceleration) is above the zero line. The convention for numbering the power bursts is to use the initial for the joint followed by a sequential numbering of the bursts beginning at the onset of the gait cycle. With use of that convention, the graph shows that second rocker (A1) is purely eccentric and third rocker (A2) is purely concentric.

Kinetics may well prove to be the most useful measurement for gait analysis in that it provides information about the cause of a movement disorder, points to the source of power for movement, and provides some information about net energy consumption at individual joints. With use of moment graphs, the activity time of a particular muscle group can be estimated, as the period of electromyographic activity should be roughly equal to the period of the internal moment depicted on the moment graph. Inspection of power graphs allows a determination of the mode of action of a particular muscle group—that is, whether the action is eccentric, concentric, or isometric. Individual joints can also be looked at as torque generators, and integration of power curves enables the estimation of the magnitude of eccentric or concentric work done in joules per kilogram (Fig. 7). If a moment is present without any generation of power, the joint must obtain its stability either from ligaments—that is, the plantarflexion-knee extension couple—or by isometric contraction of muscle. With this background, this lecture will discuss how these concepts can be used to understand the dynamics of both normal and pathological gait.

The graphs that illustrate the kinematics and kinetics of normal gait in the sagittal plane will now be considered (Fig. 8). Now that the kinematics and kinetics of the ankle have been explained, the hip and knee kinematics should be fairly self-explanatory. There are two bursts of concentric power in the hip. The former corresponds to an extensor moment and the latter, to a flexor moment. This means that the hip extensors generate power during the first half of stance and the hip flexors generate power in pre-swing and in initial swing. These two power bursts, plus the large power burst at the ankle, provide the propulsive power for walking. Which muscle groups are supplying this power can be determined from the moment graphs. For example, the first burst of concentric power at the hip coincides with an extensor moment and the second burst, with a flexor moment. Therefore, the first burst of energy is concentric and is provided by the hip extensors, whereas the second burst of energy is eccentric and represents energy absorption by the hip flexors. Similarly, at the ankle, the burst of concentric

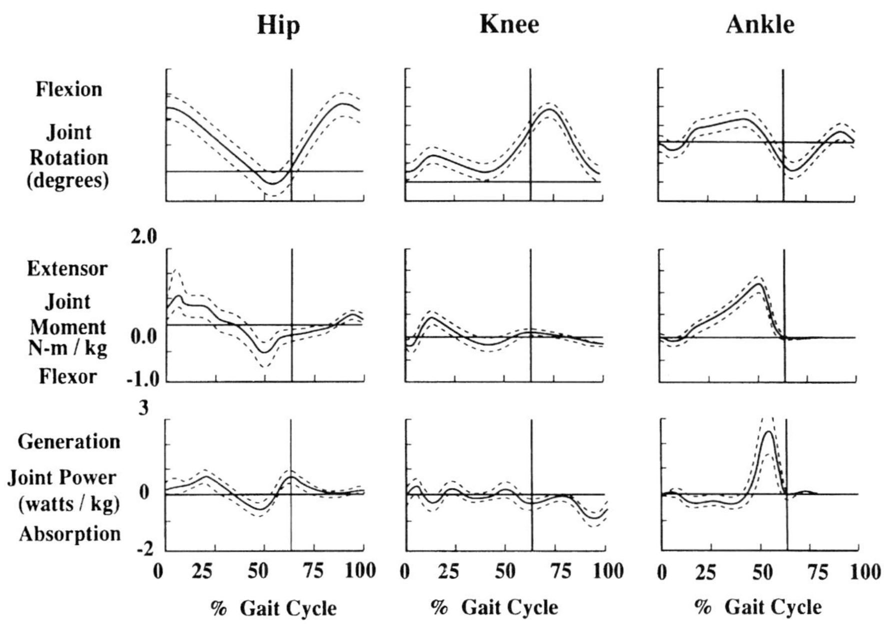

Fig. 8 The graphic output of sagittal plane moments and powers used at Newington and Gillette Children's Hospitals. From left to right, the top row shows the kinematics of the hip, the knee, and the ankle with the gait cycle displayed on the axis and the degrees of motion, on the abscissa. The middle row displays the moment of force around each of these joints in N·m/kg, and the bottom row displays the joint power in watts/kg, which is the product of the moment of the joint multiplied by its angular velocity. The solid curves represent the mean and the dotted curves show one standard deviation. (Adapted with permission from Gage JR (ed): *Gait Analysis in Cerebral Palsy*. London, UK, Mac Keith Press, 1991, p 162.)

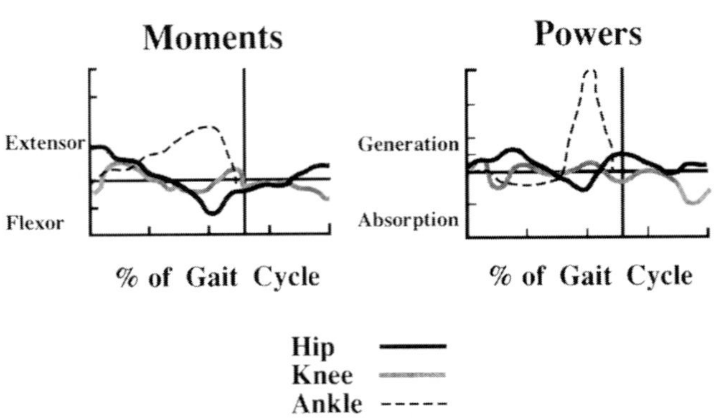

Fig. 9 Graphs of the sagittal kinetics of the hip, the knee, and the ankle, overlaid. There is an extensor moment that begins at the hip and travels sequentially down the limb to the knee and the ankle. The power graph indicates that, as the extensors contract, they generate a burst of concentric power (acceleration) at each of the joints.

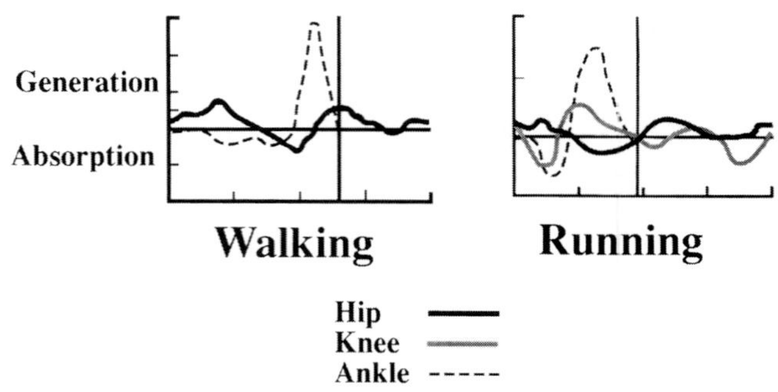

Fig. 10 Walking and running power graphs. The magnitude of the powers during running is much greater than during walking, but since the sequencing of their action, and not their magnitude, is of interest, they have been graphed to the same scale. Notice the sinusoidal nature of the hip and the knee power curves during running.

power coincides with a plantarflexion moment. Thus, the power needed for propulsion during walking comes primarily from the hip and the ankle. If the area under each of the curves is integrated, it can be determined that about 45% of the power required for walking comes from the ankle plantar flexors; 30%, from the hip extensors; and 20%, from the hip flexors.[3] It must be remembered that this power is being contributed bilaterally and that the timing is such that the power of the plantarflexion of the ankle of the trailing limb comes just slightly before the power of the hip extension of the front limb. Thus, the pushing power of the trailing limb is augmented by the pulling power of the front limb. Furthermore, the acceleration of the hip flexors, which, along with the plantarflexion burst, launches the trailing limb into swing phase, occurs concomitantly with the acceleration of the hip extensors on the front limb.

Overlaying of moment and power curves can provide additional information about normal walking, such as the way that the body controls the limbs, the support strategy for the lower limbs, and the power flow during the gait cycle. For example, overlaying of the graphs of the sagittal plane moments and powers of the hip, the knee, and the ankle reveals that there is a flow of power that starts with the hip extensors, moves down to the knee extensors (quadriceps), and finally reaches the ankle plantar flexors (Fig. 9). The support strategy for the lower limb can be seen in this wave as these are all antigravity muscles, and this bipedal flow allows the limbs to support the trunk and to avoid collapse while still delivering the smooth flow of energy that is needed for propulsion during gait. This power flow is even more apparent if these graphs are overlaid for running, because, in running, there is a more distinct contribution of power from the knee (Fig. 10). The graphs also show the sinusoidal nature of the hip and knee curves during the swing phase of running. By inspecting the moment graphs to determine which muscle group is dominant and examining the power graphs to determine whether the muscle is working eccentrically or concentrically, it can be determined that, during initial swing, there is an eccentric extensor moment at the knee and a concentric flexion moment at the hip, whereas, in late swing, there is an eccentric flexion moment at the knee and a concentric extensor moment at the hip. What these graphs show is that there is a transfer of energy from the knee to the hip during both initial and terminal swing. The body uses the two-joint muscles to accomplish this. Hence, during initial swing, the rectus femoris is contracting eccentrically at the knee and concentrically at the hip, whereas, during terminal swing, the hamstrings are contracting eccentrically at the knee and concentrically at the hip. Because the contraction is eccentric at one end of the muscle and concentric at the other, the muscles probably remain relatively isometric with respect to net length. In both cases, however, these biarticular muscles essentially work as energy-transfer straps and act to harness the energy of the shank and carry it proximally to the hip, where it can be used to augment hip flexion. Yack and Winter[6] estimated that the energy transfer of the biarticular muscles reduces the energy cost of walking by about 22%.

Illustrative Case Report

These tools will now be used to look at pathologic gait in a child who had a severe right spastic hemiplegia secondary to an embolus of the middle cerebral artery, which occurred after a cardiac procedure. The preoperative photograph of the child walking showed that the knee was flexed to about 45° in terminal swing and the foot was in mild equinus so that, at initial contact, there was a toe-toe gait on the right side as well as an extremely short step-length (Fig. 11, *left*).

The postoperative photograph showed nearly full knee extension; however, there was still mild equinus (Fig. 11, *right*). Thus, the patient was positioned to come down with a longer step-length than he had had preoperatively and with a foot-flat gait. The preoperative sagittal-plane kinematics of the hip, the knee, and the ankle (Fig. 12) showed that there was excessive lumbar lordosis and hip flexion. The knee was continuously flexed during stance with a restricted range of flexion-extension during swing. The pattern of ankle motion was interesting in that the range of motion was normal but the movement pattern was not. Maximum dorsiflexion was reached early in stance, followed by a biphasic thrust into equinus and a persistent foot drop in swing. Preoperative ankle kinetics (Fig. 13) revealed a biphasic moment and two distinct bursts of concentric power. Evaluation of the kinetics shows that the progressive dorsiflexion that normally occurs during second rocker was interrupted by a premature burst of power of the ankle plantar flexor. If the sagittal plane kinematics are examined, it is seen that, at initial contact, the knee was flexed approximately 45° and the foot was in approximately 10° of equinus. Thus, the fast-twitch, biarticular gastrocnemius was stretched from the moment of initial contact whereas, in normal gait, this muscle would not come under stretch until midstance. In addition, the muscle was spastic because, on clinical examination, ankle clonus on the hemiplegic side could be evoked easily. Finally, the monarticular soleus could have neither a static nor a dynamic contracture as the ankle allowed normal dorsiflexion.

Therefore, the most likely explanation for the double burst of power of the ankle plantar flexor was that the gastrocnemius displayed dynamic clonus during gait. In light of this information, lengthening of the Achilles tendon would not have been reasonable because this procedure would have lengthened both the gastrocnemius and the soleus. Consequently, I elected to do a Strayer-type gastrocnemius recession to address the contracted gastrocnemius and, at the same time, to preserve soleus function. In the actual analysis of the gait of this child, I also used the sagittal and coronal plane kinematics and kinetics of the hip and the knee, which are not included here. With the use of gait analysis in conjunction with a clinical examination, the patient was classified as having a type-IV hemiplegia with associated femoral anteversion.[7]

On the basis of these data, the child had a single-event surgery on the hemiplegic side that consisted of an intertrochanteric derotational femoral osteotomy, an intramuscular psoas tenotomy, lengthening of the medial hamstring, transfer of the distal end of the rectus femoris to the intramuscular stump of the gracilis, and a Strayer-type recession of the gastrocnemius. Twelve months later, the patient had postoperative gait analysis (Figs. 12 and 13). Comparison of the graphs of the preoperative and postoperative kinematics with

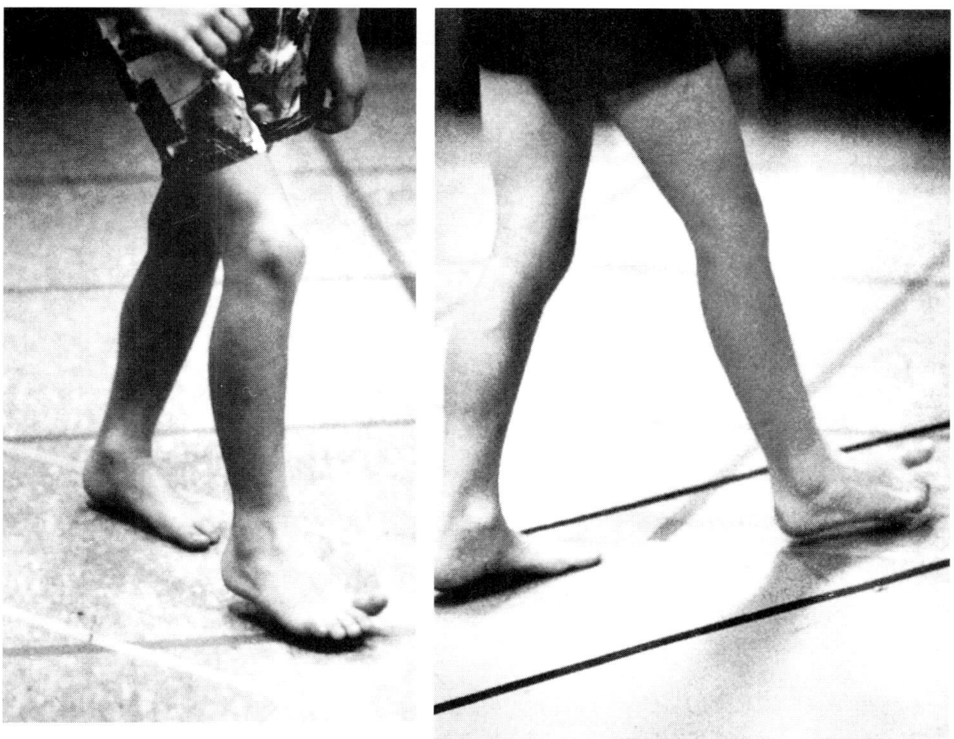

Fig. 11 Preoperative (**left**) and postoperative (**right**) photographs of a child who had a severe right spastic hemiplegia preoperatively while walking.

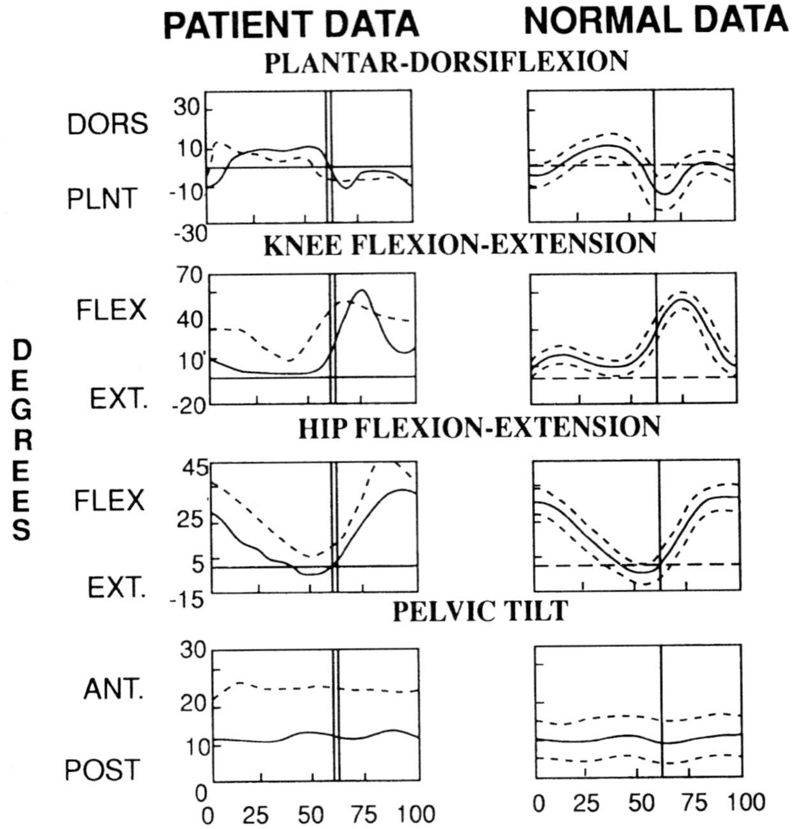

Fig. 12 Preoperative (dotted curve) and postoperative (solid curve) sagittal-plane kinematics of the patient compared with normal data demonstrate functional improvements at the ankle, the knee, the hip, and the pelvis. Kinematics provides objective evidence of the motions that occur at each individual joint and is, therefore, an excellent tool for evaluation of surgical outcomes.

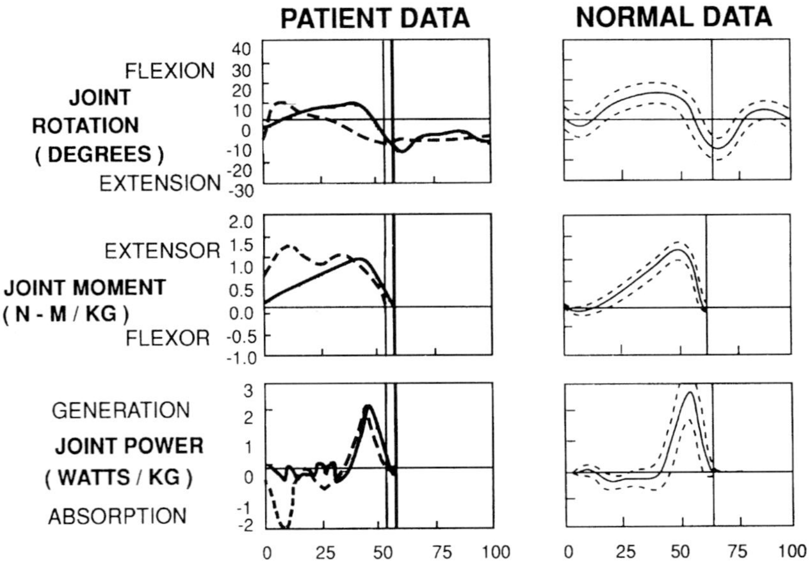

Fig. 13 Preoperative (dotted curve) and postoperative (solid curve) ankle sagittal-plane kinetics of the patient compared with normal data. Preoperatively, the ankle moment was biphasic and there was a double burst of power. Postoperatively, both the moment and the power curves closely approximated normal. (See text for explanation.)

normal graphs revealed that there had been a reduction of lordosis and that the kinematics of the hip, the knee, and the ankle were all much closer to normal. Inspection of the kinetics of the ankle showed that the postoperative plantar-flexor moment had also normalized and that there was only a single burst of power that

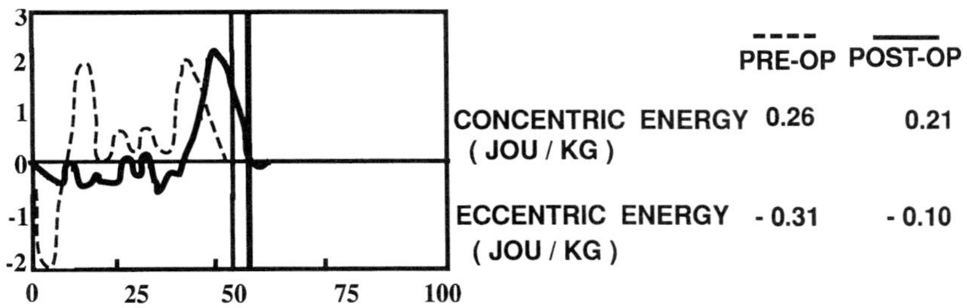

Fig. 14 By integration of the power curves, the work of the ankle plantar flexors during one gait cycle can be estimated in joules per kilogram. Preoperatively (dotted curve), the patient had an abnormal power burst in mid-stance; the abnormal burst was no longer present after the operation. The concentric energy was 0.26 joule per kilogram preoperatively compared with 0.21 joule per kilogram postoperatively. The eccentric energy was -0.31 joule per kilogram preoperatively compared with -0.10 joule per kilogram postoperatively. Since the patient was walking at approximately the same velocity preoperatively and postoperatively, the less work done in the postoperative period indicates that the ankle was functioning more efficiently.

was equal to or slightly greater in magnitude than the second preoperative burst.

Integration of the preoperative and postoperative power curves for the patient (Fig. 14) gives an estimation of the work done at the ankle during a single gait cycle in joules per kilogram of body weight.[8] Both concentric and eccentric work were reduced postoperatively. Preoperatively, the concentric work was evenly distributed between the two power bursts. The timing of the second burst was such that it contributed to forward propulsion, but the first burst was simply wasted work. Postoperatively, all of the concentric work contributed to propulsion. Since the primary goal of an operation is to make walking more energy efficient, this type of information is very useful in assessing postoperative outcomes as it provides very specific information about the effect of surgical treatment.

Finally, it is useful to compare the overlaid moments and powers of a normal profile (Fig. 9) with the postoperative moments and powers of the patient (Fig. 15). Even in the hemiplegic limb, there was a progression of extension moments that began at the hip and traveled down the limb to the ankle. Although the flow in the hemiplegic limb was not quite as smooth, it was otherwise not unlike that in the normal limb. The power bursts, on the other hand, were much more abnormal in that they were not as acutely timed or as smooth, and there were large bursts of eccentric energy, particularly at the knee, that were clearly abnormal. If this information is combined with preoperative and postoperative linear measurements (stride length, cadence, velocity, and so on) and energy costs (milliliters of oxygen used per kilogram of body weight per meter traveled), the effectiveness of the operative intervention can be assessed very critically.

Before the development of kinetics, only descriptive information could be gathered with regard to gait. With this tool, information about cause can begin to be acquired. With use of the data acquired from these new methods of investigation, important advances in the treatment of cerebral palsy have already begun.

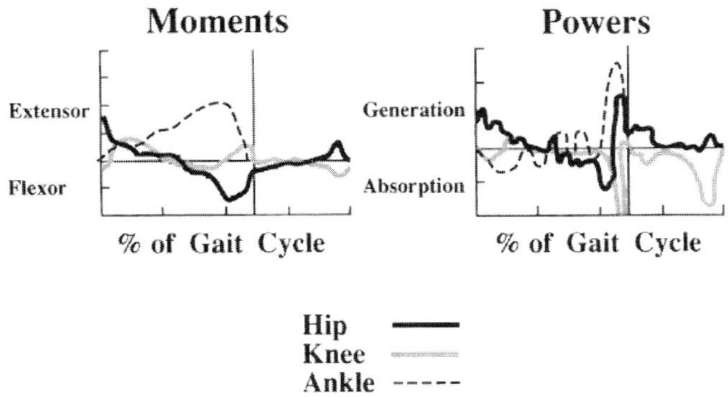

Fig. 15 Postoperative graphs of the sagittal kinetics of the hip, the knee, and the ankle of the patient, overlaid. Unlike the normal sagittal kinetics shown in Fig. 9, the extensor moments at the ankle and the hip began simultaneously at initial contact, disrupting the orderly power flow that should have been present. The power graph indicates that although the normal accelerations at the hip, the knee, and the ankle were present, they were very irregular and disorganized. Despite this, the postoperative gait was much smoother, and the patient thought that his ability to walk was greatly improved.

References

1. Winter DA: *The Biomechanics and Motor Control of Human Gait.* Waterloo, Ontario, Canada, University of Waterloo Press, 1987, pp 29-43.
2. Davis RB III, Tyburski DJ, Ounpuu S, et al: The determination of joint moments: Methodology verification, in *Proceedings of the Fifth Biennial Conference of the Canadian Society for Biomechanics.* 1988, pp 52-53.
3. Ounpuu S, Gage JR, Davis RB: Three-dimensional lower extremity joint kinetics in normal pediatric gait. *J Pediatr Orthop* 1991; 11:341-349.
4. Winter DA: *The Biomechanics and Motor Control of Human Gait: Normal, Elderly and Pathological,* ed 2. Waterloo, Ontario, Canada, University of Waterloo Press, 1991, pp 35-49.
5. Perry J (ed): The gait cycle, in *Gait Analysis: Normal and Pathological Function.* Thorofare, NJ, Slack, Inc, 1992, pp 3-7.
6. Yack HJ, Winter DA: Economy of two-joint muscles, in *Proceedings of the Fifth Biennial Conference of the Canadian Society for Biomechanics.* 1988, pp 180-181.

7. Winters TF Jr, Gage JR, Hicks R: Gait patterns in spastic hemiplegia in children and young adults. *J Bone Joint Surg* 1987;69A:437-441.

8. Gage JR (ed): Hemiplegia, in *Gait Analysis in Cerebral Palsy*. London, Mac Keith Press, 1991, pp 132-150.

Computers

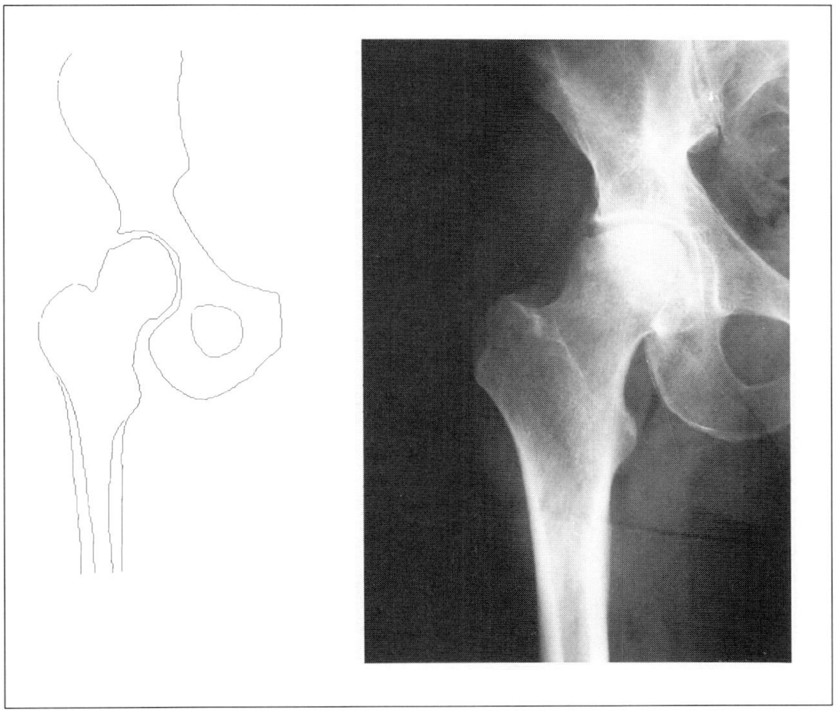

CHAPTER 46

Computer Applications for Orthopaedic Surgeons: CD-ROM and Beyond

Robert Poss, MD
Mark Koris, MD
Richard Santore, MD
Howard Mevis

As a result of advances in technology, our society is changing very rapidly. A number of recent technological advances have had a profound impact on our culture. Like the automobile and the airplane, the information age ushered in by the computer has profoundly changed our lives.

For orthopaedic surgeons, advances in computer technology are creating new benefits in an era when "keeping up" is next to impossible. The profusion of print media is overwhelming. Take a moment to think about the journals and books you read or refer to routinely. It is likely an impressive list. Searching several journals or texts to find information can be a laborious and time-consuming task. Just knowing where to start may be a problem and, sometimes, even though the information may be at our fingertips, we can't seem to put our hands on it. By comparison, the computer is a tool we can use to search and retrieve relevant information in just a few minutes.

In this chapter, we will discuss how the computer is making an impact on orthopaedic surgeons in education, information sharing and retrieval, and surgical planning. The computer is an important tool that can help us enhance patient care.

For some, purchasing a computer is a relatively easy task. For others, it can be very difficult. The key is to purchase as much technology as you can afford. The rule of thumb is to buy today's best technology. Computer system specifications are changing every month. However, if you purchase the top of the line, whether PC/AT or Macintosh, you will have technology that is likely upgradeable to the next generation of computers and will be able to operate the software you use for several years. The Academy maintains up-to-date, specifications recommendations for members who are interested in buying a personal computer.

Postgraduate Orthopaedic Continuing Medical Education (CME)

In the past, orthopaedic surgeons gained new information from a variety of sources, including reading, attending CME courses, and taking part in discussions with colleagues. Our files became filled with notes from each of these learning experiences. Finding the information after it had been filed became very difficult even for the most organized individual. Now, however, computer technology has created the capability to organize our files in large, searchable databases, which makes access much easier.

With the advent of CD-ROM technology it is now possible to store as many as 300,000 pages of text on one disc. Using a state-of-the-art searching software, information stored on these discs can be retrieved in seconds. Mastery of the techniques of searching enables the searcher to save time and find the needed information. For example, the Academy's *Orthopaedic Knowledge Update on CD-ROM* includes more than 2,500 pages of text and 3,000 images from four OKU publications, plus the full text of more than 1,200 journal articles. The computer searches these data in seconds; an individual searching the print volumes of this material would require hours to find the same information.

The approaches used to search a database include key word, table of contents, and domains. Most search/retrieval software programs use search operators to find information. An understanding of searching techniques is critical to maximizing results. For example, in the *OKU on CD-ROM* database, information retrieval changes as we change operators. The following examples show how search results may be narrowed to a manageable list of records. Hip or Fractures retrieves 1,009 records. Hip and Fractures retrieves 410 records. Hip adjacent Fractures retrieves 97 records.

Further words can be grouped or strung together to narrow or broaden the search focus. These two examples show how this is done. Ulnar "adj" nerve "adj" entrapment retrieves 5 records. Ulnar adj (nerve or entrapment) retrieves 98 records.

Some software programs will allow the user to enter the database through a traditional table of contents format. First, the searcher chooses the book or journal volume, then the chapter or publication number, and, finally, the chapter or article based on title.

Databases are set up in fields. This system allows the user to search for information using one or more of these fields. Typical fields from book or journal publications include title, author, abstract, date of publication, and affiliations. The database administrator establishes the fields.

Orthopaedic surgeons can maximize their use of a CD-ROM database by gaining skill in these techniques of searching for information. The Academy distributes a videotape demonstration program describing the techniques of searching a database. A software tutorial program is in development.

Postgraduate Orthopaedic CME (Interactive Education)

The advent of graphical user-interface software triggered a tremendous explosion in software development. There are hundreds of available educational CD-ROM programs, ranging from encyclopedias to games to medical case presentations. These programs combine media formats on the compact disc and are described as multimedia software programs. Although most of these programs can be operated on slower speed computers, optimum performance is achieved by using an operating system with fast data processing capabilities.

Multimedia includes text, still images, video, sound, animation, and more in a simple or complex format. Any media combination is possible. These programs require significant planning to develop, but they are relatively simple to use. Most programs require the user to point and click with a mouse at navigational arrows or 'hot spots.' In a medical presentation, these hot spots may highlight anatomy, additional detailed information, or graphics. Navigating through a program requires little, if any, use of the keyboard, once the program is installed on the computer's hard drive.

Interactive programs can range from simple to complex. More complex programs have several branches and sub-branches, with significant depth and breadth of content. Programs with video sequences require significant storage. Video is usually compressed (at ratios of up to 200:1) so that the CD-ROM can store the data. For example, in an uncompressed format, a 4-minute segment of video may require more than 50 megabytes of storage at high resolution rates. Compressing the video enables the disc to hold much more.

Interactive educational programs present great promise for medical education at all levels; medical school, residency, and postgraduate. Orthopaedic surgeons will need to ensure that their computing power is sufficient to operate these programs. Additionally, the display of video at high resolution will probably require installation of a special video processing board to use these programs.

Telecommunications: Going On-Line

In the past 10 years, the capabilities of electronic communication devices have evolved from the telephone, to the fax system, through modem-based telecommunications, to cable and optical fiber based networks. In the next few years, it seems likely that local cable companies, which already connect an estimated 60 million U.S. homes, will be among the forerunners in bringing high-volume, real-time information access to the general population. Today we must ask ourselves as orthopaedic surgeons and health-related professionals how best to use this new technology, the Information Superhighway, to facilitate medical practice in the future.

Computer communication performance jumps have kept pace with the leaps in speed and throughput that have occurred in today's computer systems. With the consequent advent of both multimedia computer systems and high-speed computer links, the potential for accessing data and images interactively from local sites as easily as from computers located on other continents has become reality. Information can now be transmitted rapidly enough to make it practical to expect the development of remote imaging based facilities.

At present, computer communications are transmitted over two types of data pathways: telephone links with modems and direct connections that use optical fiber, radio links, or coaxial cable (as in ethernet). In fact, both kinds of information access can be used to transmit the information, and the two can be used simultaneously.

Computer-based telecommunications, which refers specifically to inter-computer communications transmitted over telephone lines, is a subset of networking. Networking involves hardware and software used to facilitate access by a computer or computers to other remote computers via the telephone system or other specific dedicated network lines. Literature-search databases, bulletin boards for information acquisition and travel planning, and teleconsultation are examples of services that can be accessed by the orthopaedic surgeon who has access to a personal computer and a modem.

On-Line Databases

Many orthopaedic surgeons are already familiar with the use of CD-ROM-based literature-search applications and also the use of telecommunications through a modem to access such literature-search databases as MEDLINE and other online databases. MEDLINE, which is prepared by the National Library of Medicine, contains medical references from all major medical resources from 1966 to the present. The literature-search operation can be performed efficiently from the surgeon's office and provides the capacity to cross-reference information more quickly and more accurately than by a physical search through *Index Medicus.*

MEDLINE, which runs as a time-shared service from a mainframe computer system with an enormous storage capacity, requires individual users to be registered with the system and to obtain an entry code before logging on to the system. Charges are assessed for computer connect time, as well as telephone access rates. Software packages such as Paperchase, Grateful Med, and BRS Colleague are specific for Macintosh or PC/AT based platforms. These packages allow the user to customize their access to the on-line medical data bases. Some, however, have more sophisticated data-transfer algorithms, are easier to use, or can be programmed off-line for a specific search. Each program has its own advantages, and these should be considered in light of the user's specific requirements when selecting a new telecommunications package.

Bulletin board systems have now become popular in many computer-related fields, including industry and research. These systems usually consist of a single dedicated computer that is remotely accessible through one or more telephone lines. This computer provides a caller equipped with a personal computer, modem, and telecommunication software package with the ability to download files (transmit files from the remote bulletin board system to the individual's computer), join discussion groups, and leave messages for other users. Product manufacturers incorporate simple bulletin boards to provide 24-hour help facilities, user group discussions, software updates, and other support.

Discussion forums dedicated to specific topics in industry or research are clearinghouses for up-to-date information. These forums, which are frequently directed by subject matter experts in the focus topic, often invite open participation by bulletin-board users. Models for bulletin-board systems that are specific for orthopaedic surgery may be useful to practicing orthopaedic surgeons. Ongoing panel discussions on controversial topics in orthopaedic surgery could no doubt serve to summarize a topic, stimulate research, and provide a resource for practitioners with clinical questions. The technology now exists to include digitized images as well as text for discussion. With appropriate patient confidentiality, cases, complete with radiographs and photographs, could be submitted for review and comment by participants. Ultimately, the level of interest in the orthopaedic community, and the ease with which important information can be obtained, will determine acceptance and use of these bulletin board systems.

Following sections will cover the specifics of modems, communications software, network terminology, hardware and software, and reasons for their use.

Technical Considerations

Telephone Systems

The media for modem communication is the telephone system, or Public Switched Telephone Network (PSTN). This vast worldwide hardware system, which consists of hardwire, fiberoptic, microwave, and satellite links, can route information to specific locations with a minimum of effort. The system was primarily designed to reproduce information in a sound spectrum (bandwidth) that covers the frequencies encompassed by the human voice (0 - 20,000 Hz, or cycles per second). Despite its limited bandwidth and noisy lines, the telephone system does provide significant bandwidth for literature search, electronic bulletin board, and remote access applications. Voice access through wider bandwidth systems is more expensive, and has not been widely implemented. Computers, which have the potential to communicate at higher speeds, could use the extra bandwidth if it were available. Dedicated network lines, described later in this article, can provide much higher bandwidths and allow computers to communicate more rapidly.

Modems

Modems are used to send data over voice-grade telephone lines on the telephone system in order to convert the data to the analog voice-like sound that the telephone network was designed for, and then to convert these analog wave forms back to their digital counterparts for use at the receiving end. The term modem is an acronym for *mo*dulator-*dem*odulator. Each computer in communication with another requires a modem at its end of the telephone line. A modem, transmitting data, takes serial digital information representing a state of 0 or 1, as input from the first computer, and produces and transmits a unique output tone corresponding to the 0 or 1. This is considered a form of discrete frequency *mo*dulation. The receiving modem hears two discrete tones, representing a 0 or 1, from the other modem and reproduces the 0 or 1 as input to the second computer; *dem*odulating it. If data are being sent and received simultaneously in sequence across the telephone line, the channel is said to be full duplex. Four discrete tones are required to avoid confusion when full-duplex communication is occurring. Unidirectional communication is referred to as half-duplex. Although more sophisticated communication techniques are currently available, this chapter describes the basic concept presently employed in many devices. Finally, the speed of information transmission is described in terms of baud rate. Although they are technically different, one baud is roughly equivalent to one bit (a 0 or 1) per second (bps). For purposes of discussion, we will use the terms baud and bps interchangeably. Typical transmission speeds range from 300 baud to 28,800 baud.

Like personal computers, modem technology has improved steadily since it was introduced in the early 1980s. The minimum speed that exists in wide use today is 2,400 bps. Modems of 9,600 bps are rapidly becoming the accepted standard for personal computer communications via the telephone line, and 28,800 bps modems are presently available. In practice, 28,800 bps modem technology approaches the maximum capacity of the voice-grade telephone lines on the PSTN. Speed is limited by the bandwidth of the channels on the network and the relatively low signal-to-noise ratio that can be achieved. Most telecommunications programs/modems will allow you to select the baud rate of transmission.

Telephone line noise and poor transmission parameters can cause the modem to misrecognize transmitted information which introduces errors into the transmitted data. Two low-level mechanisms have been designed into the communications protocol to catch and/or correct these errors; *Parity* and *Cyclical Redundancy Check (CRC)*.

Parity

Serial data are organized into defined groups (typically 7 or 8 bits = 1 byte) that are transmitted with no intervening spaces. The first bit may or may not be designated a parity bit. The last 1 or 2 bits are usually designated stop bits. The remaining 5 to 7 bits carry the data. The originating computer assembles each 7 or 8 bits of output data into a byte. If parity has been specified in the communications protocol, it sets the first bit to 0 or 1 based on standardized parity rules applied to the pattern of the remaining bits. The receiving computer reconstructs the incoming serial bits into a string of seven or eight, and again applies the same parity rules to their pattern. If the parity bit in the received data string matches the value predicted by the parity rules in the receiving computer, the 7 or 8 bit string (byte) is accepted; otherwise, the sending computer is requested to re-send the last byte.

Cyclical Redundancy Check (CRC)

CRC error correction, an example of more sophisticated error detection and correction protocols, works in a manner similar to parity correction. By convention, most data protocols organize data bytes into blocks of 128, 256, 512, or 1024 bytes for transmission. If CRC has been requested in the communication protocol, the last byte sent may contain a CRC character, which is 7 or 8 bits set by the originating computer based on standardized CRC rules applied longitudinally to the whole data block. Similarly, the receiving computer checks the incoming data block and determines its theoretical CRC character. The block is accepted if the CRC character matches. If there is no match, retransmission is requested.

Both Parity and CRC algorithms are examples of techniques used in digital communications to ensure accurate transmission of data. Modems are available today that have more sophisticated data pre-processing, including data compression and error recovery. These techniques, usually indicated on the modem, after the product name, by characters such as CCITT (International Telegraph and Telephone Consultative Committee) V.22, V.32, and V.42, have been standardized so that modems made by different manufacturers can work together. Modems of this type allow faster throughput of data without increasing the baud rate, or bandwidth. The CCITT standard followed by *bis* indicates second version; *ter* means third. The standard for 2400 baud communications is V.22 bis, the standard for 9600 baud communications is V.32, the standard for 14,400 baud communications is V.32 bis.

Most modems are sold "bundled" with software that uses the modem to dial out to an external number, to connect to a computer with a modem at that number, to transfer data, and to answer an incoming call from another modem. These applications typically allow the user to specify the parity, number of bits per byte, number of stop bits, and the type of error checking to use when communicating with the remote computer, although the default settings are usually adequate. Communications packages today provide a large number of added features that enhance both their function and their complexity. The user should select an appropriate package based on computer type and communications needs. Useful additions include the ability to specify the file transfer protocol, the ability to function as a stand-alone bulletin board, and the ability to access remote networks and use their protocols.

Modems can be purchased for personal computers as either external or internal devices. The advantage of the internal device is that it takes up no desk space; the disadvantage is that the internal modem occupies one of the limited number of expansion slots in the personal computer. The advantages of the external modem are the visibility of status lights on the device (valuable for diagnosing problems) and the capacity to use the device with multiple computers, without having to open up the computer to set it up. The disadvantages are that it takes desk space and costs more.

Another feature that is gaining popularity among modem users is the integrated fax/data modem. In addition to all the capabilities of the data modems discussed above, this modem is also able to send, and sometimes receive, standard facsimile (fax) transmissions.

Recommendations A top of the line fax and data modem today should have the following description: 'FaxModem 14,400Snd/Rcv CCITT V.32bis/V42.bis compliant with the AT command set.' This configuration provides top speed with all the latest standards and protocols, and can be purchased without fax functionality if it is not required. Prices are in the $150 to $400 range and are still falling at this time.

Networking

Networking provides the user with resources similar to those available through telephone connections. However, the rate of information transfer and ease of interconnectivity are significantly increased. These improvements are gained at the expense of additional hardware, additional software, and a hard-wired interconnect between computers.

True personal computer-based networks have developed as a response to increasing needs for data and resource sharing. Expensive peripherals, such as printers, mass storage memory devices (disc and tape drives), and data-base functions can be made available at a lower cost per user. The simplest, slowest, and most common form of communication between computers, sometimes referred to as "sneaker net," allows the transport of information between computers, without any cost other than the price of a floppy disc. Although this system is the least expensive, it is usually the most time consuming, because writing out data to floppy disc is one of the slowest operations a computer does. This system also becomes outmoded quickly as the distance between computers increases and the need for sharing data grows.

From its inception, the Macintosh system was designed to allow "plug and play" networking capabilities. The simplest network on the Macintosh system consists of a single computer and a peripheral device such as a printer. The internal computer hardware and cable system that provide the communication between the Macintosh and the printer or another Macintosh is called Localtalk. Localtalk has a relatively slow data transmission rate (400,000 bps), and is barely acceptable for large volume data transfers. The software protocol that defines how data is handled on the network is called Appletalk. Each Macintosh is built with all the hardware and software it needs to communicate with other Macs. A single cable, similar to a telephone cable with special connectors, is all that is required to link two Localtalk compatible computers.

Macintosh systems and AT-format PCs with higher data transfer rates than are available on Localtalk can be configured to run on faster environments. Ethernet, a LAN (local area network) hardware configuration developed by Digital Equipment Corporation, Intel Corporation, and Xerox Corporation, provides for data transmission rates of up to 10 million bps and is commonly used in most personal computer local area networks. Macintosh computers that use Ethernet use a protocol similar to Appletalk, known as Ethertalk, to transfer data. PC/AT format computers, DEC, SUN, and other computers that use Ethernet use a variety of protocols, including Banyan, Novell Netware, DecNet, and TCP-IP.

Standard network services on both Localtalk and Ethernet local area networks include filesharing, disc sharing, remote access, printer/peripheral device sharing, electronic mail, and centralized backup. The specific details of the sharing and backup functions usually depend on the network protocol. These functions, which are essential to the user for routine local data handling, word processing, and data-base activities, become familiar through repeated use. Electronic mail and remote access functions enhance the orthopaedic surgeon's abilities to access or provide data and to communicate with the outside world.

Table 1
Typical pricing for 3 E-Mail packages

E-Mail Software	Average Price for 5 Users
QuickMail 2.5.1	$249.00
Microsoft Mail 3.0	$269.00
WordPerfect Office	$290.00

Electronic Mail

Electronic mail is an application that runs on the network and allows a network user to send messages or memos to one or more other users. Each network user is identified by a specific "address", that may include the network identifier, the computer on the network, and the specific user on the computer. Memos sent to other users are usually routed to one computer on the network, which performs the function of a mail server. The server is usually a dedicated computer that runs continuously, storing incoming messages in the user's mailbox, and providing access to these messages on request. It also can perform utility functions such as automated deletion of old messages and conservation of space. The computer that provides the function of the mail server may also function as a file server; sharing files and disc space with all computers on the network.

The ability to attach a text, data, program or image file to a memo is a useful addition for the orthopaedic surgeon but is not available on all E-Mail applications. Files can be transferred between users automatically. The originator generates the memo, defines the recipient and the file to be sent, and starts the transfer. The recipient reads the memo and saves the enclosed file to disc for later use. Potential users should require their E-Mail software to include this. Some E-Mail packages provide for telephone book-like lists of users in large network environments. Also, some systems provide formatted memos that can be made to resemble office paperwork.

E-Mail packages that are compatible with most network systems include: Quick-mail, Inbox Plus, cc:Mail, Microsoft Mail, and WordPerfect Office. Most systems can be obtained with multiple user licenses. Prices vary widely. Table 1 shows some common E-Mail packages and prices for each at the time of this printing.

The introduction of high-speed fiber-optic networking has brought about some real and some potential breakthroughs in the field of computer communications. One example of the tremendous benefit accrued through the use of increased speed and global connectivity is the growth of wide-area computer networking. Internet is an excellent example of an aggregated large wide-area network (WAN). First implemented in 1969 by the Defense Advanced Research Projects Agency (DARPA) to foster cross-platform computer interaction, the Internet now provides a link among diverse computers systems across the United States and throughout the world. It is commonly carried on Ethernet hardware, and uses a TCP-IP network protocol. The growth of this system has been tremendous. By January 1992, over 730,000 host computers were linked to Internet. As of July 1992 the number had grown to nearly 1 million. This growth helps meet the increasing need to transfer information reliably, inexpensively, and rapidly.

Many large computer systems on Internet allow remote logins on their system for anonymous File Transfer Protocol (FTP). FTP permits users to browse large libraries of programs and selectively download individual programs to their personal computer. Anonymous FTP servers on Internet are commonly set up for a login name, ANONYMOUS, and a password, GUEST. In this mode, user access status is limited by the host system security to file transfers, participation in discussion groups, and specialized database searches. Keyboard interactions using FTP on remote systems with data transmission rates of 10 million bps on lightly loaded host systems appear instantaneous. File transfers appear to occur at local disc transfer speeds.

Technical Considerations

Localtalk

Although Localtalk's information transfer rate is faster than telephone line transfers, it leaves much to be desired for data-transfer intensive applications (about 400,000 bits per second). It is an excellent example of a local area network (LAN). Because of the hardware, speed, and distance limitations, un-enhanced Localtalk networks, and LANs in general, are restricted to a limited number of computers and a relatively small physical area. Most cannot work with a cable length of greater than 1,000 feet. Third party vendors have developed additional hardware and software to permit IBM PS2 series and PC Clones to interact with Localtalk networks.

Ethernet

Ethernet is an excellent example of a commonly used protocol that facilitates data transfer rates of up to 10 megabits per second. It requires special cable to communicate at these rates. Three types that are currently in use are listed chronologically in order of their development: thick wire, thin wire, and 10-base-t are the most common forms of cabling for this type of network. The first two are coaxial cable, which is similar to that used for cable television. The third type, 10-base-t, is a form of paired twisted wire similar to telephone cables. The special cables are required to pass the higher speed digital signals with less loss than is possible with conventional cables. One advantage to the lower losses, besides higher transmission speeds, is that, with these lines, the distance between computers can be greater.

Network Design

Users interested in starting a new network system should first consider the predominant platform (computer type: ie, Macintosh, IBM, and PC Clone) to be used on the network. Once the computer platform is determined, a network protocol can be chosen, with the assistance of a network planner. A selection can be made based on the type of data to be transferred, the other computer types that will need to function on the network, the projected number of users, and the desired network functionality. Most network protocols provide E-Mail, peripheral resource sharing (eg, printing), file sharing, remote access, and some form of centralized access for network administrative duties such as disc/file backup and recovery. Any new network system should now include these functions as a minimum.

Internet

Internet is for information what world wide air and sea routes, superhighways, highways, side roads, backroads, and cul-de-sacs are for travel. Governments, institutions, industries, school organizations, and individuals can exist at individual addresses along these roads. At present, data, files, and images travel down its lanes. The future may include video, entertainment channels, and video-telephone systems. To traverse these paths, the user must have a vehicle (computer with associated communication hardware), an on-ramp (the internet physical access), communication software, and a map—the search facilities that are being developed on the Internet.

Physical connection to Internet can be made through a modem link to a computer already on Internet (telnet, bitnet, America On Line, Compuserve, Delphi, etc). This access is limited by the modem speed/telephone line bandwidth considerations discussed previously. More commonly, a direct connection is made by linking a LAN to a subnet on Internet. Data transmission speeds are limited by the LAN hardware, but they can be up to 10 million bytes per second. Most major teaching institutions, major businesses, and government contractors should already have access, and only the logistics of the interconnect need to be worked out. Hospital access can usually be obtained through the local Medical Information Systems department.

The core speed of the Internet is phenomenal. At present, the main trunk of the network is running at 45 million bps, as compared to 9600 bps on a modem. The

Congress of the United States recently passed a bill to implement, within the next 3 years, a speed increase on the network to over 3 billion bps. In comparison, most PC and Mac Ethernet networks rarely go faster then 10 million bps. At 3 billion bps, the integration of data, voice, and computer information becomes a reality.

Internet Address Terminology

Internet extends network services like Electronic mail and remote access. Standard LAN E-Mail memos and enclosures are routed through a series of control points on the network to the final destination. Similar to a user address on a LAN, an Internet Protocol Address (IP Address), which identifies the unique location of the intended recipient of the message, is permanently assigned to the user by the local Internet network systems operator. Another representation of the IP Address is the Host Name. Each sub-network, for example, a user's LAN, is linked to a controlling computer known as a Domain Name Server. A domain is a collection of LANs under the administration of a single name server. The domain name server maintains a list of host names, and their equivalent IP Addresses for each LAN in its domain. A computer system performing a network access to a specific host name will go to its Domain Name Server and look up the IP Address associated with that host name. For example: to find the IP Address of someone with the host name John Smith.ORTHO.BWH.HARVARD.EDU the Internet access software would find the computer that was designated as the domain name server, (the computer equivalent of a human telephone operator) and then would look up the IP address that corresponded to that host name. Note that the host name used in this example consists of several connected parts separated by periods. The whole name represents a specific location on Internet; the parts represent a shorthand map for finding that location. In this example, within the domain EDU there exists a network called HARVARD. A sub-network of HARVARD is called BWH. On the network BWH, there exists a sub-network ORTHO, which is the home of John Smith's computer. Thus, the complete host name or IP Address must be known to send E-Mail or to access any remote computer that is part of Internet. Remote access may also require knowledge of a password, or the possession of a pre-arranged system account.

Assuming you have a "vehicle," an Internet on-ramp can be purchased through an Internet service provider, or a local dial-up service (Delphi, Prodigy, Compuserve, America On Line, and others yet to come). The costs depend on the speed, and capacity of the on-ramp you need. Individual users will soon be able to purchase Internet software packages in the range of $150, and pay a $25/month fee for dial-up access. The cost for connecting your local area network to Internet via a dial-up system costs about $1000 for the first year, and $720 for subsequent years. Direct connection to Internet with a low level institutional link-up costs more, because of increased data capacity needs. A higher capacity system for the individual or groups costs about $9,000 for the first year, and $3,000 for each subsequent year. A very high capacity connection suitable for institutional access, usually a direct connection to a side road on Internet, costs about $45,000, with subsequent annual costs of $14,000. For purposes of comparison, the low capacity system has about 1,000× less capacity than the midrange capacity link, and about 5,000 to 8,000× less capacity than the institutional correlation.

Early users of Internet were often computer experts or hackers, who considered themselves "cybernauts," that is, explorers of "cyberspace"; a new virtual space created by Internet. It was the virtual equivalent to entering a vast library, without knowing the filing system, in search of a particular book. They often found interesting things, and stopped to browse, but it was difficult to find specifically what they were looking for. Currently, FTP and Telnet are programs that allow users to browse the aisles, and check out books. Users still need to know the part of the library the books are in. Gopher and Mosaic are newer software packages that permit the user to search most of the library, and then retrieve the desired information. FTP, telnet, Gopher, and Mosaic run on Macintosh, IBM personal computers, and other platforms, and now have easy-to-use graphical interfaces. Mosaic is based on the hypertext concept, also used in the OKU CD-ROM Program. The searcher clicks on a reference phrase and is rapidly transported to the appropriate part of the text (OKU CD-ROM or internet computer mosaic), where the search is begun.

Assuming you've made the jump, and invested in the vehicle and the on-ramp, what can you do on the information highway? First, it's important to realize that, like any highway, it carries things you don't necessarily want along with those you are looking for. From our point of view, it currently provides worldwide electronic mail, Medline access, National Library of Medicine bibliographic information, NIH clinical alerts and guides, cancer treatment protocols, and access to manufacturers. It also contains vast libraries of scientific data, art, history, music, weather, photographs, and a myriad of other things.

Table 2 is a partial list of potential applications that can or could exist on Internet. Before long, it should be possible to have a conference call and interactively edit a document or examine a radiograph, face to face with colleagues from around the world. Currently, it should be possible to coordinate multi-center studies in real time, or access a teleconsultation or teleradiology service about an emergency case. Basically, the information superhighway can increase your diagnostic and

Table 2
Common Ethernet cable characteristics

IEEE Name	Common Name	Connector	Maximum Distance
10BASE-5	Thick, or Regular	AUI	500 meters
10BASE-2	Thin	BNC	185 meters
10BASE-T	Twisted Pair	RJ-45	100 meters

therapeutic options, at the same time making you more efficient.

The Future

Internet is paving the way for the information age and the free exchange of information in many fields. The potential exists to use Internet, or similar wide-area network aggregates to communicate, transfer radiographs and other images, and construct or obtain access to clinical and research databases. Developments are also taking place in the field of integration of video/voice and computer information. Products now available for the Macintosh allow conferencing with other Macintosh or PC clones across the country. These systems incorporate slow video, voice, and data information. In the short term, as network speeds increase and issues of high volume radiographic digitization and storage are resolved, online digital radiography will almost certainly become a reality. Realtime video imaging should follow suit, and teleconsulting may be just around the corner.

The American Academy of Orthopaedic Surgeons' current involvement in computer communications as well as in computer-based education (CD-ROM) products insures that orthopaedic surgeons will continue to have sophisticated information-handling tools on their desktop, and that these tools will enable them to enhance patient care through self education, access to clinical data, and open dialog with their peers. The Academy is currently planning an Internet server for use some time in 1995-1996. Planned options include distribution of Academy announcements and products, course signup, E-mail, and consultation services.

Macintosh, IBM and PC clones require some additional work to allow them to interface with the Ethernet network environment. The user must install a specific networking card to allow the host computer to communicate on the network. The installation process usually requires some specific information about the existing hardware and software configuration of the host computer, in terms of interrupt allocation and software memory configuration. Software network drivers must be added to permit the operating system to access the new hardware. Because it is likely that an inexperienced user will fail to achieve a working system in a new hardware installation of a network card, we recommend that installation of any new system (other than a "plug and play" type) be done only by an experienced network manager, systems operator, or a trained computer technician.

Other network communications protocols have become popular, especially with IBM and PC clone-based systems. Novel Netware now controls the greatest share of the market, followed by Banyon. Users interested in linking to a pre-existing network should have a less difficult time if they can obtain the hardware and software specifics from the systems operator responsible for network maintenance.

CHAPTER 47

Computers for Surgical Planning of Orthopaedic Procedures

Richard F. Santore, MD

The development of applications software that enables surgeons to use personal computers to plan orthopaedic surgical procedures has added enormously to the surgeon's decision-making capabilities. The advent of this technology allows effective cross-comparison of proposed surgical solutions and virtually eliminates the need for intraoperative trial-and-error methodology.

Although computers are not necessary for the planning of orthopaedic procedures, they do improve on conventional drawings or tracer-paper techniques in the following areas: (1) Magnification errors can be eliminated. (2) Cross-comparison of competing viable options can be performed easily. (3) There is an accurate integration of angulation and linear measurements. (4) Implant fixation devices and/or prostheses can be stored in the memory and accurately superimposed on bone images.

These advantages can be seen in case no. 1, an example of a 23-year-old adult male with segmental osteonecrosis. In this case, future total hip replacement is planned at the same time as the osteotomy. This type of planning assures that the interfragmentary relationships established at the time of osteosynthesis are compatible with insertion of the stem into the upper femur, if and when that becomes necessary. In the past, the planning of interfragmentary relationships has been based primarily on concerns regarding the mechanical axis at the knee level. It is much more important to assure straightforward conversion to total hip replacement, and the mechanism by which this is accomplished is demonstrated in the following series of computer images and corresponding radiographs (Figs. 1-3).

The close correlation between preoperative plan and postoperative appearance of the bone in both the anteroposterior and lateral projections is also demonstrated. This type of careful planning ensures that the operative events are carefully controlled based on a step-by-step blueprint established by the preplanning process.

Computer Planning Methodology

The images depicted were created by tracing the outline of the preoperative images onto a digitizer board, which entered the image into the Orthographics Software program. A magnification marker present on the radiographs, in the plane of the bone, permitted the computer to control for the magnification effect inherent in plain radiographic processes.

Basic computer planning uses plain radiographs with a magnification marker placed in the plane of the bone at the time of the radiograph. This device effectively permits calculation by the computer of the magnification factor. However, it does limit planning to a single-plane, two-dimensional image.

Three-dimensional software is available. However, it requires a CT or MRI tape for input, and manipulations are complex and consume enormous amounts of memory. Creation of the images needed for osteotomies and wedges is extremely difficult. Furthermore, it is extremely difficult intraoperatively to correlate the three-dimensional rearrangement with the three-dimensional plan.

Advantages and Disadvantages

Additional limitations of computer planning include its cost and the learning curve for proficiency. A considerable investment of time is necessary to acquire ease of use of computer planning software. It is not an exaggeration to state in general terms that acquisition of proficiency in the use of virtually any software system, whether it be a new program for word processing or a new program for CAD-CAM design, demands substantial time and patience during the learning-curve phase. Once basic skills have been acquired, however, the added benefits usually justify the investment of time and effort. Additional advantages of computer planning are that hard copies can be generated for use in the operating room, for the study of clinical outcomes, and as documentation for billing purposes.

Computer images can also be down-loaded to film recorders for generation of slides, and files can be transferred from standard footprint personal computers to lap-top or notebook computers for portability. Furthermore, data can be transmitted via modem to PCs in the operating room or in the office of a colleague or a consulting physician.

System Costs

The cost in dollars can be significant, ranging from $5,000 to $7,000 for a basic system and software package to $50,000 or more for sophisticated systems. In early 1994, a basic system included a minimum 286 processor at 16 megahertz, a color printer, color monitor, digitizer board, a mouse, appropriate application software, and a math coprocessor. More sophisticated systems include tower personal-computer architecture with a Pentium chip (Intel), which operates at a speed of 66 megahertz or more. Optical disks of 1.2-gigabyte-size are desirable for acquisition and retention of memory-intensive x-ray and other video images. Images can be loaded by a digitizer board, high-resolution video camera, or optical scanner, all of which can be simultaneously connected to the system. Monitors include high-pixel-density gray scale monitors and high-pixel-density color monitors, two types of monitors that serve separate purposes. Printers include a large-carriage color printer for generation of real-size, non-compressed documents, as well as a conventional black-and-white laser printer. A film recorder is attached to the main system for immediate generation of slides. Such systems are also accompanied by slots for a high-speed CD-ROM, an internal tape back-up, and a high-speed FAX/modem.

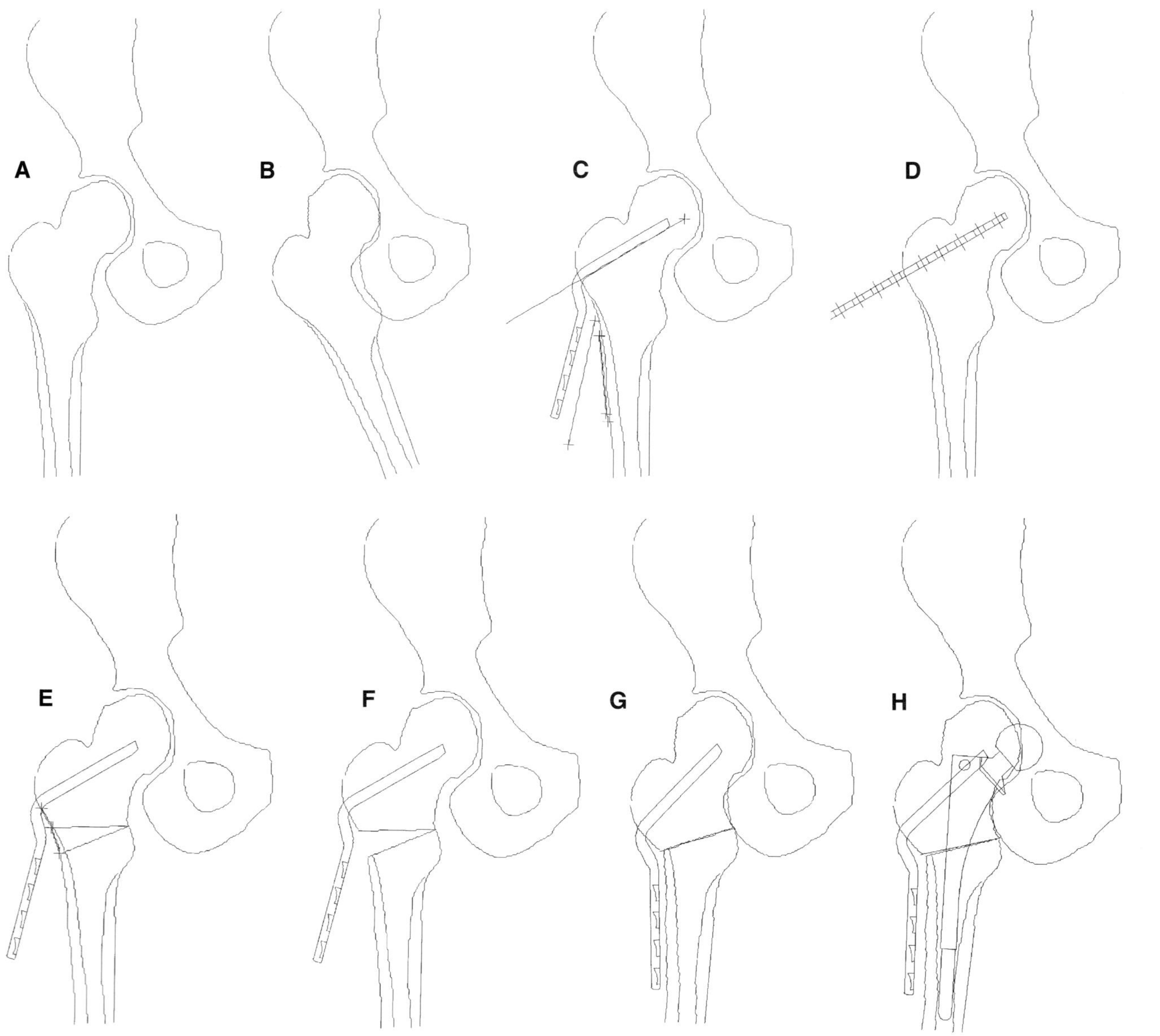

Fig. 1 **A,** The unmanipulated, unaltered presurgical image, entered into the computer through a digitizer board (boundary tracing). **B,** Computer performing 20° adduction of the femur. **C,** A 130° blade plate inserted into the femur at an angle of 70° between the line extended from the blade of the blade plate and a line parallel to the lateral cortex of the femur. This corresponds to an angle of 20° between the lateral cortex of the femur and the side arm of the blade plate. These two angular measurements confirm the planning of a 20° valgus osteotomy achieved by inserting a 130° plate in this fashion. **D,** A seating chisel replica without the blade plate. **E,** A 20° wedge with its apex at the upper border of the lesser trochanter medially, and the upper portion of the base at a point 15 mm below the lower portion of the seating chisel. This 15-mm distance between seating chisel and upper level of osteotomy is a regular part of every plan; it is important to maintain adequate strength of the lateral bridge. A full wedge was planned in this case to avoid lengthening of the limb during the valgus osteotomy. **F,** The wedge removed from its site. **G,** A simple hinge at the apex of the wedge has been performed. When osteotomies are performed in this fashion, the center of the femoral shaft is displaced medially in an unphysiologic fashion, which would complicate total hip stem placement in the future. **H,** For this reason, a total hip stem is brought up from the memory bank of the computer. In this case, an AML stem is used to depict a straight stem option.

Software required includes the application program for planning, computer graphics, slide graphics, data management, outcomes research, text-video-graphics merge, communications software, on-line databases, and Internet access.

A practical problem has been the difficulty in recovering reimbursement for time devoted to surgical planning. The federal government recently issued guidelines that approve reimbursement for computer-based planning with appropriate documentation. These

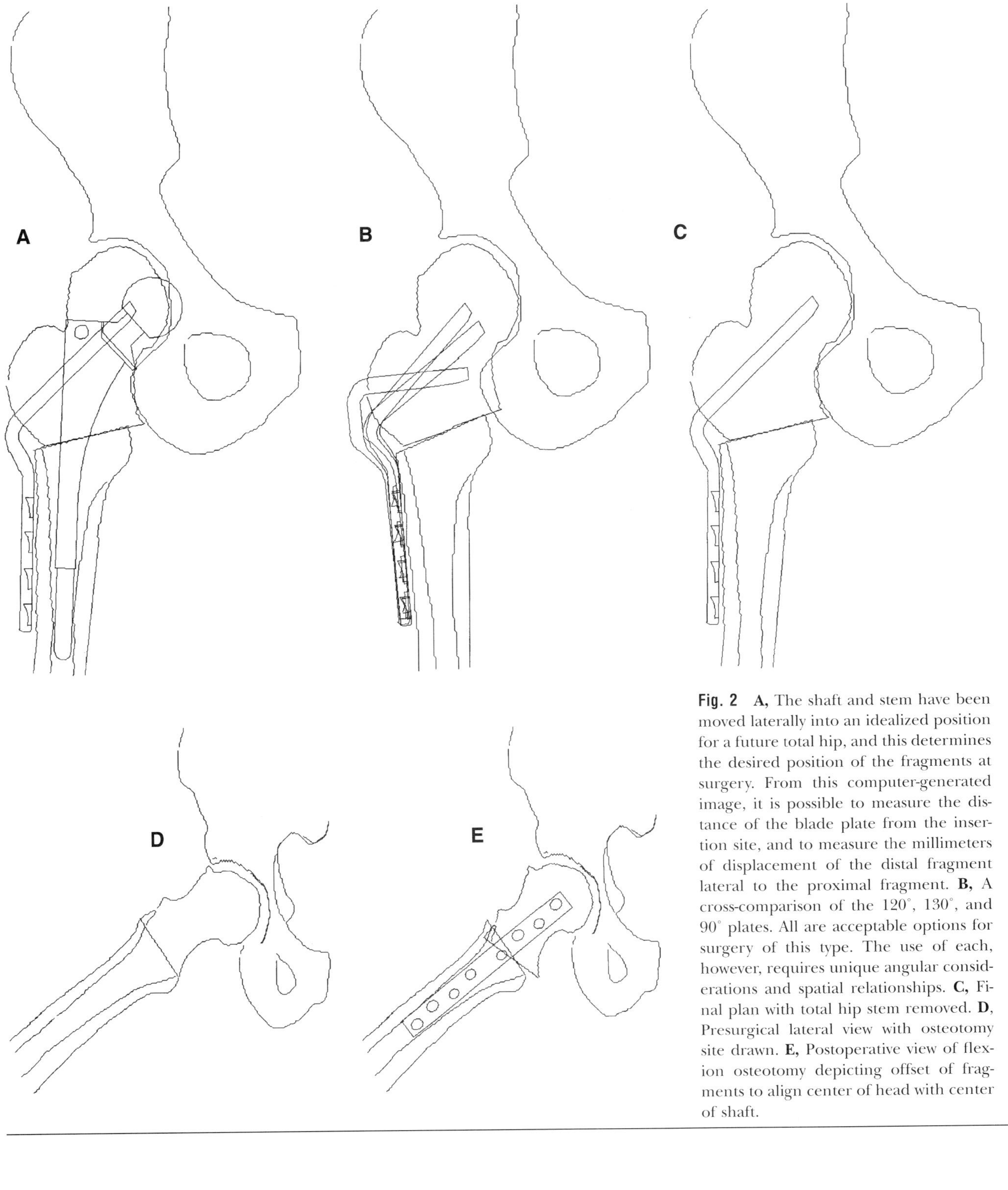

Fig. 2 **A,** The shaft and stem have been moved laterally into an idealized position for a future total hip, and this determines the desired position of the fragments at surgery. From this computer-generated image, it is possible to measure the distance of the blade plate from the insertion site, and to measure the millimeters of displacement of the distal fragment lateral to the proximal fragment. **B,** A cross-comparison of the 120°, 130°, and 90° plates. All are acceptable options for surgery of this type. The use of each, however, requires unique angular considerations and spatial relationships. **C,** Final plan with total hip stem removed. **D,** Presurgical lateral view with osteotomy site drawn. **E,** Postoperative view of flexion osteotomy depicting offset of fragments to align center of head with center of shaft.

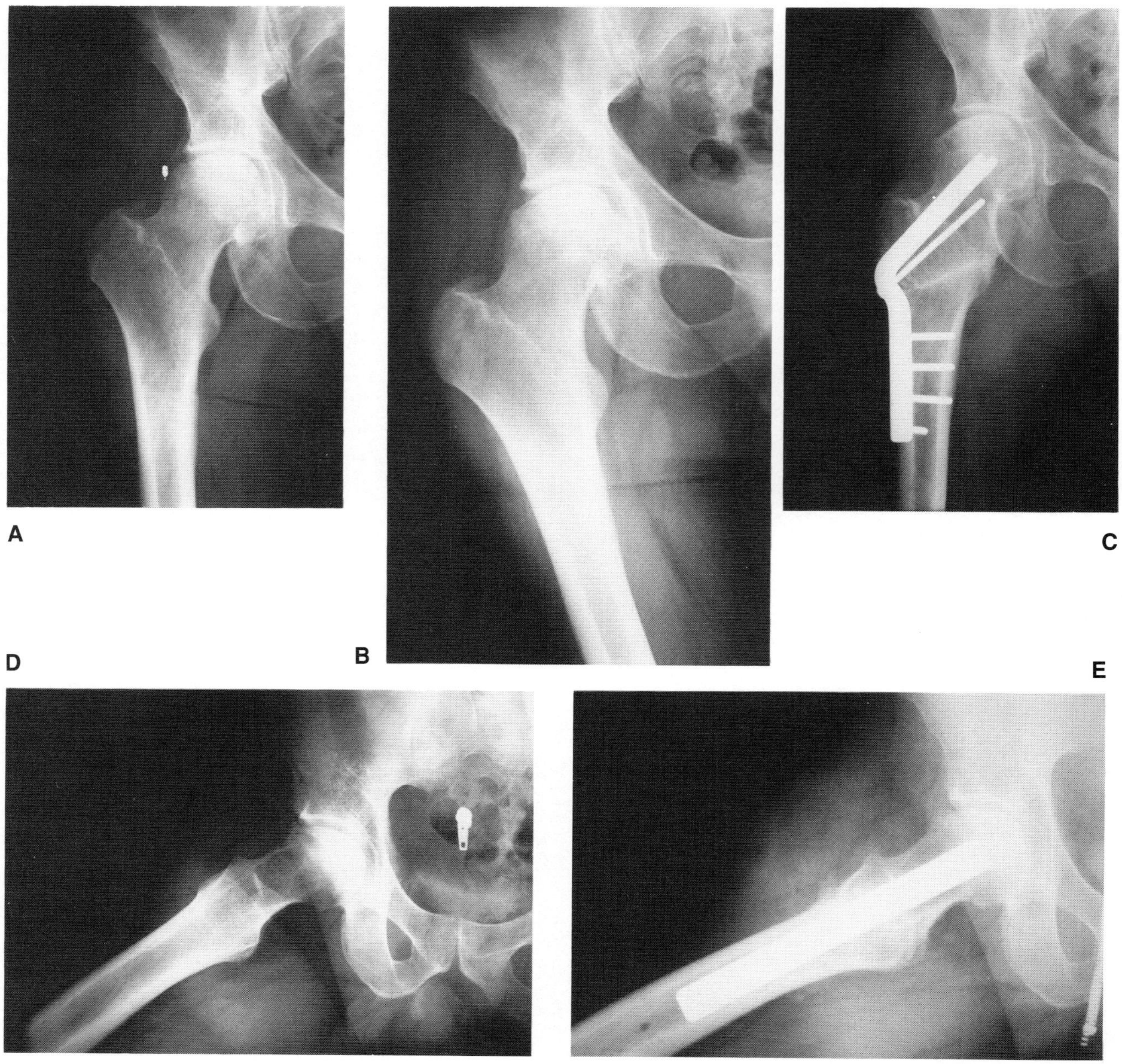

Fig. 3 **A,** Radiograph of presurgical hip. This corresponds to computer image of Fig. 1A. **B,** Anteroposterior view in adduction corresponds to Fig. 1B. **C,** Postoperative anteroposterior view corresponds to Fig. 2C. **D,** Preoperative lateral view corresponds to Fig. 2D. **E,** Postoperative lateral view corresponds to Fig. 2E.

guidelines are expected to facilitate the recovery of expenses allocated to this technology in non-capitated reimbursement environments.

Future Applications

Future applications for this technology include direct up-loading to the PC in the operating room and up-loading of information directly onto a digital fluoroscope for intraoperative image utilization.

The specific mechanics of image acquisition involve three basic options—digitized entry, video-capture, and use of an optical scanner. Digitization requires manual tracing of the outlines of a radiograph, including the outlines of the magnification marker. The advantages of manual entry include the elimination of unwanted background images, the ability to load full-length, long radiographs, and the ease of post-entry manipulation. This type of entry is clearly the best for planning of osteotomy and total knee surgery.

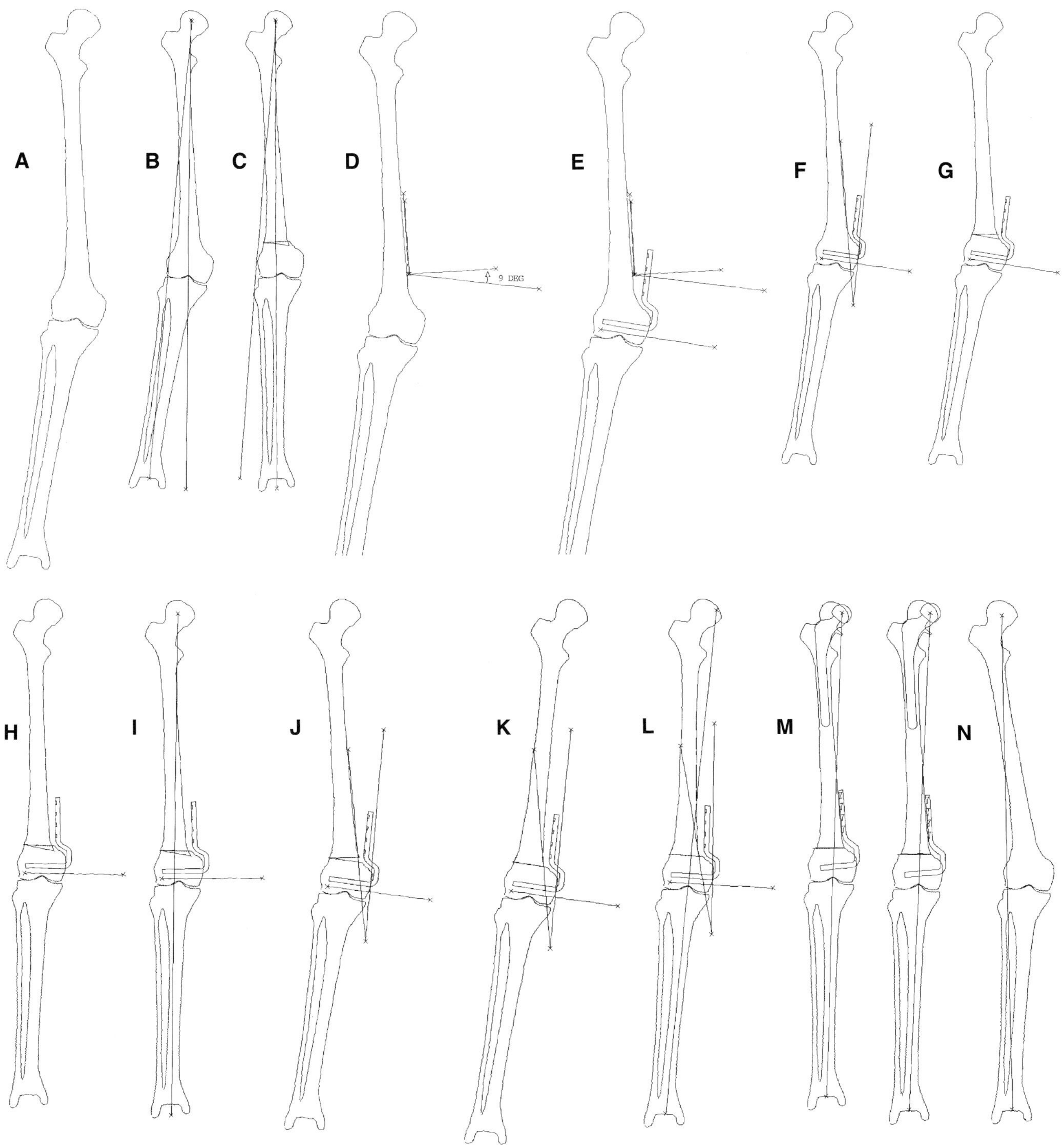

Fig. 4 **A,** Presurgical computer image prior to any displacements or angulations. **B,** The presurgical mechanical axis is passing through the lateral border of the bones at the knee level (severe grade II lateral shift of mechanical axis). The proposed postoperative mechanical axis passes through the center of the knee. **C,** The computer has shifted the lower bones below the osteotomy site until they intersect the proposed new mechanical axis; 9° of correction occurred in order to intersect the mechanical axis correctly, determining the magnitude of correction at 9°. **D,** The planning for a 9° osteotomy to achieve centralization. This depicts the angle of insertion of a 90° blade to achieve a 9° correction. **E,** The blade is shown parallel to the line of insertion. **F,** A 9° angle is shown parallel to the medial border of the femur and the side arm of the blade plate, confirming accuracy of placement. **G,** A medially-based closing wedge with an apex laterally. **H,** Straight hinging at the lateral cortex without displacement or wedge resection. Note the large gap between plate and femur. **I,** Mechanical axis in the unmodified simple hinged osteotomy. Note the residual lateral position of the mechanical axis. Such an observation mandates displacement of the fragments to achieve proper centralization of the mechanical axis. **J,** Resection of the wedge. **K,** Closing the simple hinge with full wedge resection. **L,** Confirmation of all angles in the full wedge resection example. **M,** Placement of a total hip replacement in the early arthritic hip in order to allow creation of the mechanical axis at the knee in the position of the anticipated center of rotation after total hip replacement. The fragments have been displaced appropriately to achieve normalization of the mechanical axis and intimate apposition of the plate. **N,** Comparison of the proposed plan and the preoperative status.

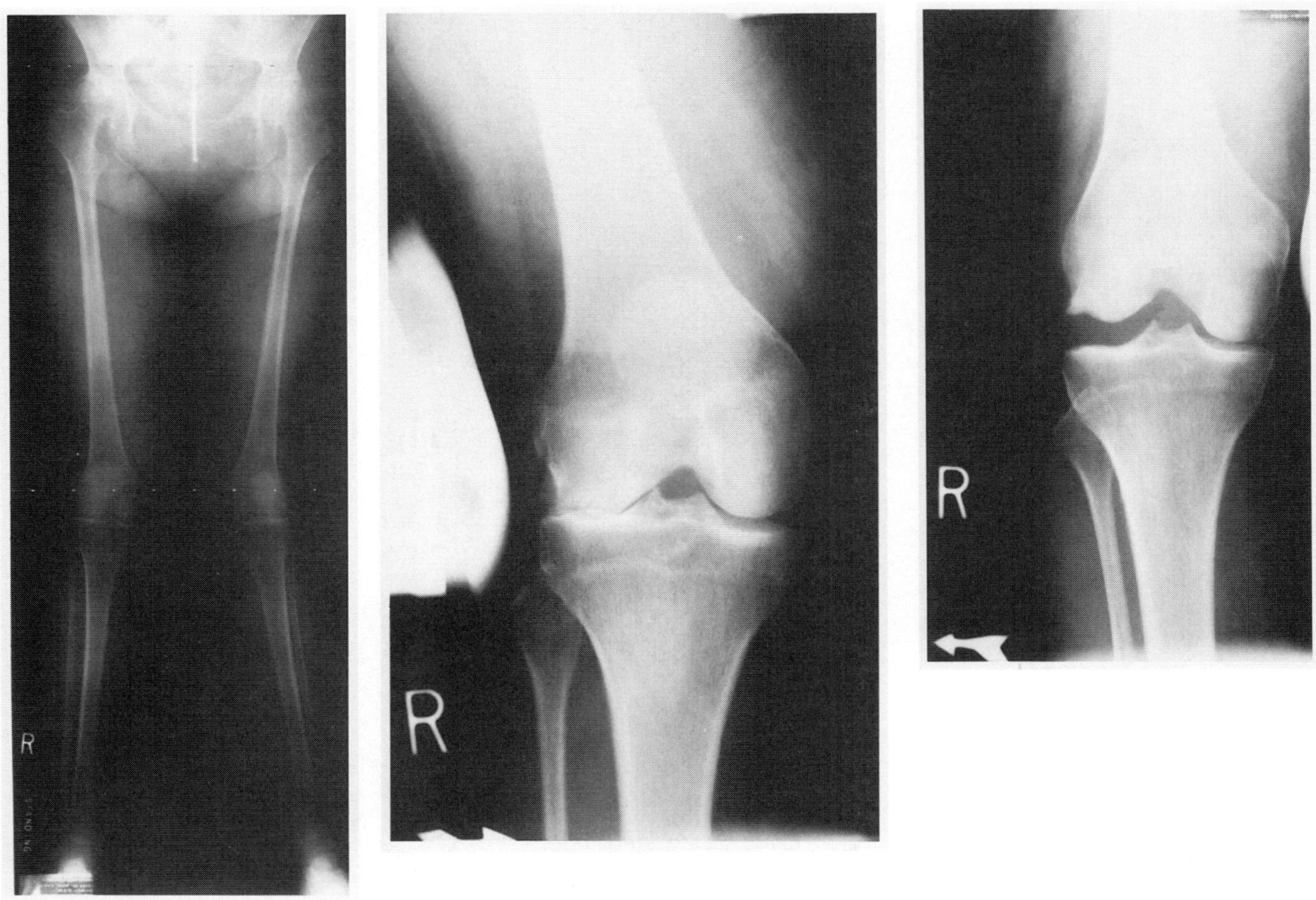

Fig. 5 **Left,** Radiograph of 69-year-old woman's knees before surgery. **Center,** Valgus stress view showing marked narrowing of the lateral joint space. **Right,** Excellent maintenance of joint space medially on varus stress view, confirming the rationale of osteotomy or lateral compartment hemiarthroplasty, as opposed to total knee replacement in such a case.

Case no. 2 demonstrates the step-by-step process of planning a varus producing supracondylar osteotomy of the distal femur in the management of acquired valgus deformity of the knee in a patient with lateral compartment osteoarthritis. There is also a coxa valga deformity of the upper femur, and future total hip replacement is anticipated.

This case demonstrates not only the step-by-step process of planning the supracondylar osteotomy, but also the technique for anticipating and predicting the future mechanical axis of the total hip that will supersede the mechanical axis of the unoperated hip.

This patient was a 69-year-old woman with primary lateral compartment osteoarthritis, who is now five years post osteotomy of the knee, and three years post total hip replacement (Figs. 4-6).

Video-capture allows a quick and high-quality entry of radiographic and other visual inputs into the computer. This is particularly useful for slide documentation, archiving of information, and enhancement of images with text overlays. It is very useful for planning and follow up of total hip procedures, which do not require long films.

The most sophisticated form of image capture is through an optical scanner. The scanner itself, however, can cost up to $40,000, take several minutes per image, and occupy a considerable amount of space. Its primary use would be for research work that requires assessment of fine detail of trabecular bone, etc.

Conclusion

Overall, the advantages of computer-based planning are numerous and significant. Most importantly, it allows the surgeon to integrate variables of displacement offset, linear measurement, angulation measurement, and implant selection accurately in advance of surgery, and equips the surgeon with hard copies of the plan to guide surgery, analogous to the blueprints of an architect and builder.

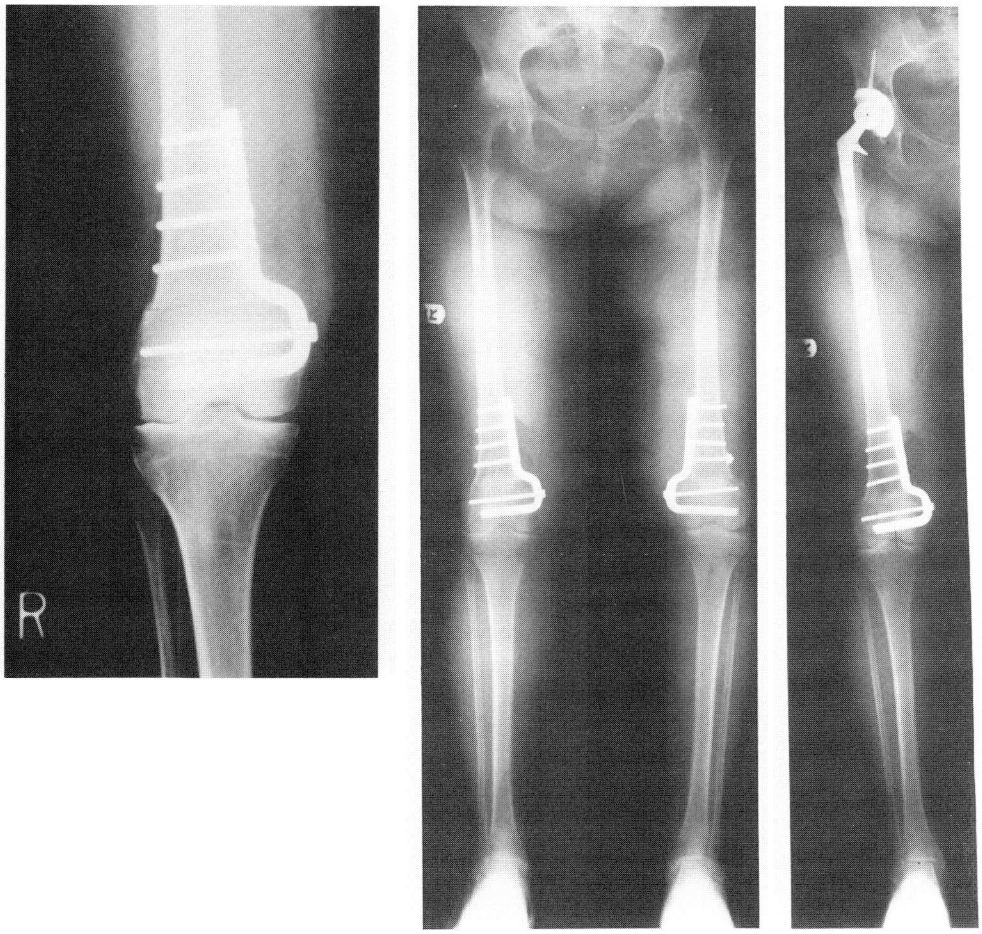

Fig. 6 **Left,** Postoperative appearance of the knee after osteotomy of 9°. This corresponds to Fig. 4M. **Center,** Status after bilateral supracondylar osteotomies. **Right,** Mechanical axis of the right knee passing through the center of the mechanical axis after total hip replacement.

C H A P T E R 4 8

Database Construction and Use Issues

Mike Ward
John Glaser

Introduction

The patient care, administrative, or research analysis needs of an orthopaedic surgeon may be satisfied through the construction and use of a database. A database is a collection of well-defined and organized data that is managed by a database management system (DBMS). The DBMS is a software application that supports data queries, report generation, data reorganization, database backup, and security. Popular DBMS's include Paradox, Access, dBase, and Oracle. The construction of a database can be time consuming and expensive. Improper construction and use of the database can mislead the analysis, lead to rework to correct data deficiencies, or necessitate re-creation of the database.

This chapter discusses several issues and makes recommendations for those who wish to construct and use a database. Specifically, it reviews five problems that haunt database construction and use, provides a database construction checklist, and suggests ways to improve your ability to enlist the help of your organization's information systems department.

Five Problems

Five common problems can haunt the construction and use of the database. These problems can make the constructed database less useful than it should be. Correcting these problems can be time consuming, and it is sometimes necessary to start the construction all over again. These problems are discussed below.

Inadequate Statement of Questions or Analysis

Database constructors often begin the construction by using a series of questions or an analysis that they would like the database to answer or support. Problems occur when the questions or analysis lack specificity or fail to consider the second and third order questions or analysis.

The following are examples of questions that lack specificity. What is the productivity of my practice? How many of my patients are hypertensive? Where do my patients come from? Ways in which lack of specificity can cause problems in the construction of the database include the following. The wrong data are collected, for example, the patient's country rather than zip code for patient origin. Data are collected in a format that limits use, for example, if hypertension is recorded as a characteristic of a patient rather than as a problem noted at a visit. Data needed to answer subsequent questions, for example, "Who is the most productive provider?" are not collected.

Poor Data Quality

Data, particularly if received from another computer system in a download, may be of poor quality. Data edit checks of allowable ranges may be incomplete, dictionaries of allowable data values may be improperly constructed, and internal consistency checks between data may be ignored. Database constructors may discover these limitations during analysis or they may not.

Database constructors can also develop poor edits of information that is being entered directly into their database. The following types of edits should be present: allowable range of the data item; dictionaries of allowable data values; internal consistency checks, for example, between zip code and city and state; and checks for alphabetic or numeric characteristics. Constructors of databases should review their proposed edits and the edits of data they are receiving from other computer systems.

Lack of Support

Sooner or later, something will go wrong. The personal computer or the DBMS will have problems. Questions about system capabilities may not have ready answers in the manual. In addition, questions regarding the data may arise; some data values or the results of an analysis may not look right. The constructors of the database must know who to call if problems occur with the computer, the software, or the data.

Differences in Data Definitions

There can be serious differences in the ways people interpret a data element. For example, does the field "service" in a casemix system refer to the service of the admitting physician, the service to which a patient was admitted, or the discharge service? Does an admission occur when the patient has been hospitalized for longer than 4 hours or when the patient occupies a bed at midnight? Misinterpretation of meaning can clearly lead to incorrect analysis or misleading query results.

Two or more physicians may compare the results of analysis performed on independent databases that purport to capture the same data that has the same meaning. Unless the definitions and mode of collection of the data for different databases are explicitly understood there is no guarantee that the data fields with the same name mean the same thing.

Too Much, Too Soon

In constructing databases, the attempt is often made to gather all of the data that might possibly be used and to gather it as quickly as possible and in the richest and most complex manner. This grandiose approach can overwhelm the construction effort.

In an effort to get everything, insufficient attention is often paid to detail and to getting the basics done correctly. Unanticipated roadblocks can occur, for example, poor speed of database retrieval due to its size or difficulty in obtaining a particular portion of the data. In addition, support from other groups, such as the information systems department, can be exponentially harder to obtain as the project effort grows larger.

This problem may be avoided by starting with the smallest core of data that allows the project to be "whole." Concentrate on obtaining this core data and on ensuring that the mechanisms for obtaining the core are solid and correct. After a successful, fully operational first phase, the size and scope of the database can be expanded.

Database Checklist

To avoid being plagued by the problems described above, the constructors of databases should use the following checklist. The checklist makes a series of recommendations that, if followed, should greatly minimize problems with database construction and use.

Make Sure You Know Who to Call

Make sure you know who you will call when (and it is not a question of if): the hardware or the software fails to work; the manuals are not helpful; you find something wrong or confusing with the data; you want to have someone else review your analysis plans; you want someone else to review the computer edits you have developed; or you don't know what's wrong or who to call. The database constructor should verify that the person to be called is (1) willing to take the time to respond to the call and (2) has the expertise necessary to provide effective assistance.

Ask Someone Else to Review Your Objectives and Approach

Database construction and use represent significant expenditures of time and money. Before initiating construction, it is a good idea to review your objectives and approaches with someone who is knowledgeable about your domain and who can point out potentially significant acts of commission or omission.

Ask Someone Else to Review Your Data Entry Edits and Consistency Checks

Correction of data that has become corrupted through erroneous entries, poor or incomplete codification, or misunderstanding of meaning can be very expensive and, in some cases, impossible. Unfortunately, these problems are often discovered after the effort to construct the database has been completed.

Invaluable review of the data entry edits and consistency checks can be provided by professional programmers and information systems staff who are familiar with the data. Their expertise and insight can be illuminating. For example, in most hospital information systems, the letter "A" is a legitimate code for a newborn's gender. It means "Ambiguous" and occurs when the genitalia for both genders is present in the newborn.

Ask Someone Else to Review Your Use of the Data

After use of the database has begun, ask someone else to review the specifics of your analysis and analysis results. This review can be particularly invaluable when held with the generators of the data. They know how and why the data were collected. This knowledge can suggest that certain analytical conclusions are inappropriate.

Know Where the Data Comes From and How It is Collected

Database constructors need to know where the data comes from and how it is collected. The source and the manner of collection clearly influence the meaning and quality of the data. For example, if you assumed that trained medical records professionals code outpatient diagnoses you would be wrong most of the time. This task is often performed by accounts receivables clerks.

Make Sure Your Data Matches That Which You Care Most About Matching

If the database being constructed parallels another database to any degree or is a shadow of another database and if a comparison of the two databases is to be done, it is necessary to ensure that the common data come from the same source for both databases. For example, a comparison of visit totals derived from data gathered from the clinic's schedules and visit totals derived for the billing system will often have discrepancies in the totals and subtotals. If there is a significant need to match with other databases, the data should come from the same source.

Know What the Data Means

The database constructor must understand the definition, source, edits, and other uses of the data gathered.

Know How to Get Downloads of Data

Obtaining downloads of the data from other systems can greatly ease the cost and time of collection and reduce the error associated with reentry of data.

Downloads can create problems, however, such as merging disparate downloads, receiving incorrectly coded or poor quality data, or having the download request wait in an information systems programming queue. The need, cost, and efficacy of a download should be discussed with the technical staff responsible for the source database. If the download is needed periodically, rather than only once, the database constructor needs to ensure that they can get the download on demand.

How to Improve Your Ability to Get the Information Systems Department to Help You

The information systems department of your hospital or group practice can be very helpful in guiding the database constructor through the questions and issues discussed above. However, because the department's workers are often burdened by many demands for their time, they may view your needs as being of relatively low importance. Several strategies can improve their responsiveness and make them more attentive to your needs and questions.

Use Technologies They Support and Understand

If the information systems department has expertise and supports IBM personal computers but would not recognize a SUN workstation, they will be less willing and able to provide assistance if your database is based on a SUN workstation. Even if the database constructor believes that the supported and understood technologies are inferior, the tradeoffs between superior technology and the availability of assistance should be weighed carefully.

Take Training Classes They Offer

Most organizations offer training classes in personal computer use and applications. The database constructor should attend these. These classes address problems that are often encountered, and they provide information regarding organizational support venues. The classes also give the database constructor an opportunity to establish a working relationship with the course trainer, who can provide support later, and with other class attendees, with whom ideas can be shared.

Understand and Leverage the Mechanisms That Guide Priority Setting

Organizations have management mechanisms to set priorities for the information systems department. An information systems steering committee is one such mechanism, or a department head may be designated to set priorities for a particular area of responsibility. The database constructor who is in need of information systems support needs to understand the management mechanisms that set priorities, as well as the individuals who set priorities, and must know how the relative merits of various projects are determined. This information puts the database constructor in a position to champion his or her needs.

Take Advantage of Friends Who Have Power

Despite the presence of formal, objective, priority-setting mechanisms, information systems departments perform projects because someone with power asked or told them to do so. Priority setting is, to a large degree, a political activity; it is an ongoing negotiation about the use of scarce resources.

Keep the Scope Doable

Projects or needs are often presented in their full grandeur and scope. This can lead to concern on the part of the information systems department personnel that they will be overwhelmed. In addition, the demands of such projects usually exceed the ability of the database constructor to manage all aspects of the project at once. Information systems departments are often willing to fit a small-scale project into their project list, but, if the project appears to be too big, the project proponent may be asked to use the formal priority-setting process or may be told that the project will take too much effort and is not worth it.

Projects should start small. Smaller projects are easier to manage, and they increase the likelihood that the information systems department will be receptive. Once the early phases have been completed, the project can grow in scope.

It Helps if Information Systems Likes You and the Project

Information systems staff, being human, are much more willing to squeeze projects into their work list or to work off-hours on the database constructor's project if they like the database constructor and think the project is interesting or has value. Establishing a rapport with key members of the information systems staff and presenting the project in terms that are appealing can greatly increase the probability of information systems support. To the extent that the project makes the world a better place, this should be emphasized.

Allow Them to Solve It Their Way if Possible

Information systems staff are systems analysts and programming professionals. Let them use their experience and judgment. Their ideas and approach are based on a multitude of experiences, and they bear the scars of mistakes. The database constructor should avoid micro-managing their efforts. The information systems professional should focus on your problem and goals, not on your preferred solution. This does not remove the need for the information systems professionals to explain what is being done and why. Neither does this mean that you, the customer, cannot express your pleasure or dissatisfaction with their approach or progress.

Conclusion

Database construction and use is a time consuming task and is often expensive. A carefully planned approach to construction and use is invaluable. The recommendations discussed above are based on dozens of projects, and the database constructor is advised to heed them. The database constructor should make every effort to use the talents and efforts of the information systems department, whose members bring years of experience to the discussion.

Index